Mario Campanacci
Bone and Soft Tissue Tumors

Co-authors of the Soft Tissue Section:
Franco Bertoni and Patrizia Bacchini

Foreword by William F. Enneking
Translated by Sylvia Notini

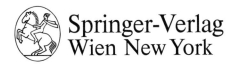 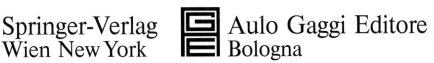

Springer-Verlag
Wien New York

Aulo Gaggi Editore
Bologna

Mario Campanacci, M.D.

Orthopaedic Surgeon, Professor of Pathological Anatomy and Histology and Clinical Orthopaedics, University of Bologna;
Director of the 1st Orthopaedic Clinic, Rizzoli Orthopaedic Institute, Bologna;
Director of the Graduate School of Orthopaedics;
Director of the Tumor Centre, Rizzoli Orthopaedic Institute, Bologna

Franco Bertoni, M.D.

Chief-of-Staff of the Department of Pathological Anatomy, M. Malpighi Hospital, Bologna;
Pathological Anatomy Consultant at Rizzoli Orthopaedic Institute, Bologna

Patrizia Bacchini, M.D.

Attending-Staff, Department of Pathological Anatomy, M. Malpighi Hospital, Bologna

William F. Enneking, M.D.

Eugene Jewett Professor of Orthopaedic Surgery and Pathology;
Distinguished Service Professor, College of Medicine, University of Florida

Sylvia Notini, M.D.

Professor at University, Bologna

Translation from the Italian edition
Tumori delle Ossa e delle Parti Molli
© 1986 by Aulo Gaggi Editore, Bologna
ISBN 88-7744-010-4

Printed in Italy by Litosei, via Bellini 22/4, Pianoro (Bologna)

Sole distribution rights: Springer-Verlag Wien - New York

With 881 Figures

Library of Congress Cataloging - in - Publication Data: Campanacci, Mario. [Tumori delle ossa e delle parti molli. English] Bone and soft tissue tumors/Mario Campanacci: foreword by William F. Enneking: translated by Sylvia Notini. p. 1142 cm. 5.8 Translation of: Tumori delle ossa e delle parti molli. Includes bibliographical references. Includes index, ISBN 3-211-82186-4 (Springer-Verlag). — ISBN 0-387-82186-4 (Springer-Verlag). — ISBN 8877440155 (Aulo Gaggi Editore) 1. Musculoskeletal System — Cancer. I. Title. [DNLM: 1. Bone Neoplasms. 2. Soft Tissue Neoplasms. WE 258 C186t] RC 280. M83C3613.1990.619.99'271 — dc20

ISBN 3-211-82186-4 Springer Verlag Wien-New York
ISBN 0-387-82186-4 Springer-Verlag New-York Wien
ISBN 88-7744-015-5 Aulo Gaggi Editore, Bologna

CONTENTS

TUMORS OF BONE

PSEUDOTUMORS OF BONE

TUMORS OF THE SOFT TISSUES

PSEUDOTUMORS OF THE SOFT TISSUES

To Giuliana

FOREWORD

This is an extraordinary book by an extraordinary author. Mario Campanacci first published three volumes on musculoskeletal neoplasms and other tumor-like processes in bone and soft parts in Italian in 1981-1985. This book is an update and expansion of that book, published for the first time in English. In this book Dr. Campanacci brings to the readers the vast experience in musculoskeletal oncology of the Rizzoli Orthopaedic Institute in Bologna where he has been head of the Oncology Unit for many years. As such, he has had at his disposal the patient records, radiographs and pathologic material dating back to 1905. In fact, a visitor to the Institute will be shown the radiograph made of the first tumor case on records — that of a giant cell tumor of the distal femur. The wealth of clinical material that has accumulated at the Rizzoli Institute, with exquisite documentation and maintenance is a unique resource and testimonial to not only the author but his predecessors. Under Dr. Campanacci's leadership, the Institute has provided care to the majority of patients with neoplasms throughout Italy. Over the past two decades a treatment team with extraordinary ability in radiology, imaging, pathology, chemotherapy, as well as orthopedic surgery has been assembled. The institute has been a major contributor to the literature of musculoskeletal oncology, has played an important role in the Musculoskeletal Tumor Society of North America, and taken a leadership role in the establishment of the European Musculoskeletal Oncology Society. This book brings to the reader an almost unparalleled experience from one of the leading centers of musculoskeletal oncology in the world.

The book first deals with the general principles of musculoskeletal oncology in an exemplary fashion as befits their experience. It then presents an extensive series of chapters, each devoted to a particular entity. Within each chapter the lesion in question is clearly defined in its frequency, sexual predilection, age of occurrence, and the anatomic localization with a detailed discussion of each point. Figures quoted are those derived from the experience at the Institute. The reader is then presented with the clinical picture and symptoms, the imaging characteristics of the lesion, and the gross and histopathologic features, all beautifully illustrated. Following this, the differential diagnosis is discussed in detail. Next, the clinical course without treatment is outlined. The next section of each chapter is a discussion of the treatment of the lesion in question and includes both surgical, chemotherapeutic and radiotherapeutic modalities. The final portion of each chapter is devoted to a discussion of the prognosis as it is currently known. Each chapter is beautifully illustrated with exceptional clarity that allows the reader an accurate portrayal of the lesion under discussion.

The manuscript is not simply a translation from Italian into English, rather an expansion of the previous text written in English. It retains the author's clarity of thought, conciseness, and sharp focus on the important issues, and, in this context, brings to the reader an exceptionally cosmopolitan international view of this subject. This book is a must for all those involved in the care of patients with musculoskeletal neoplasms regardless of their medical speciality. To those students, residents and fellows in orthopaedic surgery, radiology, medical oncology, pathology and radiation oncology, it will provide an invaluable resource and inspiration. We are greatly in Dr. Mario Campanacci's debt for the prodigious effort this singularly authored authoritative text has required.

W.F. ENNEKING

PREFACE

At the Istituto Ortopedico Rizzoli the interest on bone tumors was pioneered by V. Putti, who created a pathology laboratory and museum, successfully performed extraarticular resection of the proximal femur and acetabulum in 1914, devised and widely used a technique of resection/arthrodesis of the knee (1923) whose principles have been in use until our days. His pupil, O. Scaglietti, fostered the laboratory of pathology and the study of bone tumors up to 1941. F. Delitala introduced in 1945 the replacement of large segmental resections with original stainless steel articular endoprostheses, which functioned for decades. In 1950 R. Zanoli used intercalary massive xenografts. I.F. Goidanich founded in 1955 the Tumor Centre at the Institute, reviewing and redefining all previous cases according to the new concepts introduced by H. Jaffe in those years. I started working with Goidanich both in orthopaedic surgery and in pathology in 1958 and shortly after studied with L. Lichtenstein in San Francisco. To both those admired and beloved teachers I am indebted for everything I have been able to do thereafter and for this book.

Today the Tumor Centre of the Institute records about 15,000 cases, complete with clinical charts, original X-ray and histological slides. More than 90% of those cases have been treated at the Institute, the remaining are consultation cases.

The experience with these cases constitutes the matter of this book. Any case where diagnosis was debatable was excluded. No mention will be made of exceptional lesions which we never saw, nor of lesions of the jaws, with which we have hardly any experience. Also clinical data, surgical and gross pathologic findings, surgical techniques, as well as complications and results are entirely driven from personal experience. Some illustrations will present cases where the treatment adopted is incorrect according to our present standards; those cases are decades old.

We think that a book has to be simple to be readable. We therefore avoided all unnecessary details and not well-established facts. The bibliography has also been limited to the most significant and recent publications.

Musculo-skeletal oncology is a multidisciplinary speciality. Our work and consequently this book would not have been possible without the joint effort of the pathologists (P. Bacchini, F. Bertoni, P. Picci), the medical oncologist (G. Bacci), the general surgeons (A. Briccoli, N. Guernelli), the orthopaedic surgeons (S. Boriani, R. Capanna, A. Giunti, F. Gherlinzoni, A. Guerra, C. Leonessa, M.

Mercuri, G. Padovani, A. Toni). To all these friends I am greatly in debt because I profited greatly from their work, enthusiasm and ingenuity. A special aknowledgement to doctors M. Laus, E. Lorenzi, P. Ruggieri, and N. Fabbri for their precious and essential help in the preparation of the pictures.

M. CAMPANACCI

INTRODUCTION

TERMINOLOGY

Hyperplasia

This is constituted by an accumulation of cells due to either accelerated proliferation or slowed maturation and degeneration. The hyperplasia is caused by a stimulus, and it ceases when the stimulus is exhausted. The hyperplasia is functional: as such, it tends to be characterized by an organized or organoid structure, with cells and structures that differentiate and mature completely, and which are accompanied by blood vessels according to a specific spatial order. Typical examples of hyperplasia are exuberant bone calluses, tumor-like muscular and periosteal ossifications, brown tumors in hyperparathyroidism osteosis, and, probably, aneurysmal bone cyst, pigmented villonodular synovitis, synovial chondromatosis.

Hamartoma

During the development of the embryo (or later, in the course of body growth) an island of tissue may be excluded from regional organization, and left unused. This congenital error is known as **hamartia**. Hamartia may continue to grow independently and without having a structure aimed at a definite function, precisely because the embryonic tissue constituting it is subtracted from any kind of rule or regulation, and from any functional activity. The product of this growth, which is similar to a neoplasm, is known as **hamartoma**. Like hyperplasia, hamartoma has a relatively orderly structure, and it often tends to exhaust its growth and mature completely during adult age. Examples of hamartoma include exostoses, angiomas, neurofibromatoses, chondromas, fibrous dysplasia, hystiocytic fibromas of the skeleton. Another feature of hamartoma is that it may be multicentric or diffused, often prevalently occurring in one half of the body, as may in fact be the case in all of the examples listed above.

Neoplasm

This neoformation derives from the cells of one or more tissues and it is atypical, autonomous, and progressive.

Benign neoplasm

Its growth is autonomous, but it is much slower than that of malignant neoplasms. Cellular morphology is typical, tissue structure tends to be less disorderly and more organoid than that of malignant tumors. The cells tend to differentiate, and to mature, and they often preserve a considerable amount of their specific function. Growth is expansive, thus, the benign neoplasm is evidently limited in relation to the surrounding tissues, and it is often capsulated. It does not recur after it has been removed completely, and it does not metastasize. Examples: giant cell tumor, osteoblastoma, chondroblastoma, chondromyxoid fibroma, and, in the soft tissues, lipoma, neurinoma, myxoma.

Low-grade malignant neoplasm

Its growth is rather slow, but much more progressive than that of benign neoplasms, as it may even become of enormous size. Growth is partially invasive, thus, the limits of the tumor are less well-defined than those of benign neoplasms. If surgical removal is not truly complete, including a layer of healthy surrounding tissue, the neoplasm recurs. It infrequently metastasizes; nonetheless, both the original tumor and its local recurrence may manifest progressive malignancy in time, becoming a neoplasm with a higher degree of malignancy. Examples: grades 1, 2 chondrosarcoma, grades 1, 2 parosteal osteosarcoma, and, in the soft tissues, dermatofibrosarcoma protuberans, low-grade liposarcoma.

High-grade malignant neoplasm

Its growth is generally rapid and indefinite in time. Cellular morphology is atypical, tissue structure anarchical. The cell's differentiation, maturation and specific function are absent or decreased, and more or less anomalous. Growth is invasive and infiltrative, thus the neoplasm is not characterized by well-defined boundaries with the surrounding tissues. It locally recurs if removal does not include a wide layer of healthy surrounding tissue, or the entire original anatomical compartment, and it tends to metastasize. Examples: classic osteosarcoma, Ewing's sarcoma, grade 3 chondrosarcoma, and, in the soft tissues, high-grade liposarcoma, malignant fibrous histiocytoma, rhabdomyosarcoma, synovial sarcoma.

These definitions are schematic and approximate. At times it is impossible to define the limits between hyperplasia, hamartoma, and benign tumor. A hamartoma of the skeleton may, even after many years, constitute the site where malignant tumors originate (see exostosis, chondroma, fibrous dysplasia). There are benign tumors (such as desmoid tumor of the soft tissues) which have infiltrative growth. On the contrary, some malignant tumors are characterized by slow growth; others remain small and clearly circumscribed, but they nonetheless metastasize; others still achieve a high degree of cellular differentiation (some types of chondrosarcoma); others, finally, have an organoid structure (alveolar sarcoma of the soft tissues).

CLASSIFICATION

The basis for classification is histological and, more precisely, histogenetic. Thus, tumors are distinguished according to the cellular type by which they are composed, and thus, from which they probably derive (histogenesis). If a tumor is made up of fibroblasts-fibrocytes and collagenous fibers, it is a fibroma or a fibrosarcoma; if it is made up of chondroblasts-chondrocytes and cartilaginous substance it is a chondroma or a chondrosarcoma; if it is made up of osteoblasts-osteocytes and osteoid substance it is an osteoblastoma or an osteosarcoma; if it is made up of angioblastic-endothelial cells forming vascular canals it is an angioma, an angioendothelioma, or an angiosarcoma. And so on.

Identification is generally easy in benign tumors, the cells of which tend to be characterized by diffused and considerable morpho-functional differentiation. It may be less easy in malignant tumors, where the cells may differentiate (thus, allowing for their strain of origin to be identified, based on form and function) only in sporadic sites of the tumor and, even in these, in a vague and anomalous manner. One contribution towards establishing or confirming the histogenesis of a tumor may be constituted by histochemistry and immunohistochemistry, and by electron microscopy.

When different aspects or stages of differentiation are observed in a tumor, it is the one which is most evolved that defines the tumor. This may occur in many tumors, whether benign or malignant, but it is a particularly frequent occurrence in malignant tumors. In most types of sarcoma, for example, there may be areas composed of tumor fibroblasts. This depends on the fact that nearly all mesenchymal cells (histiocytes, lipoblasts, myoblasts, angioblasts, osteoblasts, chondroblasts) may, both in vivo and in vitro, assume the appearance and the function of fibroblasts: facultative fibroblasts (Stout and Lattes, 1967). If a sarcoma is characterized by fibrocellular neoplastic areas together with chondroblastic and osteoblastic ones, then it is an osteosarcoma. If there are fibroblastic fields alongside other lipoblastic areas, then it is a liposarcoma. If the malignant tumor is made up of undifferentiated mesenchymal areas and angioblastic areas, then it is an angiosarcoma. As previously stated, a partial fibroblastic differentiation with the production of collagenous fibers is common to many different types of sarcoma. Thus, only those tumors where there is fibroblastic differentiation alone in the entire neoplasm, and during its entire course, may be called fibrosarcomas.

A reliable classification must distinguish between types of tumors which have their own well-defined features, not only of a histogenetic and histological nature, but also of a clinical, radiographic, macroscopic, prognostic and therapeutic nature. In truth, the classification used is based on the combination of all of these elements, even if the histological and histogenetic picture is the most important one. Parosteal osteosarcoma, for example, must be distinguished from classic osteosarcoma not only because their histological features differ, but also because their clinical, radiographic and prognostic behaviors clearly differ. The same may be said for the distinction between Ewing's sarcoma and primary lymphoma of the skeleton. The distinctions made between central, peripheral and periosteal chondrosarcoma, and between osteoid osteoma and osteoblastoma are based on clinical, radiographic and prognostic differences more than on histological differences, which are relatively minor or non-existent.

On the contrary, it would not be justified to separate tumor varieties with the same histogenetic, clinical, radiographic, and prognostic features on the basis of histological features alone. Thus, for example, the hemorrhagic variety of osteosarcoma, which histologically appears to be quite different from common osteosarcoma, has no clinical, radiographic or prognostic differences sufficient to justify a classification as a category in itself.

What must also be taken into account is that a histological examination routinely reveals only an area of the tumor, removed at a certain stage in its evolution. If we could have a microscopic vision of the entire tumor, and follow the changes that occur as it develops, then histological classification would probably be exact and self-sufficient.

Finally, as correctly affirmed by Jaffe (1958), each tumor must be considered an anatomical and clinical entity in itself. In other words, the fact that some tumors have the same histogenetic basis does not at all mean that they must have other features in common. Thus, for example, osteoid osteoma has nothing in common with osteosarcoma, and it never becomes an osteosarcoma. Among tumors of the cartilaginous series, there is a relationship between chondromas and exostoses on one hand, and chondrosarcomas on the other; but there is no relationship between chondroblastoma and chondrosarcoma, nor between chondromyxoid fibroma and chondrosarcoma. The same may be said for angioma, which has nothing in common with angiosarcoma, for hystiocytic fibroma of the bone in relation to fibrosarcoma and malignant fibrous histiocytoma, and so on.

However, it is practical and traditional to group tumors together according to their histogenetic basis. The classification proposed here, with some minor changes, is that of the World Health Organization by Schajowicz et al. (1972) for tumors of the skeleton, and by Enzinger and Weiss (1983) for those of the soft tissues (Tables 1 and 2).

Mention has repeatedly been made of the soft tissues. What is meant by this is the synovial membrane and the joint capsule, as well as all of the non-skeletal tissues of the limbs, trunk, neck and head, excluding the internal organs, the periosteum, the lymph nodes and the skin.

Our classification includes neoplasms and possible hamartomas. We do not see any reason to exclude lesions such as fibrous dysplasia (as do Lichtenstein, 1965; Dahlin, 1967; Spjut et al., 1971; Schajowicz et al., 1972) or histiocytic fibroma (Spjut et al., 1971; Schajowicz et al., 1972), as it would

Table 1
BONE TUMORS

Differentiation or histogenesis	Benign	Low-grade malignancy	High-grade malignancy
Fibrous and histiocytic	Histiocytic fibroma Benign fibrous histiocytoma Giant cell tumor Desmoid fibroma	Grades 1, 2 fibrosarcoma	Grades 3, 4 fibrosarcoma Malignant fibrous histiocytoma
Cartilaginous	Exostosis Hemimelic epiphyseal dysplasia Chondroma Chondroblastoma Chondromyxoid fibroma	Grades 1, 2 central chondrosarcoma Peripheral chondrosarcoma Periosteal chondrosarcoma Clear cell chondrosarcoma Fibrocartilaginous mesenchymoma	Grade 3 central chondrosarcoma Mesenchymal chondrosarcoma
Osseous	Osteoma Osteoid osteoma Osteoblastoma Fibrous dysplasia Osteofibrous dysplasia	Parosteal osteosarcoma Periosteal osteosarcoma Low-grade central osteosarcoma	Classical osteosarcoma Hemorrhagic osteosarcoma Small cell osteosarcoma Osteosarcomatosis
Emopoietic			Lymphoma Plasmacytoma (Leukemia, Hodgkin)
Vascular	Hemangioma Lymphangioma	Low-grade hemangioendothelioma Hemangiopericytoma	High-grade hemangioendothelioma Hemangiopericytoma
Nervous	Neurinoma Neurofibroma		Ewing's sarcoma (?)
Adipose	Lipoma		Liposarcoma
Mixed		Adamantinoma (?)	Malignant mesenchymoma
Notochordal		Chordoma	

then be appropriate to exclude exostoses, chondromas, and angiomas, too.

Some tumors are labeled as having an uncertain or presumed histogenesis, such as Ewing's sarcoma, adamantinoma and, in the soft tissues, alveolar sarcoma and epithelioid sarcoma.

Table 2
SOFT TISSUE TUMORS

Differentiation or histogenesis	Benign	Low-grade malignancy	High-grade malignancy
Fibrous	Fibromatosis (subdermic, digital, aponeurotic, congenital) Desmoid tumor	Grades 1, 2 fibrosarcoma Infantile fibrosarcoma	Grades 3, 4 fibrosarcoma
Fibrohistiocytic	Benign fibrous histiocytoma	Dermatofibrosarcoma protuberans Atypical fibroxanthoma	Malignant fibrous histiocytoma (pleomorphic storiform, myxoid, giant cell, angiomatoid, histiocytic)
Adipose	Lipoma (angiolipoma, spindle-cell, pleomorphic, lipoblastoma, lipoblastomatosis, intranervous, lipomatosis, hibernoma)	Liposarcoma (well-differentiated, myxoid)	Liposarcoma (pleomorphic, round cell, dedifferentiated)
Smooth muscular	Leiomyoma (vascular, deep)	Grades 1, 2 leiomyosarcoma	Grade 3, 4 leiomyosarcoma
Striated muscular	Rhabdomyoma (adult, fetal, genital, cardiac)		Rhabdomyosarcoma (embryonal, alveolar, pleomorphic)
Vascular	Angiomas and angiodysplasias Glomus tumor Epithelioid hemangioma Hemangiopericytoma	Low-grade hemangioendothelioma Kaposi's sarcoma Hemangiopericytoma	High-grade hemangioendothelioma Kaposi's sarcoma Hemangiopericytoma
Synovial			Synovial sarcoma
Nervous	Heurinoma Neurofibroma		Malignant neurinoma Peripheral neuroepithelioma
Cartilaginous		Myxoid chondrosarcoma Synovial chondrosarcoma	Mesenchymal chondrosarcoma

Table 2
Soft tissue tumors (continued)

Osseous			Osteosarcoma
Uncertain	Intramuscular myxoma Granular cell tumor		Malignant granular cell tumor Ewing's sarcoma Alveolar sarcoma Epithelioid sarcoma Clear cell sarcoma of the tendons and apo-neurosis

Along with tumors, there are so-called **tumor-like** lesions known as such because they may resemble tumors, and are often involved in a discussion of differential diagnosis. These forms are generally dysplastic or hyperplastic, and etiology may or may not be known. They include:

in the bone:

— bone cyst;
— aneurysmal bone cyst;
— mucous cyst;
— progressive telangiectatic osteolysis;
— histiocytosis X;
— osteosis due to primary hyperparathyroidism;
— giant cell reparative granuloma;
— tumor-like periosteal ossifications.

In the soft tissues:

— palmar and plantar fibromatosis;
— nodular fasciitis;
— proliferative fasciitis and proliferative myositis;
— elastofibroma;
— xanthoma;
— infantile xanthogranuloma;
— mucous cyst;
— amputation neuroma, Morton's neuroma;
— synovial chondromatosis;
— tumoral calcinosis;
— tumor-like muscular ossifications;
— pigmented (villo-) nodular synovitis.

FREQUENCY

Bone tumors

Tumors of the bone are not a frequent occurrence. Statistics from the United States indicate an incidence of about 10 cases of primary malignant bone tumor/million population/year. If we consider the fact that there are more than thirty varieties, then only large specialized centers may have had enough experience with some of them. Some varieties, such as hemangioendothelioma, angiosarcoma, hemangiopericytoma, mesenchymal chondrosarcoma, desmoid fibroma, adamantinoma of the long bones, are so rare that their clinical and prognostic features still cannot be accurately defined.

Among benign tumors, those most frequently observed are histiocytic fibroma and exostosis, followed by chondroma, giant cell tumor, osteoid osteoma, and fibrous dysplasia.

Among malignant tumors, that most frequently observed is plasmacytoma, followed by osteosarcoma. These are followed by chondrosarcoma, and Ewing's sarcoma. Malignant fibrous histiocytoma, lymphoma and chordoma occur infrequently.

Vascular tumors and adamantinoma are rare. Tumors which derive from the nervous and fatty tissues are exceptionally rare.

The most frequent among tumor-like lesions is bone cyst, followed by the relatively frequent occurrence of histiocytosis X and aneurysmal bone cyst.

Tumors of the soft tissues

In tumors of the soft tissue benign neoformations (most of which are left unoperated) are more frequent than sarcomas (10/1 according to Enzinger and Weiss, 1983). Sarcomas of the soft tissues occur approximately twice as often as skeletal ones, thus about 20 cases/million population/year.

Among benign tumors, lipoma and histiocytoma occur frequently, and angioma and desmoid tumor relatively frequently.

Among sarcomas, those most frequently observed are liposarcoma and malignant fibrous histiocytoma.

DIAGNOSIS

It has become common-place to affirm that diagnosis must be based on a combination of clinical, radiographic, macroscopic and histological data. This affirmation, which is as boring as all common-place sayings, is however a categorical one. To repeat it with emphasis is not useless, as there are radiologists and surgeons who presume that they may make a diagnosis and establish treatment without obtaining histological confirmation, just as there are pathologists who sign their histologic reports having no knowledge of the clinical, radiographic or anatomo-surgical data.

The errors which this type of behavior may produce occur frequently, and may be the cause of irreparable consequences. A few examples in our constant and recent experience follow.

To venture a diagnosis on the basis of the **radiographic picture alone** may lead to mistaking an osteomyelitis for an Ewing's sarcoma, or vice versa, an

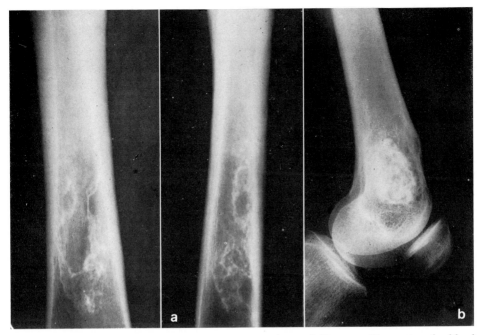

FIG. 1. - (a) Diaphyseal skeletal infarction in a male aged 42 years. The patient had had two episodes of air (decompression) embolia 19 and 13 years earlier. (b) Female aged 59 years. Chance radiographic finding. Biopsy carried out with histological finding of osseous necrosis.

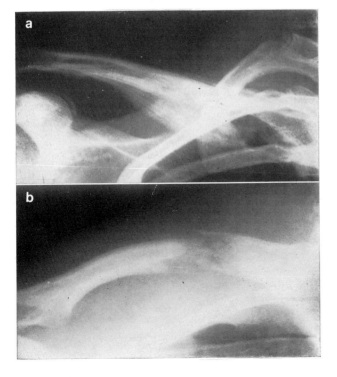

FIG. 2. - (a) Osteitis of the clavicle in a child aged 11 years. Onion-skin reactive periostosis suggested Ewing's sarcoma. (b) Osteitis of the clavicle in a female aged 42 years. The faded osteolysis with interruption of the cortex and pathologic fracture simulated an osteolytic malignant tumor, primary or metastatic.

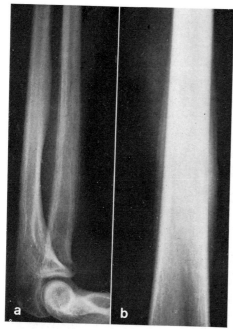

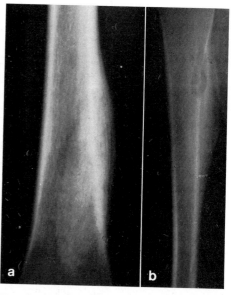

FIG. 3. - (a) Osteomyelitis of the radius in a male aged 31 years. The periosteal reaction with superimposed layers, rather faded, associated with «moth-eaten» features in the cortex, simulated an Ewing's sarcoma. (b) Osteomyelitis of the femur, in a boy aged 15 years. Again, the layered periosteal reaction suggested Ewing's sarcoma.

FIG. 4. - (a) Osteoperiostitis of the femur in a boy aged 12 years. The onion-skin periostosis is too circumscribed and mature to be an Ewing's sarcoma, and not compact enough to be an osteoid osteoma. (b) Brodie's abscess in a female aged 4 years in the proximal humerus. The osteolytic cavity has an elongated and irregular shape, which distinguishes it from osteoid osteoma.

aneurysmal bone cyst for a malignant tumor, an epithelial metastasis of the bone for a primary skeletal tumor, or vice versa, a chronic abscess of the bone or an eosinophilic granuloma or a lesion from hyperparathyroidism for a tumor.

To base diagnosis **exclusively on biopsy** may lead to mistaking a «myositis ossificans» for an osteosarcoma, an osteosarcoma for an osteoblastoma, a chondromyxoid fibroma for a chondrosarcoma, a chondosarcoma for a chondroma, a lesion from hyperparathyroidism for a giant cell tumor, a hemorrhagic osteosarcoma for an aneurysmal bone cyst, a synovial chondromatosis for a chondrosarcoma.

There are only a few types of bone tumor where the radiographic picture is so typical that biopsy is usually not required. Examples are histiocytic fibroma, exostosis, chondroma, fibrous dysplasia.

For example, let us observe the diagnostic and prognostic importance of various elements that must be associated with the histological evaluation. The latter is, nonetheless, the most important and accurate means of diagno-

FIG. 5. - (a) Chronic osteitis of the calcaneum in a female aged 28 years. Bone sclerosis suggests osteoid osteoma, even if a nidus is not observed. (b) Brodie's abscess of the calcaneum in a male aged 24 years. The osteolytic cavity, centered by a small sequester and surrounded by a halo of hyperostosis, is too irregular in shape to be an osteoid osteoma.

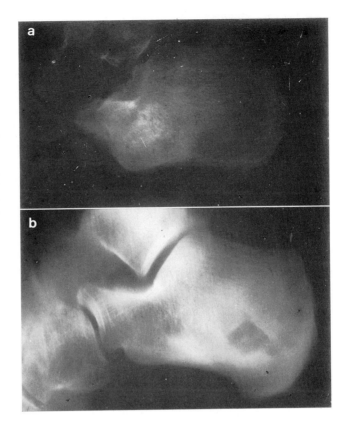

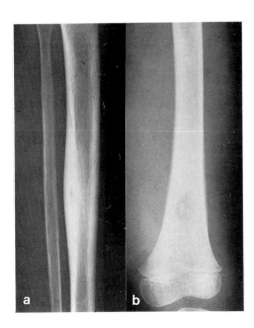

FIG. 6. - (a) Intracortical Brodie's abscess of the tibial diaphysis in a boy aged 10 years. It considerably resembles osteoid osteoma. (b) Brodie's abscess of the femur in a boy aged 7 years. The osteolytic cavity is centered by a small sequester; there is a thin line of immature periosteal reaction. It superficially resembles osteoid osteoma.

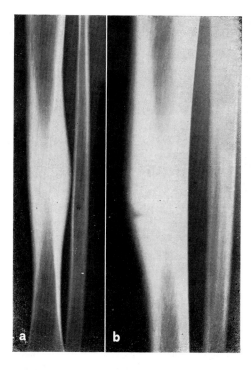

FIG. 7. - (a) Chronic sclerosing osteope-riostitis in a boy aged 6 years. The picture is very similar to that of an osteoid osteoma, except that there is no nidus. (b) Fatigue fracture of the anterior tibial cortex in a recruit aged 20 years. The fracture is surrounded by intense hyperostosis and periostosis and is only evident with tomography. Cases of this type have sometimes been needlessly biopsied.

sis. Illustrations (Figs. 1-18) pertain to some non-tumoral lesions that may, radiographically, simulate a tumor.

History and clinical features

Age may be a determining factor. A giant cell tumor, for example, is a rare occurrence prior to puberty. A chondrosarcoma is nearly unknown in the child. Ewing's sarcoma is rare before 5 years of age (metastatic neuroblasto-

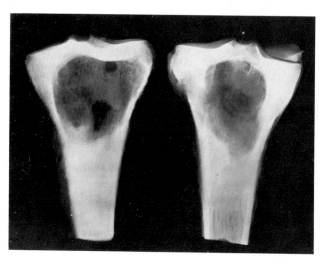

FIG. 8. - Chronic abscess of the bone in a male aged 29 years. The radiographic picture was interpreted as giant cell tumor. Nonetheless, the well-defined borders of the osteolytic area and the surrounding sclerosing bone, in addition to the central location of the lesion, contrast with this diagnosis (radiography of resected specimen).

FIG. 9. - Tubercular osteo-arthritis of the ankle joint in a male aged 39 years. The meta-epiphyseal osteolytic cavities were filled with granulation tissue and pus. The radiographic picture could suggest a tumor, but it is not typical of any particular tumor. Furthermore, there is a small area of subchondral osteolysis in the fibula. The clinical picture decidedly indicated the inflammatory nature.

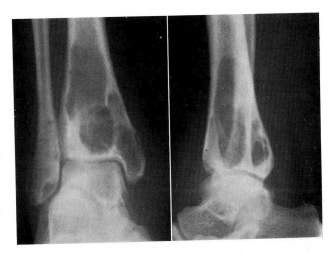

ma is more probable) and after 30 years of age (lymphoma is more probable). Plasmacytoma and chordoma are observed nearly exclusively during adult age, as is metastasis due to carcinoma. Among tumors of the soft tissues, some fibromatoses occur exclusively during childhood, and rhabdomyosarcoma is prevalently infantile. Synovial sarcoma and fibrosarcoma are usually observed during young adult age, while liposarcoma and malignant fibrous histiocytoma prevail in advanced adult age. Soft-tissue fibrosarcoma has a

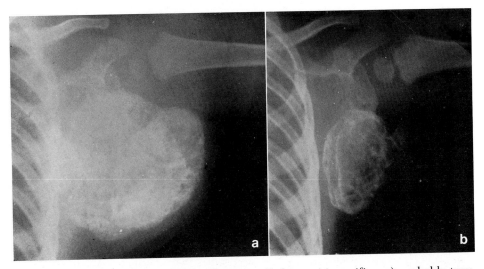

FIG. 10. - (a) Myoperiosteal ossification (so-called myositis ossificans) probably traumatic in a female aged 7 months. A parascapular mass adhering to the scapula occurred at 3 months, growing rapidly. The parents were told that it could be a malignant neoplasm. The radiogram was diagnostic and corresponded to advanced maturation of the ossification which, at this stage, had already decreased in volume. (b) After 11 months, and with no therapy, the mass has decreased in volume, it has further matured, and shoulder function is normal.

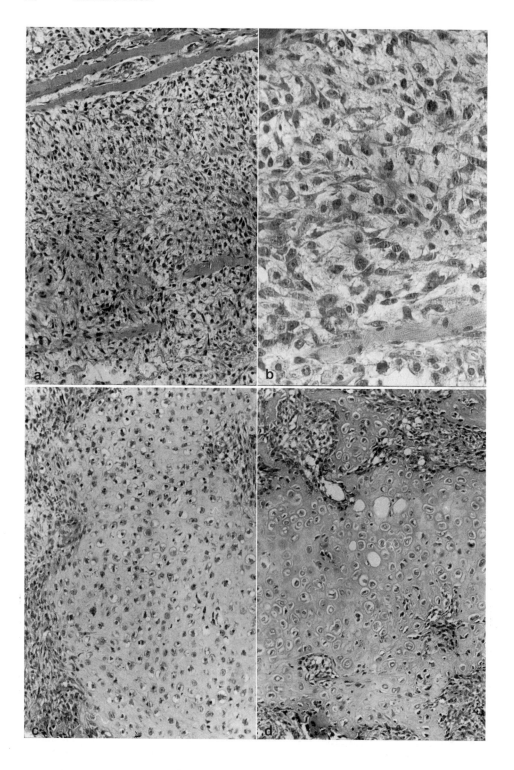

FIG. 11.

FIG. 12. - (a) «Brown tumor» due to primary hyperparathyroidism in a female aged 49 years, one year after excision of the parathyroid adenoma. The enormous tumor-like mass extensively ossified after removal of the adenoma. The resulting radiographic picture suggests a tumor, but it is very difficult to interpret. (b) Paget's osteopathy. The intense osteolysis was produced by immobilization consequent to pathologic fracture. The radiographic picture corresponds to removal of plaster and could suggest a neoplasm. (c) The same skeletal segment 14 months later resumed the more usual appearance of Paget's osteopathy.

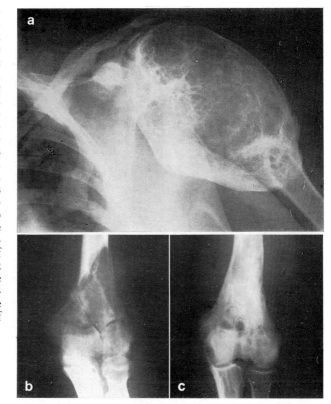

better prognosis when it occurs during childhood than when it occurs during adult age.

The **speed of the growth** of the tumor; if a doubt should arise, for example, between a usual osteosarcoma and a parosteal osteosarcoma, a history of symptoms dating back several years would indicate the second rather than the first. In sarcomas of the soft tisssues, the presence of a relatively static mass, even for several years, does not contradict malignancy, as may occur in the case of synovial sarcoma. In each sarcoma, however, rapid growth and early local recurrence are unfavorable prognostic signs.

Pain facilitates the diagnosis of osteoid osteoma and glomus tumor. The occurrence of pain in a central chondroma which has always been asymptomatic, and in the absence of fracture, leads us to suspect the insurgence of a malignant tumor. Among sarcomas of the soft tissues, pain is rather characteristic of synovial sarcoma.

◀

FIG. 11. - Histological pictures of muscular ossification. (a) Intense histiofibroblastic proliferation between residues of muscular fibrocells. (b) The actively proliferating cells are large, with slightly hyperchromatic nuclei, and frequent mitotic figures. (c) and (d) Cartilaginous and osteocartilaginous production during the early stage of ossification. This cartilage also has actively proliferating and hypertrophic cells. Histological pictures of this type were mistaken for sarcoma, particularly osteosarcoma (*Hemat.-eos.*, 125, 300, 125, 125 x).

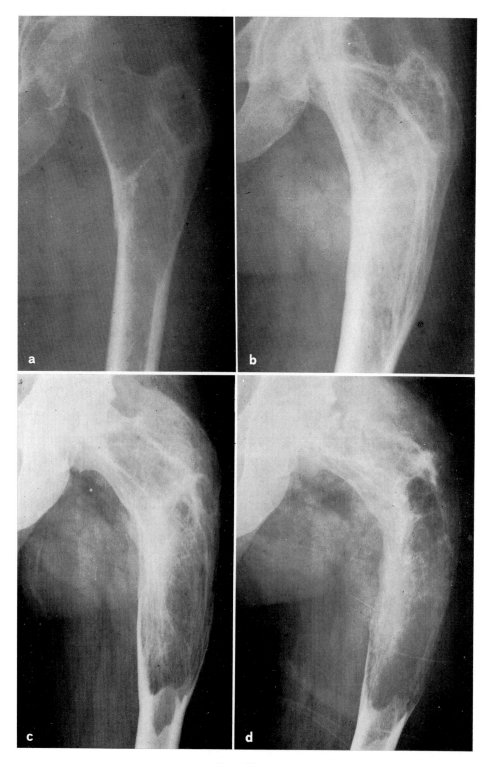

FIG. 13.

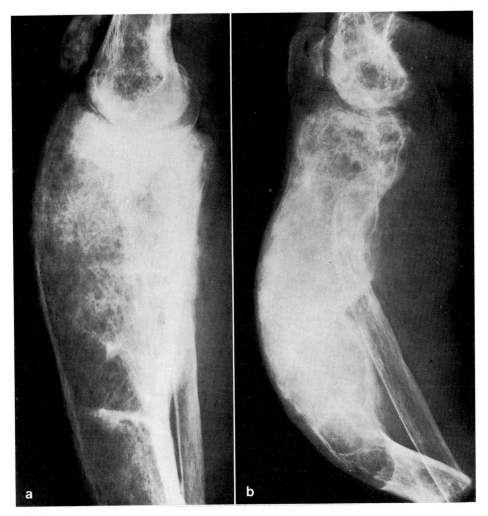

FIG. 14. - (a) Familiar osteolytic and expanding Paget's disease in a male aged 56 years. (b) Familial Paget's disease, severely osteolytic in a brother of the patient in (a), male aged 49 years. Radiography of the anatomical specimen. This patient was submitted to amputation of the thigh as a result of the deformity and repeated fractures and presumption of tumor lesion. A histological examination of the amputated specimen was erroneously interpreted as fibrous dysplasia.

The presence of **fever** and the young age of the patient tend to diagnose Ewing's sarcoma, rather than lymphoma.

An **accurate history** may be a determining factor, for example, in the case of epithelial metastasis of the skeleton and of bone lesions due to hyperpara-

◀

FIG. 13. - (a) Paget's osteopathy of the proximal femur in a male aged 36 years. (b) Extension and evolution of the lesion after 5 years. (c) After 4 more years. (d) After 7 more years. In this case the osteopathy has spontaneously become very osteolytic. The lesion in (d) was biopsied as it was presumed that there was a tumor.

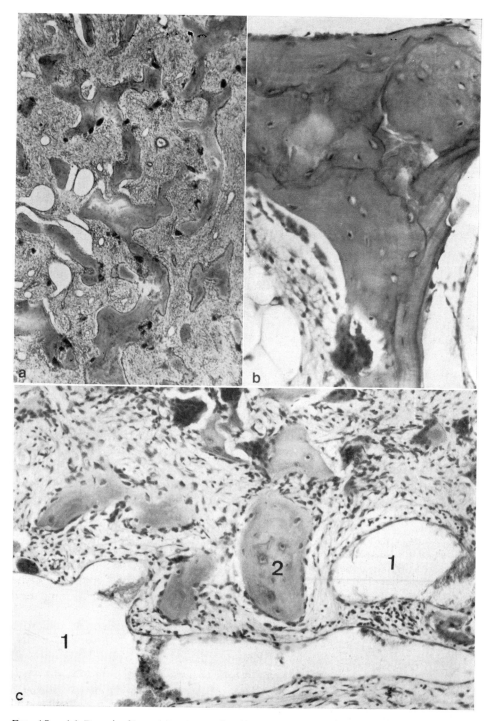

FIG. 15. - (a) Paget's disease in a prevalently osteolytic area. This picture was at times confused with fibrous dysplasia. (b) The larger skeletal trabeculae reveal the mosaic structure. (c) Detail illustrating the ample sinusoids (1), the newly-formed trabeculae (2), the loose fibrous tissue and the numerous osteoclasts (*Hemat.-eos.*, 50, 300, 125 x).

FIG. 16. - (a) Echinococcus cyst extended to most of the femur in a male aged 52 years. The lesion may suggest a tumor, but it is not typical of any tumor in particular. In 1 there is interruption of the cortex. (b) Echinococcus cyst of the fourth lumbar vertebra in a female aged 36 years. Partial destruction of the vertebral body with areas of increased radiopacity and uninjured disc space strongly suggest a malignant neoplasm.

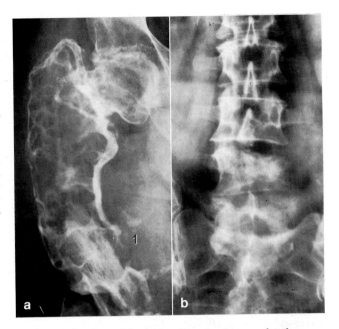

thyroidism. A family history may also be of help in diagnosing multiple exostosis and neurofibromatosis.

The **site and localization of the tumor** are of considerable importance. Giant cell tumor is nearly always located in the meta-epiphysis or in the meta-apophysis, and usually occurs when the growth cartilage has disappeared. A metaphyseal tumor where the growth cartilage is present is generally not a giant cell tumor. Chondroblastoma is nearly always localized in the epiphysis or in the apophysis abutting on or trespassing the fertile cartilage. Tumors of cartilaginous origin are not observed in the cranial bones. Adamantinoma is nearly exclusively observed in the tibia or in the ulna; chordoma, in the cranial base, in the sacrum, or in the vertebral column.

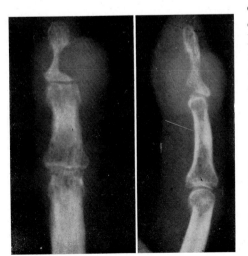

Faced with the histological slide of a tumor which is formed by hyalin cartilage, depending on whether it is localized in the bones of the hand, or in another area of the skeleton, the diagnosis could be chondroma and

FIG. 17. - Epidermoid cyst in a male aged 30 years. The nodular mass deprived of radiopacity in the soft tissues is evident. The bone of the distal phalanx appeared to be eroded from the outside. These elements distinguish it from a chondroma of the distal phalanx.

respectively low-grade chondrosarcoma. If the chondromatous tissue derives from the uppermost part of an exostosis in a child, from a periosteal chondroma, or from a synovial chondromatosis, the histological criteria of malignancy will change once again. It is a general rule that periosteal tumors are less malignant than their equivalents, originating within the bone (central): this is true for osteosarcoma, and chondrosarcoma. Some tumors are less malignant in certain sites than in others, as is the case of osteosarcoma of the jaw bones.

Synovial sarcoma is nearly always localized in the proximity of the joints, particularly, in the knee or foot; neurinoma is related to a nerve trunk. Sarcomas of the soft tissues nearly always have a deep, subfascial site; a subcutaneous mesenchymal tumor is rarely malignant, and when it is, its tendency to metastasize is less than in its deep counterpart. All sarcomas, whether of the bone or of the soft tissues, occur rarely in the hand; epithelioid sarcoma, however, shows predilection for the hand and forearm.

Radiographic features

The radiogram is an indispensable element in the diagnosis of skeletal tumors. It provides a negative image of the tumor, and reveals its aggression to the host bone. Essentially, there are two changes in bone tissue as a result of the tumor: osteolysis and reactive osteogenesis.

A massive osteolysis, with undefined borders, where the cortex is surpassed or destroyed by the tumor, with scarce reactive peritumoral osteogenesis, indicates a tumor which is rapidly aggressive. An osteolysis with well-defined borders, having a hyperopaque rim of peritumoral reactive osteogenesis, with a cortex which is well-preserved, or a continuous bony shell as a result of periosteal osteogenesis, indicates that there is a slow-growing and non-permeative tumor.

Radiograms which are repeated in time document the progression or quiescence of the tumor.

It should be stressed how much can be learned from a careful and analytical study of radiograms, which must be of excellent quality, taken in several views, and sometimes completed by tomograms. A rather instructive exercise in diagnosis is the attempt to make one or more preventive diagnoses based on radiograms, arranging them in order of probability, and then comparing them with the macroscopic picture as well as with the histological diagnosis.

The radiographic picture is a guide to biopsy and an essential complement to the histological examination. A histological diagnosis should never be made without first having seen the radiograms. Not infrequently the study of the radiograms leads the pathologist to change his first histological impression. In cases such as those involving parosteal osteosarcoma, peripheral chondrosarcoma, tumor-like muscular and periosteal ossifications, hyperparathyroidism osteosis, the radiographic picture may be of diagnostic value which is equal to or greater than that of the biopsy.

In tumors of the soft tissues a radiographic examination is of much less diagnostic importance. Nonetheless, the presence of intratumoral calcifications may direct diagnosis towards the probability of synovial sarcoma. Typical intra-articular calcifications-ossifications are very indicative of synovial chondromatosis. Images of phleboliths are pathognomic of angiomas.

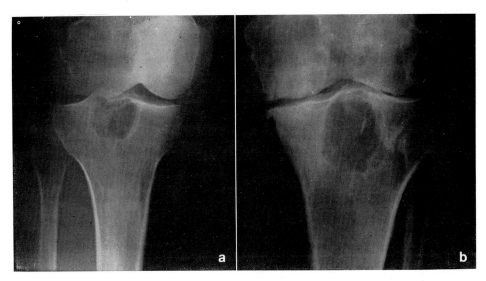

FIG. 18. - (a) and (b) In both cases the osteolytic cavity corresponds to an osteoarthritic cyst, in a woman aged 56 years and in a man aged 64, respectively.

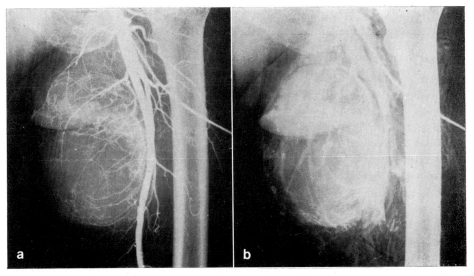

FIG. 19. - Female aged 80 years. Arteriography: (a) arterial phase; (b) venous phase. Histological diagnosis: high grade fibrosarcoma. In this case, because of the relationships with the large vessels, wide excision should include the vessels themselves in the resection.

Angiography

Arteriography is of considerable value in defining the boundaries of the tumor in its three dimensions, as well as its relationship with the principal vessels. To this purpose, arteriography must be obtained **in two orthogonal views**.

Angiography has to large extent been substituted by CAT and MRI for tumors of the skeleton and of the soft tissues. The diagnostic value of angiography is mainly restricted to tumors of a vascular nature, such as angiomas. It is, however, important in planning therapy, when, for example, a principal vascular bundle must be resected with the tumor, and a by-pass is required (Fig. 19), or when a vascularized skeletal or myocutaneous transplant is performed, or during selective arterial embolization. It is also indicated prior to extensive surgery for vertebral tumors, to show the arteries supplying the spinal cord and the vertebral arteries. Venous phase of the arteriography or phlebography may be indicated to discover venous neoplastic plugs. Arteriography is also employed when doing preoperative intra-arterial chemotherapy.

In skeletal tumors and in those of the soft tissues, **arteriographic images of malignancy** are: intense hypervascularity of the tumor; vessels which are anomalous, tortuous, ectatic, varicose, and cavernous; cloudy diffusion of contrast medium in the tumor site; indirect signs of arteriovenous shunt. Nonetheless, there are areas deprived of vessels in malignant tumors as well: chondosarcoma, necrotic, hemorrhagic, cystic areas.

Lymphography is, although rarely, indicated in demonstrating lymph node metastasis, possibly as a guide to biopsy of the lymph nodes (Ewing's sarcoma, lymphoma, rabdomyosarcoma, synovial sarcoma).

Isotope bone scan

This is carried out with technetium 99, which is fixed (early phase) where the blood supply to the bone is higher and (late phase) where Ca salt crystals are formed, that is, in areas of osteogenesis. Any process that is accompanied by vivid osteogenesis produces a «hot» area in bone scan: bone tumors with neoplastic or reactive osteogenesis, tumors of the soft tissues located near the bone, enough to induce a reaction of the bone itself, fracture, infection, rheumatoid arthritis, arthrosis, Paget's disease.

Bone scan is a useful technique for the following reasons: 1) it constitutes an index of quiescence or activity (for example, in exostoses, in «myositis ossificans»). 2) With a single examination, the entire skeleton may be explored, and, as such, it is particularly useful in histiocytosis X, skeletal metastasis, plasmacytoma, Ewing's sarcoma, lymphoma; but it is also potentially useful in the staging of each neoplasm, whether of the bone or of the soft tissues, which may metastasize to the skeleton. 3) It may reveal bone tumor localizations which are hardly or not at all visible on radiogram (osteoid osteoma, small metastatic deposits). 4) It may reveal the actual extent of the tumor along the bone, and its medullary canal; at times it reveals «skip metastases». 5) It reveals skeletal reaction to an adjacent tumor of the soft tissues, thus indicating the need to include parts of the bone in surgical excision. 6) It may be useful in periodical monitoring of the patient after treatment. 7) It constitutes an indication of the response of the tumor to chemotherapy. To this end quantitative or dynamic bone scan is used.

Computerized axial tomography (CAT)

This often constitutes the most important examination. It should be performed with contrast medium (in order to visualize the main vessels and any uptake of contrast medium by the neoplasm), including for comparison the

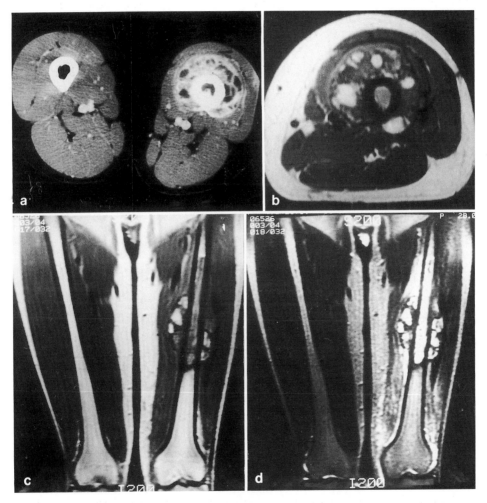

FIG. 20. - Male aged 25 years: hemorrhagic osteosarcoma of the diaphysis of the left femur. (a) CAT with contrast medium revealing the major vessels and the extraosseous part of the tumor. (b) MRI of a corresponding section. (c) and (d) MRI in the coronal plane, weighed in T_1 and T_2, respectively. The extent of the tumor in the medullary canal of the diaphysis is accurately visualized.

two halves of the body or the two limbs, using windows for the bone and/or for the soft tissues (Figs. 20, 21).

In tumors of the skeleton it helps to visualize: 1) the extent of the tumor in the medullary canal, thus establishing the site of resection, or distinguishing a periosteal or parosteal form from a central one, for example, in osteosarcoma; 2) the extent of the tumor towards the soft tissues and in the various muscular compartments and extracompartmental spaces; 3) its relationship with the main vascular bundle, the nerves, the internal organs; 4) the relationship between the tumor and the joint cavity and the capsulo-synovial insertions, in order to establish whether resection should be intra- or extra-articular.

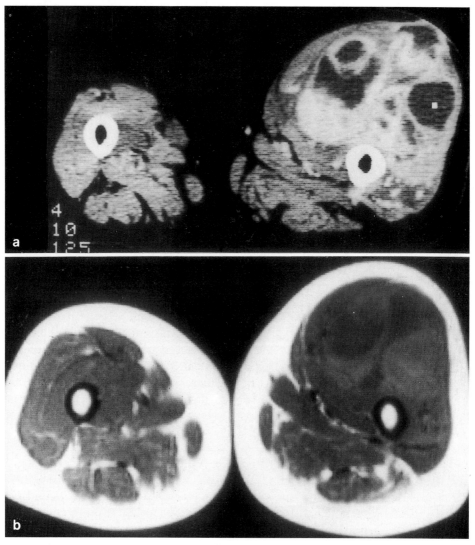

FIG. 21.

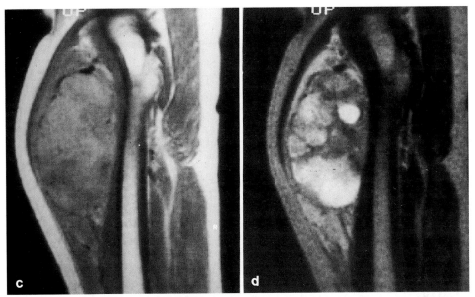

FIG. 21. - Female aged 51 years: malignant fibrous histiocytoma of the soft tissues. (a) CAT with contrast medium revealing the vessels and solid and hypervascularized parts of the tumor. (b) MRI of a corresponding section. (c) and (d) MRI in the sagittal plane, weighed in T_1 and T_2.

Similarly, in tumors of the soft tissues CAT reveals the location and extent of the tumor in the suprafascial and muscular compartments, in the extracompartmental spaces, and its relationships with the vessels, the nerves, the skeleton, the internal organs. Furthermore, it reveals whether the tumor is adipose, parenchymatous or liquid.

CAT is also useful in demonstrating the effect of radiation or chemotherapy, and it may be indispensable when monitoring local recurrence after skeletal or soft tissue resections.

CAT is also widely used to demonstrate pulmonary metastasis, for which its sensitivity is greater than that of traditional tomography.

CAT does not obtain good images when metal is involved (endoprosthesis, plates, screws): but this drawback is now dealt with by improved technique and by MRI. At times CAT may provide false positives: for example, the extent of the tumor along the medullary canal may be simulated by edema or hemorrhage of the bone marrow, and pulmonary metastases by nodules of atelectasia or fibrosis.

Magnetic resonance imaging (MRI)

It has several advantages as compared to CAT: views of longitudinal planes in addition to transverse ones, better differentiation between various tissues. It is particularly useful in measuring the extent of the tumor in the bone and along the medullary canal. Furthermore, it does not require contrast medium and is harmless for the patient (Figs. 20, 21).

Laboratory tests

These are often of determining importance for a diagnosis of plasmacytoma (monoclonal proteins), in metastases due to neuroblastoma (metabolites of the catecholamines), hyperparathyroidism osteosis (metabolism of Ca and serum PTH). In cases of osteosarcoma, serum alkaline phosphatase, and in cases of Ewing's sarcoma, lactate dehydrogenase (LDH) are of diagnostic and prognostic value.

Various types of primary tumors, in both the skeleton and the soft tissues, may exceptionally cause a hypophosphatemic and vitamin D resistant **osteomalacia**, which regresses when the tumor is eradicated. These are benign tumors, and ones which are very vascularized: in the bone, osteoblastoma, chondroblastoma, hemangiopericytoma, giant cell tumor; in the soft tissues, hemangioma and hemangiopericytoma.

Gross pathologic features

Many bone tumors, such as exostosis, histiocytic fibroma, fibrous dysplasia, osteoid osteoma, chondroma and chondrosarcoma, and in the soft tissues, desmoid tumor, angioma, lipoma, and, sometimes, liposarcoma, have a rather typical macroscopic picture. Some tumor-like lesions also have a very typical macroscopic picture, such as bone cyst, aneurysmal bone cyst, eosinophilic granuloma, mucous cyst, pigmented villo-nodular synovitis, synovial chondromatosis.

In addition to providing indications on the nature of the lesion, the macroscopic picture offers essential data on its aggression, particularly expressed by permeation and destruction of the cortex and cancellous bone, surpassing the periosteum, and invasion of the soft tissues.

It is very instructive for the surgeon to compare the macroscopic appearance in vivo and the anatomical specimen with the histological picture. By doing so he will learn to recognize the aspects of the various tumoral tissues, the areas of dry or colliquative necrosis, the hemorrhagic and cystic areas; and he will learn to distinguish healthy tissues from those modified by vicinity to the tumor (reactive bone, reactive muscle, reactive fibrous tissue), and from actual neoplasm. Needless to say, this ability to judge is of paramount importance in performing biopsy and conservative surgery of the tumor.

Histological evaluation

Rules cannot be dictated for diagnosis under a microscope, which constitutes the automatic synthesis of innumerable analytical perceptions. However, it may be recommended that a specimen be first observed under small enlargement, to then move onto the details, only after the general structure and the relationships of the tumor have been viewed. Another good habit is that of always running over the entire extent of the specimen, even when the diagnosis appears to be clear at a first glance, and the case seems to be an evident one. Vital areas of the tumor should be searched for, rather than those altered by necrosis, hemorrhage, calcification, and other regressive or reactive phenomena.

When a histological picture resembles a specific pathological process without totally identifying with it, all of the possible diagnostic alternatives are spread out on the field, radiograms are studied further, the clinical and laboratory data are examined once again, complementary sections and stains are carried out, as, quite often, the true diagnosis is not that suggested by the first microscopic impression. Although it may seem paradoxical, it is our conviction that histology is a nearly exact science. If the specimens are representative of a pathological process, if they are abundant, and technically good, the histological picture is generally that which it must be, and not another.

Long-term follow-up of patients

There is only one way to know the true biological behavior of the tumor, its gradient of aggression towards the host, its malignancy: and that is, by seeing how it evolves. This has been done, and is currently being done, by following-up an ever-increasing number of patients for many years after treatment. In this manner, the prognosis of most tumors of the skeleton is known. For some rare forms, such as skeletal hemangioendothelioma, prognosis still needs to be worked on by collecting more cases.

Sarcomas of the soft tissues have not generally been studied with the same completion and depth as tumors of the skeleton, so that some still need to be better defined in terms of their anatomo-clinical features, biological behavior, development and prognosis.

The limits of time required to be able to consider a malignant tumor to be healed is not 5 years (as is continued to be upheld arbitrarily), but rather at least 10 years after treatment.

Long-term follow-up of patients constitutes a final confirmation of the diagnosis formulated, as well as a confirmation of the validity of the classification system adopted. In fact, each oncotype has a typical prognosis.

We have said that time is the only means of establishing the aggressiveness of tumoral categories. Traditional cytological criteria for malignancy (giantism, pleomorphism, hyperchromia, mitoses) are in fact of relative value for each tumoral entity. Frequent mitotic figures may be observed in giant cell tumor, aneurysmal bone cyst, and in muscular ossifications. Cellular pleomorphism may be observed in chondromyxoid fibroma and in synovial chondromatosis. Sporadic giant bizarre cells are to be found in osteoblastoma and in neurinoma. These are all benign lesions. On the contrary, in some types of chondrosarcoma, in very sclerotic areas of usual osteosarcoma, in vast areas on parosteal osteosarcoma, the cytological aspects of malignancy may be scarce, or they may not be evident at all. And yet, these are malignant tumors.

The evolution of the tumor in the weeks following biopsy may at times correct a diagnosis which was incorrect due to underestimation. Let us recall one case, histologically diagnosed as aneurysmal bone cyst, which one month after biopsy proved to be a hemorrhagic osteosarcoma. Another case, diagnosed as osteoblastoma, was observed once again after two months, and was also revealed to be an osteosarcoma.

BIOPSY

Biopsy may be carried out using any one of five methods: using a thin needle (needle-aspiration); using a trocar (a carrot of tissue is removed); open removal of the entire tumor (excisional biopsy); open removal of a sample of tumor (incisional biopsy); open removal of a sample of tumor, with immediate diagnosis on frozen sections.

Thin needle biopsy

Needle-aspiration allows for a cytological examination on a freshly stained smear or after fixation. The disadvantage to using this method consists in the fact that diagnosis is incomplete and at times unsafe because it is based on the observation of only a few sparse cells. In tumors of the soft tissues, where for surgical indication may be sufficient a general diagnosis of sarcoma based on the demonstration of anaplastic cells, some authors recommend the use of aspiration biopsy with a thin needle. This may also be used to simply confirm clinical-radiographic diagnosis of local recurrence of a tumor whose histology is already known.

Trocar biopsy

This may be performed under local anesthesia, or it may require general anesthesia. It involves removal of one or more carrots of tissue 2-3 mm in diameter. It has the advantage of minimizing trauma, risk of infection, skin surface and underlying tissues to be sacrificed with definitive surgery, and of allowing immediate radiation therapy or chemotherapy, when indicated. It cannot be carried out in osteo-sclerotic bone tumors or in those contained by a thick layer of compact bone. Nowadays when many therapeutic protocols involve preoperative chemotherapy, trocar biopsy is used widely, thus avoiding an operation.

Trocar biopsy is particularly useful in cases where diagnosis is facilitated by the clinical-radiographic picture, such as in the case of giant cell tumor, or osteosarcoma. It is also indicated for osteolytic lesions of the vertebral body under x-ray or CAT monitoring (Fig. 573). The disadvantages of using this type of biopsy are constituted by the fact that as the specimen is scarce, diagnosis may be uncertain or impossible. Should this be the case, it is necessary to repeat the trocar biopsy or to resort to an incisional biopsy.

Excisional biopsy

Sometimes, after exposing a tumor of unknown nature, the surgeon does not limit his work to taking a bioptic sample, rather he excises the lesion (curettage of the skeletal cavity and/or dissection of the tumor from the surrounding soft tissues). This kind of blind operation (particularly practiced in tumors of the soft tissues) is dangerous, and generally irrational. If successive histological examination reveals the tumor to be malignant, excision is often followed by local recurrence. When a malignant tumor is intralesionally or marginally excised, even if it appears to be circumscribed or capsulated, some traces of the tumor are nearly always left in situ. At the periphery of a sarcoma, the compressed and reactive adjacent tisssues form a fibrous or bony pseudocapsule. Nonetheless, this delimitation of the tumor is apparent, as the pseudocapsule is nearly always permeated by a spray of tumor cells.

After an excisional biopsy for a malignant tumor, it is therefore indicated to return to the surgical wound in order to perform wide excision of the surrounding tissues. Such excision, however, is usually imprecise and hazardous, because a) the tumor is no longer there to spot the place, and b) it is not known if and where the previous surgery may have contaminated tissues with dissection, hematoma, or driving intramedullary nails. Sometimes, after a wrong excisional biopsy, the only sound procedure would appear to be amputation.

In conclusion, **excisional biopsy must be strictly limited to those cases in which the benignity of the tumor is absolutely certain, even before a histological examination** is carried out, based on clinical, radiographic and macroscopic intraoperative data (histiocytic fibroma, exostosis, bone cyst, osteoid osteoma, aneurysmal bone cyst, fibrous dysplasia, chondroma, and, in the soft tissues, angioma, lipoma). Among malignant tumors, an exception may be made for tumors where excision is in any case indicated, such as in some peripheral chondrosarcomas, in some skeletal lesions which are definitely metastatic or systemic and painful, in excision of neoplastic lymph nodes, in neoplastic lesions in sites which would not otherwise be operable except with partial or subtotal excision, and where the compressed nervous structures must be released, such as in the vertebral column.

In all other cases, when the nature of the tumor is even slightly uncertain, and a surgical solution may vary depending on the histological diagnosis, **excisional biopsy must be avoided**.

Incisional biopsy

This may above all be used in malignant tumors or ones which are suspected to be malignant.

When definitive surgery involving either bone resection or excision of the soft tissues is foreseen, **the incision of the biopsy must be made along the same line of the incision that will be used for surgery**. Furthermore, the bone will have to be approached by passing through the muscular fibers, not through the interstice between the muscles (for example, for a tumor of the proximal humerus, through the fibers of the deltoid; for a tumor of the distal femur, through the fibers of the quadriceps. In this manner, during resection such muscle will be excised en bloc together with the tumor). The muscle fibers will carefully be sutured on the biopsy. During definitive surgery the scalpel must not re-open the bioptic incision, rather it must excise it widely, including the skin and underlying tissues en bloc with the tumor. If the bioptic incision is wrongly located one of two alternatives may be chosen: to either perform definitive surgery using an atypical incision, which may be technically awkward, difficult, or impossible, and make nutrition of the skin and muscular flaps precarious, and cause necrosis; or to not excise the bioptic incision, which may cause local recurrence. The bioptic access must never cross an extracompartmental space, nor must it isolate a major neurovascular bundle.

When amputation is a possibility, the bioptic incision must be situated so as not to interfere with the pattern of the amputation flaps.

While biopsy is being carried out, the tumor must in no way be manipulated, nor must it be squeezed by Esmarch's bandage.

The soft tissues located around a malignant tumor often reveal increased or congested collateral circulation, as the tumor acts as an arteriovenous shunt. Incision of the tumor itself may produce severe hemorrhaging, when the tumoral tissue is intensely vascularized, or when it contains vascular lacunae without a wall of their own (angioblastic tumors, osteoblastoma, aneurysmal bone cyst, non-cartilaginous sarcomas, metastases due to hypernephroma). In cases such as these, the application of a hemostatic sponge, bee's wax, or prolonged compression are generally capable of controlling the hemorrhage. Nonetheless, this type of hemorrhage must be feared and possibly avoided, and the scalpel used with care.

Biopsy is performed with a scalpel, removing an entire sample of neoplastic tissue approximately 1 cubic cm in size. In central skeletal lesions an osteotome, scalpel or curette may be used, taking care to remove the block of pathological tissue with a single clean cut, delicately, without fragmenting it, crushing it, or disseminating it.

If the tissue removed appears to be necrotic or hemorrhagic, sampling should be extended until neoplastic tissue which is better-preserved is found.

After biopsy it is a good idea to seal the residual cavity (in the bone) with a block of acrylic cement or (in the soft tissues) with a hemostatic sponge, after using an electrocoagulator to generously cauterize the walls and the borders. Hemostasis must be painstaking and complete. Drainage is not used.

Incisional biopsy, with preparation of the specimens by inclusion and delayed histological diagnosis, is mainly indicated in the following: a) cases in which it is evident prior to biopsy that treatment will not be surgical: Ewing's sarcoma and lymphoma in non-surgical sites, metastases, unoperable and systemic lesions; b) cases in which a generous sample and an accurate study of the histological and cytological details is desirable (difficult tumors, such as round-cell sarcomas, sarcomas of the soft tissues, low-malignancy tumors or tumors of doubtful malignancy, rare tumors); c) cases where the tissue is completely ossified and which thus cannot be frozen-sectioned (rare cases of parosteal osteosarcoma or other eburneous tumors); d) cases in which a trocar biopsy or a frozen section specimen did not allow an accurate interpretation.

Frozen section biopsy (intraoperative)

This is an incisional biopsy, as described in the previous section. The unfixed tissue is immediately cut under the cryostat microtome (as long as it is a soft tissue, neither heavily calcified nor ossified) and stained. Modern cryostats produce excellent specimens, not much inferior to those by inclusion, in approximately 10 minutes. According to our experience, a safe diagnosis may be made — at least safe enough to answer the surgeon's question — in 9 cases out of 10. Surgery may either proceed according to a pre-established plan, or according to a different one, depending on the intraoperative histological examination.

Frozen section biopsy constitutes a rather useful method in the diagnosis of both benign and malignant tumors, with the exception of those listed in the previous section.

The method is still not routinely applied, due to the fact that it comes up against the reluctance of the surgeon and of the pathologist. The surgeon does not like to plan surgical treatment and obtain the authorization of the patient or of the family prior to knowing the histological diagnosis. The pathologist, in turn, prefers to take time to base his diagnosis on histologial specimens that are more familiar to him, rather than getting involved in a quick diagnosis made on less orthodox specimens.

It goes without saying that should histological diagnosis be uncertain on frozen sections, it will be postponed, and with it, surgery, until more extensive and clearer slides by inclusion are available.

What are the advantages of using frozen section biopsy? In benign tumors, such as giant cell tumors, chondroblastoma, osteoblastoma, aneurysmal bone cyst, it allows for the exclusion of unsuspected malignancy, thus permitting completion of treatment in one-stage surgery. In the case of ablative surgery for sarcomas, the amputation is performed immediately after the biopsy, thus avoiding two-stage surgery, and shortening the amount of time required for hospitalization.

If surgery involves resection of the skeletal segment, or en bloc excision of a tumor of the soft tissues, frozen section biopsy immediately followed by definitive surgery is considerably advantageous. In fact, operations of this kind imply that neoplastic cells are not disseminated in the surrounding tissues, and require clean cleavage planes, ones which are not modified by hematoma, edema, the onset of adherences, subsequent to biopsy performed a few days previously. Previous biopsy obliges us to remove the biopsy track widely en bloc with the tumor. Furthermore, skeletal resection (which generally involves the use of large bone grafts or endroprostheses) after previous incisional biopsy has an increased risk of infection.

Extemporaneous biopsy may also indicate whether the material removed is suited to diagnosis (and is not instead constituted by reactive, necrotic or hemorrhagic tissue), thus avoiding having to repeat the biopsy.

Finally, when in doubt, surgical margins may be monitored, thus constituting a precious means of monitoring and guiding the execution of surgery.

HISTOLOGY

In order to obtain a good histological specimen the first condition is good fixation. Some surgeons use rubbing alcohol which does not work particularly well, and which does not always provide good specimens. Formalin is more of a preservative than a fixative. It obtains good specimens, it hardens less than alcohol, but it penetrates slowly: to fix specimens of average size several days are required. Specimens are preserved in formalin for years. Thus, it may be used for the fixation of skeletal tissue, of specimens where a rapid histological preparation is not required, and which must be preserved; furthermore, it is used if staining is required for fats, eosinophilic granulocytes, for the argyrophilous reticulum. In order to make a more rapid diagnosis, to obtain better specimens and histochemical stainings, small specimens (0.5 cm in thickness) are fixed in Carnoy's or Bouin's fluid. At 58 degrees C Bouin's fluid acts as a bland decalcifier. Thus, a histological specimen may be obtained for fragments of soft tissue or for tissue which is slightly calcified (osteoid) in 24 to 48 hours.

When the specimen includes bone and soft tumor tissue, it is best to separate a fragment of soft tissue and to process it without decalcification; the non-decalcified specimen, in fact, better preserves the cytological details (for example, the staining ability of eosinophilic granulocytes). Furthermore, decalcification may lose the evidence of important details, such as pericellular calcar incrustations in chondroblastoma.

Decalcification of the bone may be obtained by using different types of acid, or with chelating substances, with or without an electrolytic method. All of these sytems are good ones, as long as they do not exceed the right point of decalcification; if this does occur, the cells lose their staining affinity and the skeletal tissue disintegrates. The best decalcifiers include formic and hydrochloric acid, ethylenediamine- tetra- acetic acid (EDTA).

Hematoxylin-eosin staining is in most cases the only one necessary. At times, however, supplementary staining is required. **P.A.S.-diastases for glycogen** is necessary in round-cell sarcomas, in order to distinguish Ewing's sarcoma (P.A.S. positive) from neuroblastoma and lymphoma (usually P.A.S. negative). In rhabdomyosarcoma, as well, both embryonal and alveolar, the cytoplasms are P.A.S. positive. In pleomorphic malignant tumors, P.A.S. positiveness allows for the exclusion of malignant fibrous histiocytoma and tends towards a diagnosis of another sarcoma or of a carcinoma. In spindle-

Table 3

GLYCOGENIC CONTENTS IN PRINCIPAL MALIGNANT TUMORS OF THE SKELETON AND SOFT
TISSUES (from Enzinger and Weiss, 1983, modified)

Usually present	Variable	Usually absent
Ewing's sarcoma Osteosarcoma Chondrosarcoma Clear cell chondrosarcoma Rhabdomyosarcoma Leiomyosarcoma Clear cell sarcoma Mesothelioma Melanoma	Carcinoma Liposarcoma Epithelioid sarcoma Angiosarcoma	Lymphoma Neuroblastoma Malignant fibrous histio- cytoma Fibrosarcoma Synovial sarcoma Malignant neurinoma

cell sarcomas, P.A.S. positiveness tends towards a diagnosis of leiomyosarcoma rather than malignant neurinoma (Table 3).

Argentic impregnation for reticular fibers is useful in distinguishing Ewing's sarcoma from lymphoma, synovial sarcoma from fibrosarcoma, hemangioendothelioma from hemangiopericytoma.

Trichromic staining for connective tissue (Mallory, Masson) is useful in cases of metastatic carcinoma, and hemagioendothelioma, in order to better distinguish the cords and tubules (epithelial and endothelial, respectively) from the support connective tissue. Masson's fuchsin is also useful, as is iron hematoxylin, and phosphotungstic acid-hematoxylin (PTAH), in order to reveal striations in the rhabdo- and leiomyosarcomas. Masson-Fontana staining is useful for melanin, in cases of skeletal or extraskeletal metastasis due to melanoma. Staining, on a fresh frozen section, for fats (Sudan III, Nile blue, Congo red) is positive in liposarcomas, but it is also positive in many other sarcomas and carcinomas; thus, it is not of considerable diagnostic value.

Staining for **hyaluronic acid and mucopolysaccharides** (alcian blue with varying pHs, mucicarmine, colloidal iron, toluidine blue) with and without hyaluronidase, may contribute to differentiate between myxoid tumors, such as myxoid liposarcoma, malignant fibrous histiocytoma in the myxoid variety, myxoid chondrosarcoma of the soft tissues, chordoma, intramuscular myxoma (Table 4).

Immunohistochemistry (peroxidase-antiperoxidase method) may be used to confirm or assess a doubtful diagnosis, by revealing the markers of epithe-

Table 4

STAINING FOR HYALURONIC ACID AND MUCOPOLYSACCHARIDES

Staining annulled by hyaluronidase	Not annulled by hyaluronidase
Myxoid liposarcoma Myxoid malignant fibrous histiocytoma Myxoma	Myxoid chondrosarcoma Chordoma

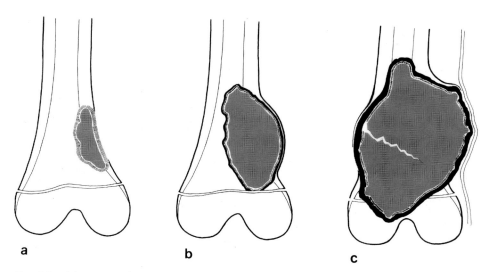

F$_{IG}$. 22. - (a) Inactive benign tumor (Stage 1). The tumor, its growth minimal or ended, is contained by an actual capsule of mature tissue (fibrous or osseous). (b) Active benign tumor (Stage 2). The tumor, which is in moderate growth, is surrounded by a thin capsule and by a thicker immature pseudocapsule. (c) Benign aggressive tumor (Stage 3). The tumor grows in a lively manner, the pseudocapsule is very immature and the tumor penetrates it with short digitations.

lial cells, endothelial cells (factor VIII), neurogenic cells (S100, Neurone specific enolase), rhabdomyoblasts (actine), and so on.

Electron microscopy is of moderate diagnostic value in tumors of the bones and soft tissues. Nonetheless, it may be useful, for instance, for a differential diagnosis of round-cell sarcomas: neuroblastoma (granules of neurosecretion), rhabdomyosarcoma (myofilaments and striations), Ewing's sarcoma (glycogene).

A histochemical demonstration of intense alkaline phosphatase activity may help to distinguish osteoid from fibrohyalin collagen production, and thus between osteoblastic tumors and fibroblastic ones. To this same aim, **tetracyclines** may be used. Marking with tetracycline, administered orally during the three days prior to surgery, corresponds to marking with radioactive isotopes. Tetracyclines are deposited electively in the newly-formed bone tissue, to which they confer yellow-orange staining under Wood lighting. Bone marked as such may be examined macroscopically, or, in non-decalcified sections, microscopically. This examination helps to better define the boundaries of the tumor, marked by a ring of reactive bone, or to reveal skip metastasis.

SURGICAL TREATMENT

Surgery of tumors of the locomotor apparatus currently offers considerable possibilities, as long as it is rational.

a) The surgeon must collaborate closely with the radiologist, the patholo-

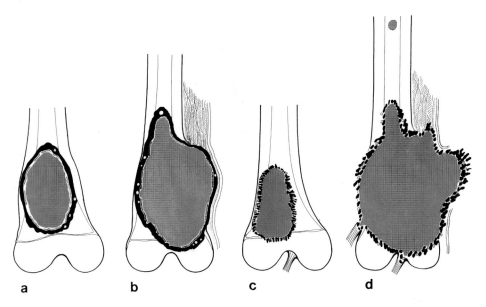

FIG. 23. - (a) and (b) Low-grade malignant tumor (Stage I A and B). The tumor does not grow very rapidly; it is surrounded by an immature pseudocapsule. It resembles a benign aggressive tumor but, unlike this, it usually presents small tumoral nodules in the pseudocapsule, knows as «satellites». (c) and (d) High-grade malignant tumor (Stage II A and B). The tumor grows rapidly. In some areas the pseudocapsule does not have enough time to form and is very thin. It is very immature, soft, edematous, very hyperemic and fragile throughout. The borders between healthy tissue, pseudocapsule and tumor are rather indistinct. The pseudocapsule is permeated by satellite tumoral nodules. Finally, the tumor may — rarely — present one or more nodules separated from the main tumoral mass, in the same or adjacent anatomical compartment, known as «skip» metastases.

gist, the chemotherapist, and he must possess a sufficient knowledge of oncology. In fact, the planning and execution of surgery requires an accurate study and correct interpretation of radiograms, CAT, MRI, bone scans and angiograms; correct biopsy and exact histological diagnosis; good experience with intraoperative macroscopic pictures; knowledge of the biological behavior of the tumor, and prognosis of the specific case; simultaneous planning of chemo- and radiation therapy. If radiation therapy is required, for example, biopsy must be carried out according to specific rules (short incision, far from bone, avoiding weakening the bone through generous sampling, accurate suturing). If radiation therapy is required, neither bone grafts nor, within certain limits, endoprostheses may be used (risk of infection, no incorporation of grafts, secondary radiation caused by metal).

b) The orthopaedic surgeon may at times be required to operate together with a general surgeon, vascular surgeon, neurosurgeon, or micro-plastic surgeon, when a pleura or a peritoneum need to be opened, when blood vessels and internal organs need to be detached or sutured, when a large vessel requires ligature or resection, when vascular grafting is required, when dealing with important nervous structures, when vascularized grafts of bone, muscle and skin are needed.

c) Surgery of tumors is a complex procedure, as it must be adapted, and, at times, invented, depending on the individual case, and because some of the operations involved are exhausting for both the surgeon and the patient. But the surgeon must not give up easily, when faced with the prospect of prolonging the life of the patient, or curing him.

Correct treatment of tumors of the locomotor apparatus may be carried out only at specialized centers. Education and the national health policy must be such that at the first diagnostic suspicion, the patient is envoyed to these centers. If the first diagnostic ascertainment and the first choices of treatment are not correct ones, the outcome of treatment and the life of the patient may be compromised.

The greatest possibilities for treatment are in the hands of the surgeon who touches the tumor for the first time. Local recurrence, for example, constitutes a severe occurrence, or one which is irremediable, and which might have been avoided.

Staging of tumors

If treatment of the tumor is not to be left up to chance, if the reason for the results obtained is to be understood, if the work done at the many centers is to be compared by means of a common language, if we wish to progress in the difficult task of healing tumors, it is necessary to classify each oncological case according to its stage.

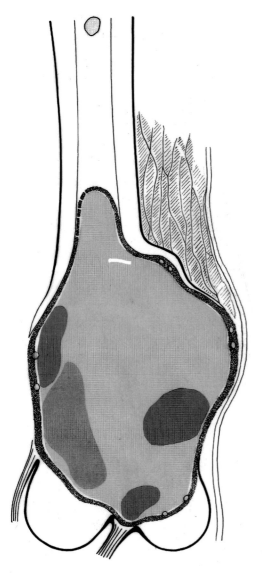

FIG. 24. - A high-grade malignant tumor (Stage II-B) which responded well to preoperative chemotherapy substantially changes its features. The tumoral mass (necrotic) often hardens (osteosarcoma) and slightly decreases in volume. The pseudocapsule (compare this with Fig. 23 d) matures. The surrounding tissues are evidently demarcated from the tumor and from its pseudocapsule. Most or all of the «satellites» have disappeared.

This signifies considering the main prognostic factors and, based on these, defining progressive stages of risk of local recurrence and metastasis. Given the considerable number of prognostic factors, as well as the variety of tumors and individual «terrain», a complete staging system, one which is accurate and relatively simple for practical use, does not exist. The system which is most used is that of Enneking *et al.* (1980), the same for benign and malignant tumors of both the skeleton and soft tissues.

This staging system is based on three elements.

1) **The grade (G) of the tumor**. Histologically, benign tumors are G_0, those of low-grade malignancy G_1 (grades 1 and 2 according to Broders), those of high-grade malignancy G_2 (grades 3 and 4 according to Broders). The grade is not based on histology alone, but on clinical and radiographic data, as well (angiograms, bone scan, CAT, MRI).

2) **The anatomical situation (T) of the tumor**. T_0 is a benign tumor which is completely surrounded by a true capsule of mature fibrous or bone tissue. T_1 is a tumor which penetrates by means of short digitations (benign), or has small satellite nodules (malignant) in the reactive layer surrounding it (pseudocapsule), but it originates within an anatomical compartment and has not exceeded the natural barriers of the compartment. T_2 is a tumor (benign or malignant) which originated extracompartmentally, or is extended beyond the barriers delimiting the original compartment, either due to

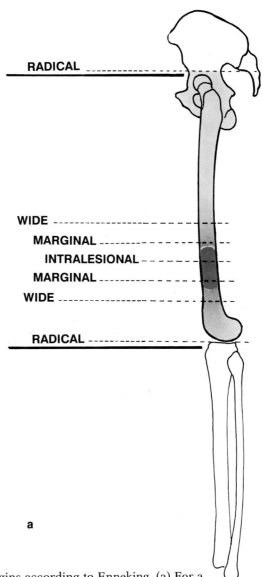

a

FIG. 25. - Definition of surgical margins according to Enneking. (a) For a tumor of the skeleton; (b) for a tumor of the soft tissues.

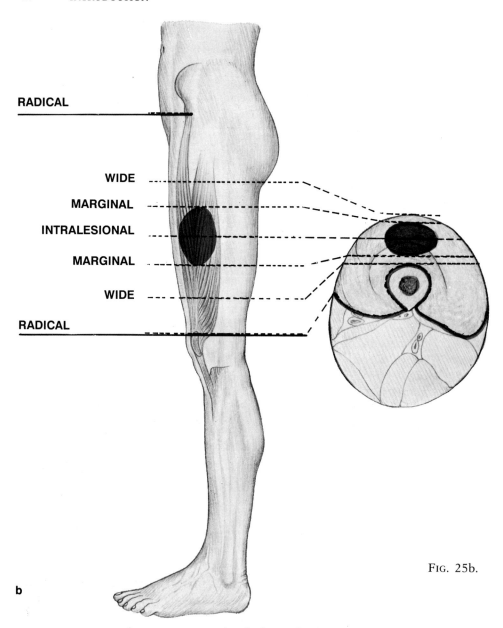

RADICAL

WIDE

MARGINAL

INTRALESIONAL

MARGINAL

WIDE

RADICAL

b

FIG. 25b.

spontaneous growth, or to trauma (pathologic fracture), or to surgery-related trauma (biopsy, intralesional or marginal excision). By compartment we mean: a bone within the periosteum; a joint within the capsule; subcutaneous tissue outside the fascia; the muscle (quadriceps, sural triceps) or muscles contained in a principal fascia of the limbs. The definitions according to Enneking are reported in Table 5.

3) Whether (M_1) or not (M_0) there are metastases, regional or distant.

With these three elements (G, T, M) Enneking (1983) devised a staging of benign (Table 6) and malignant (Table 7) tumors of the skeleton and soft tissues (Figs. 22, 23).

Table 5
ANATOMICAL SITUATION (T)

Intracompartmental (T$_1$)	Extracompartmental (T$_2$)

Intraosseous
Intra-articular
Superficial to deep fascia
Parosteal
 	
Intrafascial compartments:
   Ray of the hand or foot
   Sura
   Anterolateral leg
   Anterior thigh
   Medial thigh
   Posterior thigh
   Buttock
   Anterior forearm
   Posterior forearm
   Anterior arm
   Posterior arm
   Periscapular
	→extended to the periosteal soft tissues
	→extended to the periarticular soft tissues
	→penetrating the deep fascia
	→penetrating the skeleton or external to
	   the fascia
	Extrafascial planes or spaces:
	   Mid- or hindfoot
	   Popliteal
	   Inguinofemoral triangle
	   Intrapelvic
	   Mid hand
	   Anterior fossa to the elbow
	   Axilla
	   Paraspinal
	   Head and neck

As may be observed, in benign tumors the histological picture is always the same (G$_0$) and the distinction between stages 1, 2, and 3 is above all based on clinical and radiographic data. In malignant tumors, instead, there is a histological distinction (G$_1$ and G$_2$), but clinical and radiographic data are again of value for a differentiation between G$_1$ and G$_2$ forms, and both of these from benign tumors (G$_0$).

This staging system has its limits. For example, it is not clear just when forms with a histological grade 2 according to Broders may be considered G$_1$ and when G$_2$. For the sake of classification, we consider them all to be G$_1$. There are some rare cases where the histological picture is characterized by high-grade malignancy (G$_2$), but the symptomatology is scarce and the radiographic picture is that of a low-grade malignancy lesion or even a benign one. In cases such as these, it is our belief that the histological grade has priority, dictating classification to be stage II.

Definition of surgical margins (Enneking, 1983)

The margins involved in surgical dissection may be of four types. 1) **Intralesional**: the dissection penetrates the tumor. 2) **Marginal**: the tumor is removed whole, incising along the capsule or pseudocapsule; tumor islands may remain in the pseudocapsule (satellites) or farther away in the same compartment (skip). 3) **Wide**: dissection is intracompartmental, but the tumor is removed en bloc with a layer of healthy tissue at every part of its border; skip metastases may remain. 4) **Radical**: dissection is extracompart-

Table 6
STAGES OF BENIGN TUMORS *(from Enneking, 1983)*

Stage	1 (inactive)	2 (active)	3 (aggressive)
Grade	G_0	G_0	G_0
Anatomical site	T_0	T_0	T_{1-2}
Metastasis	M_0	M_0	M_{0-1}
Clinical course	Asymptomatic, does not grow, tends to repair spontaneously	Symptomatic, increases, expands to the surrounding tissues	Aggressive, invades the surrounding tissues
X-ray grade	I	II	III
Bone scan	Negative	Positive in the lesion	Positive beyond the borders of the lesion
Angiography	No neovascular reaction	Moderate neovascular reaction	Considerable neovascular reaction
CAT, MRI	Clear margins, thick capsule, homogeneity	Clear margins but expanded, thin capsule, homogeneity	Unclear margins, no capsule, dishomogeneity

Table 7
STAGES OF MALIGNANT TUMORS *(from Enneking, 1983, modified)*

Stage	IA	IB	IIA	IIB	IIIA	IIIB
Grade	G_1	G_1	G_2	G_2	G_{1-2}	G_{1-2}
Anatomical site	T_1	T_2	T_1	T_2	T_1	T_2
Metastasis	M_0	M_0	M_0	M_0	M_1	M_1
Clinical course	slow	slow	rapid	rapid	—	
Bone scan	positive	positive	positive beyond limits of x-ray les.	positive beyond limits of x-ray les.	(skeletal metastases)	
X-ray grade	I	II	III	III	II	III
Angiography	moderate neovascular reaction	moderate neovascular reaction (involves the n.v. bundle)	marked neovascular reaction	marked neovascular reaction (involvement of n.v. bundle)	(hypervascular lymph nodes)	
CAT, MRI	unclear margins, but intracompartmental	extracompartmental origin or expansion	unclear margins, but intracompartmental	extracompartmental origin or expansion	pulmonary nodules or metastatic lymph nodes	

mental, the tumor is removed en bloc with the entire compartment(s) containing it; in a longitudinal direction, the surgical dissection passes through or beyond the proximal and distal joints of the bone affected, the proximal and distal muscular insertions of the muscles affected; in a transverse direction, dissection goes beyond the fascial planes bordering on the compartment, and in bone tumors, beyond the periosteum; there are no residual local tumor foci (Fig. 25).

Now that the margins have been defined, surgery itself may be determined as intralesional, marginal, wide, radical. Observe that the definition does not depend on the thickness of the healthy tissue removed: a margin may be radical and be 2 cm thick, another margin (for example, removal of a tumor from the quadriceps muscle) may be wide and be thicker. The quality of the margin is just as important as its thickness: an aponeurosis of muscular covering or a joint capsule, 1 or 2 mm thick, constitute a safer margin than 4 or 5 mm of adipose tissue in the medullary canal or extracompartmental, or of reactive tissue. Furthermore, the definition is irregardless of whether surgery is conservative or ablative; an amputation may be marginal or even intralesional if the scalpel brushes up against or incises the tumor, a scapulectomy or an excision of the entire quadriceps from insertion to insertion may be radical (Table 8).

For a subcutaneous tumor, that is, one which originates in a compartment which is bordered by the deep fascia but not in other directions, the margin is wide when the excision includes the deep fascia and less than 5 cm of skin and subcutaneous fat around the tumor; radical means when it includes more than 5 cm.

During surgery, if the tumor tissue is uncovered, grazed, broken or penetrated, the wound is contaminated and all of the surrounding tissues exposed to the risk of local recurrence. If these tissues are not removed, surgery is considered to be intralesional. If these tissues are removed, surgery is wide or radical, but **contaminated**.

The definition of surgical margins must be made after every therapeutic operation by both the surgeon and the pathologist. The surgeon will note down any intraoperative contamination and sample areas of doubtful tissue

Table 8
DEFINITION OF SURGERY

Margin	Conservative surgery	Ablative surgery
Intralesional	Curettage or removal in pieces	Amputation with dissection through the tumor
Marginal	Marginal resection or excision	Amputation with dissection by the tumor
Wide	Wide resection or excision	Wide amputation
Radical	Radical resection or excision	Radical disarticulation or amputation

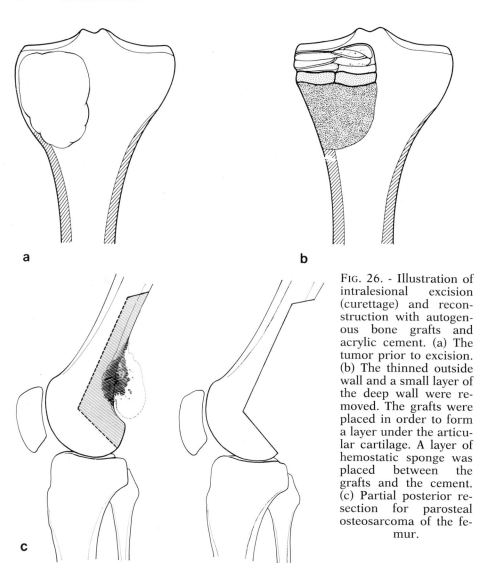

a

b

c

Fig. 26. - Illustration of intralesional excision (curettage) and reconstruction with autogenous bone grafts and acrylic cement. (a) The tumor prior to excision. (b) The thinned outside wall and a small layer of the deep wall were removed. The grafts were placed in order to form a layer under the articular cartilage. A layer of hemostatic sponge was placed between the grafts and the cement. (c) Partial posterior resection for parosteal osteosarcoma of the femur.

from the operative wound to be used for a histological examination, whether extemporaneous or by inclusion. At the end of surgery, the surgeon will examine the resected specimen, on the surface of which he will recognize the risk areas, that is, where the margin is not obviously wide, indicating those to the pathologist. The pathologist will stain these areas with Indian ink and make numerous histological sections perpendicular to the surface. A histological examination will define the margin, in this manner. If there is a normal layer of tissue between the china ink and the tumor, the margin is wide; if there is only a pseudocapsule, it is marginal; if there is nothing, it is intralesional.

This histological definition of the margins is indispensable, if we wish to evaluate the results, compare the different case series, and learn to progress in the surgery of these tumors.

Therapeutic indications in relation to the staging

For every stage of the tumor, every different surgical margin involves a risk of local recurrence, which ranges from 0 to 100%. Since the Enneking classification has been in use for only a short amount of time, accurate statistics are still not available. Indications for treatment must firstly take into account this risk of local recurrence, with the awareness that in high-grade malignant tumors **local recurrence definitely increases the risk of metastasis**. Furthermore, the indication must take into account the age of the patient, residual function at surgery, the work and life habits of the patient. Finally, the surgical indication also depends on local and general adjuvants. Our method of evaluating surgical indications based on the stage of the tumor and on the risk of recurrence is, in turn, based on the work done by Enneking (1983).

Benign tumor stage 1 (inactive). These are generally non-neoplastic lesions, for example, bone cyst, histiocytic fibroma, chondroma, exostosis, fibrous dysplasia and, in soft tissues, mucous cyst, pigmented nodular tenosynovitis, subcutaneous lipoma. Most of these lesions, which are either hardly progressive or already extinguished (in the adult), nearly entirely or entirely asymptomatic, do not require any type of surgical treatment. If surgery is indicated, an **intralesional excision** involves less of a risk of recurrence, as these lesions tend to stop growth spontaneously. In some particular cases (exostosis, fibrous dysplasia of a rib, lesions of the soft tissues) **marginal excision** will be indicated, and there will be hardly any or no risk of recurrence.

Benign tumor stage 2 (active). Examples of this tumor include, in the skeleton, osteoid osteoma, many cases of chondroblastoma and osteoblastoma, chondromyxoid fibroma, aneurysmal bone cyst, some giant cell tumors; in the soft tissues, lipoma, angioma, glomus tumor. A **marginal excision** involves a minimal risk of recurrence as the lesion is by definition intracapsular.

However, when en bloc excision could involve difficulties or surgical risks, or when it would result in considerable functional deficit, an **intralesional excision** is preferred, even if it involves a higher risk of local recurrence. In order to decrease this risk local adjuvants are used, such as phenol, cementation with methyl-methacrylate (which causes thermal and perhaps chemical necrosis) and repeated freezing-thawing with liquid nitrogen and warm physiological solution (which breaks the cellular membranes). These last two adjuvants have proven to be effective in extending the surgical margins by several millimeters, thus making curettage (intralesional) equal to a marginal excision.

Benign tumor stage 3 (aggressive). These tumors have an extracapsular extent (T_1) or even an extracompartmental one (T_2). Examples of these in the skeleton are several giant cell tumors, some chondroblastomas, osteoblastomas and aneurysmal bone cysts; in the soft tissues, desmoid tumor. **Intralesional surgery** has a considerable or high risk of recurrence. Adjuvants such as cement and liquid nitrogen may be used to decrease this risk. **Marginal**

excision also involves a moderate to high risk of local recurrence. Radiation therapy might be effective, and is sometimes used as a postoperative adjuvant when **wide excision** is not possible. Wide resection constitutes the surgery of choice as it guarantees a very low risk of local recurrence. In cases where the tumor is extremely expanded (T_2) and in those of extracompartmental or disseminated local recurrence, **wide amputation** may be the only indication.

Malignant tumor stage I-A. Examples include, in the skeleton, grades 1 and 2 chondrosarcoma, grades 1 and 2 parosteal osteosarcoma, chordoma, adamantinoma; in the soft tissues, grades 1 and 2 liposarcoma, dermatofibrosarcoma protuberans, some types of hemangiopericytoma. Because of the tendency of these tumors to have satellite micronodules in the pseudocapsule, intralesional surgery is nearly always, and marginal surgery very often, followed by local recurrence. The type of surgery guaranteeing a minimum risk of recurrence is wide surgery. Based on the intracompartmental situation of the tumor, this involves a **limb-salvaging procedure**.

Malignant tumor stage I-B. In this case, as well, a wide margin is necessary and sufficient. The extracompartmental extent of the tumor makes wide excision more difficult and not always possible, and, at times, **wide amputation** is required.

Malignant tumor stage II-A. This is an infrequent situation, as, particularly in the skeleton, most types of high-grade sarcoma are extracompartmental on diagnosis. Examples of these types of sarcoma are, in the skeleton, classical osteosarcoma, Ewing's sarcoma, grade 3 chondrosarcoma, malignant fibrous histiocytoma; in the soft tissues, grades 3 and 4 liposarcoma, malignant fibrous histiocytoma, rhabdomyosarcoma, synovial sarcoma. These types of sarcoma, in addition to having peritumor satellite nodules, are characterized by an incidence of skip metastasis which may not be overlooked. For this reason, the margin which involves the smallest risk of local recurrence is **radical or compartmental**. This margin is used willingly when it does not involve very severe functional deficit, such as in a scapulectomy or excision of a muscle from insertion to insertion. In other cases, a wide margin is usually preferred: because of the intracompartmental state of the tumor, this may be obtained by conservative surgery: **wide resection of bone or of the soft tissues**. Wide surgery is often associated with adjuvants: chemotherapy in osteosarcoma.

Malignant tumor stage II-B. The extracompartmental state of this tumor often makes radical or wide surgery ablative: **wide or radical amputation or disarticulation**. Nonetheless, the use of preoperative chemotherapy or radiation therapy leads to an extent of the indication for **limb-saving wide or radical resection**.

Preoperative chemotherapy, widely used in the treatment of osteosarcoma and Ewing's sarcoma, is capable of modifying the stage of the tumor, and, therefore, the surgical indication and the risk of local recurrence. When the tumor responds positively to chemotherapy (in osteosarcoma, tumor necrosis greater than 90% of the cells) its growth ends. The pseudocapsule has time to mature and it is transformed into a layer of well-differentiated bony or fibrous tissue (Fig. 24). Hypervascularity and edema of the surrounding tissues regress or disappear. These become distinct and mobile as compared to the pseudocapsule which adheres to the tumor. Thus, conservative surgery often becomes possible, because it is technically facilitated and because marginal surgery involves a lower risk of local recurrence.

What follows is that in stage II tumors treated with preoperative chemotherapy, the risk of local recurrence depends on the response to chemotherapy (percentage of chemo-induced necrosis) as well as on the surgical margin.

Malignant tumor stage III. Therapy in this case is often only palliative. The encouraging results obtained, with considerable percentages of five-year survival rate, using aggressive chemotherapy and thoracotomy, nonetheless increasingly lead to an evaluation of energetic and combined treatment of the primary tumor and its metastases.

Curettage of a skeletal cavity and bone grafting or acrylic cement

When performing curettage of a tumoral skeletal cavity (intralesional excision) the periosteum may be preserved when the skeletal wall is whole; more often it must be removed en bloc with the attenuated skeletal wall (Fig. 26a, b).

Many surgeons routinely make an operculum in the cortex, and through this, use a curette to empty the cavity, then filling it with bone chips. This practice is generally incorrect. The cortical wall of the cavity (tumoral or cystic) must be removed more generously, 1/2 or more of the circumference of the bone, so as to completely uncover the cavity. This allows for total excision of the tumor or cystic membrane, and removal not only of all or nearly all of the thinned cortical wall, but also of a layer of the deep cancellous bone wall. The bone grafts are small and cancellous if mechanical function is not required; otherwise, they may be larger and cortico-cancellous. There must not be large empty spaces, but the grafts must not be too crowded either, which would obstruct connective-vascular rehabitation. When the cortical wall is widely removed, widely uncovering the cavity, the grafts may be better revascularized.

After such widened intralesional excision, electrocauterization is used to cauterize the entire margin of the excision, and the residual skeletal bed may be repeatedly brushed with **phenol** 85%, subsequently washing with alcohol. In order to remove detritus, marrow or any tumoral cells, a pressure jet may be used to irrigate with physiological solution.

Acrylic cement may constitute a local adjuvant, which is characterized by thermal action that necrotizes several millimeters of the cavity wall. This is filled with cement. Moreover, the cement immediately provides a more effective stability than that of the grafts. If the stability is sufficient, the implant may be left in site permanently; otherwise, in time, it may be removed and substituted with bone grafts. Should local recurrence occur, this would soon be visible on radiograms as a result of osteolysis of the normal bone, which is clearly distinguished from the radiopaque cement.

The quality of the grafts (fresh autogenous or perfrigerated allografts) influences the rapidity and the completeness of their incorporation; if this need not be rapid and total, the latter are just as effective as the former. It must be recalled that from a mechanical point of view bone grafts go through a critical stage during rehabilitation. For this reason, as well, the association of a solid osteosynthesis is recommended when secondary fracture is feared (wide skeletal cavity with thinned or lacking cortex, particularly in the lower limb and vertebral column). Again, for mechanical reasons, in addition to the insertion of bone grafts in the cavity, the application of cortical or corticocancellous slabs on the skeletal surface may be indicated.

Osteosynthesis whether or not associated with curettage, and the use of acrylic cement

This method is widely used, particularly in the treatment of skeletal metastases and plasmacytoma.

Simple osteosynthesis is above all used as closed intramedullary (sometimes locked) nailing for diaphyseal lesions of the femur, humerus and tibia, or as screwed plates for lesions to the metaphysis. Often, however, wide osteolysis does not allow for a sufficiently solid osteosynthesis, enough to immediately and durably restore function to the limb operated. In cases such as these, when there are metastases (where skeletal repair of the osteolysis will not occur) the osteolytic lesion is exposed and excised, the cavity is filled, and the missing skeletal wall is reconstructed using acrylic cement, associating osteosynthesis with intramedullary nailing or a screwed plate. The use of cement often obtains rigid osteosyntheses and, thus, immediate or early functional recovery of the limb.

Skeletal resections

Skeletal resection may be: 1) **hemicylindrical** in a long bone (Fig. 26c); 2) of a **complete segment of a long bone**, **intra-articular** or **diaphyseal**; 3) of two skeletal segments making up a joint, **extra-articular** resection; 4) of a part of or all of a **flat or short bone**.

Resections such as these generally aim at a wide surgical margin, rarely a radical one (scapulectomy, resection of an entire humerus or femur); at times they only obtain a marginal margin.

Resection must be performed with an extraperiosteal approach and, when the tumor permeates the cortex, with the largest possible layer of surrounding soft tissues. If the tumor is external to the skeletal surface (peripheral chondrosarcoma, parosteal osteosarcoma, periosteal tumors) it must be removed, without exposing it, with a layer of healthy tissue coating it and with the underlying bone.

As a result of the most common site of tumors requiring resection, this is usually performed on the skeleton of the trunk or on a meta-epiphyseal skeletal segment. Some joint segments (shoulder, hip and knee) may be substituted with an endoprosthesis and arthroprosthesis; when this is the case, the age of the patient will be taken into account in view of the presumed duration of the prosthesis. Resection of a segment of the diaphysis, preserving the epiphysis will less frequently be required.

Skeletal resection is easier when the segment to be resected is solid and compact, with no adherences to surrounding healthy tissue (tumors which are well-contained by a solid cortex, peripheral chondrosarcoma, parosteal osteosarcoma, osteosarcoma or Ewing's sarcoma after there has been good response to preoperative chemotherapy). It is more difficult when the segment to be resected is made soft and fragile by the tumor, when there is hypervascularity, when it is adherent to the surrounding soft tissues (even due to previous surgery and/or previous radiation therapy). When there is **pathologic fracture** of the segment to be resected, it may be best to wait a few weeks for partial consolidation of the fracture and demarcation of the tumor with reactive tissue in the fractured area, prior to performing surgery.

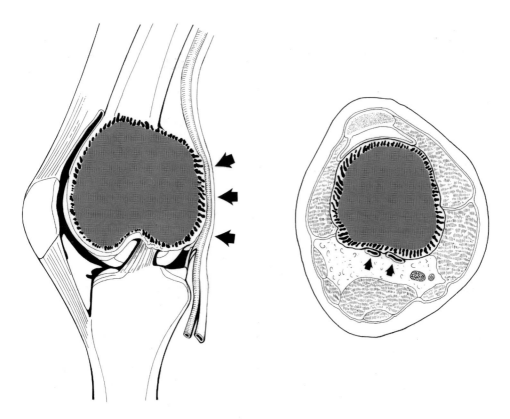

FIG. 27. - When the tumor displaces and compresses the large vessels, the adventitia becomes a part of the pseudocapsule of the tumor. Thus, if the surgeon resects the tumor isolating it from the vessels, a marginal or intralesional margin will result. In order to obtain a wide margin it is necessary to include the vessels in the resection block, or to amputate.

Risk areas in skeletal resection

In skeletal resections for sarcoma the following are considered to be risk areas. 1) Biopsy. 2) Extent of the tumor along the diaphyseal medullary canal. 3) Adherence of the tumor to the large vessels. 4) Extent of the tumor in the venous branches as neoplastic thrombi. 5) Extent of the tumor in the joint tissues. 6) Contamination (hematoma) of the joint cavity or of the extraskeletal compartmental and extracompartmental spaces.

1) **Biopsy**. The approach used for incisional or trocar biopsy must be widely excised en bloc with the tumor, including any trace of hematoma.

2) Extent of the tumor along the **diaphyseal canal**, as digitation or as skip

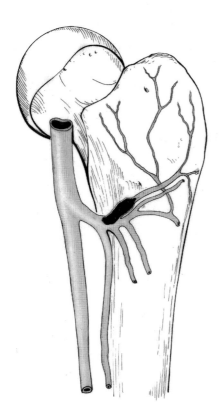
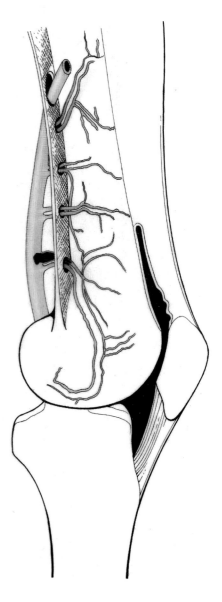

FIG. 28. - Rarely, the venous trunks connecting the tumor to the principal vein of the limb are occluded by a neoplastic thrombus. If this occlusion does not reach as far as the principal vein it is impossible for it to be revealed prior to surgery. During surgery it may be necessary to resect a segment of the principal vein en bloc with the tumor, or to transform the planned resection into amputation.

metastasis may generally be determined prior to surgery with imaging methods (x-rays, bone scan, CAT, MRI, angiography). In case of doubt, a supplementary biopsy may be carried out. The level of transection of the bone may thus be planned accurately.

3) Adherence of the tumor to the **large vessels** (Fig. 27). This especially happens when the tumor, growing outside the bone, displaces and compresses the large vessels. It may be determined preoperatively by CAT, MRI and angiography. If there is healthy tissue between the vessel and the pseudocapsule, the vessel is easily dissociated and may be preserved, with a good chance of obtaining a wide surgical margin. If, instead, there is no healthy tissue between the vessel and the tumor, the vascular adventitia is part of the pseudocapsule and dissection of the vessel from the surface of the tumor is more difficult (reactive scarring adherence). As dissection is carried out in the thickness of pseudocapsule a marginal surgical margin results. In cases such as these, if a wide margin is desired, a choice must be made between en bloc resection of the vessels with the tumor and amputation.

4) Extent of the tumor in the venous branches as **neoplastic thrombi** (Fig. 28). When a skeletal segment containing the tumor is resected the small periosteal and parosteal veins and those that run in the tumor pseudocapsule are removed en bloc. Instead, it will be necessary to ligate and divide the larger venous branches which go from the bone to the principal venous trunk. It rarely occurs that these venous branches and, at times, even the principal vein are obstructed and hardened by neoplastic thrombi. It is difficult to predict this event preoperatively, even if at times it may be demonstrated or suspected with CAT, MRI, or angiography. When it does occur, whether or not it has been predicted prior to surgery, a choice may be made between vascular resection and amputation.

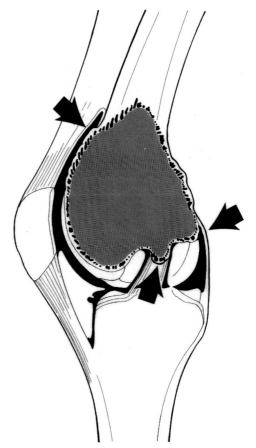

FIG. 29. - A metaepiphyseal tumor may invade the joint capsule and/or the ligaments where they are inserted in the bone. And it may invade the synovial membrane where it covers the bone. These invasions may be suspected preoperatively with imaging and they may require extra-articular resection.

5) The extent of the tumor in the **joint tissues** (Fig. 29). If the tumor involves the epiphysis, it may invade the skeletal insertions of the capsule, the joint ligaments and the synovial membrane. This invasion may be revealed by CAT or MRI. At times the invasion may indicate extra-articular resection.

6) Contamination (hematoma) of the **joint cavity** or of the **extraskeletal compartmental and extracompartmental spaces** (Fig. 30). These hematomas originate from a biopsy or a pathologic fracture. They are revealed by a history of the patient or by a clinical examination, by CAT or by MRI. Intra-articular hematomas may be resolved by extra-articular resection; muscular hematomas, by resection including one or more muscular compartments. At times, particularly if the contamination is extracompartmental or located around the neurovascular bundle, they require amputation.

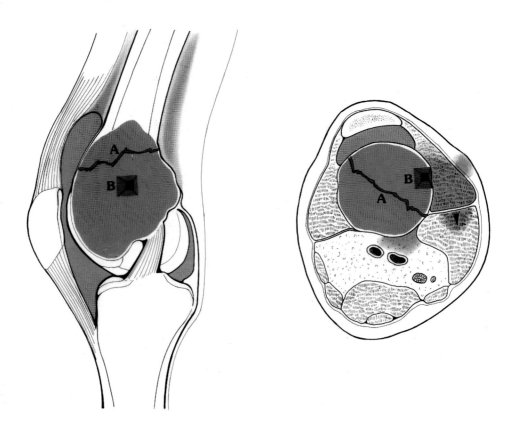

FIG. 30. - The joint cavity and/or the muscular compartments may be contaminated by a hematoma secondary to a pathologic fracture (A) or a biopsy (B). These contaminations require resection of vast muscular parts and/or extra-articular resection. If the contamination involves more than one muscular compartment or the extracompartmental spaces around the neurovascular bundle amputation may be required.

Scapulectomy

This type of surgery is of considerable efficacy in an oncological sense, as the scapula is entirely covered by a good muscular layer.

Partial scapulectomy makes sense particularly when it allows us to save the glenoid cavity. After scapulectomy the head of the humerus is suspended at the clavicle, the insertion of the trapezius is sutured to the extrarotator cuff and the deltoideus, and the tendon of the long head of the biceps is inserted to the clavicle.

Total scapulectomy involves considerable functional deficit of the shoulder, which is minor in the child than in the adult.

En bloc resection of the scapulohumeral joint

In cases of scapulohumeral tumor which invades or comes very close to the joint, the scapula (or its glenoid cavity) the lateral end of the clavicle, and the proximal end of the humerus may be resected en bloc (Fig. 31). The joint is thus removed in toto with an extracapsular approach. The humeral segment is substituted by an endoprosthesis and suspended.

This type of operation is quite effective, as the skeletal segment is resected en bloc with the joint capsule and with large layers of muscle.

The skin incision follows the external half of the clavicle, the acromion, to then descend posteriorly equidistant from the two margins of the scapular

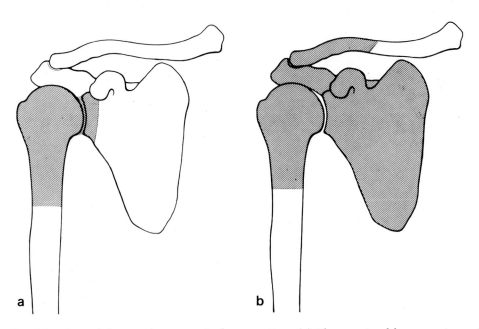

a   b

FIG. 31. - Scapulohumeral extra-articular resection. (a) The proximal humerus is resected, without opening the joint capsule, with the glenoid cavity of the scapula. (b) Included in the resection block are the proximal humerus, the entire scapula and the lateral part of the clavicle (Tikoff-Linberg procedure).

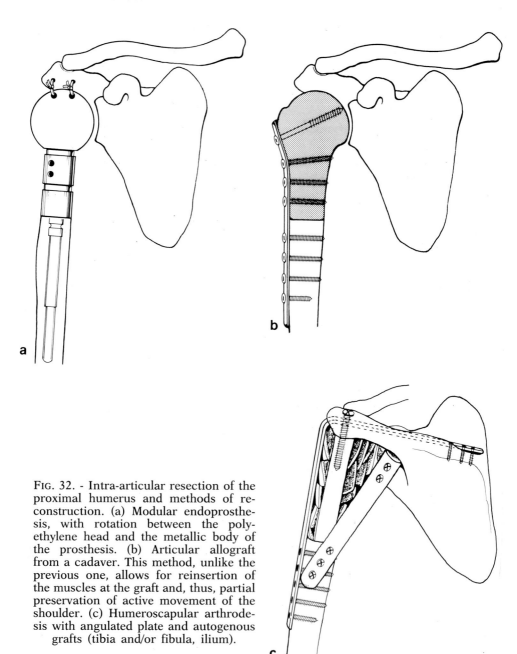

FIG. 32. - Intra-articular resection of the proximal humerus and methods of reconstruction. (a) Modular endoprosthesis, with rotation between the polyethylene head and the metallic body of the prosthesis. (b) Articular allograft from a cadaver. This method, unlike the previous one, allows for reinsertion of the muscles at the graft and, thus, partial preservation of active movement of the shoulder. (c) Humeroscapular arthrodesis with angulated plate and autogenous grafts (tibia and/or fibula, ilium).

body. From the acromion a second external or anterior longitudinal incision branches out prolonged as far as the insertion of the deltoid muscle to the humerus. The skin and subcutaneous flaps are developed, revealing the deltoid and the scapular muscles. The clavicle and proximal humeral diaphysis are transected. The following muscles are sectioned near the humeral insertion: deltoid, latissimus dorsi, teres major, pectoralis major. The following muscles are transected at the scapular insertion: pectoralis minor, short head of biceps, coraco-brachialis, long head of biceps, long head of triceps, latissimus dorsi, trapezius, elevator and rhomboid muscles, serratus anterior.

Resection of the proximal humerus

The resected segment is substituted with an endoprosthesis; acrylic cement is used to stabilize the stem in the medullary canal (Fig. 32a).

Even if the muscles are reinserted at the prosthesis with non-resorbable material, their functional capacity is nearly null, and, when possible, it is best to resect the diaphysis proximal to the insertion of the deltoid, suturing the external rotators and subscapularis to the deep aspect of the deltoid, and preserving the axillary nerve. But this condition occurs in rare cases of tumor, which is nearly limited to the epiphysis. The tendon of the long head of biceps is usually transected at the musculotendinous union suturing the distal end to the short head of the biceps.

Although from a cosmetic point of view the patient is relatively satisfied with the results, the function of the shoulder is severely reduced. At times a major part of the shoulder muscles must be removed with the bone;

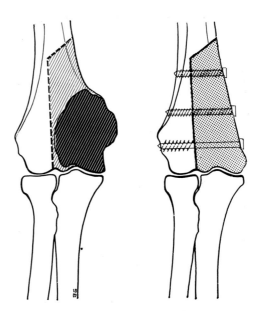

FIG. 33. - Partial resection of the distal humerus and reconstruction with a shaped autogenous graft taken from the iliac crest.

the prosthesis must be anchored to the acromion and to the glenoid cavity as it will tend to dislocate anteriorly.

We use a pivot shoulder prosthesis where the epiphyseal sphere freely rotates on the body of the prosthesis. The prosthesis is available in different modular segments (epiphyseal sphere in various diameters, metal cylinder in various lengths, diaphyseal stem in various calibers) which are chosen and assembled on the operating table depending on the size required. After scarring has occurred, the rotatory movements of the arm take place on the pivot of the prosthesis, rather than on the epiphysis, which remains nearly immobile. Thus, dislocation of the prosthesis is less frequent and rotatory stresses at the cement-to-diaphyseal bone interface are reduced. Furthermore, rotatory movements of the arm are smooth and wide, which is not the case when other types of prosthesis are used.

An alternative to prosthesis is constituted by an articular allograft of proximal humerus, or by a composite endoprosthesis plus allograft, with accurate reinsertion of all of the scapulo- and thoraco-humeral muscles at the graft (Fig. 32b). This procedure, indicated mainly in benign and low-grade tumors where it is possible to preserve most of the scapulohumeral muscles and the axillary nerve, allows for the recovery of good function of the shoulder.

Otherwise, scapulohumeral fusion may be used, with two fibular autografts stabilized to the humeral diaphysis and to the scapular glenoid cavity (Fig. 32c); this type of operation aims at obtaining some function of the shoulder, by taking advantage of the movements of the scapula on the thorax.

Resection of the distal humerus, the proximal ulna or radius

The distal humerus may be substituted with an endoprosthesis, or, better yet, with an articular allograft (Fig. 397).

In order to substitute approximately half of the distal metaepiphysis of the humerus, we used an autograft (whole thickness-iliac crest) suitably shaped, where the cranial surface becomes joint surface (Fig. 33). In order to allow for extension of the elbow a suitable olecranic fossa must be reproduced in the graft.

No reconstruction is required in resection of the proximal radius. After surgery the elbow must be kept in a supine position, so that, the supinator having been removed, the prevalence of the pronator muscles does not cause contracture in pronation.

In resection of the proximal ulna the distal end of the humerus may be placed on the anterior aspect of the neck of the radius, just behind the insertion of the biceps. The tendon of the triceps is sutured to the radial head (Enneking, 1983).

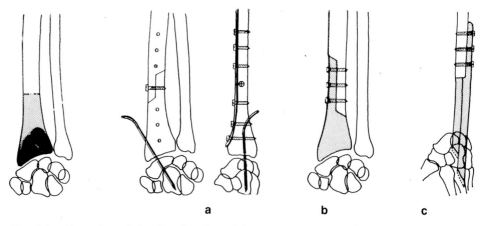

a   b   c

FIG. 34. - Resection of the distal radius. (a) Reconstruction with the proximal autogenous fibula. (b) Substitution with an allograft using an identical radial segment. (c) Fusion with autogenous tibial grafts.

Resection of the distal radius

The rare attempts at reconstruction using endoprosthesis have failed, generally causing a stiff and painful wrist.

Excellent results may be obtained by substituting the distal radius with the proximal end of the autogenous ipsilateral fibula (Fig. 34a), or an articular allograft using an identical radial segment (Fig. 34b), in order to partially preserve movement.

If movement is already severely compromised, if there are changes in the joint and/or in the soft tissues, reconstruction/arthrodesis with bone grafts is indicated (Fig. 34c).

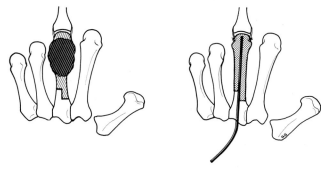

Resection of a metacarpus

FIG. 35. - Resection of a metacarpus and substitution with the third autogenous metatarsus.

This may be substituted with an articular autograft using the third or fourth metatarsus (Fig. 35), or an articular allograft. The graft is stabilized with intramedullary Kirschner wiring. The autograft fuses particularly well. The most frequent complications are joint stiffness and/or metacarpo-phalangeal subluxation, which may be avoided by preserving and suturing the collateral ligaments.

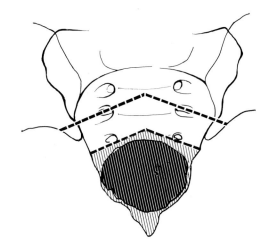

FIG. 36. - Partial resection of the sacrum, through the third foramen and through the second sacral foramen.

Resection of the sacrum

This type of surgery is indicated, and may be resolutive, in cases of chordoma, more rarely in those of chondrosarcoma, giant cell tumor. Resection of the sacrococcyx below the second sacral foramen may involve a posterior stage alone (Fig. 36). Sacrifice of the 4th and 5th sacral nerves bilaterally and of the 3rd nerve on one side only does not involve sphincter disorders, but rather (if the 3rd nerve is sacrificed on one side) perineal hypoesthesia alone.

The incision is posterior, longitudinal or like an overturned Y (Mercedes-like). The posterior aspect of the sacrum and the coccyx and the lateral margins of the sacrum are completely exposed as far as the caudal end of the sacroiliac joint, which corresponds to the lower border of the second sacral foramen (bilaterally dividing the insertion of the gluteus maximus, the sacroischiatic ligaments and the belly of the piriformis; during this stage it is important to identify and ligate branches of the gluteal vessels and to spare the pudendal nerves). Laminectomy of the sacrum is performed, the nerve roots are identified, the dural sac is ligated at the level desired, and it is turned upwards. At this point the cleavage plane between the anterior aspect of the sacrum and the retrorectal space is determined and, with the protection of a long sponge inserted from the sciatic notches and passed transversally before the sacrum, an osteotome is used to transect the entire sacrum, proceeding first from a sacral margin and then from the other margin. If the transection of the sacrum must be more cranial, it is initiated laterally to the sacro-iliac joint, from the iliac bone from both sides. After the sacrococcygeal segment has been mobilized, it is removed en bloc with the tumor, dissecting the anterior aspect from the rectal wall. The residual space is partially covered by suturing what remains of the glutei.

For resection at or above the second sacral foramen, a first anterior stage is required, which may be either transperitoneal or extraperitoneal, in order

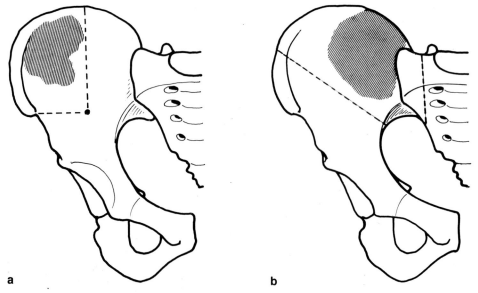

a   b

FIG. 37. - (a) Wedge resection of the ilium without interruption in the pelvic ring. (b) Resection of the ilium, of the sacroiliac joint, and of the sacral wing, with interruption of the pelvic ring.

to bilaterally ligate the internal iliac arteries and veins (thus avoiding danger-ous hemorrhage caused by laceration of an iliac vein which could occur if the resection is done directly from the posterior approach), and initiate osteo-tomy on the anterior aspect of the sacrum. After the abdomen has been closed up, surgery is completed with a posterior approach. Permanent sphinc-teric disorders and in erection will ensue, progressively more severe in rela-tion to the sacrifice of the sacral nerves above S_4.

Resection of the pelvis

In theory, an entire hemipelvis, from the sacro-iliac joint to the pubic symphisis, may be resected. In truth, this is hardly ever necessary. Unlike the scapula, the pelvis is a fixed skel-etal segment, which must be resected by means of osteotomies, or through division of either the pubic sym-phisis or the sacro-iliac synchondrosis. Such osteotomies are located as it is neces-sary in order to ob-tain wide surgical margins. It is impor-tant to preserve a part of the pelvis, in order to reconstruct continuity and a support for the femur.

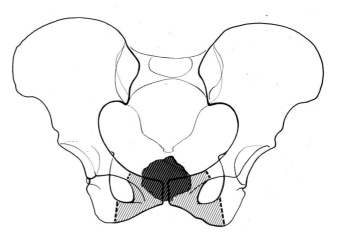

FIG. 38. - Resection of the anterior pelvic arch.

There are three types of pelvic resection.

1) **Resection of the iliac bone (extra-acetabular)**. This may save the great-er sciatic notch, removing only a section of the iliac wing and preserving the continuity of the pelvic ring (Fig. 37a); or cutting the entire ilium, from the greater sciatic notch, and interrupting the pelvic ring. In both cases, resec-tion may either save the sacroiliac joint or disarticulate it, or remove it by vertically cutting the sacral wing (Fig. 37b).

2) **Resection of the anterior pelvic arch (extra-acetabular)**. This may be unilateral or bilateral (Fig. 38) and it may include the anterior and caudal portion of the acetabulum, which involves temporary dislocation of the fe-moral head, but does not compromise joint stability of the hip, as the bottom and the roof of the acetabulum are preserved (Fig. 39).

3) **Resection of the acetabulum**. This may be **intra-articular** (with disloca-tion of the femoral head), or **extra-articular** (with resection of the proximal femur, removed en bloc with the acetabulum without opening the joint).

Type 3 resection may be associated with 1) or 2) (Fig. 40).

The most frequent indication is in chondrosarcomas; this if followed by

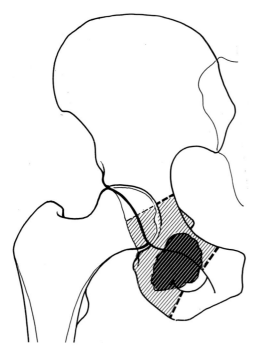

FIG. 39. - Resection of the anterior pelvic hemiarch including the caudal part of the acetabulum, for an expanded tumor in the area of the obturator foramen.

osteosarcomas and Ewing's sarcoma (after chemo- and, at times, radiation therapy). It is rare in high grade chemoresistant sarcomas, in aggressive and recurring benign tumors, in systemic tumors and in metastases. In general, the indication is made when it is believed that an adequate margin may be obtained without sacrificing the sciatic nerve (the tumor does not invade the sacroiliac joint or the greater sciatic notch) and, in malignant tumors, when it is judged that the margin to be obtained with resection is nearly the same as that which may be obtained with hindquarter amputation.

The main surgical approach (Enneking and Dunham, 1978) starts from the posterosuperior iliac spine (or the caudal end of the sacroiliac joint), following the crest of the ilium, runs medial to the anterosuperior iliac spine, then is prolonged in a half circle along the thigh and ends on its posterolateral aspect, just distal to the femoral insertion of the gluteus maximus. The

▶

FIG. 40. - Periacetabular resections and possible reconstructions. (a) Intra-articular resection of the acetabulum with anterior pelvic arch. Reconstruction with metallic wires between the femoral epiphysis and the neck of the ilium, aimed at arthrodesis or pseudarthrosis. (b) and (c) Similar resection, but extra-articular (including the head and the neck of the femur). An iliofemoral arthrodesis with limb shortening is used for reconstruction (b), or the length is maintained with an intercalar bone graft (c). The latter procedure is particularly necessary in patients who are still growing. A bent plate is used. (d) Incomplete articular part of the acetabulum remains, ischiofemoral arthrodesis with screws in compression and bone grafts is obtained. (e) and (f) The same resection, extra-articular. Even in this case, ischiofemoral arthrodesis is attempted, however it is difficult to obtain. The base of the neck may be brought close to the ischium with screws in compression, or the femur may be resected between the two trochanters, the diaphysis may be medialized and an ischiofemoral Küntscher nail used. (g) Intra-articular resection of the acetabulum, of the anterior pelvic arch, and of most of the ilium. The residual part of the iliac wing is not sufficient for an arthrodesis; thus, iliofemoral pseudarthrosis is attempted. (h) If the ischium and the insertions of the quadratus femoris remain, limiting uprising of the femur, and resection is extra-articular, reconstruction may be avoided, leaving the femoral stump free. These flail hips nonetheless, like ischiofemoral pseudarthroses, provide the worst functional results.

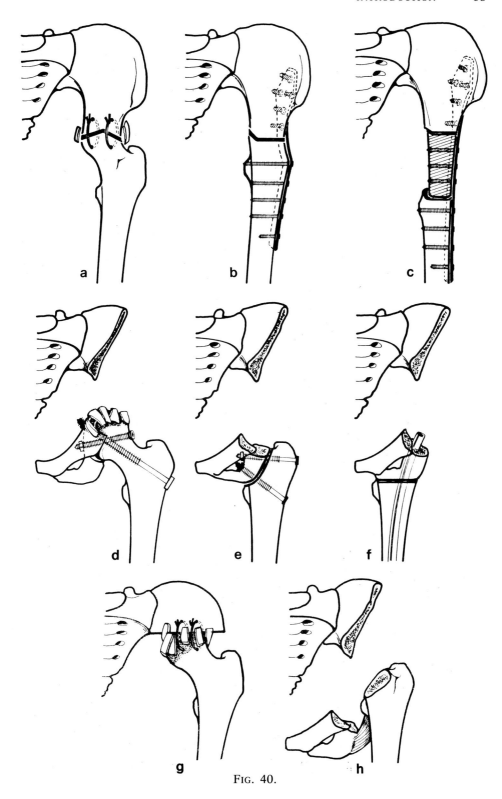

FIG. 40.

gluteal muscles are detached from the ilium (at times they are instead removed en bloc with the tumor), the tensor fasciae latae is divided in line with the skin incision, the femoral tendon of the gluteus maximus is divided, the trochanteric insertions of the glutei are detached, or the greater trochanter is osteotomized at the base, the external rotator muscles and piriformis are divided at the trochanter. Thus, a large myocutaneous flap is mobilized, exposing the entire lateral aspect of the ilium and of the acetabulum, the gluteal vessels, the sciatic nerve, the posterior aspect of the sacroiliac joint, the ischium and — crucial sites — the ischiatic insertions of the sacrospinous and sacrotuberous ligaments.

In intra-articular resections of the acetabulum the capsule is incised circularly and the femur dislocated; in extra-articular resections the femoral neck is transected at the base, or the femoral shaft is osteotomized distal to the trochanters, without opening the joint.

Divided at their insertions to the pelvis are the sartorius, the rectus anterior, and the abdominal muscles. The iliopsoas is detached from the lesser trochanter. Lifting the femoral nerve, the belly of the psoas is transected at its entry into the pelvis, generally removing the pelvic part of the muscle en bloc with the tumor. The iliac vessels are identified and protected, but not isolated if this is not required by their proximity to the tumor or by the presence of pathologic lymph nodes. The roots of the sciatic nerve are tended anterior to the

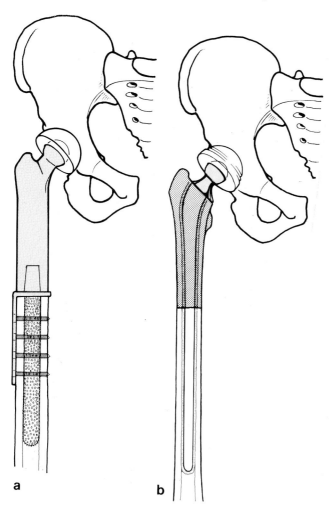

a   b

Fig. 41. - Resection of the proximal femur. (a) Substitution with a cementless modular endoprosthesis. (b) Substitution with a composite of an allograft containing a long-stem cemented prosthesis.

caudal part of the sacroiliac joint, and they may be partially sacrificed in order to widely resect the sacroiliac joint itself.

For anterior pelvic arch resection, an anterior incision is made along the upper border of the pubis, from which an incision is made at a right angle, parallel to the genitocrural plica, which reaches the ischial tuberosity. In bilateral resections of the anterior arch this incision will be bilateral. In resections of the acetabulum with part of the anterior pelvic arch, a lateral incision must be associated with an anterior one. Through the anterior incision all the muscles inserted to the pubis and ischium are divided. The femoral nerve and vessels are either moved externally or dissected out.

In order to mobilize the pelvic segment to be resected, the following is required: 1) complete division of the muscles covering the segment, which at times must be removed en bloc with the segment itself; 2) osteotomy or complete disarticulation at the two levels pre-established along the pelvic ring; 3) transection of the sacrospinous, sacrotuberous, and iliolumbar ligaments.

Methods of reconstruction. Extra-acetabular resections 1 and 2 do not generally require any reconstruction. At times, in wide iliac resections and in children — in whom deformity of the pelvic ring may become more severe — it is best to wedge a bridge graft between the sacrum and the supra-acetabular region. In type 3) resections — acetabular — femoroiliac pseudarthrosis may be obtained with simple metallic wiring, or femoroiliac arthrodesis with a screwed plate, or femoroischiatic arthrodesis may be attempted (Fig. 40).

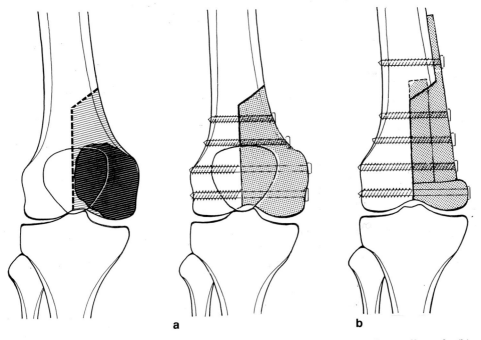

FIG. 42. - Partial resection of the distal femur. (a) Substitution with an allograft. (b) Substitution with the patella removed from the same knee and autogenous cortico-cancellous bridging graft.

A flail hip (without reconstruction) and femoroischiatic pseudarthrosis obtain the worst functional results, and must be avoided. Reconstruction with pelvic allografts and with endoarthroprosthesis are methods which continue to involve many complications, and which must be considered to be experimental.

Resection of the proximal femur

This is reconstructed by an endoprosthesis which is custom-made or modular, cemented or cementless, or by a composite of a cemented prosthesis associated with allograft (Fig. 41). As the muscular insertions are missing, the main early complication involved is that the prosthesis may dislocate. In order to prevent this, the prosthesis should not be shorter than the segment resected, rather, it should be a few millimeters longer. Furthermore, the acetabular component will be applied with an exaggerated degree of varus (20 to 30 degrees to the horizontal line) and considerable anteversion (in order to avoid dislocation in flexion). The limb will be immobilized in plaster or the patient confined to bed for 20 to 30 days, after which movement and weight-bearing will be allowed with great care. Instead of an arthroprosthesis, an endoprosthesis with a double or triple sliding surface may be used. An endoprosthesis has less of a tendency to dislocate.

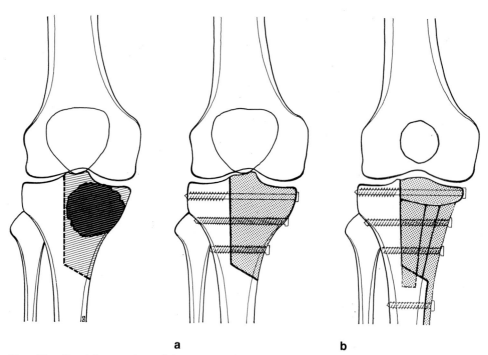

a   b

FIG. 43. - Partial resection of the proximal tibia. (a) Substitution with an allograft. (b) Substitution with the patella from the same knee and autogenous corticocancellous grafts.

Partial resection of the distal femur or proximal tibia

For rare tumors which are eccentric and not very expanded (particularly low-grade malignant tumors) only one of the two femoral or tibial condyles may be resected. In this resection the capsuloligamentous structures (medial or lateral) must be preserved as much as possible and reinserted in tension at the end of the operation. The posterior cruciate ligament must be preserved or reinserted stably.

For reconstruction, an articular allograft may be used, which is wedged in and stabilized with screws (Figs. 42a, 43a). The relatively small size of the graft and the existence of a vast cancellous contact surface between the host bone and the graft facilitates rapid consolidation and good incorporation. A very solid osteosynthesis is required, so that movement may be initiated as soon as possible.

The patella of the same knee may be used (Figs. 42b, 43b). The joint surface of the patella is of a shape and size which come very close to those of the

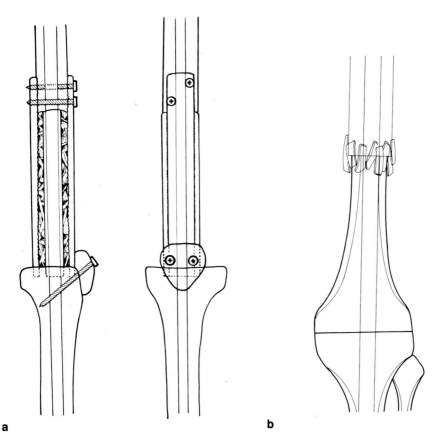

a   b

FIG. 44. - (a) The arthrodesis method used for resections of the distal femur (or of the proximal tibia) involves autogenous bone grafts removed from the homolateral fibula, contralateral tibia, and ilium. The skeletal ends of the resection are left intact, except for removal of the joint cartilage. (b) A massive allograft can be used.

joint surface of a tibial plate, while the anterior convex surface of the patella is suited to substituting the joint surface of a femoral condyle. The patella is adapted in a correct position, and then stabilized with two transverse screws. The empty space between the patella and the transverse resection line of the diaphysis is then filled with cortical and cancellous grafts taken from the tibia and/or from the ilium and stabilized with screws. Movement of the knee may be initiated after 20 days, while weight-bearing must be avoided for at least 6 months. The mobility obtained ranges from 60 to more than 90 degrees, with mild instability in flexion.

In case of parosteal osteosarcoma, typically localized in the popliteal region, the posterior half of the distal femur may be resected, preserving the epiphysis and the cruciate ligaments (Fig. 26c). Surgery involves two incisions, medial and lateral, with enlarged access to the knee. The bellies of the vastus medialis and vastus lateralis are dissected from the medial and lateral intermuscular septa; these aponeurotic septa are divided at a certain distance from the linea aspera, thus obtaining access to the popliteal space. The femoropopliteal vessels are accurately dissociated from the surface of the tumor, ligating the joint and bone branches departing from them.

Complete resection of the distal femur or of the proximal tibia, intra- or extra-articular

Resection removes the joint segment of the femur or of the tibia (**intra-articular**); or, if the tumor has penetrated into the joint, resection is **extra-articular**, removing the joint intact with the patella and a joint segment of both the femur and the tibia. Generally, this is a longer segment for the bone that hosts the tumor, and a short segment, limited to the joint surface as far as the insertion of the capsule, for the opposite bone.

Reconstruction may be obtained by aiming for fusion of the knee, or the preservation of movement.

Fusion involves considerable functional limitation, particularly in a sitting position (sedentary work, rest, driving an automobile). It may also be a complex operation, with a fair incidence of complications, and a long period of immobilization in plaster. However, once it is consolidated, it has the advantage of supporting any functional stress and lasting a life-time. Fusion is indicated for either resection of the femur or of the tibia, whatever the extent of the muscular sacrifice, in particular of the extensor apparatus.

The fusion method derived from Putti and Juvara modified by Merle d'Aubigné was used for a long time. This method presents numerous complications, consequent to wide and prolonged skeletal exposure, devascularization of the femur and tibia as a result of the taking of vast grafts, and insufficient stability of the osteosynthesis. In fact, these complications essentially consist in infection and pseudarthrosis. For this reason we have abandoned this method, taking grafts from the homolateral fibula, the contralateral tibia, and the ilium, leaving the femur and the tibia intact, just as they are after resection. Thus, the surgical exposure time of the knee affec-

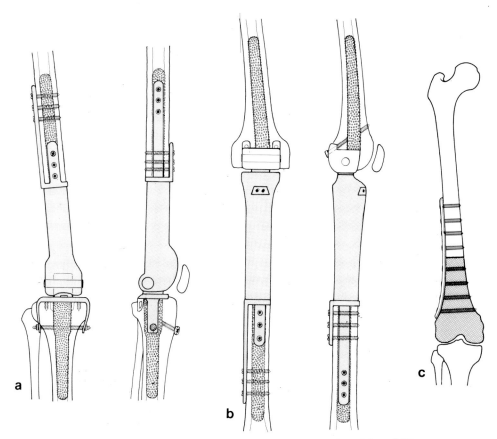

FIG. 45. - Resection of the distal femur or of the proximal tibia. (a) and (b) Reconstruction by cementless modular arthroprosthesis (Kotz). (c) Reconstruction with an articular allograft.

ted with the neoplasm is reduced and, above all, the vascularization of the diaphysis and of the epiphysis is not touched, and stability of the osteosynthesis is improved (Fig. 44a). A considerable amount of stability and mechanical resistance may be obtained when a stiff and threaded intramedullary nailing is used (Enneking and Shirley, 1977), or a locked nail of the Grosse-Kempf type. The fusion method which is currently preferred, however, involves intercalar allograft (Fig. 44b).

Reconstruction with an **articular allograft** (Fig. 45c) is perhaps the operation of choice in more fortunate cases, but it continues to involve a high incidence of complications. These include infection, fracture of the grafted epiphysis, joint instability, joint stiffness. Moreover, this method is less appealing than endoprosthetic replacement, when the patient is treated by aggressive chemotherapy.

Prosthetic replacement is a simpler procedure (Fig. 45a, b), involving minimal immediate complications, and leaving good function of the knee, even if the quadriceps has been partially resected; the procedure may substitute

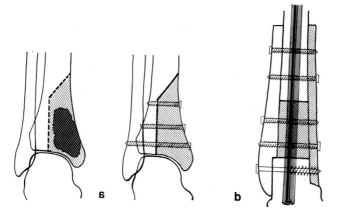

FIG. 46. - (a) Partial resection of the distal tibia and substitution with allograft. (b) Arthrodesis with an autogenous fibula, corticocancellous grafts and locked nail inserted in the talus.

very long segments of femur or tibia. But functional stress must be reduced to that of a nearly sedentary life, if the risk of mobilization or breakage of the prosthesis is to be reduced, and its duration cannot be predicted, nor is it unlimited.

Arthroprostheses are hinged, custom-made or modular, cemented or cementless. In prosthetic replacement of the proximal tibia, the patellar tendon may be reinserted on the gastrocnemius transported forward, or on the head of the fibula moved forwards by double osteotomy of the fibular diaphysis.

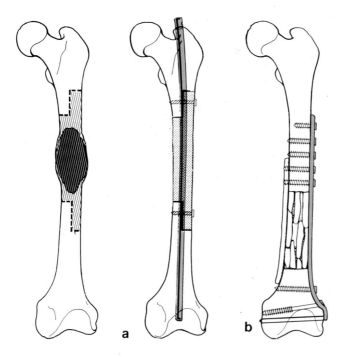

FIG. 47. - Resection of a diaphyseal segment and reconstruction with an intercalary allograft and an intramedullary nail (a) or with autogenous grafts and angulated plate (b).

Resection of the distal tibia

If resection is partial, and a tibial corticocancellous wall may be preserved, then allograft may be used (Fig. 46a). Generally, fusion is preferred, using the fibula and autografts or allografts, with a locked nail inserted in the talus (Fig. 46b).

Resection of diaphyseal segments

This may be required in cases of adamantinoma, chondrosarcoma, parosteal osteosarcoma, periosteal osteosarcoma, metastasis; or (after chemotherapy) in cases of classic osteosarcoma or Ewing's sarcoma which do not involve the epiphysis. The resected segment is substituted with auto- or allografts stabilized with an intramedullary nail or a plate (Fig. 47). It is essential that the contact areas between host bone and allograft be perfect, that around the contact areas there be abundant autogenous cancellous bone, that internal fixation be very solid, that, finally, for the lower limb, weight-bearing be allowed cautiously. Allografts are rehabited with difficulty and slowly; fractures and pseudarthrosis may occur even two or three years after surgery. As an alternative, autogenous cortical bars and cancellous bone may be used. In the case of the humerus and, for example, metastatic lesion, the diaphysis may simply be shortened and osteosynthesis used to stabilize the two segments.

When a graft is used (particularly an allograft) to substitute a femoral diaphyseal segment, intense scarring reaction and a long period of immobilization may cause extensive adherence of the quadriceps to the graft and make further myolysis surgery necessary (Judet) in order to mobilize the knee. Currently, titanium fiber-coated endoprostheses are being experimented with for substitution of a diaphyseal segment (Andersson *et al.*, 1978).

Finally, there are skeletal segments that may be **resected with no**

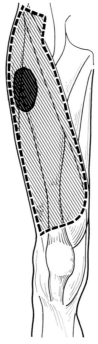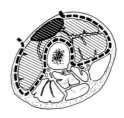

FIG. 48. - Radical excision for a malignant tumor of the soft tissues. Excision includes a skin strip and the entire quadriceps muscle, including the aponeurosis, the intermuscular septa, and the periosteum.

need for substitution, such as the proximal end of the fibula, the distal end of the ulna, the proximal end of the radius, an intermediate metatarsus, the ribs, the sternum including the manubrium, and, as we have seen, wide parts of the pelvis.

Vascularized skeletal and myocutaneous transplants

The use of microsurgery in skeletal and myocutaneous transplants is becoming more and more indispensable.

Among the skeletal transplants which are most used is that of the vascularized fibula, more rarely a rib or segment of iliac crest. These skeletal segments are removed from the same patient with their periosteum and nutritious vessels, which are then sutured to a branch (arterial and venous) of the recipient bed. As the transplant is vascularized, and therefore vital, consolidation of the transplant is rapid, functional stress on the transplant produces early hypertrophy, fractures of the transplant consolidate. Furthermore, the transplant may also be used in a bed which is altered by previous infection or irradiation.

The disadvantages to using the procedure are constituted by the limited volume and strength of the skeletal transplant and by the fact that it must be stabilized with minimum osteosynthesis, so that vascularization is not compromised, and hypertrophy under mechanical stress not obstructed. At times, vascularized skeletal transplants are combined with bone allografts.

Often, in oncological surgery of the locomotor apparatus, we are forced to sacrifice part of the skin surface, either because it is adherent, or because it is invaded by the tumor, or because it is traversed by a previous biopsy, or because it is infected or necrotic, or because it has been altered by radiation. In many cases, repair of the loss of skin substance by direct suturing of the margins, or by sliding flaps, or rotation flaps, is impossible. This is particularly true in regions where the skin is close to the skeletal plane (elbow, wrist, hand, knee, ankle, foot). Moreover, in osteoarticular reconstruction with endoprosthesis and allografts, it is particularly essential that these extraneous materials be covered by a sheath of soft tissues and thick skin, which is abundant and well-vascularized.

In cases such as these free vascularized myocutaneous flaps are used. Those most commonly used are the latissimus dorsi, the rectus abdominis, and the sartorius muscles. When surgery is ablative and there is not enough soft tissue and skin to cover the stump, a free vascularized myocutaneous flap taken from the amputated limb may be used.

Wide or radical excision of tumors of the soft tissues

This procedure is indicated in benign or low-grade malignant tumors, such as desmoid tumor, myxoid liposarcoma. Furthermore, it may be used in high-grade malignant tumors, if they are observed at a stage which is not too advanced, and as long as it is possible to remove the tumor with a layer of healthy tissue surrounding it, at least 1-2 cm in thickness, or with an aponeurosis of compartmental delimitation. At times it is best to remove in toto entire muscle groups, from insertion to insertion. The latter method may provide oncological results which are similar to those of an amputation (Fig. 48). Excision must remove the tumor in toto and intact. The surgical tools must not touch the neoplasm, the surgeon must not be able to see it. During excision the tumor is removed delicately, making contact with and cutting only those tissues which are definitely healthy, widely to the outside of the tumor pseudocapsule.

In tumors characterized by low-grade malignancy en bloc excision is usually attempted (except for exceptional cases with large expansion, with involvement of the large vessels and major nerve trunks) as local recurrence does not involve the risk of metastasis. In high-grade malignant sarcomas, on the contrary, wide or radical excision must be limited to selected cases.

Surgical behavior may be modified by adjuvant therapy. Preoperative radiotherapy, for example, may extend indications to conservative surgery.

The decision to use either excision or amputation is a difficult one to make, and it is of great importance as the life of the patient may depend on it. A decision such as this one must be based on the vast specific experience of the surgeon, the radiologist and the pathologist, as well as on an accurate clinical examination, imaging and histological staging.

Biopsy may involve a thin needle, with the advantage of not contaminating the entire anatomical compartment hosting the tumor. For a sarcoma of the vastus lateralis, for example, previous incisional biopsy would necessarily require resection of most of the quadriceps, while biopsy with a thin needle would allow for resection of the vastus lateralis alone (Stener, 1984). For these same reasons, intraoperative frozen section biopsy may be useful. Traditional incisional biopsy might be preferable when preoperative radiotherapy or chemotherapy is used because an accurate histological diagnosis on the resected specimen might not be possible.

For excision to have a high probability of success, the tumor must be of moderate size, not recurring, and preferably not submitted to previous biopsy, single, circumscribed, surrounded entirely by tissue which may be removed en bloc. If it is adherent to a nerve trunk, this must be resected and, if necessary, substituted with a graft; if it adheres to the large vessels, they must be resected and substituted by prosthesis or vascular grafts. It may be preferable to risk secondary amputation due to vascular disorder rather than local recurrence. When a truly wide or radical excision in high-grade malignant tumor of the soft tissues is not possible, amputation must be opted for.

We insist on these concepts, as sarcomas of the soft tissues are generally treated inadequately, moreso than bone sarcomas. In fact, the aggressive extent of bone sarcomas is made manifest by the radiographic picture; on the other hand, resection of a skeletal segment is often technically difficult, also because it poses the problem of the reconstruction of the resected segment. For these reasons, when first suspected, bone sarcomas are often sent to specialized centers. The opposite occurs for sarcomas of the soft tissues. In fact, marginal excision of a mass in the soft tissues is a rather simple procedure and one which does not compromise function of the limb. The problem is that most surgeons perform this type of excision following the border or the pseudocapsule of the tumor, at times without any knowledge as to the type of tumor (excisional biopsy). That is why patients affected with sarcoma of the soft tissues often come to specialized centers after one or more attempts at excision have been made. Recurrence is often the result, and if the tumor is of low-grade malignancy this makes further wide excision difficult, while if the tumor is of high-grade malignancy, it increases the probability of metastasis.

Amputations and disarticulations

When planning these procedures the direction and position of the incision required to obtain cover flaps must be taken into account. In fact, if this type of incision passes near the immediate vicinity of the tumor the procedure would be nearly equal to a marginal resection, and it could very easily be followed by local recurrence. These problems usually occur in tumors near the limb girdles, as a level higher than that of forequarter or hindquarter amputation cannot be selected.

Amputations may be performed with atypical flaps (Fig. 49). For example, an amputation at the mid third of the thigh for sarcoma of the sciatic nerve may be obtained by using a long anterior musculocutaneous flap which descends as far as the patella, and instead removing all of the posterior soft tissues and the skin as far as the gluteal plica. Similarly, for skeletal or soft tissue sarcomas involving the gluteus maximus, hemipelvectomy may be performed with an anteromedial skin and muscular flap of the thigh, used to cover the entire gluteal region removed up to the iliac crest.

Esmarch's bandaging should not be used in proximity of the tumor area. A hemostatic tourniquet may be placed at the root of the limb and, when possible (tumor of the tibia, for example) a second tourniquet may be placed above the knee, in order to interrupt any venous communication between the tumor site and the amputation site.

The latter will have to be chosen based on the imaging, keeping in mind the expansive features of the tumor along the medullary canal (see, for example, medullary extension of central chondrosarcoma, skip metastasis in osteosarcoma).

Interscapulothoracic (forequarter) amputation

This is above all indicated in malignant tumors of the proximal third of the humerus and of the soft tissues of the shoulder compromising the neurovascular bundle or those extensively reaching the skin plane. It is rarely indicated in tumors of the scapula, as scapulectomy or extra-articular resection

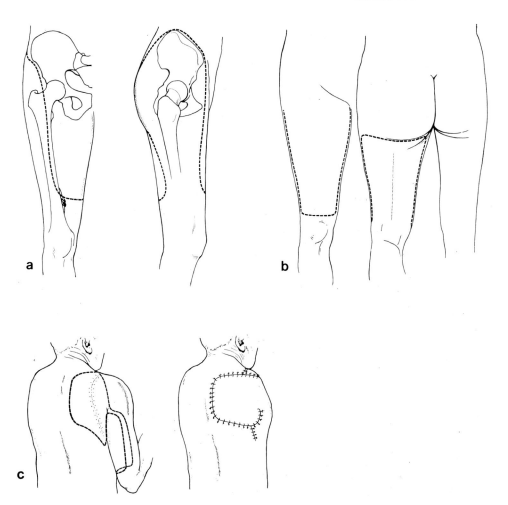

FIG. 49. - Amputation with atypical myocutaneous flaps. (a) Interilioabdominal amputation with removal of the entire gluteal region (muscles and skin included) and covering with an anteromedial myocutaneous flap from the thigh. The femoral vessels are ligated at the distal part of the thigh. (b) Midthigh amputation with removal of all of the posterior region of the thigh as far as the gluteal fold and covering with an anterior flap of the thigh. (c) Interscapulothoracic amputation with removal of all of the scapular region and covering with a medial arm flap.

of the scapula and of the proximal humerus have approximately the same effectiveness.

Interscapulothoracic amputation is more frequently indicated than disarticulation of the shoulder. Tumors of the humerus, in fact, are nearly always localized in the proximal metaepiphysis. Disarticulation of the shoulder for a malignant tumor of the proximal end of the humerus or of the surrounding soft tissues is not indicated, as the flap descends nearly as far as the humeral insertion of the deltoid; thus, it does not respond to the purpose of making the cut far away from the tumor, and it would more or less be the same performing a resection of the skeletal segment. Disarticulation of the shoulder should be limited to tumors of the humeral middle diaphysis or of the soft tissues of the arm.

Interilioabdominal (hindquarter) amputation

This procedure is particularly indicated in malignant tumors of the proximal third of the femur and of the soft tissues of the proximal thigh. For malignant tumors of the pelvis interilioabdominal amputation is indicated more rarely: particularly when the stage of the tumor would require sacrificing the sciatic nerve and the iliofemoral vessels.

The cover flaps of the interilioabdominal amputation is constituted by the gluteus maximus; thus, surgery will require an atypical flap (antero-medial of the thigh) if the gluteus maximus is invaded by the tumor or if a previous biopsy or other surgery has been performed through the buttock (Fig. 49a).

For the same reasons given for interscapulothoracic amputation, interilioabdominal amputation is more frequently indicated than hip disarticulation. The latter, in fact, is limited to tumors of the femoral mid-diaphysis and to those of the soft tissues of the mid-thigh.

Interilioabdominal amputation is often a type of surgery which is not more traumatic than hip disarticulation, as in the latter all of the muscles around the coxofemoral joint must be cut, while in the former the iliopsoas, the adductor muscles are cut, the gluteus maximus and extrarotator muscles are detached from the femur, and the muscular insertions from the iliac crest.

Furthermore, after ligating the external iliac vessels, there is only a small amount of blood loss. Disarticulation at the sacroiliac joint and/or at the pubic symphisis is often not required. Usually, it is enough to transect the ilium at the uppermost part of the greater sciatic notch and the branches of the pubis at the mid-point of the obturator foramen. When these osteotomies are done, care must be taken to remain strictly subperiosteal in order not to injure the obturator vessels (horizontal branch of the pubis), the pudendal ones (ischiopubic branch) and the superior gluteal ones (ilium at the greater sciatic notch). These vessels, particularly the gluteal ones, are of considerable caliber and, if inadvertently opened during surgery, because of their course, which is close to the bone, and their retraction within the pelvis, it is difficult to see them and to ligate them prior to removing the limb.

Rotationplasty

When a malignant tumor is located in the distal femur in a child aged under 12 years, segmental articular resection involves difficult problems to be solved in terms of reconstruction. A prosthesis may not be applied, or fusion be performed, and acceptable functional results still hoped for. Amputation of the thigh remains, with all of the severe deficit involved. In cases such as these rotationplasty may be indicated, widely resecting the distal femur and

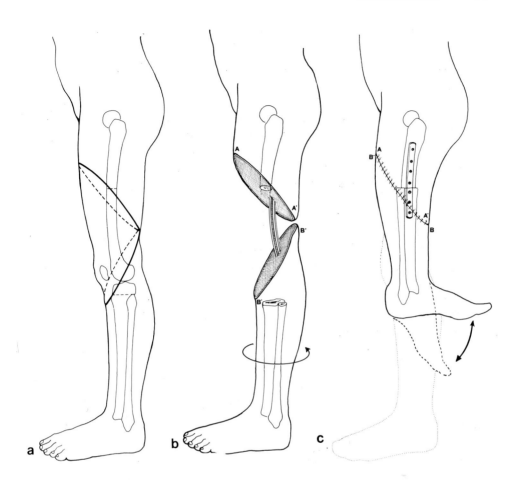

FIG. 50. - Rotationplasty. (a) Rhomboid skin incision, resection of the distal femur and of the tibial epiphysis distal to the growth cartilage. (b) The leg remains connected to the thigh only by the neurovascular bundle. If the vessels are included in the pseudo-capsule of the tumor they may be resected en bloc with the tumor, and reunited by termino-terminal suturing. The leg is extrarotated 180 degrees. (c) Reconstruction with a compression plate. The calcaneus is in the place of the patella, but it is more distal in order to compensate for the predicted growth.

the entire knee joint, providing functional results at the end of growth which are similar to those of a below-knee amputation (Fig. 50).

The procedure consists in amply resecting the distal femur and the proximal epiphysis of the tibia with all of the muscles and the skin covering them, saving the femoral vessels and the sciatic nerve. If the vessels are adherent to the tumor, they may be removed to be followed by termino-terminal suturing of the artery and vein. The leg residual to this resection is rotated 180 degrees and the proximal diaphysis of the tibia osteosynthesized at the residual diaphysis of the femur. What results from this is a shortening of the limb with the foot at the level of the knee and rotated 180 degrees. The length is calculated so that at the end of growth the foot of the limb operated on is at the level of the contralateral knee. The ankle functions as a knee and allows for controlling of a prosthesis of the lower limb, as effectively as that of a leg amputee.

In some rare cases, rotationplasty has been used for tumors of the proximal femur and of the proximal tibia.

Surgery for the treatment of pulmonary metastases

This is without a doubt indicated and often curative in cases of metastases due to non-malignant tumors, such as giant cell tumor, or low-grade malignant tumors such as chondrosarcoma, chordoma, adamantinoma. It may also be indicated in the treatment of high-grade malignant tumors, such as osteosarcoma. In the latter, more or less wide pulmonary exeresis is indicated for circumscribed metastases, which are located far from the hilum and not very progressive. With this procedure, which

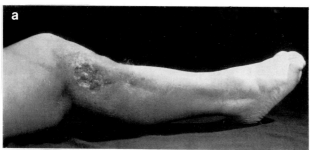

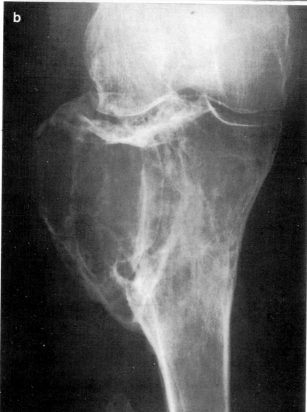

FIG. 51. - Giant cell tumor of the proximal tibia submitted to curettage and irradiated 20 years previously in a female aged 53 years. (a) Irradiation caused deformity in flexion of the knee, intense fibrous retraction in the soft tissues, torpid skin ulceration, severe joint stiffness, chronic edema in the leg, deformity and stiffness of the foot. Because of these radiation-induced lesions, the patient was amputated at the thigh, despite the fact that radiation had controlled the tumor (b).

may even be repeated several times, long periods of survival or cure may be obtained.

RADIATION THERAPY

The effects of radiation on the tumor as well as on the soft tissues and bone must be taken into account. Radiodermitis may occur at an early stage (during the first week), as far as necrosis of the borders of the surgical wound or skin, with a torpid bottom. After a few months, there may be radiation fibrosis, with brownish discoloring of the skin, adherence of the skin to the underlying planes, transformation of the soft tissues in a rather tenacious fibrous scar, one which is poorly vascularized, compact, adherent and retractive. This fibrosis may cause several drawbacks, such as making further surgery difficult, favoring dehiscence and necrosis of the surgical wound, obstruct rehabilitation of bone grafts, produce chronic distal edema due to venous and lymphatic circulatory obstruction, produce a decrease in joint mobility or fixed deformities due to joint contracture (Fig. 51).

Bone tissue is among the most resistant to radiation. At very high doses, however, radiation may cause bone necrosis, with the possibility of spontaneous fracture or fracture due to mild trauma, which is difficult to consolidate. After high doses of radiation, the irradiated skeletal segment should be considered to be more fragile than normal, and the surgeon should act accordingly.

There may also be injury to the brain and spinal cord due to irradiation to the cranium and to the vertebral column, as well as injury to the bladder and gonads due to irradiation to the pelvis.

Finally, radiation may, although rarely, cause radiation-induced sarcoma, in the bone and in the soft tissues (see specific chapter).

When radiation therapy must be used, some rules for biopsy should be followed: 1) incision should be as short as possible; 2) the window in the cortex should be as limited as possible; 3) incision should be made where the bone is covered with a good layer of soft tissues; 4) suturing should be very accurate. These rules help to initiate radiation therapy early, to avoid necrosis and dehiscence of the wound, and to reduce the risk of pathologic fracture.

Some general principles are recommended by radiotherapists, with the purpose of minimizing some of the adverse effects indicated above: the surgical wound should be scarred prior to initiating radiation therapy; all irradiation fields should be treated each day; immobilization of the joint located near the area treated should be used often, alternating it with active mobilization; marginal and compensatory filters, multiple and complex fields are often indicated; electron beam therapy should be included if possible; exclude the skin above the patella, tibial crest, or other skeletal protuberances, the skin in the area of Scarpa's triangle from the volume irradiated as much as possible; for the first 5000 rads apply a thin layer of bolus on the scar; do not apply either heat or cold to the area treated.

If chemotherapy is associated, it is usually necessary to reduce the dose of irradiation, as tissue tolerance decreases.

For some soft tissue tumors, preoperative or postoperative radiation therapy is used. **Preoperative** radiation therapy has the advantage of irradiating a well-defined mass, reducing successive surgical dissemination, of making surgery easier on a mass which is reduced in volume, hardened, more delimited, with less bleeding; the main disadvantage is constituted by possible necrosis and dehiscence of the surgical wound.

Postoperative radiation therapy could have the advantage of being proportional to the operation performed; but it involves several disadvantages, such as delay in execution, the need to irradiate a wider and poorly-defined area because of the surgical dissection, and, finally, the fact that as a hypoxic tumor cell requires a higher dose of radiation, any residual tumor foci in the surgical scar could require a higher dose than that held to be adequate for the primary tumor.

CHEMOTHERAPY

In some neoplasms of the locomotor apparatus chemotherapy has become a part of the initial therapeutic protocol, in association with surgery and/or radiation therapy. This type of chemotherapy, which is known as complementary or adjuvant, is not without dangers, even severe ones, both immediate and late. Its use is thus justified only in tumors in which experience teaches us that metastasis will occur frequently and shortly. Typical examples include osteosarcoma, Ewing's sarcoma, rhabdomyosarcoma, forms in which there is nearly constantly at the time the diagnosis is first made dissemination of micrometastases which cannot be observed by routine methods of investigation (radiological and scintigraphic). In neoplasms such as these, adjuvant chemotherapy has proven to significantly increase the percentage of long-term disease-free survival.

Adjuvant chemotherapy is generally conducted by using several drugs in sequential associations, in an attempt to strengthen the effect of the single chemotherapies, in terms of pharmacodynamics (vincristine, for example, facilitates the penetration of methotrexate in sarcomatous cells), and in terms of cellular kinetics (synchronization and recruitment). Adjuvant chemotherapy must be carried out according to rational protocols and ones which are scrupulously respected in every detail. Generally, it is carried out in intermittent cycles with constant periodicity, protracted for several months. It is very important that these cycles be initiated as early as possible, particularly after surgery. Tolerance is generally good, particularly in young patients. Naturally, systematic and routine monitoring of the following is essential during the entire treatment period: renal function (creatinemia), cardiac function (ECG), and medullary function (hemochrome and platelet count) and, at times, the hematic levels of the drug (methotrexate at high doses).

Even if it seems that adjuvant chemotherapy carried out in an intermittent manner does not determine important immunodepressive phenomena, it must be remembered that it may favor the development of infections. This must be taken into account when planning surgery.

More recently, chemotherapy has been used prior to surgery and intraarterially, as well as intravenously. This type of chemotherapy has the advantage of acting immediately after diagnosis on both the primary tumor and on any micrometastasis; moreover, it has completely overturned the relationship between conservative treatment and amputation in osteosarcoma; it has allowed for an extended use of surgery and, at times, abolition of radiation therapy in Ewing's sarcoma. Finally, a histological study of chemotherapeutically induced necrosis on the primary tumor constitutes a test of in vivo chemosensitivity that is of important prognostic value, and that allows for the adjustment of postoperative chemotherapy.

This preoperative chemotherapy/surgery/postoperative chemotherapy protocol is also known as neoadjuvant chemotherapy. It is used to treat osteosarcoma, Ewing's sarcoma, and, in some centers, highly-malignant sarcomas of the soft tissues.

REFERENCES

1954 SCHAJOWICZ F., CABRINI R. L.: Histochemical studies of bone in normal and pathological conditions, with special reference to alkaline phosphatase, glycogen and mucopolysaccarides. *Journal of Bone and Joint Surgery*, **36-B**, 474-489.

1958 JAFFE H. L.: *Tumours and tumorous conditions of the bones and joints*. Lea & Febiger, Philadephia.

1958 SISSONS H. A.: Malignant tumours of bone and cartilage. In Raven R. W.: *Cancer*, **II**, 324-343, Butterworth & Company, London.

1962 FRANCIS K. C., WORCESTER J. N. Jr.: Radical resection for tumors of the shoulder with preservation of a functional extremity. *Journal of Bone and Joint Surgery*, **44-A**, 1423-1430.

1965 LICHTENSTEIN L.: *Bone tumors*. Mosby, St. Louis.

1965 MERLE D'AUBIGNÉ R., MÉARY R., THOMINE J. M.: Résection dans les tumeurs des os. *Revue de Chirurgie Orthopédique*, **51**, 305-324.

1966 ENNEKING W. F.: Local resection of malignant lesions of the hip and pelvis. *Journal of Bone and Joint Surgery*, **48-A**, 991-1007.

1966 FOSS O. P., BRENNHOUD I. O., MESSELT O. T., EFSKIND J., LINERUD R.: Invasion of tumor cells into the bloodstream caused by palpation or biopsy of the tumor. *Surgery*, **59**, 691-695.

1966 MERLE D'AUBIGNÉ R., ALEXANDRE G.: Reconstruction condylienne fémorale par greffe rotulienne pediculée. *Revue de Chirurgie Orthopédique*, **52**, 611-633.

1966 PARRISH F. F.: Treatment of bone tumors by total excision and replacement with massive autologous and homologous grafts. *Journal of Bone and Joint Surgery*, **48-A**, 986-990.

1967 STOUT A. P., LATTES R.: *Tumours of the soft tissue*. Atlas of Tumor Pathology, 2nd series, fascicle 1, Armed Forces Institute of Pathology, Washington.

1967 SWEETNAM R., ROSS K.: Surgical treatment of pulmonaty metastases from primary tumors of bone. *Journal of Bone and Joint Surgery*, **49-B**, 74-79.

1968 AGOSTINO D.: Sono effettivamente dannose le biopsie dei tumori maligni? *Archivio di Ortopedia*, **81**, 73-79.

1968 SCHAJOWICZ F., DERQUI J. C.: Puncture biopsy in lesions of the locomotor system. Review of results in 4050 cases, including 941 vertebral punctures. *Cancer*, **21**, 531-548.

1969 ENZINGER F. M., LATTES R., TORLONI H.: *Histological typing of soft tissue tumors*. World Health Organization, Geneva.

1971 Spjut H. J., Dorfman H. D., Fechner R. E., Ackerman L. V.: *Tumors of bone and cartilage.* Atlas of Tumor Pathology, 2nd series, fascicle 5, Armed Forces Institute of Pathology, Washington.

1972 Bingold A. C.: Prosthetic replacement of a chondrosarcoma of the upper end of the femur. *Journal of Bone and Joint Surgery,* **54-B**, 139-142.

1972 Contreras E., Ellis L. D., Lee R. E.: Value of the bone marrow biopsy in the diagnosis of metastatic carcinoma. *Cancer,* **29**, 778-783.

1972 Janecki C. I., Nelson C. L.: En bloc resection of the shoulder gerdle: technique and indications. Report of a case. *Journal of Bone and Joint Surgery,* **54-A**, 1754-1758.

1972 Perez C. A., Bradfield J. S., Morgan H. C.: Management of pathologic fractures. *Cancer,* **29**, 684-693.

1972 Schajowicz F., Ackerman L. V., Sissons H. A.: *Histological typing of bone tumours.* World Health Organization, Geneva.

1973 Hall A. J., Mackay N. N. S.: The results of laminectomy for compression of the cord or cauda equina by extradural malignant tumor. *Journal of Bone and Joint Surgery,* **55-B**, 497-505.

1973 Murray R. O.: The radiological appearance of lesions resembling malignant bone tumors. Price C. H. G., Ross F. G. M.: *Bone - Certain aspects of neoplasia.* Butterworths, London.

1973 Nilsonne U.: Homologous bone and joint transplantation in bone tumour resection. Price C. H. G., Ross F. G. M.: *Bone - Certain aspects of neoplasia,* Butterworths, London.

1973 Parrish F. F.: Allograft replacement of all or part of the end long bone following excision of a tumour. *Journal of Bone and Joint Surgery,* **55-A**, 1-22.

1973 Stener B., Magnusson A., Sundin T., Höök O., Grimby G., Nordin M.: Rehabilitation after hemicorporectomy for chondrosarcoma. Price C. H. G., Ross F. G. M.: *Bone - Certain aspects of neoplasia.* Butterworths, London.

1973 Suit H. D., Russel W. O., Martin R. G.: Management of patients with sarcoma of soft tissue in an extremity. *Cancer,* **31**, 1247-1255.

1973 Van Rjissel Th. G.: Progression in bone tumors. Price C. H. G., Ross F. G. M.: *Bone - Certain aspects of neoplasia.* Butterworths, London.

1973 Vidal J., Goalard C.: Normalisation d'une prothése de toute l'extremité superieure du femur. *Revue de Chirurgie Orthopedique,* suppl. 1, 248-252.

1973 Walcher K., Dern W.: Die operative Behandeung der Spontan Fracturen. *Archiv für Orthopädische und Unfallchirurgie,* **77**, 315-319.

1973 Wanebo H. J., Shah J., Knapper W., Hajdu S., Booher R.: Reappraisal of surgical management of sarcoma of the buttock. *Cancer,* **31**, 97-104.

1974 Sim F. M., Daugherty Th. W., Ivins J. C.: The adjunctive use of methylmethacrilate in fixation of pathological fractures. *Journal of Bone and Joint Surgery,* **56-A**, 40-48.

1975 Becker F. F.: *Cancer. A comprehensive treatise.* Plenum Press, New York, London.

1975 Burrows H. J., Wilson J. N., Scales J. T.: Excision of tumours of humerus and femur, with restoration by internal prostheses. *Journal of Bone and Joint Surgery,* **57-B**, 148-159.

1975 Galasko C. S. B.: Pathological basis for skeletal scintigraphy. *Journal of Bone and Joint Surgery,* **57-B**, 353-359.

1975 Lunseth P. A., Nelson L. C.: Longitudinal amputation for the treatment of soft tissue fibrosarcoma. *Clinical Orthopaedics,* **109**, 147-151.

1975 Wara W. M., Phillips T. L., Sheline G. E., Schwade J. G.: Radiation tolerance of the spinal cord. *Cancer,* **35**, 1558-1562.

1976 Erikson U., Hjelmstedt A.: Limb-saving radical resection of chondrosarcoma of the pelvis. *Journal of Bone and Joint Surgery,* **58-A**, 568-570.

1976 Gui L., Manes E., Luppino D.: Innesti ossei massivi ed emiarticolari. *Giornale Italiano di Ortopedia e Traumatologia,* **2**, 151-162.

1976 Guntemberg B.: Effects of resection of the sacrum. *Acta Orthopedica Scandinavica,* suppl. **162**.

1976 Harrington D., Sim F. H., Enis J. E., Johnston J. O., Dick M., Gristina A. G.:

Methylmethacrylate as an adjunct in internal fixation of pathological fractures. *Journal of Bone and Joint Surgery*, **58-A**, 1047-1055.

1976 LOUIS R., CASANOVA J., BAFFERT M.: Techniques chirurgicales des tumeurs du rachis. *Revue de Chirurgie Orthopedique*, **62**, 57-70.

1976 MERLE D'AUBIGNÉ R., MAZAS F.: *Nouveau traité de technique chirurgicale*. Masson, Paris.

1976 MICKELSON M. R., BONFIGLIO M.: Pathological fractures in the proximal part of the femur treated by Zickel-Nail fixation. *Journal of Bone and Joint Surgery*, **58-A**, 1067-1070.

1976 RYAN J. R., ROWE D. E., SALCICCIOLI G. G.: Prophylactic internal fixation of the femur for neoplastic lesion. *Journal of Bone and Joint Surgery*, **58-A**, 1071-1074.

1976 SIMON M. A., ENNEKING W. F.: The management of soft-tissue sarcomas of the extremities. *Journal of Bone and Joint Surgery*, **58-A**, 317-327.

1976 THOMAS G.: Greffes homoplastiques (allogènes) des articulations du genou et de la hanche. *Revue de Chirurgie Orthopedique*, **62**, 295-307.

1977 ENNEKING W. F., SHIRLEY P. D.: Resection-arthrodesis for malignant and potentially malignant lesions about the knee using an intramedullary rod and local bone grafts. *Journal of Bone and Joint Surgery*, **59-A**, 223-236.

1977 FELD R., BODEY G. P.: Infection in patients with malignant lynphoma treated with combination chemotherapy. *Cancer*, **39**, 1018-1025.

1977 SALZER M., KNAHR K., SARZER-KUNTSCHIK M.: Indicazione alla resezione di tumori maligni delle ossa e risultati ottenuti. *Giornale Italiano di Ortopedia e Traumatologia*, **3**, 155-166.

1977 TEFFT M., CHABORA B. McC., ROSEN G.: Radiation in bone sarcomas. A reevaluation in the era of intensive systemic chemotherapy. *Cancer*, **39**, 806-816.

1978 ANDERSSON G. B. J., GAECHTER A., GALANTE J. O., ROSTEKER W.: Segmental replacement of long bones in baboons using a fiber-titanium implant. *Journal of Bone and Joint Surgery*, **60-A**, 31-40.

1978 BORIANI S., CAMPANACCI M.: Osteoblastoma e osteomalacia. Presentazione di un caso e revisione della letteratura. *Giornale Italiano di Ortopedia e Traumatologia*, **4**, 375-378.

1978 CAMPANACCI M., GIORDANO L., MASETTI G.: L'amputazione interileoaddominale. *Giornale Italiano di Ortopedia e Traumatologia*, **4**, 297-301.

1978 DAHLIN D. C.: *Bone tumors*. Charles C. Thomas, Springfield, Illinois.

1978 ENNEKING W. F., DUNHAM W. K.: Resection and reconstruction for primary neoplasms involving the innominate bone. *Journal of Bone and Joint Surgery*, **60-A**, 731-746.

1978 LAMBERT P. M.: Radiation myelopathy of the thoracic spinal cord in long term survivors treated with radical radiotherapy. *Cancer*, **41**, 1751-1760.

1978 SCHUMACHER T. M., GENANT H. K., KOROBKIN M., BOVIL E. G. Jr.: Computed tomography. Its worth in space-occupying lesions of the musculoskeletal system. *Journal of Bone and Joint Surgery*, **60-A**, 600-607.

1978 STEEL H. H.: Partial or complete resection of the hemipelvis. An alternative to hindquarter amputation for periacetabular chondrosarcoma of the pelvis. *Journal of Bone and Joint Surgery*, **60-A**, 719-730.

1978 STENER B., GUNTERBERG B.: High amputation of the sacrum for extirpation of tumors. Principles and technique. *Spine*, **3**, 351-366.

1978 TOMENO B., ISTRIA R., MERLE D'AUBIGNÉ R.: La résection-arthrodèse du genou pour tumeur. *Revue de Chirurgie Orthopédique*, **64**, 323-332.

1979 CAMPANACCI M., COSTA P.: Total resection of distal femur or proximal tibia for bone tumours. *Journal of Bone and Joint Surgery*, **61-B**, 455-463.

1979 CAMPANACCI M., LAUS M., BORIANI S.: Resezione dell'estremità distale del radio. *Giornale Italiano di Ortopedia e Traumatologia*, **5**, 153-160.

1979 DE SANTOS L. A., MURRAY J. A., AYALA A. G.: The value of percutaneous needle biopsy in the management of primary bone tumors. *Cancer*, **43**, 735-744.

1979 EILBER F. R., GRANT T. T., SAKAI D., MORTON D. L.: Internal hemipelvectomy-excision of the hemipelvis with limb preservation. *Cancer*, **43**, 806-809.

1979 SIM F. H., CHAO E. Y. S.: Prosthetic replacement of the knee and a large segmental of the femur or tibia. *Journal of Bone and Joint Surgery*, **61-A**, 887-892.

1979 HAJDU S. I.: *Pathology of soft tissue tumors*. Lea e Febiger, Philadelphia.

1980 BORIANI S.: L'ascesso di Brodie. Studio di 181 osservazioni con particolare riferimento ai criteri di diagnosi radiografica. *Giornale Italiano di Ortopedia e Traumatologia*, **6**, 367-378.

1980 MIRRA J. M.: *Bone tumors. Diagnosis and treatment*. Lippincott, Philadelphia.

1982 CAMPANACCI M., CAPANNA R., STILLI S.: Posterior hemiresection of the distal femur in parosteal osteosarcoma. *Italian Journal of Orthopedics and Traumatology*, **8**, 23-28.

1982 CAMPANACCI M., CERVELLATI C., GHERLINZONI F., CAPANNA R.: Endoprosthesis of the humerus: description of a new model and its application. *Italian Journal of Orthopedics and Traumatology*, **8**, 59-65.

1982 GIUNTI A., LIJOI F., INNAO V.: Il trattamento chirurgico delle metastasi ossee. *Giornale Italiano di Ortopedia e Traumatologia*, **8**, 247-257.

1982 KOTZ R., SALZER M.: Rotation-plasty for childhood osteosarcoma of the distal part of the femur. *Journal of Bone and Joint Surgery*, **64-A**, 959-969.

1982 ROSEN G., CAPARROS B., HUVOS A.G., WOSLOFF C., NIRENBERG A., CACAVIO A., MARCOVE R.C., LANE J.M., MEHTA B., URBAN C.: Preoperative chemotherapy for osteogenic sarcoma: selection of postoperative adjuvant chemotherapy based on the response of the primary tumor to preoperative chemotherapy *Cancer*, **49**, 1221-1230.

1982 WILNER D.: *Radiology of bone tumors and allied disorders*. W.B. Saunders, Philadelphia.

1983 AYALA A. G., ZORNOSA J.: Primary bone tumors: percutaneous needle biopsy. Radiologic-pathologic study of 222 biopsies. *Radiology*, **149**, 675-679.

1983 AZZARELLI A., GENNARI L., BONFANTI G., AUDISIO R., QUAGLIUOLO V.: Intra-arterial adriamycin for limb sarcomas. *Recent Results Cancer Research*, **86**, 218-21.

1983 BRAAT R. P., WIEBERDINK J., VAN SLOOTEN R., OLTHUIS G.: Regional perfusion with adriamycin in soft tissue sarcomas. *Recent Results Cancer Research*, **86**, 260-3.

1983 BUCK J., HEUCK F. H., REICHARDT W., ULBRICHT D.: Benign disorders of soft tissue on the roentgen computer tomogram. *Radiology*, **23**, 485-90.

1983 CAMPANACCI M., CAPANNA R., CERVELLATI C., GUERRA A., CALDERONI P.: Modular rotatory endoprosthesis for segmental resection of the proximal humerus. Experience with thirty-three cases. In «*Tumor prostheses for bone and joint reconstruction*», edited by E.U.S. Chao and J. C. Ivins. Thieme Stratton, New York.

1983 CAPANNA R., BACCI G., BERTONI F., CALDERONI P., CERVELLATI C., GHERLINZONI F., GIUNTI A., GUERNELLI N., GUERRA M., MERCURI M., PICCI P., CAMPANACCI M.: Endoprostheses for resections of the proximal humerus. In «*Modern trends in orthopaedics surgery*», edited by M. Campanacci *et al.* A. Gaggi Ed., Bologna.

1983 CAPANNA R., BACCI G., BERTONI F., CALDERONI P., CERVELLATI C., GHERLINZONI F., GIUNTI A., GUERRA A., GUERNELLI N., MERCURI M., PICCI P., CAMPANACCI M.: Resections of the pelvic bones. In «*Modern trends in orthopaedic surgery*», edited by M. Campanacci *et al.* A. Gaggi Ed., Bologna.

1983 CASTRUP H. J.: Surgery of malignant soft tissue tumors. *Chirurg*, **54**, 639-42.

1983 CERVELLATI C., BACCI G., BERTONI F., CALDERONI P., CAPANNA R., GHERLINZONI F., GIUNTI A., GUERNELLI N., GUERRA A., MERCURI M., PICCI P., CAMPANACCI M.: Patellar autograft for resection of one femoral or one tibial condyle at the knee. In «*Modern trends in orthopaedics surgery*», edited by M. Campanacci *et al.* A. Gaggi Ed., Bologna.

1983 CERVELLATI C., BACCI G., BERTONI F., CALDERONI P., CAPANNA R., GHERLINZONI F., GIUNTI A., GUERNELLI N., GUERRA A., MERCURI M., PICCI P., CAMPANACCI M.: Autografts arthrodesis for resection of the distal femur or proximal tibia. In «*Modern trends in orthopaedic surgery*», edited by M. Campanacci *et al.* Aulo Gaggi, Ed. Bologna.

1983 ENNEKING W. F.: *Musculoskeletal tumor surgery*. Vol. I e II. Churchill Livingstone, Edimburgh-London.

1983 ENZINGER F. M., WEISS S. W.: *Soft tissue tumors*. Mosby, St. Louis.

1983 FRIEDLAENDER G.E., MANKIN H.J., SELL K.W.: Osteochondral allografts. *Biology, banking and clinical applications*. Little Brown and Co., Boston/Toronto.

1983 GIUNTI A., BACCI G., BERTONI F., CALDERONI P., CAPANNA R., CERVELLATI C., GHERLINzoni F., Guernelli N., Guerra A., Mercuri M., Picci P., Campanacci M.: Endoprostheses and artroprostheses for resection of the proximal femur. In «*Modern trends inorthopaedic surgery*», edited by M. Campanacci *et al.* A. Gaggi, Bologna.

1983 Giunti A., Bacci G., Bertoni F., Calderoni P., Capana R., Cervellati C., Gherlinzoni F., Guenelli N., Guerra A., Mercuri M., Picci P., Campanacci M.: Resection of the sacrum. In «*Modern trends in orthopaedic surgery*», edited by M. Campanacci *et al.* A. Gaggi, Bologna.

1983 Guerra A., Bacci G., Bertoni F., Calderoni P., Capanna R., Cervellati C., Gherlinzoni F., Giunti A., Guernelli N., Mercuri M., Picci P., Campanacci M.: Resection and temporary stabilization with Kuntscher rod (or plate, or external fixation) and acrylic cement. In «*Modern trends in orthopaedic surgery*», edited by M. Campanacci *et al.*, A. Gaggi, Bologna.

1983 Hossfeld D. K., Lempidakis S., Seeber S.: Chemotherapy of malignant soft tissue tumors. *Chirurg*, **54**, 649-51.

1983 Kadir S., Ernst C. B., Hamper U., White R. I. Jr.: Management of vascular soft tissue neoplasms using transcatheter embolization and surgical excision. *American Journal of Surgery*, **146**, 409-12.

1983 Larson D. L., Liang M. D.: The quadriceps musculocutaneous flap: a reliable, sensate flap for the hemipelvectomy defect. *Plast. Reconstr. Surg.*, **72**, 347-354.

1983 Lawrence W. Jr., Neifeld J. P., Terz J. J.: *Manual of soft tissue tumor surgery*. Springer, New York.

1983 Melanotte P. L., Esposito C., Mercuri M., Calderoni P.: Resezioni diafisarie. In «*Modern trends in orthopaedic surgery*», edited by M. Campanacci *et al.* A. Gaggi Ed., Bologna.

1983 Mercuri M., Bacci G., Bertoni F., Calderoni P., Capanna R., Cervellati C., Gherlinzoni F., Giunti A., Guernelli N., Guerra A., Picci P., Campanacci M.: Fibular autograft for distal radius resection. In «*Modern trends in orthopaedic surgery*», edited by M. Campanacci *et al.* A. Gaggi Ed., Bologna.

1983 Monticelli G., Santori F. S., Ghera S., Folliero A.: Resection and reconstruction of the distal end of the femur of proximal end of the tibia after radical excision of diaphyseal and epiphyseal segments. *Italian Journal of Orthopedics and Traumatology*, **9**, 427-37.

1983 Rydholm A.: Management of patients with soft-tissue tumors. Strategy developed at a regional oncology center. *Acta Orthopedica Scandinavica*, Suppl. **203**, 13-77.

1983 Rydholm A., Berg N. O., Persson B. M., Akerman M.: Treatment of soft-tissue sarcoma should be centralised. *Acta Orthopedica Scandinavica*, **54**, 333-9.

1983 Scales J. T.: Bone and joint replacement for the preservation of limbs. *Br. J. Hosp. Med.*, **30**, 220-232.

1983 Schajowicz F.: *Tumors and tumorlike lesions of bone and joints*. Mosby, St. Louis.

1983 Schauer A., Altmannsberger H. M.: Pathology of malignant soft tissue tumors. *Chirurg.*, **54**, 629-38.

1984 Arnoldi C., Johansen H., Mouridsen H. T.: Soft tissue sarcomas in adults. Surgical, radiologic and cytotoxic treatment. *Acta Radiologica*, **23**, 169-75.

1984 Boriani S., Ruggieri P., Sudanese A.: La biopsia: considerazioni sulla tecnica chirurgica dedotte da 749 casi di tumore osseo. *Giornale Italiano di Ortopedia e Traumatologia*, **10**, 497-507.

1984 Eilber F. R.: Soft tissue sarcomas of the extremity. *Curr. Probl. Cancer*, **8**, 3-41.

1984 Eilber F. R., Eckhardt J., Morton D. L.: Advances in the treatment of sarcomas of the extremity, current status of limb salvage. *Cancer*, **54**, 2695-701.

1984 Eilber F. R., Morton D. L., Eckarat J., Grant T., Weisenburger Th.: Limb salvage for skeletal and soft tissue sarcomas. *Cancer*, **53**, 2579-2584.

1984 Enjoji M., Hashimoto H.: Diagnosis of soft tissue sarcomas. *Pathol. Res. Pract.*, **178**, 215-26.

1984 Eusebi V., Bondi a., Rosai J.: Immunohistochemical localization of myoglobin in nonmuscular cells. *American Journal of Surgical Pathology*, **8**, 51-5.

1984 Ghussen F., Nagel K.: Regional hyperthermic cytostatic perfusion as an alternative in the treatment of malignant soft tissue tumors of the extremities. *Chirurg.*, **55**, 505-7.

1984 Heiken J. P., Lee J. K., Smathers R. L., Totty W. G., Murphy W. A.: CT of benign soft-tissue masses of the extremities. *American Journal Röntgenology*, **142**, 575-80.

1984 Kirchner P. T., Simon M. A.: The clinical value of bone and gallium scintigraphy for soft-tissue sarcomas of the extremities. *Journal of Bone and Joint Surgery.*, **66-A**, 319-27.

1984 Marcove R. C.: *The surgery of tumors of bone and cartilage.* 2nd Ed. Grune-Stratton, Orlando.

1984 Mizuta H., Yamasaki M.: Nuclear magnetic resonance studies on human bone and soft tissue tumors. *Nippon Seikeigeka Gakkai Zasshi*, **58**, 97-106.

1984 Reiser M., Rupp N., Heller H. J., Allgayer B., Lukas P., Lange J., Pfafferott K., Fink U.: MR-tomography in the diagnosis of malignant soft-tissue tumours. *European Journal of Radiology*, **4**, 288-93.

1984 Rydholm A., Berg N. O., Gullberg B., Thorngren K. G., Persson B. M.: Epidemiology of soft-tissue sarcoma in the locomotor system. A retrospective population-based study of the inter-relationships between clinical and morphologic variables. *Acta Pathol. Microbiol. Immunol. Scand.*, **92**, 363-74.

1984 Rosemberg S. A.: Prospective randomized trials demonstrating the efficacy of adjuvant chemotherapy in adult patients with soft tissue sarcomas. *Cancer Treat. Rep.*, **68**, 1067-78.

1984 Stehlin J. S. Jr., Giovanella B. C., Gutierrez A. E., de Ipolyi P. D., Greeff P. J.: 15 years experience with hyperthermic perfusion for treatment of soft tissue sarcoma and malignant melanoma of the extremities. *Front Radiat. Ther. Oncol.*, **18**, 177-82.

1984 Stener B.: Musculoskeletal tumor surgery in Göteborg. *Clinical Orthopedics*, **191**, 8-20.

1984 Tonak J., Hohenberger W., Göhl J.: Hyperthermic isolation perfusion of the extremities in malignant melanomas and soft tissue sarcomas. *Chirurg.*, **55**, 499-504.

1984 Trojani M., Contesso G., Coindre J. M., Rouesse J., Bui N. B., de Mascarel A., Goussot J. F., David M., Bonichon F., Lagarde C.: Soft-tissue sarcomas of adults; study of pathological prognostic variables and definition of a histopathological grading system. *International Journal of Cancer*, **33**, 37-42.

1985 Basso-Ricci S., Bartoli C.: Cutaneous carcinomas and soft tissue sarcomas induced by ionizing radiation therapy. Presentation of a series of 42 cases. *Tumori*, **71**, 29-33.

1985 Bendix-Hansen K., Myhre-Jensen O., Enzyme histochemical investigations on bone and soft tissue tumours. *Acta Pathol. Microbiol. Immunol. Scand.*, **93**, 73-80.

1985 Bramwell V. H., Crowther D., Deakin D, P., Swindell R., Harris M.: Combined modality management of local and disseminated adult soft tissue sarcomas: a review of 257 cases seen over 10 years at the Christie Hospital & Holt Radium Institute, Manchester. *British Journal of Cancer*, **51**, 301-18.

1985 Campanacci M., Cervellati C., Donati U.: Autogenous patella as replacement for a resected femoral or tibial condyle. A report on 19 cases. *Journal of Bone and Joint Surgery*, **67-B**, 557-563.

1985 Capanna R., Rock M., Giunti A., Picci P., Campanacci M.: Femoral megaprosthesis in the management of bone tumors. A study of 49 cases. *J. West Pac. Orthop. Ass.*, **22**, 33-43.

1985 Capanna R., Guerra A., Ruggeri P., Biagini R., Campanacci M.: Le protesi modulari di Kotz nelle resezioni osteoarticolari massive per tumore osseo. *Giornale Italiano di Ortopedia e Traumatologia*, **11**, 281-291.

1985 D'Angiò G.J., Evans A.E.: *Bone tumors and soft tissue sarcomas.* Arnold, London.

1985 Dick H.M., Malinin T.I., Mnayneh W.A.: Massive allograft implantation following radical resection for high-grade tumors requiring adjuvant chemotherapy treatment. *Clinical Orthopaedics*, **197**, 88-95.

1985 Donaldson S. S.: The value of adjuvant chemotherapy in the management of sarcomas in children. *Cancer*, **55**, 2184-97.

1985 Goodnight J. E. Jr., Bargar W. L., Voegeli T., Blaisdell F. W.: Limb-sparing surgery for extremity sarcomas after preoperative intraarterial dozorubicin and radiation theraphy. *American Journal of Surgery*, **150**, 109-13.

1985 GUERRA A., BRICCOLI A., CAPANNA R., GUERNELLI N., PICCI P., CAMPANACCI M.: Les resections avec conservation du membre inferieur dans le chondrosarcome du bassin. *Revue Chirurgie Orthopedique*, **71**, 493-501.

1985 GUERRA A., CAPANNA R., BIAGINI R., RUGGIERI P., CAMPANACCI M.: Resezione extrarticolare della spalla (Tikoff-Linberg). *Giornale Italiano di Ortopedia e Traumatologia*, **11**, 157-163.

1985 HANCOCK B.W., WARD A.M.: *Immunological aspects of cancer*. Martinus Nijhoff Publ., Boston.

1985 HUDSON T.M., HAMLIN D.J., ENNEKING W.F., PETTERSON H.: Magnetic resonance imaging of bone and soft tissue tumors: early experience in 31 patients compared with computed tomography. *Skeletal Radiology*, **13**, 134-146.

1985 LYNGE E.: A follow-up study of cancer incidence among workers in manufacture of phenoxy herbicides in Dermark. *British Journal of Cancer*, **52**, 259-70.

1985 MALININ T.T., MARTINEZ O.V., BROWN M.D.: Banking of massive osteoarticular and intercalary   bone allografts. 12 years' experience. *Clinical Orthopaedics*, **197**, 44-57.

1985 MUCHMORE J. H., CARTER R. D., KREMENTS E. T.: Regional perfusion for malignant melanoma and soft tissue sarcoma: a review. *Cancer Invest.*, **3**, 129-43.

1985 MURRAY M. P., JACOBS P. A., GORE D. R., GARDNER G. M., MOLLINGER L. A.: Functional performance after tibial rotation plasty. *J. Bone Joint Surg.*, **67-A**, 392-399.

1985 PETTERSSON H., HAMLIN D. J., MANCUSO A., SCOTT K. N.: Magnetic resonance imaging of the musculoskeletal system. *Acta Radiol. Diagn.*, Stockh. **26**, 225-34.

1985 SHAFFER J.W., FIELD G.A., GOLDBERG V.M., DAVY D.T.: Fate of vascularized and non-vascularized autografts. *Clinical Orthopaedics*, **197**, 32-43.

1985 TEPPER J. E., SUIT H. D.: Radiation therapy of soft tissue sarcomas. *Cancer*, **55**, 2273-7.

1985 WEEKES R. G., McLEOD R. A., REIMAN H. M., PRITCHARD D. J.: CT of soft-tissue neoplasms. *American Journal Röntgenology*, **144**, 355-60.

1985 WEIDNER N., BAR R.S., WEISS D., STROTTMAN M.P.: Neoplastic pathology of oncogenic osteomalacia/rickets. *Cancer*, **55**, 1961-1705.

1986 AISEN A.M., MARTEL W., BRAUNSTEIN E.M., MC MILLIN K.I., PHILLIPS W.A., KLING T.F.: MRI and CT evaluation of primary bone and soft tissue tumors. *American Journal of Radiology*, **146**, 749-756.

1986 BOHNDORF K., KAISER M., LOCHNER B., FRAUX DE LACROIX W., STEINBRICH W.: Magnetic resonance imaging of primary tumors and tumor-like lesions of bone. *Skeletal Radiology*, **15**, 511-517.

1986 COTTON G.S., VAN PUFFELEN P.: Hypophosphatemic osteomalacia secondary to neoplasia. *Journal of Bone and Joint Surgery*, **68**, 129-133.

1986 ENNEKING W.F.: A system of staging musculoskeletal neoplasms. *Clinical Orthopaedics*, **204**, 9-24.

1986 GITELIS S., RYAN W.G., ROSENBERG A., TEMPLETON A.C.: Adult-onset hypophosphatemic osteomalacia secondary to neoplasm: a case report and review of pathophysiology. *Journal of Bone and Joint Surgery*, **68-A**, 133-138.

1986 HAJDU S.E.: *Differential diagnosis of soft tissue and bone tumors*. Lea & Febiger, Philadelphia.

1986 SUNDARAM M., MC GUIRE M.H., HERBOLD D.R., WOLVERSUN M.K., HEIBERG E.: Magnetic resonance imaging in planning limb-salvage surgery for primary malignant tumors of bone. *Journal of Bone and Joint Surgery*, **68**, 809-819.

1986 VAN OOSTEROM A.T., VAN LUNNIK J.A.M.: *Management of soft tissues and bone sarcomas*. Raven Press, New York.

1987 ARLEN M., MARCOVE R.C.: *Surgical management of soft tissue sarcomas*. Saunders, Philadelphia.

1987 CONTESSO G., ZAFRANI B., MAZABRAUD A., LACOMBE M.J., ZEMOURA L., GENIN J., MISSENARD G., DUBOUSSET J.: Place de l'anatomopathologiste dans le traitement des sarcomes ostéogènes. *Revue de Chirurgie Orthopédique*, **73**, 293-296.

1987 COOMBS R., FRIEDLAENDER G.: *Bone tumor management*. Butterworths, London.

1987 COURTHEOUX P., THERON J., MANI J.: L'embolisation préopératoire des lésions tumorales ostéo-muscolaires en dehors des localisations rachidiennes. *Revue de Chirurgie Orthopédique*, **73**, 293-296.

1987 ENNEKING W.F.: *Limb salvage in musculoskeletal oncology*. Churchill Livingstone, New York.

1987 FARLEY F.A., HEALEY J.H., CAPARROS-SISON B., GODBOLD J., LANE J.M., GLASSER D.B.: Lactate dehydrogenase as a tumor marker for recurrent disease in Ewing's sarcoma. *Cancer*, **59**, 1245-1248.

1987 FRAGER D.H., GOLDMAN M.J., SEIMON L.P., ELKON C.M., CYNAMON J., SCHREIBER K., HABERMANN E.T., FREEMAN L.M., LEEDS N.E.: Computed tomography guidance for skeletal biopsy. *Skeletal Radiology*, **16**, 644-646.

1987 FRIEDLAENDER G.E.: Bone grafts. The basic science rationale for clinical applications. *Journal of Bone and Joint Surgery*, **69-A**, 786-790.

1987 HIDDEMANN W., ROESSNER A., WÖRMANN B., MELLIN M., KLOCKENKEMPER B., BÖSING T., BÜCHNER T., GRUNDMANN E.: Tumor heterogeneity in osteosarcoma as identified by flow cytometry. *Cancer*, **59**, 324-328.

1987 HUDSON T.H.: *Radiologic-pathologic correlation of musculoskeletal lesions*. Williams & Wilkins, Baltimore.

1987 LAVAL-JEANTET M., ROGER B., DELEPINE G., BUY J.N.: Apport de l'imagerie par résonance magnétique (I.R.M.) dans l'explorations des tumeurs osséuses malignes. *Revue de Chirurgie Orthopédique*, **73**, 72-75.

1987 TOMENO B.: Procédés de reconstruction après résection totale ou partielle d'un hemibassin dans le traitement des tumeurs malignes de l'os iliaque. A propos des 33 cas. *Revue de Chirurgie Orthopédique*, **73**, 95-98.

1987 TOMENO B., GERBER CH.: Les résections-reconstitutions diaphysaires des grands os des membres en pathologie tumorale. A propos de 23 cas. *Revue de Chirurgie Orthopédique*, **73**, 131-136.

1987 XIANG J., SPANIER S.S., BENSON N.A., BRAYLAN R.C.: Flow cytometric analysis of DNA in bone and soft-tissue tumors using nuclear suspensions. *Cancer*, **59**, 1951-1958.

1988 BAUER H.C.F., KREICBERGS A., SILVERSWARD C., TRIBUKAIT B.: DNA analysis in differential diagnosis of osteosarcoma. *Cancer*, **61**, 2532-2540.

1988 CHALMERS J.: Tumours of the musculoskeletal system. Clinical presentation. *Current Orthopaedics*, **2**, 135-140.

1988 DELEPINE G., DELEPINE N.: Résultats préliminaires de 79 allogreffes osséuses massives dans le traitement conservateur des tumeurs malignes de l'adulte et de l'enfant. *International Orthopaedics*, **12**, 21-29.

1988 ENNEKING W.F., MAALE G.E.: The effect of inadverted contaminations of wounds during the surgical resection of musculoskeletal neoplasms. *Cancer*, **62**, 1251-1256.

1988 GALASKO C.S.B.: Tumors of the musculoskeletal system: principles of management of metastatic disease. *Current Orthopaedics*, **2**, 158-167.

1988 MANKIN H.J., GEBHARDT M.C., SPRINGFIELD D.S.: Tumors of the musculoskeletal system. Investigations. *Current Orthopaedics*, **2**, 141-144.

1988 NILSONNE U.: Tumours of the musculoskeletal system: principles of management of metastatic disease. *Current Orthopaedics*, **2**, 158-167.

1988 OKAJIMA K., HONDA I., KITAGAWA T.: Immunohistochemical distribution of S-100 protein in tumors and tumor-like lesions of bone and cartilage. *Cancer*, **61**, 792-799.

1988 SOUHAMI R., CRAFT A.: Progress in management of malignant bone tumors. *Journal of Bone and Joint Surgery*, **70-B**, 345-347.

1988 STOKER D.J.: Tumors of the musculoskeletal system: imaging. *Current Orthopaedics*, **2**, 145-152.

1988 SUDANESE A., TONI A., BALDINI N., TIGANI D., CAMPANACCI M.: Partial resection of distal humerus and reconstruction using autogenous iliac bone graft. *International Orthopaedics*, **12**, 115-118.

1988 SUNDARAM M., MC GUIRE M.H.: Computed tomography or magnetic resonance for evaluating the solitary tumor or tumor-like lesions of bone? *Skeletal Radiology*, **17**, 393-401.

1988 UYTTENDAELE D., DE SCHRYVER A., CLAESSENS H., ROELS H., BERKVENS, MONDE-

LAERS: Limb conservation in primary bone tumors by resections, extracorporal irradiation and re-implantation. *Journal of Bone and Joint Surgery*, **70-B**, 348-353.

1988 YOSHIKAWA M., TAKAOKA K., MASUMARA K., ONO SAKAMOTO Y.: Prognostic significance of bone morphogenetic activity in osteosarcoma tissue. *Cancer*, **61**, 569-573.

1989 BERQUIST Y.H.: Magnetic resonance imaging of musculoskeletal neoplasm. *Clinical Orthopaedics*, **244**, 101-118.

1989 CAPANNA R., BIAGINI R., RUGGIERI P., BETTELLI G., CASADEI R., CAMPANACCI M., Temporary resection-arthrodesis of the knee using an intramedullary rod and bone cement. *International Orthopaedics*, **13**, 253-258.

1989 CHAO E.Y.S.: A composite fixation principle for modular segmental defect replacement (SDR) prostheses. *Orthopaedic Clinics of North America*, **20**, 439-453.

1989 FINN H.A., SIMON M.A.: Staging systems for musculoskeletal neoplasms. *Orthopaedics*, **12**, 1365-1371.

1989 GHELMAN B.: Radiology of bone tumors. *Orthopaedic Clinics of North America*, **20**, 287-312.

1989 HAUSMAN M.: Microvascular application in limb sparing tumor surgery. *Orthopaedic Clinics of North America,* **20**, 427-437.

1989 HEARE T.C., ENNEKING W.F., HEARE M.M.: Staging techniques and biopsy of bone tumors. *Orthopaedic Clinics of North America*, **20**, 273-285.

1989 JAFFE N.: Chemotherapy for malignant bone tumors. *Orthopaedic Clinics of North America*, **20**, 487-503.

1989 KALNICKI S.: Radiation therapy in the treatment of bone and soft tissue sarcomas. *Orthopaedic Clinics of North America*, **20**, 505-512.

1989 LANGLAIS F., VIELPEAU C.: Allografts of the hemipelvis after tumour resection: technical aspects of four cases. *Journal of Bone and Joint Surgery*, **71-B**, 58-62.

1989 MIRRA J.M., PICCI P., GOLD R.H.: *Bone tumors. Clinical radiologic and pathologic correlations*. Lea & Febiger,Philadelphia/London.

1989 MNAYMNEH W., MALININ T.: Massive allografts in surgery of bone tumors. *Orthopaedic Clinics of North America*, **20**, 455-467.

1989 TAKAOKA K., YOSHIKAWA H., HASUHARA K., SUGAMOTO K., TSUDA T., AOKI Y., ONO K., SAKAMOTO Y.: Establishment of a cell line producing bone morphogenetic protein from a human osteosarcoma. *Clinical Orthopaedics*, **244**, 258-264.

1990 CARTER S.R., EASTWOOD D.M., GRIMER R.J., SNEATH K.S.: Hindquarter amputation of the musculoskeletal system. *Journal of Bone and Joint Surgery*, **72-B**, 490-493.

1990 DE BOER H.H., WOOD M.B., HERMANS J.: Reconstruction of large skeletal defects by vascularized fibula transfer. Factors that influenced the outcome of union in 62 cases. *International Orthopaedics*, **14**, 121-128.

1990 EXNER G.U., VON HOCHSTETTER A.R., AUGUSTINY N., VON SCHULTHESS G.: Magnetic resonance imaging in malignant bone tumors. *International Orthopaedics*, **14**, 49-55.

1990 GEBHARDT M.C., ROTH Y.F., MANKIN H.J.: Osteoarticular allografts for reconstruction in the proximal part of the humerus after excision of a musculoskeletal tumor. *Journal of Bone and Joint Surgery*, **72-A**, 334-345.

1990 KNOP J., DELLING G., HEISE U., WINKLER K.: Scintigraphic evaluation of tumor regression during preoperative chemotherapy of osteosarcoma. Correlation of 99mTc-methylene diphosphonate parametric imaging with surgical histopathology. *Skeletal Radiology*, **19**, 165-172.

1990 MC DONALD D.J., CAPANNA R., GHERLINZONI F., BACCI G., FERRUZZI A., CASADEI R., FERRARO A., CAZZOLA A., CAMPANACCI M.: Influence of chemotherapy on peroperative complications in limb salvage surgery for bone tumors. *Cancer*, **65**, 1509-1516.

1990 MERKEL D.E., MC GUIRE W.L.: Ploidy, proliferative activity and prognosis: DNA flow cytometry of solid tumors. *Cancer*, **65**, 1194-1205.

1990 O'CONNOR M., SIM F.H.: Salvage of the limb in the treatment of malignant pelvic tumors. *Journal of Bone and Joint Surgery*, **71-A**, 481-494.

1990 POITOUT D., GAUJOUX G., LEMPIDAKIS M.: Réconstructions iliaques totals ou partiellas à l'aide d'allogreffes de banque. *International Orthopaedics*, **14**, 111-119.

1990 SHIMIZU T., CHIGIRA M., NAGASE M., WATANABE H., UDAGAWA E.: HLA phenotypes in patients who have osteosarcoma. *Journal of Bone and Joint Surgery*, **72-A**, 68-70.

1990 WUISMAN P., ENNEKING W.F.: Prognosis for patients who have osteosarcoma with skip metastasis. *Journal of Bone and Joint Surgyer*, **72-A**, 60-68.

TUMORS OF BONE

HISTIOCYTIC FIBROMA
(Synonyms: fibroma, non-ossifying fibroma, non-osteogenic fibroma, fibrous defect of the cortex, fibrous metaphyseal defect, fibrous xanthoma, histiocytic xanthogranuloma)

DEFINITION

It is a metaphyseal hamartoma, made up of histio-fibroblasts; it is generally small in size and ephemeral; at times it is larger, but even when this is so it is rarely symptomatic, and exceptionally persistent. The first variety was named «fibrous defect of the cortex» or «fibrous metaphyseal defect», while the second was named «non-ossifying or non-osteogenic fibroma». This is actually the same lesion, and the only differential criteria consists in its size.

FREQUENCY

H.F. occurs very frequently, and it is probably present in 20-30% of all children aged from 4 to 10 years. Its actual incidence cannot be evaluated, as almost all cases of H.F. are asymptomatic and ephemeral.

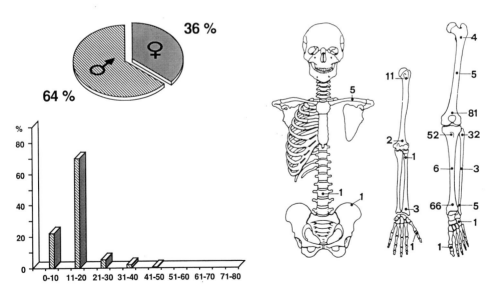

Fig. 52a. (legend on the following page).

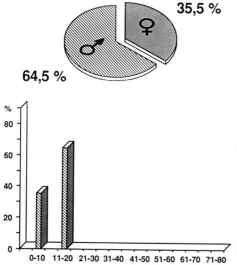

35,5 %

64,5 %

FIG. 52. - (a) Sex, age and localization in 281 cases of histiocytic fibroma. These cases were all submitted to histological assessment as they were operated and sent for consultation. Thus, the series includes fibromas of larger size. In most of the cases surgery was superfluous. The localization indicated refers to the largest fibroma, as in many cases there were more than one. Diffused multicentric histiocytic fibroma were not taken into consideration here (16 cases). (b) Sex and age in 16 cases of diffused multicentric histiocytic fibroma.

FIG. 52b.

SEX

There is predilection for the male sex, at a ratio of 1.5:1 (Fig. 52).

AGE

H.F. is typical of childhood and adolescence. It is rarely observed prior to the age of 5 and after the age of 20 (Fig. 52). The smallest H.F. are generally observed prior to 10 years of age, as many of these regress thereafter, while some progress. On the contrary, H.F. which are more expanded and those which are (although very rarely) symptomatic prevail after 10 years of age.

HEREDITY

There is a significant familial tendency.

LOCALIZATION

Most cases of H.F. are located in the long bones of the lower limbs, prevalently around the knee (Fig. 52). The most frequent site is the distal metaphysis of the femur (particularly in the posterior and medial aspects). This is followed by the proximal metaphysis and the distal metaphysis of the tibia, and then by the proximal metaphysis of the fibula. It is more rarely located in the proximal metaphysis of the femur and in the upper limb (humerus, ulna, radius). Solitary H.F. is nearly unknown in the short and flat bones, and in the tubular bones of the hand or foot.

Quite frequently, two or three H.F. may be observed in the same lower limb or in both lower limbs. In exceptional cases, **multiple H.F. of considerable size** may be observed, with a sui generis radiographic picture. These may extend to one or both of the lower limbs (at times involving the pelvis), or spread to all four limbs with hemisomic prevalence.

H.F. is generally localized in the metaphysis. At the onset it is close to the growth cartilage and it is subperiosteal or intracortical. Thereafter, as the limb grows in length, it may move towards the diaphysis and, in progressive forms, it may expand to much of or even to all of the section plane of the metaphysis or diaphysis.

SYMPTOMS

Most cases of H.F. are and remain completely asymptomatic. In more expanded forms, which occur rarely, there may be mild pain, which is at times related to trauma and, although rarely, pathologic fracture. In exceptional cases a «giant» H.F. expands the cortex, and causes moderate swelling of the bone.

In the rare cases of **diffused multiple H.F.** pigmented skin spots may be observed as well as congenital anomalies, such as mental retardation, cryptorchidism, ocular alterations, aortic stenosis (cfr. neurofibromatosis) (Fig. 53).

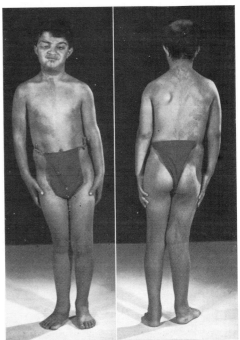

FIG. 53. - Male aged 11 years, affected with multicentric histiocytic fibroma (see Fig. 65). There are areas of pigmented skin, particularly in the right hemisoma, alopecia, leg length discrepancy, right palpebral ptosis. The patient was also severely mentally retarded.

RADIOGRAPHIC FEATURES

The radiographic picture is so typical that one may nearly always rely on a radiographic diagnosis without obtaining a histological confirmation (Figs. 54-62).

Initially, the osteolytic defect is small, metaphyseal, eccentric and superficial. In one of the two radiographic projections it may even appear to be central, but the other always shows that it is intracortical or subperiosteal (Fig. 54). Its major axis is oriented according to the length of the bone, and its form is generally polycyclical. Its boundaries toward the underlying cancellous bone or the medullary canal are always clear-cut and often marked by a thin radiopaque rim of reactive hyperostosis.

The osteolytic image may appear to be cloistered, due to the presence of parietal crests, or, rarely, to continuous bony septa. The cortex that generally encloses the fibroma is attenuated, at times slightly expanded. Some of the smaller H.F. appear to be subperiosteal and dig into the cortex from its surface.

The small H.F. that regress spontaneously are close to the metaphysis and contained within the cortex, which progressively thickens and narrows around the fibroma, until its image is completely obliterated. At the end, there may be a knot of focal thickening of the compact cortical bone, and no further traces of the H.F.

Lasting longer in time, progressive forms of the disease are more often shifted towards the diaphysis. They nearly always appear to be enclosed by a layer of thin cortex, which is often slightly expanded. They may extend to the entire section of the bone, which is particularly the case in the thinner bones, such as the fibula and the bones of the upper limb. At times an image of pathologic fracture is associated. These more expanded forms, as well, stop growing at the end of body growth and tend to ossify during adult age (Figs. 61, 62).

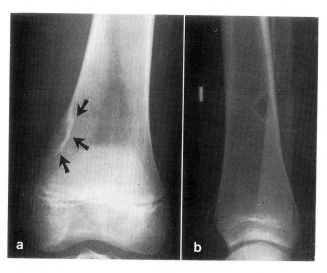

FIG. 54. - Small intracortical histiocytic fibromas at the age of 12 years (a) and at 10 years (b).

Multicentric diffused forms of H.F. are characterized by a specific radiographic picture. Osteolyses are contained at the surface by a thin layer of bone or by the periosteum alone, while they are demarcated towards the inside of the bone by a clear-cut thickened hyperostotic layer, with narrowing of the medullary canal. Osteolyses which originate at the metaphysis may extend along much of the diaphysis and they are often singularly symmetrical when they involve the limbs bilaterally, they are more frequent in

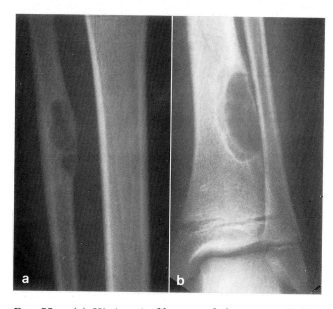

FIG. 55. - (a) Histiocytic fibroma of the peroneal diaphysis at the age of 9 years. (b) Histiocytic fibroma of fair size in a female aged 8 years. Pathologic fracture may be observed in the upper part of the photograph.

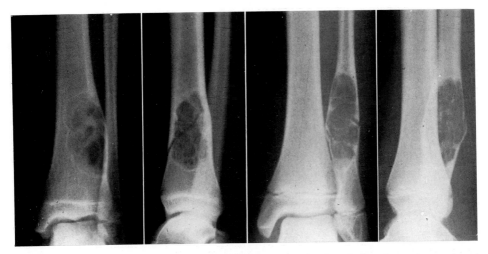

FIG. 56. - Histiocytic fibromas of considerable size in the distal tibia (age 12 years) and in the distal fibula (age 11 years). In both cases the fibroma was revealed by pathologic fracture visible on radiograms.

the upper limb than is the case in common H.F., and they may cause pathologic fracture, particularly in the lower limb (Figs. 65, 66).

GROSS PATHOLOGIC FEATURES

The tissue is typical. It is compact, of soft gummy consistency, and as for color it either tends towards leathery-yellow or is definitely rusty-brown. It may not be uniform, rather variegated by darker areas (due to

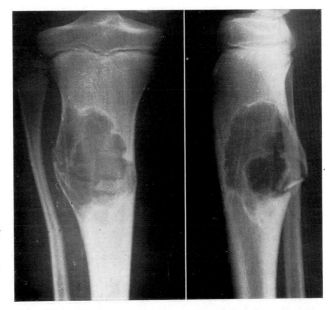

FIG. 57. - Histiocytic fibroma of considerable size in a male aged 8 years, expanding the cortex and complicated by pathologic fracture.

hemosiderin contents) and by yellow areas (due to lipoid accumulation).

In smaller and initial forms, the tissue is often subperiosteal. In more expanded and advanced forms, it is enclosed in a layer of cortex and it may be separated by means of bony walls in distinct loculi.

In particularly expanded forms, within the tissue there may be numerous cysts containing serohematic fluid.

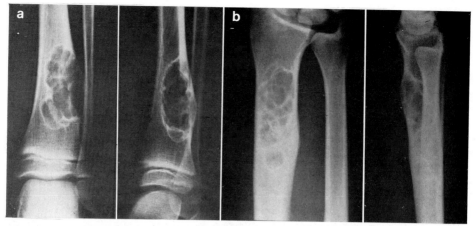

FIG. 58. - (a) Histiocytic fibroma of considerable size in a male aged 6 years. (b) A rare example of isolated histiocytic fibroma of the upper limb in a male aged 20 years. The lesion was discovered by a casual radiographic examination.

HISTOPATHOLOGIC FEATURES

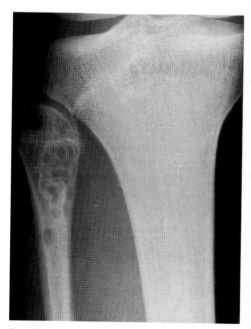

FIG. 59. - Histiocytic fibroma in a boy aged 15 years, chance radiographic finding.

Histopathological findings are also characteristic, and they remain the same whatever the size of the H.F. There is compact histio-fibroblastic tissue in bundles which are imbricated and whorled (storiform pattern), disseminated by few giant cells, which are small and elongated. Granules of intra- and extracellular hemosiderin pigment constitute a nearly constant feature. Occasionally, there may be areas of foam cells, more rarely (in older forms) bunches of cholesterin crystals are observed (Figs. 63, 64).

In initial or progressive forms the tissue is richly cellular. The nuclei may appear to be slightly plump, well-stained, and they may show some mitotic figures. The collagen is delicate and scarce. In forms of the disease where growth has ended, and in which regression is underway, the cells are less numerous, in the form of more mature fibroblasts or fibrocytes, and the collagenous bundles become pre-eminent. The number of giant cells and the hemosiderin contents also decrease, while the areas of foam cells and cholesterin

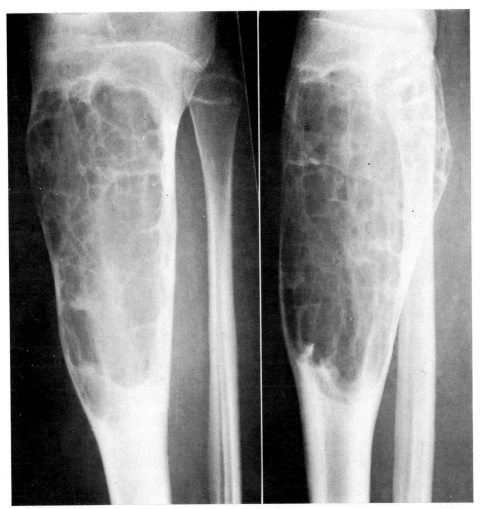

FIG. 60. - Histiocytic fibroma of enormous size in a male aged 15 years. The size of this fibroma is absolutely exceptional. The contents of the cavity was partially cystic; but its tissue, sampled in several sites, showed the histological features of histiocytic fibroma throughout.

crystals increase. These lipoid accumulations express the regressive phenomena of the tumor.

H.F. has no osteogenic properties. Considerable reactive and repair osteogenesis may instead be observed during the regression and ossification stages of H.F.

HISTOGENESIS AND PATHOGENESIS

H.F. is clearly a hamartoma. This is shown by age, site, familiarity, multiplicity, course, its rare association with pigmented skin spots and with other

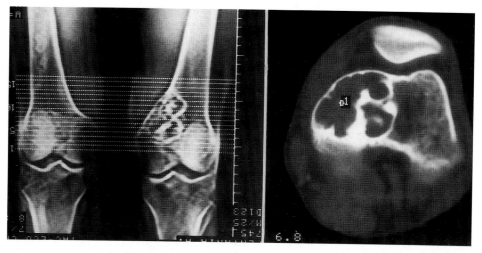

FIG. 61. - Histiocytic fibroma in a male aged 25 years, observed radiographically by chance. CAT reveals evident demarcation with sclerotic rim.

congenital anomalies (cfr. neurofibromatosis). It apparently originates from an area of histio-fibroblastic tissue which is isolated in the process of the formation of the metaphyseal cortical bone during growth. Its cellular composition (histiocytes, «facultative» fibroblasts, macrophages with hemosiderin or lipids, giant cells) and structure (in whorls) indicate a histiocytic derivation and the fact that H.F. belongs to the group of histiocytomas.

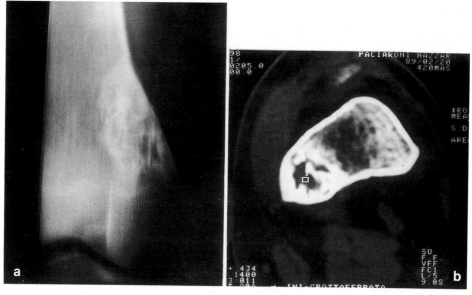

FIG. 62. - Histiocytic fibroma in a male aged 28 years, observed radiographically by chance. (a) Tomography. (b) CAT. Observe the advanced ossification of the fibroma, which proceeds from the rim and the cloisters of osteosclerosis.

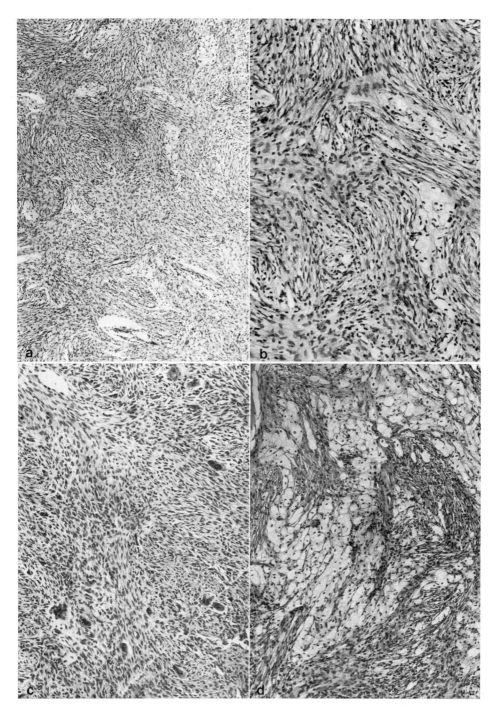

FIG. 63. - Histological picture typical of histiocytic fibroma. (a) and (b) Different enlargements show the compact and richly cellular tissue, the storiform structure of the tumor, its scarce vascularity, the foci of foam cells. (c) Small sparse multinucleate giant cells may be observed. A color photograph would also show a fair amount of hemosiderin pigment. (d) Area with abundant foam cells (*Hemat.-eos.*, 50, 125, 125, 125 x).

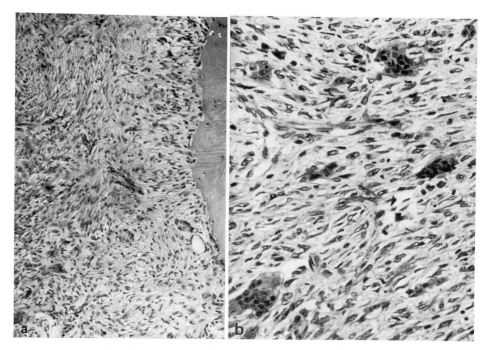

FIG. 64. - (a) The fibroma abruptly borders on the surrounding bone tissue. (b) Higher power view of the stromal cells and giant cells (*Hemat.-eos.*, 125, 310 x).

DIAGNOSIS

In most cases diagnosis is based on a radiogram obtained for unrelated reasons, generally trauma, as H.F. is asymptomatic and is not treated surgically. This does not, however, mean that diagnosis is doubtful, as the radiographic picture is absolutely typical.

If a child or adolescent complains of pain in the knee, the ankle or the hip, and the radiograms reveal H.F., it is generally wrong to attribute symptomatology to H.F. and submit the patient to surgery, as H.F. is nearly always asymptomatic.

When H.F. is expanded or extends to most or all of the metaphysis or diaphysis, a radiographic diagnosis may not be so easy. There may be some doubt as to whether one is dealing with **fibrous dysplasia, chondromyxoid fibroma** or **bone cyst**. In cases such as these, surgery will reveal the typical yellow-brown tissue and a histological assessment will leave no room for doubt.

In exceptional **severe polyostotic forms** of the disease, the radiographic picture is quite characteristic, and it may generally be distinguished from that of **fibrous dysplasia**. What may nonetheless contribute to confusing H.F. with fibrous dysplasia is the possible presence, in both forms, of café-au-lait spots, and the fact that in some areas fibrous dysplasia may have a histological picture which is the same as that of H.F. As previously stated, the differ-

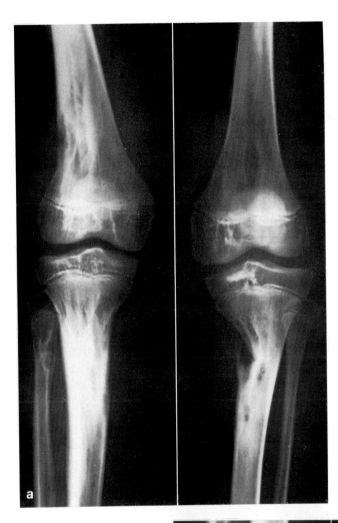

FIG. 65a. (legend on page 105).

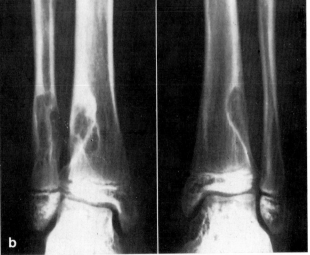

FIG. 65b.

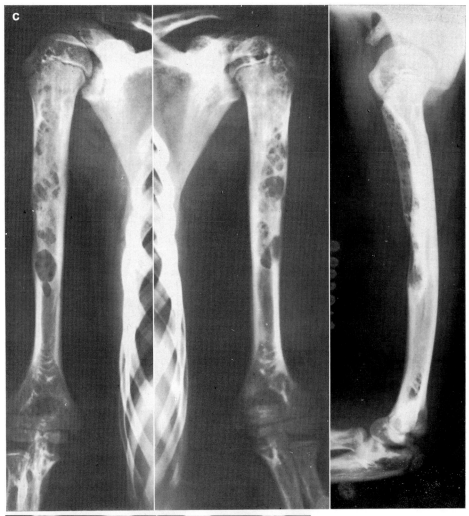

FIG. 65c.

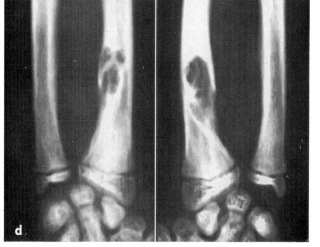

FIG. 65d.

FIG. 65. - Diffused multicentric histiocytic fibromas in a male aged 11 years (the same case as Fig. 53). (a) Diffused histiocytic fibromas are nearly symmetrical in the metadiaphyses around the knee. Note the peculiar image of subperiosteal osteolysis, which is particularly marked in the left tibia, with pathologic fracture. (b) The same nearly symmetrical images may be noted in the distal metadiaphyses of the leg. (c) Intracortical and bubbling osteolytic images in the two humeri, extended to most of the diaphysis. The lateral view clearly shows the intracortical nature of the osteolysis, with endosteal thickening and narrowing of the medullary canal. (d) Symmetrical, intracortical osteolysis in the distal diaphysis of the radius. (e) Changes in the skull with a peculiar image of depression.

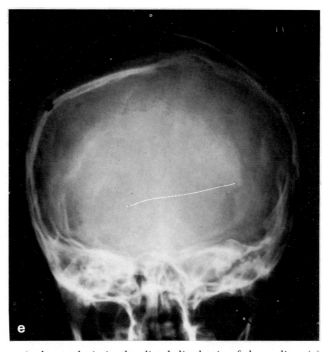

ence lies in the radiographic picture, and in the fact that multiple H.F. does not seem to present in any site the woven bone production which is instead typical of fibrous dysplasia.

Histologically, forms of H.F. which are densely cellular and characterized by plump nuclei could momentarily suggest **well-differentiated fibrosarcoma**; but the whorling of the cellular bundles, the scarcity of collagenous fibers, the absence of anaplasia and cellular atypia, the presence of small giant cells and of hemosiderin pigment, are all rather typical elements of H.F. Without considering the importance of the radiographic and gross pathologic features.

The histological picture rarely suggests a diagnosis of **giant cell tumor**, when the multinucleate elements are numerous and the stromal cells quite plump. In addition to the clinical and radiographic features of the disease, its storiform structure, the fact that there are more spindle cells, the greater amount of collagenogenesis, the smaller giant cells, will dispel any doubts. Instead, the histological picture is the same as that of **benign fibrous histiocytoma** (see specific chapter).

COURSE

Most cases of H.F. occur after 5 years of life; they achieve small or modest size, and then regress spontaneously after a period of time ranging from 1 to 10 years. H.F. rarely achieves considerable size (Figs. 57, 60). Even in cases where this does occur, any growth is nearly always arrested after puberty, and H.F. tends to ossify during adult age. Diffused multicentric H.F. also stop growing after puberty.

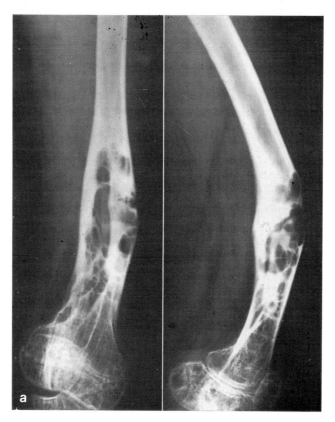

FIG. 66a.

FIG. 66. - Diffused multicentric histiocytic fibromas in a male aged 8 years. In this case café-au-lait spots, mental and physical retardation, and bilateral cryptorchidism are associated. (a) Bubbling osteolysis of the femoral diaphysis, evidently intracortical and subperiosteal towards the metaphysis. Pathologic fracture. (b) Nearly symmetrical osteolyses of the two humeri. To the right a swollen osteolysis of the proximal ulnar metaphysis may be observed. To the left, the lateral view shows the intracortical nature of the osteolyses of the humerus. (c) Osteolyses in the right forearm, with the usual characteristics (intracortical onset, bubbling, covered by a layer of very thin cortex or by periosteum alone, with evident demarcation and a hyperostotic rim towards the inside of the bone and the medullary canal).

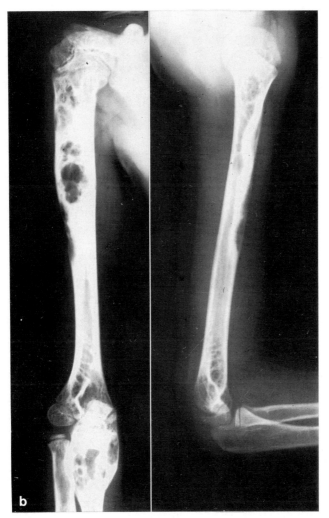

FIG. 66b.

TREATMENT AND PROGNOSIS

Asymptomatic H.F. requires no treatment. In most cases, the work of the specialist, which is consulted for a small skeletal lacuna unexpectedly observed at a radiographic examination carried out for other reasons, is limited to reassuring the parents of the patient, who are often worried by more alarming conjectures and by the idea of a «tumor». Rare symptomatic forms of the disease, and those which are rather expanded, enough to constitute a danger of fracture, should be submitted to curettage and bone grafting. In some cases of H.F. of the fibula, subperiosteal resection may be a good method to use. Healing is constant.

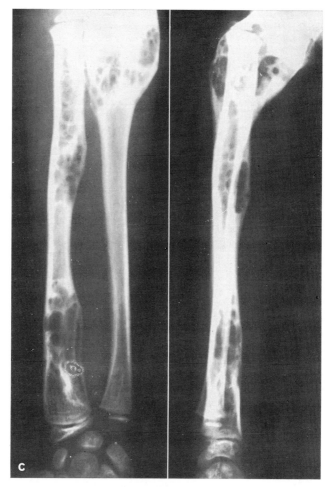

FIG. 66c.

REFERENCES

1942 JAFFE H. L., LICHTENSTEIN L.: Non osteogenic fibroma of bone. *American Journal of Pathology*, **18**, 205-221.

1945 HATCHER C. H.: The pathogenesis of localized fibrous lesions in the metaphyses of long bones. *Annals of Surgery*, **122**, 1016-1030.

1949 PONSETI I. V., FRIEDMAN B.: Evolution of metaphyseal fibrous defects. *Journal of Bone and Joint Surgery*, **31-A**, 582-588.

1951 KIMMELSTIEL P., RAPP I. H.: Cortical defect due to periosteal desmoids. *Bulletin of the Hospital for Joint Diseases*, **12**, 186-297.

1955 CAFFEY J.: On fibrous defects in cortical walls of growing tubular bones. *Advances in Pediatry*, **7**, 13-51.

1955 MAREK F. M.: Fibrous cortical defect and periosteal desmoid. *Bulletin of the Hospital for Joint Diseases*, **16**, 77-87.

1956 CUNNINGHAM J. B., ACKERMAN L. V.: Methapyseal fibrous defects. *Journal of Bone and Joint Surgery*, **38-A**, 797-808.

1961 SELBY S.: Metaphyseal cortical defects in the tubular bones of growing children. *Journal of Bone and Joint Surgery*, **43**-**A**, 395-400.

1964 MORTON K. S.: Bone production in non-osteogenic fibroma. An attempt to clarify nomenclature in fibrous lesions of bone. *Journal of Bone and Joint Surgery*, **46**-**B**, 233-243.

1966 BERKIN C. R.: Non ossifying fibroma of bone. *British Journal of Radiology*, **39**, 469-471.

1966 BHAGWANDEEN S. B.: Transformation of a non osteogenic fibroma of bone. *Journal of Pathology and Bacteriology*, **92**, 562-564.

1967 MAGLIATO H. J., NASTASI A.: Non-osteogenic fibroma occurring in the ilium. Report of a case. *Journal of Bone and Joint Surgery*, **49**-**A**, 384-386.

1972 DENIS B., DRENNAN J. J., FAHEY, DONALD J. MAYLAHN: Fractures through large non ossifying fibromas. The operative and non-operative course to healing. *Journal of Bone and Joint Surgery*, **54**-**A**, 1794.

1974 STEINER G. C.: Fibrous cortical defect and nonossifying fibroma of bone: a study of the ultrastructure. *Archive of Pathology*, **97**, 205-210.

1978 EVANS G. A., PARK W. M.: Familial multiple non-osteogenic fibromata. *Journal of Bone and Joint Surgery*, **60**-**B**, 416-419.

1979 LAUS M., VICENZI G.: Fibroma istiocitico dell'osso. Studio di 170 osservazioni. *Giornale Italiano di Ortopedia e Traumatologia*, **5**, 359-365.

1980 DESTOUET J.M., KYRIAKOS M., GILULA L.: Fibrous hystiocitoma (fibroxanthoma) of a cervical vertebra. *Skeletal Radiology*, **5**, 241-246.

1981 ARATA M., PETERSON H.A., DAHLIN D.C.: Pathological fractures through non-ossifying fibromas. *Journal of Bone and Joint Surgery*, **63**-**A**, 980-988.

1982 HERRERA G.A., REIMANN B.E.F., SCULLY T.J., DIFIORE R.J.: Non-ossifying fibroma. *Clinical Orthopaedics*, **167**, 269-276.

1982 MIRRA J.M., GOLD R.H., RAND F.: Disseminated non-ossifying fibromas in association with café-au-lait spots (Jaffe-Campanacci Syndrome). *Clinical Orthophaedics*, **168**, 192-205.

1983 CAMPANACCI M., LAUS M., BORIANI S.: Multiple non-ossifying fibromata with extraskeletal anomalies: a new syndrome? *Journal of Bone and Joint Surgery*, **65**-**B**, 623-627.

1987 MOSER R.P., SWEET D.E., HASEMAN, MADEWELL J.: Multiple skeletal fibroxanthomas. Radiologic-pathologic correlation of 72 cases. *Skeletal Radiology*, **16**, 353-359.

1988 BLAU R.A., ZWICK D.L., WESTPHAL R.A.: Multiple non-ossifying fibromas. *Journal of Bone and Joint Surgery*, **70**-**A**, 299-304.

1988 RITSCHL P., KARNEL F., HAJEK P.: Fibroma, metaphyseal defects. Determinations of their origin and natural history using a radiomorphological study. *Skeletal Radiology*, **17**, 8-15.

1989 RITSCHL P., HAJEC P.C., PECHMANN U.: Fibrous metaphyseal defects. Magnetic resonance imaging appearances. *Skeletal Radiology*, **18**, 253-259.

BENIGN FIBROUS HISTIOCYTOMA
(Synonyms: xanthoma, fibroxanthoma)

It is a benign tumor which originates from histiocytes and is somewhat similar to histiocytic fibroma and giant cell tumor.

It occurs **rarely** and, up until the present, very few cases have been reported, so that it is difficult to indicate predilection for **sex, age** and **localization** (Fig. 67). However, it does seem to prefer adult age and the metaepiphyses of the long bones. It has also been observed in the sacrum, in the ilium, and in the mandible.

Symptoms, which are moderate and long-lasting, consist in pain and swelling (when it develops in the superficial bones).

Radiographically there is pure osteolysis (Fig. 68, 69). If it is situated in a large metaepiphysis, it appears to be roundish, eccentric, with clear boundaries at times demarcated by a thin line of osteosclerosis, with thinning and, at times, slight expansion of the cortex. In the smaller bones, such as the fibular head, it occupies the entire section of the bone, expands and at times partially cancels the cortex. There is no periosteal reaction.

Macroscopically, the periosteum and the connective parostal tissue are

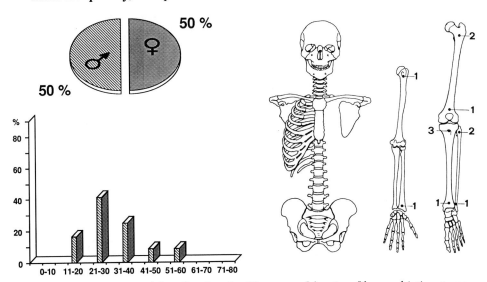

FIG. 67. - Sex, age, and localization in 12 cases of benign fibrous histiocytoma.

normal, at times the cortex is also continuous although attenuated (Fig. 68b). The tumor is compact, of gummy or slightly fibrous consistency, leathery-yellow in color, at times it has bright-yellow spots. Alongside this tissue there may be a softer one, light brown or reddish-brown in color, the same as that of giant cell tumor. The boundaries with the surrounding bone are clear cut.

Histopathologically, there is a dense cellular and collagenous pattern with a constant and diffused whorled structure (storiform). The cells have roundish-oval nuclei, which may be elongated in the direction of the fibers. Large foam cells abound, which may be isolated or in groups. The giant multinucleate cells are sparse and small, mitotic figures are rare. In other fields (corresponding to the macroscopic picture indicated as being the same as that of giant cell tumor) a structure which is the same as that of a giant cell tumor may be observed (Figs. 70, 71).

The histogenesis of B.F.H., similar to that of histiocytic and fibro-histiocytic tumors of the soft tissues, derives from the histiocyte which evolves in

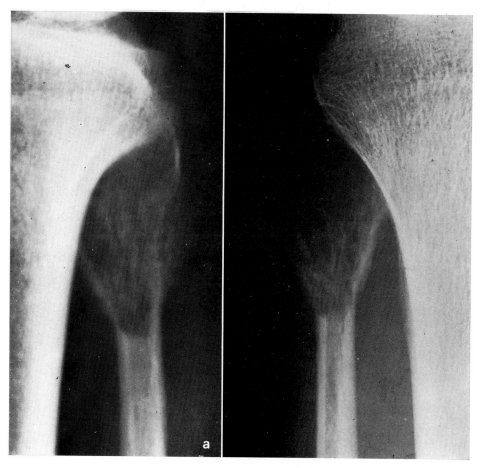

FIG. 68a.

FIG. 68. - Benign fibrous histiocytoma. (a) and (b) Male aged 38 years. Osteolysis of the proximal fibula.

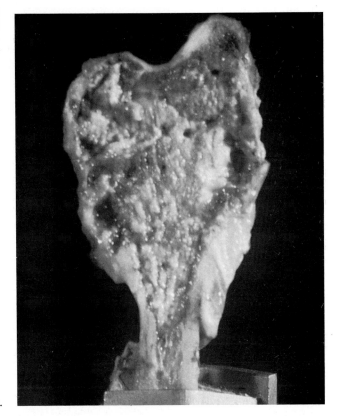

FIG. 68b.

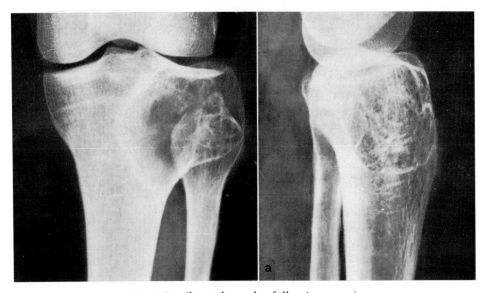

FIG. 69a. (legend on the following page).

FIG. 69. - Benign fibrous histiocytoma. (a) Female aged 34 years. Osteolysis of the proximal tibia. Pain and swelling for the past 2 years. The lesion is clearly delimited, and has a bony wall which is perfectly continuous and relatively hard. (b) Resection of the tibial condyle (preoperative diagnosis, not totally disproven by frozen section biopsy, giant cell tumor) was excessive. Curettage would have been appropriate. No recurrence after 8 years.

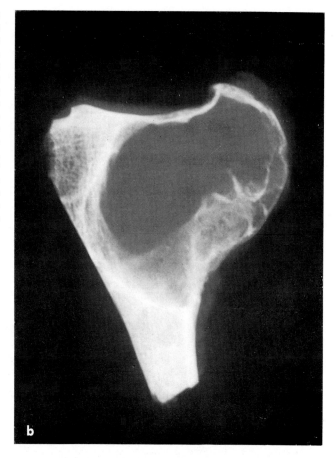

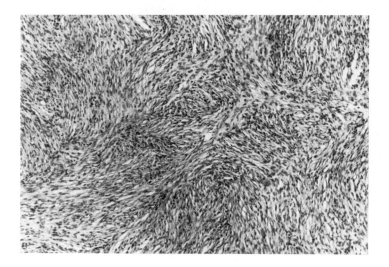

FIG. 70. - Benign fibrous histiocytoma with typical storiform structure (*Hemat.-eos.*, 125 x).

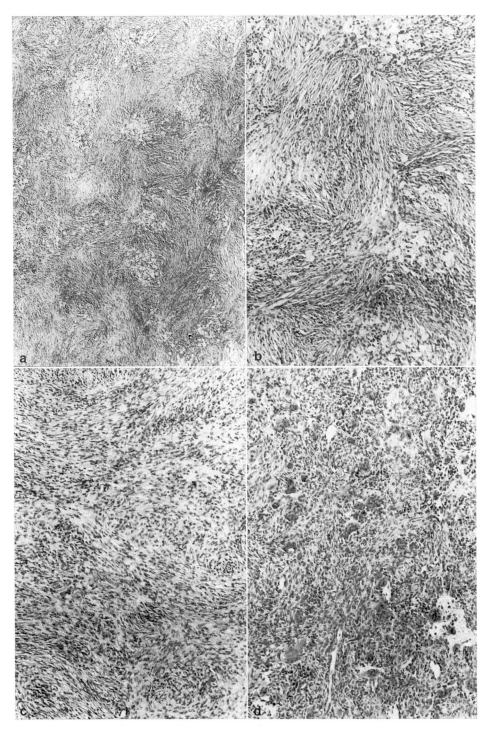

FIG. 71. - (a) and (b) Benign fibrous histiocytoma with storiform structure and nests of foam cells. (c) and (d) Other case of benign fibrous histiocytoma which, in certain sites, contains numerous giant cells (d). (*Hemat.-eos.*, 50, 125, 125, 125 x).

its various forms of histiocytary cell, macrophage, foam cell, giant cell and «facultative fibroblast».

Differential **diagnosis** involves histiocytic fibroma and giant cell tumor. B.F.H. differs from **histiocytic fibroma** in that it grows and is symptomatic during adult age; it may involve the epiphysis or a flat bone; it may have a histological picture which is decidedly more histiocytary with a more evident and diffused storiform structure, more macrophagic activity, a larger quantity of foam cells; finally, it may have aspects of transition with the giant cell tumor. When compared to **giant cell tumor** B.F.H. has grown less aggressively, its radiographic boundaries are better defined, it is characterized by osteo-periosteal walls which are better preserved in relation to the size of the tumor, a different macroscopic picture, a different histological picture, probably less of a tendency to recur. However, it has been observed that within the same tumor there may be areas resembling B.F.H and others resembling giant cell tumor.

The **course** of B.F.H., as previously stated, is slow. **Treatment** involves surgery, and is that which is generally indicated for a benign tumor stage 2 (active): curettage with local adjuvants. If excision is complete, healing seems to be constant.

REFERENCES

1977 DAHLIN D. C., UNNI K. K., MATSUNO T.: Malignant (fibrous) histiocytoma of bone. Fact or fancy? *Cancer*, **39**, 1508-1516.
1978 DAHLIN D. C.: *Bone tumors*. Charles C. Thomas, Springfield, Illinois.
1981 SCHAJOWICZ F.: *Tumors and tumor-like lesions of bone and joints*. Springer Verlag, New York.
1983 BERTONI F., CAPANNA R., CALDERONI P., BACCHINI P.: Case report 223. Benign fibrous histiocytoma. *Skeletal Radiology*, **9**, 215-217.
1986 BERTONI F., CALDERONI P., BACCHINI P., SUDANESE A., BALDINI N., PRESENT D., CAMPANACCI M.: Benign fibrous histiocytoma of bone. *Journal of Bone and Joint Surgery*, **68-A**, 1225-1230.
1988 HERMANN G., STEINER G.C., SHERRY H.: Case report 465. *Skeletal Radiology*, **17**, 195-197.

GIANT CELL TUMOR
(Synonym: osteoclastoma)

DEFINITION

G.C.T. is a central neoplasm of the bone, which probably originates from histio-fibroblastic elements, and is constituted by basic cells that tend to fuse into multinucleate giant cells.

What differentiates this tumor from all of the numerous skeletal lesions (neoplastic or non-neoplastic) containing giant cells, even in a large number, is the fact that in G.C.T. these cells are an integral and constant part of the neoplastic proliferation, moreover, they are its characteristic element. On the contrary, in all of the other aforementioned skeletal lesions, giant cells constitute occasional reactive elements, assigned the function of resorbing hematic effusion, calcium deposits, osseous or cartilaginous substances [1].

In addition to this precise histological identity, G.C.T. presents rather distinct clinical, topographical, and anatomo-radiographical features. Its most important and singular aspect is its biological behavior, characterized by considerable local aggression which is not very predictable, as well as rare progression to malignancy. In fact, G.C.T. may become sarcoma (fibrosarcoma, osteosarcoma, or malignant fibrous histiocytoma). Sarcomatous transformation may only be recognized if there are previous bioptic findings of a genuine G.C.T., or where there are areas of benign G.C.T. alongside sarcomatous areas in the same specimen. The transformation of G.C.T. in sarcoma is favored by radiation therapy.

FREQUENCY

G.C.T. occurs relatively frequently. Transformation in sarcoma is rare: less than 5% of all G.C.T.

----

[1] At one time the label «giant cell tumor» covered a wide range of differing tumoral and non-tumoral forms, among which aneurysmal bone cyst, histiocytic fibroma, chondroblastoma were the most common. But at times also included were brown tumors due to hyperparathyroidism, epulis tumors, and others.

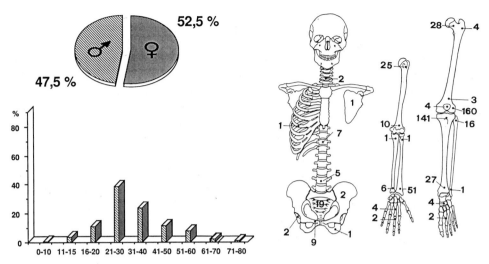

FIG. 72. - Sex, age and localization in 539 cases of giant cell tumor.

SEX

There is slight predilection for the female sex (Fig. 72).

AGE

G.C.T. is characteristic of young adult age. In most cases it is manifested between 20 and 40 years of age. Not rarely is it observed between 15 and 20 years of age, and between 40 and 50 years of age. The observation of G.C.T. prior to puberty is instead exceptional, that is, prior to closure of the growth cartilage; it is also rarely observed after 50 years of age (Fig. 72).

LOCALIZATION

In 90% of the cases it is observed in the long bones, where it is nearly always localized in a meta-epiphyseal segment. In exceptional cases, in which the tumor develops before closure of the growth cartilage, it originates in the metaphysis (Fig. 84). In the adult, when the growth cartilage has disappeared, the metaphysis and the epiphysis are no longer two anatomically separate regions, and the tumor tends to involve both. Our impression is that it generally initiates in the metaphysis, adjacent to the old physis, and that, as this is already fused, it extends to the epiphysis (or the apophysis)[1].

---

[1] In the adult, as well, cases with purely metaphyseal localization are observed rarely. Instead, we have never observed a G.C.T. exclusively localized in the epiphysis or in the apophysis, without involving the metaphysis.

The two meta-epiphyses which are preferred by the tumor are the distal femur and the proximal tibia (Fig. 72). More than half of all cases of G.C.T. are located in the knee area. These are followed by, and in this order, the distal radius(¹), proximal femur, distal tibia, proximal humerus. The tumor is rare in the elbow (distal humerus, proximal radius and ulna), in the proximal fibula, in the distal ulna, and in the tubular bones of the hand and foot where it is usually oriented towards the only epiphysis but, given the small size of the bone, it is extended to much of the diaphysis.

Apart from the long bones, G.C.T. is less rare in the sacrum and in the pelvis (where it may affect the ilium, the ischium or the pubis), in the other vertebrae and in the tarsus; it is extremely rare in the remaining short and flat bones. A lesion similar to G.C.T. may be observed in the cranium, but exclusively as a complication of Paget's disease (see specific chapter).

There are exceptional cases of multicentric G.C.T. Before accepting

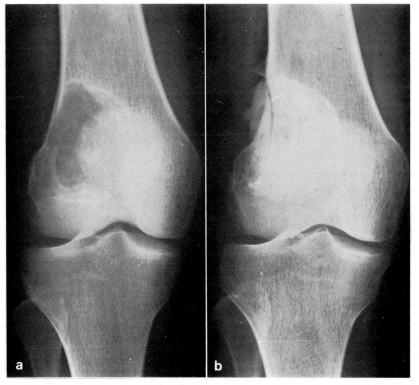

FIG. 73. - Female aged 19 years. (a) Quiescent radiographic variety. (b) Healing 3 years after curettage and bone grafting.

(¹) This localization certainly cannot be compared for frequency to that of the knee, nor does it much exceed that in other metaepiphyses, as it occurs in approximately 10% of all cases of G.C.T. Nonetheless, what is important is that all other tumors are rare in the distal radius (and ulna) and that, as a result, a tumor of the metaepiphyses of the wrist is, in 8 cases out of 10, a G.C.T.

such an extraordinary event, primary hyperparathyroidism must obviously be excluded.

SYMPTOMS

The most important elements for a clinical evaluation are age, site, duration of symptoms, any signs of expansion of the cortical bone and in the soft tissues.

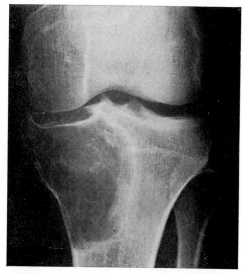

FIG. 74. - Male aged 33 years. Quiescent radiographic variety but one which is rather expanded. The osteolysis widely reaches as far as the articular cartilage. Cured 22 years after resection-arthrodesis.

The main symptom is pain, which is often felt in the joint. The proximity of the tumor to the joint cavity (from which it is often separated by the cartilaginous layer, rarely does the tumor grow within the joint capsule or the synovial membrane, or perforate the cartilage) often causes functional limitation and effusion in the joint. In the superficial bones and in those of small diameter (proximal tibia, distal radius and ulna, fibular head, metacarpals and phalanges) expansion of the bone often produces visible swelling. Microfracture and pathologic fracture, particularly in the lower limb, easily occur due to thinning of the cortex, thus increasing pain and functional deficit. If the tumor is very expanded and has worn down the cortex abutting in the soft tissues, there is soft swelling, peritumoral edema, and the evidence of superficial venous reticulum.

RADIOGRAPHIC FEATURES

In its entirety, it is quite characteristic. Practically speaking, an evaluation of the clinical and radiographic elements often allows for diagnosis to be made prior to biopsy.

The radiographic picture is that of a tumor which is generally eccentric, and which occupies the meta-epiphyseal region; it has throughout the radio-transparence of the soft tissues and is expanded circularly in all directions. G.C.T. demonstrates intense osteolytic properties and with the same facility cancels cancellous and cortical bone. Although its growth is usually neither rapid not permeative, reactive hyperostosis of either the endosteum or the periosteum is quite scarce (Figs. 73-83).

At the onset there is an image of round-oval osteolysis, which is frequently eccentric, in the passage area between the metaphysis and the epiphysis.
The osteolysis is homogeneous and contains neither ossification nor calcification. Its boundaries with the cancellous bone are regular and clearly defined or slightly faded, like those of water on sand (the tumor is not permeative, rather it is expansive), but they generally do not have that clear outline

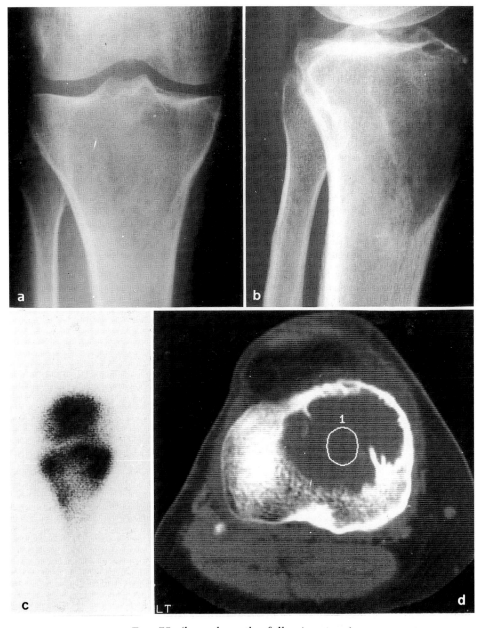

FIG. 75. (legend on the following page).

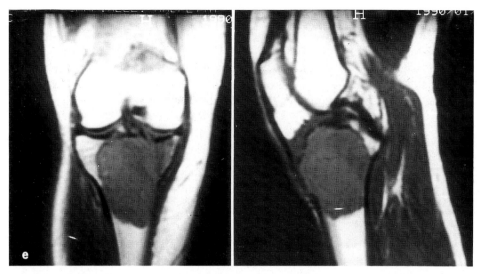

FIG. 75. - Giant cell tumor in a female aged 45 years with pain for the past 6 months. Imaging reveals the typical aspect of radiographically active lesions.

deriving from a radiopaque rim of reactive hyperostosis. The tumor often extends **as far as the joint cartilage**; this aspect is important when choosing a type of surgery (see further on). The cortex above the tumor is attenuated early and diffusedly. When the tumor is more expanded, it may extend to most of the meta-epiphysis and, on the surface, completely cancel the cortex. In tubular bones of smaller diameter (radius, ulna, fibula) all of the meta-epiphysis and, at times, the entire diaphysis (metacarpals, phalanges) are invaded and the bone may be considerably expanded.

Because of the moderate osteogenetic reaction that is expressed at the periphery of the tumor by scarce osteoid tissue, which is not very mature and which is quickly resorbed, in the area where the tumor expands the skeletal perimeter there is at most a thin layer, which may be discontinuous, of slight and faded radiopacity. Even the pathologic fractures of this layer cause a minimal formation of repair callus.

For all of these reasons it may be understood how the radiographic image of G.C.T. is rarely and scarcely compartmentalized. Some images of pseudo-sepimentation may derive from the fact that the tumor, in its expansion, saves some parietal bony crests. If this aspect is clear and dominant, it indicates slower and less expansive growth than usual (Fig. 83a).

At times there are signs of more rapid growth and aggressiveness. The osteolytic area expands rapidly and its boundaries with the cancellous bone are decidedly unclear. At times, the entire meta-epiphysis is invaded, the bone is expanded, the cortex is cancelled, and the tumor mass protrudes amply in the soft tissues, deprived of any radiographically visible delimitation.

Depending on the radiographic picture, it is customary to distinguish G.C.T. in three categories, which correspond to Enneking's stages for benign tumors.

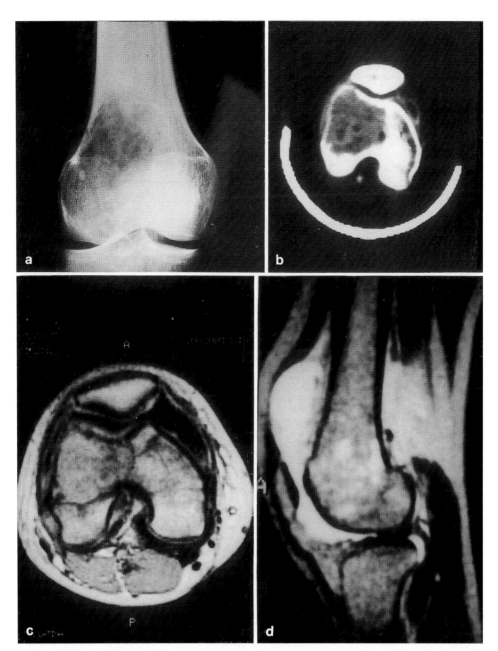

FIG. 76. - Giant cell tumor in a female aged 20 years. (a) Active radiographic stage. (b) CAT. (c) MRI revealing pathologic fracture. (d) MRI in the sagittal plane revealing joint effusion consequent to fracture. Treated with needle biopsy, curettage, bone grafts and cement.

1) «Quiescent» radiographic variety (Figs. 73, 74, 96).

The cortical bone is whole, or slightly thinned and not expanded. The osteolysis has well-defined limits, marked by a rim of slight peritumoral

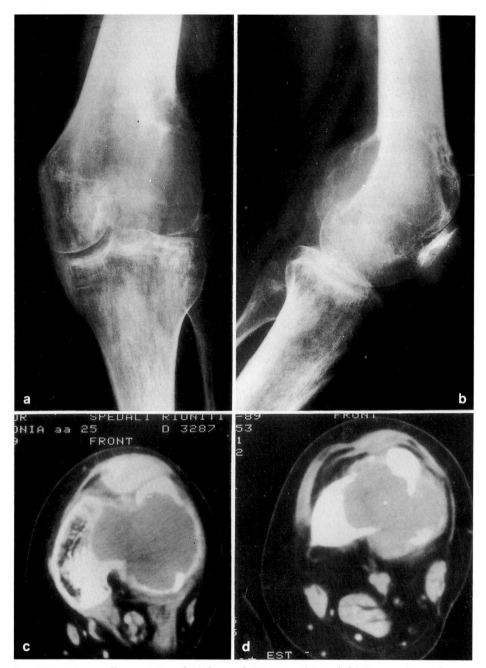

FIG. 77. - Giant cell tumor in a female aged 25 years. (a) and (b) Aggressive radiographic stage. (c) and (d) CAT reveals reactive and discontinuous bone shell. The patient was treated with needle biopsy, marginal resection and endoprosthesis.

hyperostosis. At times there is an image of pseudosepimentation. The tumor is not very large and it does not reach the articular cartilage, unless it has been there for a long time. In cases monitored over a long period of time,

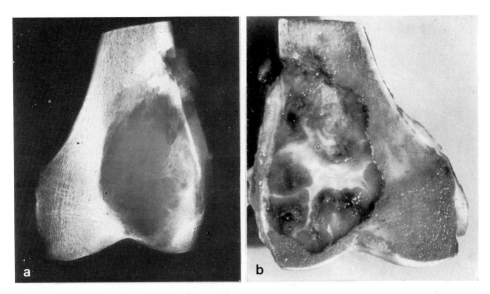

FIG. 78. - Male aged 23 years. (a) Radiograph of the resected segment. Active radiographic variety. (b) Photograph of the same segment. Note the clear-cut limits of the tumor. Interruption in the cortical bone in the upper part of the photograph corresponds to the biopsy performed one month prior to resection. The patient is cured 18 years after surgery.

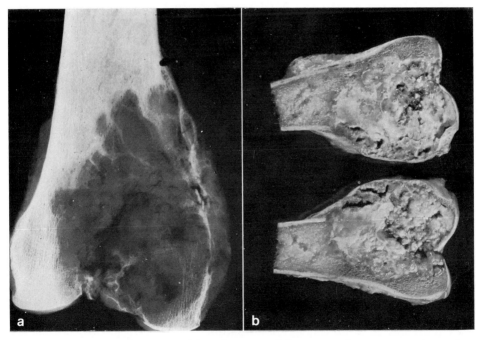

FIG. 79. - Female aged 39 years. (a) Radiogram of the resected segment. Active radiographic variety. Observe how the osteolysis reaches the articular cartilage in the intercondylar notch, where it invades the insertion of the cruciate ligaments. (b) Photograph of the same segment. Observe the continuity of the periosteum. The patient is cured 9 years after resection.

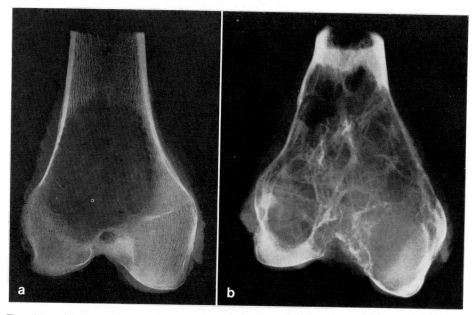

FIG. 80. - (a) Female aged 23 years. Resected segment. Active radiographic variety. N.E.D. 5 years after resection. (b) Female aged 21 years. Resected segment. Active radiographic variety rather extensive. The patient is N.E.D. 8 years after resection.

slow expansion of the tumor is observed. This variety is the most rare and corresponds to stages 1-2.

2) «Active» radiographic variety (Figs. 75, 76, 78, 79, 80, 98, 102).

This is the most characteristic and frequent form. The cortex is very thinned, at times it is nearly cancelled, but the tumor is clearly bordered by the periosteum; in fact, any expansion is continuous with the outline of the bone. The osteolysis has somewhat unclear boundaries and it often comes very close to or actually reaches the articular cartilage. Often, the tumor is considerably expanded or, in any case, when there are successive radiograms, it reveals lively growth. It corresponds to stage 2.

3) «Aggressive» radiographic variety (Figs. 77, 81, 82, 86, 99).

The cortex appears to be cancelled, with expansion towards the soft tissues of a globose tumor mass having no radiopacity. This mass is not contained by the periosteum as it does not respect the outlines of the bone and it does not show any radiopaque delimitation. When there are successive radiograms, the rapid and aggressive expansion of the tumor is observed, involving most or all of the epiphysis, and always reaching the articular cartilage. The aggressive variety is rarely observed as an initial picture, less rarely in cases of recurrence. It corresponds to stage 3.

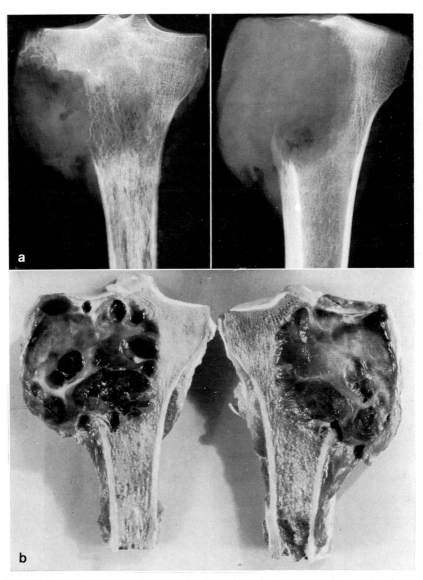

FIG. 81. - Male aged 35 years. Amputation based on the incorrect diagnosis of sarcoma. (a) Section of the anatomical specimen. Aggressive radiographic variety. Histologically, typical G.C.T. (b) Photograph of the same specimen. The tumor surpasses the periosteum and invades the muscles. The patient was N.E.D. 14 years after amputation.

The quiescent and active radiographic forms of the tumor never correspond to a sarcomatous transformation, the radiographic picture of which is always aggressive. But only few aggressive radiographic forms become sarcomas. Many radiographically aggressive tumors are, histologically, typical G.C.T., which may thus be successfully treated by marginal or even intralesional surgery, with local adjuvants, even if a wide surgical margin is that of choice.

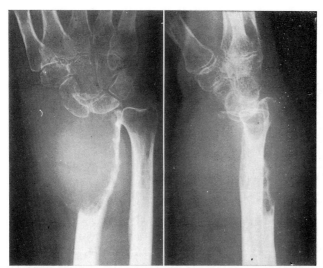

FIG. 82. - Female aged 30 years. Treated 8 years previously by curettage, bone grafting and radiation therapy. For the past 3 years there had been signs of local recurrence. Aggressive radiographic variety. Histologically, typical G.C.T. Patient submitted to resection and arthrodesis, and cured 17 years after surgery.

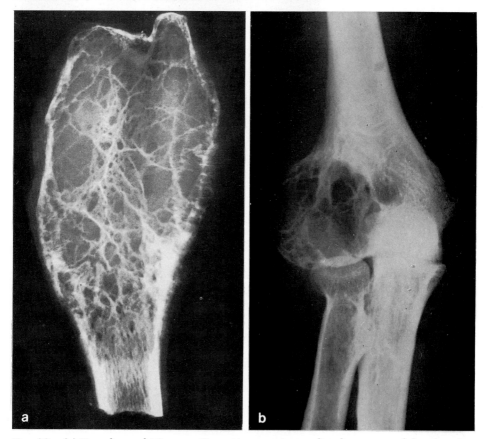

FIG. 83. - (a) Female aged 29 years. Resection specimen, distal segment of the ulna. Active radiographic variety. Cured 7 years after resection. (b) Male aged 27 years. Patient had been submitted to curettage and bone grafting 1 year earlier. Extensive local recurrence. Active radiographic variety. Patient submitted to partial resection of the articular segment. N.E.D. 6 years after surgery.

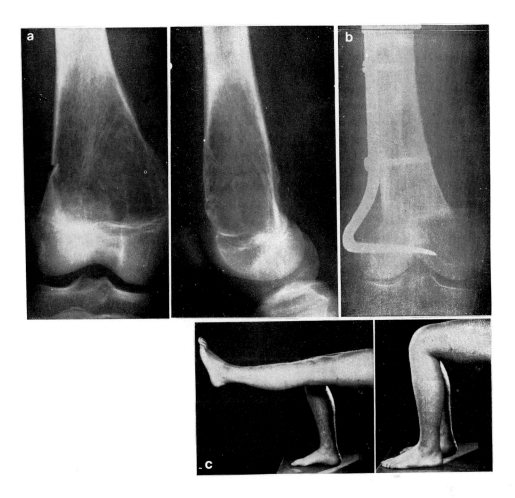

FIG. 84. - Male aged 14 years. (a) Exceptional example of G.C.T. occurring when the growth cartilage is still fertile and, thus, not extended to the epiphysis. Active radiographic variety. (b) En bloc resection of the metadiaphyseal segment, preserving the epiphysis, and reconstruction with allo- and autogenous bone grafts. Good fusion of the grafts after 2 years. (c) N.E.D. with excellent function of the knee after 18 years.

In some cases osteolysis of the tumor extends to the nearby bone: for example, to the fibula from a tumor of the proximal or distal tibia (Fig. 85), or to the ulna from a tumor of the distal radius. This occurs when the tumor propagates along the joint capsule, the ligaments, or the synovial membrane, and may thus reach as far as and dig into the adjacent bone. Exceptionally, by means of this route, the tumor may surpass the main joint, for example extending to the patella or the tibia from the distal femur, to the acetabulum from the proximal femur, to the carpus from the distal radius.

The recurrence of G.C.T. in the soft tissues as a result of surgery often has a peripheral layer of ossification.

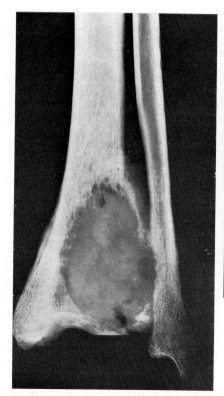 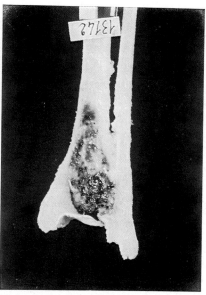

FIG. 85. - Female aged 23 years. Transected amputation specimen. There was local recurrence after previous curettage and bone grafting. Aggressive radiographic variety.
Histologically, «aggressive» G.C.T. Observe how the tumor invades the medial cortex
of the fibula. The patient was submitted to amputation and is N.E.D. after 10
years.

GROSS PATHOLOGIC FEATURES

When the tumor is not altered it is compact, light brown or reddish-
brown in color; it is uniformly parenchymatous, soft, and has a smooth surface. There is no visible trace of either bone or calcification within the tumor.
Its boundaries with the cancellous bone, the medullary canal and the attenuated cortex or the periosteum are relatively clear cut, but there is neither fibrous nor hyperostotic demarcation (Figs. 78, 79, 81).

Generally, the tissue is not so uniform. It may appear to have whitish
veins branching through it (the expression of fibrosis secondary to regressive
phenomena of the tumoral cells), or variegated by yellow-ochre areas (the result of lipoid accumulation). Often it is marked by hemorrhagic areas; at
times hyperemic-hemorrhagic alteration is considerably diffused and the entire tumor resembles a sponge full of blood. At times it contains areas of necrosis, greyish-yellow in color, dry or colliquative. Finally, there may be cystic
cavities, of hemorrhagic or necrotic origin.

Even if the cortex is completely resorbed, in radiographically active forms

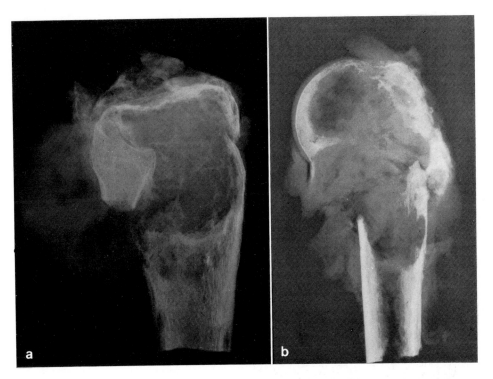

FIG. 86. - (a) Male aged 28 years. Symptoms for the past 4 years. Treated by radiation therapy. Over the last 3 months swelling had increased. Biopsy revealed areas of typical G.C.T. next to others of high-grade fibrosarcoma. Thigh amputation (X-ray of the amputation specimen.) The patient died of pulmonary metastases after 2 years. (b) Male aged 61 years. Three years earlier, submitted to biopsy (histologically, typical G.C.T.). Treated with radiation therapy (5000 r). Symptoms progressed over the last 6 months. Patient submitted to resection-endoprosthesis. (X-ray of the resected specimen.) Histologically, malignant fibrous histiocytoma. After 3 months pulmonary metastases occurred, treated by lobectomy. After 6 months skeletal metastases occurred. The patient died after 1 year.

the tumor is well-circumscribed by the periosteum. In aggressive forms, instead, the neoplastic mass that comes out of the cortex may not be delimited by the periosteum, thus, it may expand, even with multiple knots, in the soft tissues and muscles, delimited by a thin pseudocapsule, which may be veiled and difficult to see (Fig. 81). At times the tumoral tissue **penetrates the joint capsule, the ligaments, the synovial membrane, and it may reach as far as the adjacent bone** (Fig. 85). More rarely, it surpasses the joint cartilage.

When a G.C.T. which is quite expanded is exposed surgically, intense hyperemia in the surrounding soft tissues and in the periosteum is observed, with large ectatic vessels and increased intravenous pressure. When the tumor is incised, considerable hemorrhaging may be provoked.

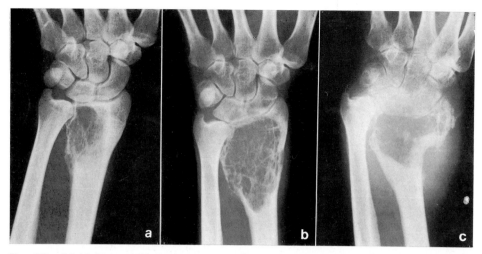

FIG. 87. - (a) Male aged 30 years. Active radiographic variety. (b) After 15 months, the tumor expanded, again in the active variety. At this stage the patient was submitted to curettage, the histological picture was that of typical G.C.T. Tumor recurred and was irradiated. (c) Three years after curettage and 2 years after radiation therapy, the radiographic aspect was considerably aggressive. Histologically, high-grade fibrosarcoma. Amputation. The patient died 1 year later due to pulmonary metastases.

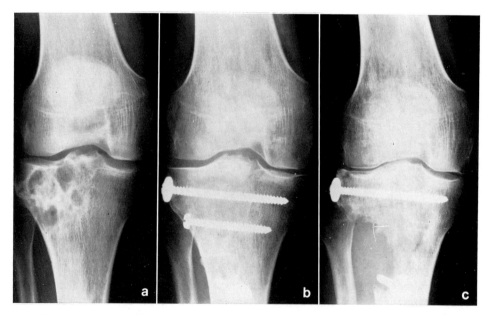

FIG. 88. - Male aged 23 years. (a) G.C.T. recurring afterf curettage and bone grafts carried out 1 year earlier. Radiographically active, histologically «aggressive». (b) Partial resection of the meta-epiphysis and substitution with unicondylar articular allograft. Excellent consolidation and preservation of the graft after 8 months. (c) Thirteen months after resection there was recurrence with a radiographically aggressive aspect. Biopsy showed grade 3 fibrosarcoma (see Fig. 94). Thigh amputation. The patient is N.E.D. after 6 years.

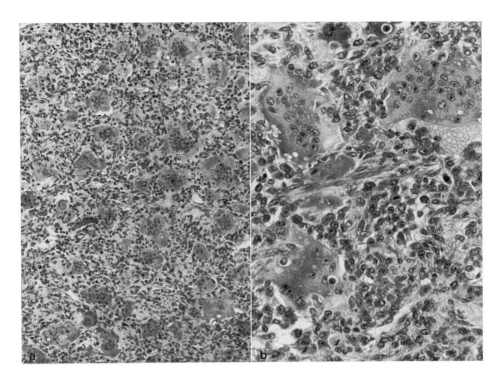

FIG. 89. - Typical G.C.T. This is the usual aspect of G.C.T. The nuclei of the basic cells are not very large, they do not considerably differ in size, nor is there hyperchromia. Frequent mitotic figures are observed. The giant cells are numerous throughout, they are large and have many nuclei. (*Hemat.-eos.*, 125, 310).

HISTOPATHOLOGIC FEATURES

The histological picture is made up of a dense population of cells of average size and with a single nucleus, constellated nearly everywhere by a large number of multinucleated giant cells. The cells with a single nucleus, which we shall call basic cells, are globose, oval, or spindle-shaped. The nuclei are rounded or oval, well-colored, with an outline which is slightly notched and very marked, at times conferring on the nuclei a somewhat vesicular aspect. Often one or more evident nucleoli are observed. A moderate amount of pleomorphism-polydimensionality in the nuclei and frequent mitotic figures are the norm (Figs. 89, 90).

The giant cells have ample cytoplasm which may be vacuolated, and a large number of nuclei (even 50-100 in the section plane) gathered at the center. The nuclei are the same as those of the basic cells.

Among the basic cells are reticular and collagen fibers which may be scarce and thin or more evident. Blood vessels are numerous, often in the form of wide sinusoids, and the lumen may contain some giant cells. Plugs of neoplastic tissue may be observed inside some of the venules in the pseudo-capsule of the tumor.

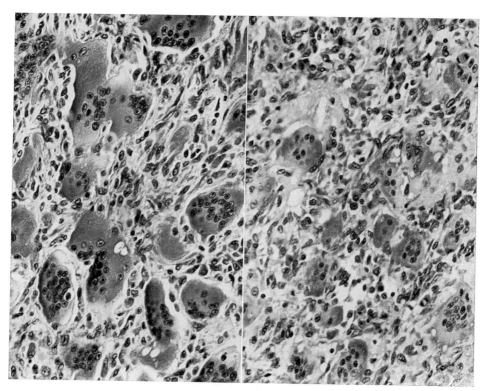

FIG. 90. - Typical G.C.T. (*Hemat.-eos.*, 310, 310x).

Regressive aspects are frequent. The giant cells, which constitute the most ephemeral elements, often contain pyknotic nuclei. Elsewhere, the entire tumoral tissue may appear to be undergoing necrosis or in total necrosis. Also frequent are aspects of scarring repair in the form of strands of fibrous tissue. Despite the fact that G.C.T. is osteolytic par excellence, thin osteoid trabeculae may be observed, particularly at the periphery of the tumor and under the periosteum, but also within the neoplasm. This osteoid tissue is in part reparative, and produced by peritumoral tissue, but it may also be partially produced by the cells of the tumor themselves. Hemorrhaging is also a frequent occurrence, at times diffusedly interstitial, at times producing hematic cavities similar to those of aneurysmal bone cysts (Fig. 95). Consequent to hemorrhaging, necrosis, and repair phenomena, accumulation of foam cells, batches of cholesterin crystals, granules of hemosiderin may be observed.

What is stated above is proof of the fact that in order to make a histological evaluation of G.C.T. wide and numerous specimens must be taken, so as to collect vital and not altered areas of the tumor. But better yet, the **observation of wide tumoral areas is indispensable for a histological evaluation** of any sarcomatous transformation. In fact, as is the case in all neoplasms demonstrating progression in malignancy (cfr. chondroma and chondrosarcoma, hemangioendothelioma, parosteal osteosarcoma), the aspects of any ma-

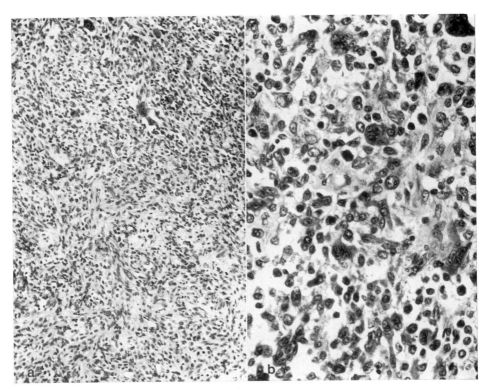

FIG. 91. - G.C.T. with «aggressive» histological aspects. (a, b) Under higher power, the stromal cells show evident anisocytosis (some nuclei are 3-4 times larger than others) and a certain amount of nuclear hyperchromia. The giant cells are small and scarce. (This tumor, in a female aged 30 years, was located in the proximal tibia, it was radiologically aggressive, and it was recurring after curettage and radiation therapy carried out 2 years previously). The patient was N.E.D. 26 years after en bloc resection (*Hemat.-eos.*, 125, 310x).

lignant proliferation may be limited to specific areas of the tumor.

At one time, in accordance with Jaffe and Lichtenstein, G.C.T. was divided into three histological grades of increasing aggressiveness. This grading was abandoned because it did not correspond to the clinical behavior of the tumor, and was thus useless. **Nowadays, G.C.T. is only distinguished from sarcoma, into which it may be transformed**[1]. This is generally a fibrosarco-

---

[1] Between G.C.T. and sarcoma there could exist a form of transition which we have temporarily called aggressive G.C.T. In this form of the disease, the nuclei of the basic cells are large, with a considerable amount of polydimensionality, tending towards a vesicular aspect, are somewhat hyperchromatic, with a large nucleolus. Furthermore, there are spindlecellular currents with a fibrosarcomatoid aura (not to be confused with areas of scarring fibrosis). The number of mitotic figures is of little importance. The giant cells are less numerous and smaller as compared to those of a typical G.C.T. (Figs. 91, 92, 93).

This aggressive G.C.T. is rare, and seems to have a local aggression which is greater

ma (Fig. 94), an osteosarcoma, or a malignant fibrous histiocytoma. In these cases the diagnosis of a sarcomatous transformation of G.C.T. evidently presupposes a previous histological picture of G.C.T., or the histological finding of areas maintaining the structure of G.C.T. alongside sarcomatous areas.

HISTOGENESIS

Recent studies in electron microscopy indicate that the basic cells have two different aspects: one is fibroblastic and the other is histiocytary. Thus, the hypothesis that the tumor derives from histio-fibroblasts would be confirmed. Giant cells originate from the fusion of basic cells. The histochemical and electronmicroscopic features do not allow for a distinction to be made between these giant neoplastic cells and normal osteoclasts, or reactive giant cells present in many other lesions in the skeleton.

DIAGNOSIS

Among clinical and radiographic elements, of considerable aid to diagnosis are the age of the patient and the site of the tumor. We have seen how there exist exceptional cases of G.C.T. occurring prior to closure of the growth cartilage and circumscribed to the metaphysis. Nonetheless, when dealing with a **metaphyseal tumor with growth cartilage which is still open**, one must be very careful before accepting a diagnosis of G.C.T., as this diagnosis is usually erroneous[1]. If the growth cartilage is still present, and the tumor extends both in the epiphysis and the metaphysis (but prevalently in the epiphysis), then we are quite certainly dealing with a chondroblastoma. **When the cartilage has disappeared** (post-puberal age) and the osteolytic tumor involves the epiphysis and the metaphysis, **radiographic differential diagnosis** may be made with numerous other osteolytic lesions, including: chondroblastoma, chronic abscess of the bone, brown tumor from hyperparathyroidism, chondrosarcoma, fibrosarcoma, osteolytic osteosarcoma, epithelial metastasis, solitary plasmacytoma.

Chondroblastoma. The osteolytic area has better defined borders, marked by a thin rim of hyperostosis; at times it contains images of intratumoral calcification/ossification.

---

than that of typical G.C.T., but with a scarce tendency to produce metastasis. We never forget to search for and note these histological aspects; but it must be admitted that generally the clinical-radiographic picture is pre-eminent in a therapeutic and prognostic evaluation. In exceptional cases, this «aggressive» G.C.T. or even a typical G.C.T. may be transformed into a sarcoma which maintains a structure similar to that of G.C.T. These would be actual «giant cell sarcomas», which, on the other hand, may also be considered malignant fibrous histiocytomas.

[1] These are generally aneurysmal bone cysts or histiocytic fibromas.

Chronic abscess of the bone. This is more central, it has a more irregular shape and its limits are marked by a halo of increased radiopacity (Fig. 8).

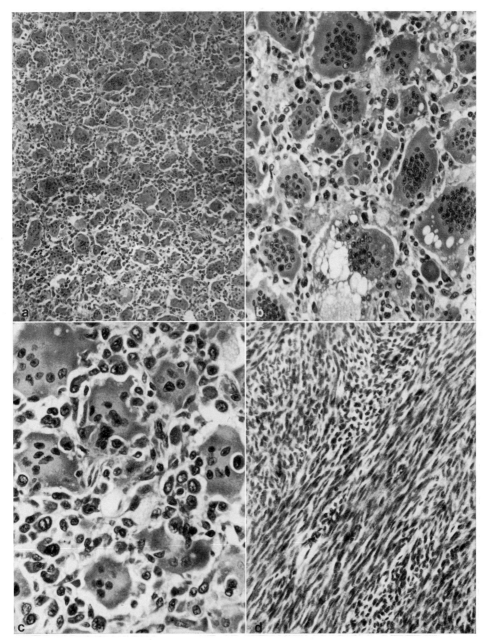

FIG. 92. - (a) and (b) Typical G.C.T. (c) In the same tumor some areas present more plumpness and pleomorphism of the nuclei of the basic cells. (d) Other areas have a spindle-cellular structure with a fibrosarcomatoid aura. This G.C.T. was histologically considered to be «aggressive»; localized in the proximal humerus in a female aged 55 years, it was treated by resection-endoprosthesis and was cured 6 years after surgery (*Hemat.-eos.*, 125, 310, 350, and 310 x).

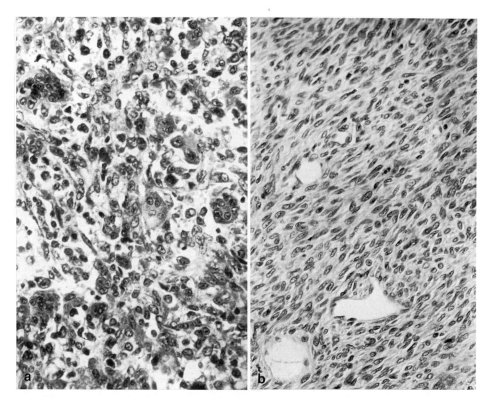

FIG. 93. - G.C.T. with «aggressive» histological aspects. (a) A fair amount of pleomorphism and hyperchromia in the nuclei of the basic cells. The giant cells are scarce and
small. (b) In some fields the cells are spindle-shaped, with a fibrosarcomatoid aura. (a, b)
refers to a male aged 28 years, operated on 6 months previously with curettage of an active G.C.T. of the proximal humerus. The histology represented here comes from a very
aggressive local recurrence, submitted to wide resection and endoprosthetic replacement. The patient is N.E.D. 20 years later (*Hemat.-eos.*, 310, 310 x).

It may contain the radiopaque image of small sequesters. It never thins the cortex, which may instead appear to be thickened.

   Brown tumor from hyperparathyroidism. When it is solitary and it involves the epiphysis (more often it is meta-diaphyseal) it may have a radiographic aspect which is very similar to that of a G.C.T. Nonetheless, the bone
surrounding the «tumor» generally reveals typical lacunar osteoporosis of
hyperparathyroidism.

   Central chondrosarcoma. The cortex may be interrupted, or thickened;
there is intratumoral calcar radiopacity, greater osteogenetic reaction of the
periosteum. In the epiphysis, the «clear-cell» variety of chondrosarcoma
may occur, and radiographically mimick G.C.T.

   Fibrosarcoma. Its boundaries are usually faded, and it is more invasive.
Nonetheless, radiographic distinction may not be possible. As compared to
the sarcomatous transformation of a G.C.T. there is no difference. The distinction is based on the patient's history, on previous radiograms (which may re-

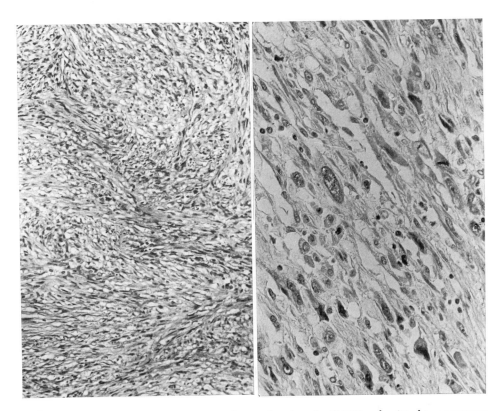

FIG. 94. - Grade 3 fibrosarcoma occurring at the site of a G.C.T. submitted to curettage and then en bloc resection. (Same case as Fig. 88). (*Hemat.-eos.*, 125, 310 x).

veal the aspects of a G.C.T.), and particularly on the histological finding of previous or coexisting G.C.T.

Osteolytic osteosarcoma. In exceptional cases, an osteosarcoma which is nearly deprived of osteogenetic properties (for example, a hemorrhagic osteosarcoma) may present an initial radiographic picture which is difficult to distinguish from that of G.C.T.

Epithelial metastasis. Radiographically, it may simulate a G.C.T. It has rather faded boundaries, and it interrupts the cortex at an early stage. A distinction may be attempted, in some cases, also based on the patient's history and on the duration of the symptoms.

Solitary plasmacytoma. Often it is characterized by expansion, or by bubbling pseudosepimentation, in other cases it is very destructive and it has rather faded boundaries; but in exceptional cases it may be radiographically nearly the same as a G.C.T.

Histological differential diagnosis. In our experience, there is but one lesion which may appear to be the same as a G.C.T. and that is a **brown tumor due to hyperparatyroidism** (see specific chapter). On the contrary, there are rare cases of hemorrhagic G.C.T. where it may be very difficult to distinguish it histologically from an **aneurysmal bone cyst**. Finally, there are exceptional

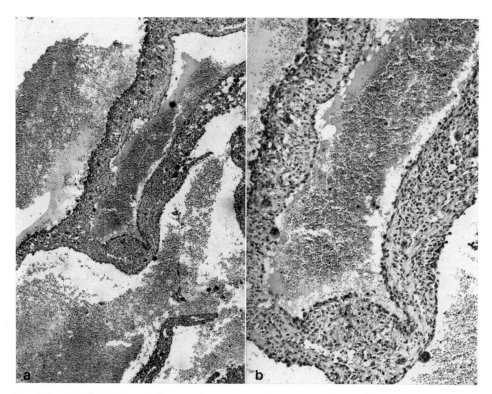

FIG. 95. - G.C.T. with cystic-hemorrhagic areas the same as those of an aneurysmal bone cyst. In other areas the histological structure was that of a typical G.C.T. The lesion was located in the proximal tibia of a female aged 63 years. (*Hemat.-eos.*, 50, 125 x).

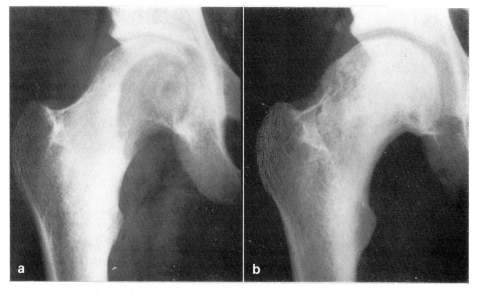

FIG. 96. - (a) Male aged 23 years. Active radiographic variety. (b) Patient submitted to curettage and bone grafts, cured after 7 years.

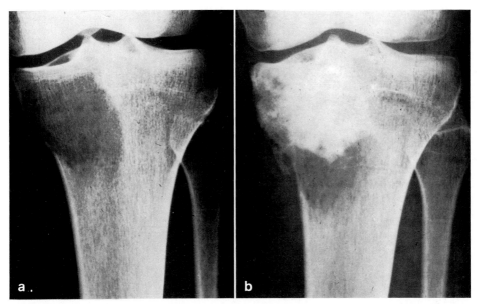

FIG. 97. - Female aged 25 years. (a) Active radiographic variety. Submitted to curettage and bone grafts. (b) After 2 months, tumor resumes expansion to its distal pole. Histologically, «aggressive» G.C.T. The patient was submitted to en bloc resection and arthrodesis. There were no signs of recurrence after 5 years.

observations of **bone metastasis due to carcinoma** (of the thyroid, pancreas, lung) histologically simulating a G.C.T. Apart from these rare exceptions, the histological picture of G.C.T. cannot be mistaken. Here and there it may resemble a **chondroblastoma**, a **histiocytic fibroma**, an **osteoblastoma**. But these are superficial resemblances and/or ones circumscribed to some areas of the tumor (see specific chapter). As for differential diagnosis with **benign fibrous histiocytoma** see specific chapter.

COURSE

The course of the tumor varies and is unpredictable. We have already discussed the meaning of the radiographic pictures quiescent, active and aggressive, which correspond to different courses of the neoplasm. There is also a certain relationship between the course of the neoplasm and the histological picture, in the sense that G.C.T. which is histologically aggressive seems to have a more rapid course, not to speak of sarcomas. Nonetheless, even a histologically typical G.C.T. may have a rather rapid and aggressive expansion. In conclusion, this is an absolutely unreliable tumor: at times it grows slowly and remains well-contained for years, while at times it becomes very invasive in just a few weeks.

Recurrence of the tumor, occurring after incomplete excision, is nearly always manifested within 3 years of surgery. In exceptional cases it may occur after more than 3 years. G.C.T. may also grow in the soft tissues. The obser-

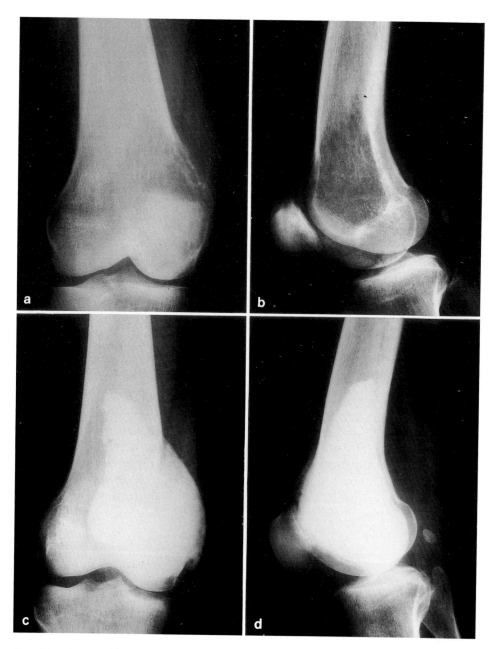

Fig. 98. - Giant cell tumor in a female aged 33 years. (a) and (b) Active radiographic stage. Treated with frozen section biopsy, curettage, and cement. (c) and (d) Cured after 5 years.

vation of extraskeletal recurrence, in the surgical wound (often ossifying), or in the site from which bone grafts have been removed (for example, the iliac wing) is not exceptional.

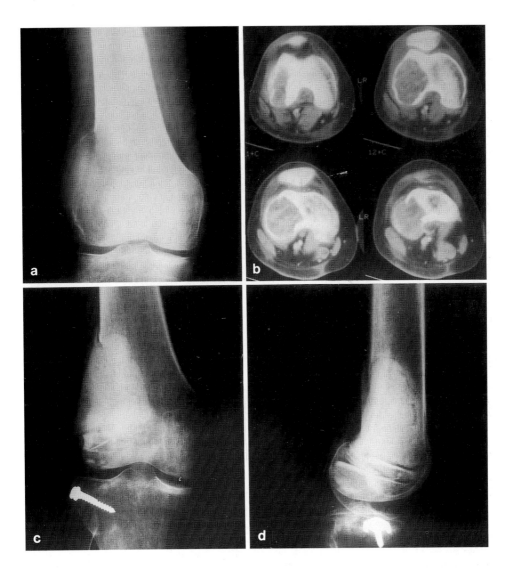

FIG. 99. - Giant cell tumor in a female aged 21 years. (a) Aggressive radiographic stage. (b) CAT. Treated with frozen section biopsy, curettage, autogenous subchondral cortico-cancellous grafts and cement. (c) and (d) The patient healed locally after 3 years. At the same time (3 years after surgery) there was a single pulmonary metastasis which was excised and confirmed histologically.

In 1-2% of all cases, a histologically typical G.C.T. produces pulmonary metastases which are histologically the same as the primary tumor. These metastases often have a slow course and, even if not removed or removed only partially, they may allow for a long survival rate or even healing. Metastasis due to a G.C.T. in the regional lymph nodes is an exceptional occurrence, but it has been observed, for example, in the popliteal region.

The sarcomatous transformation of a G.C.T. may be manifested in three

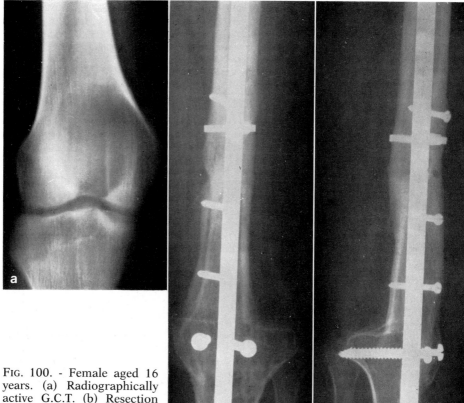

FIG. 100. - Female aged 16 years. (a) Radiographically active G.C.T. (b) Resection and arthrodesis using autogenous grafts. N.E.D. after 18 years.

different conditions: a) due to the spontaneous transformation of a G.C.T. left untreated. This is certainly a rare occurrence, but it is also particularly difficult to demonstrate. b) In the local recurrence of a G.C.T. operated and not irradiated. This occurrence is also rare, but well-proven (Figs. 88, 94). c) In the area of a G.C.T. previously operated and irradiated. This is the most frequent occurrence accounting for more than half of the cases of secondary sarcoma (Figs. 86, 87).

Thus, it may be concluded that sarcomatous evolution is an infrequent occurrence (less than 5% of all G.C.T.) and that it is favored by radiation therapy.

When G.C.T. has been irradiated the question arises whether the sarcoma derives from the evolution of the G.C.T., or whether it is a radiation-induced sarcoma (see specific chapter) independent of the G.C.T. The distinction could be based on the following facts. 1) **Sarcoma due to progression of the malignancy of the G.C.T.**: like the recurrence of a G.C.T. this is manifested less than 2-3 years after roentgentherapy. At times there are radiographic

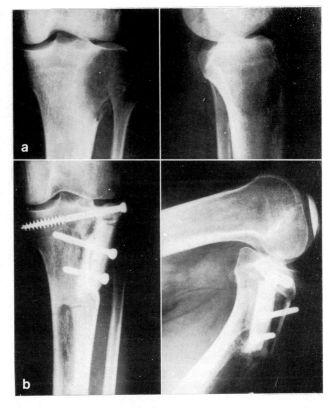

FIG. 101. - (a) G.C.T. in a male aged 19 years. (b) Result 4 years after resection of the tibial condyle, grafting of the patella and autogenous grafting from the diaphysis of the tibia. Mobility of the knee normal. N.E.D. after 10 years.

(signs of the activity of the primary G.C.T. which has never ceased. 2) **Radiation sarcoma**: this is manifested more than 3 years after irradiation, in the site of a G.C.T. which for all of that time had radiographically appeared to be «sterilized». The frequency of sarcoma in irradiated G.C.T. (more than 20% of all of the cases irradiated with more than 3-4000 r) is much higher than that of radiation-induced sarcoma. Thus, it may be admitted that radiotherapy favors the progression of the malignancy of G.C.T. The risk dose seems to be that which exceeds 3-4000 r.

TREATMENT AND PROGNOSIS

Until recently G.C.T. treated by intralesional excision (curettage) had a high percentage (approximately 40%) of local recurrence. This was due to the fact that there was no accurate staging of the tumor, to the fact that curettage was carried out through a limited window in the wall, and not in a sufficiently accurate manner, and to the fact that local adjuvants were not used. Thus, en bloc resection was used frequently. As the resected skeletal segment was generally part of an important joint (knee, shoulder, hip, wrist, ankle) complex reconstruction and/or important functional deficit were the result.

The current orientation is clearly more conservative; **intralesional exci-**

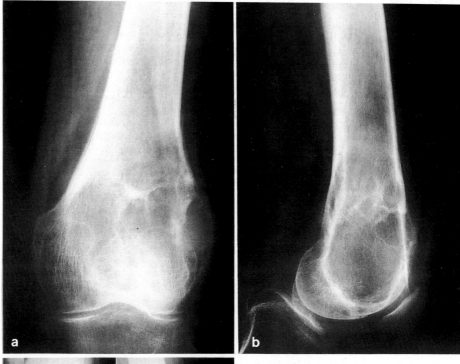

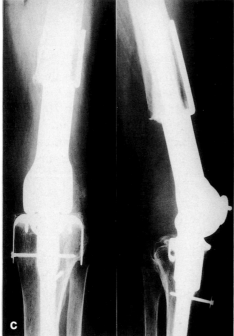

FIG. 102. - Giant cell tumor in a male aged 53 years. (a) and (b) Active radiographic stage recurring after curettage performed one year earlier. The patient was submitted to marginal resection and endoprosthesis. (c) Healed after 7 years.

sion has become the treatment of choice. The indication is for primary tumors at stages 1, 2 or even 3, when enough bone is preserved to allow for a reconstruction which is biologically and mechanically effective. The entire cortical wall thinned by the tumor and which may be exposed surgically will have to be removed en bloc and by an extracapsular approach (marginal or wide margin). The surrounding surgical field is protected by moist sponges. Curettage is completed until normal bone has been reached, making use of a high-velocity burr drill, as well. Electrocoagulation is used to

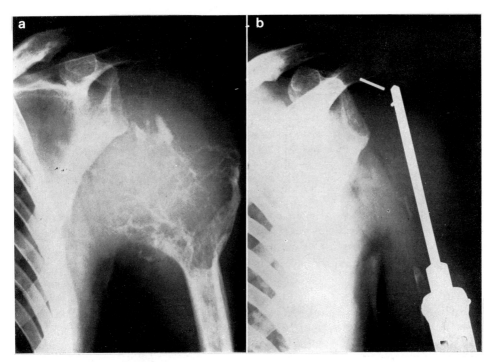

FIG. 103. - Male aged 28 years. (a) Radiographically aggressive G.C.T. and very expanded. (b) Resection-endoprosthesis. N.E.D. after 12 years.

cauterize the attenuated walls which cannot be removed. The walls are washed
with physiological solution under pressure. They are then soaked with 80% phenol, alcohol, and physiological solution. This is repeated 3 times. Finally, the cavity is filled with compressed acrylic cement.

When the tumor has reached the articular cartilage, in order to keep the
cement from coming into contact with the cartilage, and in order to keep the
cartilage from leaning up against avascular and rigid material, a layer of approximately 2 cm of autogenous cortico-cancellous bone chips is placed under the cartilage, and under this layer, protected by a thin hemostatic
sponge, the cement is applied (Figs. 26a, b, 99).

The association of cement cement/bone grafting and internal osteosynthesis is rarely indicated.

When the localization of the tumor (proximal femur) or the extent of the
osteolysis do not allow us to obtain a mechanically valid solution with cement, reconstruction is carried out using autogenous (Fig. 96) and allografts,
generally associated with internal osteosynthesis.

Some authors have suggested that cement be used initially, and, in time,
when it is ascertained that local recurrence has not occurred, that it be substituted by bone grafts. But this practice is generally not necessary as, with
the correct indication, the cement is well-tolerated, and guarantees complete
permanent stability.

In addition to being an effective local adjuvant, the cement provides the advantage of early radiographic evidence of local recurrence. For this reason radiopaque cement is used (Fig. 98).

By using this method, the incidence of local recurrence decreased to less than 10%.

Local recurrence may still be treated by curettage and local adjuvants, based on the stage of the recurrence.

En bloc **resection** (marginal or wide) of the articular skeletal segment (Figs. 100, 102, 103) is restricted to cases of very extensive G.C.T. (particularly at stage 3), where the bone is nearly completely destroyed (a frequent occurrence in the distal radius, in the tubular bones of the hands and feet); to expendable bones (proximal fibula, anterior pelvic arch, ilium); to rare cases with invasion of the capsule, ligaments or joint cavity. For local recurrence in the soft tissues, as well, marginal or wide excision will be used.

After marginal or wide resection which is not contaminated (including the track of the previous biopsy or surgery) the incidence of local recurrence is nearly zero.

Vertebral localizations (and in the first two sacral segments) may be treated by curettage and internal osteosynthesis. As curettage cannot be as accurate in these localizations as it is in those of the limbs, and as local adjuvants are not used routinely, curettage may be followed by precautional radiation

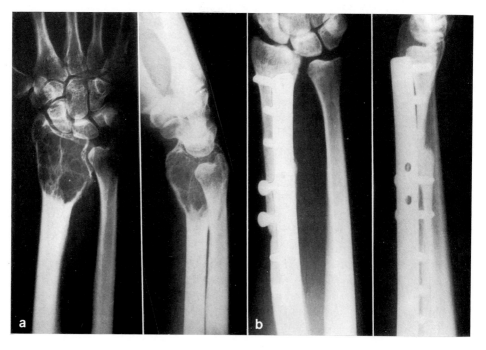

FIG. 104. - (a) Female aged 39 years. G.C.T. of the distal radius. (b) Six years after resection and autogenous proximal fibular (non-vascularized) grafting. The wrist was stable and painless, mobile in flexion at 20 degrees, extension 45 degrees, laterality and pronosupination half of normal.

therapy. This will be carried out approximately 6 months after surgery, if bone grafts were used, and it must not exceed 4000 r administered at high energy and in concentrated doses.

In exceptional cases of G.C.T. with wide invasion of the soft tissues and of the neurovascular bundle amputation is required.

Pulmonary metastases must be treated surgically, when possible, otherwise by radiation therapy. Chemotherapy seems to have little or no effect. In most cases pulmonary metastases may be treated successfully; rarely they may progress and result in death.

Sarcomas occurring on G.C.T. are treated by wide or radical surgery, usually ablative, combined with chemotherapy. Prior to the use of chemotherapy, the survival rate was approximately 20%. As these types of sarcoma are rare, we do not know whether and how much the survival rate has indeed increased as a result of chemotherapy.

Local recurrence and metastases of G.C.T. occur exceptionally after more than 3 years postsurgery. Thus, the site of the primary tumor and the pulmonary fields must be monitored particularly during the first 3 years.

Those cases of G.C.T. which result in death are inoperable ones in sites such as the vertebrae or the sacroiliac joint, those (exceptional) that produce uncontrollable pulmonary metastases, and many of those on which sarcoma has occurred. Since the use of radiation therapy, favoring sarcoma, has been reduced to a minimum, these G.C.T. resulting in death are probably less than 5%.

REFERENCES

1940 JAFFE H. L., LICHTENSTEIN L., PORTIS R. B.: Giant cell tumor of bone. His pathologic appearance, grading, supposed variants and treatment. *Archives of Pathology*, **30**, 993-1031.

1956 MURPHY W. R., ACKERMAN L. V.: Benign and malignant giant-cell tumors of bone. A clinical-pathological evaluation of thirty-one cases. *Cancer*, **9**, 317-339.

1961 SCHAJOWICZ F.: Giant-cell tumor of bone (osteoclastoma). A pathological and histochemical study. *Journal of Bone and Joint Surgery*, **43-A**, 1-29.

1961 SHERMAN M., FABRICIUS R.: Giant-cell tumor in the metaphysis in a child. Report of an unusual case. *Journal of Bone and Joint Surgery*, **43-A**, 1225-1229.

1962 HUTTER R. V. P., WARCESTER J. N. Jr., FRANCIS K. C., FOOTE F. W. Jr., STEWART F. W.: Benign and malignant giant cell tumors of bone. A clinico-pathological analysis of the natural history of the disease. *Cancer*, **15**, 653-690.

1963 SILVERBERG S. G., DE GIORGI L. S.: Osteoclastoma like giant cell tumor of the thyroid. *Cancer*, **31**, 621-625.

1964 JEWELL J. H., BUSH L. F.: Benign giant-cell tumor of bone with a solitary pulmonary metastasis. A case report. *Journal of Bone and Joint Surgery*, **46-A**, 848-852.

1964 MNAYNNEH W. A., DUDLEY H. R., MNAYNNEH L. G.: Giant-cell tumor of bone. An analysis and follow-up study of the forty-one cases observed at the Massachusetts General Hospital between 1925 and 1960. *Journal of Bone and Joint Surgery*, **46-A**, 63-75.

1964 PAN P., DAHLIN D. C., LIPSCOMB P. R., BERNATZ P. E.: Benign giant cell tumor of the radius with pulmonary metastasis. *Mayo Clinic Proceedings*, **39**, 344-349.

1967 RILEY L. H., HARTMANN W. H., ROBINSON R. A.: Soft-tissue recurrence of giant-cell tumor of bone after irradiation and excision. *Journal of Bone and Joint*

       Surgery, **49-A**, 365-368.

1968 MERLE D'AUBIGNÉ R., THOMINE J. M., MAZABRAND A., HANNOUCHE D.: Evolution spontanée et post-opératoire des tumeurs à cellules géantes. *Revue de Chirurgie Orthopedique*, **54**, 689-714.

1968 ROSAI J.: Carcinoma of pancreas simulating giant cell tumor of bone. Electron-microscopic evidence of its acinar cell origin. *Cancer*, **22**, 333-344.

1969 JOHNSON K. A., RILEY L. H. Jr.: Giant cell tumor of bone. An evaluation of 24 cases treated at the Johns Hopkins Hospital between 1925 and 1955. *Clinical Orthopaedics*, **62**, 187-191.

1970 DAHLIN D. C., CUPPS R., JOHNSON E. W.: Giant-cell tumor: a study of 195 cases. *Cancer*, **25**, 1061-1070.

1970 GOLDENBERG R., CAMPBELL C. J., BONFIGLIO M.: Giant cell tumor of bone. An analysis of two-hundred and eighteen cases. *Journal of Bone and Joint Surgery*, **52-A**, 619-664.

1970 HANAOKA H., FRIEDMAN B., MACK R.: Ultrastructure and histogenesis of giant-cell tumor of bone. *Cancer*, **25**, 1408-1423.

1972 STEINER G. C., GHOSH L., DORFMAN H. D.: Ultrastructure of giant cell tumors of bone. *Human Pathology*, **3**, 569-586.

1973 CAMPBELL C. J., BONFIGLIO M.: Aggressiveness and malignancy in giant-cell tumors of bone. PRICE C. H. G., ROSS F. G.M.: *Bone - Certain aspects of neoplasia*, Butterworths, London.

1973 KOSSEY P., CERVENANSKY J.: Malignant giant-cell tumours of bone. PRICE C. H. G., ROSS F. G. M.: *Bone - Certain aspects of neoplasia*, Butterworths, London.

1973 SYBRANDY S., DE LA FUENTE A. A.: Multiple giant-cell tumor of bone. Report of a case. *Journal of Bone and Joint Surgery*, **55-B**, 350-356.

1975 CAMPANACCI M., GIUNTI A., OLMI R.: Giant-cell tumours cf bone. A study of 209 cases with long-term follow-up in 130. *Italian Journal of Orthopaedics and Traumatology*, **1**, 153-180.

1975 CAMPBELL J. C., AKBARNIA B. A.: Giant cell tumor of the radius treated by massive resection and tibial bone graft. *Journal of Bone and Joint Surgery*, **57-A**, 982-986.

1975 LARSSON S. E., LORENTZON R., BOQUIST L.: Giant-cell tumors of the spine and sacrum causing neurological symptoms. *Clinical Orthopaedics*, **111**, 201-211.

1975 TORNBERG D., DICK H., JOHNSTON A.: Multicentric giant-cell tumors in the long bones. A case report. *Journal of Bone and Joint Surgery*, **57-A**, 420-422.

1977 DAHLIN D. C.: Giant cell tumor of vertebrae above the sacrum. A review of 31 cases. *Cancer*, **39**, 1350-1356.

1977 OYASU R., BATTIFORA H. A., BUCKINGHAM W. B., HIDVEGI D.: Metaplastic squamous cell carcinoma of bronchus simulating giant cell tumor of bone. *Cancer*, **39**, 1119-1128.

1978 MARCOVE R. C., WEIS L. D., VAGHAIWALLA M. R., PERSON R., HUVÒS A. G.: Cryosurgery in the treatment of giant cell tumors of bone. A report of 52 consecutive cases. *Cancer*, **41**, 957-969.

1979 NASCIMENTO A. G., HUVOS A. G., MARCOVE R. C.: Primary malignant giant cell tumor of bone. A study of eight cases and review of the literature. *Cancer*, **44**, 1393-1404.

1981 SCHAJOWICZ F.: *Tumors and tumor-like lesions of bone and joints*. Springer Verlag, New York.

1983 ENNEKING W.F.: *Musculoskeletal tumor surgery*. Churchill Livingstone, New York.

1983 MALONEY W.G., VAUGHAN L.M., JONES M.H., ROSS J.: Benign metastasizing giant-cell tumor of bone. Report of three cases and review of the literature. *Clinical Orthopaedics*, **243**, 208-215.

1983 PICCI P., MANFRINI M., ZUCCHI V., GHERLINZONI F., ROCK M., BERTONI F., NEFF J.R.: Giant-cell tumor of bone in skeletally immature patients. *Journal of Bone and Joint Surgery*, **65-A**, 486-490.

1983 VANEL D., CONTESSO G., REBIBO G., ZAFRANI B., MASSELOT J.: Benign giant-cell tumors of bone with pulmonary metastases and favourable prognosis. Report of 2 cases and review of the literature. *Skeletal Radiology*, **10**, 221-226.

1984 ROCK M.G., SIM F.H., UNNI K.K.: Metastases from histologically benign giant-cell tumor of bone. *Journal of Bone and Joint Surgery*, **66-A**, 269-274.

1985 BERTONI F., PRESENT D., ENNEKING W.F.: Giant-cell tumor of bone with pulmonary metastases. *Journal of Bone and Joint Surgery,* **67-A**, 890-900.

1986 BORIANI S., SUDANESE A., BALDINI N., PICCI P.: Sarcomatous degeneration of giant cell tumors. *Italian Journal of Orthopaedics and Traumatology,* **12**, 191-199.

1986 ECKARDT J.J., GROGAN T.J.: Giant-cell tumor of bone. *Clinical Orthopaedics,* **204**, 45-58.

1986 GOLDRING S.R., SCHILLER A.L., MANKIN H.J., DAYER J.M., KRANE S.M.: Characterization of cells from human giant-cell tumors of bone. *Clinical Orthopaedics,* **204**, 59-75.

1987 CAMPANACCI M., BALDINI N., BORIANI S., SUDANESE A.: Giant-cell tumor of bone. *Journal of Bone and Joint Surgery,* **69-A**, 105-114.

1987 HERMANN S.D., MESGARZADME M., BONAKDARPOUR A., DALINKA M.K.: The role of magnetic resonance imaging in giant-cell tumor of bone. *Skeletal Radiology,* **16**, 635-643.

1987 LACKMAN R.D., MC DONALD D.J., BECKENBAUGH R.D., SIM F.H.: Fibular reconstruction for giant-cell tumor of the distal radius. *Clinical Orthopaedics,* **218**, 232-238.

1987 OSAKA S., TORIYAMA S.: Surgical treatment of giant-cell tumor of the pelvis. *Clinical Orthopaedics,* **222**, 123-131.

1988 BERTONI F., PRESENT D., SUDANESE A., BALDINI N., BACCHINI P., CAMPANACCI M.: Giant-cell tumor of bone with pulmonary metastases. Six case reports and a review of the literature. *Clinical Orthopaedics,* **237**, 275-285.

1989 AOKI J., MOSER R.P., VINH T.N.: Giant-cell tumor of the scapula. A review of 13 cases. *Skeletal Radiology,* **18**, 427-434.

1989 CARRASCO C.H., MURRAY J.A.: Giant-cell tumors. *Orthopaedic Clinics of North America,* **20**, 395-405.

1989 LADANYI M., TRAGANOS F., MUVOS A.G.: Benign metastasizing giant-cell tumors of bone: a DNA flow cytometric study. *Cancer,* **64**, 1521-1526.

1990 BRIDGE J.A., NEFF J.R., BHATJA P.S., SINGER W.G., MURPHEY M.D.: Cytogenetic findings and biologic behaviour of giant cell tumors of bone. *Cancer,* **65**, 2697-2703.

1990 GITELIS S., WANG J., QUAST M., SCHAJOWICZ F., TEMPLETON A.: Recurrence of a giant-cell tumor with malignant transformation to a fibrosarcoma twenty-five years after primary treatment. *Journal of Bone and Joint Surgery,* **71-A**, 757-761.

1990 WRAY C.C., MACDONALD A.W., RICHARDSON R.A.: Benign giant-cell tumor with metastases to bone and lung. *Journal of Bone and Joint Surgery,* **72-B**, 486-489.

DESMOID FIBROMA
(Synonym: desmoplastic fibroma)

DEFINITION

It is a mature fibroma, similar to desmoids of the soft tissues and, like these, it easily recurs.

GENERALITIES

The tumor occurs rarely. Its predilection for sex is not known. It has been observed at every age: nonetheless, 90% of the cases was aged under 30 years at diagnosis. As it is a slow-growing tumor and symptoms are observed late, it may be considered to initiate nearly always during adolescence or youth. It does not seem to have a predilection for site, as it has been observed through-out the skeletal system. In the long bones (particularly the femur, the humerus and the tibia) it is more often observed in the meta-diaphysis, but it may be diaphyseal (Fig. 105). During adult age it usually extends to the epiphysis.

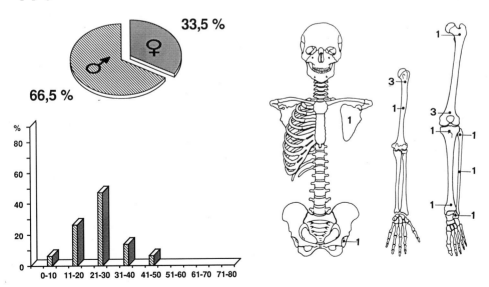

FIG. 105. - Sex, age and site in 15 cases of desmoid fibroma.

SYMPTOMS

Symptoms are mild and occur late (the tumor grows slowly and is not very vascularized). Symptoms consist in moderate pain, pathologic fracture, and at times there is considerable expansion of the bone.

RADIOGRAPHIC FEATURES

D.F. has often achieved considerable extension when the first radiograms are obtained, because of the scarcity of symptoms. The radiographic picture consists in osteolysis, at times uniform, at times cloistered and bubbling due to the presence of parietal bone crests (Figs. 106, 107). The cortical bone may be thinned eccentrically, or throughout the entire circumference of the bone.

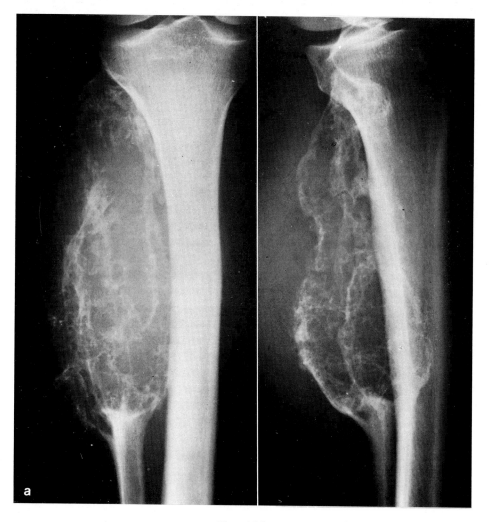

FIG. 106a.

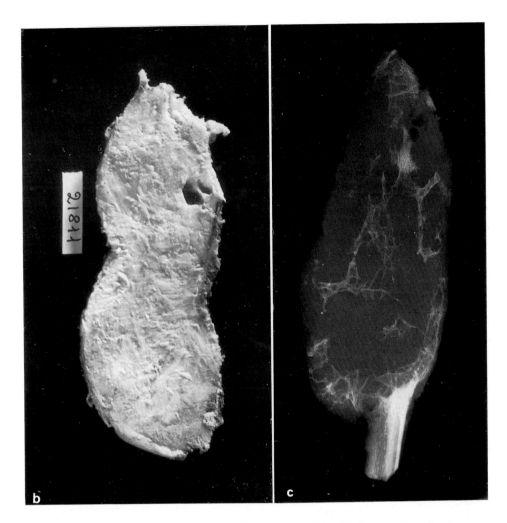

FIG. 106. - (a) Male aged 32 years. Desmoid fibroma of the fibula. Swelling for the past 15 years, which slowly increased and is painless. Resection. There are no signs of recurrence after 12 years. (b) and (c) Photograph and x-ray of the resected segment in the same case.

At times there is reactive hyperostosis at the boundaries of the tumor, and a radiopaque rim is produced. In some cases the cortex is destroyed by the tumor, which produces an image of total osteolysis.

D.F. takes the contrast dye on arteriography only moderately and diffusedly, and it appears relatively «cold» on bone scan.

GROSS PATHOLOGIC FEATURES

It is typical of desmoids; compact tissue, lucent tendinous-white, in bundles and whorls, with an apparently well-defined boundary (Fig. 106b).

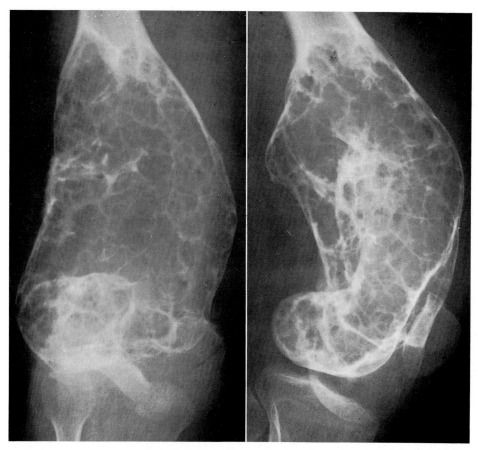

FIG. 107. - Male aged 24 years. For the past 3 years there was pain, swelling and progressive deformity. Histologically desmoid fibroma. Patient submitted to resection-
endoprosthesis and after 6 months amputated as a result of infection. No signs of recurrence or metastasis after 26 years.

HISTOPATHOLOGIC FEATURES

It is a fibrous tissue which is to a greater or lesser extent compact and mature, varying from field to field with regard to the proportion between fibroblasts and collagenous fibers (Fig. 108). However, the fibroblasts-fibrocytes
are never very numerous, they are small, more or less mature, without considerable plumpness of the nuclei, or hyperchromia, rare or no mitotic figures.
The collagenous fibers are abundant and they often form undulated bands or
even compact areas of hyaline aspect. The outside boundaries of the tissue
are not as well-defined as they may have appeared to be on gross examination, rather they tend to fade into the surrounding tissues.

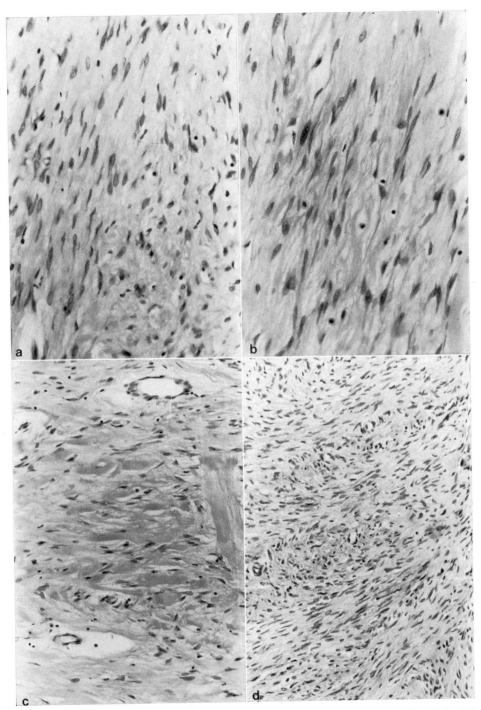

FIG. 108. - Histological picture of desmoid fibroma (*Hemat.-eos.*, 310, 310, 125, 125 x).

DIAGNOSIS

Preoperative diagnosis may be suspected when dealing with an osteolytic tumor of long duration, large size, which is cloistered and ballooning, and having no features of malignancy. Histologically, it must be distinguished from a **grade 1 fibrosarcoma**, which is more cellular, has more plump and pleomorphic nuclei, and more frequently has mitotic figures. In some cases the distinction may be difficult to make: in truth, D.F. and low-malignancy fibrosarcoma fade into one another without a clear demarcation (Fig. 108).

COURSE

Growth of the tumor is slow or very slow, it may even take several years, prior to causing considerable symptoms. It never metastasizes.

TREATMENT AND PROGNOSIS

After curettage has been performed, there is recurrence in approximately half of the cases. Treatment of choice is thus en bloc resection with a marginal or wide margin. When treated in this manner, even the most expanded forms heal.

REFERENCES

1958   JAFFE H. L.: *Tumors and tumorous conditions of the bones and joints*. Philadelphia, Lea & Febiger.

1960   GOLDENBERG R. R.: Well-differentiated fibrosarcoma of the calcaneus. Report of a case treated by resection. *Journal of Bone and Joint Surgery*, **42-A**, 1151-1155.

1960   WHITESIDES T. E. Jr., ACKERMAN L. C.: Desmoplastic fibroma. A report of three cases. *Journal of Bone and Joint Surgery*, **42-A**, 1143-1155.

1964   DAHLIN D. C., HOOVER N. W.: Desmoplastic fibroma of bone. Report of two cases. *Journal American Medical Association*, **188**, 685-687.

1966   ROSEN R. S., KIMBAL W.: Extra-abdominal desmoid tumors. *Radiology*, **86**, 534-540.

1967   HARDY R., LEHRER H.: Desmoplastic fibroma. A desmoid tumor of bone. Two cases illustrating a problem in differential diagnosis and classification. *Radiology*, **88**, 899-901.

1968   RABHAN W. N., ROSAI J.: Desmoplastic fibroma. Report of ten cases and review of the literature. *Journal of Bone and Joint Surgery*, **50-A**, 487-502.

1969   HINDS E. C., KENT J. N., FECHNER R. E.: Desmoplastic fibroma of the mandible. Report of a case. *Journal of Oral Surgery*, **27**, 271-274.

1969   NILSONNE U., GOTHLIN G.: Desmoplastic fibroma of bone. *Acta Orthopedica Scandinavica*, **40**, 205-216.

1976   SUGIURA I.: Desmoplastic fibroma. Case report and review of the literature. *Journal of Bone and Joint Surgery*, **58-A**, 126-130.

1981   SCHAJOWICZ F., *Tumors and tumor-like lesions of bone and joints.* Springer Verlag, New York.

1984   BERTONI F., CALDERONI P., BACCHINI P., CAMPANACCI M.: Desmoplastic fibroma of bone. A report of 6 cases. *Journal of Bone and Joint Surgery*, **66-B**, 265-268.

1988   YOUNG J.W.R., AISNER S.C., LEVINE A.M., RESNIK C.S., DORFMAN H.D.: Computed tomography of desmoid tumors of bone: desmoplastic fibroma. *Skeletal Radiology*, **17**, 333-337.

FIBROSARCOMA

DEFINITION

It is a sarcoma the cells of which tend to differentiate exclusively in fibroblasts, and which produce reticular and collagen fibers.

FREQUENCY

It definitely occurs infrequently, at least ten times less frequently than
osteosarcoma.

SEX

It shows no predilection for sex, or rather, there is only a slight predilection for the male sex (Fig. 109).

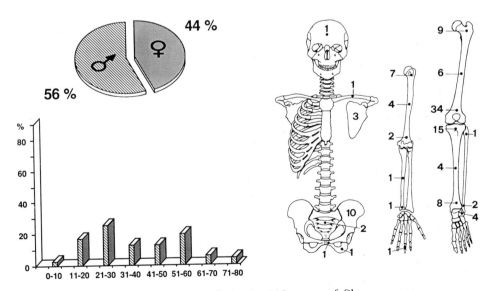

FIG. 109. - Sex, age and site in 118 cases of fibrosarcoma.

AGE

It may be observed at any age, indifferently distributed from 15 to 60 years. Only in exceptional cases does it occur before puberty (Fig. 109).

LOCALIZATION

There is predilection for the following sites, in decreasing order: the distal femur, the proximal tibia, the proximal femur, the proximal humerus, and the pelvis. Nearly half of all cases of F.S. are localized around the knee; nearly 20% in the proximal limbs; approximately 20% in the skeleton of the trunk. It very rarely occurs in the hand or in the foot (Fig. 109).

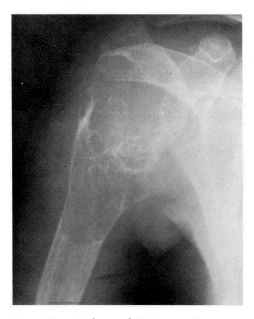

In the long bones, the tumor is generally located towards one end of the diaphysis or in the meta-physis and, as we are dealing with adults, it often invades the epi-physis. Purely diaphyseal localiza-tions are observed infrequently.

In rare cases F.S. is multiple on diagnosis, generally located in one or more bones of the same limb; in other cases, which are also rare, skeletal localization is associated with, or in time it is followed by, lo-calization in the soft tissues.

FIG. 110. - Male aged 22 years. One year earlier pathologic fracture. Histologically, grade 1 fibrosarcoma. Resection and graft-ing with an autogenous fibula. After 5 years extensive local recurrence. Shoulder disarticulation. The patient died after 28 years for reasons unrelated to the tumor.

SYMPTOMS

Pain is the main symptom. Swelling is absent, or mild and late in low-grade F.S.; instead, it occurs earlier when F.S. is more aggressive. Pa-thologic fracture is a frequent occurrence (Fig. 112).

At times evidence of a pre-existing skeletal lesion is shown by the patient's history or by radiographic and anatomical signs (see secondary F.S.).

RADIOGRAPHIC FEATURES

The radiographic picture is dominated by osteolysis (any neoplastic osteogenesis, by definition, is absent). The picture varies and is not very char-acteristic. It also depends on the aggressiveness of the tumor. Often osteo-lysis is massive, with fuzzy borders, interruption of the cortex, and invasion

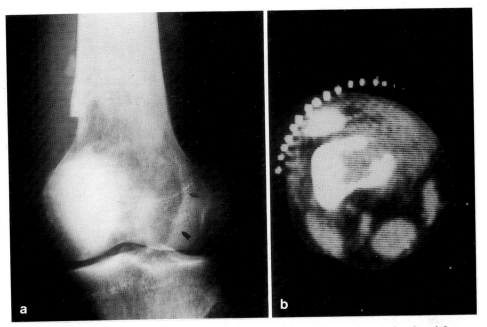

FIG. 111. - Male aged 35 years. Onset of symptoms 3 years earlier in the distal femur. Two years earlier radiation therapy. For the past 15 days pathologic fracture. There was a second osteolytic localization of the ipsilateral proximal femur. Histologically grade 2 fibrosarcoma. Hip disarticulation. The patient died after 5 months of pulmonary metastases.

of the soft tissues. The osteogenetic reaction of the periosteum is scarce or totally absent. In other cases the tumor may permeate the cancellous and cortical bone, causing «moth-eaten» images and areas of osteolysis which are either sparse or confluent (Figs. 110-115).

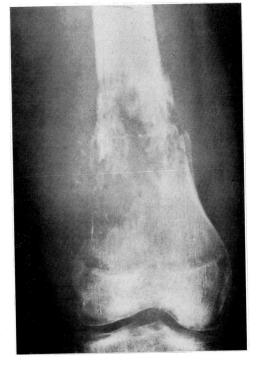

FIG. 112. - Female aged 23 years. One month earlier pathologic fracture. The vast amount of swelling formed within 3 months. Histologically, grade 4 fibrosarcoma. Thigh amputation. After 3 years recurrence on the stump. After 3 more months the patient died of pulmonary metastasis.

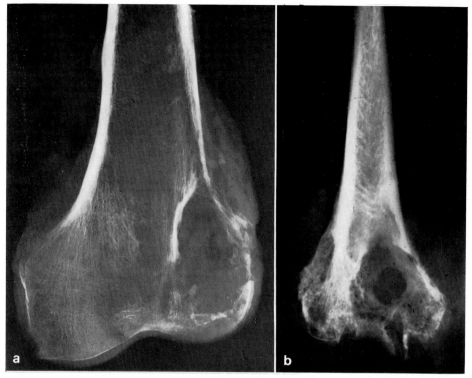

FIG. 113. - (a) Male aged 52 years. Pain for the past 8 months. Histologically, grade 2 fibrosarcoma. Amputation. After 1 and 1/2 years the patient died of skeletal metastases.
(b) Female aged 45 years. Histologically, grade 3 fibrosarcoma. Amputation and chemotherapy. The patient died after 11 months of pulmonary and costal metastases.

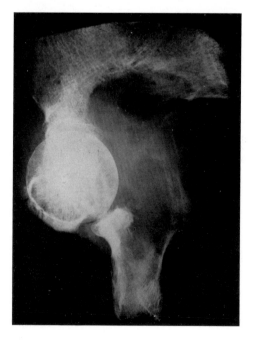

FIG. 114. - Female aged 41 years. Pain
for the past 4 months. Histologically,
grade 3 fibrosarcoma. En bloc resection
of the hip joint. Resection segment. After 6 months there was local recurrence
and after 1 year the patient died of diffused metastases.

FIG. 115. - Boy aged 15 years. Pain for the past 3 months. Histologically grade 2 fibrosarcoma. Amputation. X-ray of arterially injected anatomical specimen. The tumor seems to have an intra-cortical or periosteal development. No signs of recurrence or metastasis after 30 years.

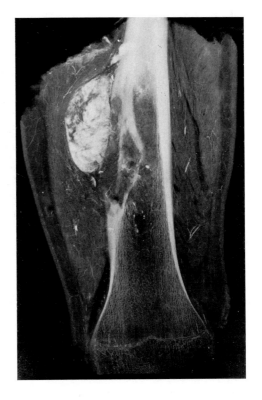

GROSS PATHOLOGIC FEATURES

In more differentiated and colla-genized forms, the tissue appears to be whitish, compact, of rather firm consistency. In less differentiated forms it is softer, juicy, and hyper-emic, due to the prevalence of cells over fibers and due to the fact that it is more vascular. Color ranges from white to pinkish, to grey. The aspect may be parenchymatous or decidedly encephaloid (Fig. 116). Hemorrhagic, necrotic, or cystic areas are observed frequently. At times there are areas of myxoid aspect.

HISTOPATHOLOGIC FEATURES

Skeletal F.S. may be distinguished in grades of increasing malignancy and decreasing differentiation. This distinction evidently has unclear and subjective boundaries, but it has bearing on prognosis and treatment.

Generally, the grade of histological differentiation is uniform throughout the tumor and does not change with recurrence or metastasis. This finding is the same as that of F.S. of the soft tissues and contrasts with that of some types of chondrosarcoma and parosteal osteosarcoma. In truth, F.S. shows little or no tendency towards progression of malignancy.

Grade 1 F.S.

This is differentiated from desmoid fibroma (although not always clearly) by a greater cellularity, plumper nuclei, mild hyperchromia and pleomor-phism, some mitotic figures. Collagen fibers are abundant (Fig. 117).

Grade 2 F.S.

The tissue is compact and rather uniform throughout the tumor. Its structure is characterized by bundles and currents, typically arranged in a herring-bone pattern. Generally, the cells are numerous, relatively large and spindle-shaped. The nuclei are plump and hyperchromatic. Generally, pleomorphism is scarce. Mitotic figures are frequently observed, and they may be anomalous. The collagen fibers are often relatively scarce or very scarce. The argyrophilic reticulum is always abundant and diffused, nearly around each cell (Fig. 118). At times, instead, the fibers form large bundles and areas of hyalin collagen around the tumoral cells, which remain embedded. The vessels are relatively numerous, nearly always provided with their own continuous wall. At times, imbibition of the stroma produces aspects of the myxoid type.

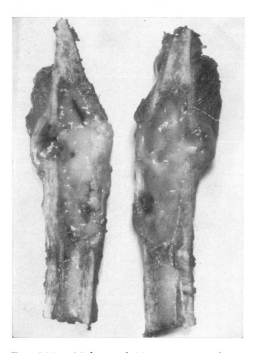

FIG. 116. - Male aged 35 years. Osteolytic lesion of the ulna. Histologically, grade 3 fibrosarcoma. The patient was submitted to en bloc resection and autogenous graft. There are no signs of the disease after 15 years. Observe the soft, encephaloid aspect of the tumor.

Grade 3-4 F.S.

The collagen fibers become rather scarce. The structure characterized by bundles and currents in herring-bone pattern is less prominent. The cells dominate the picture and are large; they are considerably pleomorphic. The nuclei are very hyperchromatic, bizzarre, infrequently monstruous or multiple. Mitotic figures are a frequent occurrence and generally anomalous (Fig. 119). The vessels may have a cavernous shape or be deprived of their own wall.

In F.S. of any grade benign (reactive) multinucleate giant cells and inflammatory infiltration, particularly of lymphocytes, may be observed.

HISTOGENESIS AND PATHOGENESIS

F.S. maintains its exclusively fibroblastic morpho-functional composition **throughout and during its entire course**. Otherwise, as previously stated, it is not a F.S.

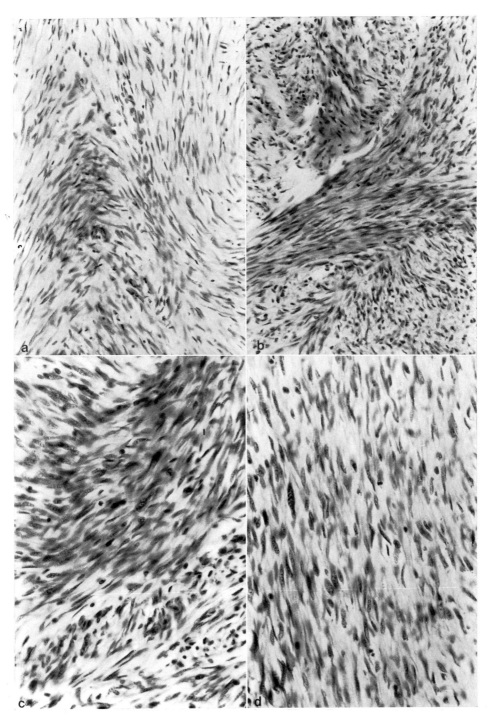

FIG. 117. - Histological aspects of grade 1 fibrosarcoma. In cases such as this one, it is sometimes difficult to make a distinction with desmoid fibroma (*Hemat.-eos.*, 125, 125, 310, 310 x).

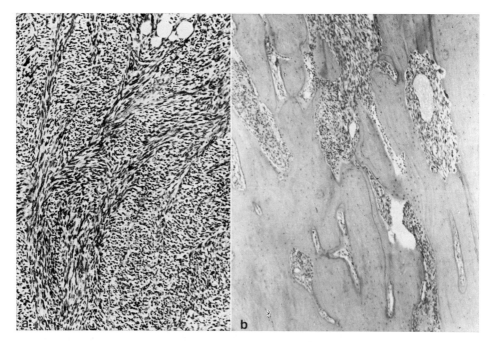

FIG. 118. - (a) Grade 2 fibrosarcoma. Note the herring bone pattern. (b) The same tumor infiltrates the medullary spaces. Aspects such as this one could be confused with parosteal osteosarcoma (*Hemat.-eos.*, 125, 50 x).

Several F.S. are **secondary** as they occur on pre-existing skeletal lesions. Some are secondary to a giant cell tumor, whether or not irradiated. Other F.S. occur in the site of a pre-existing chondroma or chondrosarcoma, exceptionally at the top of an exostosis. There are F.S. on irradiated bone, on pagetic bone, in an area of fibrous dysplasia, in an area of bone infarct and, finally, on a chronic osteomyelitis (see specific chapters).

The aforementioned possibility of multiple F.S. in several bones, or in the bone and in distant soft tissues, along with the observation of frequent local recurrences on the amputation stump and of frequent skeletal metastases even in the absence of pulmonary metastases, seem to suggest the possibility of a multicentric origin of the tumor, in addition to a frequent loco-regional dissemination and a tendency towards skeletal metastases.

DIAGNOSIS

A radiographic diagnosis of F.S. cannot constitute more than a hypothesis. A F.S. may provide images similar to those of any primary or metastatic malignant osteolytic tumor in the adult.

Thus, diagnosis must rely on pathology. Histologically, a grade 1 F.S. may be difficult to distinguish from **desmoid fibroma**. In F.S. the nuclei are more numerous, larger, and plump, with mild hyperchromia and a fair

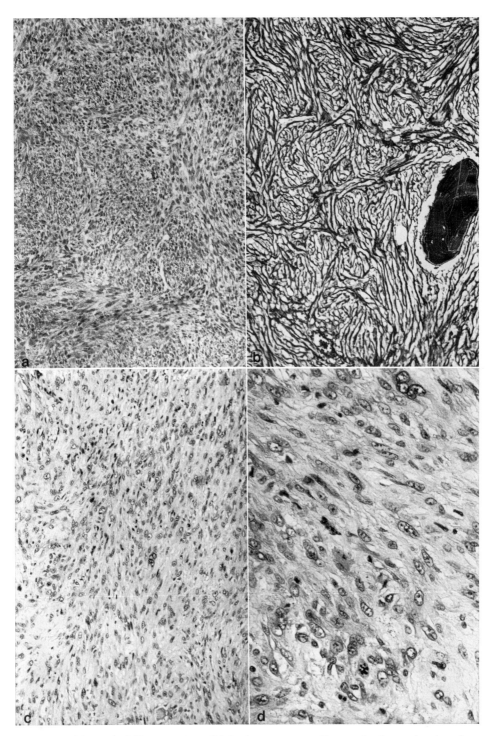

Fɪɢ. 119. - (a) Grade 3 fibrosarcoma. (b) In the same case silver stain shows the abundant pericellular reticulum. (c) and (d) Grade 4 fibrosarcoma. Observe the greater amount of anaplasia and of cellular pleomorphism (*Hemat.-eos.*, 125, 125, 125, 310 x).

amount of pleomorphism, with the presence of mitotic figures; moreover, the collagen component is less dense and mature. A histological distinction with benign forms such as histiocytic fibroma or fibrous dysplasia is easier to make. Apart from the absence of any feature of malignancy, **histiocytic fibroma** has a more whorled structure, it has hemosiderin pigment, and giant cells, at time it has foam cells. **Fibrous dysplasia** is less fasciculated and contains characteristic islands of woven bone.

Genuine grade 3-4 F.S. occur rarely: when faced with a sarcoma having gigantic cells, bizarre nuclei, and scarce or moderate fibroblastic differentiation, it is best to extend histological observation to numerous specimens, to evaluate radiographs properly, to study any recurrence or metastasis, as we may be dealing with osteosarcoma or malignant fibrous histiocytoma. **Osteosarcoma** may be extensively fibroblastic; at times there may be scarce hyaline material between the cells which is difficult to judge to be osteoid or collagen. Positive staining for alkaline phosphatase and positive marking with tetracycline indicate its osteoid nature. **Malignant fibrous histiocytoma** has a storiform structure, cells with a great deal of cytoplasm which is deeply stained, histioid nuclei, mono-and multinucleated giant cells, foam cells, a lesser amount of pericellular reticulum.

Finally, at times, F.S. may reveal cords of cells embedded in a dense fibro-hyaline substance, so much so as to cause one to suspect **hemangioendothelioma** or **epithelial metastasis**. On the contrary, there are epithelial metastases, particularly due to undifferentiated carcinoma of the kidney, which have spindle-shaped cells. In cases such as these, trichromic staining for the connective tissue, silver impregnation for the reticulum, and immunohistochemical methods can be useful.

COURSE

Grades 1-2 F.S. grow more slowly; grades 3-4 grow more rapidly. On the average the course is slower as compared to that of osteosarcoma.

Grades 2-4 F.S. frequently cause metastases by hematic route. Metastases, particularly if the tumor is well-differentiated, may occur even after several years. In addition to pulmonary metastases, bone metastases occur frequently; in the lymph nodes they occur only in exceptional cases.

TREATMENT

Wide resection is indicated in grade 1 F.S. In grades 2-4 F.S. resection may be indicated in selected cases, when the anatomical site of the tumor and its expansion make it possible to perform a rather wide resection. In most cases of F.S., particularly those classified as grades 3-4, amputation is required. As there is considerable expansion of the tumor in the bone at surgery (perhaps due to the scarcity of symptoms, so that surgery is performed later) and the consequent frequency of recurrence on the stump, the amputation site must be carefully determined, with the aid of arteriography, bone scan, CAT, MRI. In any case, the site must be quite distant from the tumor. When F.S. is located in the femur, for example, amputation will have to be very high and at times hip disarticulation or an interilioabdominal amputation will be required, more frequently than is the case with osteosarcoma.

F.S. is known to be radio-resistant. Radiation therapy is indicated only as a palliative, in forms which cannot be operated. Preoperative chemotherapy is of little effect and, thus, it is not used routinely. Cyclical and combined chemotherapy, prolonged after wide surgery, using the same protocols as those used for osteosarcoma, may be attempted — we still do not know what the results are — in high-risk cases, and in younger subjects.

It is worth it to surgically remove pulmonary metastases, whenever indicated and feasible.

PROGNOSIS

There seems to be a relationship between histological grading and prognosis. Grade 1 F.S. has a relatively good prognosis. On the average, grades 2-4 F.S. allow for a survival rate after 10 years, which is about 30% in cases in which adequate surgical treatment may be used.

We still do not know whether the association of adjuvant chemotherapy is capable of increasing these percentages.

REFERENCES

1944 STEINER P. E.: Multiple diffuse fibrosarcoma of bone. *American Journal of Pathology,* **20,** 877-893.

1958 GILMER W. S. Jr., MAC EVEN G. D.: Central (medullary) fibrosarcoma of bone. *Journal of Bone and Joint Surgery,* **40-A,** 121-141.

1960 FUREY J. G., FERRER-TORRELS M., REAGAN J. W.: Fibrosarcoma arising at the site of bone infarcts. A report of two cases. *Journal of Bone and Joint Surgery,* **42-A,** 802-810.

1962 NIELSEN A. R., POULSEN H.: Multiple diffuse fibrosarcomata of the bones. *Acta Pathologica Microbiologica Scandinavica,* **55,** 265-272.

1966 DORFMAN H. D., NORMAN A., WOLFF H.: Fibrosarcoma complicating bone infarction in a caisson worker. A case report. *Journal of Bone and Joint Surgery,* **48-A,** 528-532.

1968 CUNNINGHAM M. P., ARLEN M.: Medullary fibrosarcoma of bone. *Cancer,* **21,** 31-37.

1969 DAHLIN D. C., IVINS J. C.: Fibrosarcoma of bone. A study of 114 cases. *Cancer,* **23,** 35-41.

1969 EYRE-BROOK A. L., PRICE C. G. H.: Fibrosarcoma of bone. Review of fifty consecutive cases from the Bristol bone tumor registry. *Journal of Bone and Joint Surgery,* **51-B,** 20-37.

1974 NILSONNE W., MAZABRAUD A.: Les fibrosarcomes des l'os. *Revue de Chirurgie Orthopedique,* **60,** 109-122.

1975 HUVOS A. G., HIGINBOTHAM N. L.: Primary fibrosarcoma of bone. *Cancer,* **35,** 837-847.

1976 HERNANDEZ F. J., BALBINO F. B.: Multiple diffuse fibrosarcoma of bone. *Cancer,* **37,** 939-945.

1976 LARSSON E. S., LORENTZON R., BOQUIST L.: Fibrosarcoma of bone. *Journal of Bone and Joint Surgery,* **58-B,** 412-617.

1977 CAMPANACCI M., OLMI R.: Fibrosarcoma of bone. A study of 114 cases. *Italian Journal of Orthopaedics and Traumatology*, **3**, 199-206.
1983 SIM F.H.: *Diagnosis and treatment of bone: a team approach.* Mayo Clinic Monograph, New Jersey.
1989 MARKS K.E., BAUER T.W.: Fibrous tumors of bone. *Orthopaedics Clinics of North America*, **20**, 377-393.

MALIGNANT FIBROUS HISTIOCYTOMA

This is a sarcoma of histiocytary origin, which is rarely constituted by histiocytes (histiocytoma) in its entirety, generally by histiocytes and fibroblasts (fibrous histiocytoma).

It is not a rare tumor.

There seems to be predilection for the male **sex**; there is predilection for adult and adult-to-advanced **age**.

It is most commonly **localized** in the long bones, the femur, the tibia and the humerus, in this order (Fig. 120). Like osteosarcoma, it occurs more frequently in the distal femur and in the proximal tibia. Unlike osteosarcoma, it extends more easily from the metaphysis or metadiaphysis to the diaphysis and, as we are generally dealing with adults, even to the epiphysis. At times, it is only diaphyseal, or it may be observed in the short and flat bones.

The **symptoms** (pain and swelling) are usually of short duration at diagnosis, but at times they have been present for more than 1-2 years.

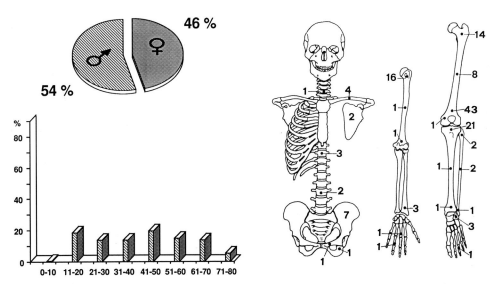

FIG. 120. - Sex, age and localization in 142 cases of malignant fibrous histiocytoma.

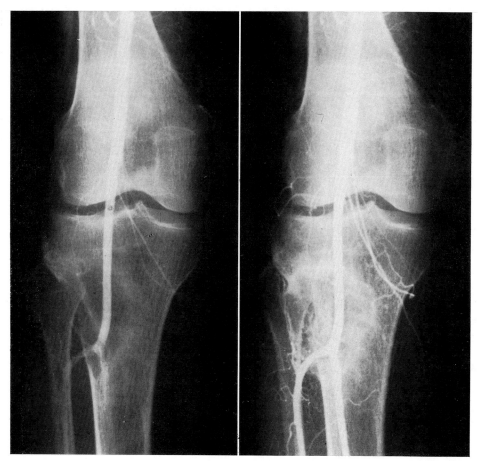

FIG. 121. - Female aged 53 years. Malignant fibrous histiocytoma. The cortex is nearly completely cancelled. Arteriography shows expansion of the tumor towards the soft tissues.

The **radiographic picture** is more similar to that of fibrosarcoma than to that of osteosarcoma (Figs. 121-127). It is a pure osteolysis, with confluent spots, or rather massive, with fuzzy borders. Relatively frequently, certainly more than is the case in osteosarcoma, the cortex appears to be attenuated, but not surpassed by the tumor. This may partially be a false radiographic impression, disproved by angiography, CAT, MRI and by surgical findings, or due to a lack of neoplastic osteogenesis and reactive periosteal osteogenesis. Reaction of the periosteum is rarely observed (mainly in diaphyseal localizations and in younger subjects).

Macroscopically, there is usually interruption of the cortex. The tumoral tissue is either encephaloid or it is harder and whitish (collagenized areas), with frequent yellow areas due to lipoid accumulation or necrosis, or yellowish-brown ones due to the hemosiderin contents.

Histologically, there are areas with a prevalently histiocytary structure, and others with a prevalently fibrocytary one (Figs. 128, 129). Rarely, the for-

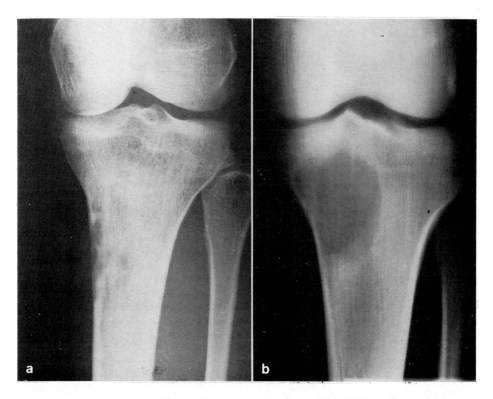

F<small>IG</small>. 122. - Two malignant fibrous histiocytomas of the tibia. (a) Female aged 44 years. (b) Male aged 36 years (stratigraphy). In both cases, the cortex is attenuated but it does not seem to be interrupted. Macroscopically the tumor, however, invaded the soft tissues.

mer are nearly exclusive (histiocytoma), generally the two are associated (fibrous histiocytoma). The histiocytary aspect is constituted by large cells, ones which are globose, oval or slightly spindle-shaped, with extensive cytoplasm which is intensely colored, eosinophilic, without clear boundaries; moreover, there is a large nucleus with an irregular outline, a thick nuclear membrane, clear-cut chromatin lumps, a voluminous nucleolus. Some cells have very extensive cytoplasm, which is well-colored and finely granulous, with an eccentric nucleus, enough to recall rhabdomyoblastic elements. Gigantic cells are constant with several atypical nuclei (sarcomatous giant cells), and frequently there are multinucleate giant cells having no nuclear atypia (reactive). Often there are tumoral cells in macrophagic activity (hemosiderin pigment, erythrocytes) and tumoral cells with foam cytoplasm. Where these histiocytary aspects prevail the tissue is richly cellular, with severe pleomorphism, gigantism, nuclear monstruosity, frequent atypical mitotic figures. In other areas, the aspect is prevalently or totally spindle-cellular, at times rather collagenized. Here the cells tend to be more sparse, with nuclei which are sharper, and dense chromatin; whorled or storiform structure prevails. Frequently there are areas of necrosis and there is constant

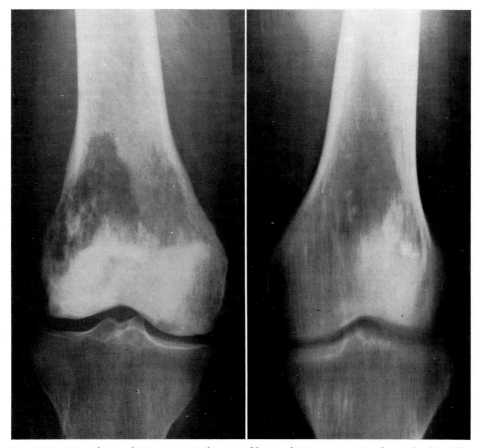

FIG. 123. - Female aged 70 years. Malignant fibrous histiocytoma in the right distal femur, on bone infarct. Symmetrical infarct (ascertained histologically) is present in the contralateral femur (stratigraphy).

lymphocytary infiltration (granulocytes are more rare), particularly at the periphery of the tumor.

In short, the histological elements of M.F.H. are as follows: histiocytary-like or epithelioid cells; spindle cells (facoltative fibroblasts) with fibrogenesis; storiform structure; malignant giant cells; benign (reactive) multinucleate giant cells; foam cells; inflammatory cells (usually lymphocytes); anaplasia and frequent mitotic figures (normal or atypical). Nearly all M.F.H. are of high histological grade (3-4). Nonetheless, there are exceptional cases where the grade is lower or very low (2-1). In truth, these have faded boundaries with giant cell tumor or benign fibrous histiocytoma.

Histogenesis goes back to the histiocyte, of which the fibrocyte is a morpho-functional modulation which is common in tumors belonging to this series (facultative fibroblast).

As for **pathogenesis**, M.F.H. of the bone is frequently **secondary**: it may be on meta-diaphyseal infarct (usually of the femur); on irradiated bone; on

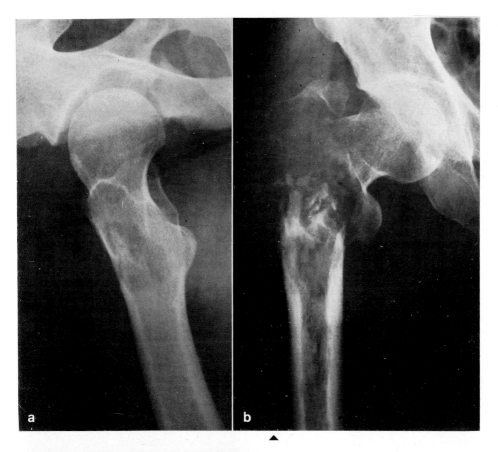

FIG. 124. - Two malignant fibrous histiocytomas of the proximal femur. (a)
Male aged 30 years. Here, too, the cortex seems to be continuous. (b) Male
aged 45 years. Wide destruction of the
cortex and pathologic fracture. In both
cases there was no periosteal reaction.

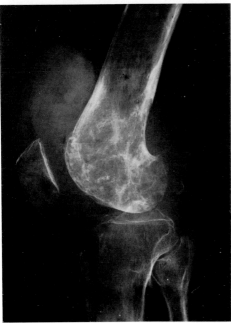

FIG. 125. - Male aged 61 years. Malignant fibrous histiocytoma. Amputation
specimen. Observe the spotted invasion
of the epiphysis. Despite this, interruption of the cortex is not clearly visible;
there is, however, a large neoplastic
mass deprived of calcification in the suprapatellar soft tissues.

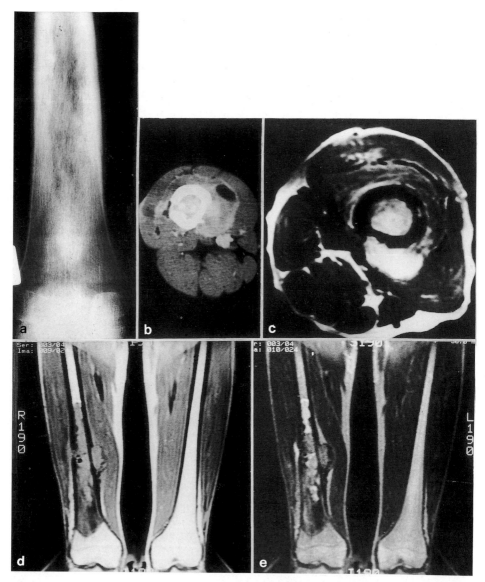

FIG. 126. - Malignant fibrous histiocytoma in a male aged 18 years. Diaphyseal localization. While the radiogram (a) does not reveal vast interruption in the cortex, CAT (b)
and MRI (c-e) show considerable invasion of the soft tissues. CAT clearly shows the
relationship with the large vessels (b). MRI (d,e) shows the extent of the tumor along
the medullary canal and towards the metaphyseal cancellous bone. For this purpose,
magnetic resonance is the most significant examination.

pagetic bone; on old chondromas or chondrosarcomas; on giant cell tumors;
on chronic osteomyelitis.

Differential radiographic **diagnosis** particularly involves fibrosarcoma,
osteolytic osteosarcoma, lymphoma, osteolytic metastasis; histological diagnosis involves fibrosarcoma (diffusedly spindle cells, herring-bone struc-

ture) and osteosarcoma (neoplastic osteogenesis). To this regard, it is best to recall that areas similar to M.F.H. may be observed in fibrosarcoma and in osteosarcoma. Thus, the identity of M.F.H. is still somewhat uncertain or at least it is unclear, and diagnosis must be based on ample and numerous histological sections. Histological differential diagnosis may also involve metastases due to carcinoma: these may have elongated cells arranged with a vaguely storiform structure; on the contrary, the histiocytes of M.F.H. may have an epithelioid aspect and be grouped in alveoli.

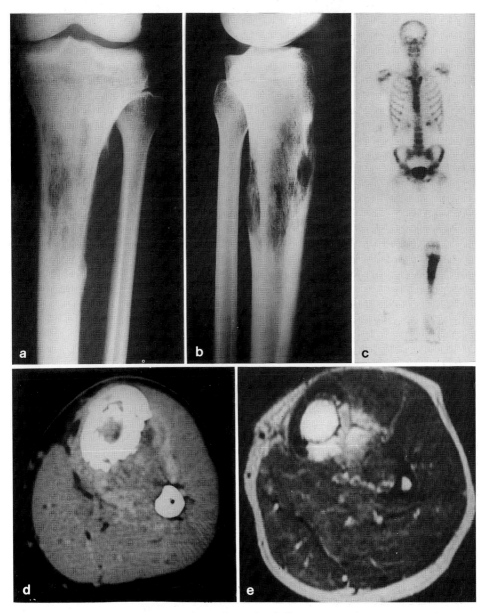

FIG. 127. (legend on the following page).

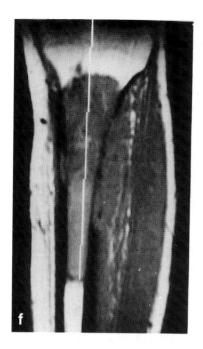

FIG. 127. - Male aged 19 years. Malignant fibrous histiocytoma. Observe how CAT (d) shows involvement of the medullary canal. MRI (e, f) more clearly reveals the extent of the tumor in the soft tissues and in the medullary canal; the latter may be more accurately measured as compared to bone scan (c). The patient was treated with preoperative chemotherapy, wide resection and endoprosthesis.

The **course, prognosis and treatment** of M.F.H. seem to be similar to those of grades 3-4 fibrosarcoma and those of osteosarcoma. Like fibrosarcoma, M.F.H. may at times be multiple in the skeleton and, in particular, it tends towards local recurrence even after removal with a very wide margin. Preoperative chemotherapy, which is the same as that used for osteosarcoma, obtains a good response in nearly half of all cases. With postoperative chemotherapy used for osteosarcoma, survival is evidently improved. Thus, M.F.H. is treated like osteosarcoma (see specific chapter). We emphasize that surgical margins in the treatment of M.F.H. must be particularly wide or radical, even moreso than in osteosarcoma.

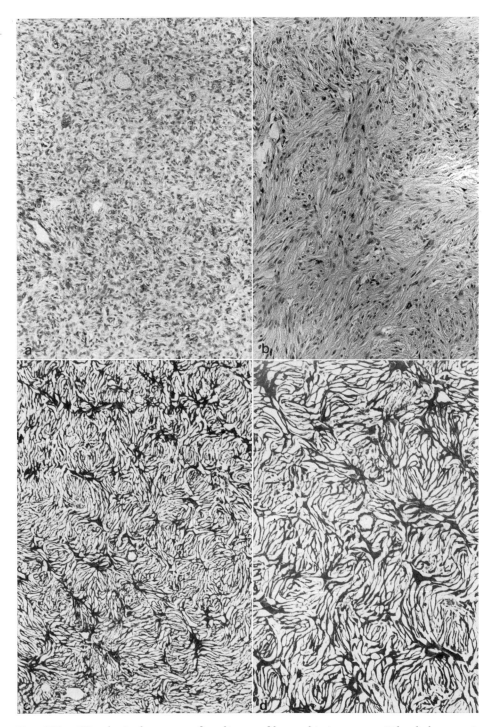

FIG. 128. - Histological aspects of malignant fibrous histiocytoma. Whorled or storiform structure. (a) and (b) *Hemat.-eos.*, 125 x. (c) and (d) *Silver stain*, 80 and
125 x.

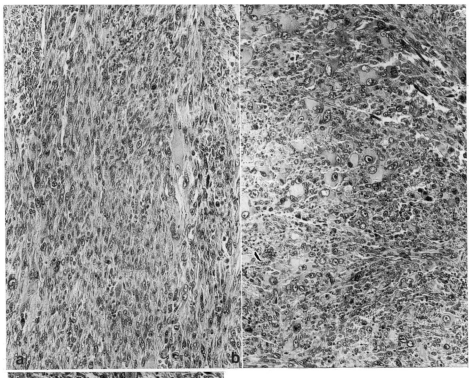

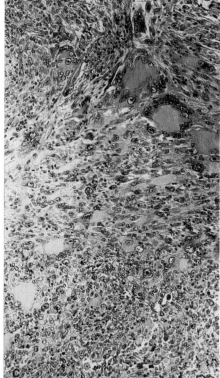

FIG. 129. - Histological aspects of malignant fibrous histiocytoma. (a) Large spindle-shaped cells, some with extensive cytoplasm. (b) Large histiocytes, some with large granulous cytoplasm, large nucleoli. (c) Giant multinucleate sarcomatous cells (*Hemat.-eos.*, 125, 125, 125 x).

REFERENCES

1974 MIRRA J. M., BULLOUGH P. G., MARCOVE R. C., JACOBS B., HUVOS A. G.: Malignant fibrous histiocytoma and osteosarcoma in association with bone infarcts. *Journal of Bone and Joint Surgery*, **56-A**, 932-940.

1975 NEWLAND R. C., HARRISON M. A., WRIGHT R. G.: Fibroxanthosarcoma of bone. *Pathology*, **7**, 203-208.

1975 SPANIER S. S., ENNEKING W., ENRIQUEZ P.: Primary malignant fibrous histiocitoma of bone. *Cancer*, **36**, 2084-2098.

1976 HUVOS A. G.: Primary malignant fibrous histiocytoma of bone: clinicopathologic study of 18 patients. *New York State Journal Medicine*, **76**, 552-559.

1976 MICHAEL R. H., DORFMAN H. D.: Malignant fibrous histiocytoma associated with bone infarcts. Report of a case. *Clinical Orthopaedics*, **118**, 180-183.

1977 DAHLIN D. C., UNNI K. K., MATSUNO T.: Malignant (fibrous) histiocytoma of bone. Fact or fancy? *Cancer*, **39**, 1508-1516.

1977 MIRRA J. M., GOLD R. H., MARAFIOTE R.: Malignant (fibrous) histiocytoma arising in association with a bone infarct in sickle-cell disease: coincidence or cause and effect? *Cancer*, **39**, 186-194.

1977 TAXY J. B., BATTIFORA H.: Malignant fibrous histiocytoma. An electron microscopic study. *Cancer*, **40**, 254-267.

1978 BERTONI F., DE SANCTIS E., LAUS M., SANCHEZ FERNANDEZ BRAVO J.: Istiocitoma fibroso maligno dell'osso. *Giornale Italiano di Ortopedia e Traumatologia*, **4**, 365-374.

1978 CHEN K. T. K.: Multiple fibroxanthosarcoma of bone. *Cancer*, **42**, 770-773.

1978 GALLI S. J., WEINTRAUB H. P., PROPPE K. H.: Malignant fibrous histiocytoma and pleomorphic sarcoma in association with medullary bone infarcts. *Cancer*, **41**, 607-619.

1978 KAHN L. M., WEBBER B., MILLS E., ANSTEY L., HESELSON N. G.: Malignant fibrous histiocytoma (malignant fibrous xanthoma, xanthosarcoma) of bone. *Cancer*, 640-651.

1983 HELESON N.G., PRICE S.K., MILLS E.E.D., CONWAY S.S.M., MARKS R.K.: Two malignant fibrous histiocytomas in bone infarcts Case report. *Journal of Bone and Joint Surgery*, **65-A**, 1167-1171.

1983 URBAN C., ROSEN G., HUVOS A.G., CAPARROS B., CAVAVIO A., NIRENBERG A.: Chemotherapy of malignant fibrous histiocytoma of bone. A report of 5 cases. *Cancer*, **51**, 795-802.

1983 WEINER M., SEDLIS M., JOHNSTON A.D., DICK H.M., WOLFF J.A.: Adjuvant chemotherapy of malignant fibrous histiocytoma of bone. *Cancer*, **51**, 25-29.

1984 CAPANNA R., BERTONI F. BACCHINI P., BACCI G., GUERRA A., CAMPANACCI M.: Malignant fibrous histiocytoma of bone. The experience at the Rizzoli Institute. Report of 90 cases. *Cancer*, **54**, 177-187.

1984 LEE Y., PHO R., NATER A.: Malignant fibrous histiocytoma at site of metal implant. *Cancer*, **54**, 2286-2289.

1985 HUVOS A.G., HEILWELL M., BRETSKY S.S.: Malignant fibrous histiocytoma of bone. A study of 130 patients. *American Journal of Surgical Pathology*, **9**, 853-871.

1985 ROHOLL P.J.M., KLEIJNE J., VAN BASTEN C.D.H., PUTTE J., UNNI K.K.: A study to analyse the origin of tumor cells in malignant fibrous histiocytomas. A multiparametric characterization. *Cancer*, **56**, 2809-2815.

1986 BOLAND P.J., HUVOS A.G.: Malignant fibrous histiocytoma of bone. *Clinical Orthopaedics*, **204**, 130-134.

1987 BACCI G., SPRINGFIELD D.S., CAPANNA R., PICCI P., BERTONI F., CAMPANACCI M.: Adjuvant chemotherapy for malignant fibrous histiocytoma in the femur and tibia. *Journal of Bone and Joint Surgery*, **67-A**, 620-625.

1987 LECOMTE-MOUCKE M., PARENT M.: L'histiocytofibrome malin osseux. *Revue de Chirurgie Orthopédique*, **73**, Suppl. 2, 81-86.

1988 RADIO S.J., WOOLBRIDGE T.N., LINDER J.: Flow cytometric DNA analysis of malignant fibrous histiocytoma and related fibrohistiocytic tumors. *Human Pathology*, **19**, 74-77.

SOLITARY EXOSTOSIS
(Synonyms: osteocartilaginous exostosis, osteochondroma)

DEFINITION

It is a hamartoma of the skeleton which derives from an aberrant sub-periosteal germ of the fertile cartilage; it grows mainly during the period of skeletal growth and it matures according to normal enchondral ossification.

FREQUENCY

After histiocytic fibroma it is the most frequent benign tumor of the skeleton. Some cases of E. are not observed as they are asymptomatic.

SEX

There is predilection for the male sex, with a ratio of 1.5-2:1 (Fig. 130).

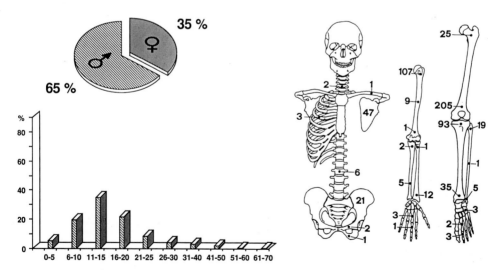

FIG. 130. - Sex, age and localization in 615 cases of solitary exostosis (allegedly solitary, such as in most cases radiographic examination did not extend to the entire skeleton). These are exclusively cases which were operated and verified histologically and thus mainly exostoses of fair size and/or symptomatic.

AGE

The tumor is rarely observed before 8 to 10 years of age, as it does not show any symptoms until it becomes of considerable size. As its growth is similar to that of the skeleton, it is at its largest around puberty. Thus, most cases of E. show signs between 10 and 18 years of age, and rarely afterwards (Fig. 130).

As we shall see, the age factor is of diagnostic and prognostic importance. In fact, up until puberty, it is normal for E. to grow, and it is nearly impossible for it to produce a peripheral condrosarcoma. On the contrary, an E. which resumes growth during adult age has nearly certainly transformed into chondrosarcoma.

LOCALIZATION

As the tumor originates from the growth cartilage on the metaphyseal side, E. is not observed either in a bone with direct ossification (the cranium, the face), or in an epiphysis, or in a bone of the carpus and tarsus, except for the calcaneus. Nearly 90% of all cases of E. are developed in the long bones of the limbs, in the proximity of a metaphysis.

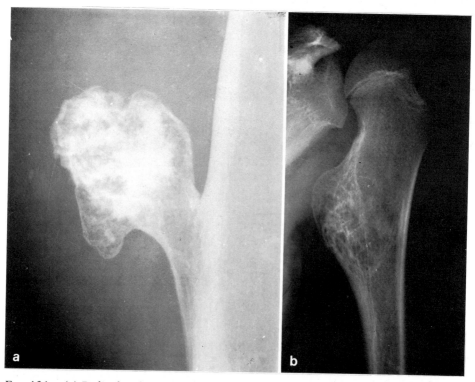

FIG. 131. - (a) Pediculated exostosis of the distal femur in a boy aged 14 years. (b) Sexile exostosis in a boy aged 10 years. The medial aspect of the proximal humerus is a site of election for these sexile exostoses.

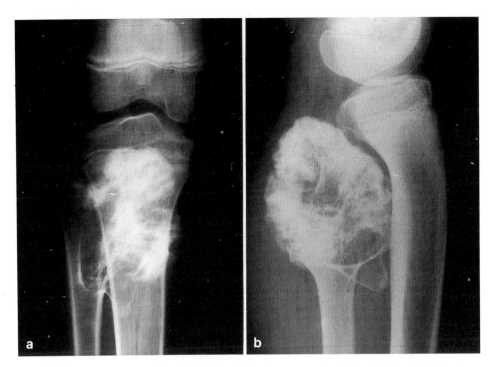

FIG. 132. - Exostosis in a boy aged 11 years. The exostosis deformed the tibia by compression. These exostoses also easily cause compression on the large vessels and on the popliteal nerve. For this reason, removal is often indicated even during childhood.

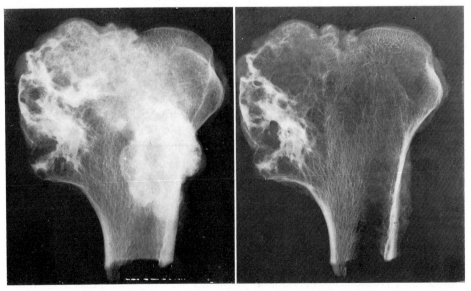

FIG. 133. - Large exostosis of the proximal humerus in a male age 39 years. Because of the size and the radiopacity of the tumor, this exostosis was believed to be in malignant transformation and operated by resection of the proximal humerus. The macroscopic and microscopic examinations instead indicated that it was simply a benign exostosis.

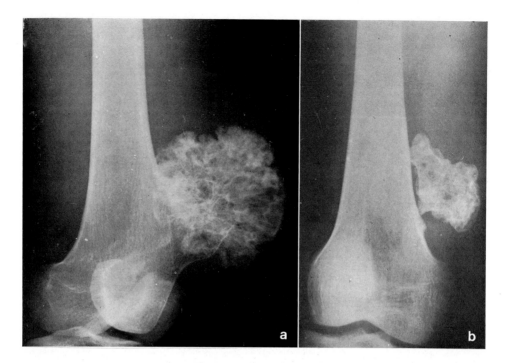

FIG. 134. - (a) Radiographic pictures of a large exostosis of the distal femur in a male aged 23 years. Despite the size and the radiopacity of the tumor, this exostosis did not show any histological signs of evolution in chondrosarcoma. (b) A rare example of pe-diculated exostosis in a male aged 31 years, with traumatic fracture of the pedicle of the exostosis.

The metaphyses which are most frequently involved are those close to the knee (particularly, the distal femoral) and the shoulder (proximal humerus). These are followed by the ankle, the proximal femur, the wrist, in this order. E. occurs less frequently in the skeleton of the trunk, and it is particularly ob-served in the scapula, the pelvis (where it is prevalently implanted on the ilium), the vertebral column (posterior arch). Only exceptionally is it observed in the tubular bones of the hand and foot. Some cases of E. localized in the deep sites, such as the vertebral and iliac sites, go unobserved, as they are asymptomatic (Fig. 130).

SYMPTOMS

Nearly the only symptom is a painless skeletal excrescence which slowly increases in volume during skeletal growth. E. is one with the skeletal plane from which it originates and it does not adhere to the soft tissues. In some sites E. is completely asymptomatic and it is visualized in a radiographic ex-amination carried out for other reasons (Fig. 138a). Most patients turn to a physician either for cosmetic reasons, or fearing that they have a «tumor», or

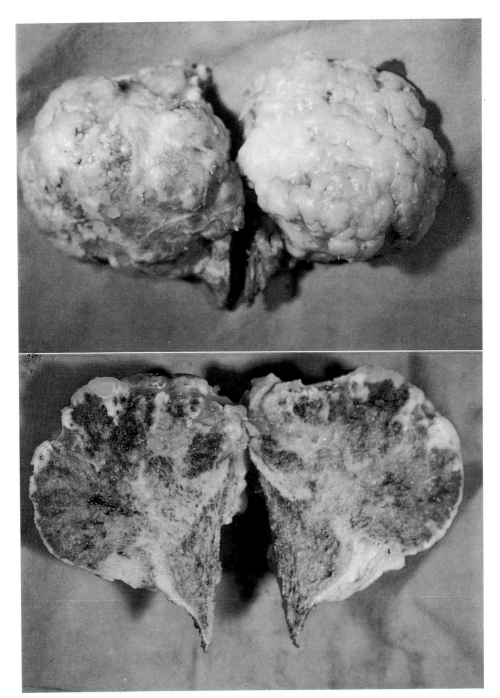

FIG. 135. - Macroscopic features of the exostosis illustrated in Fig. 134a.

because E. is a nuisance during specific movements and when the muscles are exerted, or because E. (located close to the knee) causes one knee to rub up against the other, or (E. located in the ankle) because problems arise

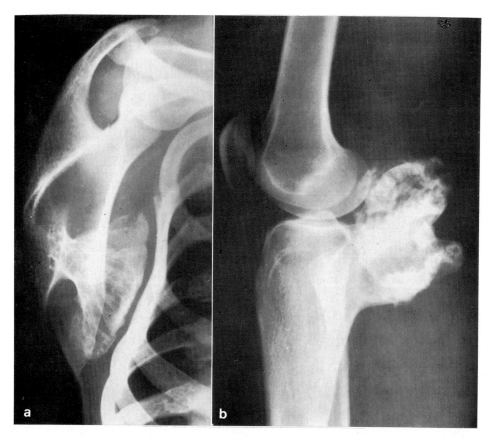

FIG. 136. - (a) Exostosis of the scapula in a female aged 15 years. The surface of the exostosis and the costal plane were modelled by the reciprocal contact. (b) Large exostosis of the proximal tibia in a female aged 18 years. This exostosis caused limited joint function.

when wearing shoes. A particular phenomenon may be caused by scapular E. as a result of contact with the costal plane during movements of the scapula: trigger scapula, which may be painful (Fig. 136a). At times, E. produces attrition phenomena with the muscular, aponeurotic, and tendinous structures covering it. When this is the case, a mucous bursa often forms on the surface of the E. Rarely, due to repeated trauma, serous or serohematic collection is manifested in this bursa. In similar conditions, the site of E. may become moderately painful and there may be rapidly increasing swelling. This is no cause for alarm because — as shown by the radiograph as well — it is not caused by an increase in the E.

In exceptional cases, juxtaepiphyseal E. and large-sized E. may interfere with joint function (Fig. 136b). Equally exceptionally, E. may compress a nerve trunk or the dural sac, or a large artery, thus causing neurological or vascular symptoms, for example, popliteal aneurysm.

In exceptional cases, as a result of traumatic fracture of its pedicle, E. be-

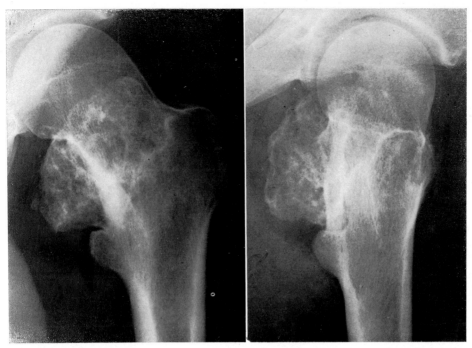

FIG. 137. - Intra-articular exostosis of the proximal femur in a male aged 29 years. The patient complained of some pain, and minor limitation of joint function.

comes painful and mobile in relation to the skeletal plane, clinically simulating muscular ossification or a loose joint body (Fig. 134b).

RADIOGRAPHIC FEATURES

The radiographic picture is absolutely typical, so much so that diagnosis is nearly always certain, even when there is no anatomo-pathological evidence. Nonetheless, radiograms must be obtained in at least two views and, in some sites (such as the vertebral column and the pelvis), CAT may be carried out in order to reveal the implant base of the tumor (Fig. 139). In fact, a radiographic view which shows E. from the front may give the false impression of a central lesion of the bone.

The pathognomonic radiographic feature of E. is that the cortex of the host bone is evaginated, like the finger of a glove, to become the cortex of the E. The cancellous bone of the E. continues directly with the cancellous bone of the metaphysis. Thus, the E. is an excrescence of the bone and it is made up as follows: 1) by a thin external cortex; b) by an internal cancellous bone; c) by a summit which is expanded and bumpy, more rarely sharp. The radiographic boundaries of E. in relation to the soft tissues are always well-defined (Figs. 131-141).

The internal structure of the E. is that of mature cancellous bone, but it is

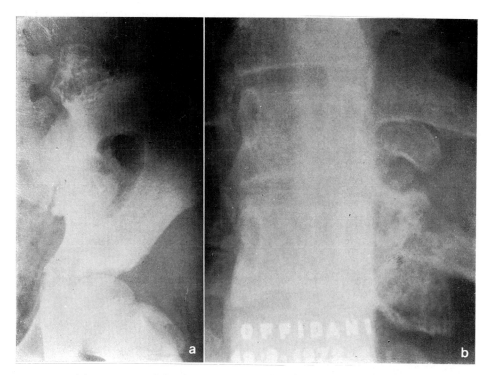

FIG. 138. - (a) Exostosis of the ilium, occasional radiographic finding in a boy aged 9 years. (b) Exostosis of the transverse apophysis of the 9th thoracic vertebra in a female aged 20 years. The patient had observed hard and painless swelling.

neither regular not orderly according to stress lines (as it is a useless structure, like all hamartomas). Moreover, a cancellous bone with very wide and very irregular mesh is observed. Due to the fact that it develops by enchondral ossification, and this ossification often proceeds irregularly, the E. may contain included cartilaginous islands that tend towards calcification, and focal thickening of bone trabeculae. This gives rise to radiographic images of intensely radiopaque clots within the E. At times these radiopaque clots are diffused and confluent (Figs. 131a, 132, 133). This finding was erroneously considered to be a sign of suspected malignant evolution: perhaps because it is generally observed in large-sized E. and because it recalls the radiopacity of some peripheral chondrosarcomas. On the contrary, if it

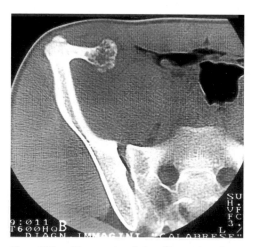

FIG. 139. - Exostosis of the iliac wing in a female aged 25 years.

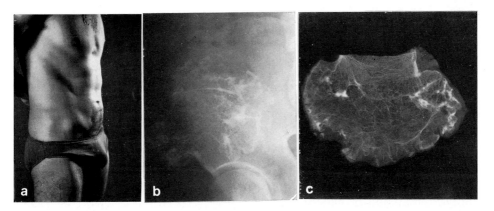

FIG. 140. - (a) Male aged 23 years who for the past 7 years had noted a hard and bumpy mass in the iliac fossa to the right. (b) Radiographic aspect of the large iliac exostosis. (c) Section of the excised exostosis. The macroscopic and microscopic examinations showed no signs of malignancy.

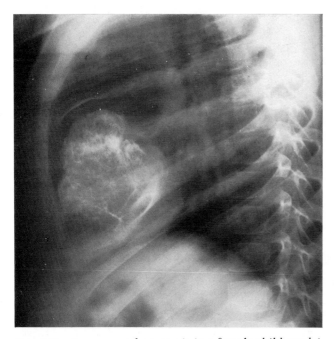

FIG. 141. - Large costal exostosis in a female child aged 6 years. The exostosis, which was resected with the implant rib, showed no histological signs of malignancy.

is contained within certain limits, it is not alarming (see peripheral chondrosarcoma).

The shape of E. varies, like its size. Some are pediculated, with a stem that expands in a globose and bumpy summit, or ends in a sharp horn-like extremity. Others are sexile, that is, having a large implant base; from here the E. may expand like a very large globose and bumpy mass; or it may only represent a moderate hilliness of the surface of the host bone. Finally, when E. is pediculated, it is usually inclined towards the diaphysis, escaping the epiphysis. It is oriented depend-

ing on the tension lines of the regional muscles.

CAT (MRI, angiography) is indicated in cases of suspect malignant transformation, or as a guide for surgery (shifting of the neurovascular bundle). It emphasizes any anomalous thickness of the cartilaginous cap and any fluid collected in E. with bursitis.

Bone scan is considerably positive in active E. in the child, while it is weakly positive or negative in inactive E. in the adult.

GROSS PATHOLOGIC FEATURES

The summit of E. is covered by a cartilage cap. This varies according to age. If the E. is observed during the very first years of life, which is hardly ever the case, it would appear to be prevalently constituted by cartilage, the initial ossification of which fuses with the fringe of the newly-formed bone trabeculae of the metaphysis. In the child, the cartilaginous cap still covers the entire summit of the E. It is a white to light blue hyaline cartilage similar to normal infantile cartilage, and its thickness ranges from a few millimeters to 1 centimeter or more (Fig. 142b). As age advances the cartilaginous cap (which, like growth cartilage, tends to exhaust its fertility) decreases in thickness and in many sites it disappears. Thus, during adult age, all that is usually left of the primary cartilaginous cap are a few lenticular residues, the thickness of which does not exceed a few millimeters (Figs. 135, 142c). In order to evaluate the malignant evolution of an E. during adult age, the thickness and the aspect of the cartilaginous cap are important (see Peripheral chondrosarcoma).

On the cut surface, located under the cartilaginous cap there is cancellous bone with irregular mesh, yellow marrow and — here and there — red marrow as well. Peninsulas of cartilage may go down from the superficial sheath for a short distance, or islands of cartilage may have remained included within the E. As the years go by, both appear to be heavily calcified and/or ossified, like yellowish-white clots which are rather hard and gritty.

The periosteum continues to coat the entire E. from the metaphysis, adhering to the cartilaginous cap as well. On the summit of the E. a mucous bursa may be observed, at times having pseudosynovial coating. Rarely (in the adult) this bursa may contain serous or serohematic effusion, or loose osteocartilaginous bodies.

HISTOPATHOLOGIC FEATURES

During the growth phase of E. the cartilage cap presents the same aspects of normal growth cartilage, although they are less regular. Starting from the surface, the proliferative, columned, hypertrophic and calcified layers may be recognized. These are followed by bone trabeculae formed by enchondral ossification, which are very irregular in distribution, direction and shape, occasionally containing islands of included cartilage. In the adult, the discontinuous and thin cartilage cap resembles mature hyaline cartilage, similar to articular cartilage (Fig. 143).

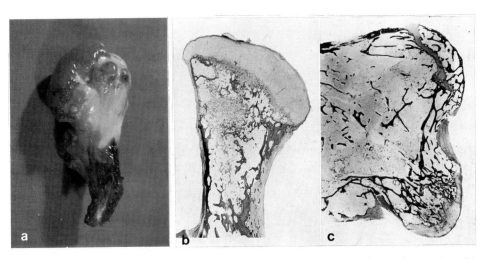

FIG. 142. - (a) Macroscopic aspect of pediculated exostosis in a male aged 12 years. (b) Histological picture under small enlargement of the same. (c) Histological aspect under small enlargement of sexile exostosis in a female aged 32 years.

The intensely radiopaque foci of E. appear to be constituted by islands of calcified cartilage, clumped and necrotic bone trabeculae, calcar precipitations in the necrotic intertrabecular connective tissue (Fig. 144). These phenomena seem to be correlated to a local defect in blood supply. In fact, they are particularly observed in large-sized E. The bone marrow is mostly fibroadipose but also, in certain areas, hemopoietic.

Practically speaking, the only thing of importance in the histological examination of E. is the verification that there are no histological aspects of a sarcomatous transformation in the cartilage (see peripheral chondrosarcoma).

HISTOGENESIS AND PATHOGENESIS

All of the descriptive elements recalled up to here show that E. is a hamartoma originating from an aberrant island of fertile cartilage, which remained excluded at the surface of the bone.

In the child, the occurrence of typical E. **after radiation therapy** on a bone of enchondral origin has been observed. In cases such as these, radiation was always used in children under 3 years of age, for different conditions, such as eosinophilic granuloma, metastases due to neuroblastoma, Wilms' tumor. The doses ranged from less than 1000 to more than 6000 R, and the interval of time between irradiation and the exostotic manifestation was from 1 and 1/2 to 9 years. E. appeared in the metaphyseal site of the long bones, but also in the scapula, ribs, iliac bone. They always developed within the limits of the irradiated areas, having anatomical features which were the same as those of common E. In one case, radiation-induced E. were multiple and one of these was transformed into chondrosarcoma. Evidently, the action of the rays,

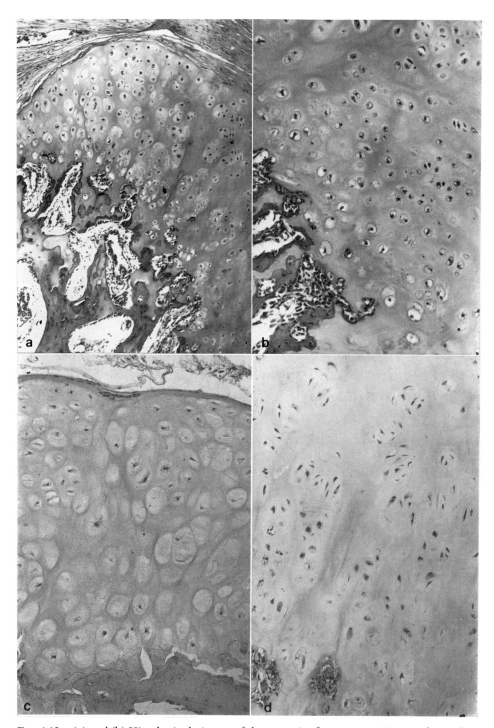

FIG. 143. - (a) and (b) Histological picture of the summit of an exostosis in a male aged 15 years. (c) In a female aged 22 years. (d) In a female aged 12 years. During childhood signs of vivid proliferation (dense cellularity, plump nuclei, some double nuclei) are normal in the cartilage of the exostosis (*Hemat.-eos.*, 50, 125, 125, 125 x).

partially arresting and disorganizing the proliferation of the fertile cartilage, favored the isolation of a fertile cartilaginous island from which the E. originated.

DIAGNOSIS

As previously stated, diagnosis is easy and nearly always possible based solely on clinical and radiographic elements. The only problem in diagnosis may be a differentiation between benign E. and **E. in sarcomatous transformation**. This problem is solved by evaluating all of the clinical, radiographic, scintigraphic, macroscopic and histological features (see peripheral chondrosarcoma).

Rarely, and only superficially, the radiographic aspect of an E. could suggest **parosteal osteosarcoma**. Any doubts could however be dispelled by a knowledge of the patient's history (E. is present without revealing much of an increase since adolescence), by the clear radiographic boundaries of the surface of the E., and, above all, by the fact that the E. is not fused to the surface of the cortical bone, rather representing an evagination of this (Fig. 136b).

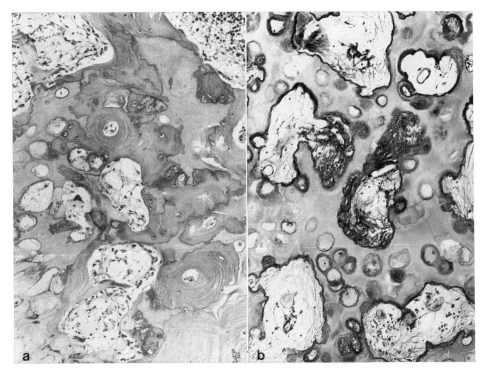

Fig. 144. - (a) In this area of focal bony thickening at the center of an exostosis observe the necrotic osteocartilaginous remnants and the disorderly bone deposit. (b) Area of necrosis of the cartilage and necrosis of the medullary connective tissue with calcar incrustations at the center of an exostosis (*Hemat.-eos.*, 125, 125 x).

So-called **subungueal exostosis** of the hallux and many parosteal ossifications of the tubular bones of the hand have nothing in common with actual E. (see pseudotumoral ossifications).

COURSE

The growth of E., whether it is large or small, continues for as long as the body grows. Then, it is completely exhausted. Thus, an E. which resumes growth during adult age must be considered in all probability to be a peripheral chondrosarcoma (cases of E. which continue to grow even in adult age are very rare, and if they do, their growth is only scant).

The transformation of solitary E. into peripheral chondrosarcoma is a rare occurrence. The incidence of this transformation is not known, but it certainly varies depending on the site of the E. In fact, E. localized in the skeleton of the trunk (pelvis, vertebrae, scapulae, ribs) may turn into chondrosarcoma with a frequency which probably comes close to 10%. Among E. of the long bones, sarcomatous transformation is rare, but it may occur for those localized towards the limb girdles (proximal femur and proximal humerus); while it is rare in the knee, it is nearly unknown in E. of the more distal segments. The development of a chondrosarcoma on an E. does not occur before puberty.

The patient affected with E., particularly if localized in the skeleton of the trunk or at proximal limbs, must be warned that if E. grows during adult age medical supervision will be promptly required.

TREATMENT AND PROGNOSIS

In most cases it is not worth removing the E. The patient must be told that he may live with the E. for the rest of his life. Nonetheless, when the E. is localized in the skeleton of the trunk, and even if it is asymptomatic, it may be removed as a preventive measure against a not very uncommon transformation in chondrosarcoma (Figs. 140, 141).

Apart from these considerations, surgery is indicated only with a cosmetic purpose or when the E. causes symptoms. Like in all hamartomas, it is best not to operate during childhood: this is because it is difficult to evaluate indications for surgery before the E. has grown completely, and because excising it in the child could lead to the manifestation of a local recurrence. Nonetheless, there are rare cases in which it is best to anticipate indications for surgery to childhood: when the E. is the cause of considerable functional deficit, or deformity, or when it grows near a neurovascular bundle (popliteal region-Fig. 132, axilla).

The E. must be removed in its entirety and with its capsule (marginal excision) in order to avoid leaving fragments of the cartilaginous cap, which could again grow. In the adult, it is not necessary to remove the stem and the base of the E. as far as the root, as the bony part has no proliferative potential; and even an intracapsular excision of the summit of the exostosis is generally not followed by recurrence. In the child, instead, excision must be completely extracapsular and even the base of the E. and the periosteum surrounding it must be removed, as they may contain fertile cartilaginous germs, the cause of possible recurrence.

When there is clinical and radiographic suspicion of an initial sarcomatous transformation, excision must be rigorously extracapsular, marginal or wide, avoiding peeling the cartilaginous surface of the E. of its capsule and breaking the E. during removal.

MULTIPLE HEREDITARY EXOSTOSES

DEFINITION

These are characterized by three main aspects: a) heredity; b) association with skeletal shortening or deformity; c) considerable frequency of transformation in peripheral chondrosarcoma.

FREQUENCY

The frequency ratio of M.E. to solitary E. is approximately 1:10. Thus, it is an infrequent condition.

AGE

Due to the multiplicity of the E., they are manifested earlier than solitary E., generally before 10 years of age (Fig. 145). It is difficult to discover the E. by obtaining radiographs of the newborn children of a family affected with the disease (Fig. 148). There are mild forms (particularly in females) in which the disease remains clinically latent for life.

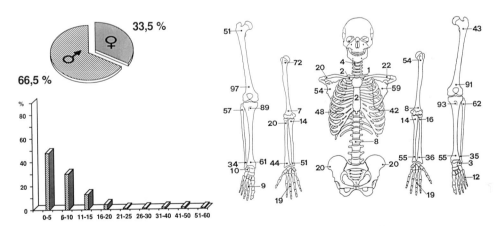

FIG. 145. - Sex, age and site in 120 cases of multiple exostoses (with a total of 1533 exostoses).

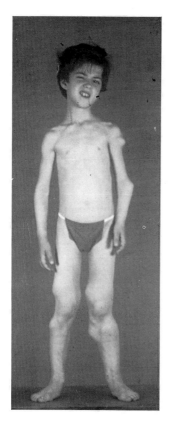

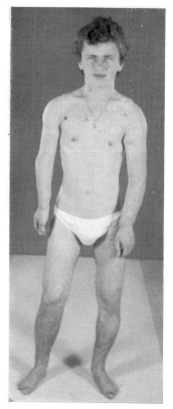

FIG. 146. - Boy aged 9 years affected with hereditary multiple exostoses.

FIG. 147. - Male aged 15 years affected with hereditary multiple exostoses.

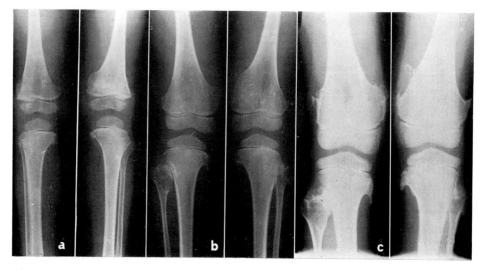

FIG. 148. - (a) Hereditary multiple exostoses in a boy aged 3 years. (b) At 6 years of age. (c) At 9 years of age.

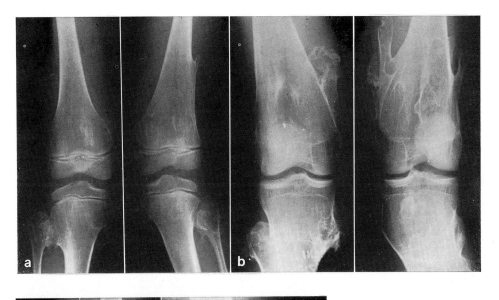

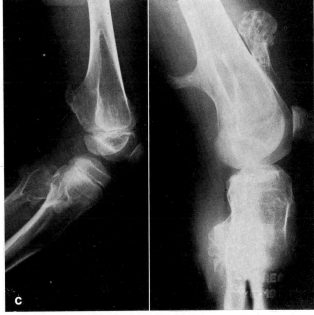

FIG. 149. - (a) Hereditary multiple exostoses in a boy aged 8 years. (b) The same patient at 16 years of age. (c) The same patient at 8 and 16 years of age, respectively.

SEX

There is evident predilection for the male sex (2:1) (Fig. 145).

HEREDITY

Heredity is manifested in nearly 2/3 of all cases. If one of the two parents is affected with M.E., approximately half of the children will inherit the disease.

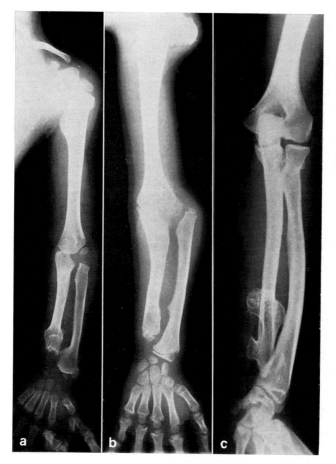

FIG. 150. - (a) Hereditary multiple exostoses in a boy aged 3 years. (b) The same limb at the age of 9 years. Observe how relative shortening of the ulna caused dislocation of the radial head. (c) Hereditary multiple exostoses in a boy aged 16 years. The relative shortening of the ulna caused bowing of the radius (pseudo-Madelung).

As previously stated, this prevails among males; if the male in a family affected with the disease is normal, he will not transmit the disease to his descendents. On the contrary, a female in the same family may transmit the disease even if she is normal. In other words, in males the disease and the ability to transmit it are both manifest; in females, the disease may be latent or not apparent, but it may nonetheless be transmitted to the descendents. These facts must be acknowledged for the purposes of matrimonial prevention.

LOCALIZATION

M.E. are generally diffused and relatively symmetrical (Fig. 145). All of the bones preformed in cartilage may be the site of E. Nonetheless, E. are more frequent, more numerous, and larger in the metaphyses of the long bones, particularly those close to the knee, the shoulder, the hip, the wrist, and the ankle. More rarely and to a milder degree is the elbow involved. In other

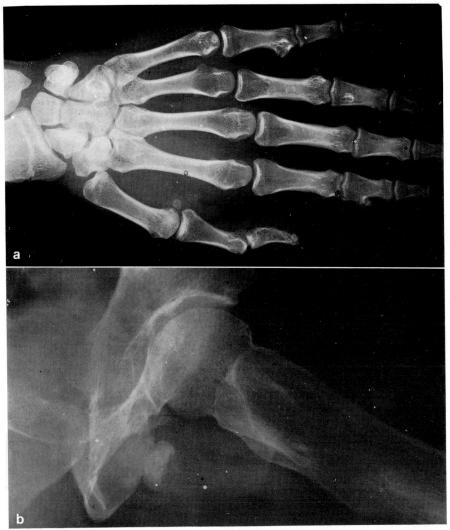

FIG. 151. - (a) Hereditary multiple exostoses in a boy aged 16 years. Small exostoses may be observed in the tubular bones of the hand. (b) Hereditary multiple exostoses in a male aged 40 years. Exostosis in a rare site like the ischium.

words, while E. develop in all of the metaphyses in the lower limb — although there is prevalence in the knee where skeletal growth is livelier — in the upper limb they clearly predominate near the shoulder and the wrist. They are also frequently observed in the bones of the trunk. In this site they develop in proximity of the secondary or apophysary centers of ossification. In the scapula, near the vertebral margin and the lower angle, the acromion, the glenoid and the coracoid; in the pelvis particularly along the iliac crest; in the vertebral column particularly in the spinous and transverse apophyses; in the ribs more often in the osteochondral junction or in the posterior extremity. Instead, they do not occur in the bones of either the carpus or the tarsus (except for the calcaneus which has a secondary nucleus of ossification), which develop in the same manner as the epiphyses. They may be observed in the clavicle which partially originates from enchondral ossification.

SYMPTOMS

Multiple skeletal excrescences may be observed and palpated which are often rather symmetrical. In relatively severe forms of the disease the aspect of the patient is so characteristic that diagnosis is made on first sight (Figs. 146, 147). In more severe forms, shortening of the limbs is associated. At times it is so marked and so diffused that it resembles that of achondroplasia. Nonetheless, there are no achondroplastic stigmata. In fact, shortening is not due to an anomaly in the growth cartilage, which functions normally, but rather to the fact that the proliferative potential of this cartilage is dissipated in external ramifications (E.) instead of being used in lengthening the bone. As this external dispersion is not uniform in either the perimeter of the metaphysis or the two bones making up the forearm and the leg, shortening may be associated with deformity, such as valgus or varus of the knee, the ankle, the elbow, the wrist. The most typical deformity is that of the forearm and wrist. Due to that fact that E. occur more frequently and are more extended to the wrist than to the elbow, and as 3/4 of the lengthening of the ulna occurs in its distal segment, while 4/5 of that of the radius occurs in the proximal segment, the ulna remains shorter than the radius. Thus, the radius is curved with lateral and dorsal convexity, the hand deviates ulnarly, at times the radial head is dislocated (Fig. 150).

RADIOGRAPHIC AND GROSS PATHOLOGIC FEATURES

M.E. are the same in structure as solitary E. The difference resides in the number. Subsequently, the metaphyses from which they originate are often widened and deformed (Figs. 148-152).

The periosteum covering the metaphyses and the E. is thickened, particularly in the recesses and depressions, and it is strongly adherent to the affected bone and to the E.

HISTOPATHOLOGIC FEATURES

These are the same as those of solitary E. Jaffe (1958) observed foci of cartilage in the deep layer of periosteum in proximity of the E.

PATHOGENESIS

Heredity and the diffused distribution of M.E. show its congenital, hamartomatous genesis.

FIG. 152. - X-ray of an anatomical specimen in hereditary multiple exostoses.
Male aged 42 years disarticulated for
peripheral chondrosarcoma of the proximal femur. Observe metadiaphyseal
deformity associated with exostoses.

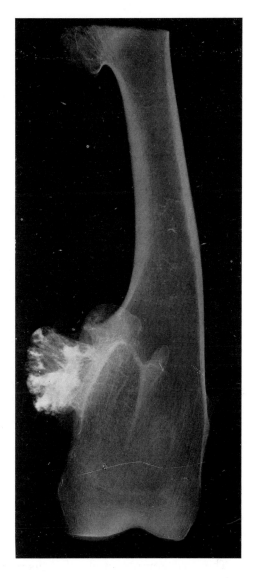

DIAGNOSIS

Diagnosis is easy and leaves no
doubts. There are no problems with
regard to differential diagnosis. At
one time M.E. was confused with
chondromatosis (Ollier's disease),
but these two forms are so different
that it is impossible to mistake one
for the other. In exceptional cases, a
chondroma in Ollier's disease may
grow at the surface of the bone, but
its radiographic features are different from those of an E. (Fig. 183).
Practically, M.E. are never associated with enchondromas; in the ge-
nealogical trees of M.E. there have
never been any cases of chondromatosis. The latter is more rare and
does not show any heredity.

COURSE

Like solitary E., M.E. practically
stop growing (with rare exceptions)
when body growth has ended. The considerable growth of an E. in adult age
is usually a sign of sarcomatous transformation. There is a high risk of one of
the M.E. transforming into peripheral chondrosarcoma. The incidence is approximately 25% in Jaffe's (1958) and Dahlin's (1978) cases; it is around 20%
in ours. If we consider the fact that sarcomatous transformation is a possibility from 15 years of age onwards, it is evident that its true incidence could
only be evaluated if we were to monitor those affected for their entire lives.
In exceptional cases two chondrosarcomas may derive from two different E.
in the same patient.

TREATMENT AND PROGNOSIS

Given the multiplicity of the E., not all of them may be removed. Generally, only the largest ones are removed, and those which cause the greatest problems.

At times osteotomy is indicated in order to correct axial deviation of the limb.

Prognosis is always reserved due to the risk of malignant transformation. The patient must be taught to request medical supervision should an E. grow considerably during adult age (see peripheral chondrosarcoma).

REFERENCES

1958 JAFFE H. L.: *Tumors and tumorous conditions of the bones and joints*. Lea & Febiger, Philadelphia.

1964 SOLOMON L.: Hereditary multiple exostosis. *American Journal of Human Genetic*, **16**, 351-363.

1968 CHRISMAN O. D., GOLDENBERG R. R.: Untreated solitary osteochondroma. Report of two cases. *Journal of Bone and Joint Surgery*, **50-A**, 508-512.

1969 ANDERSON B. R. L., POPOWITZ L., J. K. H. L. I.: An anusual sarcoma arising in a solitary osteochondroma. *Journal of Bone and Joint Surgery*, **51-A**, 1199-1204.

1969 KATZMAN H., WAUGH T., BORDON W.: Skeletal changes following irradiation in childhood tumors. *Journal of Bone and Joint Surgery*, **51-A**, 825-842.

1972 HERSHEY S. L., LADSDEN F. T.: Osteochondromas as cause of false popliteal aneurysms. Review of the literature and report of two cases. *Journal of Bone and Joint Surgery*, **54-A**, 1765-1768.

1973 PARSONS T. A.: The snapping scapula and subscapular exostoses. *Journal of Bone and Joint Surgery*, **55-B**, 345-349.

1978 DAHLIN D. C.: *Bone tumors*. Charles C. Thomas, Springfield.

1979 SHAPIRO F., SIMON S., GLIMCHER M.: Hereditary multiple exostoses. Anthropometric, roentgenographic and clinical aspects. *Journal of Bone and Joint Surgery*, **61-A**, 815-825.

1981 SCHAJOWICZ F.: *Tumors and tumor-like lesions of bone and joints*. Springer-Verlag, New York.

1981 VOEGELI E., LAISSUE J., KAISER A., HOFER B.: Case report 143: multiple hereditary osteocartilaginous exostosis affecting right femur with an overlying giant cystic bursa (exostosis bursata). *Skeletal Radiology*, **6**, 134-137.

1983 MILGRAM J.W.: The origins of osteochondromas and enchondromas: a histopathologic study. *Clinical Orthopaedics*, **174**, 264-284.

1984 HUDSON T.M.: Benign exostoses and exostotic chondrosarcomas: evaluation of cartilage thickness by CT. *Radiology*, **152**, 595-599.

1984 LANGE R., LANGE T., BHASKARA K.R.: Correlative radiographic, scintigraphic and histological evaluation of exostosis. *Journal of Bone and Joint Surgery*, **66-A**, 1454-1459.

1987 FANNEY D., TEHRANZADEH J., QUENCER R., NAJDI M.: Case report 415: osteochondroma of the cervical spine. *Skeletal Radiology*, **16**, 170-174.

1987 UNGER E., GILULA L., KYRIAKOS M.: Case report 430: ischemic necrosis of osteochondroma of tibia. *Skeletal Radiology*, **16**, 416-421.

1989 PETERSON H.A.: Multiple hereditary osteochondromata. *Clinical Orthopaedics*, **239**, 222-230.

1990 LIU S., THACHER C.: Case report 622. *Skeletal Radiology*, **19**, 383-385.

HEMIMELIC EPIPHYSEAL DYSPLASIA
(Synonyms: tarso-epiphyseal aclasia*;
dysplastic epiphyseal osteochondromas)

This is constituted by the anomaly of the growth and enchondral ossification of one or more epiphyses and/or tarsal bones, is infantile and monomelic, characterized by the development of tumorlike osteocartilaginous masses

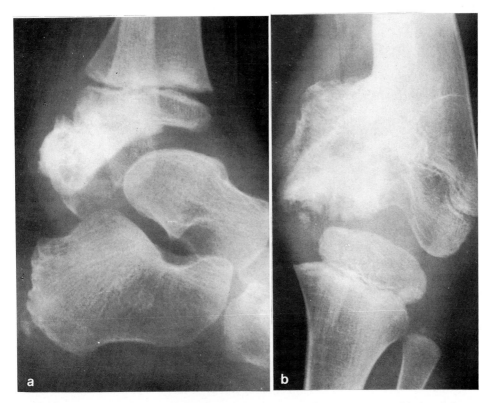

FIG. 153. - (a) Boy aged 6 years. Hard and bumpy swelling was noticed behind the tibial malleolus. (b) Boy aged 4 years. There was varus of the knee and considerable bulging on the medial side, with a decrease in joint movement.

---

* From the Greek *a-clasia* = absent destruction.

from the epiphyseal surface. It is defined hemimelic as it involves (not always) only one half of one or more epiphyses of the limb.

It is a **very rare** condition. There is no familiarity. There is evident predilection for the male **sex**. The lesion occurs during **childhood**, generally between 2 and 8 years of age.

H.E.D. nearly always involves only one lower limb (in exceptional cases one upper limb, or two lower limbs). It may be single or multiple, but generally it is limited to only one half of the epiphysis or tarsal bone, more often the medial half. The epiphysis which is preferred is the distal one of the femur, followed by the astragalus. The proximal epiphysis of the femur is hardly ever involved and in association with more distal lesions. Neither the proximal fibular epiphysis nor the patella are ever involved.

The first **symptom** is usually swelling of skeletal consistency, which is articular, on one side of the knee, ankle or foot, and which increases gradually. Pain is not constant, it occurs late and is mild. Frequently, instead, there is joint functional limitation (at times loose bodies) and joint axial deformity, for example varus or valgus of the knee. Growth of the limb is not compromised in a significant manner.

The **radiographic aspect** is characteristic (Figs. 153, 154). The change is strictly epiphyseal, rather hemiepiphyseal, and/or tarsal. From the surface of a hemiepiphysis a bumpy mass expands externally; the mass is irregular, and it is first formed by cartilage containing different centers of ossification. Subsequently, these tend to merge, and the entire mass appears to be bony,

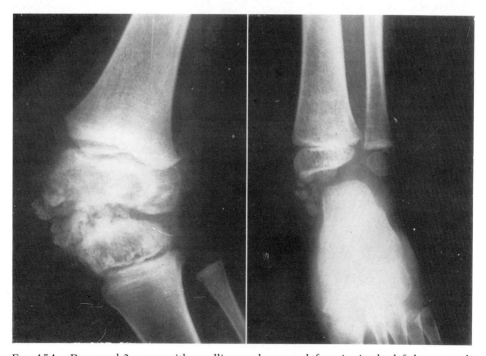

FIG. 154. - Boy aged 3 years with swelling and severe deformity in the left knee; swelling and deformity in valgus in the left ankle.

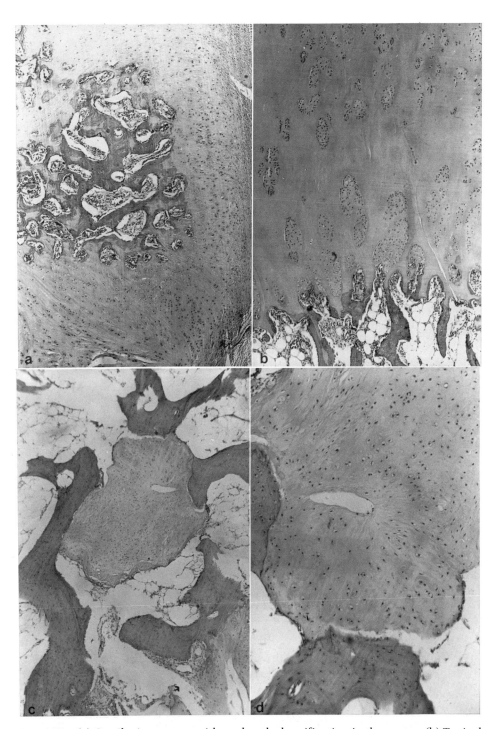

FIG. 155. - (a) Cartilaginous area with enchondral ossification in the center. (b) Typical aspect of cartilage with enchondral ossification. (c) and (d) Two images under different enlargements of a cartilaginous nodule, included in cancellous bone (*Hemat.-eos.*, 50, 50, 50, 125 x).

with irregular trabeculation. Expansion of the tumor causes deformity of the joint surface and may involve a part of the metaphysis, altering the adjacent growth cartilage. These aspects explain the deficit observed in joint function, as well as the axial deformity.

Macroscopically, the newly-formed mass appears to be round-topped, with a surface of cartilaginous aspect. Within there is normal cancellous bone, with an irregular structure. At times loose articular bodies become detached from the main mass.

The **histological picture** recalls that of exostosis. On the surface there is a sheath of hyaline cartilage, lower down there is cancellous bone. Between the two tissues the usual aspects of enchondral ossification are observed. However, this histological pattern is never as simple and as regular as it is in exostoses, as the ossification centers are different and they are scattered irregularly in the proliferating cartilage. The result is a disorderly alternation of osseous, cartilaginous and even fibrous tissue. The aspect is always hyperplastic, it is never neoplastic nor is it pathognomonic. If we histologically examine the fragments of tissue without taking the clinical and radiographic data into account, we might be led to imagining the existence of an exostosis or of a repair osteocartilaginous callus (Fig. 155).

It is believed that H.E.D. is caused by a **congenital alteration in the development of the epiphysis and the bones of the tarsus**. Normally, the cartilage which covers an epiphysis (or tarsal bone) during growth has its proliferative layer just under the surface. From this layer, if we proceed towards the center of epiphyseal ossification, those of the columned, hypertrophic and calcified cartilage are observed. On the contrary, if we go back up towards the surface, the cartilage cells of the proliferative layer give rise to elements which are increasingly mature, as well as small and flat. The more superficial cells end up flaking and falling in the joint cavity. In H.E.D. the cartilaginous cells do not follow this normal process of evolution, rather they behave at the surface as they do deep inside the epiphysis. In other words, they continue to proliferate even towards the outside of the epiphysis, forming cartilaginous protruberances within which (as occurs in the center of the epiphysis) numerous centers of ossification subsequently occur. Thus, the alteration is not unlike that of hamartomas and exostoses. Hemimelic distribution may be somewhat related to the vascularization of the epiphysis, which occurs by means of two distinct vascular pedicles, each for one epiphyseal half (Trevor, 1950).

H.E.D. **evolves** progressively during the first years of life. At the same time as tumoral growth joint deformity is observed. Towards 6-7 years of age, the mass usually achieves its largest size and its centers of ossification fuse together. After which the lesion may be considered stabilized.

Surgical **treatment** must be early, in order to prevent deformity and joint stiffness as much as possible. It consists in total removal of the exuberant mass remodelling the epiphyseal surface. There are no recurrences (except in youngsters), but morphology and joint function cannot be gained back completely.

REFERENCES

1950   TREVOR D.: Tarso-epiphyseal aclasis: a congenital error of epiphysial develop-
       ment. *Journal of Bone and Joint Surgery*, **32-B**, 204-213.
1953   INGELRANS P., LACHERETZ M.: A propos d'un cas de chondrodystrophie épiphy-
       saire. *Revue de Chirurgie Orthopédique*, **39**, 242-248.
1969   CAMPANACCI M., GIUNTI A.: Displasia epifisaria emimelica. *Chirurgia degli
       degli organi di Movimento*, **58**, 330-341.
1972   VERNON LUCK J., SMITH C. F.: Dysplasic epiphysealis osteochondromata. Twen-
       ty-two cases correlated with seventy cases in medical literature. *Journal of
       Bone and Joint Surgery*, **54-A**, 1351-1532.
1974   HENZINGER R. N., COWELL H. R., RAMSEY P. L., LEOPOLD G. R., Familial dyspla-
       sia epiphysealis hemimelica, associated with chondromas and osteochon-
       dromas. Report of a case with variable presentations. *Journal of Bone and
       Joint Surgery*, **56-A**, 1513-1519.
1978   FINIDORI G., RIGAULT P., PADOVANI J. P., NAOURI A.: Dysplasie épiphysaire hé-
       mimélique (tarsomégalie). Aspects cliniques, radiologiques et évolutifs, trai-
       tement chirurgical. A propos de huit observations. *Revue de Chirurgie Ortho-
       pédique*, **64**, 367-374.

SOLITARY CHONDROMA
(Synonym: enchondroma)

DEFINITION

This is a benign intraosseous tumor, made up of well-differentiated cartilage. It is probably a hamartoma originating from included cartilaginous
germs.

FREQUENCY

It occurs rather frequently. In terms of incidence, it is second only to histiocytic fibroma and exostosis.

SEX

There is no predilection for sex (Fig. 156).

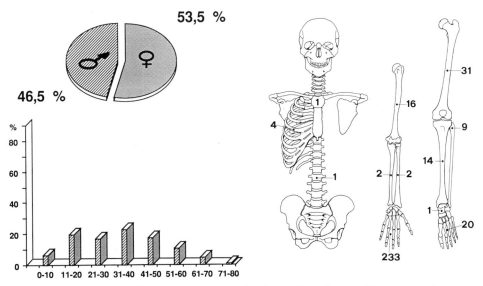

FIG. 156. - Sex, age and site in 334 cases of solitary chondroma. These are only cases
which were operated and verified histologically.

AGE

If we consider it to be a hamartoma, it may be presumed that C. initiates its development during childhood. Nonetheless, the first diagnosis is made at any age, and more often from 10 to 50 years of age (Fig. 156). This, at least in part, depends on the fact the C. remains for a long time — and at times for an entire life-time — completely asymptomatic.

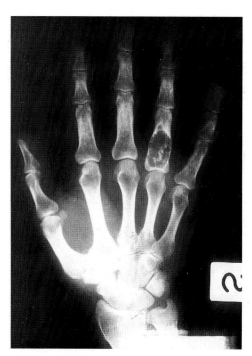

FIG. 157. - Chondroma of the first phalanx in a male aged 67.

LOCALIZATION

C. occurs only in bones which are preformed in cartilage. Its distribution is very characteristic. Two-thirds of the cases are observed in the tubular bones of the hand: more often the first phalanx, followed, in this order, by the metacarpals, second phalanx, and terminal phalanx. C. constitutes the tumor which occurs most frequently in the bones of the hand. More rarely, it may be observed in the tubular bones of the foot. Here, the incidence does not surpass that observed in many other parts of the skeleton. In exceptional cases, it may be observed in the bones of the carpus and tarsus (Fig. 163b).

Many of the remaining C. are distributed in the long bones of the limbs, with evident preference for the femur and humerus. Last in order of frequency is localization in the skeleton of the trunk (Fig. 156). The incidence of C. in the long bones of the limbs and in the skeleton of the trunk is much greater than that which has been ascertained, as most cases of C. in these sites remain asymptomatic for the entire life-time.

It is interesting to compare the skeletal distribution of C. with that of central chondrosarcoma. In some ways they are antithetical. Nearly all cartilaginous tumors of the hand are benign. Most cartilaginous tumors of the skeleton of the trunk and cranio-facial bones are malignant. Finally, in the long bones of the limbs, central chondrosarcomas are probably just as frequent as C.

In the phalanges and in the metacarpals C. is generally formed in proximity of the fertile cartilage. Thus, it is usually (but not always) oriented towards the proximal part of the phalanges and towards the distal part of the metacarpals. In the hand, the tumor may extend to the entire diaphysis. In the long bones it may be metadiaphyseal or diaphyseal, probably as a result of a migration in the course of bone growth. In both the hand and in the long bones, C. may involve the epiphysis when the growth cartilage has disappeared; but it may also have an epiphyseal origin (like chondroblastoma) (Figs. 163a, 164).

SYMPTOMS

C. is a tumor which grows slowly; it is small in size and it is nearly avascular. Thus[1] it often remains asymptomatic. If it does cause symptoms, it is because localized in small and superficial bones such as the tubular bone of the hand, it easily provokes expansion of the bone and visible and bothersome swelling, or because a painful pathologic fracture intervenes. This second possibility is also more common in the bones of the hand, where the cortex is considerably thinned and made fragile even by a small tumor. In the long bones of the limbs, instead, most C. remain indefinitely asymptomatic and are discovered by chance, when an x-ray is obtained for some other reason, or a pathologic fracture occurs.

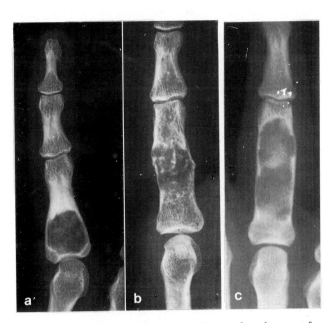

FIG. 158. - Three examples of solitary chondroma of a phalanx of the hand in adults. In (b) observe the pathological fracture.

When pain occurs, in a cartilaginous tumor of the long bones of the limbs or of the skeleton of the trunk, in the absence of a pathologic fracture, malignancy is suspected.

RADIOGRAPHIC FEATURES

C. appears as an osteolytic area with well-defined boundaries, at times

---

(1) As may easily be deduced if we think of angiomas, osteoid osteoma, glomus tumor and other richly vascularized tumors, the variations in tension connected to an intense hematic irroration and the presence of nerves in the walls of the blood vessels cause pain even in tumors of slow and limited growth.

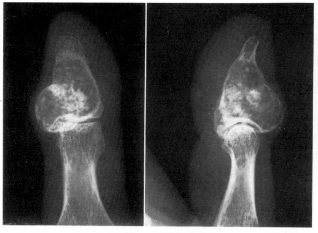

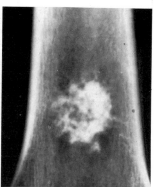

Fig. 160.

Fig. 159.

Fig. 159. - Chondroma of the terminal phalanx of the thumb with considerable expansion of the bone in a female aged 42 years.

Fig. 160. - Old calcified chondroma in the distal diaphysis of the femur in a male aged 48 years. Radiographs were obtained for unrelated reasons.

polycyclical due to the lobulated structure of the tumor cartilage. As the tumor grows slowly, its limits are often marked by a thin rim of reactive osteosclerosis (Fig. 167).

It must be recalled that C. is always a tumor of **small or moderate size**. If a very large tumor is observed, it is not a C. or it is a C. which has changed into a chondrosarcoma.

Often, C. is central and does not expand, or expands only slightly, the cortex without attenuating it excessively. In other cases, particularly in the hand, it is eccentric and considerably expands the cortex, which may be very thin, or, at times, nearly absent. Evidently, because of the small diameter of the tubular bones of the hand, even a C. of modest size may cause considerable expansion of the cortex (Figs. 158-167).

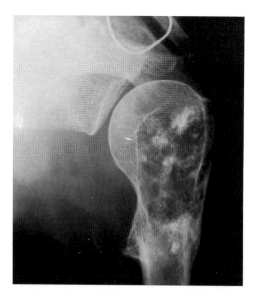

Fig. 161. - Chondroma in a female aged 54 years, chance radiographic finding while treating a fracture of the proximal humerus with acromioclavicular dislocation. The chondroma is completely asymptomatic and radiographically stabilized.

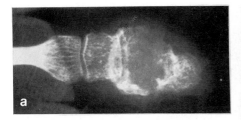

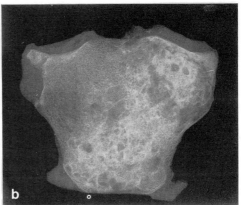

FIG. 162. - (a) Chondroma of the second phalanx of the third toe in a female aged 28 years. (b) Chondroma of the sternal manubrium in a female aged 20 years (Resected specimen).

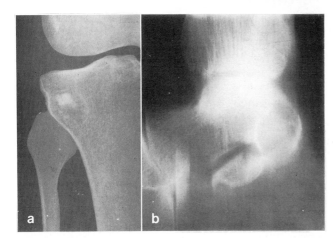

FIG. 163. - (a) Metaepiphyseal chondroma in a female aged 30 years. Casual radiographic finding. (b) Chondroma of the astragalus in a male aged 33 years, who complained of mild pain (stratigraphy).

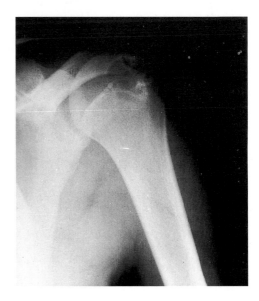

FIG. 164. - Chondroma of the humeral epiphysis in a boy aged 16 years complained of pain for the past 10 months. Age, symptoms, site and radiographic picture were all typical of chondroblastoma.

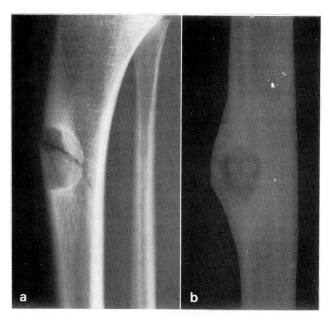

FIG. 165. - (a) Intracortical chondroma of the tibial diaphysis in a male aged 10 years, with pathologic fracture. (b) Intracortical chondroma of the humeral diaphysis in a female aged 17 years.

Often C. contains minute radiopaque granules, which are the expression of calcifications of the tumoral cartilage. In other cases, there are intratumoral gross areas and radiopaque bands due to calcification and ossification. C. which have aged, particularly in the long bones of the limbs, often manifest an intense and diffused radiopacity in bumpy and notched spots, expressing the extensive calcification and ossification of a cartilage which is no longer fertile and for the most part necrotic. C. which are intensely and diffusedly calcified are in fact observed during adult age. These images of calcification, when they are present, constitute the most characteristic, and practically pathognomic radiographic feature of C. (Fig. 160, 161).

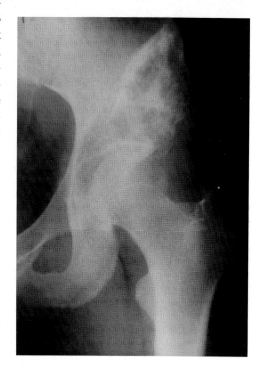

FIG. 166. - Chondroma of the iliac wing in a female aged 33 years, chance radiographic finding.

GROSS PATHOLOGIC FEATURES

The macroscopic picture is very characteristic because it has the aspect of hyaline cartilage. The tumor is made up of packed and faceted lobuli of white-to-light blue and semi-translucent cartilage. The tissue is obviously nearly deprived of blood. The tumoral cartilage is frequently altered by regressive phenomena and thus it may appear to be softer, white-opaque, resembling boiled rice, or in some areas it may have a mucoid aspect. The areas of calcification-ossification resemble opaque yellowish-white clots, they are chalky, granulous and hard.

The limits of C. are irregular, as lobules of cartilage push towards the mesh of the cancellous bone and within niches excavated in the cortical bone. This finding is interesting because it implies that the curettage of a C. may easily leave residues of cartilage in situ.

Bone scan captation may vary; it may even be decidedly increased, without signifying a diagnosis of chondrosarcoma.

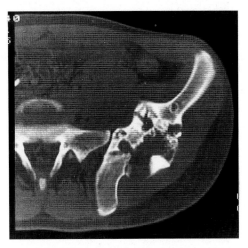

HISTOPATHOLOGIC FEATURES

This is a rather well-differentiated and mature cartilaginous tissue. The chondrocytes are sparse, with small round, dense and deeply stained nuclei, of relatively uniform size. At times the cells are clustered in isogenous groups, more often they are isolated. Cells having

FIG. 167. - Chondroma of the iliac wing in a boy aged 17 years, asymptomatic: chance radiographic finding. Incisional biopsy revealed chondroma. The lesion remained stable at clinical and radiographic monitoring three years after biopsy.

double nuclei are rare (at most not more than 1-2 per microscopic field under medium enlargement) (Fig. 168-170). In some areas the tissue has a myxoid aspect, with spindle-stellate cells and an essentially fluid ground substance. In others, calcification and/or ossification of the cartilage may be observed. The presence of cartilaginous lobuli slightly penetrating the host bone at the periphery of the tumor does not indicate malignancy.

HISTOGENESIS AND PATHOGENESIS

Several different elements (site, age, anatomical features, course) lead us to believe that C. is a hamartoma originating from an island of fertile cartilage, which is quite often detached from the growth cartilage. Similar cartila-

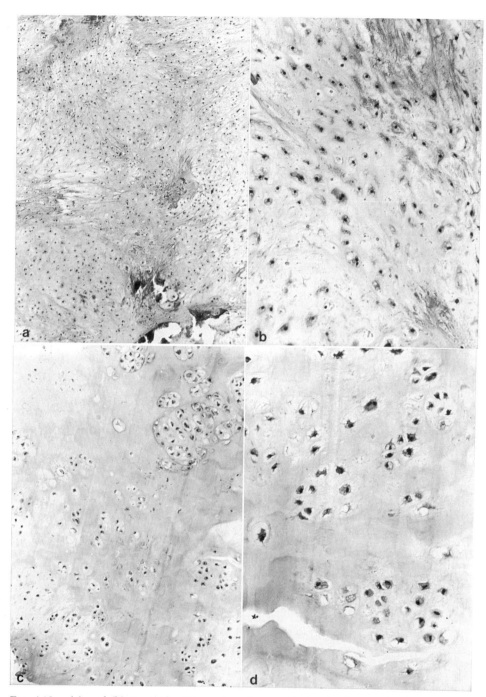

FIG. 168. - (a) and (b) Typical solitary chondroma. Under the largest enlargement (b) two cells with a double nucleus are observed. (c) and (d) Chondroma of the hand. By comparison with (a, b) (the enlargements are the same) observe greater anisocytosis with a fair frequency of binucleate cells. These aspects do not have an unfavorable prognostic meaning, when dealing with a chondroma of the hand (*Hemat.-eos.*, 80, 200, 80, 200 x).

ginous remains (hamartiae) have rarely been observed in the metaphyseal areas systematically sectioned on autopsy in individuals having a normal skeleton (Jaffe, 1958).

DIAGNOSIS

The problem of diagnosis is certainly not that of recognizing C., also because — apart from the clinical and radiographic features — the hyperplastic cartilage (for example, bone callus or synovial chondromatosis) has a different histological aspect. The problem is that of histologically evaluating whether there are signs of malignancy. The limits separating C. from grade 1 chondrosarcoma are not sharp. To this purpose, diagnostic conclusions must be based on a microscopic examination of the vital and non-calcified areas of the tumor (calcification is associated with changes in the chondrocytes which do not allow for an evaluation to be made). Clinical features are also of considerable diagnostic importance (pain, growth of the tumor), as well as radiographic and scintigraphic data (signs of activity). Finally, the area from which the tumor originates must be taken into account. If the C. is located in the hand, if it is a C. in Ollier's chondromatosis (see further on), or a periosteal C. (see further on), fair aspects of proliferative vivacity are compatible with complete benignity (Fig. 168b, c). If instead it is a central cartilaginous

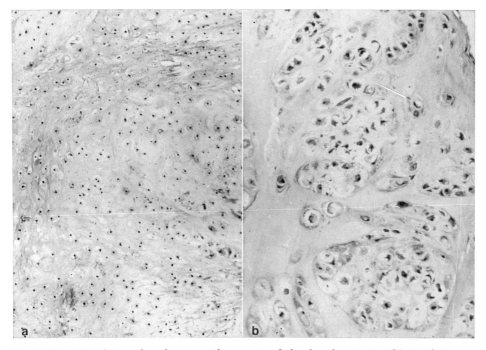

FIG. 169. - (a) Solitary chondroma with aspects of absolute benignity. (b) Grade 1 central chondrosarcoma of the humeral diaphysis: the same case as Fig. 210a. The two microphotographs are at the same enlargement (*Hemat.-eos.*, 200, 200 x).

tumor of the long bones or the skeleton of the trunk, in an adult, the same histological aspects signify low-grade malignancy (Figs. 169, 170). For the differential histological features for benignity and malignancy, see central chondrosarcoma.

Problems of differential diagnosis with non-cartilaginous lesion may occur only in terms of the radiographic picture, as the macroscopic and histological pictures leave no doubts as to the cartilaginous nature of the tumor. Radiographically, a C. of the hand is difficult to confuse with another lesion, and only if there is no intratumoral calcification. **Giant cell tumor** which is rare in the metacarpals and even more rare in the phalanges, always involves the epiphysis and is more expansive. **Giant cell reparative granuloma** lacks calcifications, at times expanding the bone. **Fibrous dysplasia**, when it involves the hand, is nearly always polyostotic (see differential diagnosis of chondromatosis).

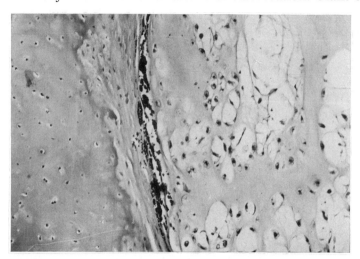

FIG. 170. - Solitary chondroma of a rib. To the left, normal costal cartilage. To the right, tumoral cartilaginous tissue. This chondroma, even in consideration of its site, must be considered borderline between benign and malignant or suspected of malignant evolution (*Hemat.-eos.*, 200 x).

Epidermoid cyst (Fig. 17) produces an osteolytic lacuna, but it is exclusive of the last phalanx and, eroding the bone from the outside, it always causes a saucerlike lysis of the cortical bone. The same may be said for subungueal **glomus tumor**.

In the long bones, if C. is metaepiphyseal and not-calcified, it may be similar to **giant cell tumor** or **chondroblastoma**. If it is diaphyseal and not calcified, it may be difficult to distinguish from a **localized fibrous dysplasia** or a **bone cyst**.

Finally, a classic radiographic differential diagnosis is that between calcified C. of the long bones in the adult and **metadiaphyseal bone infarct**. Despite a certain resemblance, the distinction may be made based only on the radiographic evaluation (Figs. 1 and 160, 161). The radiopaque spots of C. are small, rounded, ammassed in a circumscribed area, at times alternated with or surrounded by areas of osteolysis, and they never fuse with the trabeculae of the surrounding bone. The radiopacity of infarct, instead, is more like bands of smoke, and in any case it is fused with the surrounding cancellous and cortical bone (thickened). Histologically, the difference is clear: in chondroma, however intensely calcified and ossified, there are always cartilaginous remnants.

COURSE

C. grows rather slowly. Probably, growth tends to be exhausted at the beginning of adult age, as generally occurs in hamartomas. C. which are asymptomatic and intensely calcified in the adult in fact constitute tumors which are extinguished and amply necrotic.

Nonetheless, as is the case in exostoses, probably the quiescent cartilaginous remains in the adult may give origin to a chondrosarcoma or another type of sarcoma. We say «probably» because it is very difficult to demonstrate this transformation. When there is a chondrosarcoma, it is nearly always impossible to exclude whether we are dealing with a chondrosarcoma from the very beginning; if there is another type of sarcoma (fibrosarcoma, malignant fibrous histiocytoma, osteosarcoma), occurring on a pre-existing and asymptomatic cartilaginous tumor, the latter usually has some atypical histological aspect, enough to have to be classified as grade 1 or 2 central chondrosarcoma (see so-called dedifferentiated chondrosarcoma).

TREATMENT

C. located in the hand which do not cause any symptom may be left in situ; otherwise, curettage and bone grafting are used. In these cases, a histological examination is carried out after curettage; that is, excisional biopsy is carried out. Curettage often leaves some traces of the tumor in situ, and thus it is advisable to treat the walls with burr drill and phenol. Only in rare cases, in which rapid growth and the large size of the cartilaginous tumor of the hand lead one to suspect its malignancy, incisional biopsy will be required, ascertaining malignancy, and thus, if necessary, a more aggressive type of treatment may be resorted to (see chondrosarcoma).

Calcified and asymptomatic C. of the long bones do not require any type of treatment. The patient will have to be advised to report any pain occurring in the area of the C. In the case of osteolytic and/or symptomatic C. of the long bones, treatment is obviously surgical. Even if the clinical, radiographic and macroscopic pictures do not indicate any malignancy, histological confirmation may be obtained with an incisional biopsy. It is, however, necessary after curettage has been performed, to histologically examine the entire tumor. In fact, a limited sampling could delete those tumoral areas in which initial malignant transformation may have taken place. The walls are treated with burr drill and phenol and the cavity is filled with bone grafts. If the histological examination of the entire tumor should reveal any signs of suspected initial malignancy, the patient will have to be carefully monitored, as recurrence will be possible. If recurrence should be manifested, a more drastic form of treatment will be used, with resection of the skeletal segment.

In cartilaginous tumors of the skeleton of the trunk, the fact that most of these cases are chondrosarcomas must be taken into account. Thus, care must be taken in bioptic evaluation and surgery must be adequately planned and preferably result in wide margins.

PROGNOSIS

C. of the hand nearly always heal, even if curettage leaves some traces of the tumor in situ. At times, there may be limited recurrence, but exceptionally will further surgery be required. If a second operation is performed, the histological aspect of the recurrence is generally not different from that of the original tumor. Nonetheless, there are very rare cases in which the cartilaginous tumor of the hand is or becomes a chondrosarcoma.

Even most cases of C. of the long bones heal with curettage. Those which recur often reveal histological signs of low-grade malignancy.

PERIOSTEAL CHONDROMA
(Synonym: juxtacortical chondroma)

It is a variety of C. which develops at the surface of the bone, under the periosteum or in the insertion sites of the tendons and ligaments. In this latter localization the definition of juxtacortical chondroma used by Jaffe (1958) appears to be the most appropriate.

P.C. occurs rarely, it is observed at **ages** varying from childhood to maturity and it is **localized** in the metaphyseal or metadiaphyseal regions of the long bones, particularly in the proximal humerus (Fig. 171).

Clinically, it causes moderate swelling which grows slowly and it may become of fair size. Swelling has little or no pain.

Radiographically, there is saucerlike excavation of the cortex, which is rather superficial, at times mildly polycyclical, marked by a rim of osteosclerosis. Generally, there is no penetration in the medullary canal. The lenticular or hemispherical chondromatous mass has a radiotransparence which is similar to that of the soft tissues, and which at times contains radiopaque granules and spots expressing calcification and/or ossification of the cartilage. Along the perimeter of the C. the periosteum may produce a bone spur which

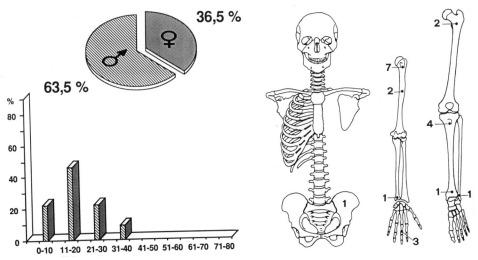

FIG. 171. - Sex, age and site in 22 cases of periosteal chondroma.

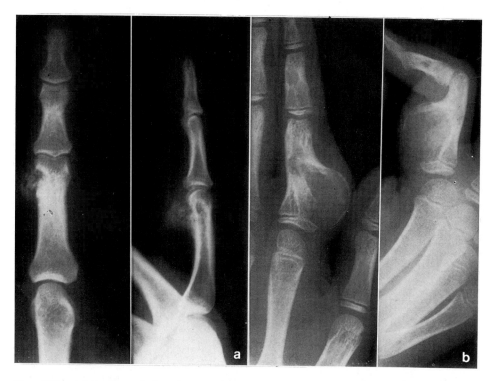

FIG. 172. - (a) Periosteal chondroma of a phalanx in a female aged 15 years. (b) Chondroma with prevalently peripheral development of the phalanx in a girl aged 8 years.

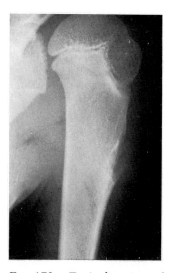

FIG. 173. - Typical periosteal chondroma in a boy aged 10 years.

is elevated from the cortex, and which embraces the base of the tumor (Figs. 172-174).

Macroscopically, the tumor is composed of packed lobuli of compact hyaline cartilage.

Histologically, as compared to central C., it is generally more cellular. The cells also tend to be larger, at times with some polydimensionality of the nuclei, plump nuclei, some binucleated cells. Thus, it is «normal» to find numerous cells, plump nuclei, mild pleomorphism, a few double nuclei, and it does not have the same prognostic meaning that it would have in a central cartilaginous tumor of the long bones or the trunk.

If the P.C. is asymptomatic and does not grow in time (as it usually does not grow after body growth has ended), periodical monitoring will suffice, and surgery is not required. If it is submitted to surgery, en bloc excision, marginal or wide, guarantees healing; but complete intralesional removal also has a high success rate.

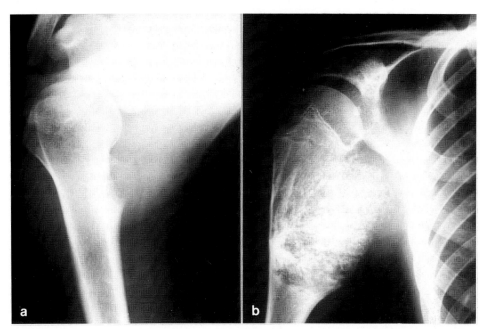

FIG. 174. - (a) Periosteal chondroma of the proximal humerus in a female aged 25 years. Lesion characterized by slight pain, submitted to marginal excision. (b) Periosteal chondroma in a boy aged 13 years. Biopsy showed a cartilaginous tumor with mild aspects of anaplasia (grade 1). Nonetheless, considering the young age of the patient, the apparently periosteal origin of the tumor, and its extent, which would have required rather invasive surgical treatment, we decided not to operate. Five years later the chondroma seemed to be substantially stabilized.

MULTIPLE CHONDROMAS
(Synonyms: chondromatosis, Ollier's disease)

DEFINITION

Unlike multiple exostoses, M.C. do not show any heredity, they are more variable in number and extent, and they tend to be prevalently localized in one half of the body. M.C. very rarely coexist with angiomas of the skin and/or of the soft tissues (**Maffucci syndrome**).

In their most typical and diffused expression, M.C. are characterized by a) peculiar radiographic and histological aspects, b) shortening and deformity of the affected bones, c) frequent transformation in chondrosarcoma.

FREQUENCY

M.C. occur ten times less frequently than solitary chondroma. Severe and diffused chondromatosis occurs rarely. Maffucci syndrome occurs in exceptional cases.

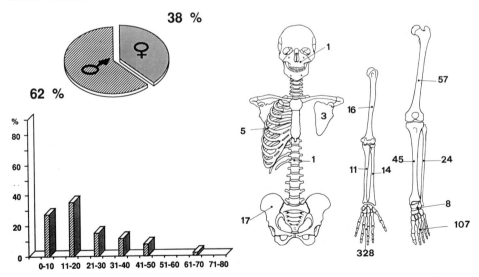

FIG. 175. - Sex, age and site in 51 cases of multiple chondromas (637 localizations).

SEX

There is evident predilection for the male sex.

AGE

Unlike solitary chondroma, M.C. do not remain asymptomatic for long. In the more diffused and severe forms, symptoms appear in early childhood (Fig. 175).

LOCALIZATION

Unlike multiple exostoses but similar to fibrous dysplasia of the skeleton and diffused angiomas of the soft tissues, M.C. tend to be exclusive or prevalent in one half of the body.

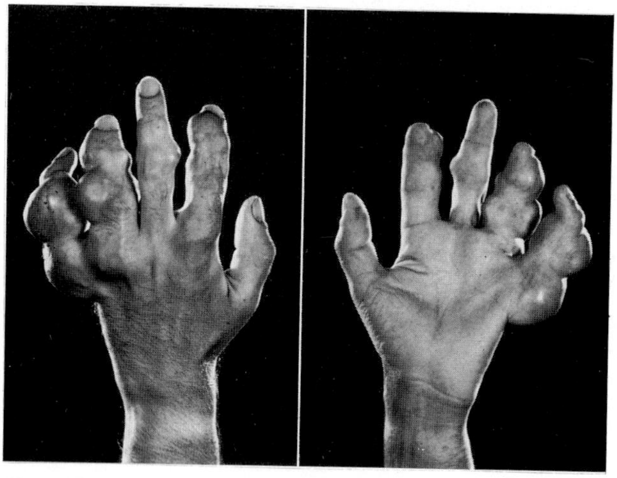

FIG. 176. - Chondromatosis in a male aged 35 years.

The diffusion of C. varies. At times there are only a few C. limited to one or two rays of the hand, rarely in the foot. At other times they are diffused to the skeleton of the hand, of the two hands, of one foot, and, possibly, to a more proximal part of the same limb. In other cases still, diffusion is hemisomic, extended to two limbs and to the skeleton of the trunk, possibly with some more limited localizations in the contralateral hemisoma. Finally, C. are rarely diffused to all four of the limbs and to the skeleton of the trunk, but always prevalently in one half of the body. The bones which are most frequently affected, after the hand, are, in this order, the tubular bones of the foot, the femur, the bones of the leg, the humerus and the bones of the forearm, and the pelvis (Fig. 175).

In the long bones, C. begin to develop in the metaphysis. From here they may extend towards the diaphysis. In the bones of the hand and foot, C. may easily involve the entire metacarpus, metatarsus, or phalanx. In more severe forms, the epiphysis may also be involved from an early age. Otherwise, the epiphyses may be involved when the growth cartilage disappears. Generally, C. are not observed in either the bones of the carpus or in those of the tarsus. The skeleton of the trunk is scarcely involved by the disease. In more extended forms of the disease, some C. may be observed in the pelvis, more rarely in the scapula, ribs, sternum, and vertebral column. The cranial base and the facial bones which are pre-formed in cartilage are hardly ever involved by C.

SYMPTOMS

As previously stated, the occurrence of symptoms is constant and even early. In fact, M.C. usually grow much more than solitary C., and they may cause shortening and axial deviations.

In the hands, they are manifested with ball-like or knot-like swelling, which is typical (Figs. 176, 180a). In more severe forms of the disease, deviations and shortening of the fingers are associated. At times the hand may be monstruously deformed. Swelling has little or no pain, unless there are pathologic fractures. In the more proximal parts of the limbs there may be mild expansion in the regions corresponding to the metaphyses and, as bone growth progresses, there may be shortening and deformity. Typically, shortening and deformity are exclusive or prevalent in one limb or in one half of the body (unlike multiple exostoses). In the upper limb, deformity of

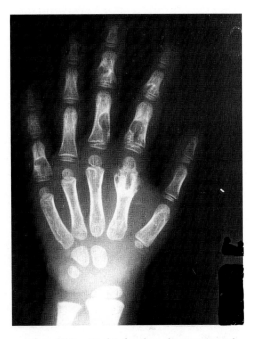

Fig. 177. - Multiple chondromas in a female aged 5 years.

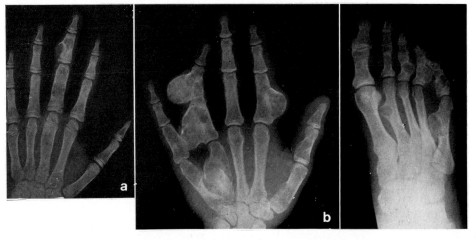

Fig. 178. - (a) Multiple chondromas of a digital ray in a boy aged 11 years. (b) Hand and foot in a case of chondromatosis. Female aged 19 years.

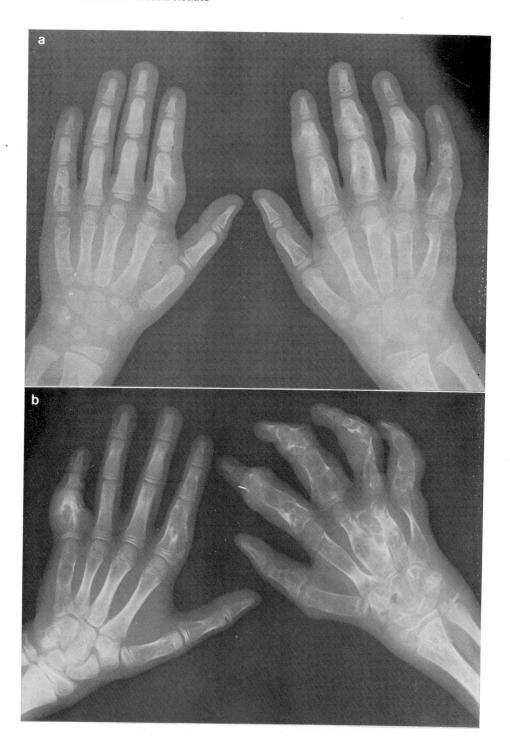

FIG. 179. - Chondromatosis associated with skin angiomas (Maffucci syndrome). (a) At 3 years of age. (b) At 9 years of age.

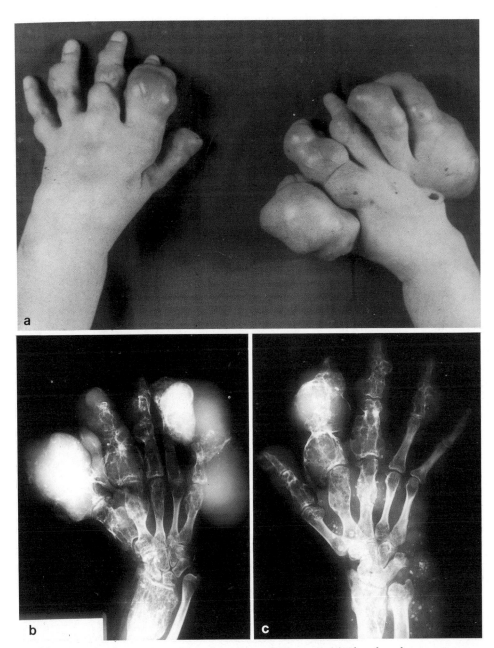

FIG. 180. - Maffucci syndrome in a female aged 30 years. (a) The chondromatous masses and the skin angiomas are observed, (b, c) Radiograms show bubbly osteolyses of the chondromas, some of which vastly invading the soft tissues. In (c) phleboliths typical of angiomas are observed.

the forearm with lateral convexity of the radius, ulnar deviation of the hand, at times dislocation of the radial head are all characteristic. This deformity, which is similar to that due to multiple exostoses, is caused by shortening of the ulna which is more severe than that of the radius, for the same reasons which are recalled with regard to multiple exostoses (see specific chapter). In the lower limb, valgus of the knee, which may be of extreme degrees, and shortening which even measures a few centimeters as early as during infancy, and which may exceed 10 centimeters during adult age, are characteristic. In rare forms of the disease, where C. achieve a maximum amount of expansion, large metaphyseal swelling may be observed.

In Maffucci syndrome (Figs. 179, 180) multiple angiomas coexist, not necessarily in the same site as the C. These are cutaneous and subcutaneous angiomas, more rarely muscular ones. At times, they are diffused angiomas, with phlebectasia. At times visceral angiomas coexist. Instead, there are no skeletal angiomas.

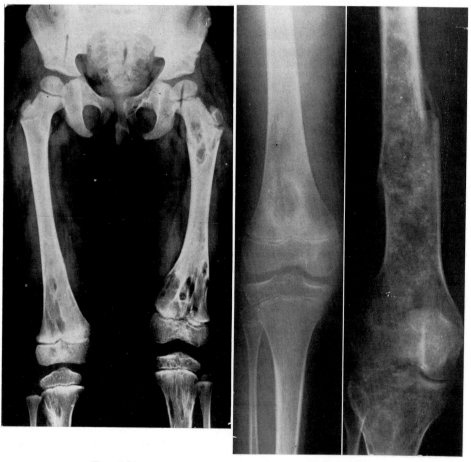

FIG. 181.   FIG. 182.

FIG. 181. - Chondromatosis in a boy aged 4 years. Observe shortening of the left femur, which is more severely involved.

FIG. 182. - Right femur in chondromatosis at ages 9 and 22. (Same case as Fig. 179).

RADIOGRAPHIC FEATURES

In its entirety it is very characteristic. Particularly in the metaphyses of the long bones (the aspect is less evident in the hand) there are images of osteolysis which are vaguely similar to large pendent drops descending from the metaphysis towards the diaphysis (Fig. 181). It may be useful to imagine the tumoral cartilage «dripping» in large sticky drops from the physis towards the diaphysis. The boundaries of these osteolytic images are quite clear, marked by a thin line of osteosclerosis. Between one «drop» and another there are shoots of ossification which may form «W» and upturned «M» images (Fig. 183). Other times, the osteolysis is concamerated and bubbling.

At times, particularly in the bones of the hand, but also in the metaphyses of the long bones, the cortex is expanded or cancelled, and the cartilaginous masses protrude towards the soft tissues (Figs. 179, 180, 183, 184). The areas of osteolysis may considerably extend towards the diaphysis. At times there are subperiosteal osteo-

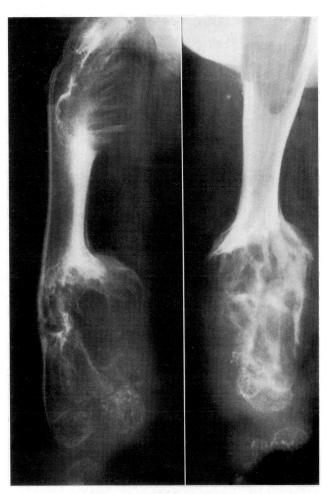

FIG. 183. - Severe case of chondromatosis in a boy aged 1 and 1/2 years.

lyses, with a radiographic aspect which is typical of periosteal C. Areolar osteolyses and calcar dotting may be observed in the epiphyses, even prior to closure of the fertile cartilage (Fig. 183).

In chondromatous masses there may be typical granular calcifications of the C. (Fig. 182).

The bone in which the C. develop is often shortened and crooked (Figs. 181-184).

GROSS PATHOLOGIC FEATURES

They are the same as those of solitary C. with the exception of extent and expansion of the cartilaginous masses and the shortening-deformity of the skeletal segments. Like solitary chondroma, M.C. are made up of lobuli which are packed and faceted, of cartilaginous aspect. In more extensive forms and in the adult, cartilaginous nodules may be diffused to the epiphysis and along the diaphysis. The cortex may appear to be expanded in certain sites and, particularly in the bones of the hand, it may be thin or absent, as C. is covered by periosteum alone.

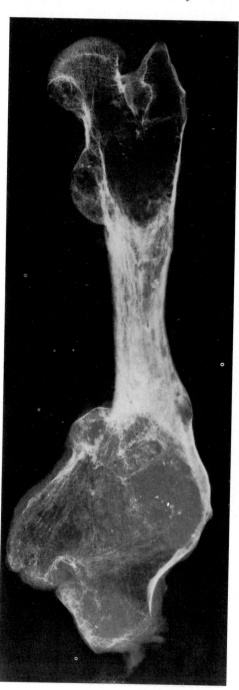

HISTOPATHOLOGIC FEATURES

The histological aspect of M.C. generally differs from that of solitary C. The tissue is more cellular, its nuclei are larger, they are less uniform, and frequently double. Frequently, it has a structure which tends towards a myxoid one, characterized by mildly spindle-stellate cells and rather fluid ground substance (Fig. 185). These histological aspects, which reveal the vivid chondromatous proliferation, agree with the clinical behavior of M.C., the growth of which is more active and more persistent than

Fig. 184. - Male aged 35 years, with severe chondromatosis. In the proximal humerus grade 2 central chondrosarcoma occurred, for which resection-endoprosthesis was performed. After 3 years, left hip disarticulation as a result of the severity of the chondromatosis which, in the lower left limb, had no histological features of malignancy. X-ray of the femur.

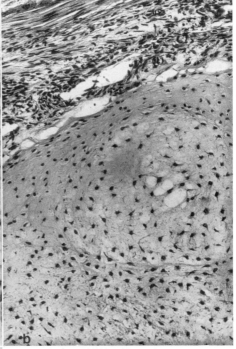

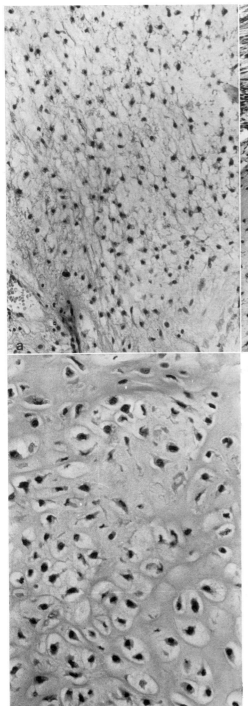

FIG. 185. - Histological aspects of chondromatosis (*Hemat.-eos.*, 200, 200, 500 x).

that of solitary C. Even if these histological aspects do not as yet indicate chondrosarcomatous transformation, they do confirm Jaffe's correct observation (1958) that M.C. constitute a pre-sarcomatous state.

PATHOGENESIS

The multiplicity of C., the prevalent hemisomic distribution, the possible association with angiomas of the soft tissues, are all elements which agree with its hamartomatous genesis. Cartilaginous hamartiae could derive from either fertile metaphyseal cartilage or the deep layer of the periosteum (Jaffe, 1958).

Of considerable importance is the fact that, unlike solitary C., exostoses, and many other hamartomas, the growth of which tends to end as body growth does, M.C. maintain considerable proliferative potential for a longer period of time, even in adult age.

DIAGNOSIS

The clinical, radiographic, and anatomical picture of M.C. is absolutely characteristic. Diagnosis is easy. The only possible confusion could involve **fibrous dysplasia**. Even fibrous dysplasia may be prevalently hemisomic and involve the skeleton of the hand. Furthermore, the tissue of fibrous dysplasia may contain cartilaginous islands. Fibrous dysplasia may be mistaken for chondromatosis if a small biopsy specimen made up of one of these cartilaginous islands is examined under the microscope, without taking the radiographic picture into account.

Vice versa, the radiographic picture of fibrous dysplasia is very different from that of chondromatosis, and a more ample histological examination will show the typical fibro-osseous tissue of fibrous dysplasia, alongside cartilaginous tissue. No mistake can be made with **multiple exostoses** (see specific chapter).

COURSE AND PROGNOSIS

As observed, M.C. tend to grow considerably, even during adult age. In other cases, the growth of C. stabilizes, as body growth ends.

In any case, transformation in sarcoma (usually chondrosarcoma, but also fibrosarcoma, malignant fibrous histiocytoma, osteosarcoma) is very frequent, probably occurring in 30 to 50% of all cases. Malignant transformation is always manifested during adult age, at times even at an advanced age. Rarely is sarcomatous transformation manifested in two different skeletal segments in the same patient, even 20-30 years between the first and the second sarcoma. Thus, as previously observed with regard to multiple exostoses, the actual incidence of chondrosarcoma could be evaluated by monitoring those affected with M.C. for their entire lifetimes. Malignant transformation does not strictly depend on the diffusion of the chondromas. It may also be observed in moderate monomelic cases. Nonetheless, as is the case for solitary C., M.C. localized in the hand are rarely transformed into sarcoma.

TREATMENT

This involves surgical treatment of those C. which cause symptoms. At times resection or amputation is required, particularly of one or more digital rays.

Skeletal deformities may be corrected by osteotomies, which consolidate relatively well.

If there should be malignant transformation, treatment is the same as that used for chondrosarcoma or for any other sarcoma present.

REFERENCES

1956 JAFFE H. L.: Juxtacortical chondroma. *Bulletin of the Hospital for Joint Diseases*, **17**, 20-29.

1957 STRINGA G.: *I condromi della mano*. Edizioni Scientifiche Istituto Ortopedico Toscano, Firenze.

1958 JAFFE H. L.: *Tumors and tumorous conditions of the bones and joints*. Lea & Febiger, Philadelphia.

1964 MARMOR L.: Periosteal chondroma (juxtacortical chondroma). *Clinical Orthopaedics*, **37**, 150-153.

1965 COWAN W. K.: Malignant change and multiple metastases in Ollier's disease. *Journal of Clinical Pathology*, **18**, 650-653.

1966 BRADDOCK G. T. F., HADLOW V. D.: Osteosarcoma in enchondromatosis (Ollier's disease). Report of a case. *Journal of Bone and Joint Surgery*, **48-B**, 145-149.

1967 MANGINI U.: Tumors of the skeleton of the hand. *Bulletin of the Hospital for Joint Diseases*, **28**, 61-103.

1969 NOSANCHUK J. S., KAUFER H.: Recurrent periosteal chondroma. Report of two cases and a review of the literature. *Journal of Bone and Joint Surgery*, **51-A**, 375-380.

1970 UNGAR F.: Revisione clinico-statistica di 187 condromi e di 94 condrosarcomi osservati nel Centro Tumori degli Organi di Movimento di Firenze. *Archivio Putti*, **25**, 257-278.

1971 JEWUSIAK E. M., SPENCE K. F., SELL K. W.: Solitary benign enchondroma of the long bones of the hand. Results of curettage and packing with freeze-dried cancellous-bone allograft. *Journal of Bone and Joint Surgery*, **53-A**, 1587-1590.

1971 ROCKWELL M. A., ENNEKING W. F.: Osteosarcoma developing in solitary enchondroma of the tibia. *Journal of Bone and Joint Surgery*, **53-A**, 341-344.

1971 TAKIGAWA K.: Chondroma of the bones of the hand. A review of 110 cases. *Journal of Bone and Joint Surgery*, **53-A**, 1591-1600.

1972 ROCKWELL M. A., SAITER E. T., ENNEKING W. F.: Periosteal chondroma. *Journal of Bone and Joint Surgery*, **54-A**, 102-108.

1973 CAMPANACCI M., LEONESSA C., BONI A.: Tumori cartilaginei dello scheletro della mano. Studio di 112 osservazioni. *La chirurgia degli organi di movimento*, **62**, 413-490.

1973 LEWIS R. J., KETCHAM A. S.: Maffucci's Syndrome: Functional and neoplastic significance. Case report and review of the literature. *Journal of Bone and Joint Surgery*, **55-A**, 1465-1479.

1975 PEYROU P. L.: *Problèmes orthopédiques des tumeurs cartilagineuses multiples, enchondromatose, maladie exostosante, syndrome de Maffucci*. Thèse médicine, Paris.

1978 BORIANI S., LAUS M.: Condromi e condromatosi. Studio di 265 osservazioni di cui 200 controllate a distanza. *Giornale Italiano di Ortopedia e Traumatologia*, **4**, 351-354.

1979 SANERKIN N. G., WOODS C. G.: Fibrosarcomata and malignant fibrous histiocytomata arising in relation to enchondromata. *Journal of Bone and Joint Surgery*, **61-B**, 366-372.

1980 MIRRA J.M.: *Bone tumors. Diagnosis and treatment*. Lippincott, Philadelphia, Toronto.

1981 SCHAJOWICZ F.: *Tumors and tumor-like lesions of bone and joints*. Springer-Verlag, New York.

1982 BERTONI F., BORIANI S., CAMPANACCI M.: Periosteal chondrosarcoma and periosteal osteosarcoma. Two distinct entities. *Journal of Bone and Joint Surgery*, **64-B**, 370-376.

1982 GARRISON R., UNNI K., MC LEOD R., PRITCHARD D., DAHLIN D.: Chondrosarcoma arising in osteochondroma. *Cancer*, **48**, 1890-1897.

1983 BORIANI S., BACCHINI P., BERTONI F., CAMPANACCI M.: Periosteal chondroma. A review of 20 cases. *Journal of Bone and Joint Surgery*, **65-A**, 205-212.

1984 HUDSON T.M., SPRINGFIELD D.S., SPANIER S.: Benign exostosis and exostotic chondrosarcoma: evaluation of cartilage thickness by CT. *Radiology*, **152**, 595-599.

1985 MIRRA J.M., GOLD R., DOWNS J., ECKARDT J.J.: A new histological approach to the differentiation of enchondroma from chondrosarcoma of the bones. A clinico-pathologic analysis of 51 cases. *Clinical Orthopaedics*, **201**, 214-237.

1985 NOJIMA T., UNNI K., MC LEOD R., PRITCHARD D.: Periosteal chondroma and periosteal chondrosarcoma. *American Journal of Surgical Pathology*, **9**, 667-677.

1985 SUN T.C., SWEE R.G., SHIVES T.C., UNNI K.K.: Condrosarcoma in Maffucci's syndrome. *Journal of Bone and Joint Surgery*, **67-A**, 1214.

1987 AZOUZ E.M.: Case report 418. *Skeletal Radiology*, **16**, 236-239.

1987 LIU J., HUDKINS P., SWEE R., UNNI K.K.: Bone sarcoma associated with Ollier's disease. *Cancer*, **59**, 1376-1385.

1987 MITCHELL M.L., ACKERMAN L.V.: Case report 405. *Skeletal Radiology*, **16**, 61-66.

1987 SCHWARTZ H.S., ZIMMERMANN N.B., SIMON M.A., WROPLE R.R., MILLAR E.A., BONFIGLIO M.: The malignant potential of enchondromatosis. *Journal of Bone and Joint Surgery*, **59-A**, 269-274.

1989 GREENSPAN A.: Tumors of cartilage origin. *Orthopaedics Clinics of North America*, **20**, 247-366.

CHONDROBLASTOMA
(Synonyms: benign chondroblastoma, epiphyseal chondroblastoma)

DEFINITION

It is a benign tumor, which may be either epiphyseal or apophyseal, usually manifested during late childhood or adolescence, and composed of cells considered to be chondroblasts.

FREQUENCY

It is an unfrequent tumor.

SEX

There is predilection for the male sex, with a ratio of 2-3:1 (Fig. 186).

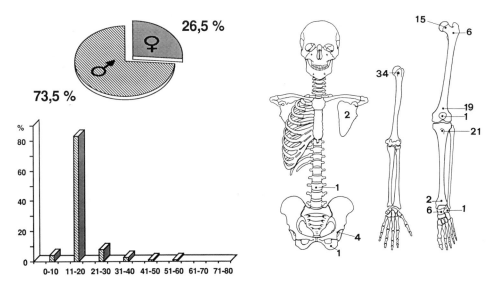

FIG. 186. - Sex, age and site in 113 cases of chondroblastoma.

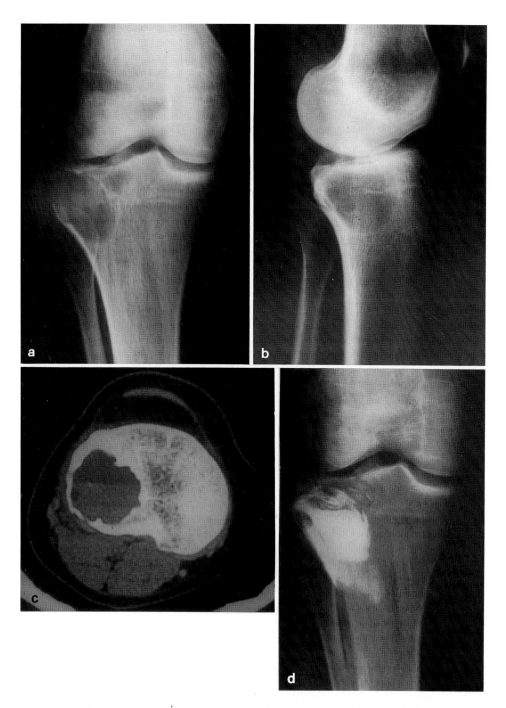

FIG. 187. - Chondroblastoma in a female aged 20 years. (a) and (b) reveal the typical localization of the osteolysis with rather evident limits marked by a thin sclerotic rim.
(c) CAT reveals a «level» image. In fact, there was a cystic cavity containing fluid. (d)
  Curettage, phenol, autogenous grafting (under the articular cartilage) and cement.

AGE

In most cases it is manifested between 10 and 20 years of age. As its growth is slow and symptoms may become consistent even several years after the onset of the tumor, it may also be observed at 25 or 30 years of age, but the evidence leads us to believe that it initiates during the period of skeletal growth. Nonetheless, only in exceptional cases is C.B. observed prior to 10 and after 20-25 years of age (Figs. 186, 193).

LOCALIZATION

Typical localization of C.B. is in an epiphysis or an apophysis in proximity of the growth cartilage. In its expansion, the tumor tends to destroy the growth cartilage, and thus it may extend from the epiphysis to the adjacent metaphysis. There are exceptional cases of C.B. developing in the opposite side of the growth cartilage, that is, in the metaphysis.

The parts of the skeleton which are most affected are the epiphysis and the apo-

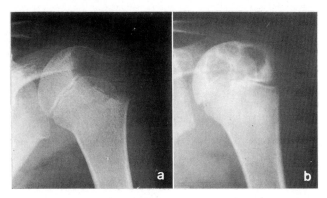

FIG. 188. - (a) Chondroblastoma in a female aged 11 years. (b) In a boy aged 10 years.

physis of the long bones, the femur, the humerus and the tibia, in that order. In the proximal femur, the tumor may originate from the epiphysis, or from the greater trochanter. C.B. of the humerus occurs in the proximal end where it often originates from the greater tuberosity. In the tibia, the most frequent localization is in the proximal end. Most cases of C.B. are localized in the knee, shoulder, and hip (Fig. 186).

More rare localizations are the pelvis (mostly around the Y-cartilage), the scapula (in the glenoid process), the talus and calcaneus, the ribs, the cranio-facial bones. These localizations (other than the epiphyses-apophyses of the long bones) are especially observed after 30 years of age (Dahlin and Ivins, 1972).

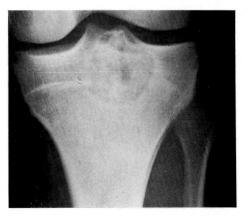

FIG. 189. - Chondroblastoma in a female aged 15 years.

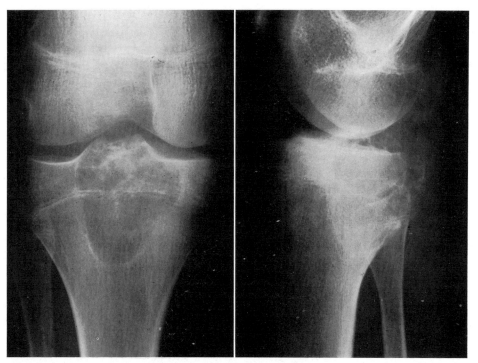

FIG. 190. - Chondroblastoma in a male aged 13 years.

SYMPTOMS

Symptoms often occur late and are mild. The tumor is usually diagnosed when symptoms have been present for months, at times, years. As the tumor is nearly always para-articular, symptoms are generally related to a joint, in this order: knee, shoulder, hip. There is a moderate pain, which may be revealed by trauma and awakened by pressure, and mild eccentric swelling of the bone may be palpated in more expansive and superficial tumors. Functional limitation of the joint, moderate joint serous or serohematic effusion, muscular hypotrophy may be observed.

As is often the case in other tumors (osteoid osteoma, osteoblastoma), C.B. may also provoke intense inflammatory reaction of the surrounding tissues, which is clinically expressed by pain, heat, edema, joint effusion, and joint stiffness; radiographically by diffused regional osteoporosis; and anatomically by hyperemia, chronic edema, muscular atrophy, osteoporosis, adherent fibrosis.

RADIOGRAPHIC FEATURES

The radiographic picture is rather typical, particularly in epiphyseal localizations of the tumor. There is an osteolytic area which, initially contained in the epiphysis, tends to surpass the growth cartilage, extending towards the metaphysis. At times, when the first radiographs are obtained, body

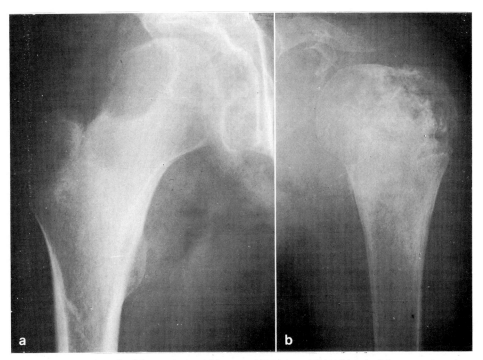

FIG. 191. - (a) Chondroblastoma in a boy aged 15 years. (b) Chondroblastoma in a boy aged 14 years. This, originating from the greater tuberosity, extended to most of the humeral head and presented considerable calcification.

growth has nearly or entirely ended, and the growth cartilage has already disappeared or is about to; in earlier observations, it may clearly be seen how the tumor destroys and surpasses a growth cartilage which is still present (Figs. 188, 192).

C.B. is a tumor of small or moderate size, which goes from a minimum of 1-2 to a maximum of 6-7 centimeters in diameter. The osteolysis is central or eccentric in relation to the epiphysis. It is often eccentric at the proximal humerus, when the tumor originates from the greater tuberosity. It is a rounded or slightly polycyclical osteolysis. Its radiolucency is not very intense and it may be veiled or spotted by nubecolae and granules of tenuous and fading radiopacity (Figs. 189, 191).

The well-defined borders of the tumor are characteristic, which may at times be marked by a thin rim of osteosclerosis (Fig. 187). In forms of the disease which are eccentric and more expansive, the cortex may be expanded and nearly cancelled (Fig. 194). The tumor may also completely cancel the subchondral bone towards the joint. In the site where the tumor expands the metaphyseal cortex, there is little or no periosteal reaction.

GROSS PATHOLOGIC FEATURES

The macroscopic picture of the tumor is compact and soft, very similar to

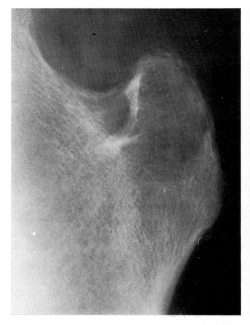

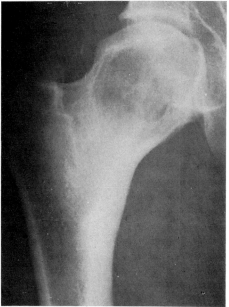

FIG. 192. - Chondroblastoma of the greater trochanter in a boy aged 17 years.

FIG. 193. - Chondroblastoma in a male aged 28 years. These forms of the disease in the adult must be distinguished from clear-cell chondrosarcoma, which they resemble radiographically.

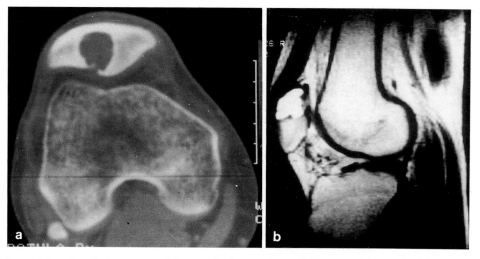

FIG. 194. - Chondroblastoma of the patella in a male aged 27 years. (a) CAT and (b) magnetic resonance.

or the same as giant cell tumor, with sharp limits in relation to the surrounding bone. In calcified areas, it looks like rough wet sawdust. Color varies from gray to reddish to brown, with small yellowish-white chalky areas

(areas of calcar impregnation) and at times whitish areas of fibrous or chondroid aspect. Hemorrhagic areas and cystic cavities are sometimes observed, which may occupy a vast part of the tumor (Fig. 187c). When C.B. has surpassed the physis and it has extended in the metaphysis, destruction of the cartilage itself may clearly be observed, some residues of which may be included in the tumor. Frequently, the tumor in the epiphysis goes as far as the joint cartilage, which thus appears to be thinned and impressible. In rare cases, the joint cartilage is also surpassed, and the tumoral tissue invades the joint.

HISTOPATHOLOGIC FEATURES

The essential histological picture in vital, unaltered areas of the tumor, is that of medium sized cells, globose and polyhedrical, with well-defined cytoplasmatic boundaries, resembling the bits of a mosaic. The nuclei are rounded, well-stained, and often have an evident nucleolus or nucleoli. Mild pleomorphism is observed, as well as some multinucleate cells (with only a few nuclei) and rare mitotic figures (Figs. 195, 196).

Between the cells there is a scarce fibrillary reticulum and even scarcer ground substance. Here and there are small foci of calcification. Calcar salts, at times in the form of fine powder, encrust the intercellular substance and the cells, forming a delicate pericellular reticulum. These calcification foci may be considered pathognomic of C.B. but they are not constant. In order to be able to discern this aspect of considerable diagnostic value, it is best to separate soft tumor from the surrounding bone and thus avoid decalcifying it. Where the cells are encrusted with calcium, they at first appear to be swollen, to then degenerate and die. These focal, sparse areas of necrosis and calcification are rehabitated by a fibrous or osseous repair tissue. Furthermore, islands of tumoral tissue which is decidedly chondroid and immature, may be observed.

In C.B. there may be multinucleate giant cells, the presence and number of which may vary. These are mostly macrophages which, like in many skeletal lesions, are reactive to hemorrhage, calcification and ossification.

Sometimes, C.B. contains large hematic or serous cavities similar to those of an aneurysmal bone cyst: cystic forms (Fig. 196d). Rarely, it presents histological aspects of transition with chondromyxoid fibroma.

HISTOGENESIS AND PATHOGENESIS

The hypothesis put forth by Jaffe and Lichtenstein (1942) that C.B. originates from chondroblasts, is supported by the morphology of the cells which, even under electron microscopy, is similar to that of chondroblasts; by the peculiar pericellular calcification characterizing chondral tissues; by the presence of evidently chondroid areas within the tumor. The constant closeness between C.B. and growth cartilage must also be taken into consideration.

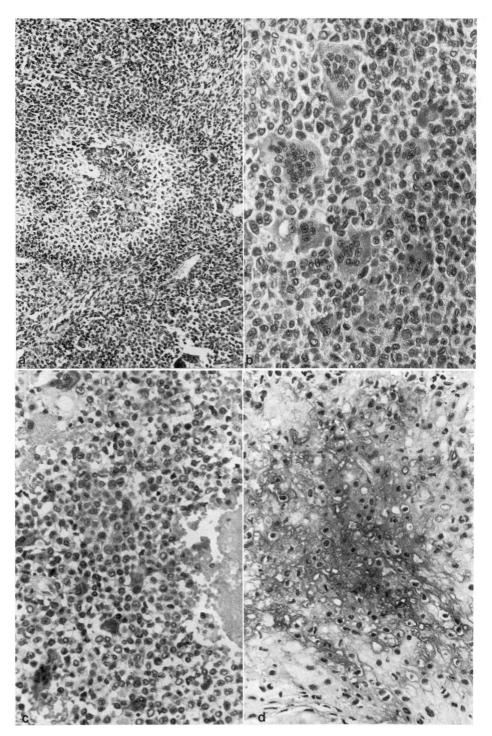

FIG. 195. - (a) Focal area of intercellular calcification. (b) and (c) Cellular areas disseminated by numerous multinucleate giant cells. (d) Calcified chondroid area (*Hemat.-
eos.*, 125, 310, 310, 310 x).

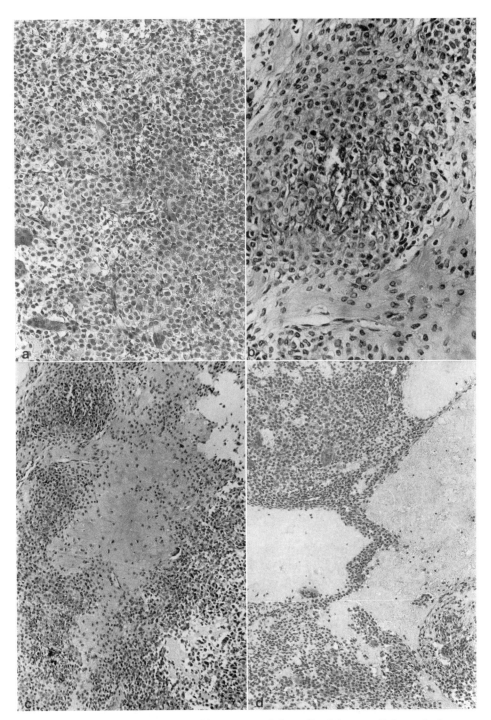

F̲ɪɢ. 196. - (a) Observe the mosaiclike aspect of the cells. (b) Pericellular calcification. (c) Area of chondroid differentiation. (d) Cystic and hemorrhagic cavity (*Hemat.-eos.*, 200, 310, 125, 125 x).

DIAGNOSIS

From a radiographic point of view, differential diagnosis may involve **giant cell tumor**, but only during adult age (as there is no giant cell tumor involving the epiphysis when the growth cartilage is still open). An important difference is that C.B. usually has clear boundaries, while giant cell tumor has boundaries which are more faded. A second difference may be the calcification nubecolae in C.B., when they are in fact present. Histologically, even in areas where calcification and chondroid differentiation are absent, and giant cells are numerous, C.B. may clearly be distinguished from giant cell tumor as the basic cells have better defined limits, somewhat resembling the pieces in a mosaic. The giant cells are distributed irregularly, above all collected in areas of hemorrhaging. Mitotic figures are more rare.

Even a **clear-cell chondrosarcoma** may be radiographically very similar to a C.B., including calcification. These chondrosarcomas are observed in the adult, however, and histologically they may clearly be distinguished from C.B.

Rarely, a **chondroma or central chondrosarcoma** localized in the epiphysis may be radiographically similar to a C.B.; the difference is macroscopic and histological.

Another radiographic differentiation involves an **inflammatory cavity**, whether specific or aspecific. This may also contain radiopaque images due to small sequesters, but its shape is more irregular and it has a wider and denser halo of peripheral osteosclerosis.

COURSE

C.B. often has slow growth. At times years go by between the first symptoms and surgical treatment. In rare cases, left alone for a long period of time or when the tumor is particularly aggressive, it may become of considerable size, destroying the entire metaepiphysis and/or widely invading the joint and even the opposite epiphysis.

Exceptional cases have been reported in which C.B. having the usual histological aspect has caused pulmonary metastases. These metastases are characterized by a slow course, like the primary tumor, and may be treated successfully.

TREATMENT

This generally consists in intralesional excision after frozen section biopsy. All of the osteo-periosteal wall and the joint cartilage attenuated by the tumor must be removed. A few millimeters of the deep bony wall are removed, and this is treated with phenol. The cavity may be filled with acrylic cement, sometimes interposing a layer of autogenous cancellous grafts between the articular cartilage and cement (Fig. 187d).

When the joint surface has to be removed, osteo-chondral bone grafts are used (homogenous head of the femur, autogenous patella).

In rare cases of very expanded tumor or extensive local recurrence, marginal or wide resection of a part or all of the articular bone segment will be required. Reconstruction will be done with allografts or autografts, to restore the articular function or to produce an arthrodesis.

Radiation therapy is contraindicated, either alone or associated with surgery, for three reasons: 1) C.B. is moderately radio-sensitive; 2) many patients are still growing; 3) exceptional cases of radiation-sarcoma in irradiated C.B. have been reported. Thus, radiation therapy must be reserved for unoperable sites.

In the exceptional case of pulmonary metastases, excision of the metastases is indicated.

PROGNOSIS

Generally, C.B. heals with curettage. If curettage is not complete, it may recur, approximately in 10% of all cases. Exceptionally, tumoral nodules may form in the soft tissues by surgical implantation. Nonetheless, recurrence may be cured with a new operation involving wider removal.

REFERENCES

1942 JAFFE H. L., LICHTENSTEIN L.: Benign chondroblastoma of bone. Reinterpretation of the so-called calcifying or chondromatous giant cell tumor. *American Journal of Pathology*, **18**, 969-991.

1959 LICHTENSTEIN L., BERNSTEIN D.: Unusual benign and malignant chondroid tumors of bone. *Cancer*, **12**, 1142-1157.

1964 WELSH R. A., MEYER A. T.: A histogenetic study of chondroblastoma. *Cancer*, **17**, 578-589.

1969 DE RUBERTIS R.: Sul condroblastoma. Rilievi clinico statistici. *Archivio Putti*, **24**, 282-295.

1969 KAHN L. B., WOOD F. M., ACKERMANN L. V.: Malignant chondroblastoma. Report of two cases and review of the literature. *Archives of Pathology*, **88**, 371-376.

1970 SCHAJOWICZ F., GALLARDO H.: Epiphyseal chondroblastoma of bone; a clinicopathological study of 69 cases. *Journal of Bone and Joint Surgery*, **52-B**, 205-226.

1972 DAHLIN D. C., IVINS J. C.: Benign chondroblastoma. A Study of 125 Cases. *Cancer*, **30**, 401-413.

1972 HUVOS A. G., MARCOVE R. C., ERLANDSON R. A., MIKE V.: Chondroblastoma of bone. A clinico-pathologic and electron-microscopic study. *Cancer*, **29**, 760-771.

1972 LEVINE G. D., BENSCH K. G.: Chondroblastoma. The nature of the basic cell. A study by means of histochemistry, tissue culture, electron microscopy, and autoradiography. *Cancer*, **29**, 1546-1562.

1973 RIDDELL R. J., LONIS C. J., BROMBERGER N. A.: Pulmonary metastases from chondroblastoma of the tibia. *Journal of Bone and Joint Surgery*, **55-B**, 848-853.

1975 GREEN P., WHITTAKER R. P.: Benign chondroblastoma. Case report with pulmonary metastasis. *Journal of Bone and Joint Surgery*, **57-A**, 418-420.

1975 MEARY R. ABELANET R., FOREST M., LE CHARPENTIER Y., TOMENO B., LANGUEPIN A., NEZELF CH., LESEC G.: Les chondroblastomes bénins des os. Etude anatomo-clinique et ultrastructurale à propos de 11 observations. *Révue de chirurgie orthopedique*, **61**, 717-734.

1977 CAMPANACCI M., GIUNTI A., MARTUCCI E., TRENTANI C.: Epiphyseal chondroblastoma. A study of 39 cases. *Italian Journal of Orthopaedics and Traumatology*, **3**, 67-74.

1979 WIRMAN J. A., CRISSMAN J. D., ARON B. F.: Metastatic chondroblastoma. Report of an unusual case treated with radiotherapy. *Cancer*, **44**, 87-93.

1983 MIRRA J.M., ULICH T.R., ECKARDT J., BHUTA S.: « Aggressive » chondroblastoma. Light and ultramicroscopic findings after en bloc resection. *Clinical Orthopaedics*, **178**, 276-284.

1985 KYRIAKOS M., LAND V., PENNING L., PARKER S.: Metastatic chondroblastoma. Report of a fatal case with a review of the literature on atypical, aggressive, and malignant chondroblastoma. *Cancer*, **55**, 1770-1789, 1985.

1985 SPRINGFIELD D.S., CAPANNA R., GHERLINZONI F., PICCI P., CAMPANACCI M.: Chondroblastoma. A review of seventy cases. *Journal of Bone and Joint Surgery*, **67-A**, 748-755.

1986 SOTELO-AVILA C., SUNDARAM M., KYRIAKOS M., GRAVIS E., TAYLOR A.: Case report 373: diametaphyseal chondroblastoma of the upper portion of the left femur. *Skeletal Radiology*, **15**, 387-390.

1987 MATSUNO T., HASEGAWA I., MASUDA T.: Chondroblastoma arising in the triradiate cartilage. Report of two cases with review of the literature. *Skeletal Radiology*, **16**, 216-222.

1988 BRECHER M.E., SIMON M.A.: Chondroblastoma. An immunohistochemical study. *Human Pathology*, **19**, 1043-1047.

1988 MOSER R.P., BROCKMOLE D.M., VINH T.N., KRANSDORF M.J., AOKI J.: Chondroblastoma of the patella. *Skeletal Radiology*, **17**, 413-419.

1989 CORSAT J., TOMENO B., FOREST M., VINH T.S.: Chondroblastomes bénins: une revue de 30 cas. *Revue de Chirurgie Orthopédique*, **75**, 179-187.

1989 KURT A.M., UNNI K.K., SIM F.H., McLEOD R.A.: Chondroblastoma of bone. *Human Pathology*, **20**, 965-976.

1989 PIGNATTI G., NIGRISOLI M.: Case report 573. *Skeletal Radiology*, **18**, 225-227.

1990 MAYO-SMITH W., ROSENBERG A.E., KHURANA J.S., KATTAPURAM S.V., ROMERO L.H.: Chondroblastoma of the rib. A case report and review of the literature. *Clinical Orthopaedics*, **251**, 230-234.

CHONDROMYXOID FIBROMA
(Synonym: fibromyxoid chondroma)

DEFINITION

It is a benign tumor, characterized by a lobulated, fibro-myxoid and chondroid histological structure.

FREQUENCY

It is rare, definitely moreso than chondroblastoma.

SEX

There is predilection for the male sex (Fig. 197).

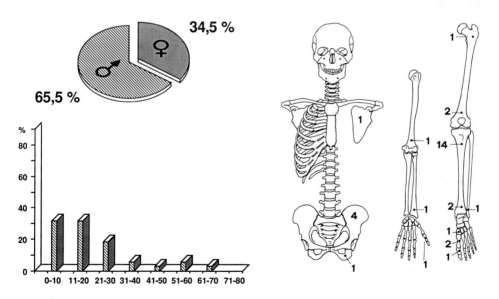

FIG. 197. - Sex, age, and site in 33 cases of chondromyxoid fibroma.

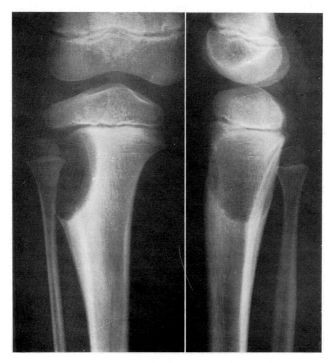

FIG. 198. - Chondromyxoid fibroma in a boy aged 6 years.

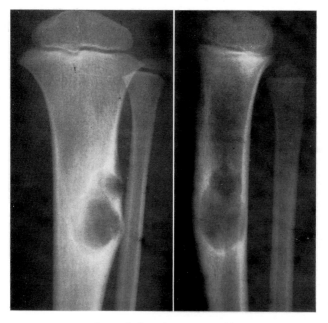

FIG. 199. - Diaphyseal chondromyxoid fibroma in a girl aged 4 years.

AGE

It is generally observed between 5 and 30 years of age. Like chondroblastoma, it is exceptional when it occurs after 30 years of age, but, unlike chondroblastoma, it is often observed prior to 10 years of age (Fig. 197).

LOCALIZATION

Evidently unlike chondroblastoma C.F. always begins (eccentric) in a metaphysis. With time it may expand and move towards the diaphysis, but usually it does not surpass the growth cartilage for as long as it is present. The epiphyseal involvement is more easily observed in the adult and the small tubular bones of the foot (Fig. 200).

C.F. is nearly always localized in the lower limb. Here, the bone which is most frequently involved is the tibia (particularly, the proximal metaphysis), followed by the femur (particularly, the distal metaphysis), the bones of the foot (metatarsals, phalanges) and the fibula (Fig. 197). In the upper limb, in

FIG. 200. - (a) Chondro-
myxoid fibroma in a fe-
male aged 29 years. (b)
Chondromyxoid fibroma
in a male aged 30 years.

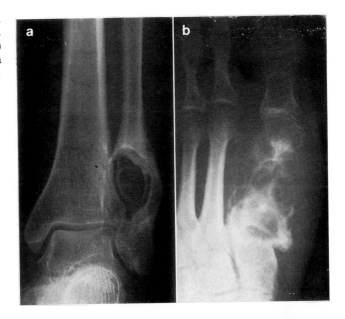

exceptional cases it may be observed in the humerus, radius, ulna, metacarpals and phalanges. Also exceptional are localizations in the skeleton of the
trunk.

SYMPTOMS

Symptoms are scarce and long-lasting, related to the slow growth of the
tumor. There is mild and discontinuous pain, the onset of which is at times
related to trauma. In more superficial and expanded forms of the disease
there may be mild swelling, which increases very slowly.

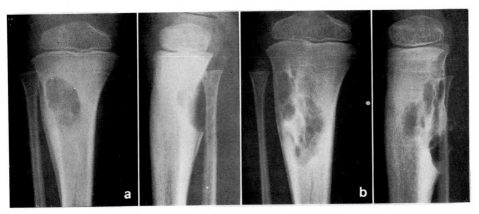

FIG. 201. - (a) Chondromyxoid fibroma in a boy aged 5 years. (b) Recurrence of the tumor one year later, after curettage.

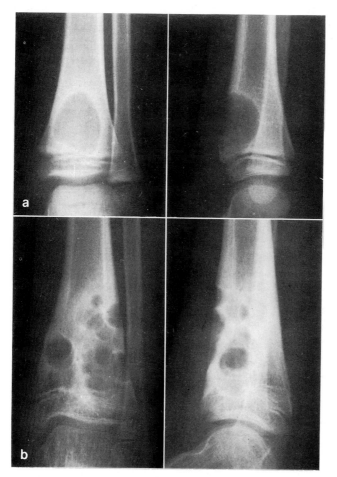

FIG. 202. - (a) Chondro-
myxoid fibroma in a boy
aged 6 years. (b) Recur-
rence and evolution of the
tumor 2 years later after
three attempts at curet-
tage and autogenous bone
grafting.

RADIOGRAPHIC FEATURES

The radiographic picture is rather typical in aspect and evolution. At
first, there is an area of metaphyseal osteolysis, which is decidedly eccentric
and superficial. It is an intensely and completely radiolucent osteolysis, of
moderate size, globose or more often oval in shape, with its major axis parallel to the length of the diaphysis. Its boundaries are relatively regular and
clear and, towards the inside of the bone, they are marked by a thin line of
osteosclerosis. As the tumor evolves, the osteolysis tends to become plurilobulated, always maintaining a globose, regular and clear outline. Thus, polycyclical or bubbling images may be obtained. Any radiographic impression
of sepimentation is false and due to multiple roundish excavations of the skeletal wall and to the interposed osseous crests. In its expansion, the tumor
may move towards the diaphysis and gain the center of the medullary canal.
In thinner tubular bones (fibula, metatarsals, metacarpals, phalanges) it easily occupies all of the bone, which in this case may appear to be consider-

ably «blown up» by the tumor. Normally, C.F. expands the cortex very little. It instead tends to considerably thin and in many cases **totally cancel** the cortex. A final radiographic element of importance is the complete absence of periosteal reaction (Figs. 198-204).

C.F. does not become of large size, at most it achieves 8-10 centimeters in diameter.

In exceptional cases and particularly during adult age, within the tumor, granules of fading radiopacity, due to calcification of the tumoral cartilage, may be observed (Fig. 204).

GROSS PATHOLOGIC FEATURES

Even when radiograms show the cortex to be totally cancelled, the tumor is always contained by the periosteum. The neoplastic tissue is compact, and soft. Its aspect varies and is variegated: reddish or pale brown where undifferentiated and vascularized areas prevail; whitish and translucent soft where chondromyxoid areas prevail. In the latter case, the macroscopic aspect may be the same as that of a chondrosarcoma (Fig. 204d): but, unlike chondrosarcoma, the limits of the tumor in relation to the bone are quite well-defined.

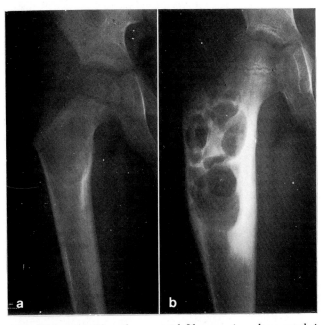

FIG. 203. - (a) Chondromyxoid fibroma in a boy aged 4 years. (b) Recurrence and evolution of the tumor 2 years later after an attempt at curettage and bone grafting.

HISTOPATHOLOGIC FEATURES

The histological aspect of C.F. is particularly evocative under a **small enlargement** (Figs. 205-208). A compact whole of rounded and confluent lobuli is observed, the center of which is lighter (chondromyxoid) and the periphery darker (because it is densely cellular). As they begin to form, the smaller lobuli are nearly entirely dark, with just a hint of a lighter center. On the contrary, the larger lobuli are nearly entirely light, the dark part being limited to a thin peripheral layer. These dark bands at the periphery of the lobuli

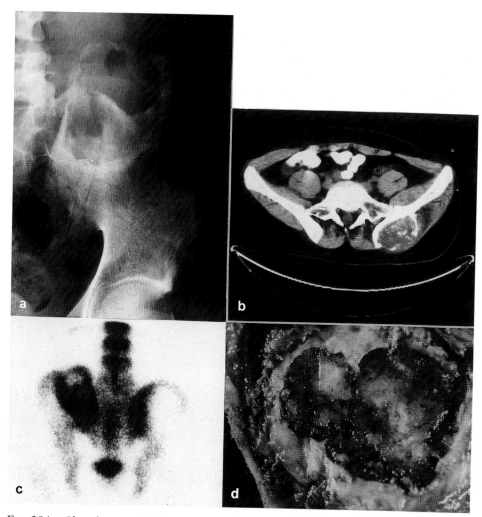

Fig. 204. - Chondromyxoid fibroma in a male aged 24 years. Pain for the past year. (a) and (b) Significant osteolysis, with well-defined boundaries, containing some calcifications, and a minimal amount of periosteal reaction. (c) Bone scan is colder at the center of the lesion, a sign of scarce vascularization. (d) The chondromyxoid gross aspect is very similar to that which may be observed in chondrosarcoma. The patient was submitted to marginal resection and is cured after 7 years.

actually form around the interlobular fibrovascular laminae, while they are absent where the lobuli fuse together without being separated by a fibrovascular lamina. The boundaries of the tumor in relation to the bone and to the periosteum are quite sharp; nonetheless, at the periphery of the tumor small nodules may penetrate between the skeletal trabeculae and be the cause of recurrence.

Under greater enlargement, it may be observed that the clear central part of the more mature lobuli is composed of spindle-stellate cells interspersed in an abundant and fluid ground substance. The cells have ossiphile cytoplasms (reddish with eosin), which are spindle and ramified. The nuclei are

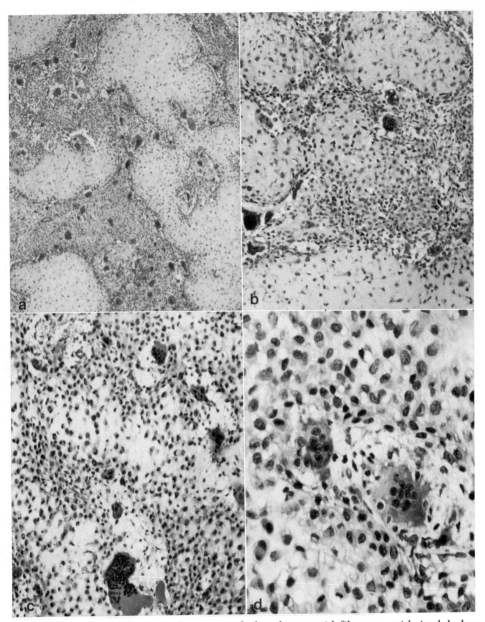

FIG. 205. - Typical histological aspects of chondromyxoid fibroma, with its lobular structure (*Hemat.-eos.*, 50, 125, 125, 310 x).

roundish, oval, triangular and polyhedrical, well-stained and fairly or considerably dismetrical and pleomorphic. The ground substance stains very light blue with hematoxylin (basophile), but it does not take on the colors of the mucin. Thus, it is a very watery ground substance, but it is not mucoid. Argentic impregnation shows that a tenuous fibrillary pattern runs through the ground substance.

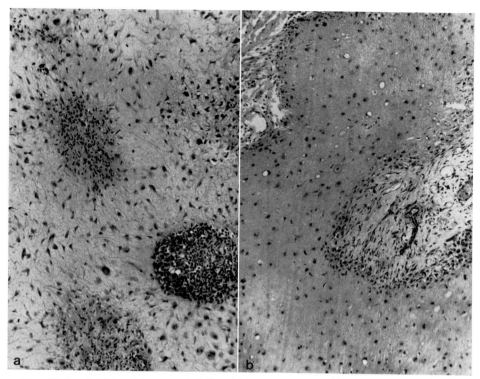

Fig. 206. - (a) Myxoid area and (b) chondroid area (*Hemat.-eos.*, 125, 125x).

Towards the periphery of the lobule the tissue becomes much more cellular, and the ground substance disappears. The band separating the two adjacent lobuli is constituted by rather densely distributed cells, with rather plump nuclei, which are well-stained and usually not very pleomorphic. Mitotic figures are quite rare. Numerous and ectatic blood vessels run through these peri- and interlobular bands (the center of the lobuli is avascular). Rarely are cystic-hemorrhagic cavities similar to those of aneurysmal bone cyst observed. Macrophages, multinucleate giant cells, hemosiderin pigment and a few lymphocytes are observed around the vessels and together with the perilobular cells, which represent the younger more proliferative and undifferentiated phase of the tumor.

In some areas and in some tumors, the «myxoid» areas become more collagenous, with a more compact, fibro-hyaline intercellular substance. Or there are many frankly chondroid and cartilaginous areas, or further cellular areas similar to those of the chondroblastoma. At times there are centers of calcar precipitation which resemble those of chondroblastoma and prevalently occurring in areas of degenerated cartilage.

▶

Fig. 207. - (a) and (b) Under different enlargements chondromyxoid centro-lobular area and peri-lobular area with giant cells. (c) and (d) Under different enlargements myxoid lobule with cellular pleomorphism (*Hemat.-eos.*, 50, 125, 50, 125 x).

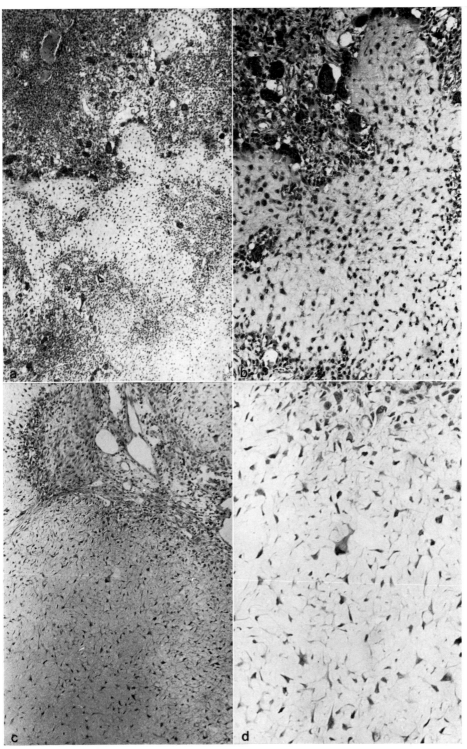

FIG. 207.

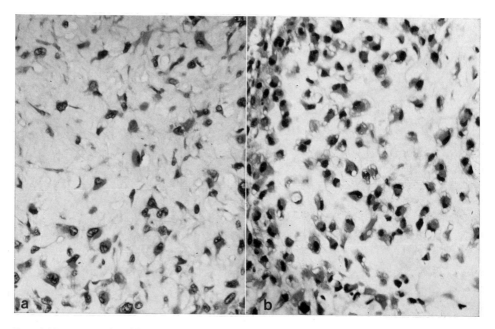

FIG. 208. - Considerable size, pleomorphism and hyperchromia of the nuclei in the chondromyxoid area. These aspects, considered by themselves, could be mistaken for a chondrosarcoma (*Hemat.-eos.*, 310, 310 x).

HISTOGENESIS

Several different histological elements suggest a fibro-cartilaginous differentiation and thus a probable chondral or fibro-chondral histogenesis. The tumor originates in the vicinity of fertile cartilage (on the metaphyseal side). It is hardly ever observed in bones that have none (cranium, carpus, tarsus except for the calcaneus).

DIAGNOSIS

As previously observed, the radiographic aspects of C.F. are rather characteristic: particularly eccentric metaphyseal osteolysis, with well-defined limits, often polycyclical, with considerable thinning or total disappearance of the cortex, with no periosteal reaction. Nonetheless, in some cases, particularly if the localization is in a non-tubular bone, the radiographic image may be less meaningful.

Histologically, C.F. is one of those tumors that is easily diagnosed as long as one has experience with it. Otherwise, one may run the risk of erroneously diagnosing a **chondrosarcoma**. This grave error was common prior to the description of chondromyxoid fibroma by Jaffe and Lichtenstein (1948) and it was justifed by the considerable pleomorphism and hyperchromia in the nuclei. In truth, if observation were limited to a detail of the tumor, overlooking its typical structure on the whole, and if one were only to focus on the cellular details, one could have an impression of malignancy.

Furthermore, as previously observed, the macroscopic aspect of C.F. may be the same as that of a chondrosarcoma. The diagnosis is based on the age of the patient (chondrosarcoma is never observed in children) and on the radiographic aspect, as well as on the histological picture.

C.F. also has a histological structure which is very different from that of **myxoma** of bone, which is practically only observed in the jaws. Myxoma of the maxillae is characterized by a histological aspect which is common to all myxomas, which are more often observed in the soft tissues.

At times, instead, C.F. may have histological aspects which are similar to or of transition with **chondroblastoma**.

COURSE

C.F. grows slowly and does not become of large size.

TREATMENT

Treatment usually consists in aggressive intralesional excision: complete extraperiosteal removal of the attenuated bony wall, excision of a good layer of cancellous bone of the deep wall, the use of local adjuvants.

Marginal or wide resection of the entire bone segment is indicated when the tumor involves it extensively, or in the case of extensive local recurrence. Radiation treatment is never indicated.

PROGNOSIS

C.F. nearly always heals with conservative surgical treatment. However, it easily recurs, if the first attempt at removal was not truly complete. Two cases have been reported (Jaffe, 1958; Dahlin, 1978) which developed a sarcoma on a typical C.F. without the latter having previously been irradiated.

REFERENCES

1948 JAFFE H. L., LICHTENSTEIN L.: Chondromyxoid fibroma of bone. A distinctive benign tumor likely to be mistaken especially for chondrosarcoma. *Archiv of Pathology*, **45**, 541-551.

1956 DAHLIN D. C.: Chondromyxoid fibroma of bone, with emphasis of its morphological relationship to benign chondroblastoma. *Cancer*, **9**, 195-203.

1958 IWATA S., COLEY B. L.: Report of six cases of chondromyxoid fibroma of bone. *Surgery, Gynecology and Obstetrics*, **107**, 571-576.

1958 JAFFE H. L.: *Tumors and tumorous conditions of the bones and joints.* Lea & Febiger, Philadelphia.

1961 SCAGLIETTI O., STRINGA G.: Myxoma of bone in childhood. *Journal of Bone and Joint Surgery*, **43-A**, 67-80.

1962   RALPH L. L.: Chondromyxoid fibroma of bone. *Journal of Bone and Joint Surgery*, **44-B**, 7-24.

1962   TURCOTTE B., PUGH D. G., DAHLIN D. C.: The roentgenologic aspects of chondromyxoid fibroma of bone. *American Journal of Roentgenology*, **87**, 1085-1095.

1964   MARCOVE R. C., KAMBOLIS C., BULLOUGH P. G., JAFFE H. L.: Fibromixoma of bone. A report of 3 cases. *Cancer*, **17**, 1209-1213.

1965   SALZER M., SALZER KUNTSCHIK M.: Das Chondromyxoidfibrom. *Langenbecks Archiv für Chirurgie*, **312**, 216-221.

1969   FRANK W. E., ROCKWOOD C. A. Jr.: Chondromixoid fibroma. Review of the literature and report of four cases. *Southern Medical Journal*, **62**, 1248-1253.

1971   SCHAJOWICZ F., GALLARDO H.: Chondromyxoid fibroma (fibromyxoid chondroma) of bone. A clinico-pathological study of 32 cases. *Journal of Bone and Joint Surgery*, **53-B**, 198-216.

1972   RAHIMI A., BEABOUT J. W., IVINS J. C., DAHLIN D. C.: Chondromyxoid fibroma: a clinicopathologic study of 76 cases. *Cancer*, **30**, 726-736.

1978   DAHLIN D. C.: *Bone tumors*. Charles C. Thomas, Springfield.

1983   GHERLINZONI F., ROCK M., PICCI P.: Chondromyxoid fibroma The experience at the Istituto Ortopedico Rizzoli. *Journal of Bone and Joint Surgery*, **65-A**, 198-204.

1987   TANG J., GOLD R.M., MIRRA J.M.: Case report 454. *Skeletal Radiology*, **16**, 675-678.

1989   ZILLMER D.A., DORFMAN H.D.: Chondromyxoid fibroma of bone: thirty-six cases with clinico-pathologic correlation. *Human Pathology*, **20**, 952-964.

CHONDROSARCOMAS

DEFINITION AND GENERALITIES

These are sarcomas the cells of which tend to differentiate into cartilage.

C.S. are classified as: **central** (originating within the bone), **peripheral** (originating outside the bone from a pre-existing exostosis) and **periosteal** (or parosteal). To these are added **mesenchymal** C.S. and **clear cell** C.S. In central and periosteal C.S. origin from a pre-existing chondroma is rare also because it is difficult to demonstrate. Peripheral C.S. originate from a pre-existing exostosis.

In C.S. there are different histological grades of malignancy, which correspond to differences in prognosis and treatment. C.S. are subject to a **progression in malignancy**: they may transform from a histological grade to a superior one (still remaining C.S.); or from a C.S. another high-grade sarcoma such as fibrosarcoma, osteosarcoma, malignant fibrous histiocytoma (so called **dedifferentiated C.S.**) may develop.

Diagnosis and histological classification of C.S. require considerable specific experience and are not reliable if clinical and anatomo-radiographic data are not taken into account.

In C.S. where the effect of radiation therapy and chemotherapy is practically null, **treatment** is exclusively surgical, offering considerable possibilities of cure (in fact, many C.S. do not metastasize, or metastases occur late). In practice, these possibilities are diminished for three main reasons. a) The most common site of C.S. (proximal limbs, pelvis, bones of the trunk, scapula) makes surgery difficult, unless at an early stage and/or in the less aggressive forms of the disease. b) The scarce symptomatology (many C.S. grow slowly, as they are not very vascularized they may cause little pain, at times they originate from an exostosis that the patient knows he has had for many years and about which he is not worried) often results in late diagnosis. c) The imperfect knowledge of the anatomo-radiographic and histological aspects of C.S. at times leads to an underevaluation of its malignancy (diagnoses of chondroma are not rare) and to inadequate treatment.

The **prognosis** of C.S. essentially depends on two conditions: the possibility of wide excision and the histological grade of malignancy. Peripheral and periosteal C.S. globally have a reduced histological grade of malignancy as compared to that of central C.S., and even when the histological grade is the same, their behavior is less malignant.

Due to the slow growth of some chondrosarcomas, local recurrence and metastases may occur even more than 10 years after removal of the primary tumor.

CENTRAL CHONDROSARCOMA

DEFINITION

It is a C.S. which originated inside the bone.

FREQUENCY

C.C.S. is fourth, after plasmacytoma, osteosarcoma and Ewing's sarcoma, among primary malignant tumors of the skeleton.

SEX

There is predilection for the male sex, at a ratio of 1.5-2:1 (Fig. 209).

AGE

The maximum incidence of the tumor is from 30 to 70 years of age. Thus, the tumor is typical of adult age, rare before 20 years of age, exceptional before puberty (Fig. 209).

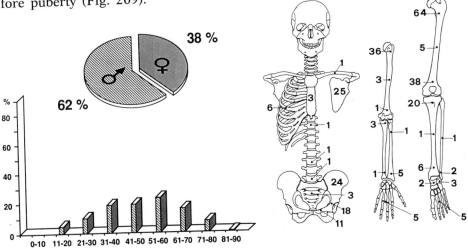

FIG. 209. - Sex, age and site in 293 cases of central chondrosarcoma (295 localizations: 2 cases of chondromatosis developed two chondrosarcomas each).

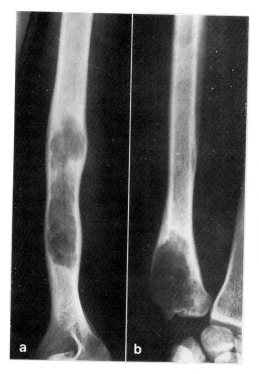

Fig. 210. - (a) Central cartilaginous tumor in a female aged 17 years. As a result of a first curettage it was interpreted as chondroma, but there were already suspicious histological signs of grade 1 chondrosarcoma. The tumor recurred 4 times (after repeated curettages) over 19 years. The first three recurrences presented a histological aspect of grade 1 chondrosarcoma (Fig. 169b). In the last recurrence, instead, the tumor surpassed the cortex and histologically it was a grade 2 chondrosarcoma. Operated by wide resection of the diaphysis, it presented neither signs of recurrence nor of metastases after 15 years. (b) Central chondosarcoma, histologically grade 1 in female aged 24 years. The patient was submitted to wide resection and healed after 25 years.

LOCALIZATION

C.C.S. reveals evident predilection, in this order, for the femur (particularly proximal), the pelvis, the proximal humerus, the scapula, the proximal tibia. Other less frequent localizations follow, including the other bones of the trunk, the radius and the ulna, the foot and the hand (Fig. 209) (chondroma frequently occurs in the hand, rarely in the trunk). It is not an exceptional occurrence when it is observed in the cranial base and in those parts of the facial bones that develop from a cartilaginous model.

In the long bones it usually originates towards one end of the diaphysis or in the metaphysis. As these are adults in whom the growth cartilage has disappeared, it frequently invades the epiphysis, at times the joint. Rarely does it originate in the intermediate part of the diaphysis. At times, on diagnosis, the tumor is extended as far as a third, half, or more, of the entire long bone. In the pelvis there seems to be predilection for the region (ilium, ischium, or pubis) surrounding the acetabulum, in the scapula for the coracoglenoid region. In the pelvis and the scapula, as well, C.C.S. may extend to most of the bone.

SYMPTOMS

Symptoms are generally characterized by their tenuity and slowness. The clinical history of the tumor is often of long duration and at times speaks of a

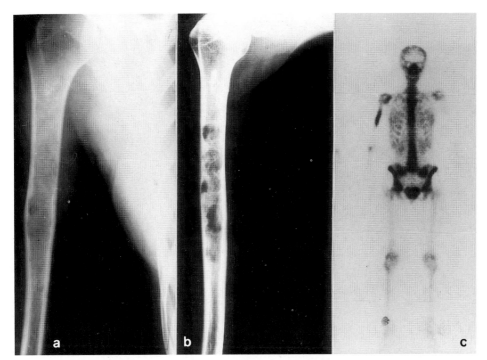

FIG. 211. - (a) Chondroma in a female aged 23 years. (b) After 10 years, during which the patient complained of occasional pain, the radiographic picture appears to have evolved with multiple scalloping of the internal part of the cortex. (c) Intensely positive bone scan. Because of the considerable extent of the chondroma, the occasional presence of pain, the slow radiographic evolution with scalloping of the cortex, clinical-radiographic diagnosis was borderline lesion between chondroma and chondrosarcoma. Thus, it was surgically treated with opening of the diaphysis in two valves, currettage and phenol. The diaphyseal half which was temporarily removed was cleansed of the tumor, treated with liquid nitrogen and placed back in site. A histological examination of the entire tumor confirmed the diagnosis of borderline chondroma-chondrosarcoma.

«chondromatous» tumor, which was operated locally and recurred. The main symptom is pain, deep, not intense, discontinuous. Often, as there is not yet considerable expansion of the tumor in the soft tissues, an extraosseous mass is not palpated; there is only slight enlargement of the bone. But at more advanced phases, large globose and extraosseous masses are formed.

There are cases, for example those with vertebral, sacral, costal, or pelvic localization, where pain is very intense, at times irradiated, due to compression on the nerve trunks.

There are cases which from the start, or secondarily, grow rapidly and invasively, with early destruction of the cortex and ample invasion of the soft tissues.

At times the tumor invades the joint from the epiphysis, causing joint symptoms. Pathologic fractures are a rare occurrence.

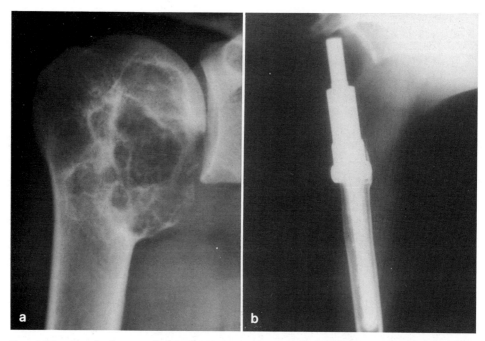

FIG. 212. - Grade 1 central chondrosarcoma in a male aged 40 years. The lobulated aspect of the osteolysis is observed; its boundaries are well-defined. The patient was submitted to wide resection and endoprosthesis, and there were no signs of disease after 4 years.

At times the recurrence of a C.C.S. which was submitted to surgery is more aggressive than the original tumor.

RADIOGRAPHIC FEATURES

The radiographic picture is that of an intraosseous, osteolytic tumor, which often grows slowly, at times rapidly, and may be impregnated with calcar salts (Figs. 210-222). In the metaepiphysis the tumor may appear to be eccentric (Figs. 212, 242a), in the diaphysis its development is central.

At times only an osteolysis with faded limits may be observed, one with or without interruption in the cortex. Often, as the cartilage tends to calcify and ossify, intratumoral radiopacities are manifested. Calcification (which often occurs at the periphery of the cartilaginous lobuli) is not structured, and characterized by an aspect of irregular «sprayed» granules, nodules or radiopaque rings (Figs. 218, 221, 239, 243).

At times there are bubbling aspects, or ones resembling bread crumbs, due to crests of the skeletal wall (Figs. 211, 212, 219b). At times the calcifications are so packed that the tumor has a metallic and nearly compact opacity (Fig. 213). Rarely, if the tumor infiltrates the medullary spaces of the cancellous bone without destroying the trabeculae, calcar precipitation and reactive hyperostosis may cause an increase in opacity of the spongy bone which is

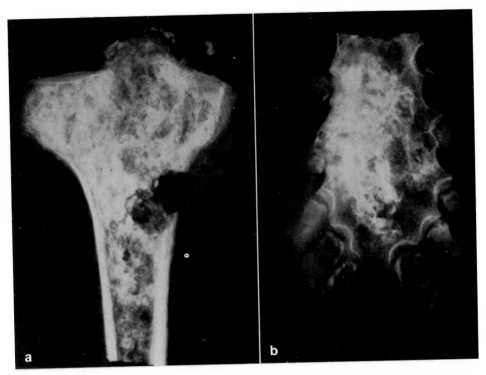

FIG. 213. - (a) Central chondrosarcoma in a male aged 70 years with symptoms for the past 2 years. The tumor was well-contained in the cortex (interruption visible corresponds to biopsy), but it invaded the joint. Histologically grade 1. No signs of either recurrence or metastasis 10 years after radical amputation. (b) Central chondrosarcoma in a male aged 50 years with pain for the past few months. Resection specimen of the sternum. Histologically grade 1. No signs of recurrence 16 years after wide resection.

nearly homogeneous (Fig. 221b). If, instead, the C.C.S. infiltrates the cancellous bone without destroying the trabeculae and it does not calcify, the intraosseous part of the tumor may remain nearly unapparent in radiograms. In this case, diagnosis may be difficult (Fig. 222) and late (Fig. 239), if bone scan, CAT and MRI (Fig. 218) are not used.

The most intense calcification is observed in well-differentiated C.C.S., while it is scarce or null in the myxoid areas, in those characterized by grade 3 malignancy, and in dedifferentiated ones.

The cortex may appear to be thinned, with **scalloping** of its internal part (Fig. 211), or interrupted in some areas. At times, due to the slow expansion of the tumor, the cortex has time to react with a hyperostosis and thus appears to be thickened. The outside surface of this thickened cortex is often characterized by a roughness which is similar to the profile of a mountain covered with trees. This radiographic aspect is rather typical of C.C.S. and indicates that the thickened cortical bone is infiltrated by the tumor (Figs. 214b, 215, 216, 217, 219a, 220, 244b).

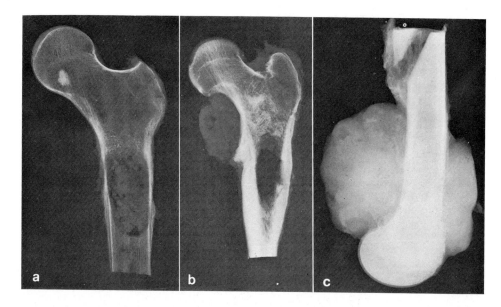

FIG. 214. - Central chondrosarcoma. Radiograms of anatomical specimens with differing anatomo-radiographic expansion of the tumor. (a) Tumor contained by the cortex (radiopaque image in the femoral neck corresponds to an island of compact). Histological grade 2. (b) A fair amount of expansion of the tumor ouside the cortex. Histological grade 2. (c) Enormous expansion of the tumor in the soft tissues. Histological grade 3.

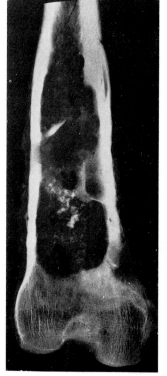

C.C.S. tends to expand in areas where there is less resistance, such as the diaphyseal medullary canal. In nearly a half of the cases radiograms show a tumor which extends as far as a third, a half, or more of the entire long bone (Figs. 211, 215, 216, 218, 219b, 220b). But from the start invasion of the medullary canal may not be visible radiographically (Figs. 218, 222). It is important to keep this in mind, in order not to risk performing inadequate surgery and having recurrence on the diaphyseal resection or amputation stump. **The extent of the tumor along the medullary canal must be studied preoperatively** by bone scan, CAT and, above all, MRI (Fig. 218d).

FIG. 215. - Radiogram of the anatomical specimen. Central chondrosarcoma, histological grade 2, in a male aged 64 years. The tumor expanded in the medullary canal nearly as far as the boundary of the specimen. Treated with amputation, the patient was well after 16 years.

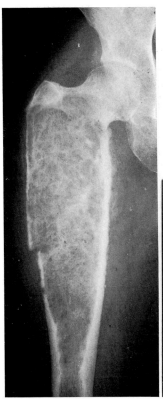

FIG. 216. - Central chondrosarcoma, histological grade 2, in a female aged 47 years who complained of pain for 2 and 1/2 years. The tumor extended for more than half of the femur without gross interruptions in the cortex. This, however, was infiltrated and, at anatomical examination, it was surpassed by the tumor in several sites. Marginal resection was followed by local recurrence after 1 and 1/2 years, and the patient died of metastases 3 years later.

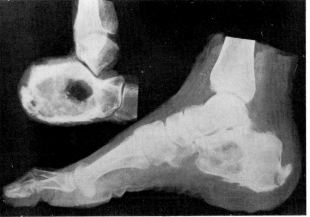

FIG. 216.   FIG. 217.

FIG. 217. - Central chondrosarcoma, histological grade 2, in a male aged 66 years. Observe thickening and peculiar roughness of the outer cortex. The patient died of metastases 3 years after amputation.

In more aggressive forms, C.C.S. interrupts the cortex early and extensively, and expands to the soft tissues with a neoplastic mass which is not very calcified. The periosteum, which is infiltrated and uplifted, may react with thin and faded radiopaque bands, perpendicular to the cortex, but neither the «tooth-comb» image nor the Codman triangle which are typical of osteosarcoma are hardly ever visualized (Figs. 214c, 218d, 220, 239).

Generally, clinical-radiographic and histological grade of malignancy correspond. Nonetheless, the radiographic picture is related not only to the grade of the tumor, but also to the duration of symptoms. Thus, in rare cases, a tumor which is radiographically still relatively contained may be observed (seen at an early stage) with elevated histological malignancy (Fig. 221b); or a tumor which is radiographically very destructive and expanded (because it is at a very advanced stage) with scarce histological malignancy (Fig. 219b).

GROSS PATHOLOGIC FEATURES

In lower-malignancy C.C.S. (grade 1) the cortex may appear to be normal, or slightly expanded but not infiltrated by the tumor. The aspect of the latter does not much differ from that of a chondroma. In more advanced forms, even grade 1 C.C.S. may surpass the cortex and grow to a large size.

In grades 2-3 C.C.S. the cortex is nearly always infiltrated or interrupted by the tumor. In forms and areas of the disease characterized by good cartilaginous differentiation, the tissue still resembles the aspect of cartilage, and tends to form lobuli which are close together and faceted. The cartilage is grayer, softer, juicier and more transparent than normal cartilage and than that of chondromas. In the myxoid areas (particularly frequent and diffused in grade 2 C.C.S.) the tissue is more or less gelatinous, grayish-white, at times there are areas of mucoid colliquation and hemorrhagic sites (Fig. 222c).

In C.C.S. the neoplastic tissue, which is compressed inside the bone and poorly blood supplied, undergoes frequent degenerative and necrotic changes. Thus, areas where the cartilage is disgregated are observed, which appear to be white, opaque, resembling boiled rice; yellowish and dry areas of

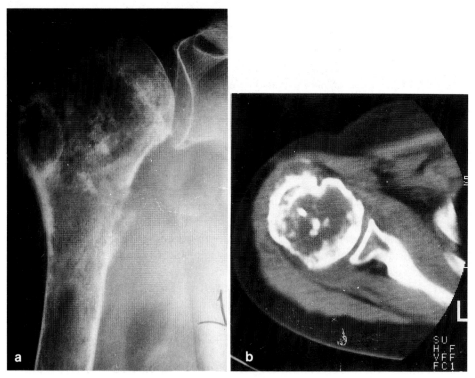

Fig. 218. - Central chondrosarcoma in a female aged 68 years. Pain for the past year. (a) X-ray with pathological fracture on an osteolytic lesion containing calcifications. (b) CAT. (c) Bone scan, like the X ray, does not reveal the actual extent of the tumor along the medullary canal, which is instead evident and able to be measured with (d). The patient was submitted to wide intra-articular resection (16 cm from the joint space). Histologically, grade 2 chondrosarcoma.

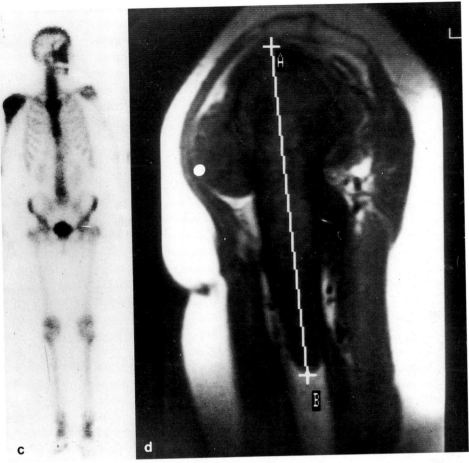

FIG. 218 c-d.

necrosis; cystic or hemorrhagic colliquations. The calcar precipitations may clearly be discerned; they have a chalky yellowish-white aspect and their consistency is hard and gritty. They are in the form of small granules or spots, isolated or confluent, at times rings corresponding to the periphery of the cartilaginous lobules.

In areas where the cortex is thickened, its external surface may appear to be rough. This aspect, for which we have described the corresponding radiographic image, depends on the infiltration of the tumor in the haversian canals, causing a chronic osteogenetic reaction of the bone.

Unlike osteosarcoma, which rapidly invades and perforates the cortex, C.C.S. often expands following the area where there is less resistance, that is, the diaphyseal canal. Thus, there may be considerable discrepancy between the radiographic picture and the anatomical one. C.C.S., which radiographically appeared to be limited to the metaepiphysis, and which hardly ever surpass the cortex, may be extended for a long distance in the the medullary canal of the diaphysis (Figs. 218d, 222).

In some cases neoplastic invasion of the joint may be observed (Figs. 213, 233, 239). This generally occurs in forms of the disease where there is considerable extension in the bone.

HISTOPATHOLOGIC FEATURES

Grade 1 C.C.S. This occurred in approximately 20% of our cases. Nearly always well-differentiated in cartilage, it rarely includes myxoid areas. The cytological signs that distinguish it from chondroma are as follows (Figs. 223a 225a, b). 1) Slightly larger nuclei. 2) The nuclei are of different size, generally maintaining their rounded shape. 3) Frequent cells with a double nuclei (in practice, at least two or three binucleated cells for each microscopic field under average enlargement). Mitotic figures are never observed (the

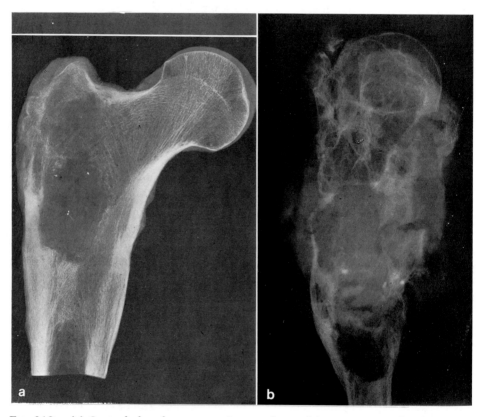

FIG. 219. - (a) Central chondrosarcoma in a male aged 34 years. Pain for the past 3 years. Histologically grade 2. Neither recurrence nor metastases 22 years after wide resection; observe the relative preservation of the cortex. (b) Central chondrosarcoma in a male aged 43 years. Onset of symptoms 10 years earlier. The patient had already been submitted to curettage twice, with recurrence. Histologically grade 1. Healed 25 years after disarticulation of the shoulder.

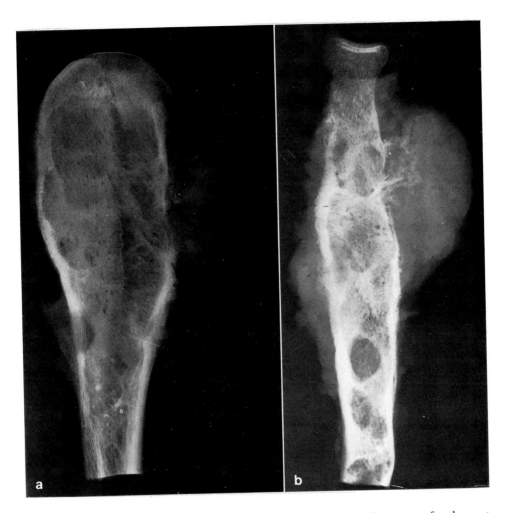

FIG. 220. - (a) Central chondrosarcoma in a male aged 31 years. Symptoms for the past 3 years. Histologically grade 2. The patient died 2 and 1/2 years after wide resection-endoprosthesis, due to metastases, but there was no local recurrence. (b) Central chondrosarcoma in a male aged 63 years. Histologically grade 2. Amputation of the arm. No signs of disease after 10 years.

cells multiply by direct division). 4) The cells are even more numerous in relation to most chondromas. However, this in itself is not a valid element. There are very cellular chondromas (particularly in chondromatosis) and there are areas of C.C.S. which are not very vital, containing few nuclei.

Grade 1 C.C.S. discretely infiltrates the medullary spaces of the surrounding bone. Nonetheless, it may be recalled that in chondroma, as well, small cartilaginous lobuli may push forward for a very limited extent in the mesh of the cancellous bone located around the tumor.

Grade 2 C.C.S. This is the most frequent variety of the tumor (approximately 60% of our cases) (Figs. 223b, 224, 225c, d). The cartilage

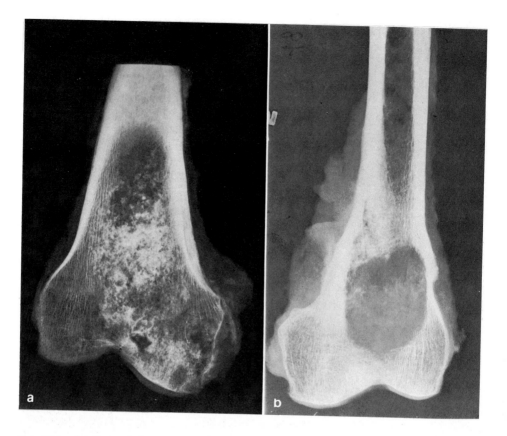

FIG. 221. - (a) Central chondrosarcoma in a male aged 48 years. Histologically grade 2. No signs of recurrence or metastasis 16 years after wide resection. (b) Central chondrosarcoma grade 3 in a female aged 53 years. Widely amputated, there were no signs of either recurrence or metastasis after 13 years.

tissue shows aspects of frank atypia. The nuclei are large, characterized by evident hyperchromia. Binucleate cells are very frequently observed, trinucleate cells rarely. Some nuclei are 4-5 times normal size and/or of bizarre shape.

In nearly half of the cases the tumor is partially or totally myxoid (Fig. 224). In the myxoid areas the cells have a spindle-stellate shape, at times it is roundish. They are dispersed, or gathered in small groups or in short cords in single file. The cytoplasm is ossiphile and is clearly visible on the rather abundant ground substance, which is semi-liquid, tenuously basophile. Nuclear pleomorphism may be scarce (at times less than what is observed in a chondromyxoid fibroma). The nuclei are fairly plump and hyperchromic, at times they are double. Exceptionally, a mitotic figure may be observed.

Grade 2 C.C.S. extensively infiltrates the medullary spaces of the host bone. This may constitute a histological element of determining importance for diagnosis in cases of extensive necrosis of the tumor, making an evaluation of its cytological features difficult. The permeated bone trabeculae may not be

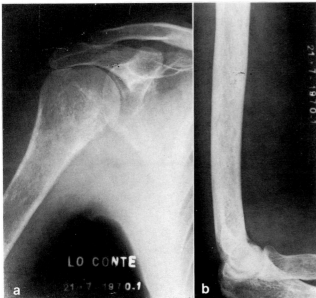

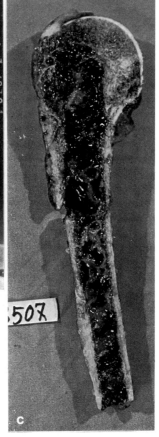

FIG. 222. - (a) Central chondrosarcoma in a male aged 43 years with pain symptoms for the past 2 years. Observe a small interruption in the medial cortex near the epiphysis. (b) The diaphysis of the same humerus is radiographically not very changed. (c) The patient was submitted to interscapulothoracic amputation following frozen section biopsy; the anatomical specimen showed that the humerus was nearly entirely invaded by the tumor which pushed into the medullary canal of the entire diaphysis. Histologically grade 2. The patient died of skeletal and pulmonary metastases 3 years after surgery.

initially destroyed. When the tumor has invaded the soft tissues it may appear to be delimited by a pseudocapsule, but this, too, is infiltrated by neoplastic satellites.

Grade 3 C.C.S. This is observed in approximately 20% of our cases. Nearly always it is well-differentiated in cartilage (Figs. 223, 226a, 227). Often, however, the periphery of the cartilaginous lobuli is made up of a thickly cellular halo of chondroblastic and undifferentiated mesenchymal elements, which are packed and deeply stained.

The cartilaginous cells are very atypical, very numerous, characterized by severe pleomorphism and intense hyperchromia of the nuclei. These are often gigantic (5-10 times normal); cells with three or more nuclei and nuclei having a bizarre shape abound. Unlike chondromas and low-grade C.S., the details of chromatin within the nuclei can be clearly recognized. Some mito-

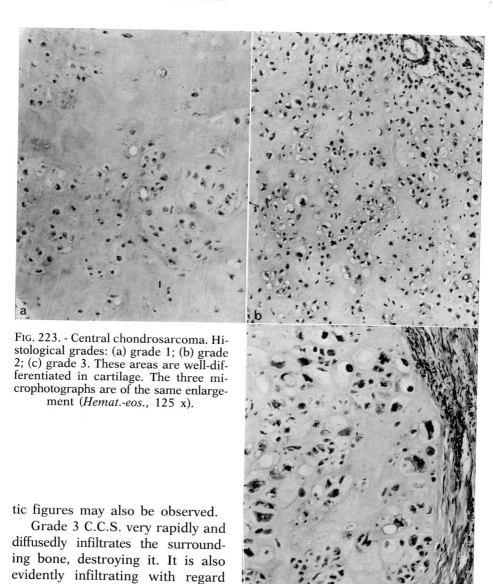

FIG. 223. - Central chondrosarcoma. Histological grades: (a) grade 1; (b) grade 2; (c) grade 3. These areas are well-differentiated in cartilage. The three microphotographs are of the same enlargement (*Hemat.-eos.*, 125 x).

tic figures may also be observed.

Grade 3 C.C.S. very rapidly and diffusedly infiltrates the surrounding bone, destroying it. It is also evidently infiltrating with regard to the soft tissues.

***

The histological classification of C.C.S., which is evidently approximate, nonetheless undoubtedly corresponds with the course and the prognosis of the tumor, and thus is of considerable value in planning treatment.

The most delicate histopathological problem is that of distinguishing a grade 1 C.C.S. from a chondroma. This distinction, like that between grades 1-2-3, cannot be made without taking into account several essential aspects of the problem.

a) Histological observation must be focused on the vital areas of the tumor, and particularly areas which are not modified by calcification-ossification of the neoplastic cartilage. In fact, the calcification-ossification of the cartilage is associated with cellular modifications (hypertrophic cartilaginous cells, swelling of the nuclei) which have nothing to do with the cytological aspects that interest us as indexes of malignancy.

b) Often the cytological signs of malignancy are not the same throughout the tumor, rather varying from zone to zone. For this reason, histological specimens must be as many as possible, and the observer must carefully examine all of the areas of the specimen. Those areas revealing the higher signs of malignancy are those which define the histological grade of the tumor.

c) The signs of cytological malignancy which we have recalled, when mild, must be interpreted in light of the clinical data, the radiographic picture, and the macroscopic aspect. For example, slightly polydimensional nuclei, plump and hyperchromic ones, cells having a double nuclei, do not signify malignancy if the chondroma is located in the tubular bones of the hand, or if it is part of a multiple chondromatosis, especially in the child (let us recall that C.S. is hardly ever manifested prior to puberty), or if it is a periosteal chondroma. Cytological aspects which are even more anaplastic (similar to those of a grade 2 C.S.) do not signify malignancy if the cartilaginous tissue originates from a synovial chondromatosis.

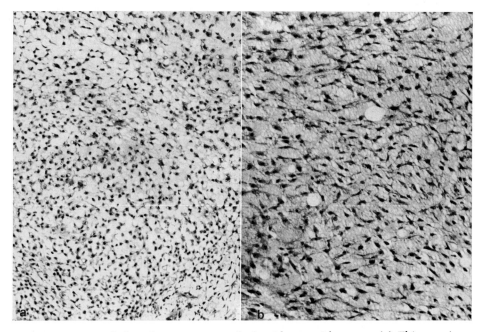

FIG. 224. - Central chondrosarcoma grade 2 with myxoid aspect. (a) This specimen corresponds to the patient in Fig. 220a, who died of metastasis. (b) This specimen corresponds to the patient in Fig. 216, who also died of metastasis. (*Hemat.-eos.*, 125, 125 x).

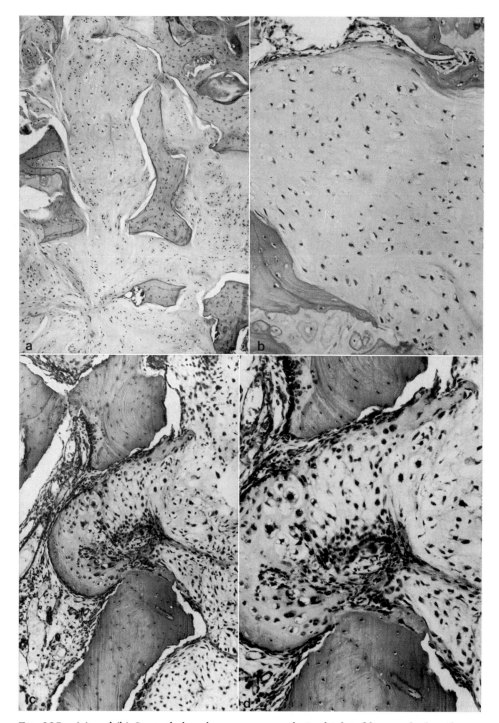

FIG. 225. - (a) and (b) Central chondrosarcoma grade 1 which infiltrates the host bone. The specimen corresponds to the case in Fig. 213a. (c) and (d) Central chondrosarcoma grade 2 which infiltrates the host bone. This specimen corresponds to the case in Fig. 219a. (*Hemat.-eos.*, 50, 125, 80, 125 x).

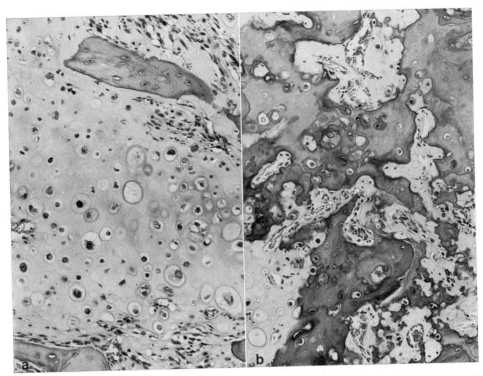

FIG. 226. - (a) Well-differentiated central chondrosarcoma grade 3. (b) Ossification of the neoplastic cartilage. This repair-reactive ossification must not be confused with neoplastic bone in an osteosarcoma (*Hemat.-eos.*, 125, 125 x).

On the contrary, if mild signs of anaplasia are observed in a cartilaginous tumor localized in a major long bone or, even moreso, in the skeleton of the trunk, the probability of local recurrence and initial evolution in malignancy must be taken into consideration (cf. Figs. 168, 169, 170, 185). Similarly, a diagnosis of C.C.S. rather than chondroma will be confirmed by the clinical and radiographic evidence of considerable growth of the tumor, pain occurring where pathologic fracture is absent, a very positive bone scan, recurrence occurring after a first removal, a tumor of large size that has scalloped, expanded, or even surpassed the cortex.

Necrosis, calcification and ossification phenomena occur frequently in all cases of C.C.S. Ossification in C.C.S. is constituted by a newly-formed bone, but one which has no features of malignancy (Fig. 226b). This is a **repair** bone, which substitutes the degenerated and calcified cartilage, or rather is formed by the endosteum and the periosteum as a **reaction** to tumoral invasion. It is never an osteoid produced directly by the mesenchymal sarcomatous cells: in this case the tumor would be an osteosarcoma.

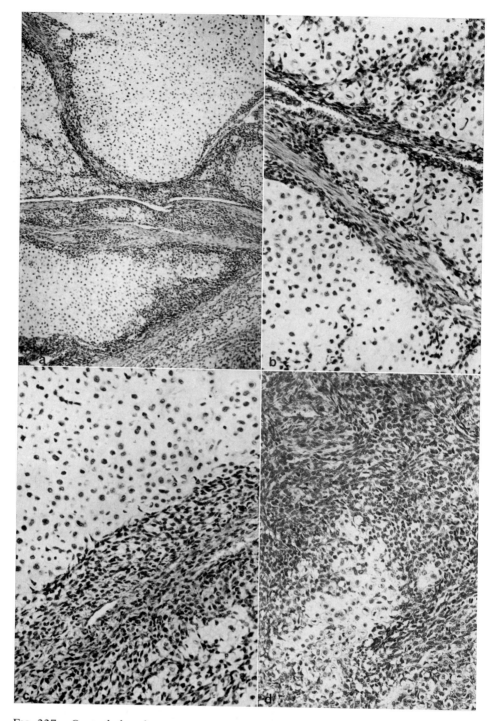

FIG. 227. - Central chondrosarcoma grade 3. Observe crowding of mesenchymal cells at the periphery of the cartilaginous lobuli. These aspects must not be confused with either dedifferentiated chondrosarcoma or with mesenchymal chondrosarcoma (*Hemat.-eos.*, 50, 125, 125, 125 x).

PROGRESSION OF MALIGNANCY
«DEDIFFERENTIATED CHONDROSARCOMA»

Progression of malignancy may be observed in recurrences and in metastases but, not rarely, also in the primary tumor when aspects of different grade of malignancy coexist (Figs. 230, 235). Progression from a chondroma to a C.C.S. is rarely observed, and almost exclusively in cases of multiple chondromas or chondromatosis. Also rare and very slow is progression from grade 1 to 2 (after 19 years in one of our cases, Fig. 210a). Thus, a grade 1 C.C.S. may remain the same even in multiple recurrences and over the course of many years. Progression from grade 2 to 3 may instead be more rapid and, thus, it is observed less rarely.

At times, generally on a grade 1 or 2 C.C.S., an aggressive tumor originates, which histologically is a malignant fibrous histiocytoma, a fibrosarcoma, an osteosarcoma, an angiosarcoma. These tumors have been defined «dedifferentiated chondrosarcomas». They would probably better be defined «high grade sarcomas occurring on chondrosarcoma».

The observation of these **dedifferentiated C.S.** is not rare: about 15% of all C.C.S. in our series. Logically, age is greater than that at which C.C.S. occurs: generally over 50 years (Fig. 231).

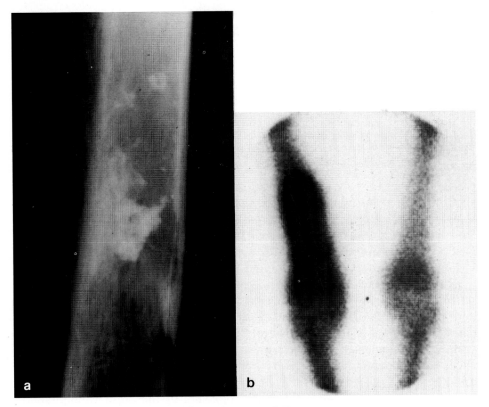

FIG. 228. (legend on the following page).

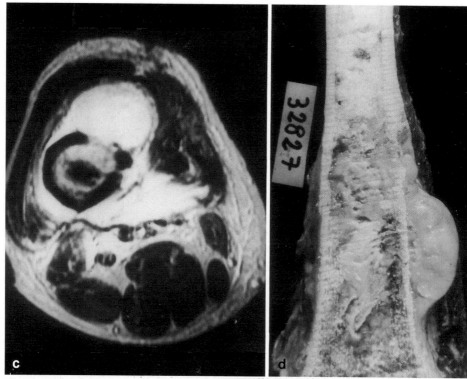

FIG. 228. - Dedifferentiated chondrosarcoma in a female aged 62 years. Pain for the past 3 months and swelling for 1. (a) X-ray shows a calcified «chondrosarcoma», surrounded by some osteolysis, but with no evident interruption in the cortex. (b) Bone scan shows intense hypercaptation extended to the distal half of the femur and overflowing the borders of the bone. (c) MRI shows the extra-cortical tumoral mass which is clearly visible in the section of the anatomical specimen (d). The patient was treated with wide resection (30 cm long) and uncemented endoprosthesis. The patient died after 10 months of pulmonary and diffused metastases. A histological examination of the segment revealed a grade 1 central chondrosarcoma side by side with a grade 4 malignant fibrous histiocytoma.

Clinically, there may be a history of long duration with moderate symptoms, and a rapid successive progression of pain and swelling, with expansion of the latter to the soft tissues. In other cases the symptoms of high-grade sarcoma initiate without any significant antecedents, or the sarcoma is manifested suddenly by pathologic fracture.

Radiographically, the old cartilaginous lesion is usually represented by moderate expansion of the outlines of the bone, with thickening of the cortex and a fair amount of bony demarcation, and by typical intratumoral calcifications. The new lesion is indicated by an aggressive osteolysis (rarely aggressive osteogenesis), which dissolves the calcifications, and tends to interrupt the cortex and invade the soft tissues (Figs. 228, 229, 233). At other times only the new aggressive tumor is observed (Fig. 232), radiographically similar to various high-grade osteolytic neoplasias in the adult (malignant fibrous histiocytoma, fibrosarcoma, lymphoma, metastasis due to carcinoma).

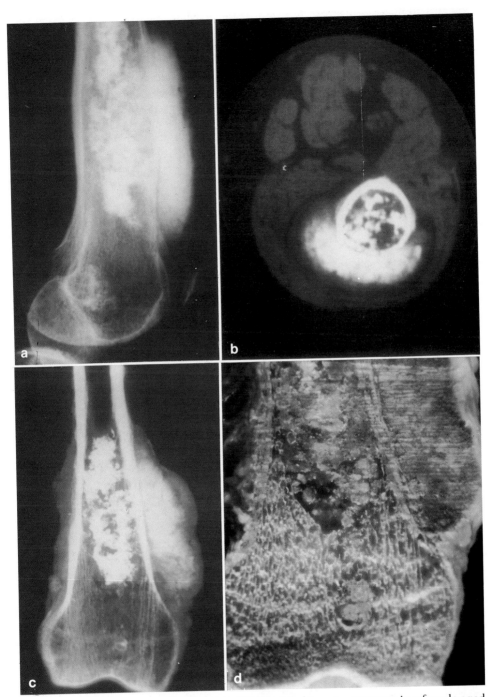

FIG. 229. - Central chondrosarcoma, dedifferentiated in osteosarcoma in a female aged 66 years. Pain for the past 6 months and swelling for the past 4. The typical aspect of a calcified cartilaginous tumor is observed inside the cortex, as is the typical aspect of sclerosing osteosarcoma outside. Histologically, grade 1 chondrosarcoma dedifferentiated in grade 4 osteoblastic osteosarcoma. The patient was submitted to wide resection and uncemented endoprosthesis.

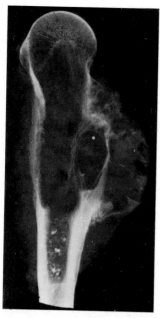

Fig. 230. - Male aged 24 years. For the past year pain and for 3 months swelling. Wide resection and endoprosthesis. No signs of recurrence after 9 years. Histologically the main part of the tumor, which surpassed the cortex, has the aspect of well-differentiated grade 2 chondrosarcoma, while the lower part, contained in the medullary canal and having calcifications, has the aspect of a grade 1 chondrosarcoma. This is an example of progression in malignancy.

Only if antecedent radiograms are available and/or a histological study of the entire tumor is carried out can traces of the pre-existing low-grade cartilaginous tumor be discovered. In other cases, on the contrary, the radiographic and macroscopic aspects are those of the usual C.C.S., and only a few limited areas will histologically reveal the new high-malignancy sarcoma (Fig. 234).

Thus, in order to diagnose dedifferentiated C.S. a macroscopic and histological evaluation of the **entire tumor** is indispensable; this must be sectioned in its various planes and the areas where the macroscopic aspect is not clearly cartilaginous must be searched for in particular.

Histologically, there are two clearly distinct tumoral tissues. One is a well-differentiated cartilaginous tumor, which may vary from case to case and, at times, within the same case, from chondroma to grade 3 chondrosarcoma. Most of our cases reveal the aspect of a grade 1 or 2 C.C.S. The other is

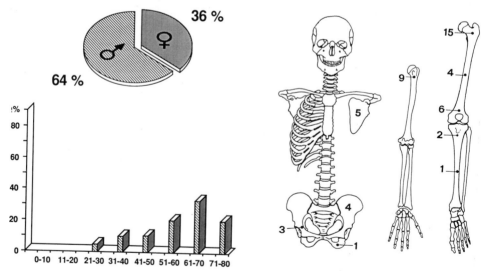

Fig. 231. - Sex, age and site in 50 cases of dedifferentiated central chondrosarcoma.

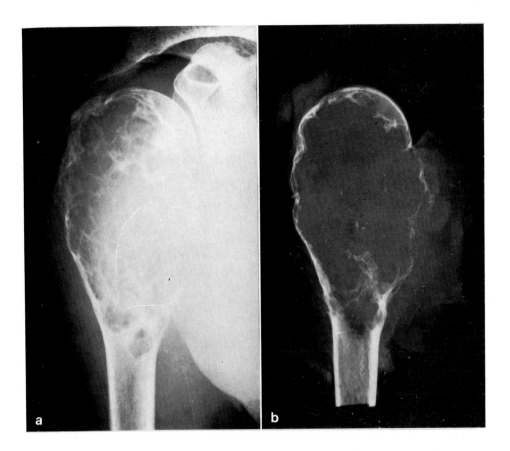

Fig. 232. - (a) Dedifferentiated chondrosarcoma in a male aged 29 years. The patient had mild symptoms for the past 4 years and over the last 2 months he had observed sudden worsening of the pain and particularly of the swelling. (a) Preoperative radiogram; (b) of the anatomical specimen. Wide expansion of the tumor in the soft tissues beyond the medial cortex is visible. Histologically grade 2 chondrosarcoma next to vast areas of poorly differentiated grade 4 fibrosarcoma. Local recurrence 1 month after marginal resection-endoprosthesis. Interscapulothoracic amputation. Recurrence on the stump after 2 months. Radiation therapy. The patient died after 1 year of pulmonary metastases.

a malignant fibrous histiocytoma, or an osteosarcoma, or a fibrosarcoma, and this is always characterized by a high grade of malignancy. The transition from one type of tissue to the other is abrupt (Fig. 236).

Dedifferentiated C.S. will have to be distinguished from grade 3 C.C.S. (Fig. 227) (with undifferentiated cells at the periphery of the lobuli, and gradual transition between these and the cartilaginous cells), as from mesenchymal C.S. (Fig. 280) (having small undifferentiated cells with sparse islands of cartilaginous differentiation).

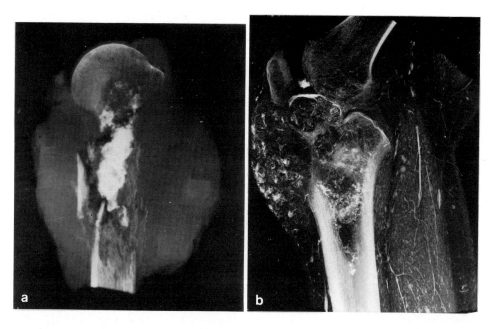

FIG. 233. - Dedifferentiated chondrosarcoma in a female aged 67 years. X-ray of the amputation specimen. An osteolytic lesion invading the soft tissues is observed, and in the center there is an old calcified cartilaginous tumor. Histologically, the latter has the aspect of a grade 1 chondrosarcoma; the remaining part of the tumor has the aspect of a prevalently fibroblastic high grade osteosarcoma. (b) Dedifferentiated chondrosarcoma in a female aged 33 years, who had been submitted to curettage 6 years before with a histological diagnosis of central chondrosarcoma grade 2. A radiograph of the amputation specimen with vascular injection revealed extensive recurrence as far as the subcutaneous plane, and invading the joint. This time, the histological aspect is of grade 2 chondrosarcoma at the center of the diaphysis; while the rest of the tumor (note its intense vascular injection) has the aspect of a malignant fibrous histiocytoma. Pulmonary metastases occurred 2 years after amputation.

HISTOGENESIS AND PATHOGENESIS

Nearly all cases of C.C.S., at least apparently, originate ex novo, as there is no indication (in the patient's history, radiographic, histological) of a pre-existing solitary chondroma.

Rarely (in 5% of our cases), C.C.S. occurs in a case of chondromatosis. The malignant transformation of chondromatosis is a frequent occurrence, but chondromatosis itself is rare. At times, in one case of chondromatosis two C.C.S. develop in different sites, and with many years in between.

DIAGNOSIS

When diagnosing C.C.S. it is important to take into account, more than ever, clinical and radiographic data. The fact that with the same histological aspect a cartilaginous tumor may be benign or malignant, depending on age,

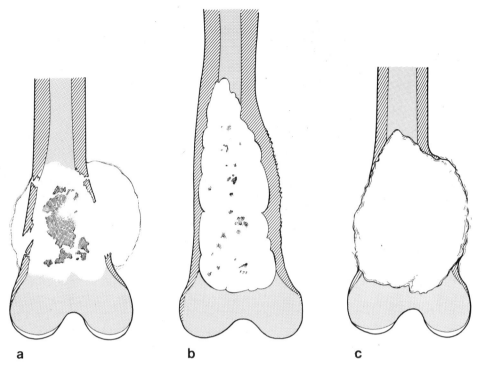

a   b   c

Fig. 234. - Different possibilities of radiographic presentation of dedifferentiated central chondrosarcoma. (a) Observe an intensely calcified veterate cartilaginous lesion, in which a new osteolytic and aggressive lesion has occurred, which tends to cancel the pre-existing calcifications and may cause pathologic fracture. (b) The aspect is that of an usual chondrosarcoma. Diagnosis of dedifferentiated chondrosarcoma is discovered by a histological study of the entire tumor, which reveals small high-grade and noncartilaginous areas of sarcoma. (c) The radiographic aspect is, on the contrary, that of any high-grade osteolytic malignancy of the adult age. In fact the «dedifferentiated» sarcoma has almost completely destroyed the preexisting chondrosarcoma. The correct diagnosis can only result from the histological study of the entire tumor (revealing a small remnant of a low-grade chondrosarcoma), or can be suspected if a cartilage tumor was apparent in previous X-rays.

site, symptoms, radiographic, bone scan, CAT features must not be overlooked. Furthermore, it must be recalled that the definition of histological grade of malignancy may be affirmed only after at least one section of **the entire** tumor has been examined.

C.C.S. often grows slowly and causes moderate symptoms, and it is often localized in cancellous bone which is difficult to explore radiographically (bones of the trunk and of the limb girdles). For all of these reasons, diagnosis is often late. There are cases of C.C.S. of the shoulder treated as for periarthritis for a long time, of the lumbo-sacroiliac region operated on the erroneous diagnosis of disc herniation, of the pelvis or proximal femur which go unrecognized for a long time. When there is persistent pain in the adult, pain which cannot be classified according to common arthralgic and neuralgic syndromes, and which does not respond to treatment, bone scan of the skeleton should be obtained and study with CAT and MRI be carried out.

As treatment of C.C.S. is exclusively surgical, and often difficult and conservative, staging of the tumor must be particularly accurate, and biopsy should be planned with great care, in order to keep therapeutic intervention from becoming difficult, risky, or ineffective.

Often, preoperative diagnosis is quite easy. Nonetheless, numerous tumoral and pseudotumoral affections may be involved in differential diagnosis. The first of these is **chondroma**, which must above all be distinguished from grade 1 C.C.S. and from borderline malignant forms of the tumor. Favoring chondroma are childhood and, in the adult, a lesion which does not grow over the years. Furthermore, chondroma is not painful, unless there is pathologic fracture, it is usually of moderate size, it does not provoke scalloping of the internal face of the cortex, it does not interrupt the cortical bone, and it does not cause swelling in the soft tissues. In short, chondroma usually leaves the cortical bone intact, except when it is localized in the small tubular bones of the hand and foot. As cartilaginous tumors of the hand are nearly always benign, in this site a diagnosis of C.C.S. will be accepted only when the clinical, radiographic, and histological signs indicate evident malignancy. On the contrary, as cartilaginous tumors of the trunk are frequently malignant, in these sites C.C.S. may be suspected, unless proven otherwise (for example, a lesion which is perfectly circumscribed and has remained un-

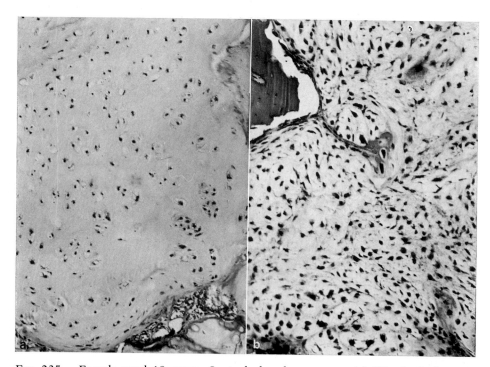

FIG. 235. - Female aged 19 years. Central chondrosarcoma. (a) Histological aspect grade 1. (b) After 8 years and after two local recurrences there is progression in malignancy to grade 2. At times histological aspects of different grades of malignancy coexist in the same tumor (*Hemat.-eos.*, 120 x).

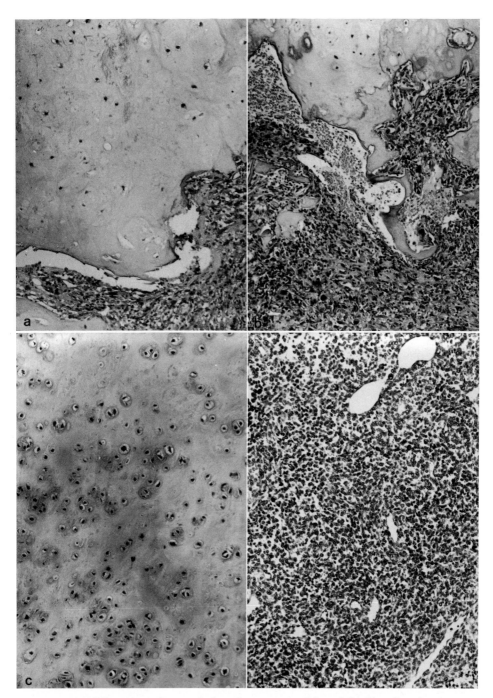

FIG. 236. - Dedifferentiated central chondrosarcoma. (a) and (b) The chondrosarcoma is of borderline malignancy. Observe the abrupt transition from well-differentiated cartilaginous tissue and the «dedifferentiated part» which has the aspect of high-grade malignant fibrous histiocytoma. (c) Area of grade 1 chondrosarcoma. (d) Area of scarcely differentiated high-grade fibrosarcoma. Between the two zones the transition was abrupt. Specimens c-d correspond to the case illustrated in Fig. 232. (*He-mat.-eos.*, 125, 125, 125, 125 x).

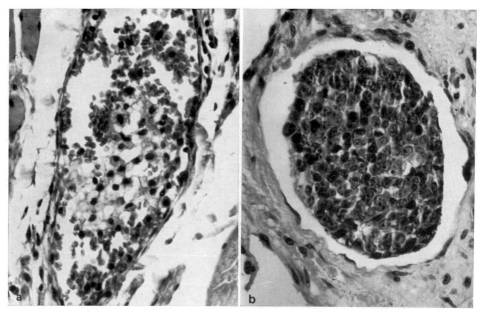

FIG. 237 (a) Intravenous neoplastic plug of grade 2 central chondrosarcoma. (b) Intravenous neoplastic plug of mesenchymal chondrosarcoma (*Hemat.-eos.*, 310, 500 x).

changed for years). In case of doubt, wide surgery will be performed.

Multiple chondromas and chondromatosis. In chondromatosis, chondromas may grow to considerable size, continue to grow even during adult age, and be characterized by histological aspects of lively proliferation. Transformation in C.C.S., which occurs frequently, will always be suspected when there is a change in symptoms and in the radiographic picture during adult age, and this will immediately be ascertained by biopsy.

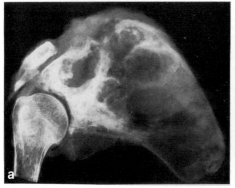
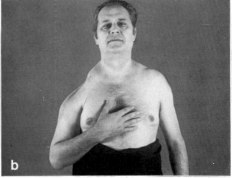

FIG. 238. - Central chondrosarcoma grade 2 in a male aged 51 years. The patient was submitted to wide resection of the scapulohumeral joint, there were no signs of either recurrence or metastases 15 years after surgery. (a) X-ray of the resected specimen. (b) Photo of the patient after surgery.

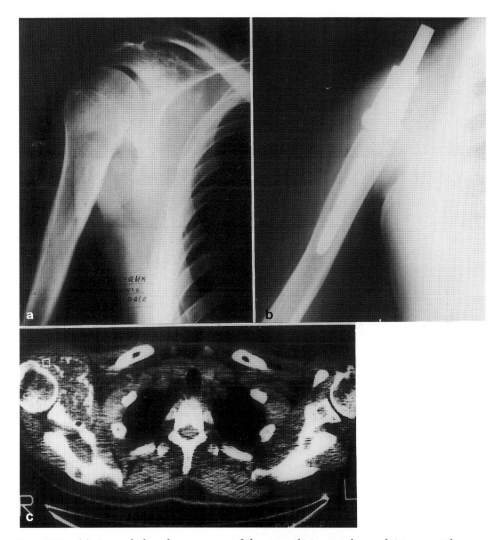

FIG. 239. - (a) Central chondrosarcoma of the scapula in a male aged 46 years. The patient complained of pain for the past 4 years and swelling for 2. The lesion went unrecognized and was treated as periarthritis. CAT (c) reveals the chondrosarcoma invading the glenoid and the joint. The patient was submitted to extra-articular resection of the shoulder (Tikhoff-Linberg) following frozen section biopsy. A histological examination of the entire resected segment showed grade 2 chondrosarcoma. Reconstruction with cemented rotatory modular prosthesis (b).

In joint **synovial chondromatosis**, at times the cartilaginous tissue forms large lobulated masses filling the joint, extensively excavating the joint bone ends, invading the capsule and soft tissues, growing around the metadiaphysis. In these cases of synovial aggressive chondromatosis, the macroscopic (soft, grayish and translucent cartilage) and histological (marked pleomorphism and dismetry of the nuclei) pictures are nearly the same as those for C.C.S. The difference lies in the intrarticular (or paratendinous) origin of

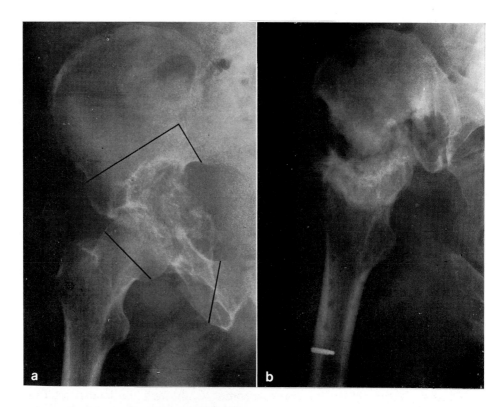

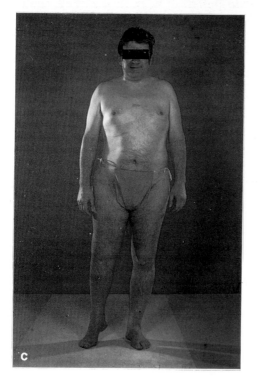

FIG. 240. - Central chondrosarcoma, histological grade 2, in a male aged 36 years. (a) Radiographic aspect of the chondrosarcoma occupying the bottom of the acetabulum. In another hospital the patient had been submitted to curettage with a posterior approach, and bone grafting. The limits of planned skeletal resection are marked. (b) Radiogram 2 years after wide resection (the plate was removed for infection, healed without osteomyelitis). An iliofemoral pseudarthrosis was produced allowing for stable and painless weight-bearing. (c) Photo of the patient 3 years after surgery N.E.D. at 12 years.

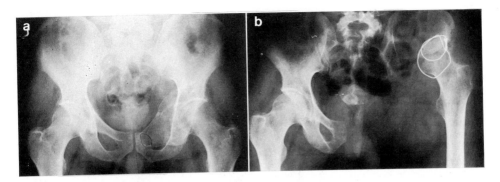

Fig. 241. - (a) Central chondrosarcoma, histological grade 2, in a male aged 46 years. Despite the radiographic aspect, the tumor had completely eroded the cortex in one area, and came into contact with the urinary bladder with several nodules covered only by a thin fibrous capsule. (b) Marginal resection of the hemipelvis and fixation of the epiphysis to the residue of the iliac wing, 2 years after surgery. Pseudarthrosis occurred which allowed for a fair amount of mobility and stable and painless loading. N.E.D. at 10 years.

the tumor, and in the bunchlike arrangement of the cartilaginous cells. Even C.C.S. may invade the joint, but it originates from the epiphysis and its cells are diffusedly distributed.

Classic (chondroblastic) osteosarcoma. Childhood indicates osteosarcoma (C.C.S. hardly ever exists prior to puberty). Even in the adult, the radiographic picture and the macroscopic aspect are generally different. But the difference lies above all in the histological examination. In osteosarcoma, even when it is mostly chondroblastic, aspects of osteoblastic differentiation and osteoid production on the part of the tumoral cells must be found; furthermore, the malignancy of the cartilaginous cells of the osteosarcoma is more elevated (grade 4) than what is observed in C.C.S. At any rate, there are rare cases where, on a limited bioptic specimen, differential diagnosis is difficult or even impossible. In cases such as these, it is best to repeat biopsy, more extensively and specifically, before deciding whether or not to use chemotherapy.

Chondromyxoid fibroma. The macroscopic aspect may be the same as that of C.C.S. and, histologically, the centro-lobular cells may suggest a grade 1 or 2 C.C.S. Chondromyxoid fibroma is distinguished by the infantile age, the radiographic aspect, and the typical histological structure.

Particular care must be taken in diagnosing **dedifferentiated C.S.** (malignant fibrous histiocytoma, osteosarcoma, high-grade fibrosarcoma). This diagnosis may be suspected based on the clinical history of the patient and radiograms. Suspicion should lead to specific biopsy and, if confirmed, treatment must be more aggressive than that of C.C.S., and prognosis is worse. At times, preoperative suspicion is not possible, and diagnosis is made only when a histological examination of the entire tumor is available, after its surgical removal (Fig. 234c).

FIG. 242. - (a) Central chondrosarcoma grade 2 in a male aged 67 years, affected with skeletal chondromatosis (25 years previously he had been amputated below the knee in the contralateral limb for chondrosarcoma of the first metatarsal). (b) Radiogram of the widely resected specimen: internal femoral condyle. (c) The condyle was substituted with the patella of the same knee and with autogenous bridging grafts. Results after 6 years. The knee is stable and mobile from 180 to 90 degrees. N.E.D. at 16 years.

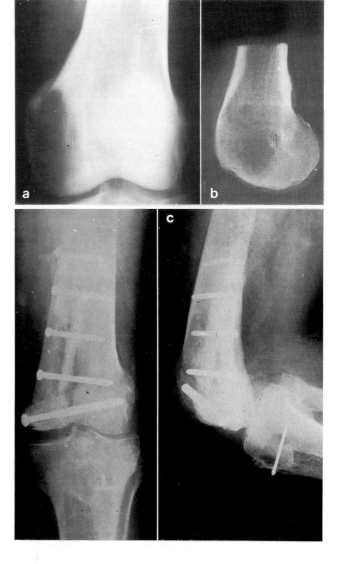

COURSE

C.C.S. generally grows more slowly than osteosarcoma. Often the interval of time between the first symptoms and diagnosis exceeds 1 year, at times 2 years, not rarely 5 and even 10. Nonetheless, it is important to distinguish between grades 1, 2, and 3 C.C.S. The latter may have a course which is as rapid as that of typical osteosarcoma. Furthermore, as previously stated, a C.C.S. may be characterized by progression in malignancy or by its becoming dedifferentiated, either within the same tumor, or within its recurrence. In the former case, the tumor which has grown slowly for months and years, is suddenly characterized by a more rapid and aggressive course. In the latter case, a few months or years after the removal of a C.C.S. which had grown relatively slowly, recurrence which is more rapidly expansive and invasive, histologically more malignant and at times dedifferentiated, occurs.

In grades 2 and 3 C.C.S., recurrence nearly always occurs within 5 years, and often within less than 1. In grade 1 C.C.S. it may be manifested even after more than 10 years. Metastases may occur after a period of time ranging from a few months to 20-25 years after the onset of symptoms, more often within 5 years.

C.C.S. metastasizes nearly exclusively by hematic route. Metastases to the regional lymph nodes occur in exceptional cases. Metastases are nearly

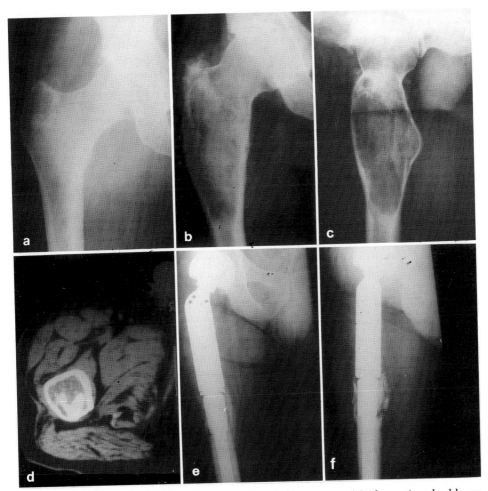

Fig. 243. - Central chondrosarcoma in a male aged 33 years. (a) The patient had been operated elsewhere by marginal resection of the greater trochanter with diagnosis of chondroma. (b), (c) and (d) Recurrence and extent of the tumor after 9 years. (e) and (f) The patient was submitted to wide resection and uncemented endoprosthesis. Histologically, extensively myxoid grade 2 chondrosarcoma. There were no signs of disease after 2 years.

always pulmonary. In some rare cases metastases may occur in the skeleton (particularly in the trunk), even when there is no radiographic pulmonary metastasis. The tissue of the metastasis may maintain cartilaginous differentiation, or it may be less differentiated.

Grade 1 C.C.S. usually do not metastasize. Grade 2 C.C.S. have a considerable tendency to metastasize, at times early, at times late. Grade 3 C.C.S. have a higher tendency to metastasize, more or less early. As the cells of C.C.S. are generally amalgamated by the ground substance, and are not in direct contact with the vascular lumi, they are not easily dispersed in the circulation. Rather, metastasis occurs when the tumor erodes the wall of the veins and forms solid intravenous plugs (Fig. 237). These neoplastic thrombi may grow within the venous tree (cases are described in which a continuous chondrosarcomatous plug went from the femoral vein to the right heart and to the ramifications of the pulmonary artery), or become detached and go as far as the lungs [1]. It is important to recall that C.C.S. with growth in the venous tree may cause severe circulatory and respiratory decompensation and result in death without any metastasis occurring in the pulmonary parenchyma. In these cases, radiograms of the thorax remain negative and only autopsy may reveal the intravenous ramification of the tumor (Lichtenstein, 1965).

TREATMENT

One must not rely on the slow growth of a C.C.S. At times, because of the progression of malignancy or «dedifferentiation», any delay may result in severe or irremediable error.

Treatment of C.C.S. is surgical and offers considerable possibilities of cure, often also by conservative means. These possibilities depend on the fact that, at first diagnosis, many C.C.S. have not as yet produced pulmonary metastases (cf. course).

A histological diagnosis may be made intraoperatively using frozen sections, particularly in cases where development is rapid, destructive and invasive. In cases characterized by lower malignancy, when a decision on performing a more or less conservative operation may also depend on an accurate histological grading of the disease, it is best to postpone surgery for a few days, while waiting for inclusional slides. While carrying out biopsy great care must be taken not to disseminate traces of neoplastic tissue in the wound, as C.C.S. may easily be implanted in the soft tissues.

Curettage is not indicated because it is hardly ever successful, whatever the grade of histological malignancy. Only in borderline cases between chondroma and grade 1 C.C.S. has aggressive intralesional excision been per-

---

[1] In one of our cases, characterized by pulmonary metastases, embolia of the femoral artery was observed to occur, evidently due to progression of a lung-left heart-aorta circulation neoplastic embolus.

formed successfully, associated with the use of local adjuvants such as phenol, cement and liquid nitrogen (Figs. 211, 244).

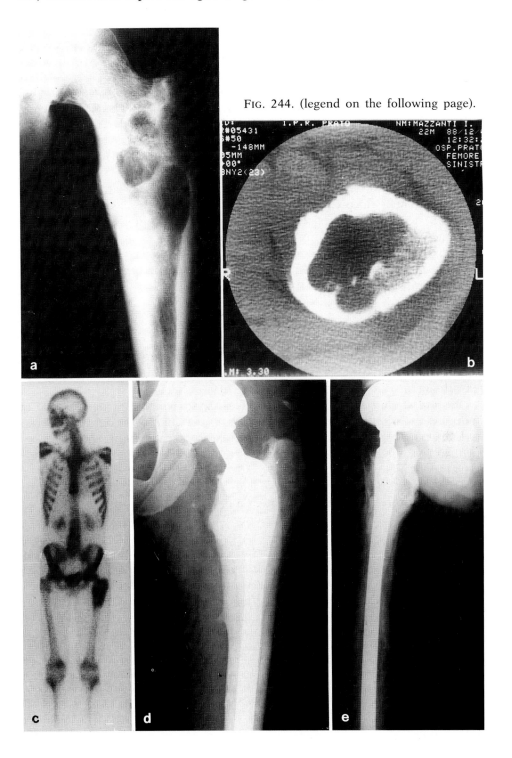

FIG. 244. (legend on the following page).

Wide or radical surgical margins must be obtained. A marginal margin is exposed to a high risk of recurrence, which increases as the grade of histological malignancy does. In many cases, conservative **resection** may be obtained by using wide margins.

Amputation is necessary in cases with large expansion in the soft tissues, particularly in grade 3 and in nearly all dedifferentiated C.S.

In planning the site of resection or amputation, it is important to study (bone scan, CAT, MRI) the extent of the tumor along the diaphyseal medullary canal, or in the spongy bone (C.C.S. of the pelvis).

When there is recurrence in the soft tissues of a resected C.C.S., it is not delimited (unlike what occurs in some cases of peripheral chondrosarcoma) and generally it cannot be resolved by en bloc excision, instead requiring ablative surgery.

Unfortunately, considerable obstacles to the surgical treatment of C.C.S. derive from their localization in the skeleton of the trunk.

C.C.S. is a radiation-resistant tumor. Radiation therapy is of minimal effectiveness, even as a palliative of pain. The same may be said of chemotherapy which is used only in some cases of dedifferentiated C.C.S.

In cases of circumscribed pulmonary metastases, resection of the metastases is indicated.

PROGNOSIS

Grade 1 C.C.S. generally do not metastasize. They recur in loco if removal was not wide. Death may result by invasion of the splanchnic cavities or vertebral canal.

Despite its slow course and histological aspect which may be deprived of the more apparent features of malignancy, **grade 2 C.C.S.** is capable of even early metastases, and locally recurs very easily. If surgical treatment is immediate and adequate (which is not always the case), the percentage of healing may be approximately 60%.

Grade 3 C.C.S. seems to have the worst prognosis: the probability of surviving would be approximately 40%.

◀

FIG. 244. - Central chondrosarcoma (grade 1) in a male aged 21 years. Discontinous pain for the past few years, which had become more continuous over the last 6 months. (a) Radiographic aspect of rounded osteolysis with excavation of the inner cortex and in other areas thickening of the cortex. (b) CAT revealed the same aspects as well as a wrinkled external surface of the cortex, and some small intratumoral calcifications. (c) Bone scan indicated the longitudinal extent of the tumor. (d) and (e) Considering the stage of the tumor (IA), we decided to attempt a rather conservative surgery. Wide intra-articular resection of the proximal femur was done. The femoral neck and the epiphysis were removed from the resected segment, curettage of the tumor performed, followed by freezing and thawing three times, by immersion in liquid nitrogen. An endoprosthesis was cemented in the resection segment and the caudal part of the stem was cemented in the residual diaphysis. Follow-up at 1 year showed excellent union of the perfrigerated autograft.

Dedifferentiated C.S. have a very poor prognosis (as is generally the case in secondary sarcomas: in Paget's disease, due to radiation); even when surgical treatment is wide or radical, metastases occur frequently and early. We still do not know how much chemotherapy may be of help (rarely used also because of the advanced age of most of these patients).

Prognosis in C.C.S. essentially depends on two factors: the histological grade of malignancy; the adequacy of surgical margins (wide or radical and not contaminated).

PERIPHERAL CHONDROSARCOMA

DEFINITION

It is a C.S. which originates outside the bone, but is implanted on the bone. Secondary origin from an exostosis may be affirmed with certainty in cases of multiple exostosis and in some P.C.S. where signs (the patient's history, radiographic and anatomical) of pre-existing solitary exostosis are observed. In the others (particularly of the proximal femur, pelvis, spine, ribs) there is no trace of exostosis, which remained asymptomatic and which the P.C.S. has completely cancelled. But in these, as well, extraosseous localization and radiographic and anatomical aspects are such that an epiexostotic origin is nearly certain.

FREQUENCY

P.C.S. occurs less frequently than central chondrosarcoma (Fig. 245).

SEX

There is predilection for the male sex at a ratio of 2:1 (Fig. 245).

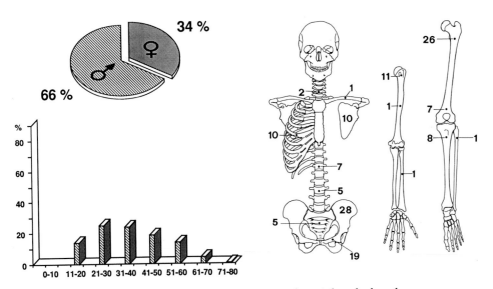

FIG. 245. - Sex, age and site in 142 cases of peripheral chondrosarcoma.

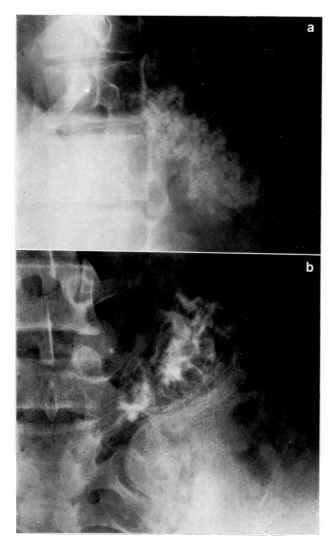

FIG. 246. - (a) Peripheral chondrosarcoma of the arch of the 12th thoracic vertebra in a male aged 40 years. Histologically grade 2. (b) Exostosis which for the past two months had increased in size and become painful in a male aged 16 years. Histologically grade 1 peripheral chondrosarcoma. No signs of recurrence 11 years after wide removal.

AGE

The tumor occurs in the adult. It is generally observed after 20 years of age, and never before puberty (Fig. 245).

An exostosis which increases in volume during childhood should not cause worry. During this age, it is normal for it to grow. On the contrary, an exostosis that resumes growth during adult age can only suggest P.C.S.

LOCALIZATION

The most frequent site in which P.C.S. occurs is the pelvis, followed by, in decreasing order, the proximal femur, vertebral column and sacrum, proxi-

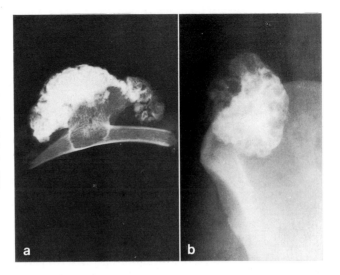

FIG. 247. - (a) Grade 1 peripheral chondrosarcoma from costal exostosis in a male aged 34 years. (b) Exostosis in initial grade 1 chondrosarcomatous transformation of the ilium in a female aged 33 years. For the past few weeks the exostosis had become painful. Transformation corresponds to the more external and radiotransparent area of the exostosis.

mal humerus, ribs, scapula, distal femur, proximal tibia. As compared to C.C.S. it has a more evident predilection for the pelvis and the skeleton of the trunk. Furthermore, **it is hardly ever observed distal to the knee and elbow** (Fig. 245).

In the vertebrae and sacrum it originates from the posterior arch; in the pelvis it more often originates from the iliac wing or from the anterior arch; in the scapula, from the body; in the long bones, from a diaphyseal end near the metaphysis (like exostosis).

The tumor expands outside the bone, invading the pre-existing exostosis and, in more aggressive and advanced forms, also the implant bone.

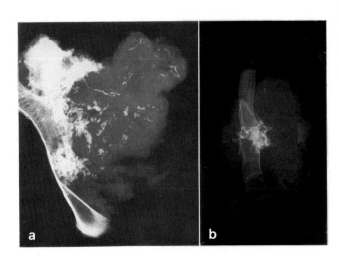

FIG. 248. - (a) Peripheral chondrosarcoma of the internal face of the iliac wing in a male aged 48 years. This chondrosarcoma had already been removed 10 years earlier. The radiogram corresponds to the wide resection specimen including the entire iliac wing and the sacroiliac joint. Histologically grade 1. No recurrence after 14 years. (b) Peripheral chondrosarcoma of the 7th rib in a female aged 55 years. Histologically grade 1. No recurrence 21 years after wide costal resection.

SYMPTOMS

The principal sign is the presence of a mass, coming from the skeletal plane, which grows slowly. The mass is contained within the soft tissues, to which it does not adhere, it is often rounded and vaguely bumpy, it is bony hard or hard-elastic.

In some cases the patient is affected with multiple hereditary exostoses. In other cases the patient was aware of the fact that he had a solitary exostosis in the site of increasing swelling. More often, instead, no trace is found in the patient's history of previous exostosis. A history of one or more surgical removals, with recurrence of the tumoral mass, is not a rare finding. In cases such as these, either a single mass or multiple nodes in the soft tissues, completely separated from the skeleton, may be observed.

At times, the neoplasm is painless, but in more than half of all cases there is pain, which is generally mild and subsequent to swelling. In P.C.S. of the pelvis, at times there are signs of compression of the lumbosacral plexus or its terminal branches. In vertebral localizations of the disease, paraplegia due to medullary compression may occur.

As P.C.S. grows slowly without causing considerable symptoms, at least for a certain period of time, and as the patient is often used to living with exostosis which he does not fear knowing that it is harmless, it often occurs that on first observation P.C.S. has grown to conspicuous size, which may even be monstruous.

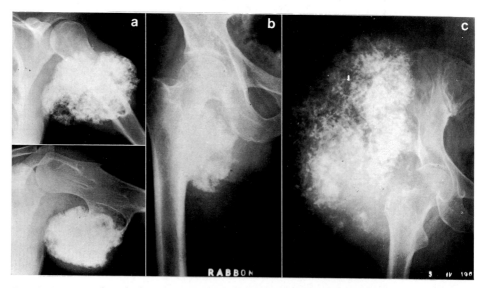

FIG. 249. - Peripheral chondrosarcoma. (a) In multiple hereditary exostoses in a female aged 29 years. Histological grade 1. (b) In a male aged 36 years. Histological grade 2. (c) In a female aged 40 years. Histological grade 2.

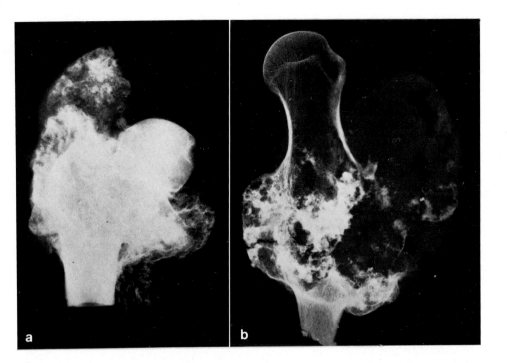

FIG. 250. - (a) Peripheral chondrosarcoma in a female aged 44 years. The lesion was discovered 1 year earlier by X-ray obtained for trauma. Resection specimen (same case as Fig. 263). Histologically grade 1. (b) Peripheral chondrosarcoma in a male aged 45 years. The patient was affected with solitary exostosis observed for the first time at 8 years of age. For the past 2 years progressive increase in swelling. Histologically grade 2. The patient was submitted to resection-endoprosthesis. No signs of recurrence or metastasis after 14 years.

RADIOGRAPHIC FEATURES

Usually, the radiographic picture cannot be mistaken for any other, so that diagnosis may be certain even before histological assessment has been carried out.

The essential radiographic element is constituted by radiopacities due to calcification-ossification of the neoplastic cartilage. In general, calcification is more constant and abundant as compared to C.C.S. In many cases, this radiopacity is diffused to nearly the entire tumor and it is rather intense (Figs. 246a, 247, 249, 254, 255b). Thus, an extraosseous mass is observed, vaguely lobulated, bumpy like a cauliflower, and intensely radiopaque. In the areas where the thickness of the mass does not cause a compact eburneous image (and, in particular, when x-raying sections of the anatomical specimen), it may be observed that the calcification is not structured and has a typical nodule, spot and ring shape (corresponding to cartilaginous lobuli and their periphery, respectively) (Figs. 247a, 248a, 250b, 255b, 257b). The superficial lay-

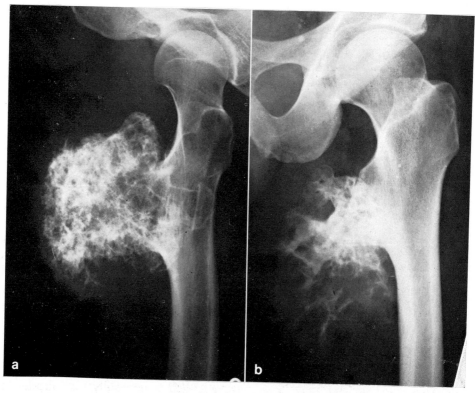

FIG. 251. - (a) Peripheral chondrosarcoma in a male aged 44 years. Histologically grade 1. The patient was submitted to marginal removal, recurrence 2 years later. (b) Peripheral chondrosarcoma in a male aged 34 years. Swelling had only been observed for the past few months. Histologically grade 2. The patient was submitted to intralesional or marginal excision, repeated eight times, with just as many recurrences, over 13 years time.

er of the tumor (of more recent formation) is less calcified and may thus reveal fuzzy boundaries towards the soft tissues.

In other cases, more or less vast parts of the tumor have no radiopacity (because they are formed by non-calcified neoplastic cartilage), with limits which are totally faded, so that they may be visualized with CAT or MRI alone (Figs. 252, 253). Nonetheless, in these cases, as well, the tumor, and particularly towards its base, is nearly always sprayed with typical radiopacities which are nodular, spotted, ringlike, popcornlike (Figs. 248, 250b).

At times, the radiopacity appears to be partially more structured (calcification is associated with ossification), with irregular and dense trabeculation, or curvilinear shoots making up bubbling images or ones resembling bread crumbs similar to those of some types of C.C.S. (Figs. 250a, 251, 265).

At times, the implant base of the exostosis is still visible, as is the typical evagination of the bony cortex (Figs. 247a, 249a, 250b, 251, 253a, 255b, 256, 262). Often, when P.C.S. surrounds the bone of origin and when it has invaded and completely cancelled the exostosis, the implant base cannot be recognized (Figs. 248, 252c), or rather the tumor may be observed to invade the host bone (Fig. 250b).

In exceptional cases, in forms which are observed at the very beginning, the radiographic aspect is still that of exostosis, and malignant evolution is manifested by CAT and MRI, and by macroscopic and histological examinations (Figs. 246b, 253). Unlike what occurs in exostosis in the adult, bone scan is intensely positive (Fig. 252b).

When P.C.S. has already been removed and local recurrence, lacking any calcification, develops in the soft tissues, the radiogram may appear to be completely negative. In cases such as these CAT and MRI are essential investigations, especially in the pelvis and in the trunk.

In the skeleton of the trunk traces of pre-existing exostosis (probably small and unrecognized) are hardly every observed.

The radiographic picture may allow us to deduce the grade of malignancy of P.C.S. If radiopacity is intense and diffused to the entire tumor, if the limits towards the soft tissues are relatively well-defined, and if there is no invasion of the implant bone, it is generally a grade 1 P.C.S. More often, what

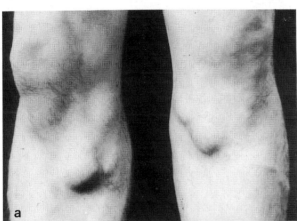

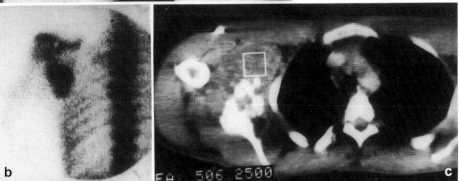

FIG. 252. - Multiple hereditary exostoses, in a male aged 24 years. For the past year pain in the right scapula irradiated along the upper limb. In the same region swelling occurred, which gradually increased. (a) Clinical aspect of multiple exostoses in the knee. (b) Intense isotope uptake (c) CAT reveals large non-calcified tumoral masses corresponding to the neoplastic cartilage. The patient was submitted to wide scapulectomy. Histological diagnosis of grade 2 peripheral chondrosarcoma. No signs of disease after 8 years.

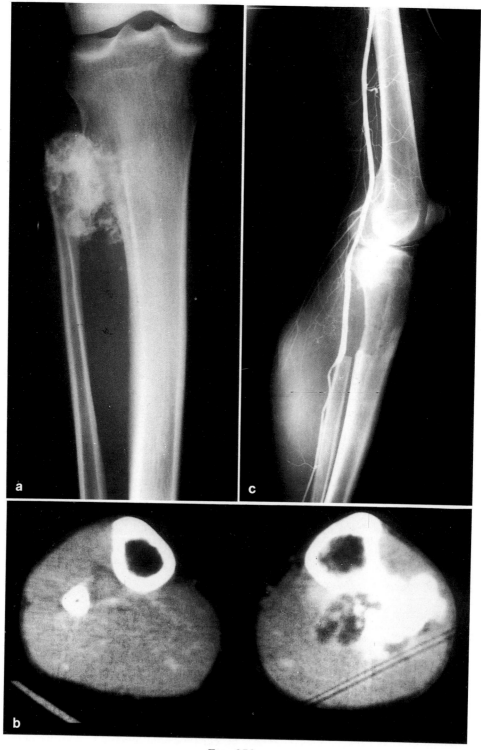

FIG. 253.

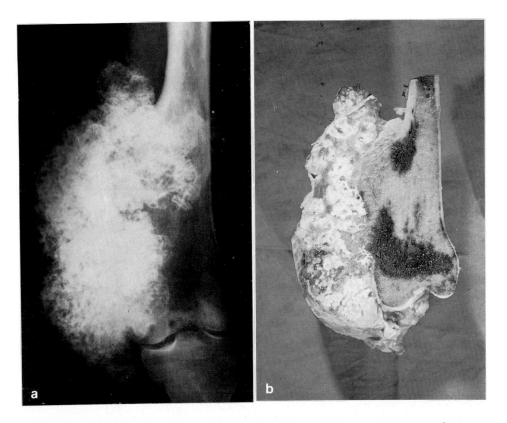

FIG. 254. - Peripheral chondrosarcoma in a female aged 25 years. At the age of 8 years an exostosis had been partially excised in the same site. Histologically grade 1. The patient was widely amputated, and is well after 19 years. (a) Radiographic aspect. (b) Macroscopic aspect. Observe lobuli of cartilage, most of which calcified, penetrating deep into the exostotic mass.

is observed is a mass with some non-calcified areas, partially faded limits, of considerable size. This radiographic aspect corresponds to a histological grade 1 or 2. Finally, in other cases, the tumor is extensively deprived of radiopacity, with limits which are extensively faded, of rather large size, at times there is invasion of the implant bone. This aspect corresponds to a histological grade 2 or 3, or to dedifferentiated P.C.S.

◀

FIG. 253. - Peripheral chondrosarcoma in a male aged 40 years. For the past 9 years pain and ischemic symptoms in the foot. The tumor surrounded the tibial nerve and peroneal nerve as well as the posterior and anterior tibial vessels. Thus, he was submitted to resection of the posterior cortex of the tibia and of the whole fibula, en bloc with the popliteal nerve and the tibial vessels. The latter were reconstructed by arterial by-pass (c). The resection was marginal and histological examination revealed a grade 2 peripheral chondrosarcoma. There were no signs of disease after 2 years.

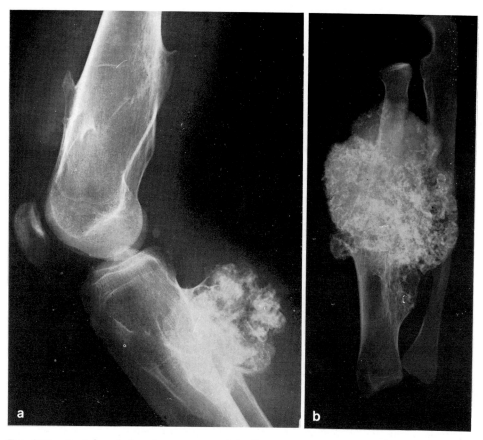

FIG. 255. - Peripheral chondrosarcoma of the forearm in a male aged 22 years affected with multiple hereditary exostoses. (a) Exostoses of the lower right limb (with no signs of malignancy). (b) Peripheral chondrosarcoma of the left radius. Histologically grade 2. No metastases 24 years after amputation.

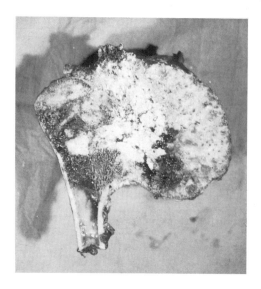

FIG. 256. - Peripheral chondrosarcoma in a female aged 28 years. Resection specimen of the proximal humerus. Histologically grade 1. No recurrence after 27 years.

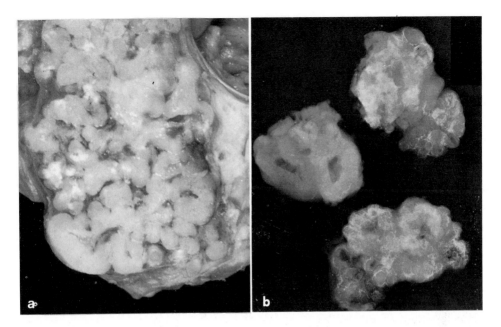

F$_{IG}$. 257. - (a) Typical macroscopic aspect of peripheral chondrosarcoma. The white spots correspond to calcification. (b) Radiogram of the cartilaginous tissue with perilobular ringlike calcification.

GROSS PATHOLOGIC FEATURES

Generally, the tumor is found to be of large size when it is exposed surgically. The surface is typically bumpy, like a cauliflower. The tumor is delimited by a fibrous pseudocapsule, which is often rather thin.

During the initial stages of malignant transformation of the exostosis it may be observed that its cartilaginous cap (which should be very thin and discontinuous during adult age) is of considerable thickness. Practically speaking, when in an adult the thickness of the cartilage of an exostosis achieves or exceeds 1-2 centimeters, malignant transformation will have to be suspected. (In the child the thickness of the cartilage may even reach 2 centimeters without this signifying malignancy). Furthermore, the cartilage tends to grow round-topped and in lobuli, both at the surface and in profundity, penetrating the spongy bone of the exostosis. Finally, this cartilage does not have the aspect of normal hyalin cartilage, rather, it is softer, juicy, grayish and translucent.

In more advanced phases of P.C.S., while the surface expands like a cauliflower or mushroom, tending to surround the base of the exostosis and the implant bone, the neoplastic cartilaginous lobuli invade the spongy bone of the exostosis and, at the end, also the host bone (Figs. 254, 256). The neoplastic cartilage has a strong tendency to calcify and ossify, which is greater in the deeper parts of the tumor, less at the surface. Calcification is manifested

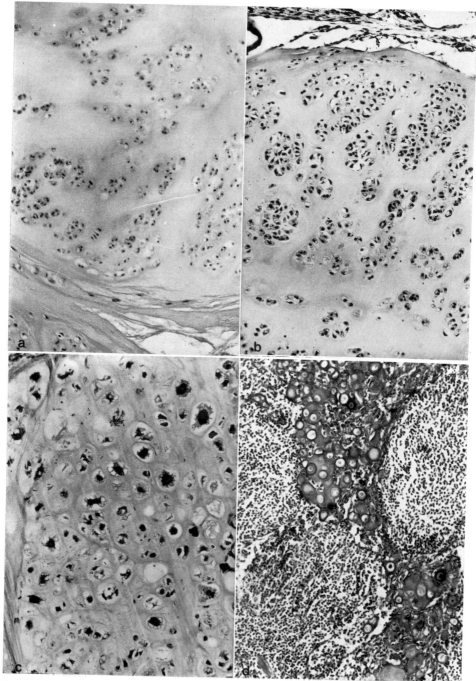

FIG. 258. - Peripheral chondrosarcoma. Histological grades: (a) grade 1, (b) grade 2, (c) grade 3. The three microphotographs are at the same enlargement. (d) Peripheral chondrosarcoma of large size of the anterior pelvic arch in a male aged 38 years. Histologically grade 2. (The patient was submitted to interilioabdominal amputation with excision of the iliac lymph nodes.) Microphotograph shows metastatic nests in a lymph node. (*Hemat.-eos.*, 125, 125, 125, 70 x).

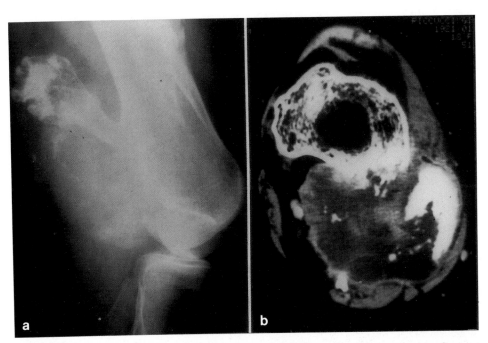

FIG. 259. - Grade 2 peripheral chondrosarcoma dedifferentiated in grade 4 malignant fibrous histiocytoma in a male aged 67 years affected with multiple exostoses in the lower limbs. For the past 2 months swelling had rapidly increased and was painful. Marginal resection of the tumor with its implant base, dissociating it from the large vessels to which it adhered. Following the histological diagnosis thigh amputation was performed. (a) and (b) Radiogram and CAT showed the osteolytic tumor adhering to the large vessels alongside a typical exostosis. The medullary canal was not involved. Diagnosis should have been suspected prior to surgery. The patient died after 1 year of pulmonary and diffused metastases.

in granules, rings, irregular spots of yellowish-white aspect, chalky and gritty, of hard consistency; ossification has the aspect of hypermic cancellous, or eburneous and whitish bone.

In less malignant forms (histological grade 1) calcification-ossification is often very intense and diffused. The entire P.C.S. has a rather hard or eburneous consistency, except for some superficial cartilaginous areas. P.C.S. which grow more rapidly (histological grades 2-3) are instead softer, made up of large lobuli of juicy, translucent cartilage. At the center of the lobuli mucoid softening is frequently observed (Fig. 257a).

The pseudocapsule of the tumor is rather thick in less aggressive forms, while it is quite thin in the others, enough to allow the color of the cartilage to appear. At times, under the capsule, there are large sacs containing mucinous liquid, in which loose cartilage bodies float. This finding may cause the clinical sensation of fluctuation and make the tumor seem larger than it appears to be radiographically.

In recurrence and, at times, even after previous biopsy, nodules of cartilage which are hardly or not at all calcified may be observed, **scattered through-**

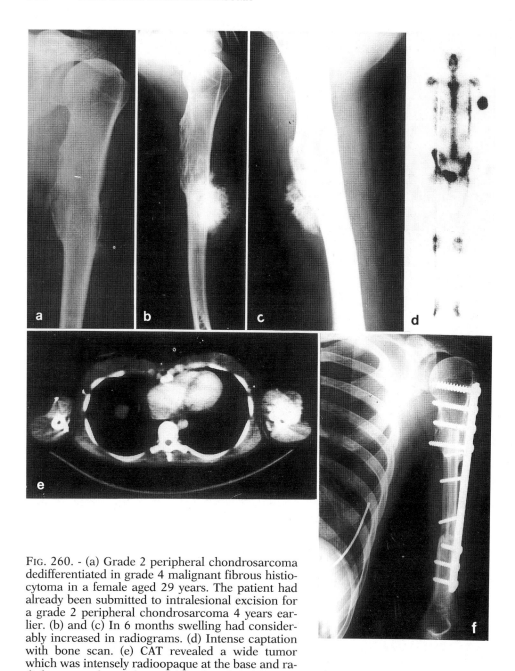

FIG. 260. - (a) Grade 2 peripheral chondrosarcoma dedifferentiated in grade 4 malignant fibrous histiocytoma in a female aged 29 years. The patient had already been submitted to intralesional excision for a grade 2 peripheral chondrosarcoma 4 years earlier. (b) and (c) In 6 months swelling had considerably increased in radiograms. (d) Intense captation with bone scan. (e) CAT revealed a wide tumor which was intensely radioopaque at the base and radiolucent at the surface with rather faded boundaries towards the soft tissues and scarce involvement of the medullary canal. The patient was submitted to wide resection of the humeral diaphysis (9 cm) following frozen section biopsy, which revealed a grade 2 chondrosarcoma. (A histological examination of the entire tumor revealed the areas of dedifferentiation in grade 4 malignant fibrous histiocytoma). (f) Reconstruction with autoplastic fibula well-consolidated after 1 year. After 3 and 1/2 years skeletal metastases in the ilium which was biopsied with a histological diagnosis of grade 4 malignant fibrous histiocytoma and treated with radiation therapy. The patient is alive with disease.

out the soft tissues and which are not visible radiographically. These, too, have clear boundaries and may be excised successfully.

HISTOPATHOLOGIC FEATURES

Histological examination must always be carried out on non-calcified cartilage. In some cases of grade 1 P.C.S., which are intensely calcified, cartilage may be very scarce, limited to a few areas at the surface of the tumor.

Unlike central chondrosarcoma, P.C.S. is nearly always composed of well-differentiated cartilage. In exceptional cases, there may be myxoid areas. Furthermore, the cartilage of P.C.S. (evidently more nourished than that of C.C.S. due to its free expansion in the soft tissues) is, particularly in the superficial lobuli, a vital and exuberantly proliferating cartilage. Based on these features, it is sometimes possible to distinguish between C.C.S. and P.C.S. under microscopy. There is ground substance which is abundant and compact, with rather numerous cells, at times gathered in thick isogenous groups. Areas of cellular necrosis are frequent in the deeper parts of the tu-

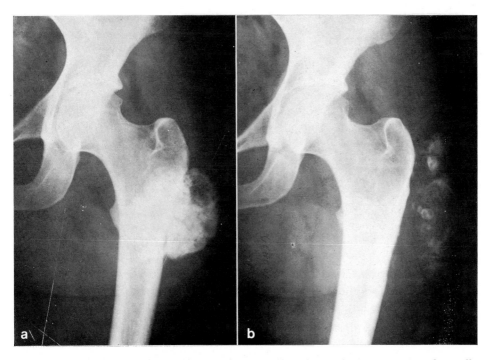

FIG. 261. - (a) Peripheral chondrosarcoma in a female aged 18 years. Histologically grade 1. The patient was submitted to intralesional excision. (b) After 7 years recurrences in the soft tissues revealed radiographically by calcification. This time the tumor was histologically grade 2. The patient was again submitted to excision, which was wide, and there was no recurrence 6 years later.

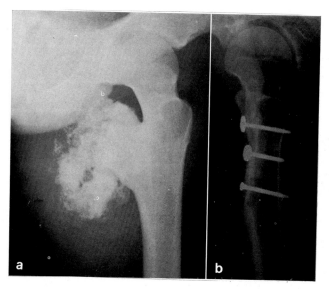

FIG. 262. - (a) Peripheral chondrosarcoma in a male aged 17 years. Progressive swelling was observed for only the past 3 months. Histologically grade 1. (b) The patient was submitted to wide excision including a large posteromedial cortico-cancellous wedge of the femur, and all of the implant base. The loss of femoral substance was filled with an autogenous iliac graft. No signs of recurrence 18 years after surgery.

mor. Three grades of malignancy are acknowledged in P.C.S., too (Fig. 258).

Histological grade 1. This is very frequent (approximately 2/3 of all cases). At times it corresponds to exostosis in initial sarcomatous evolution. However, most cases are represented by voluminous or enormous tumors where primary exostosis can no longer be recognized. Generally, the tumor is diffusedly and heavily calcified-ossified and chondrocytes are rare, due also to necrosis. Particularly in these zones, there are no cytological aspects of malignancy. In more demonstrative, superficial and non-calcified areas, the cartilage reveals numerous cells, which are fairly large and characterized by moderate polydimensionality and, frequently, double nuclei.

Histological grade 2. It is rather frequent (approximately 1/3 of all cases). Less constantly and intensely calcified-ossified than the previous type, it nearly always corresponds to a tumor which is radiographically aggressive or very aggressive. The cells clearly have large nuclei, which are hyperchromatic, polydimensional and pleomorphic, very often double.

Histological grade 3. This is observed in exceptional cases. It always corresponds to an aggressive or very aggressive radiographic picture, with scarce calcification. The tumor is again made up of cartilage which is well-differentiated throughout. The nuclei are definitely pleomorphic and hyperchromatic, at times gigantic or bizarre, often triple or multiple.

***

At the surface, the cartilaginous lobuli generally have sharp limits and are well-circumscribed by a fibrous pseudocapsule. At times, there are small nests of tumoral cells separated from the surface of the principal mass and contained in the pseudocapsule (satellites).

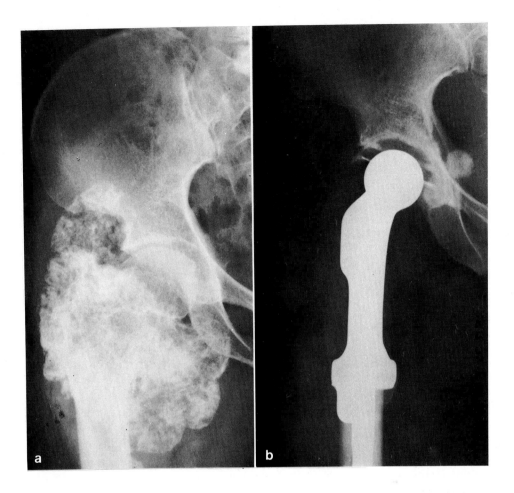

FIG. 263. - (a) Peripheral chondrosarcoma in a female aged 44 years. Histological grade 1. (b) The patient was submitted to wide resection-endoprosthesis, and there were no signs of recurrence with good function of the limb 17 years later.

The most delicate histio-diagnostic problem lies in recognizing the first signs of malignancy in an exostosis. As previously stated, clinical, radiographic and macroscopic data are of considerable importance to this regard. If the exostosis was removed in a child or an adolescent, the presence of numerous and slightly plump cartilaginous cells, some having a double nuclei, does not signify malignant evolution. On the other hand, P.C.S. never occurs before puberty. During adult age, instead, the presence of soft islands of cartilage which sink into the exostosis, the presence of numerous chondrocytes, with large nuclei, and which are slightly pleomorphic and hyperchromatic, often having a double nuclei (2-3 per microscopic field), constitute indexes of malignant evolution (see further on, under diagnosis).

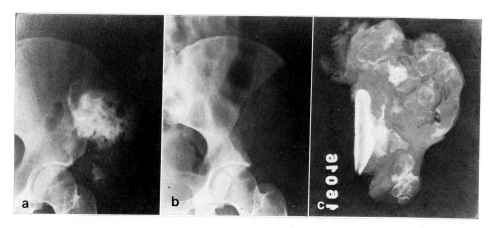

Fig. 264. - (a) Peripheral chondrosarcoma in a female aged 19 years. Histological grade 1. (b) Resection of the iliac wing. (c) X-ray of the anatomical specimen. No sign of recurrence after 17 years.

PROGRESSION IN MALIGNANCY
«DEDIFFERENTIATED CHONDROSARCOMAS»

Progression from grade 1 to 2 requires many years (20 years in one of our observations) so that it is more difficult to observe; that from grade 2 to 3 may instead occur in less time. Particularly grade 1 P.C.S., but also grade 2 P.C.S., may recur many times over 10 years or more, without revealing progression in malignancy.

Similar to what occurs in C.C.S., in P.C.S. a high-grade non-cartilaginous sarcoma may develop (malignant fibrous histiocytoma, fibrosarcoma, osteosarcoma), but more rarely (4% in our series): so-called dedifferentiated C.S. In these cases, as well, a P.C.S. is observed on which a rapidly aggressive, osteolytic sarcoma develops, invading the P.C.S. (dissolving radiopacity) and the soft tissues. Anatomically, there is evidence of pre-existing P.C.S. and/or exostosis and, side by side but without any transitional aspect, the non-cartilaginous high-grade sarcoma (Figs. 259, 260).

HISTOGENESIS AND PATHOGENESIS

Generally, P.C.S. originates from the cartilage of an exostoses during adult age. P.C.S. is frequently observed (in 20% of our cases) in multiple hereditary exostoses. In exceptional cases, two chondrosarcomas are manifested in the same patient from two different exostoses, even after many years. P.C.S. in multiple exostoses develop with equal frequency in the skeleton of the limbs and in that of the trunk.

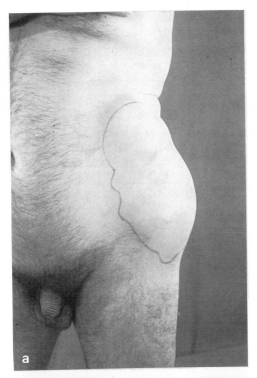

FIG. 265. - (a) Peripheral chondrosarcoma in a male aged 34 years who had
observed a progressive increase in
swelling over the last 6 years. Photo of
the patient. (b) Preoperative radiogram. (c) The patient was submitted to
wide resection of the iliac wing and did
not present signs of recurrence 15 years
after surgery. (d) Radiogram of a section of the removed specimen (weight
3500 g).

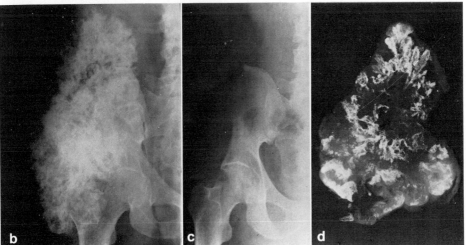

DIAGNOSIS

Diagnosis is generally easy, even when based exclusively on radiographs.
At times there may be some doubt between an **exostosis** of considerable size
and which is very radiopaque, and a P.C.S. The radiopacity of exostosis, however intense and irregular, always has perfectly sharp limits towards the

soft tissues. In P.C.S., on the contrary, the radiopacity in some areas fades towards the soft tissues. CAT and MRI are very useful in revealing the thickness of the cartilaginous cap (Fig. 252c) and in distinguishing it from any liquid effusion on the surface of the exostosis. An intensively positive bone scan also indicates P.C.S., as it is usually only weakly positive in exostosis in the adult. Another important element for the diagnosis of P.C.S. is the demonstration of the growth of the tumor during adult age, with successive radiograms in time.

As previously stated, the diagnosis of the sarcomatous evolution of exostosis is confirmed by a macroscopic and histological examination. The tumor must be transected perpendicular to its surface in those areas where the

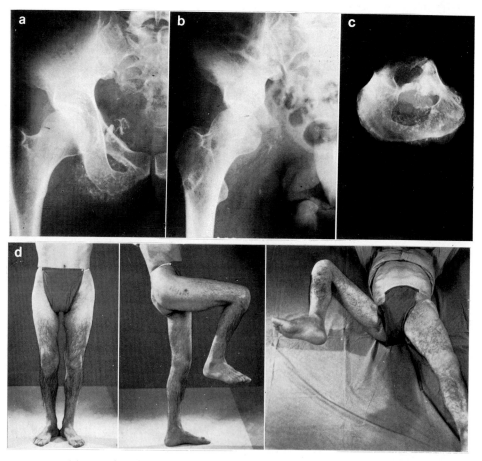

FIG. 266. - (a) Peripheral chondrosarcoma of the obturator region in a male aged 40 years. This tumor constitutes a recurrence after intralesional excision performed 2 years earlier and followed by radiation therapy. (b) Wide resection of the anterior pelvic hemiarch with disarticulation of the pubic symphysis and transection of the acetabulum under the roof. (c) X-ray of the resected specimen. (d) No signs of recurrence and good functional result 16 years after surgery.

cartilage is thicker, and these areas plus those where the cartilage penetrates inside the exostosis are studied histologically. Here, too, as in the case of chondroma/central chondrosarcoma, there are borderline cases in between exostosis and P.C.S.

Histological diagnosis must always take into account clinical, radiographic and macroscopic data. If the cartilaginous tissue being examined covers the exostosis of a child, thickness and some signs of proliferative vivacity do not at all signify malignancy. If, on the contrary, the histological examination (particularly in areas of calcified or ossified cartilage) does not show any signs of malignancy while the radiogram clearly indicates a P.C.S., further histological specimens must be examined, and diagnostic prevalence given to the radiogram. If the specimen should derive from a C.C.S., the same histological features of malignancy would have a more severe prognostic meaning.

Rarely, if there is no trace of exostosis and the tumor has extensively invaded the implant bone, some doubts may arise with regard to **central chondrosarcoma**. **Periosteal chondrosarcoma** is distinguished because it is applied on the cortex, excavating it saucer-like, with a chronic periosteal reaction surrounding it at the base. Doubts as to diagnosis may in exceptional cases arise with this tumor, as well.

Differential diagnosis is easy as regarding **parosteal osteosarcoma**. This tumor, which may have cartilaginous areas, is characterized by different elective sites, a different implant base at the bone, dense bony radiopacity, typical histology in the non-cartilaginous areas.

Finally, the tissue of a **synovial chondromatosis** may be, macroscopically and histologically, very similar to that of a grade 1 or even grade 2 P.C.S. It is distinguished mainly because it derives from the joint cavity, or from one of the tendinous sheaths and thus has rather different clinical-radiographic and gross pathologic features.

Finally, in exceptional cases, differential diagnosis may be made with **reactive or pseudotumoral osteocartilaginous callus**, where the reactive cartilage may be characterized by vivacious proliferation and hypertrophic cells (see specific chapter).

COURSE

P.C.S. grows rather slowly, on the average more slowly that C.C.S. In nearly half of all cases the duration of symptoms prior to surgery is from 2 to 5 years, and in a fourth of all cases, it is more than 5 years.

Recurrence is manifested over a wide range of time, from a few months to 10 years. In untreated cases, death may occur even 20-30 years after the onset of symptoms, generally after more than 5 years. Pulmonary metastases are infrequent (less than 20% of all cases), and generally late (Fig. 267). Metastases in the lymph nodes occur in exceptional cases (Fig. 258d).

In some cases there have been up to 5-6 recurrences after just as many operations over 10-15 or more years, with no metastases. If there is no pro-

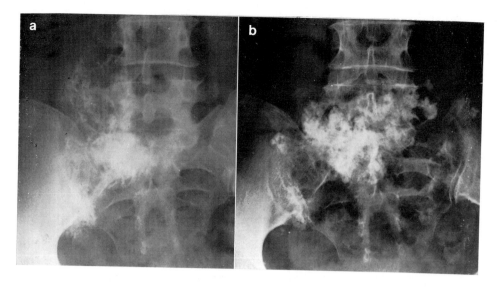

FIG. 267. - (a) Peripheral chondrosarcoma of the sacrum in a male aged 48 years. Histologically grade 1. (b) After 20 years local recurrence. During this period of time repeated attempts at surgical excision were made. The patient died after 2 more years, 22 years after the radiogram (a) was taken, affected with paraplegia due to compression on the cauda, and pulmonary metastases.

gression of malignancy beyond grade 2, recurrence may be cured by wide excision or amputation, even if repeated and performed many years after the onset of the tumor.

When the tumor is localized in the skeleton of the trunk death is often caused by compression of the internal organs or the spinal cord.

TREATMENT

It is important to obtain wide surgical margins. In grade 1 P.C.S. and borderline cases, even a marginal margin in some areas (where the tumor is covered only by the pseudocapsule) may be acceptable, because the risk of local recurrence is less high, and because any local recurrence may still be treated, often conservatively. Instead, any type of intralesional surgery is absolutely contraindicated, such as opening of the pseudocapsule, «peeling» the pseudocapsule from the cartilage, breaking the tumor.

In rare initial forms of the disease, and ones where there is not much expansion, excision of the tumor at the implant base may be performed (Figs. 249a, 262); more often, due to the large size of P.C.S. and its tendency to surround the bone of origin, the entire skeletal segment must be resected with the tumor. This may be done in the limbs, the scapula and the ribs, often in the pelvis, rarely in the vertebral column (Figs. 253, 263-266).

If P.C.S. has already been submitted to biopsy or partial removal, and in the case of local recurrence, it is important to be aware of the fact that even small and multiple neoplastic nodules may be present scattered in the soft scarring tissue, separated from the principal mass (Fig. 261). Nonetheless, recurrence is not irreparable. P.C.S. may recur even more than once, maintaining local malignancy and forming circumscribed nodules. Thus, recurrence may be operated successfully as long as it is removed with a considerable layer of healthy surrounding tissue.

Amputation is required in forms of the tumor which are so voluminous that they would otherwise be unoperable; margins should be wide. As P.C.S. prevalently occurs in the limb girdles, amputation is usually interilioabdominal or interscapulothoracic.

Radiation therapy and chemotherapy are not effective, not even as palliatives.

In order to avoid dissemination of neoplastic cells in the soft tissues, it is often best to carry out frozen section biopsy intraoperatively. On the other hand, the clinical and radiographic aspects are so typical that biopsy generally does not change the type of surgery, and it may even be omitted.

In the rare cases of dedifferentiated P.C.S. surgical treatment must be wide (Fig. 260) or radical, often ablative (Fig. 259). Adjuvant chemotherapy is associated.

PROGNOSIS

Prognosis usually depends on the possibility of wide removal and on the grade of histological malignancy. Grade 1 P.C.S. hardly ever metastasizes; grade 2 P.C.S. may metastasize, but this is exceptionally manifested within 5 years after the onset of symptoms; grade 3 P.C.S. has a greater tendency to metastasize, but in this case, as well, metastases rarely occur early.

P.C.S. is less malignant than C.C.S.: not only because the histological grade 1 forms of the tumor occur more frequently and grade 3 forms occur much more rarely; but also because, at the same histological grade, P.C.S. is less malignant than C.C.S.

In P.C.S. localized in the skeleton of the trunk (more than half of the total number), death may occur whatever the histological grade of the tumor. Nonetheless, tumors located in the ribs, pelvis, scapula heal with wide resection. Vertebral and sacral localizations rarely heal.

PERIOSTEAL AND PAROSTEAL CHONDROSARCOMA
(Synonym: juxtacortical chondrosarcoma)

It is a rare variety. Its classification as an entity in itself is justified by its anatomical-radiographic features, and above all by its prognosis, which is more favorable than that of C.C.S.

In terms of **sex and age** it does not much differ from C.C.S. (Fig. 268).

It is localized in the metaphysis or towards one end of the diaphysis of a long bone, femur, tibia, and humerus, in that order. It hardly ever occurs in a short or flat bone (Fig. 268).

Symptoms are dominated by swelling (given the subperiosteal site of the tumor), which is characterized by little or no pain.

Radiographically and macroscopically it is a globose mass, at times bumpy, lying on the outer surface of the cortex, and thus probably of periosteal or parosteal origin. Similar to parosteal osteosarcoma, the tumor, when located in the distal femur, seems to preferably develop from the posterior part towards the popliteal fossa (Figs. 269-272). Its macroscopic aspect is frankly

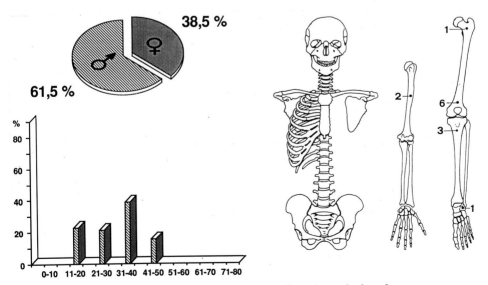

FIG. 268. - Age, sex and site in 13 cases of periosteal chondrosarcoma.

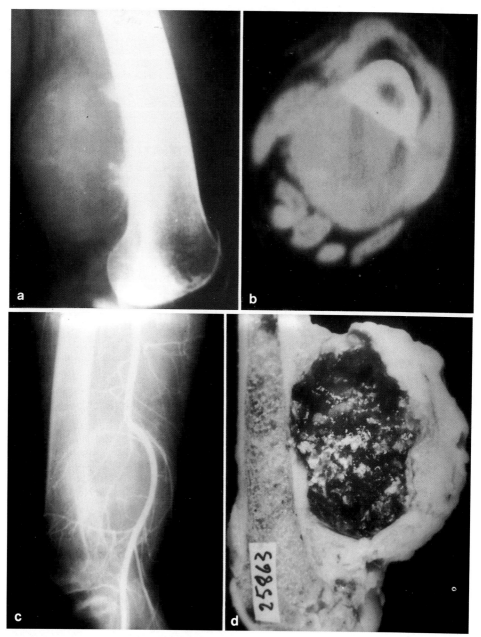

FIG. 269. - Grade 2 periosteal chondrosarcoma in a female aged 31 years. For the past 3 months pain, swelling, and a decrease in motion of the knee. (a) Radiogram shows a globose mass deprived of radiopacity attached to the posterior cortex. The cortex is slightly eroded at the center of the mass, while at the two ends of such erosion there is chronic reaction of the periosteum. (b) CAT confirms the periosteal site of the tumor and the non-involvement of the medullary canal. (c) Arteriography shows shifting of the popliteal artery which adheres to the tumor. Following incisional biopsy the thigh was amputated. (d) Transection of the anatomical specimen revealed the chondromyxoid and hemorrhagic tissue with erosion of the cortex, but no penetration of the medullary canal. The patient was free of disease after 8 years.

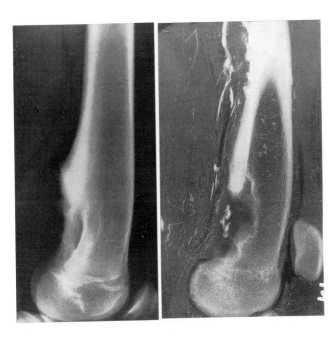

FIG. 270. - Male aged 18 years. Mild discomfort for the past 6 months. Histologically periosteal chondrosarcoma grade 2. The patient healed 30 years after amputation. This operation was definitely excessive; a resection, even a partial one of the distal femur, would have been indicated.

cartilaginous. At times the tumor is totally radiolucent (Fig. 269) and may only be clearly delineated with CAT or MRI. More often, it contains calcification granules, spots and rings (Figs. 270-272), exceptionally it contains bunches of faded ossification. The underlying cortical bone at times appears to be intact, at times superficially eroded. Erosion may be faded, but more often it is a saucer-like depression with sharp and thickened limits. At the periphery of the tumor the periosteum may react with a triangular ossification

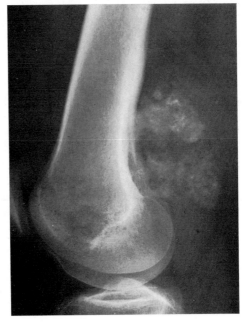

FIG. 271. - Male aged 30 years. Symptoms for the past 3 years. Periosteal chondrosarcoma, histological grade 2. The radiopacity due to calcification and ossification of the cartilage produces a radiographic aspect which is similar to that of a parosteal osteosarcoma.

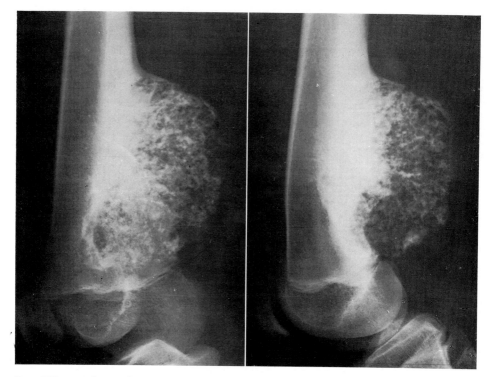

FIG. 272. - Male aged 16 years. Painless swelling for the past 2 years. Grade 2 periosteal chondrosarcoma.

(Fig. 269) which may partially embrace the base of the tumor.

Histologically, periosteal C.S., like peripheral C.S., is generally well-differentiated (Fig. 273); it rarely has a myxoid aspect. Its histological aspects and
distinction in histological grades 2 and 3 ([1]) are similar to those recalled for
peripheral C.S. As in peripheral C.S., in this case, as well, observations of
grade 3 are rare. In periosteal C.S., as well, there may be progression in
malignancy.

Differential diagnosis involves **periosteal chondroma**; radiographically,
periosteal C.S. is more expanded and more invasive of the cortical bone generally without penetrating the medullary canal. But the distinction is above
all histological. To this regard, it must be recalled that moderate signs of
anaplasia are compatible with complete benignity and, thus, with a diagnosis of periosteal chondroma, particularly during childhood. Thus, a diagnosis
of grade 1 periosteal C.S. is probably not justified. Differential diagnosis also
involves **periosteal osteosarcoma** which affects the diaphysis, radiographically presenting radiopaque spicules perpendicular to the cortex, and his-

---

([1]) If the aspect corresponds to a grade 1 C.S., it is believed to be a benign tumor
and thus considered to be a periosteal chondroma (see specific chapter).

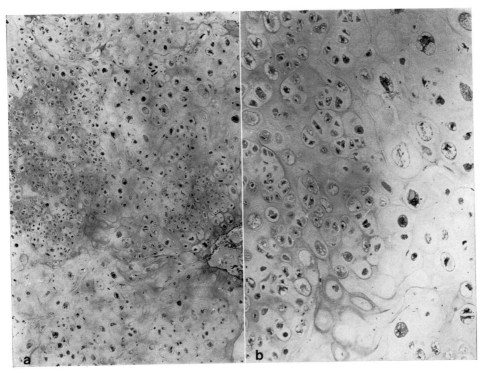

FIG. 273. - Grade 2 periosteal chondrosarcoma. The same case as that in Fig. 271. Throughout the tumor the same well-differentiated cartilaginous aspect was observed (*Hemat.-eos.*, 50, 125 x).

tologically, although extensively chondroblastic, having areas of neoplastic osteogenesis (see specific chapter).

Prognosis and treatment. Periosteal C.S. is much less malignant than central chondrosarcoma of the same histological grade. It is cured with wide surgery, usually conservative and there is little or no tendency to metastasize.

CLEAR-CELL CHONDROSARCOMA

This is a rare tumor variety (Fig. 274) which is somewhat similar to chondroblastoma and, as for malignancy, seems to be somewhere between a grade 1 and grade 2 central chondrosarcoma.

Sex and age correspond to those of chondrosarcoma. It is **localized** in the epiphysis or apophysis, generally in the proximal femur or in the proximal humerus, or in flat or short bones.

The **radiographic picture** resembles that of epiphyseal chondroblastoma, including, at least at the onset, evident demarcation of the osteolytic area (Figs. 275, 276); but the lesion may recur after curettage and, if left alone, it may take on considerably aggressive characteristics. The tumor may include calcification opacities. Growth is slow or rather slow.

The **macroscopic** aspect is that of soft tumor, which is vaguely chondroid, at times granulous (due to the presence of osteoid), often reddish or hemorrhagic.

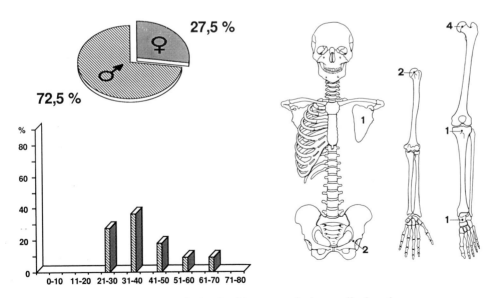

FIG. 274. - Sex, age and site in 11 cases of clear-cell chondrosarcoma.

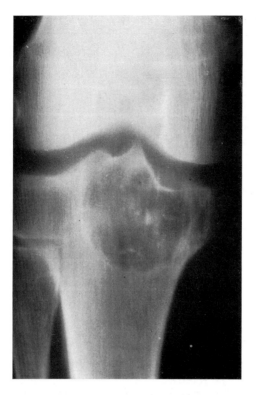

FIG. 275. - Clear-cell chondrosarcoma in a male aged 38 years. Observe the localization and the rather well-defined borders of the osteolysis, which may suggest chondroblastoma. This osteolysis was present, in a slightly smaller size, in radiograms obtained 4 years earlier. The finding had suggested a benign tumor. Finally, note the small intratumoral calcifications, which had suggested a cartilaginous tumor (stratigraphy). This patient was treated by aggressive curettage and bone grafting, and there were neither signs of recurrence nor metastasis 10 years later.

Histologically, it is a lobular tissue, with «clear» cells: central nucleus, extensively vacuolated cytoplasm, strongly P.A.S. positive (Fig. 277). There is a fair or considerable amount of pleomorphism, rare mitotic figures. At the

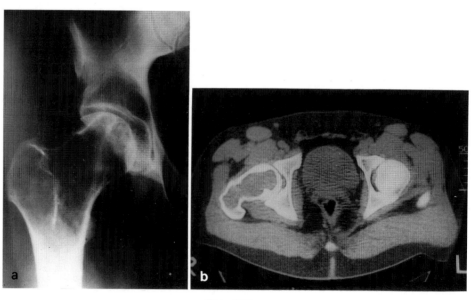

FIG. 276.

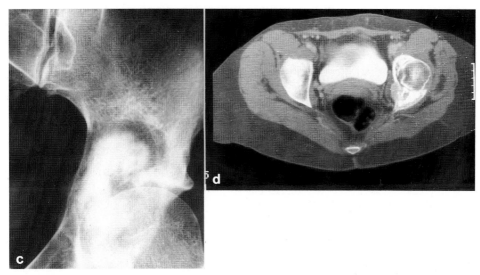

FIG. 276. - (a) and (b) Clear-cell chondrosarcoma of the proximal femur in a male aged 27 years. Occasional pain for the past few years. There was homogeneous osteolysis extended to the epiphysis and to the neck of the femur with well-defined boundaries and a well-preserved cortex. The patient was submitted to wide intra-articular resection and uncemented prosthesis. No signs of disease after 3 years. (c) Clear-cell chondrosarcoma of the ilium in a female aged 32 years. Pain for the past 2 years. There was osteolysis containing calcifications. (d) CAT revealed interruption in the cortex. The tumor reached as far as the joint cartilage. The patient was submitted to frozen section biopsy (with erroneous diagnosis of osteoblastoma) and (thus) curettage. After 9 months the patient complained of pain and there were radiographic signs of severe arthrosis, but there were no signs of recurrence of the tumor.

periphery of the lobuli the cells are more numerous and benign (reactive) multinucleate giant cells are observed. Alongside these, areas of well-differentiated C.S., histological grades 1 or 2, may be observed. At times, there is intercellular calcification (like in chondroblastoma), at times the production of osteoid (reactive), at times cystic spaces.

Treatment of choice consists in wide resection, and generally it is successful. Rarely, nonetheless, the tumor may metastasize.

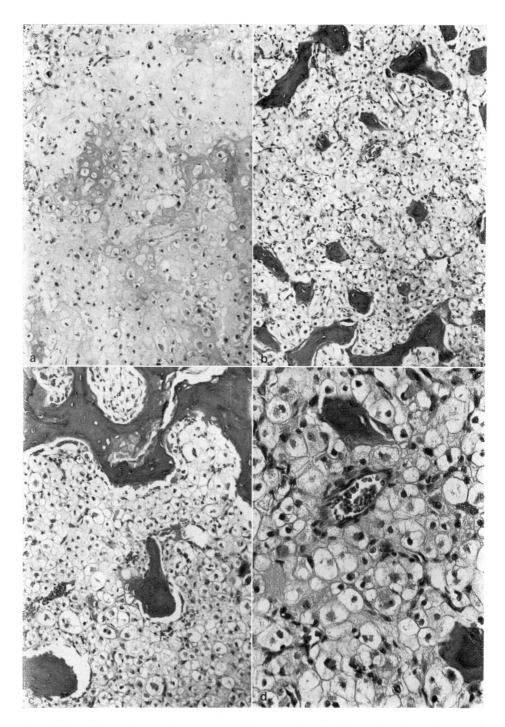

FIG. 277. - Clear-cell chondrosarcoma. (a) Area of well-differentiated cartilage with aspect of grade 1 chondrosarcoma. (b), (c), and (d) Clear-cell chondroblastic tissue. Observe the presence of small blood vessels and newly-formed reactive bone trabeculae. (*Hemat.-eos.*, 125, 125, 125, 310 x). (Specimen of Dr. D.C. Dahlin).

MESENCHYMAL CHONDROSARCOMA

This is a rather rare form. Incidence by **sex** and **age** does not much differ from that for other chondrosarcomas. As for **site**, there is predilection for the skeleton of the trunk and the cranio-facial bones; more rarely, it may be observed in the bones of the limbs (Fig. 278).

Radiographically, it is an osteolytic tumor which permeates and breaks the cortex (Fig. 279) and often contains faded images of calcification.

Histologically, it is constituted by a dense round cell proliferation, which resembles Ewing's sarcoma (the cells contain glycogen), lymphoma, and particularly hemangiopericytoma (Fig. 280). The cells may be roundish or oval in shape. Often, these small cells have a hemangiopericytoma-like or alveolar structure. Within the tissue there are small foci or larger islands of cartilage. These cartilaginous areas may not have cytological aspects of malignancy, and they often tend to calcify-ossify. Diagnosis will be wrong (possible confusion with lymphoma, hemangiopericytoma, Ewing's sarcoma) if mesenchymal C.S. is not taken into consideration, and if extensive and nu-

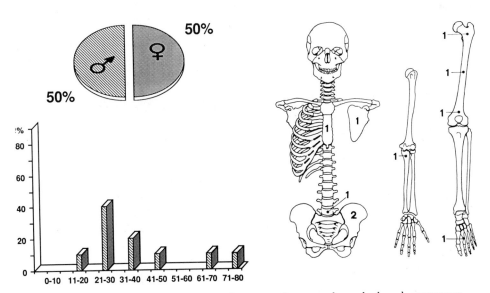

FIG. 278. - Sex, aged and site in 10 cases of mesenchymal chondrosarcoma.

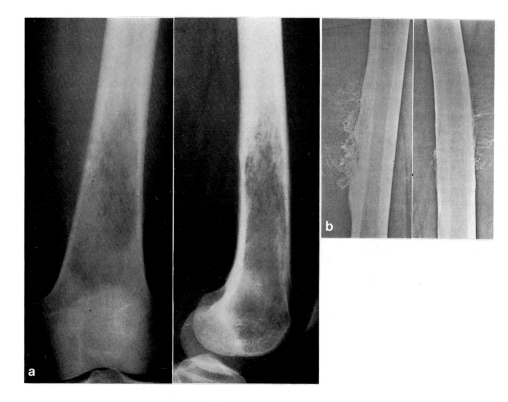

FIG. 279. - Mesenchymal chondrosarcoma. (a) Female aged 29 years. Pain and swelling for the past month. There is faded osteolysis, with a moth-eaten aspect, and surpassing the cortex with no periosteal reaction. The patient refused amputation and was thus submitted to radiation therapy. She died 4 months later of pulmonary metastases. (b) Female aged 30 years. Pain and swelling for the past 2 years. Xeroradiography reveals a periosteal mass eroding the cortical bone at the surface, but which does not penetrate in the medullary canal. Wide resection and chemotherapy. Died 3 years later of pulmonary and spread metastases.

merous samples of the tumor are not examined, in order to discover the foci of cartilaginous differentiation.

In exceptional cases, at diagnosis the tumor is multicentric in the skeleton. Most of the cases have had a fatal outcome, even several years after removal of the tumor. Thus, **prognosis** is very severe.

Treatment is based on wide or radical surgical removal. The effectiveness of chemo- and radiotherapy is not as yet known.

This is one of those tumoral forms which, because of its rarity, requires better characterization which will be possible when a more consistent number of observations has been collected.

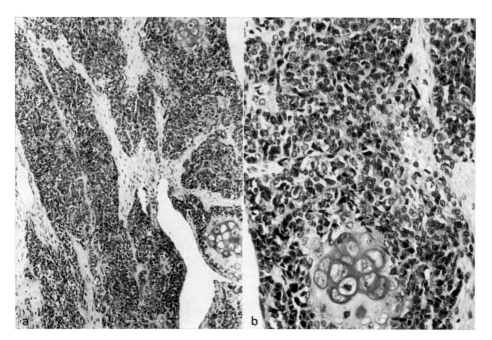

FIG. 280. - Mesenchymal chondrosarcoma (*Hemat.-eos.*, 80, 200 x).

REFERENCES

1952 LICHTENSTEIN L.: *Bone tumors*. Mosby, St. Louis.
1954 COLEY B. L., HIGINBOTHAM N. L.: Secondary chondrosarcoma. *Annals of Surgery*, **139**, 547-559.
1959 LICHTENSTEIN L., BERNSTEIN D.: Unusual benign and malignant chondroid tumors of bone. *Cancer*, **12**, 1142-1157.
1963 GOTTSCHALK R. G., SMITH R. T.: Chondrosarcoma of the hand. Report of a case with radioactive sulphur studies and review of literature. *Journal of Bone and Joint Surgery*, **45-A**, 141-150.
1963 HENDERSON E. D., DAHLIN D. C.: Chondrosarcoma of bone. A study of two hundred and eighty eight cases. *Journal of Bone and Joint Surgery*, **45-A**, 1450-1458.
1965 PADUA S., MIZZAU M.: Evoluzione maligna delle esostosi. *Archivio Putti della Chirurgia degli Organi di Movimento*, **20**, 296-308.
1967 FROIMSON A. I.: Metastatic chondrosarcoma of the hand. Report of a case. *Clinical Orthopaedics*, **53**, 155-160.
1967 McKENNA R. J., SCHNUM C. P., HIGINBOTHAM N. L.: Chondrosarcoma of bone. *Journal of Bone and Joint Surgery*, **49-A**, 1013-1013.
1967 SCHAJOWICZ F., BESSONE J. E.: Chondrosarcoma in three brothers. A pathological and genetic study. *Journal of Bone and Joint Surgery*, **49-A**, 129-141.
1968 BOSTRÖM M., EDGREN B., FRIBERG U., LARSSON K. S., NILSONNE U., WENGLE B., WESTER P. O.: Case of chondrosarcoma with pulmonary and skeletal metastases after hemipelvectomy, successfully treated with 35 S-sulfate. *Acta Orthopaedica Scandinavica*, **39**, 549-564.
1971 DAHLIN D. C., BEABOUT J. W.: Dedifferentiation of low-grade chondrosarcomas. *Cancer*, **28**, 461-466.
1971 MARCOVE R. C., HUVOS A. G.: Cartilaginous tumors of the ribs, *Cancer*, **27**, 794-801.

1971   SALVADOR A. H., BEABOUT J. W., DAHLIN A. C.: Mesenchymal chondrosarcoma. Observations on 30 new cases. *Cancer*, **28**, 605-615.

1971   STENER B.: Total spondilectomy in condrosarcoma arising from the seventh thoracic vertebra. *Journal of Bone and Joint Surgery*, **53-B**, 288-295.

1972   REITER F. B., ACKERMAN L. V., STAPLE T. W.: Central chondrosarcoma of the appendicular skeleton. *Radiology*, **105**, 525-530.

1972   MARCOVE R. C., MIKÉ V., HUTTER R. V. P., HUVOS A. G., SHOJI H.: Chondrosarcoma of the pelvis and upper end of femur. An analysis of factors influencing survival time in one hundred and thirteen cases. *Journal of Bone and Joint Surgery*, **54-A**, 561-572.

1973   STEINER G. C., MIRRA J. M., BULLOUGH P. G.: Mesenchymal chondrosarcoma. *Cancer*, **32**, 926-936.

1974   DAHLIN D. C., SALVADOR A. H.: Chondrosarcomas of bones of the hands and feet. A study of 30 cases. *Cancer*, **34**, 755-760.

1974   MIRRA J.M., MARCOVE R.C.: Fibrosarcomatous dedifferentiation of primary and secondary chondrosarcoma. *Journal of Bone and Joint Surgery*, **56-A**, 285-296.

1975   CAMPANACCI M., GUERNELLI N., LEONESSA C., BONI A.: Chondrosarcoma. *Italian Journal of Orthopaedics and Traumatology*, **1**, 387-414.

1975   CULVER J. E., SWEET D. E., McCUE F. C.: Chondrosarcoma of the hand arising from a pre-existent benign solitary enchondroma. Case report and pathological description. *Clinical Orthopaedics*, **113**, 128-131.

1975   PANDEY S.: Giant chondromas arising from the ribs. A report of four cases. *Journal of Bone and Joint Surgery*, **57-B**, 519-522.

1975   SMITH W. S., SIMON M. A.: Segmental resection for chondrosarcoma. *Journal of Bone and Joint Surgery*, **57-A**, 1097-1103.

1976   UNNI K. K., DAHLIN D. C., BEABOUT J. W., SIM F. H.: Chondrosarcoma: clear-cell variant. A report of sixteen cases. *Journal of Bone and Joint Surgery*, **58-A**, 676-683.

1977   EVANS H. L., AYALA A. G., ROMSDAHL M. M.: Prognostic factors in chondrosarcoma of bone. A clinicopathologic analysis with emphasis on histologic grading. *Cancer*, **40**, 818-831.

1977   PATEL M. R., PEARLMAN H. S., ENGLER J., WOLLOWICK B. S.: Chondrosarcoma of the proximal phalanx of the finger. Review of the literature and report of a case. *Journal of Bone and Joint Surgery*, **59-A**, 401-403.

1977   PEPE A. J., KUHLMANN R. F., MILLER D. B.: Mesenchymal chondrosarcoma. A case report. *Journal of Bone and Joint Surgery*, **59-A**, 256-258.

1977   ROBERTS P. H., PRICE C. H. G.: Chondrosarcoma of the bones of the hand. *Journal of Bone and Joint Surgery*, **59-B**, 213-221.

1977   SCHAJOWICZ F.: Juxtacortical chondrosarcoma. *Journal of Bone and Joint Surgery*, **59-B**, 473-480.

1978   POSTEL M., FOREST M., TOMENO B., LE CHARPENTIER Y., ROUX J. P., MAZABRAUD A., ABELANET R.: Une nouvelle variété de chondrosarcomes: les chondrosarcomes à cellules claires ou sarcomes chondroblastiques. Étude anatomo-clinique de 5 cas. *Revue de Chirurgie Orthopédique*, **64**, 333-348.

1979   CAMPANACCI M., BERTONI F., CAPANNA R.: Condrosarcomi dedifferenziati. *Giornale Italiano di Ortopedia e Traumatologia*, **5**, 345-357.

1979   CUVELIER C. A., ROELS H. J.: Cytophotometric studies of the nuclear DNA content in cartilaginous tumors. *Cancer*, **44**, 1363-1374.

1979   LARSSON S. E., BORSSEN R., BOQUIST L.: Chondrosarcoma. A multifactorial clinical and histopathological study with particular regard to therapy and survival. *International Orthopaedic (SICOT)*, **2**, 333-341.

1979   LE CHARPENTIER Y., FOREST M., POSTEL M., TOMENO B., ABELANET R.: Clear-cell chondrosarcoma. A report of five cases including ultrastructural study. *Cancer*, **44**, 622-629.

1979   SANERKIN N. G., GALLAGHER P.: A review of the behaviour of chondrosarcoma of bone. *Journal of Bone and Joint Surgery*, **61-B**, 395-400.

1980   CAMPANACCI M., BERTONI F., LAUS M.: Condrosarcoma a cellule chiare. *Giornale Italiano di Ortopedia e Traumatologia*, **6**, 359-366.

1980 MANKIN H.J., CANTLEY K.P., LIPIELLO L., SCHILLER A.L.: The biology of human chondrosarcoma. I. Description of the cases, grading and biochemical analyses. *Journal of Bone and Joint Surgery*, **62-A**, 160-176.

1980 MANKIN H.J., CANTLEY K., SCHILLER A.L., LIPIELLO L.: The biology of chondrosarcoma. II. Variation in chemical composition among types and subtypes of benign and malignant cartilage tumors. *Journal of Bone and Joint Surgery*, **62-A**, 176-188.

1981 ERIKSSON A.I., SCHILLER A., MANKIN H.J.: The management of chondrosarcoma of bone. *Clinical Orthopaedics*, **153**, 44-66.

1983 BERTONI F., PICCI P., BACCHINI P., CAPANNA R., INNAO V., BACCI G., CAMPANACCI M.: Mesenchymal chondrosarcoma of bone and soft tissues. *Cancer*, **53**, 533-541.

1983 HUVOS A.G., ROSEN G., DABSKA M., MARCOVE R.C.: Mesenchymal chondrosarcoma. A clinicopathological analysis of 35 patients with emphasis on treatment. *Cancer*, **51**, 1230-1237.

1984 CAMPANACCI M., GUERRA A.: Les chondrosarcomes. Traitement chirurgical. *Cahiers d'enseignement de la SOFCOT*, **20**, 55-78.

1984 JAWROSKI R.C.: Dedifferentiated chondrosarcoma. An ultrastructural study. *Cancer*, **53**, 2674-2678.

1984 ROSENTHAL D., SCHILLER A., MANKIN H.: Chondrosarcoma: correlation of radiological and histologic grade. *Radiology*, **150**, 21-26.

1985 ASTORINO R., TESLUK H.: Dedifferentiated chondrosarcoma with a rhabdomyosarcomatous component. *Human Pathology*, **16**, 318-320

1985 BERTONI F., PRESENT D., PICCI P., BACCHINI P.: Case report 301: dedifferentiated chondrosarcoma of the upper end of the humerus. *Skeletal Radiology*, **13**, 228-232.

1985 MIRRA J.M., GOLD R., DOWNS J., ECKARDT J.: A new histologic approach to the differentiation of chondroma and chondrosarcoma of the bones. A clinicopathologic analysis of 51 cases. *Clinical Orthopaedics*, **201**, 214-237.

1986 FRASSICA F., UNNI K., SIM F.: Case report 347. Dedifferentiated chondrosarcoma: grade IV arising in a grade I chondrosarcoma (femur). *Skeletal Radiology*, **15**, 77-81.

1986 HEALEY J.H., LANE J.M.: Chondrosarcoma. *Clinical Orthopaedics*, **204**, 119-129.

1986 JOHNSON S., TETU B., AYALA A., CHAWLA S.: Chondrosarcoma with additional mesenchymal component (dedifferentiated chondrosarcoma) I. A clinicopathologic study of 26 cases. *Cancer*, **58**, 278-286.

1986 TETU B., ORDONEZ N., AYALA A., MACKAY B.: Chondrosarcoma with additional mesenchymal component (dedifferentiated chondrosarcoma). *Cancer*, **58**, 287-298.

1987 HUVOS A.G., MARCOVE R.C.: Chondrosarcoma in the young. A clinicopathologic analysis of 79 patients younger than 21 years of age. *American Journal of Surgical Pathology*, **11**, 930-942.

1988 CAMPANACCI M., RUGGIERI P.: Il condrosarcoma. La diagnosi. Atti LXXIII Congresso SIOT. *Giornale Italiano di Ortopedia e Traumatologia*, **14**, Suppl., 23-25.

1988 CAPANNA R., BERTONI F., BETTELLI G., PICCI P., BACCHINI P., PRESENT D., CAMPANACCI M.: Dedifferentiated chondrosarcoma. *Journal of Bone and Joint Surgery*, **70-A**, 60-69.

1989 GREENSPAN A.: Tumors of cartilage origin. *Orthopaedic Clinics of North America*, **20**, 347-366.

1990 LEGGON R.E., UNNI K.K., BEABOUT J.W., SIM F.H.: Clear-cell chondrosarcoma. *Orthopaedics*, **13**, 593-596.

1990 MANDHAL N., HEIM S., ARHEDEN K., RYDHOLM A., WILLEN H., MITELMAN F.: Chromosomal rearrangements in chondromatous tumors. *Cancer*, **65**, 242-248.

1990 SHIVES T.C., McLEOD R.A., UNNI K.K., SCHRAY M.F.: Chondrosarcoma of the spine. *Journal of Bone and Joint Surgery*, **17-A**, 1158-1165.

FIBROCARTILAGINOUS MESENCHYMOMA

It is a tumor composed by two distinct tissues, one cartilaginous and benign resembling a growing epiphyseal plate, and the other similar to a low-grade fibrosarcoma.

This entity has been found in four cases among the 15000 problem bone tumors sent in for consultation to Dahlin and in two cases of the Rizzoli Institute. It is therefore exceedingly rare and its epidemiology, course and prognosis can only be approximately and provisionally indicated. Its gross and histological features, however, appear to be fairly distinct in all six of those cases.

Males were more frequently affected, and age ranged from 9 to 23 years (mean 13 years). Five cases out of 6 were aged under 20 years and 3 were aged under 10 years.

Location was in the metaphysis of the proximal fibula (3 cases), rib, 1st metatarsal, and proximal humerus (1 each); the epiphysis was involved only in the skeletally mature patient.

Symptoms indicate a rather slow growing tumor, of several months duration. They include slight discomfort and tenderness and (in the superficial bones) regular, firm expansion of the bony contours with sharp limits.

Radiograms show a lucent lesion abutting the growth plate, but invading the epiphysis in the adult. The contour of the bone is moderately expanded, the cortex is thinned with a scalloped or lobulated appearance. Usually, there is a small area of cortical destruction with bulging of the tumor in the soft tissues. Periosteal reaction is very scarce and of the chronic type, as the outer aspect of the thinned cortex is either smooth or slightly rough. Frequently, the tumor contains some mineralization, either granular or ringlike, thus suggestive of a cartilaginous component, or fuzzy and suggestive of an osseous component (Fig. 281).

Grossly the tumor is solid, whitish, dense and fasciculated, similar to a desmoid tumor or low-grade fibrosarcoma. This background contains cartilaginous islands, which sometimes have the peculiar shape of serpentine bands reminiscent of a growth plate (Fig. 281d, e).

Histologically there are sweeping and intersecting bundles of spindle cells and collagen fibers. This tissue is rather cellular and shows some nuclear plumpness, pleomorphism and hyperchromatism, with rare mitotic figures. This background contains well-defined islands of cartilage, which is clearly differentiated and benign. The cartilage is often remarkably similar to an epiphyseal growth plate, forming thick undulated bands, with gradual columnation, hypertrophy and enchondral ossification. In short, there is a predominant component of the tumor which is similar to a grade 1 fibrosarcoma, and a second sharply distinct component mimicking an epiphyseal line and suggesting a benign, organoid, hamartomatous feature (Fig. 282).

Radiographic **differential diagnosis** concerns several tumors. Desmoid fibroma and low-grade fibrosarcoma, however, lack any intratumoral mineralization; chondrosarcoma is extremely unlikely in skeletally immature patients. Osteoblastoma has a ground-glass or cloudy radiopacity, not a granu-

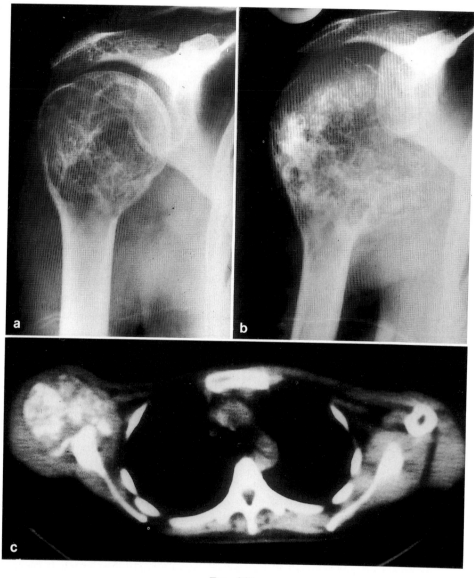

Fig. 281.

lar or ringlike one, and lacks the lobulated pattern. Giant cell tumor is rare in growing patients and lacks any mineralization. In children osteosarcoma and in adults clear cell chondrosarcoma should also be ruled out. Histologically, fibrous dysplasia with a cartilaginous component differs because the fibrous tissue is clearly benign, it includes characteristic bony islands, and the cartilage does not mimic the growth plate.

Course, treatment, and prognosis. Its course is slow but of low-grade malignancy. After intralesional excision local recurrence is common, even after a few years. The treatment of choice, both of the primary tumor and of its local recurrence, appears to be wide en bloc resection. Metastases have not been reported.

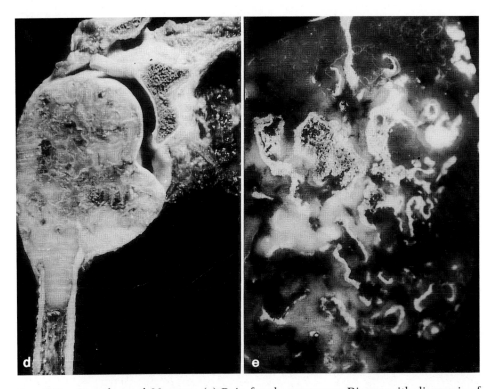

FIG. 281. - Female aged 23 years. (a) Pain for the past year. Biopsy with diagnosis of «fibroma». Curettage and bone grafts. (b) After 1 year recurrence and extension of the osteolysis, with calcifications of the cartilaginous type. (c) CAT shows expansion towards the soft tissues and around the joint. A review of the histological specimens obtained from previous surgery shows fibrocartilaginous mesenchymoma with a grade 2 fibrous component. Wide extra-articular resection was performed. (d) The transected specimen shows compact tissue of a fibrous aspect run through by wavy cartilaginous and calcar bands. (e) Detail of the same surface under Wood lighting showing tetracycline labeling of the areas of ossification. The serpent-like shape of the cartilaginous band is reproduced. The patient showed no signs of disease after 8 years.

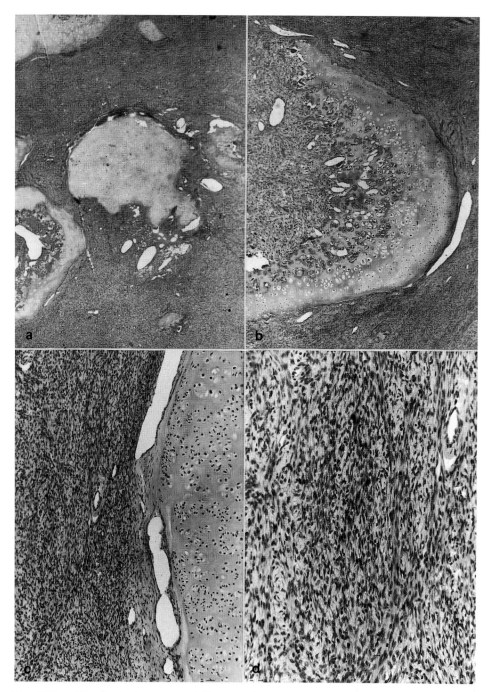

FIG. 282. - Histological aspects of fibrocartilaginous mesenchymoma. There is fibro-histiocytic tissue surrounding islands (a, b) of cartilage. These cartilaginous areas often recall the aspect of growth cartilaginous plate. The histio-fibroblastic tissue presents aspects of low-grade malignancy (c, d). (*Hemat.-eos.*, 25, 50, 100, 200x).

OSTEOMA

DEFINITION

It is a benign tumor located nearly exclusively in the cranio-facial bones (of membranous origin) and it seems to have a periosteal or parosteal origin. Multiple osteomas, associated with intestinal polyps, soft tissue desmoid tumors and epidermoid cysts, may be observed in Gardner's syndrome.

FREQUENCY

It is infrequent but not rare in otorhinolaryngology and stomatology.

SEX

There is predilection for the male sex.

AGE

It is more often observed in the adult, but as it remains asymptomatic for a long time, growing slowly, it probably initiates during childhood.

LOCALIZATION

The most frequent localization of the tumor is in the cranial sinuses, particularly the frontal one, and the maxillary sinus. Furthermore, it develops extrasinusally from the upper maxilla or from the mandible. More rarely, it originates from the external or internal cortex of the cranial bones. Generally, it has an implant base on the cortex growing externally, like a periostotic mass.

In exceptional cases, in the long bones of the limbs, a parosteal mass is observed, with a large implant base on the metaphyseal or diaphyseal cortical bone, which is radiographically eburneous (Figs. 283b, c, 284).

SYMPTOMS

O. is often and for a long time asymptomatic, until it does not alter the sinusal drainage and sinusitis occurs, or until it deforms the walls of the orbit,

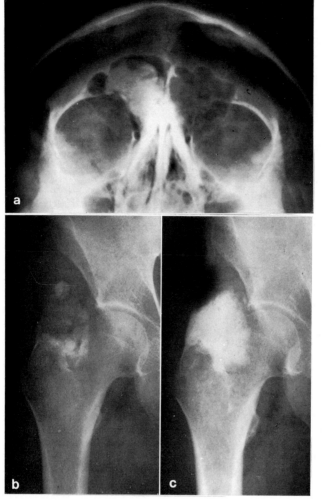

FIG. 283. - (a) Osteoma of the frontal sinus in a female aged 35 years. (b) Male aged 29 years, who for the past 2 years has complained of moderate pain, increasing over the last 6 months. Biopsy revealed newly-formed bone tissue with no sign of malignancy. (c) Four years later. A diagnosis of parostal osteosarcoma seems excluded as the tumor did not increase in volume over 4 years, and because it did not have any histological aspect of malignancy. Even more shaky and delicate is the limit between «parosteal osteoma» and myo-periosteal reactive ossification (so called myo-periostitis ossificans.)

or it protrudes under the oral mucosa or from the surface of the cranial bone. In exceptional cases, it may cause intracranial symptoms, eroding the wall of a sinus and placing it in communication with the epidural space. Exceptional cases of O. of the limbs are characterized by very slow growth and very scarce symptoms.

RADIOGRAPHIC FEATURES

The radiographic picture is usually typical and consists in a lobulated mass, which usually grows within the cranio-facial sinus, with a relatively wide implant base on the sinus wall (Fig. 283a). The density of O. is that of

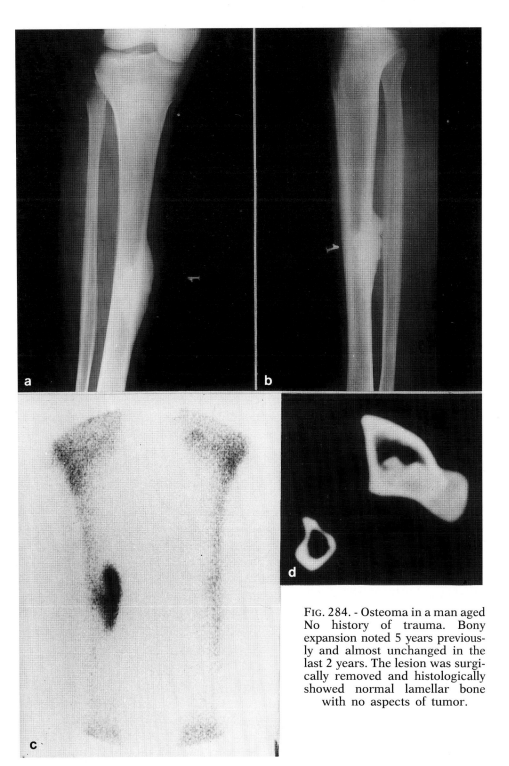

FIG. 284. - Osteoma in a man aged No history of trauma. Bony expansion noted 5 years previously and almost unchanged in the last 2 years. The lesion was surgically removed and histologically showed normal lamellar bone with no aspects of tumor.

mature bone, which varies from cancellous to eburneous. It has a rather uniform density with well-defined boundaries; nonetheless, within it faded areas of relative lucency and dots of more intense radiopacity may be observed.

GROSS PATHOLOGIC FEATURES

It is a mass characterized by a round-topped surface, smooth, covered by periosteum, and, in intrasinusal or buccal forms, by a mucosa which may be inflammed. The mass has the hardness of mature bone, at times it is more spongy, at times, compact.

HISTOPATHOLOGIC FEATURES

The most frequent aspect is that of a rather packed framework of large bony trabeculae, which are relatively mature and lamellar (Fig. 285). The number of osteocytes, the presence of osteoblasts in activity and of some osteoclasts, the aspects of remodelling (with cementing lines sometimes recalling the pagetic mosaic) vary from case to case. More or less loose collagenous tissue is observed in the medullary spaces, which is poorer in cells than what is observed in fibrous dysplasia. At times, the medullary spaces contain adipose and hemopoietic tissue, which is never observed in fibrous dysplasia. Even the presence of lamellar bone and, at times, osteoblastic rows contrasts with the histological features of fibrous dysplasia.

HISTOGENESIS AND PATHOGENESIS

Like a repair bone callus or a heterotopic ossification, O. derives from osteoforming mesenchymal cells producing bone which is normally structured and mature, having connective tissue and small blood vessels, which are equally normal and mature, in the medullary spaces. Thus, more than that of a tumor, O. has the histological features of a hyperplasia (see periosteal and muscular ossification), or a hamartoma. Nonetheless, there is no proof of a causal stimulus of hyperplasia, or of a hamartomatous nature. The exostotic development of most cases of O. would appear to suggest a periosteal or parosteal origin.

DIAGNOSIS

Distinction with regard to a solitary area of **fibrous dysplasia** is based on the clinical-radiographic and histological picture. Radiographically, fibrous dysplasia develops within the bone, whether cranial or facial, and it may cause the bone to expand as a result of intracortical expansion, not extracortical apposition. Furthermore, it nearly always presents radiolucent areas

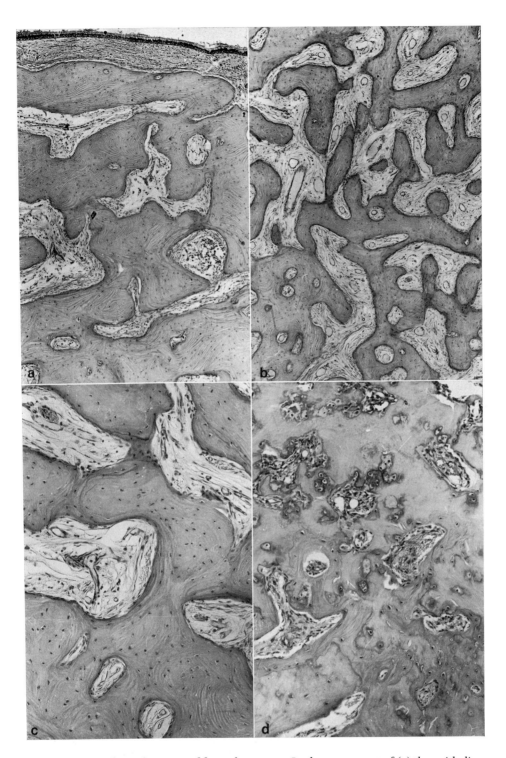

FIG. 285. - Histological aspects of frontal osteoma. In the upper part of (a) the epithelium of the sinus covering the osteoma is observed (*Hemat.-eos.*, 50, 50, 125, 125 x).

alongside cloudy images of radiopacity. Histologically, fibrous dysplasia reveals a much more cellular histio-fibroblastic production, and trabeculae of reticular, not lamellar, bone, not bordered by osteoblasts. Differential diagnosis between the exceptional occurrence of O. in the extracranial skeleton and **parosteal osteosarcoma** may be a more delicate matter (see specific chapter).

COURSE

O. grows very slowly. O. which are radiographically monitored for several years increase in volume, but their radiographic features do not change. This indicates that O. does not originate from another lesion, for example, from the «maturation» of a fibrous dysplasia.

TREATMENT

Asymptomatic O. does not require any treatment. If the O. causes important symptoms, treatment consists in surgical excision. This is not difficult, as O. is often attached to the skeletal surface with an implant base which is not very wide.

PROGNOSIS

O. does not recur after complete removal.

REFERENCES

1939 CHILDREY J. H.: Osteoma of sinuses, the frontal and the sphenoid bone. Report of fifteen cases. *Archiv of Otolaryngoiatry*, **30**, 63-72.
1950 HALBERG O. E., BEGLEY J. W. Jr.: Origin and treatment of osteomas of the paranasal sinuses. *Archiv of Otolaryngoiatry*, **51**, 750-760.
1952 SMITH A. G., ZOVALETA A.: Osteoma, ossifying fibroma, and fibrous dysplasia of facial and cranial bones. *Archiv of Pathology*, **54**, 507-527.
1969 AEGERTER E. E., KIRKPATRICK J. A. Jr.: *Tumor-like processes (osteomas)*. Orthopedic Disease 3th. ed., 569-571, W. B. Saunders Company, Philadelphia.
1981 SCHAJOWICZ F.: *Tumors and tumor-like lesions of bone and joints*. Springer-Verlag, New York.
1988 MIRRA J.M., GOLD R.H., PIGNATTI G., REMOTTI F.: Case report 497. *Skeletal Radiology*, **17**, 437-442.

OSTEOID OSTEOMA

DEFINITION

It is a benign tumor, which is always small in size and painful, often dia-physeal. It is constituted by osteoid tissue and surrounded by a halo of reactive hyperostosis.

FREQUENCY

O.O. occurs relatively frequently. Among benign tumors of the skeleton it is preceded only by exostosis and histiocytic fibroma (Fig. 286).

SEX

There is predilection for the male sex, at a ratio of 2:1 (Fig. 286).

AGE

The tumor is typical of late childhoood, adolescence and young adult age. It is rarely observed before 5 years of age and after 30 (Fig. 286).

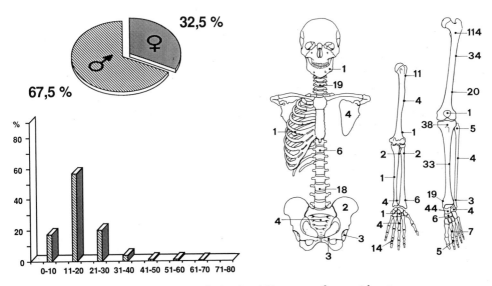

FIG. 286. - Sex, age and site in 448 cases of osteoid osteoma.

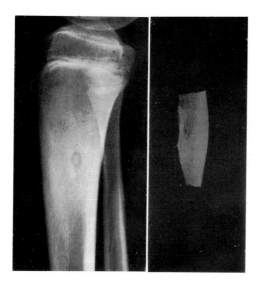

FIG. 287. - Diaphyseal osteoid osteoma in a girl aged 11 years.

LOCALIZATION

The most frequent localization is in the long bones: femur, tibia, humerus, in that order. It may occur in the diaphyseal shaft or towards the metaphysis, with considerable predilection for the proximal femur (neck and intertrochanteric region). It is observed in the short bones, particularly in the tarsus (where it prefers the talus), often in the vertebral column (where there is preference for the lumbar tract over the cervical one, and it is nearly exclusively localized in the posterior arch in the area of the pedicle), in the metacarpals, metatarsals, and phalanges. It rarely occurs in the flat bones, or in the epiphysis (Fig. 301b), and it is unknown in bones of membranous origin (cranium and clavicle).

SYMPTOMS

Pain is an almost constant and permanent symptom, and nearly the only one. Pain is of variable intensity, usually enough to require the use of analgesics. It is independent of function, nearly continuous but more intense during the night. Pain is often exacerbated when alcoholic beverages are drunk (vasodilation) and it is elicited by local pressure. Rather characteristic is the fact that pain is mitigated or regresses totally with aspirin. Pain is not always well-localized, which may lead to the attribution of symptoms to the nearby joint or to a radicular or nervous irradiation, for example sciatica. O.O. is suspected in the vertebral column when a patient aged under 30 years complains of constant back pain, when there is marked vertebral stiffness and muscular contraction, scoliotic deviation, positive Lasègue, with no signs of nerve root compression.

When O.O. is localized in a diaphysis, a slight fusiform prominence may be palpated, corresponding to the·hyperostosis, covered by normal skin. Some O.O. of the long bones, occurring during childhood, cause some considerable lengthening of the bone.

The duration of symptoms at surgery usually ranges from a few months to two years or so.

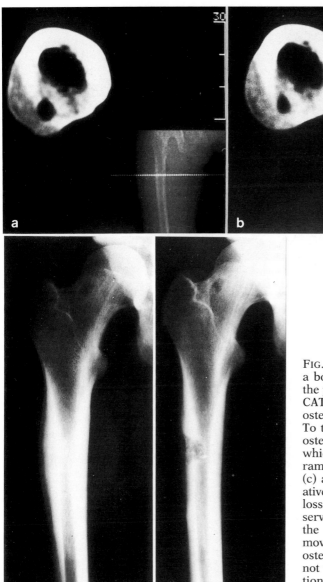

FIG. 288. - Osteoid osteoma in a boy aged 19 years. Pain for the past 14 months. (a) and (b) CAT revealed intracortical osteoid osteoma (to the left). To the right there was a small osteolytic lacuna of the cortex which corresponded to the foramen for the nutrient vessels. (c) and (d) Pre- and postoperative radiograms. The minimal loss of bone substance is observed, which was filled with the cortical bone chips removed to expose the osteoid osteoma. This method does not weaken the bone and functional recovery may be immediate. The patient is cured after 3 years.

RADIOGRAPHIC FEATURES

Generally, the radiographic picture is very characteristic. The basic element is a small or very small rounded area of osteolysis («nidus»), the diameter of which hardly ever exceeds 1 centimeter, surrounded by a regular halo of hyperostosis. Within the nidus there may be a central and irregular nucleus of bony opacity. This picture may change considerably, depending on

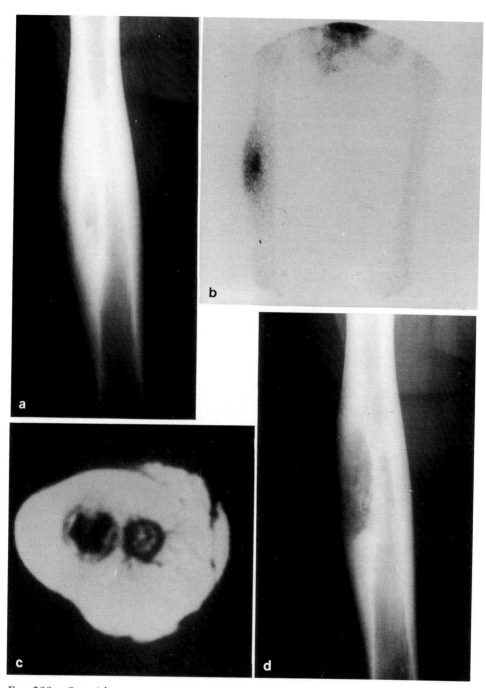

Fig. 289. - Osteoid osteoma in a boy aged 15 years. Pain for the past year and a half.
(a), (b) and (c) Typical aspect of intracortical osteoid osteoma. CAT showed the nidus
which was nearly the same size as the medullary canal and which was covered with a
thick layer of sclerosing periosteal reaction. (d) The osteoid osteoma was removed.
Only the layer of reactive bone coating it was slivered out, until the nidus appeared.
This was evident because of its reddish color against the white of the surrounding
bone. Functional recovery and healing occurred immediately (follow-up 2 years).

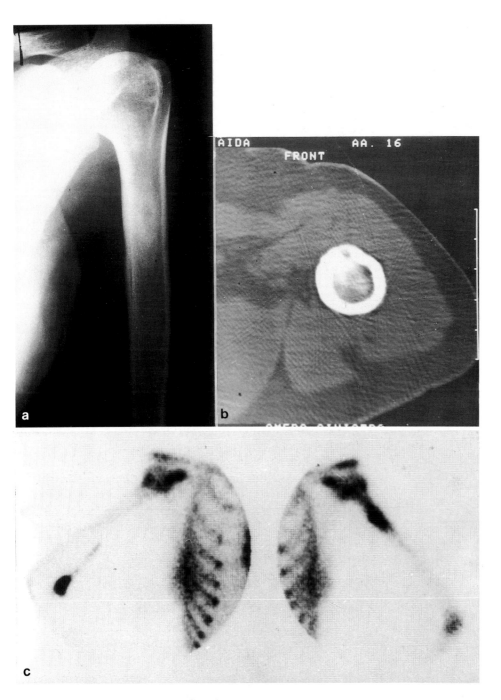

Fig. 290. - Osteoid osteoma in a female aged 16 years. Pain for the past 3 months. Two and 1/2 years earlier the patient had been submitted to surgery with temporary regression of pain. On histological examination there had been no trace of osteoid osteoma. (a), (b) and (c). Typical aspect of intracortical osteoid osteoma. The nidus was visualized and excised with minimal bone removal. Immediate functional recovery and healing (follow-up at 2 years).

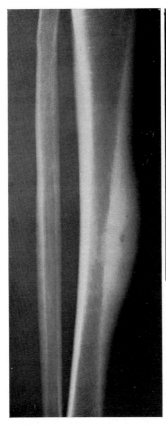

FIG. 291. - Diaphyseal osteoid osteoma in a female aged 15 years.

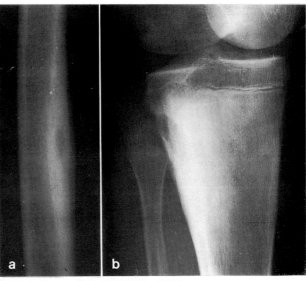

FIG. 292. - (a) Diaphyseal osteoid osteoma in a girl aged 12 years. (b) Voluminous metaphyseal osteoid osteoma in a boy aged 11 years.

the site of the tumor and on its stage of progression (Figs. 287-305).

In cortical diaphyseal localizations there is fusiform thickening of a single side of the shaft, with clean and regular surfaces, and compact and intense radiopacity. The osteolytic area of O.O. is located at the center of this thickening, generally totally contained within the primary cortex, at times oriented towards its endosteal surface, more rarely towards its external one, but

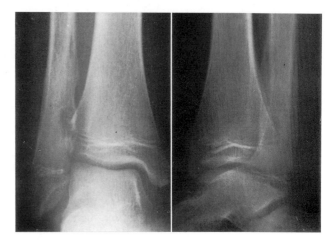

FIG. 293. - Voluminous metadiaphyseal and para-articular osteoid osteoma of the fibula in a boy aged 12 years.

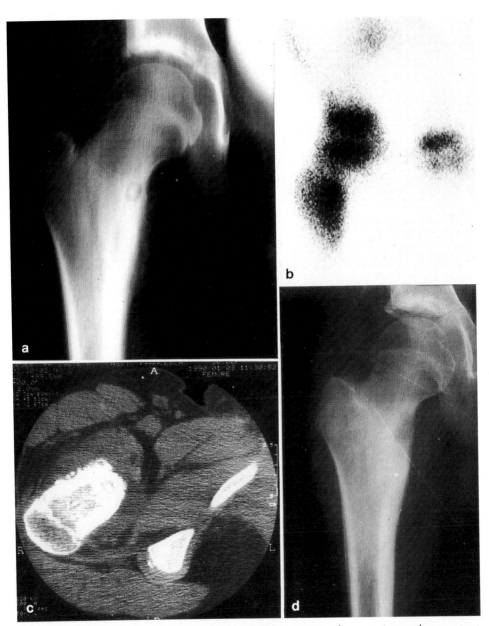

FIG. 294. - Osteoid osteoma in a female aged 10 years. For the past 6 months constant pain, especially at night. (a) and (b) Typical aspect of osteoid osteoma with tomography and bone scan. (c) CAT revealed the intracortical localization of the osteoid osteoma and indicated the surgical approach (anterior). CAT also showed reactive hyperostosis with a wrinkly surface. (d) After surgery, which consisted in removing the bone layer covering the osteoma and thus curetting the nidus, the loss of bone substance was minimal. The patient was able to move her hip and bear weight after a few days.

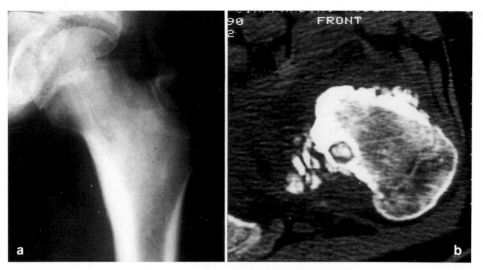

Fig. 295. - Osteoid osteoma in a boy aged 13 years, operated 8 months earlier, with no regression of pain. Surgery had been performed through a lateral approach, and the patient wore a spica cast for 5 months. (a) and (b) Radiogram and CAT showed the typical nidus and reactive capsular ossifications due to the previous operation. CAT showed the posterior localization of the osteoid osteoma which indicated a posterior surgical approach. This approach was used visualizing and curetting the nidus. Immediate functional recovery and healing (follow-up at 3 years).

always surrounded by the reactive hyperostosis. At times bony reaction is so thick and eburneous that the small nidus cannot be seen except with CAT (Fig. 288).

When the tumor is localized in cancellous bone (for example, the femoral

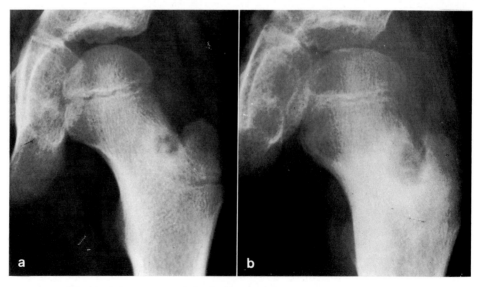

Fig. 296. - (a) Osteoid osteoma of the femoral neck in a girl aged 5 years. (b) The same case 2 years later.

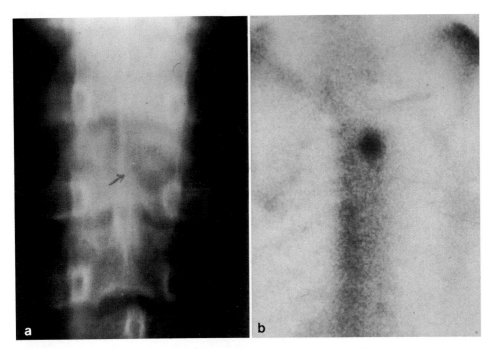

FIG. 297. - Osteoid osteoma of the 5th thoracic vertebra in a male aged 15 years. Typical aspect on radiographs (a) and bone scan (b). The nidus was contained in the vertebral lamina. The patient was cured after 2 years.

neck, the vertebrae, the bones of the tarsus), the halo of osteosclerosis may be very scarce (Figs. 293, 297); at times diffused and even intense osteoporosis may be associated (Figs. 249, 250a). In cases such as these, if the O.O. is small, it may be very difficult to reveal on radiographs, and bone scan and CAT are required. In these same sites O.O. is often nested at the surface of the

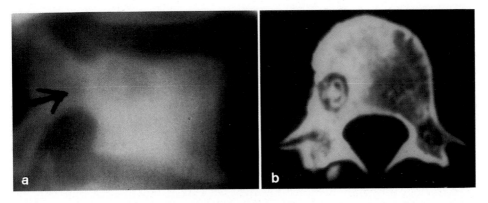

FIG. 298. - Osteoid osteoma of the 4th lumbar vertebra in a female aged 18 year. For the past year lumbar pain and for the past 6 months crural pain. (a) and (b) Typical aspect on radiographs and CAT. Localization in the vertebral body is quite rare. The osteoma was excised by extraperitoneal anterior approach. Healed at 3-year follow-up.

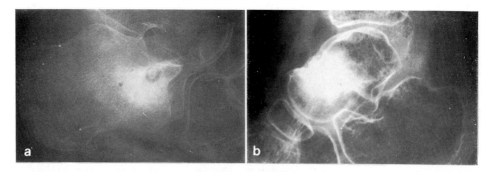

FIG. 299. - (a) Osteoid osteoma of the calcaneus in a female aged 18 years. (b) Osteoid osteoma of the talus in a boy aged 9 years. Observe the intense diffused regional osteoporosis.

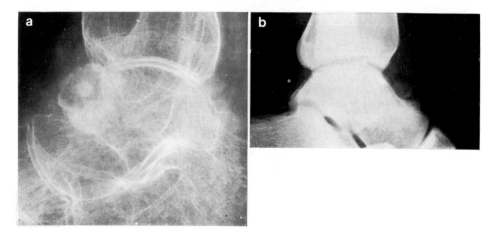

FIG. 300. - (a) Superficial osteoid osteoma of the talus in a female aged 14 years. Observe the diffused regional osteoporosis. (b) Osteoid osteoma of the talus which is completely external and lying on the surface of the bone in a female aged 15 years.

bone and appears to be a small niche of the cortex, or a rounded formation with a radiopaque central nucleus, protruding from the bone (Fig. 300).

In vertebral localizations of the tumor, there is usually a uniform and faded increase in opacity in the pedicular or isthmic area, caused by the reactive osteosclerosis, with little evidence of the nidus. At times, radiograms are nearly totally negative, as O.O. is nested at the surface of an area in the vertebral arch. Rarely, O.O. is contained in the vertebral body (Fig. 298). It usually causes scoliosis due to anthalgic contraction, which is always concave on the side where the O.O. is located.

Arteriography may demonstrate the rich vascularity of O.O. (particularly in the small bones and/or in the cancellous bone). By subtracting the image, which eliminates the radiopacity of the bone and preserves that of the contrast medium, it is possible to visualize an O.O. which is invisible on standard radiograms (Fig. 303).

FIG. 301. - (a) Osteoid osteoma of the patella in a female aged 15 years. (b) Epiphyseal osteoid osteoma (distal tibia) in a male aged 22 years. (c) Osteoid osteoma of the mandible in a female aged 17 years. (d) Osteoid osteoma of the scapula in a female aged 14 years.

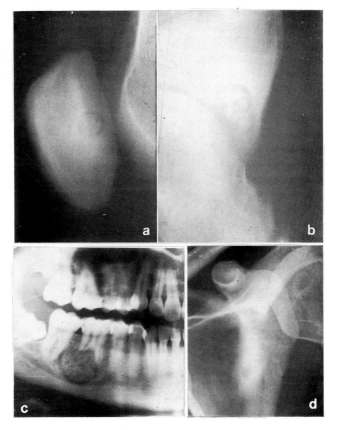

But essential tests for diagnosis are **bone scan** and **CAT**. Bone scan reveals a rounded area of intense hypercaptation, resembling a «headlight in the fog» (Figs. 290, 294, 297). If bone scan is negative, diagnosis of O.O. may be excluded. If it is positive, CAT is carried out, with a window for the bone, in the area of hypercaptation. CAT reveals the nidus and allows for accurate planning of surgery.

There are rare cases in which the tumor becomes of larger size (1-2 cm) although it has the same clinical, radiographic and histological features of O.O. («giant osteoid osteoma»: Figs. 301c, 302b, 304, 305).

GROSS PATHOLOGIC FEATURES

O.O. is a small roundish and hyperemic tumor, which is much softer than the surrounding bone, but somewhat gritty. Its consistency increases in proportion to the degree of calcification of the central part of the nidus.

When O.O. is superficial and there is less reactive hyperostosis, as may be the case in areas of cancellous bone, it may protrude at the surface of the bone;

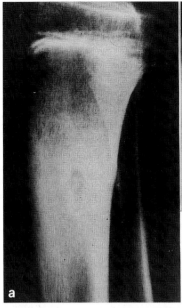
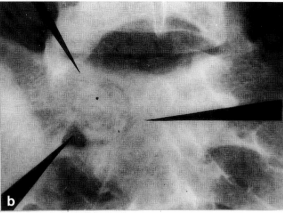

FIG. 302. - (a) Diaphyseal osteoid osteoma in a girl aged 8 years, with pain for 1 and 1/2 years. (b) Giant osteoid osteoma of the sacrum in a female aged 15 years with pain for the past year and a half.

in the vertebral site it may thus irritate and compress a nerve root. When the tumor is intraosseous or covered by a sheath of hyperostosis, such as in the diaphysis, it is clearly visualized after removal of the covering bone, due to its reddish color, on the eburneous color of the surrounding bone (Fig. 306).

Generally, O.O. is easily enucleated from its skeletal bed (Fig. 306).

The soft tissues and the synovial membrane, covering a superficial or intra-articular O.O., are often thickened, hyperemic, edematous, the same as around a chronic inflammatory process.

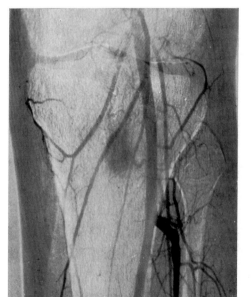

FIG. 303. - Osteoid osteoma of the proximal metaphysis of the tibia in a male aged 16 years. The osteoid osteoma was hardly visible on standard radiograms, as there was hardly any osteosclerosis around the nidus. Arteriography and image subtraction revealed the osteoma on the surrounding bone, with its intense vascular injection.

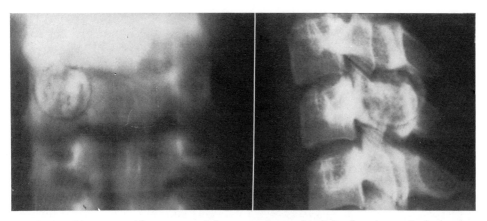

FIG. 304. - Giant osteoid osteoma of the posterior arch of the fourth cervical vertebra in a female aged 15 years.

HISTOPATHOLOGIC FEATURES

Because of its small size, O.O. is frequently observed whole, with the layer of skeletal wall containing it (Fig. 307). Thus, a packed and labyrinthlike whole of thin and contorted osteoid trabeculae is observed, immersed in a rather cellular tissue, with histio-fibroblasts, osteoblasts, osteoclasts and numerous capillaries which are dilated and filled with blood (Figs. 308, 309). At times, sparse large cells, with giant and bizarre nuclei (cf. osteoblastoma), and rare mitotic figures are observed.

The osteoid tissue is more mature at the center (the older part of the tumor) where the trabeculae merge in masses which are more compact, more calcified, poorer in cells. This thicker and more calcified center corresponds

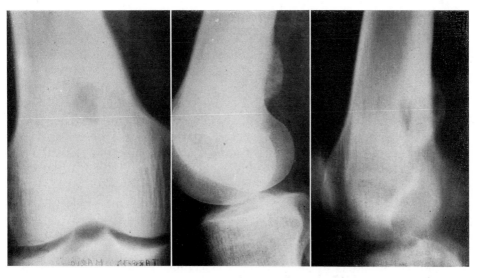

FIG. 305. - Giant osteoid osteoma in a male aged 47 years.

to the radiopaque nucleus of the nidus (Figs. 307a, 309c, d).

The border between the tumor and the surrounding bone is rather sharp (Fig. 307b). In the bone surrounding O.O. there are aspects of hyperostosis, remodelling, and medullary fibrosis. There may be some light and scattered lymphocytic infiltrations. Similar aspects of hyperplasia and reactive phlogosis, which may even be intense, with marked hyperemia and pseudo-follicular lymphocytary infiltrations, may be observed in the synovial membrane, when O.O. is juxta-articular, or in the soft tissues near the nidus.

By staining the neurofibrillae, thin nerve endings, probably accompanying the vessels, have been shown in O.O.

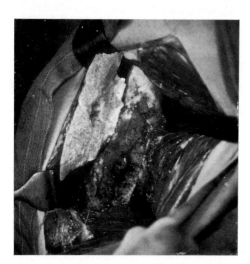

FIG. 306. - Typical surgical finding of diaphyseal osteoid osteoma.

HISTOGENESIS AND PATHOGENESIS

The inflammatory nature of O.O. is not longer asserted. It instead seems to be a benign tumor. Its smallness and close delimitation by the host bone do not oppose this interpretation. Isn't glomus tumor just as small? O.O. produces an intense hyperostotic reaction in the host bone. This, too, may partially explain the limited growth of the tumor.

DIAGNOSIS

If one waits to see the characteristic radiographic picture of O.O., in many cases diagnosis will be delayed or even missed. The first suspect must be clinical: in a child or youth who complains of sharp, continuous pain, which is more intense at night, of long duration, and which is not influenced by any kind of treatment (except for temporary relief with aspirin), in a hip, a diaphysis, the spine, a foot, O.O. is suggested. Based on this suspect, radiography and bone scan are carried out; if bone scan is positive, CAT is obtained. These last two tests will reveal O.O. even when radiography is negative or doubtful. These tests must never be omitted, not even when radiography seems to be characteristic of O.O., as they confirm diagnosis, and as CAT may be of aid to surgery.

When clinical data, bone scan and CAT are typical for O.O., diagnosis may be considered to be nearly certain, even prior to surgery.

When the tumor is localized in the long bones, radiographic differential diagnosis may be made with **Brodie's abscess**. The latter is more often

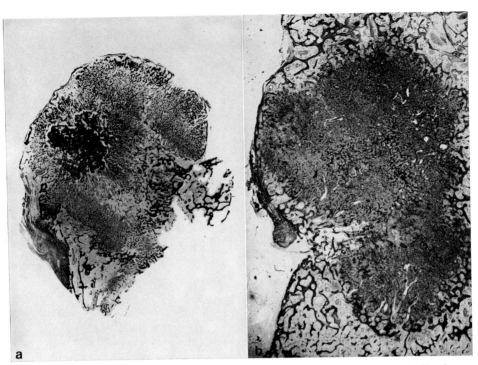

Fig. 307. - Two examples of whole osteoid osteoma photographed under small enlargement (*Hemat.-eos.*, 20 x).

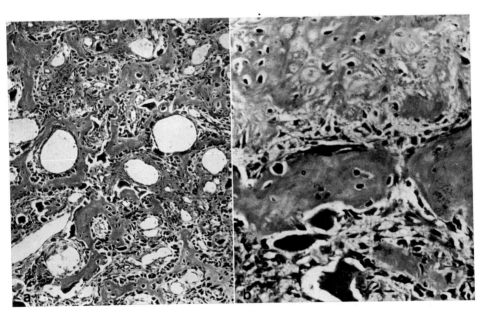

Fig. 308. - Histological aspects of osteoid osteoma (*Hemat.-eos.*, 125, 310 x).

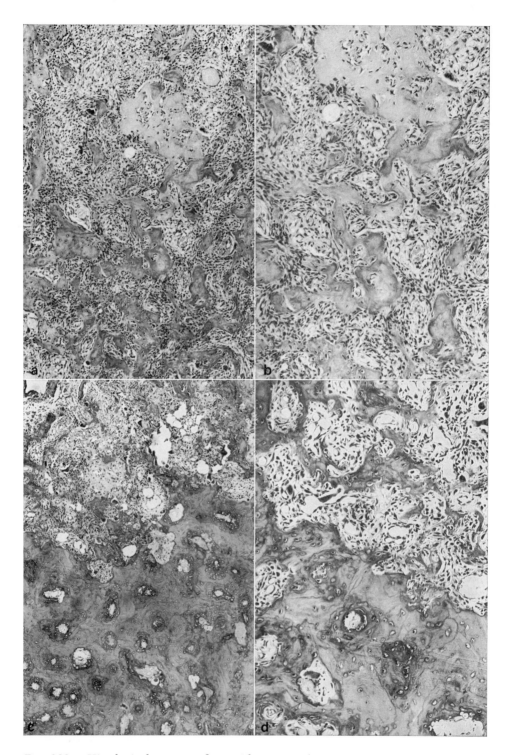

FIG. 309. - Histological aspects of osteoid osteoma (*Hemat.-eos.*, 80, 125, 50, 125 x).

metaphyseal, it has a clinical history of intermittent pain, it causes a larger and more irregular osteolysis (at times with flamelike off-shoots starting from the rounded cavity), a halo of hyperostosis which is more intense and wide in the cancellous bone, and when submitted to surgery the cavity contains pus. Nonetheless, there are exceptional cases of Brodie's abscess with rather small osteolytic lacunae, at times centered by a minute sequestrum (which may simulate the radiopaque nucleus of the nidus) and containing reddish granulation tissue. In these last cases diagnosis may solely be based on histological assessment (Figs. 5-7).

Inflammatory **sclerosing osteo-periostitis** is distinguished from O.O. because pain is less intense and is discontinuous, bone scan is less intensely positive and more diffused, and there is no nidus.

Fatigue fracture with circumscribed bone thickening is distinguished from O.O. by the patient's history (strenuous physical exercise, pain which is initially sharp to then gradually regress) and by the radiographic picture (transverse cortical fissure and band of sclerosis, no nidus) (Fig. 7b).

There may be some uncertainty as to diagnosis of an O.O. or an **osteoblastoma** (see osteoblastoma), especially when the histopathologist is availed of small fragments of tumoral tissue.

COURSE

O.O. which is left untreated increases very little in volume. Because of the phlogistic reaction which is associated, it may instead determine deformity of the metaepiphysis in growth and joint stiffness, particularly of the hip. In exceptional cases (3 in our experience) an O.O. became transformed into osteoblastoma (Figs. 318-320).

TREATMENT

Treatment consists in complete, marginal or intralesional surgical removal of the nidus. Removal of the entire area of hyperostosis or of the reactive soft tissues is instead not indicated, as these return to normal after removal of the nidus.

The problem consists in 1) reaching and clearly exposing the nidus, so that it may be completely removed; 2) removing as little surrounding bone as possible, in order to avoid weakening it (Figs. 288, 294).

The first requirement is that of planning surgery with the aid of CAT. In the femoral neck, for example, O.O. is generally superficial, more often closer to the anterior cortex, rarely to the posterior one (Fig. 295), and it is often intra-articular. Evidently, depending on the two localizations, the surgical approach and arthrotomy will be either anterior or posterior.

Once the nidus has been localized by imaging, if it is located at the surface of the bone, it is immediately visible at surgery. If, as is more often the case, it is intraosseous, it is best to shave off the bone covering it until the nidus is visualized. It will then be easy to excise it in toto with a wide, marginal or intralesional margin. Thus, excisional biopsy is carried out.

If this method is used, postoperative immobilization will not be required and restitutio ad integrum is rapid and complete.

PROGNOSIS

The surgical treatment of O.O. causes the patient to be very satisfied with the surgeon. On awakening, pain is completely and definitively regressed. In rare cases, recurrence may occur, but only if the O.O. was not totally removed.

REFERENCES

1951 MOBERG E.: The natural course of osteoid osteoma. *Journal of Bone and Joint Surgery*, **33-A**, 166-170.

1953 CARROL R. E.: Osteoid osteoma in the hand. *Journal of Bone and Joint Surgery*, **35-A**, 888-893.

1954 DAHLIN D. C., JOHNSON E. W. Jr.: Giant osteoid osteoma. *Journal of Bone and Joint Surgery*, **36-A**, 559-572.

1954 GOLDING J. S. R.: The natural history of osteoid osteoma with a report of twenty cases. *Journal of Bone and Joint Surgery*, **36-B**, 218-229.

1959 FREIBERGER R. H., LORTMAN B. S., HELGERM M., THOMPSON T. C.: Osteoid osteoma. A report on 80 cases. *American Journal of Roentgenology*, **82**, 194-205.

1959 VICKERS C. W., PUGH D. C., IVINS J. C.: Osteoid osteoma. A fifteen year follow-up of an untreated patient. *Journal of Bone and Joint Surgery*, **41-A**, 357-358.

1960 LIDBON A., LINDWALL N., SODERBERG G., SPJUT H. I.: Angiography in osteoid osteoma. *Acta Radiologica*, **54**, 327-333.

1961 SPENCE A. J., LLOYD-ROBERTS G. C.: Regional osteoporosis in osteoid osteoma. *Journal of Bone and Joint Surgery*, **43-B**, 501-507.

1966 MARCOVE R. C., FREIBERGER R. H.: Osteoid osteoma of the elbow. A diagnostic problem. Report of four cases. *Journal of Bone and Joint Surgery*, **48-A**, 1185-1190.

1966 ROSBORAUGH D.: Osteoid osteoma. Report of a lesion in the terminal phalanx of a finger. *Journal of Bone and Joint Surgery*, **48-B**, 485-487.

1967 MACLELLAN D. I., WILSON F. C. Jr.: Osteoid osteoma of the spine. A review of the literature and report of six new cases. *Journal of Bone and Joint Surgery*, **49-A**, 111-121.

1968 BYERS P. D.: Solitary benign osteoblastic lesions of bone. Osteoid osteoma and benign osteoblastoma. *Cancer*, **22**, 43-57.

1969 GALWAY R., BOBECHKO W. P., HESLIN J.: Osteoid osteoma in childhood. *Journal of Bone and Joint Surgery*, **51-B**, 196-196.

1970 DUNLOP J. A. Y., MORTON K. S., ELLIOT G. G.: Recurrent osteoid osteoma. Report of a case with a review of the literature. *Journal of Bone and Joint Surgery*, **52-B**, 128-133.

1970 LAWRIE T. R., ATERMAN K., SINCLAIR A. M.: Painless osteoid osteoma. A report of two cases. *Journal of Bone and Joint Surgery*, **52-A**, 1357-1363.

1970 SCHULMAN L., DORFMAN H. D.: Nerve fibres in osteoid osteoma. *Journal of Bone and Joint Surgery*, **52-A**, 1351-1356.

1975 DEJOUR H., LECLERC P., NOURISSAT C.: Ostéome-ostéoide du fond du cotyle. *Revue de Chirurgie Orthopédique*, **61**, 755-768.

1975 GORE D. R., MUELLER H. A.: Osteoid osteoma of the spine with localization aided by 99 mTc-polyphosphate bone scan. Case report. *Clinical Orthopaedics*, **113**, 132-134.

1975   KEIM H. A., REINA E. G.: Osteoid osteoma as a cause of scoliosis. *Journal of Bone and Joint Surgery*, **57**-A, 159-163.

1975   NORMAN A., DORFMAN H. D.: Osteoid osteoma inducing pronounced overgrowth and deformity of bone. *Clinical Orthopaedics*, **110**, 233-238.

1975   O'HARA J. P., TESMEYER C., SWEET E. D., McCUE F. C.: Angiography in the diagnosis of osteoid-osteoma of the hand. *Journal of Bone and Joint Surgery*, **57**-A, 154-159.

1975   SIM F. H., DAHLIN D. C., BEABOUT J. W.: Osteoid osteoma: diagnostic problems. *Journal of Bone and Joint Surgery*, **57**-A, 154-159.

1976   HEIMAN M. L., COOLEY CH. J., BRADFORD D. S.: Osteoid osteoma of a vertebral body. Report of a case with extension across the intervetebral disk. *Clinical Orthopaedics*, **118**, 159-163.

1977   LATEUR L., BAERT A. L.: Localisation and diagnosis of osteoid osteoma of the carpal area by angiography. *Skeletal Radiology*, **2**, 75-79.

1977   MEHTA M. H., MURRAY R. O.: Scoliosis provoked by painful vertebral lesions. *Skeletal Radiology*, **1**, 223-230.

1977   WINTER P., JOHNSON P., HILAL S., FELDMAN F.: Scintigraphic detection of osteoid osteoma. *Radiology*, **122**, 177-178.

1986   CAPANNA R., AYALA A., BERTONI F., PICCI P., CALDERONI P., GHERLINZONI F., BETTELLI G., CAMPANACCI M.: Sacral osteoid osteoma and osteoblastoma: a report of 13 cases. *Archives of Orthopaedic and Traumatic Surgery*, **105**, 205-210.

1986   HEALEY J.M., GHELMAN B.: Osteoid osteoma and osteoblastoma: current concepts and recent advances. *Clinical Orthopaedics*, **204**, 76-85.

1987   ALANI W.O., BARTAL E.: Osteoid osteoma of the femoral neck simulating an inflammatory synovitis. *Clinical Orthopaedics*, **223**, 308-312.

1987   HELMS C.A.: Osteoid osteoma: the double intensity sign. *Clinical Orthopaedics*, **222**, 167.

1988   AUGEREAU B., WIOLAND M., DE LABRIOLLE-VAYLET C., PADOVANI J.P., MARTIN TH., VERNERET C., APOIL A., MILHAUD G.: Le repérage isotopique per-opératoire des ostéomes ostéoides et autres lésions hyperfixantes à la scintigraphie. *Revue de Chirurgie Orthopedique*, **74**, 764-770.

1989   GITELIS S., SCHAJOWICZ F.: Osteoid osteoma and osteoblastoma. *Orthopaedic Clinics of North America*, **20**, 313-325.

1989   KERET D., HARCKE T., MAC EWEN D., BOWEN R.: Multiple osteoid osteomas of the fifth lumbar vertebra. *Clinical Orthopaedics*, **248**, 163-168.

1990   MOSER R.P., KRANSDORF M.J., BROWER A.C., HUDSON T., AOKI J., HUDON BERREY B., SWEET D.E.: Osteoid osteoma of the elbow. A review of six cases *Skeletal Radiology*, **19**, 181-186.

OSTEOBLASTOMA

DEFINITION

It is a benign tumor the cells of which tend to differentiate in osteoblasts, producing osteoid and bone. In most cases it is distinguished from osteoid osteoma by its clinical, radiographic, anatomical features, and by its progression. Nonetheless, there are transitional and intermediate cases located somewhere between osteoid osteoma and O.B.

FREQUENCY

O.B. occurs rarely, about 5 times more rarely than osteoid osteoma (Fig. 310).

SEX

Like osteoid osteoma, there is evident predilection for the male sex: 2/1, 3/1 (Fig. 310).

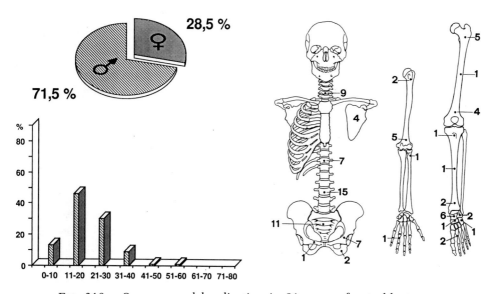

Fig. 310. - Sex, age and localization in 91 cases of osteoblastoma.

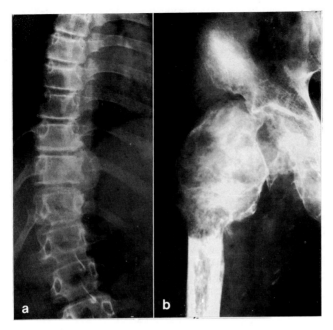

Fig. 311. - (a) Osteoblastoma of the 11th thoracic vertebra in a male aged 13 years. Observe the functional scoliosis concave on the same side as the lesion. (b) Rather expanded osteoblastoma in a male aged 28 years, with pathologic fracture.

AGE

Again, like osteoid osteoma, the tumor is typical of childhood and youth. It is rarely observed prior to 10 and after 30 years of age (Fig. 310).

LOCALIZATION

O.B. may be manifested in any area of the skeleton (Fig. 310). Nonetheless, it is the only benign tumor of the skeleton which shows evident predilection for the vertebral column and the sacrum (both the body and the posterior arch). Otherwise, it is distributed, in decreasing order, in the long bones of the limbs, in the pelvis, in the foot. It may also be observed in the craniofacial bones. When located in the long bones, O.B. is generally observed in the meta-diaphysis; more rarely, and only during adult age, it may also extend to the epiphysis. There are exceptional cases of subperiosteal O.B.

SYMPTOMS

The symptoms are those of any slow-growing benign bone tumor. It is not characterized by the sharp and typical pain of osteoid osteoma. However, it is characterized by pain, of varying intensity and of long duration; at times there is skeletal expansion; there may be pathologic fracture. In vertebral localizations, there may be signs of spinal cord compression and/or compression of the spinal nerve roots (Fig. 312). Often the amount of time between

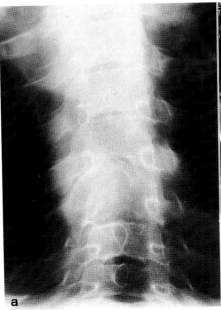

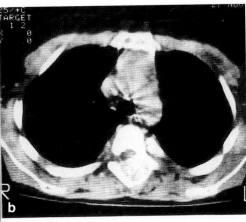

FIG. 312. - Osteoblastoma of the 4th thoracic vertebra in a male aged 14 years (a). CAT (b) revealed an osteolysis which expanded the posterior arch and narrowed the medullary canal. The osteolysis was delimited by a very thin cortex and contained cloudy radiopacity. The patient was submitted to curettage. The tumor recurred after 8 months, with sudden signs of medullary compression. Emergency curettage and medullary decompression were followed by radiation therapy. Regression of neurological signs and no signs of recurrence after 5 years.

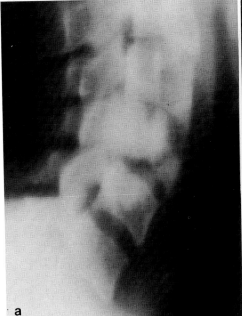

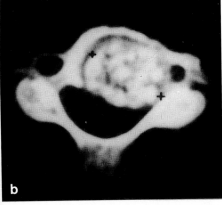

FIG. 313. - Osteoblastoma of the 4th cervical vertebra in a female aged 26 years with pain for the past 3 years and no neurological deficit. Radiogram (a) and particularly CAT (b) showed the tumor that substituted most of the vertebral body, which had well-defined boundaries and which narrowed the vertebral canal. Typical radiopacities «cotton wool» like within the tumor. The patient was submitted to curettage by anterior approach, and intersomatic arthrodesis with autoplastic bone graft. There were no signs of recurrence after 7 years.

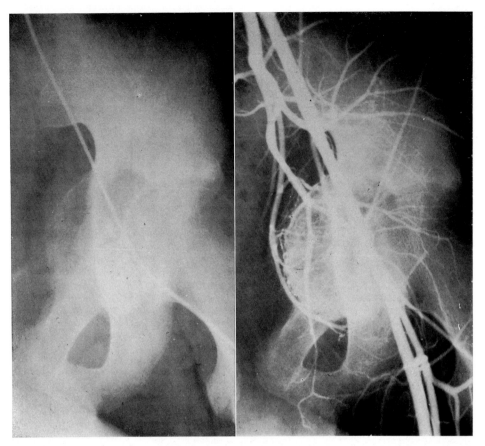

FIG. 314. - Osteoblastoma of the pelvis in a male aged 17 years. Arteriography. The patient was N.E.D. 5 years after curettage.

the first symptoms and treatment exceeds 1-2 or more years, in agreement
with the slow growth of the tumor.

RADIOGRAPHIC FEATURES

The radiographic picture may vary from case to case, and depending on
the progression of the tumor. The dominant finding is a generally single and
roundish area of osteolysis, characterized by boundaries which are not always well-defined, sometimes marked by moderate reactive osteosclerosis.
Usually, this is not as intense and extensive as in osteoid osteoma (Figs.
311-320).

O.B. may become of considerable size, up to 10 cm in diameter (Figs. 311b
315) and, whether it be central or eccentric, it tends to attenuate the cortex
and expand the bone, at times with aspects which are similar to those of
aneurysmal bone cyst (Figs. 314, 315, 316). In some cases the cortex appears
to be nearly cancelled. Sometimes the tumor remains capsulated and delimit-

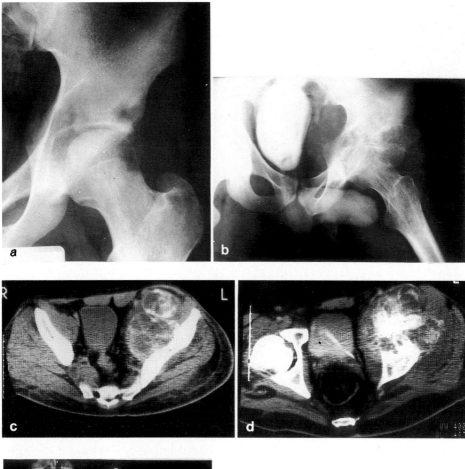

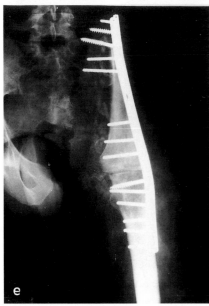

FIG. 315. - Osteoblastoma in a male aged 22 years. Pain for the past year. Radiogram obtained at that time (a) showed a small supra-acetabular osteolysis. The latest radiogram (b) showed severe extent of the osteolysis involving the joint and a contracture in flexo-abduction of the hip. CAT (c, d) showed a severely aggressive tumor (stage 3) with wide invasion of the soft tissues and containing faded radiopacities. (e) After selective arterial embolization, the patient was submitted to extra-articular marginal resection of the hemipelvis and hip and reconstruction-arthrodesis with allograft (proximal tibia). There were no signs of recurrence after 1 year.

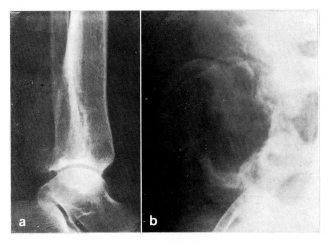

Fig. 316. - (a) Osteobla-
stoma in a female aged 47
years. No recurrence 5
years after marginal excision. (b) Osteoblastoma of
the posterior arch of the
third   lumbar   vertebra
which expands the spin-
ous process. No recur-
rence 9 years after intralesional excision.

ed in relation to the surrounding soft tissues (Fig. 318); but sometimes its limits towards the soft tissues are blurred (Figs. 315, 319). There is hardly any
or only a fair amount of periosteal reaction, of the chronic type.

In some cases the tumor appears to be totally osteolytic, even partially cystic
(Figs. 316, 318). In others it is characterized by diffused ground glass radiopacity, not unlike that of fibrous dysplasia (Figs. 311a, 312, 314, 315).

In other cases still, it is characterized by disseminated or confluent, irregular or faded nubecolae, of more intense opacity, which may even be very
intense (Figs. 311b, 313, 317b, 319). When there is radiopacity of the tumoral
tissue, it constitutes the most important radiographic feature leading to a
diagnosis of O.B. This radiopacity is the expression of the quantity and the
degree of maturation of the neoplastic osteoid substance. Thus, it changes
with the evolution and the aging of the tumor. Typically, O.B. becomes very
radiopaque after radiation therapy.

Fig. 317. - (a) Osteoblastoma with an apparently
periosteal origin from the
spinous process of the
seventh cervical vertebra
in a boy aged 9 years. (b)
Osteoblastoma in a boy
aged 8 years. In these two
cases the choice between
a diagnosis of osteoblas-
toma and giant osteoid
osteoma purely depends
on personal preferences.

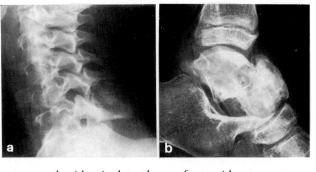

In fact histological aspects may be identical to those of osteoid osteoma.

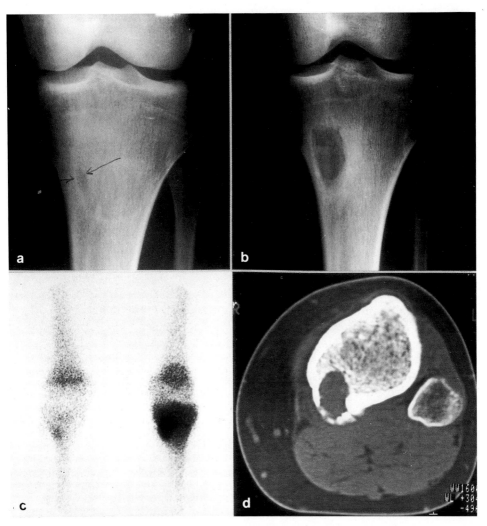

FIG. 318. - Osteoblastoma in a female aged 19 years. Pain for the past 2 and 1/2 years. Radiogram obtained at that time (a) showed a small osteolysis identical to an osteoid osteoma. The current radiogram (b) showed growth of the lesion. Bone scan was intensely positive (c). Radiogram and CAT (b, d) showed an osteolysis which was nearly deprived of radiopacity and moderate reaction of the surrounding bone.

Angiography may reveal the intense vascularity of the tumor (Fig. 314). In some cases (very painful with peritumoral inflammatory reaction) a regional osteoporosis is associated.

GROSS PATHOLOGIC FEATURES

O.B. has rather compact tissue, reddish or reddish-brown in color, of soft and granulous consistency (because of the osteoid contents). At times it contains granules, nodules or vast areas of decidedly osseous consistency.

A frequent characteristic of the tumor is intense hyperemia. As generally occurs in skeletal pathology, the hyperemia is more evident when the tumor develops in spongy bone with red marrow, such as the vertebrae, the cranium, the pelvis, the ribs. Particularly in these sites, incision of the tumor provokes hemorrhage of oxygenated blood, which is quite intense and at times slightly pulsating. Although O.B. appears to contain ectatic vessels, only

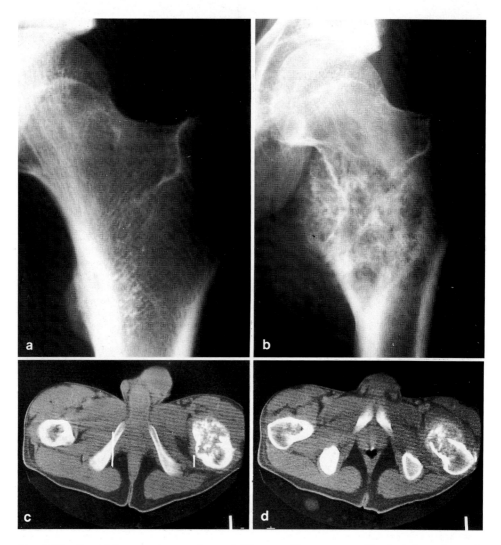

FIG. 319. - Osteoblastoma in a male aged 18 years. Two years earlier based on the typical pain and radiographic picture (a), osteoid osteoma was diagnosed and the patient was operated with no regression of pain. The latest radiograms (b) show progression in vast osteolysis which interrupts the cortex, contains faded radiopacity, and is surrounded by moderate sclerosing reaction. (c) and (d) CAT reveals an aggressive tumor (stage 3) and typical intratumoral radiopacities «cotton wool» like. The patient was submitted to wide resection and endoprosthesis and there were no signs of recurrence after 2 years.

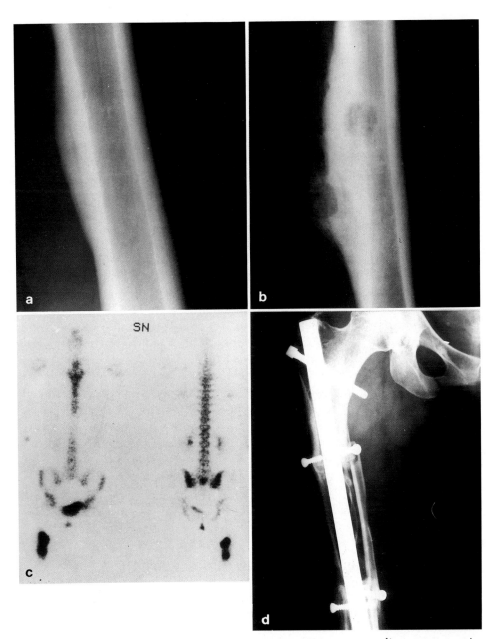

FIG. 320. - Osteoblastoma in a female aged 24 years. Two years earlier constant pain, prevalently at night, irradiated. Radiogram (a) showed typical aspect of osteoid osteoma. The patient was submitted to removal of a window of the cortex using multiple perforations to delimit the window. After a few months pain recurred. (b) Latest radiogram showed two rounded osteolytic cavities surrounded by intense sclerosing bone reaction. (c) Intense scintigraphic captation. (d) After incisional biopsy the patient was submitted to wide resection of the diaphysis and reconstruction with a locked nail and autogenous grafts from the fibula and ilium. No signs of recurrence after 3 years. (In this case the tumor, initially having all of the features of osteoid osteoma, was probably disseminated by the perforating drill and recurred in several sites assuming the features of osteoblastoma).

occasionally are wide hematic cavities typical of aneurysmal bone cyst observed.

The cortical bone is thinned and often expanded; in some areas it may be absent, the tumor abutting in the soft tissues covered by a pseudocapsule. At times there is intense peritumoral reaction, with the features of a chronic inflammatory process.

HISTOPATHOLOGIC FEATURES

The main feature of O.B. is a proliferation of mesenchymal cells which tend towards osteoblastic differentiation and which are accompanied by a rich capillary and sinusoidal vascularization (Figs. 321, 322). In areas where proliferation is more active, the osteoblasts appear to be large, with deeply stained cytoplasms and nuclei, which are slightly pleomorphic; there are rare mitotic figures. There may even be large and bizarre cells with a large blown-up nucleus and a large nucleolus (Fig. 322). But these are **sporadic** elements of the regressive type, and ones which do not signify malignancy. Furthermore, the structure of the tissue is much more regular and organoid than that of osteosarcoma. Another feature of O.B. is that the tumoral tissue tends towards progressive ossification-maturation. This is not uniform throughout the entire neoplasm, so that, alongside densely ossified and calcified areas there may be scattered foci of cellular proliferation. Hypervascularity and possible interstitial hemorrhages, together with the resorption of newly-formed bone, explain the presence of numerous multinucleate giant cells.

In many cases, the histological picture is the same as that of osteoid osteoma; at times, however, it is richer in cells and more immature.

The presence of scattered foci of cellular proliferation may give the impression that the tumor is characterized by multicentric origin in the skeletal area involved.

Rarely, the tumor contains large hemorrhagic and cystic cavities, likening it to an aneurysmal bone cyst.

HISTOGENESIS AND PATHOGENESIS

O.B. is a benign tumor mainly composed by osteoblasts. Thus, its histogenesis is similar to that of osteoma, osteoid osteoma, and fibrous dysplasia. Instead, its biological behavior, expressed by its clinical and anatomical features, differentiate it rather clearly from these other forms. As compared to fibrous dysplasia, O.B. does not have any hamartomatous features. As compared to osteoid osteoma, it has a higher growth potential, and it provokes less reactive hyperostosis of the host bone.

DIAGNOSIS

There do exist delicate problems of differential diagnosis with osteoid osteoma and — much more vital — with osteosarcoma.

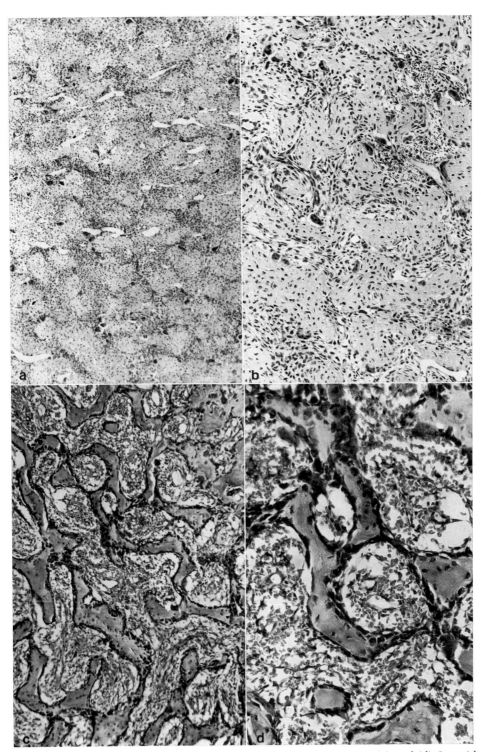

FIG. 321. - (a) and (b) Very immature osteoid. Organoid structure. (c) and (d) Osteoid trabeculae bordered by rows of large osteoblasts. Intense hyperemia (*Hemat.-eos.*, 50, 125, 125, 310 x).

Osteosarcoma. In the past some O.B. have been mistaken for osteosarcoma, resulting in the tragic consequences which may easily be imagined. This error is unacceptable; the clinical, radiographic and macroscopic pictures must be taken into account, and extensive histological specimens representative of the tumor and the peritumoral tissues must be available. In fact, O.B. is often observed in skeletal areas where osteosarcoma is an exceptional occurrence. Its growth is slower. Its radiographic and macroscopic boundaries are clearer. Histologically, its overall structure is much more orderly. It never forms neoplastic cartilage. Diffused cellular atypia is not observed (but care must be taken not to overrate O.B.'s sporadic pseudomalignant cells). The vessels have their own wall. It does not permeate the medullary spaces of the surrounding bone, nor does it present intravascular tumoral plugs. It does not cause increase in serum alkaline phosphatase.

There are instead rare cases of osteosarcoma in which it is important to be very careful not to underestimate the tumor and consider it an O.B. (see osteosarcoma and low-malignancy central osteosarcoma).

Osteoid osteoma. As compared to osteoid osteoma, O.B. has different elective localizations, it becomes much larger in size, it does not cause typical pain, its histological aspect may be more immature. Nonetheless, there are cases of transition between osteoid osteoma and O.B. By convention, osteoid osteoma is that which is less than 2 cm in diameter.

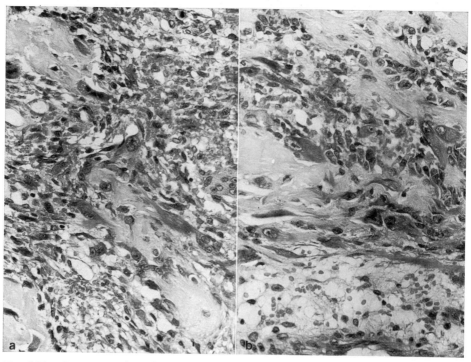

FIG. 322. - Large pseudomalignant cells with large dark cytoplasm and large nucleus with evident nucleolus (*Hemat.-eos.*, 310, 310 x).

Giant cell tumor. There are meta-epiphyseal O.B. of the adult which are totally radiolucent, and which radiographically appear to be similar to a giant cell tumor (Fig. 316a). Histologically, too, in some areas of O.B., there may be tissue similar to that of a giant cell tumor, characterized by only a small amount of osteogenesis. As limited aspects of osteogenesis may also be observed in giant cell tumor, doubt as to diagnosis is rarely legitimate; but this may be resolved by a suitable histological examination.

Aneurysmal bone cyst. Both O.B. and aneurysmal bone cyst are often observed in the vertebral column, where they may be very similar both radiographically and on surgical exposure (Fig. 316b). Furthermore, there are exceptional cases of subperiosteal O.B. which are radiographically the same as aneurysmal bone cyst; and there are cases of O.B. containing wide hemorrhagic and cystic cavities, similar to those of aneurysmal bone cyst. Differential diagnosis is based on a histological study. Even if O.B. contains hematic cysts which under small enlargement liken it to aneurysmal bone cyst, the tissue is more neoplastic, rich in immature cells, with diffuse proliferation and anomalous osteogenesis. In aneurysmal bone cyst, instead, there is histiocytary, fibroblastic, and osteoblastic tissue with features which are more hyperplastic and reparative than neoplastic.

COURSE

Although O.B. grows relatively slowly, if it is left alone it may become of considerable size and continue to grow for several years. Even if some parts of O.B. tend towards bony maturation, other proliferative foci are likely to form and then grow.

Rarely, we have observed a lesion identical to an osteoid osteoma which, spontaneously or as a local recurrence after incomplete removal, transformed into a typical O.B. (Figs. 318-320).

TREATMENT

Treatment depends on the stage and the localization of the tumor. In stage 1 (latent) or stage 2 (active) O.B., intralesional excision (curettage) may be indicated, associated with local adjuvants. Curettage will especially be used in vertebral localizations, in those in a growing metaphysis, or near a functionally important epiphysis.

In stage 3 O.B. (aggressive) marginal or wide resection is indicated. This is difficult and risky in vertebral localizations. In the latter, aggressive curettage is used, associated with internal fixation, and completed by radiation therapy, which is fairly effective.

Selective arterial embolization may also be useful immediately prior to surgery (vertebral, pelvic localizations) in order to reduce hemorrhage during surgery.

PROGNOSIS

If removal is complete, O.B. does not recur. It may recur after incomplete removal, even after several years. Cases of aggressive O.B. are described, characterized by considerable expansion and local recurrence, at times with delayed metastases. We suspect that at least those cases which metastasized were not O.B., but osteosarcomas from the start, which went unrecognized because of the low grade of malignancy (see osteosarcoma), or because they were characterized by atypical histology (Fig. 402).

REFERENCES

1956 JAFFE H. L.: Benign osteoblastoma. *Bulletin of the Hospital for Joint Diseases*, **17**, 141-151.

1956 LICHTENSTEIN L.: Benign osteoblastoma. A category of osteoid and bone-forming tumors other than classical osteoid osteoma, which may be mistaken for giant-cell tumor or osteogenic sarcoma. *Cancer*, **9**, 1044-1052.

1960 POCHACZEVSKY R., YEN Y. M., SHERMAN R. S. S.: The röntgen appearance of benign osteoblastoma. *Radiology*, **75**, 429-437.

1964 LICHTENSTEIN L., SAWYER W. R.: Benign osteoblastoma. Further observations and report of twenty additional cases. *Journal of Bone and Joint Surgery*, **46-A**, 755-765.

1967 MAYER L.: Malignant degeneration of so-called benign osteoblastoma. *Bulletin of the Hospital for Joint Diseases*, **28**, 4-13.

1968 BYERS P. D.: Solitary benign osteoblastic lesions of bone. Osteoid osteoma and benign osteoblastoma. *Cancer*, **22**, 43-57.

1969 KENT J. N., CASTRO H. F., GJROTTI W. R.: Benign osteoblastoma of the maxilla. Case report and review of the literature. *Oral Surgery*, **27**, 209-219.

1970 SCHAJOWICZ F., LEMOS C.: Osteoid osteoma and osteoblastoma. Closely related entities of osteoblastic derivation. *Acta Orthopedica Scandinavica*, **41**, 272-291.

1975 MARSH B. W., BONFIGLIO M., BRADY L. P., ENNEKING W. F.: Benign osteoblastoma: range of manifestations. *Journal of Bone and Joint Surgery*, **57-A**, 1-9.

1976 MCLEOD R. A., DAHLIN D. C., BEABOUT J. W.: The spectrum of osteoblastoma. *American Journal of Roentgenology*, **126**, 321-335.

1976 MIRRA J. M., KENDRICK R. A., KENDRICK R. E.: Pseudo-malignant osteoblastoma versus arrested osteosarcoma. A case report. *Cancer*, **37**, 2005-2014.

1976 SCHAJOWICZ F., LEMOS C.: Malignant osteoblastoma. *Journal of Bone and Joint Surgery*, **58-B**, 202-211.

1977 YOSHIKAWA S., NAKAMURA T., TAKAGI M., IMAMURA T., KAZUTOSHI O., SASAKI A.: Benign osteoblastoma as a cause of osteomalacia. A report of two cases. *Journal of Bone and Joint Surgery*, **59-B**, 279-286.

1978 BORIANI S., CAMPANACCI M.: Osteoblastoma e osteomalacia. Presentazione di un caso e revisione della letteratura. *Giornale Italiano di Ortopedia e Traumatologia*, **4**, 375-378.

1978 DAHLIN D. C.: *Bone tumors*. Charles C. Thomas, Springfield.

1984 KIRWAN E. O'G., HUTTON P.A.N., POZO J.L., RANSFORD A.O.: Osteoid osteoma and benign osteoblastoma of the spine. *Journal of Bone and Joint Surgery*, **66-B**, 21-26.

1985 BERTONI F., UNNI K.K., MCLEOD R.A., DAHLIN D.C.: Osteosarcoma resembling osteoblastoma. *Cancer*, **55**, 416-426.

1985 KENAN S., FLOMAN Y., ROBIN G., LAUFFER A.: Aggressive osteoblastoma. A case report and review of the literature. *Clinical Orthopaedics*, **195**, 294-298.

1986 CAPANNA R., AYALA A., BERTONI F., PICCI P., CALDERONI P., GHERLINZONI F., BETTELLI G., CAMPANACCI M.: Sacral osteoid osteoma and osteoblastoma: a report of 13 cases. *Archives of Orthopaedic and Traumatic Surgery*, **105**, 205-210.

1986   HEALEY J.H., GHELMAN B.: Osteoid osteoma and osteoblastoma: current concepts and recent advances. *Clinical Orthopaedics*, **204**, 76-85.

1986   PETTINE K.A., KLASSEN R.A.: Osteoid osteoma and osteoblastoma of the spine.
Journal of Bone and Joint Surgery, **68-A**, 354-361.

1989   BETTELLI G., CAPANNA R., VAN HORN J.R., RUGGIERI P., BIAGINI R., CAMPANAC-
CI M.: Osteoid osteoma and osteoblastoma of the pelvis. *Clinical Orthopaedics*, **247**, 261-271.

1989   DE COSTER E., VAN TIGGELEN R., SHAHABPOUR M., CHARELS K., OSTEAUX M.,
OPDECAM P.: Osteoblastoma of the patella: case report and review of the
literature. *Clinical Orthopaedics*, **243**, 216-219.

1989   GITELIS S., SCHAJOWICZ F.: Osteoid osteoma and osteoblastoma. *Orthopaedic
Clinics of North America*, **20**, 313-325.

1989   MORTON K.S., QUENVILLE N.F., BEAUCHAMP C.P.: Aggressive osteoblastoma.
Journal of Bone and Joint Surgery, **71-B**, 428-431.

FIBROUS DYSPLASIA
(Synonym: fibrous dysplasia of the skeleton)

DEFINITION

F.D. of the skeleton, congenital and similar to hamartomas, is an intraosseous neoformation, which may be monostotic or polyostotic, of a fibro-osseous tissue. Skeletal lesion may be associated with skin pigmentation spots, early skeletal maturity and (in females) precocious puberty. This quadruple association is known as Albright's syndrome.

FREQUENCY

F.D. is a much more frequent occurrence than what appears to be the case in reported series (including ours) because these include only those cases submitted to surgery. Monostotic forms are more frequent than polyostotic ones. The association of pigmented skin spots is observed in approximately 20% of reported cases, with a predominant incidence among polyostotic forms. Albright's syndrome is a rare occurrence (less than 5% of all cases) and it is above all observed in diffused polyostotic forms.

SEX

There is slight predilection for the female sex (Fig. 323).

AGE

In agreement with its congenital hamartomatous nature, F.D. begins during early childhood (Fig. 323). The first symptoms are usually manifested between 5 and 15-20 years of age: the more extended the dysplasia, the earlier the onset of symptoms. Circumscribed monostotic and oligostotic forms may remain asymptomatic and only be revealed by a radiographic examination obtained for other reasons during adult age.

LOCALIZATION

In **monostotic forms** the most frequent sites are, in this order: the maxil-

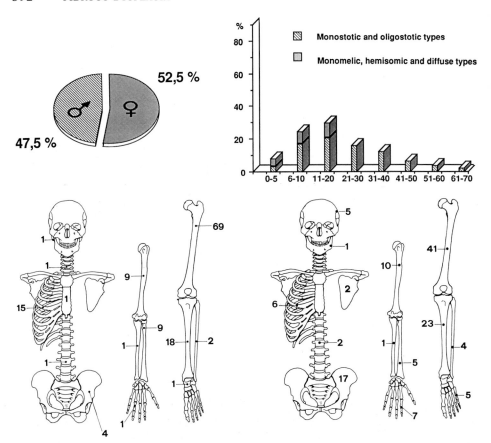

FIG. 323. - Sex, age and localization in 166 cases of fibrous dysplasia. (These are cases submitted to surgery and ascertained histologically). To the left, localization in 133 cases of monostotic fibrous dysplasia. To the right, 129 localizations in 33 cases of diffused, monomelic-hemisomic, oligostotic fibrous dysplasia.

lary bones, the proximal femur, the tibia. These are followed by the humerus, the ribs, the radius, the iliac bone.

Polyostotic forms may be distinguished as follows.

1) Oligostotic forms with few localizations, generally in the proximal femur, the ilium, some ribs, the mandible.

2) Monomelic or hemisomic forms. More often these involve the lower limb and the homolateral hemipelvis. At times they particularly involve an upper limb. In other cases, finally, they are extended to one half of the body, possibly including the cranium, the pelvis, and the ribs.

3) Generalized forms, with extension to the two lower limbs and to the pelvis, or to three or four of the limbs, the scapula, and possibly the bones of the trunk and the cranium. Nonetheless, in these cases, too, lesions tend to prevail in one half of the body.

In conclusion, some essential features concerning the distribution of the lesions may be noted. No bone is immune to F.D. **There is predilection**

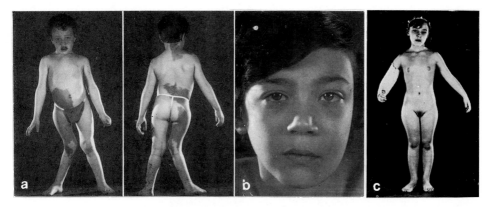

FIG. 324. - (a) Café au lait skin spots and deformities in polyostotic fibrous dysplasia in a boy aged 9 years. (b) Deformity of the facial bones due to fibrous dysplasia in a boy aged 12 years. (c) Precocious puberty in Albright's syndrome in a girl aged 6 years.

for the femur which, in circumscribed forms of the disease, is generally affected in its proximal half. Other frequent localizations are the maxillary bones, the tibia, the ribs, and the ilium. In multicentric and diffused forms of the disease, the lesions are exclusive, or they prevail in one half of the body. In the limbs, the frequency of localization decreases from the proximal parts towards the extremities: the hand and the foot are rarely involved, and only in more diffused forms of the disease. Another rare localization is the vertebral column (Fig. 323).

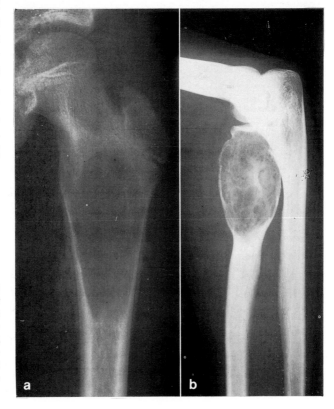

FIG. 325. - (a) Monostotic fibrous dysplasia in a boy aged 6 years. Observe the unusual finding of a periosteal reaction due to a recent pathologic microfracture. (b) Monostotic fibrous dysplasia in a female aged 29 years.

In the long bones, F.D. begins more often in a metaphysis; it may remain circumscribed, or extend to the diaphysis. Instead, it does not invade the epiphysis, as long as growth cartilage is present. Monostotic forms of the disease are generally circumscribed and metadiaphyseal; more rarely, they are centro-diaphyseal. Polyostotic forms of the disease are more often diffused to most or all of the long bone, except for the epiphyses. These may be partially invaded by the dysplastic tissue only during adult age (with rare exceptions: Fig. 338b).

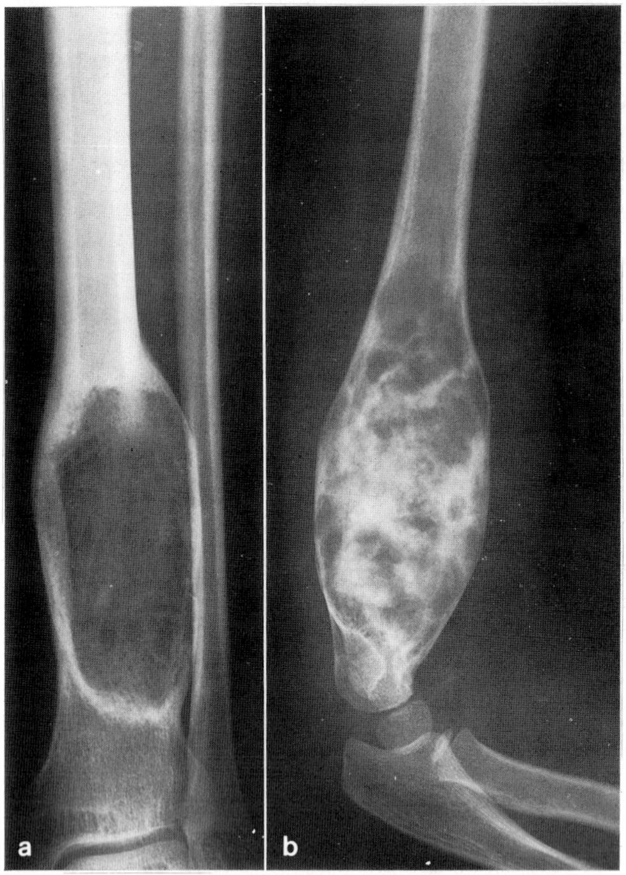

FIG. 326. - Examples of monostotic fibrous dysplasia. (a) Distal tibial lesion in a female aged 19 years. (b) Lesion of the distal humerus in a boy aged 3 years.

SYMPTOMS

In **monostotic forms** of the disease symptoms are mild and occur late, so that often it is manifested in adult age, or not at all. In the superficial bones (ribs, maxillary bones, iliac wing, tibia) there may be moderate skeletal expansion. Pain is more frequent in lesions of the lower limbs; it may be caused by frequent **microfractures and pathologic fractures**. There may be a relatively rapid increase in swelling, particularly in the ribs, during adult age; this swelling, and above all when there are no other localizations of the dysplasia, may lead to the fear of a malignant tumor. This phenomenon above all depends on hemorrhaging in the tissues of the dysplasia.

The symptoms occur earlier and are more apparent in **polyostotic forms** of the disease. Early occurrence and severity of symptoms are directly proportional to the extent of the skeletal lesions. As in monostotic forms, symptoms include skeletal expansion, pain, pathologic fracture and, furthermore, deformity. Skeletal expansion tends to be moderate and diffused to the metaphysis and diaphysis. Pain is either absent or mild and discontinuous; more often it is caused by microfractures and pathologic fractures, which occur very frequently, particularly in the tibia and femur. Deformities occur just as frequently, and they, too, dominate in the lower limb, particularly the femur. They are caused by expansion, bowing, shortening, and pathologic fractures of the bones affected. Bowing of the long bones has a long radius and involves the entire diaphysis and the metaphysis. The most typical deformities are varus of the proximal femur which may even be very severe (shepherd-crook) and, milder, varus or valgus of the tibia (Figs. 324a, 334). There may be static scoliosis, due to shortening of a lower limb. The facies may be modified by monolateral or asymmetric expansion of the cranio-facial bones (Fig. 324b). Deformity and shortening are not symmetrical, rather they are exclusive, or they prevail in one half of the body (Fig. 324a). In exceptional cases, instead of shortening, there is lengthening of the long bones affected (Fig. 338b).

Skin pigmentation (particularly in polyostotic forms of the disease) consists in melanin spots, which may be small, spraylike, or large, maplike, varying in color from yellow-brown to dull brown (Fig. 324a). Their site and extent is not related to that of the skeletal lesions.

In infrequent cases of extended polyostotic F.D. and in both sexes there may be **early growth and maturation of the skeleton**. Due to early somatic growth,

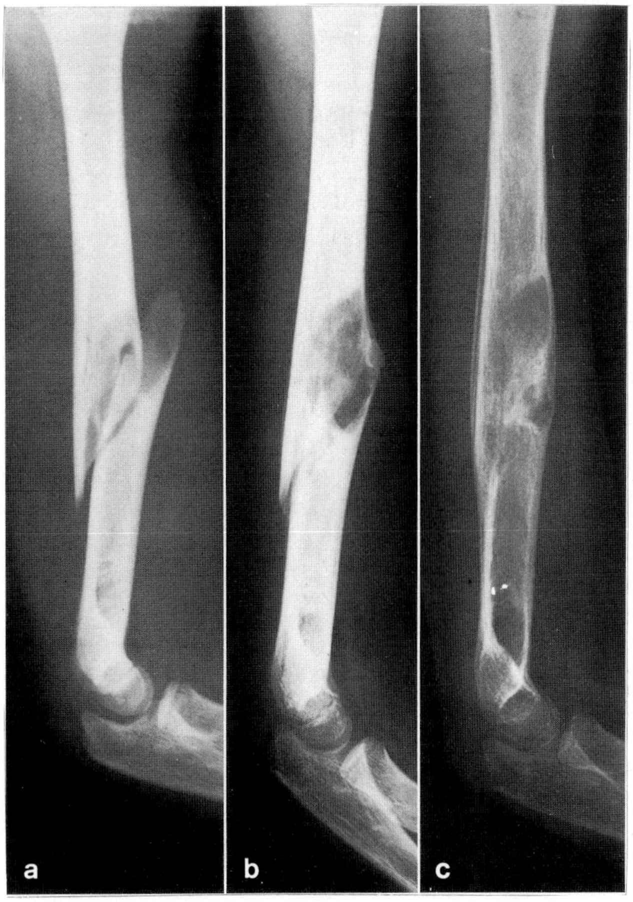

FIG. 327. - Monostotic fibrous dysplasia. (a) Fracture on a centro-diaphyseal osteolytic lesion which is just visible, in a girl aged 8 years. (b) After consolidation of the fracture, the osteolytic lesion is more evident, which on histological examination was revealed to be a fibrous dysplasia. (c) Aspect 6 months after fracture.

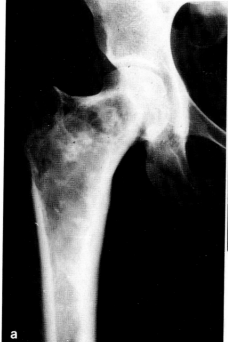
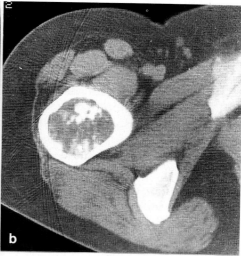

FIG. 328. - Fibrous dysplasia with cartilaginous areas in a female aged 40 years. Mild discontinuous pain. The images of intralesional calcification correspond to cartilaginous foci. Successive radiograms showed that the lesion was stabilized for a few years. Thus, surgery was not indicated. Differential diagnosis with chondrosarcoma may be resolved without biopsy because the cortex is not eroded, its external surface is perfectly smooth, and the lesion is stabilized. In this case, diagnosis was ascertained with an unnecessary biopsy.

during late childhood there may be an increase in stature as compared to what is normal. Nonetheless, at the end of growth, stature is less than the average as maturation and fusion of the growth cartilage are premature. **Precocious puberty** is rarely observed and particularly in cases of more severe and extended F.D., generally associated with skin pigmentation and early somatic development. It occurs nearly exclusively in the female sex, although it has exceptionally also been observed in the male. In the female it consists in early or very early menarches and the development of the genitals and secondary sexual features (Fig. 324c). More rarely, there are other associations, such as **multiple myxomas of the soft tissues, hyperthyroidism, diabetes mellitus, renal and cardiovascular anomalies.**

An increase in **alkaline phosphatase** is the only hematochemical finding of importance. It is not constant, nor is it very elevated, and more easily observed in extensive polyostotic forms of the disease.

RADIOGRAPHIC FEATURES

The radiographic picture is very typical in extensive and advanced forms of the disease, less typical in initial and circumscribed ones. In any case, it reveals the features of slow or exhausted growth.

FIG. 329. - Fibrous dysplasia in a female aged 63 years. Chance radiographic finding. In the adult the «mature» lesion may become intensely radiopaque.

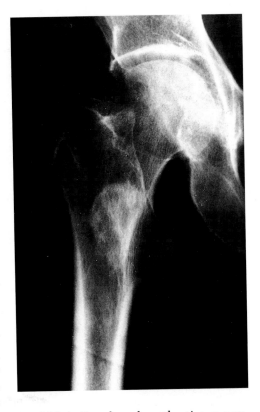

Radiographic aspects depend on two conditions.

1) On the quality of the dysplastic tissue. If it is nearly exclusively fibrous pure osteolysis is observed (Figs. 325a, 326a, 330, 336c, 337a). Radiotransparence is even more intense when the tissue contains cystic cavities. When there are abundant microscopic islands of newly-formed bone, faded radiopacity occurs, which varies from a minimum ground glass intensity (Figs. 325b, 331a, 332, 333b, 334, 338b) to a maximum intensity which may even become of eburneous aspect (particularly in the cranio-facial bones) (Figs. 326b, 331b, 332c, 338a). Rarely, when the tissue contains cartilaginous areas with calcification at the periphery of the cartilage lobules, anular radiopacities similar to those of cartilaginous tumors may be observed (Figs. 328, 333a).

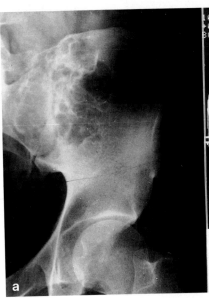

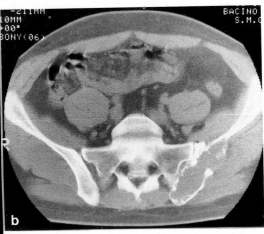

FIG. 330. - Fibrous dysplasia in a male aged 22 years. Chance radiographic finding. Lesion ascertained with biopsy.

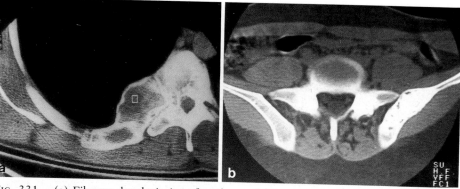

FIG. 331. - (a) Fibrous dysplasia in a female aged 27 years. Chance radiographic finding and diagnosis ascertained with biopsy. CAT showed moderate expansion of a rib and alteration in the adjacent vertebral body, as well. Observe the mild ground glass radiopacity of the lesion. In these cases radiographic examination and CAT are diagnostic. Generally, there is no indication for biopsy, or for any type of treatment. It is enough to monitor the lesion with radiograms repeated in time. (b) Fibrous dysplasia in a female aged 21 years. Chance radiographic and CAT findings revealed that the lesion was mostly ossified and sclerotic as it may occur during adult age. In this case, as well, biopsy was not required.

2) On the fact that the cortex is slowly eroded from the inside (thinned); it becomes spongy (faded radiopacity) and finally it may appear to be expanded, as endosteal resorption is associated with slow periosteal apposition.

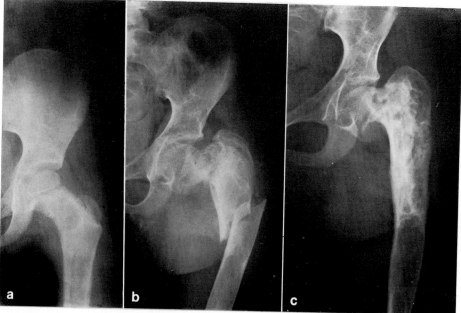

FIG. 332. - Fibrous dysplasia. (a) Initial aspect in a girl aged 5 years. (b) At 11 years of age pathologic fracture. (c) The same at 12 years of age.

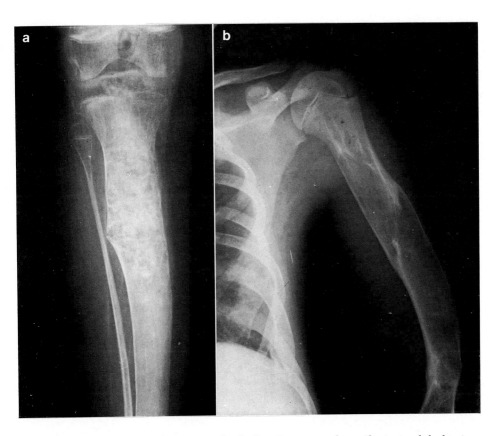

FIG. 333. - (a) Ringlike radiopacity of calcification around cartilaginous lobules in a girl aged 10 years. (b) Cloudy or ground glass radiopacity in a boy aged 13 years.

In **monostotic and localized** forms there may be a purely osteolytic area, single or polycyclical (due to the presence of parietal crests) (Fig. 336c) with clear or slightly faded boundaries. Ground glass radiopacity often occurs, which in these cases constitutes the main radio-diagnostic evidence. During early childhood the lesion may begin with a small spot of metaphyseal osteolysis which is not typical (Fig. 332a). Only when it extends (in progressive cases) does the lesion assume radiographic features which are more significant.

In forms which are **extended** to most or all of a long bone (generally polyostotic) there are more typical radiographic aspects (Figs. 332, 333, 334). Mild skeletal expansion, which is unequal and diffused; diaphyseal and metaphyseal bowing; considerable and diffused thinning of the cortex; osteolytic spots alternating with faded radiopaque cloudiness. Furthermore, the radiopacity of the cortex is decreased (because it is spongy) and is often confused with the ground glass radiopacity of the dysplastic tissue. In deformed bones the cortex is always attenuated and spongy on the convex side, while it is thicker and compact on the concave one.

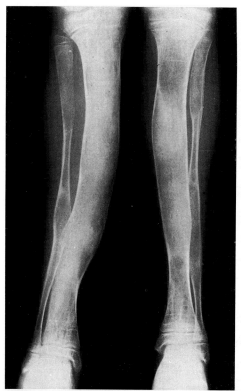

In the **cranium** there is thickening of the bone, including bubbling osteolytic cavities and faded spots of radiopacity (Figs. 335, 336a). The internal and external cortices may be thinned and spongy. Sclerosing radiographic alterations prevail in the cranial base and the facial bones (Figs. 336b, 338a) with narrowing of the corresponding sinuses. Often there is expansion of the maxillary bones.

In the **ribs** osteolytic and beehive swelling is a frequent occurrence (Figs. 331a, 336c).

The **vertebrae** are rarely involved, but they may collapse due to pathologic fracture (Figs. 331a, 337b).

The skeleton of the **hand** is also rarely involved and always in forms of the disease which are

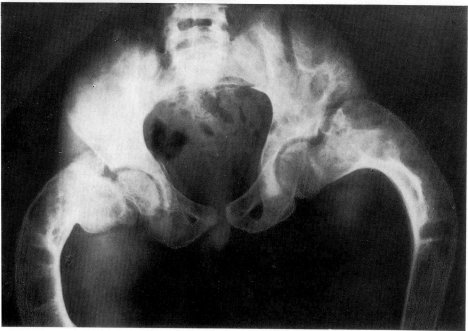

Fig. 334. - Boy aged 11 years. Diffused form with all of the most typical radiographic aspects of fibrous dysplasia: expansion, thinning and spongy transformation of the cortex, ground glass opacity, cystic images, deformities.

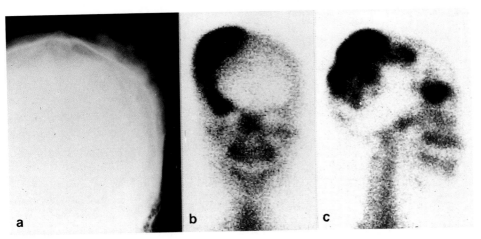

FIG. 335. - Monostotic fibrous dysplasia of the cranium in a male aged 17 years.

diffused to the entire upper limb. There is diffused enlargement (and at times lengthening) of the metacarpals and phalanges, with the usual radiographic aspects. These changes may involve the metacarpal epiphyses and the bones of the carpus (Fig. 338b).

The radiographic picture of F.D. tends to modify during **adolescence and adult age**. Lesions slow down and stop growing and extend; the walls of the osteolytic areas and the cortices tend to thicken very slowly (Figs. 329, 350). Rarely, the ground glass radiopacity increases in intensity until it becomes eburneous.

GROSS PATHOLOGIC FEATURES

Under the periosteum, which is not changed, the cortex is thinned; at times it is also spongy so that it may be incised by a scalpel. Within there is whitish compact tissue, with a particular elastic and granulous consistency. The granulosity is due to the delicate osteoid and osseous trabeculae contained in the fibrous tissue, and it varies as the quantity and the maturation of the trabeculae vary. The tissue is generally not very vascularized; nonetheless, particularly in the spongy bones (cranium, ribs, pelvis, metaphysis), it may appear to be dotted with hypervascular or hemorrhagic spots. Cystic cavities are often observed, consequent to edematous or hemorrhagic softening, and containing serous or hematic fluid. At times, particularly in monostotic forms of the disease, nearly the entire osteolytic area is reduced to a cavity of fluid contents, so that the surgical finding may be similar to that of a bone cyst.

At times the tissue contains cartilaginous islands, which are more abundant during early childhood and in the metaphyseal areas.

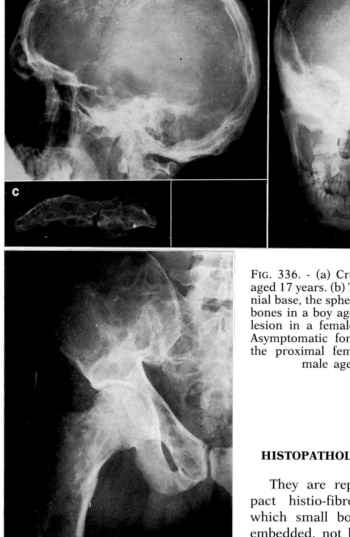

Fig. 336. - (a) Cranial lesion in a boy aged 17 years. (b) Thickening of the cranial base, the sphenoid and the ethmoid bones in a boy aged 6 years. (c) Costal lesion in a female aged 26 years. (d) Asymptomatic form of the disease in the proximal femur and pelvis in a male aged 34 years.

HISTOPATHOLOGIC FEATURES

They are represented by compact histio-fibroblastic tissue in which small bone trabeculae are embedded, not bordered by osteoblasts (Figs. 339, 340).

Generally, the histio-fibroblasts are numerous and plump, with rare mitotic figures, surrounded by a delicate collagenous fibrillary net. At times there is a whorled or storiform pattern. At times there are multinucleate giant cells, particularly surrounding hypervascular or hemorrhagic areas (particularly in the very vascularized cancellous bones, such as the ribs: Fig. 343d). In some areas the tissue is deprived of bony trabeculae and it appears to be the same as that of

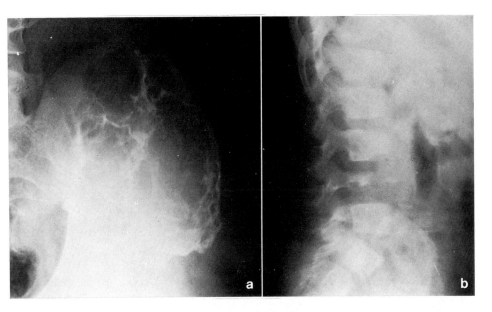

FIG. 337. - (a) Iliac lesion in a female aged 34 years. (b) Vertebral lesion in a boy aged 5 years with polyostotic form of the disease.

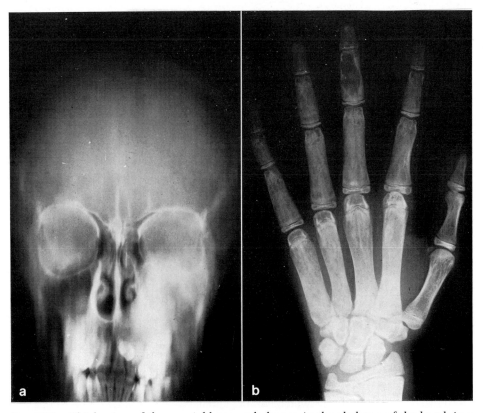

FIG. 338. - Thickening of the cranial base and change in the skeleton of the hand, in a boy aged 8 years with generalized fibrous dysplasia.

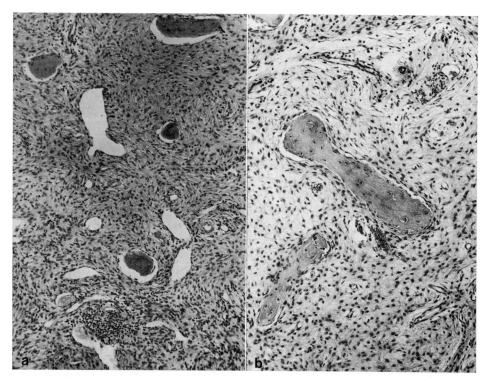

FIG. 339. - Histological aspects typical of fibrous dysplasia (*Hemat.-eos.*, 125, 125 x).

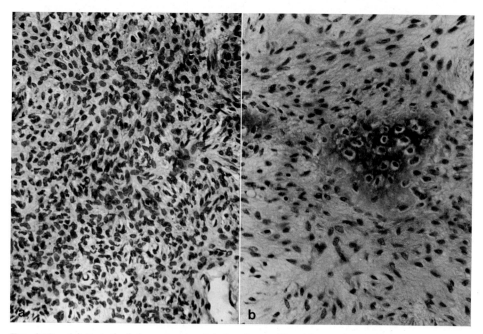

FIG. 340. - (a) Detail of the stroma, rich in plump fibroblasts. (b) Formation of osteoid substance by the stromal cells which do not assume the aspect of osteoblasts (*Hemat.-eos.*, 300, 300 x).

a histiocytic fibroma (Fig. 343a). Other times, instead, it has a myxoid aspect (Fig. 341a).

The osteoid and osseous trabeculae are generally small and sparse, shaped like Chinese ideograms, rarely larger and anastomized amongst themselves (Fig. 339). They are never bordered by rows of osteoblasts. The bone trabeculae of F.D. always have a woven structure, never a lamellar one; they may contain uneven and broken cementing lines. At times the osseous formations are small and rounded, similar to the cement bodies of the periodontal membrane (Fig. 342). This aspect is prevalently observed in the cranio-facial bones, but it may also be observed in the skeleton of the limbs.

In the tissue of F.D. the vessels are scarce and thin. At times there is a sort of vascular pedicle penetrating the lesion. Rarely, areas with abundant dilated capillaries and hemorrhagic effusion, which may be cystic, are observed.

Areas of cartilaginous tissue are sometimes observed included in the dysplastic fibro-osseous tissue (Fig. 344). These may be small or quite extended, in the form of well-circumscribed lobules, having the structure of normal hyalin cartilage. The histological aspect of these cartilaginous areas is different from that of solitary or multiple chondromas; it is instead similar to that of growth cartilage plate or hyperplastic cartilage of a repair callus.

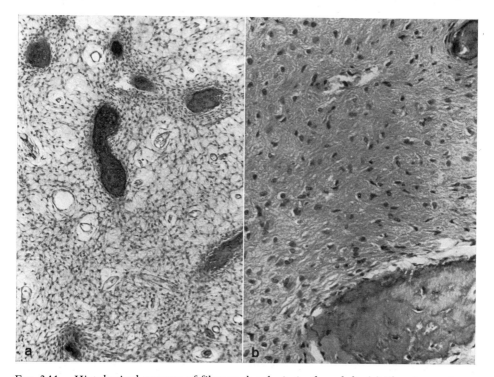

FIG. 341. - Histological aspects of fibrous dysplasia in the adult. (a) The stroma has a myxoid aspect. (b) Dense and mature collagenous stroma; mature bone trabecula, characterized by a woven structure not bordered by osteoblasts (*Hemat.-eos.*, 125, 300 x).

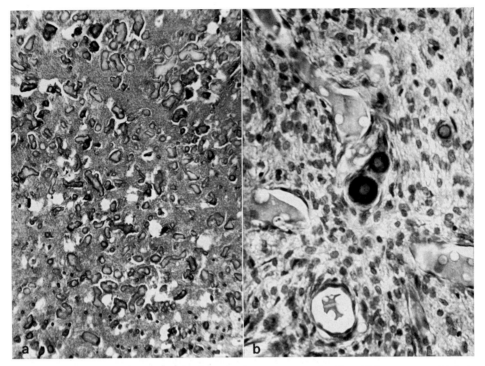

Fig. 342. - Round-oval osseous bodies similar to cement bodies. This aspect, which is more frequent in cranio-facial localizations, is rarely observed in the bones of the limbs (*Hemat. eos.*, 50, 300, x).

The abrupt demarcation between the cartilaginous areas and the dysplastic fibro-osseous tissue allows us to exclude the idea that the cartilage is formed as a result of metaplasia. In most cases, in which cartilaginous areas are observed during childhood or adolescence in the metaphysis, when there has been no previous surgery or fracture, they seem to derive from inclusions or gemmations of the growth cartilage. In some rare cases, where the cartilage is subperiosteal and where there has been a recent pathologic fracture or microfracture, or previous surgical treatment, the cartilage is instead due to a repair osteochondral callus.

The histological aspects, like the radiographic and macroscopic ones, tend to change during **adult age**. Progressively, even if in an inconstant and variable manner, the proliferative activity slows down and maturation and regressive phenomena of the dysplastic tissue are accentuated. In the fibrous tissue the cells decrease in number, mature in fibrocytes, the collagen stroma becomes denser, or it presents diffused myxoid aspects (Fig. 341), which may contain foam cells, cholesterin crystals. The bone trabeculae also tend to mature (Fig. 343b). In some cases the fibrous component prevails over the osseous one, and it contains cystic or hemorrhagic cavities. In other cases the lesion becomes densely ossified and sclerotic.

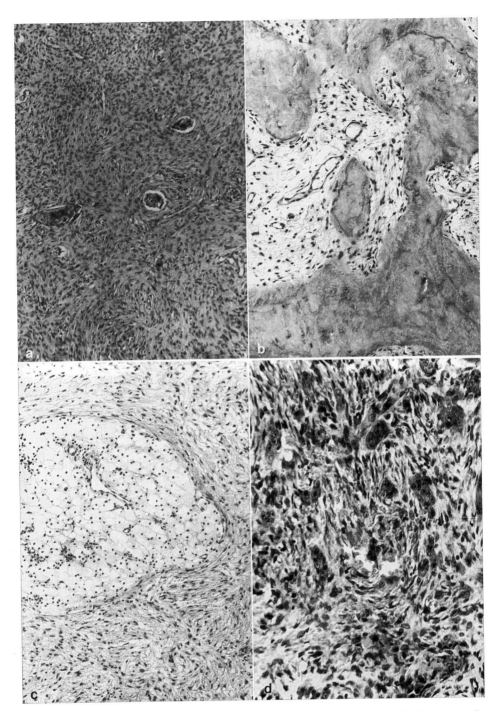

FIG. 343. - (a) The structure of the stroma is nearly the same as that of a histiocytic fi-broma. Small and rare osteoid islands are seen which, in other areas, may be entirely missing. (a) Aspects of fibrous dysplasia in the adult, with abundant woven bone tis-sue, and differentiated and mature fibrous tissue. (c) Extensive nidus of foam cells. (d) Numerous multinucleate giant cells and hemosiderin pigment (*Hemat.-eos.*, 125 x).

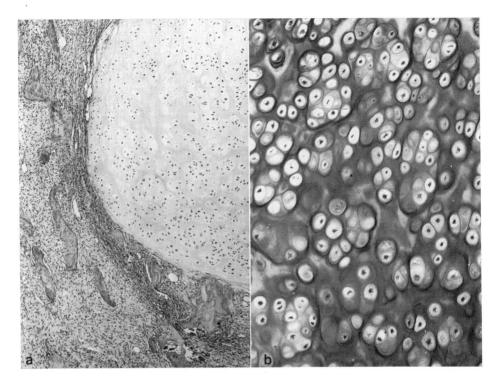

FIG. 344. - (a) Included island of cartilage, with evident demarcation, in the tissue typical of fibrous dysplasia. (b) Aspect of the included cartilage with isogenous groups of hypertrophic cells (*Hemat.-eos.*, 50, 125 x).

HISTOGENESIS AND PATHOGENESIS

Even if the cells of F.D. hardly ever take on the shape of osteoblasts, rather, that of fibroblasts or histiocytes, they undoubtedly produce osteoid substance (Fig. 340). Thus, histogenesis calls for a classification of F.D. among tumors made up of osteo-forming cells.

As for pathogenesis, F.D. seems to be a hamartoma of congenital origin, like exostoses, chondromas, angiomas, histiocytic fibroma, neurofibromas. This is shown by the age of insurgence, distribution (solitary, multiple, or diffused with hemisomic prevalence), decrease in proliferation and tendency of the tissue to mature during adult age, the association with melanin spots and with changes in skeletal growth and endocrine function, which are also congenital.

DIAGNOSIS

In extensive or diffused forms radiographic diagnosis is easy and certain. With regard to d.d. with **multiple histiocytic fibroma of the skeleton and with Ollier's chondromatosis**, see the specific chapters. There are exceptional cases of **Paget's disease** with an osteolytic mark, characterized by expansion

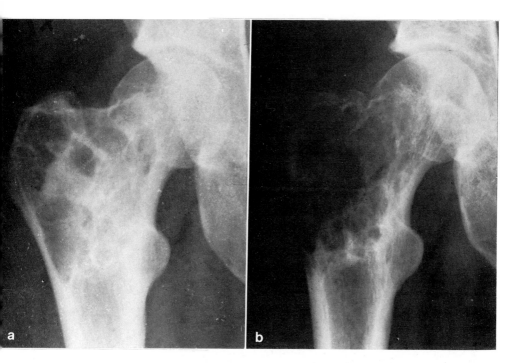

FIG. 345. - Female aged 46 years. Fibrosarcoma (b) (histologically grade 3) occurring on an area of fibrous dysplasia diagnosed radiologically (a) and histologically 30 years earlier. This fibrosarcoma was treated by intra-articular wide resection-endo-prosthesis. After 1 year, recurrence in the acetabulum with invasion of the pubis. After 3 years pulmonary metastases.

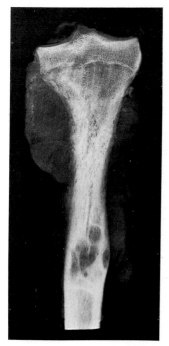

of the bone and familiarity which, radiographically, may suggest F.D. because of the skeletal swelling and the diffused osteolysis, at times a ground glass appearance (Figs. 13, 14). What defines pagetic osteopathy in cases such as these is the adult-advanced age at which symptoms begin, the possible familiarity, the presence on radiograms (at least in some areas) of a filamentous structure, the clearly pagetic aspect of other bones, or of the same bone in previous radiograms, the regional hypervascularity, the different histolo-

FIG. 346. - Male aged 16 years. Osteosarcoma (in the proximal meta-diaphysis) and area of fibrous dysplasia in the more distal diaphysis. The two different lesions were ascertained histologically and among these there was close anatomical adjacency.

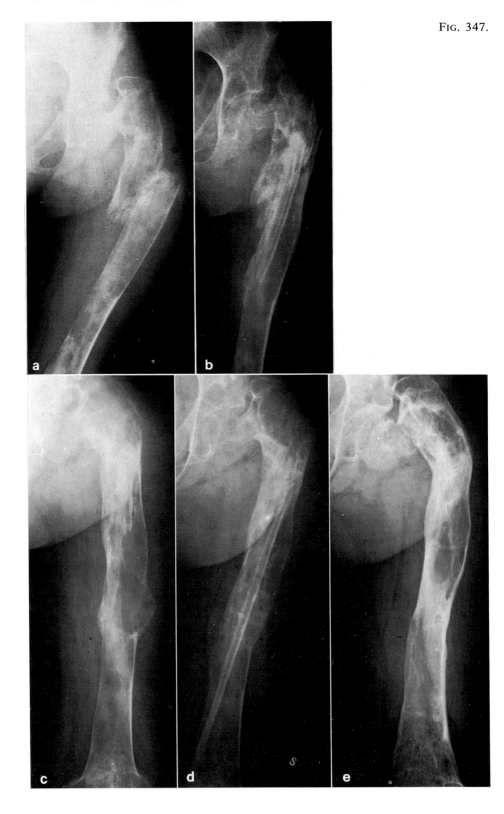

FIG. 347.

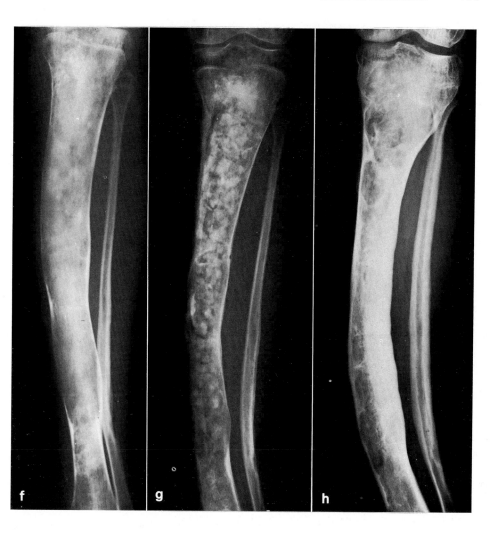

FIG. 347. - Female aged 12 years. Diffused fibrous dysplasia of the lower left limb (already submitted to curettage and grafting, had repeated pathologic fracture). (a) The patient has a new pathologic fracture. (b) The patient was submitted to reduction of the fracture, partial curettage and grafting with a homoplastic fibula. (c) After 1 year wide resorption of the grafts and expansion of the osteolysis. (d) The patient was submitted to further more extensive curettage and more abundant grafting with autoplastic cancellous bone and homoplastic fibula. (e) After 4 years the grafts appear to be mostly resorbed. Nonetheless (the patient is now 18 years old) the progression of the dysplasia has stopped and the cortical bones appear to be fairly reinforced. Pseudarthrosis of the varus femoral neck occurred. (f) In the same patient lesion of the left tibia at 12 years of age. (g) Extensive curettage carried out and homoplastic cancellous grafting. (h) After 6 years the grafts are partially resorbed but progression has arrested with considerable reinforcement of the cortex. Observe thickening of the fibula. In this case the number of operations performed was not proportional to the results, which would not have differed much if the operations had not been performed. It would have been better to deal with the varus of the femoral neck.

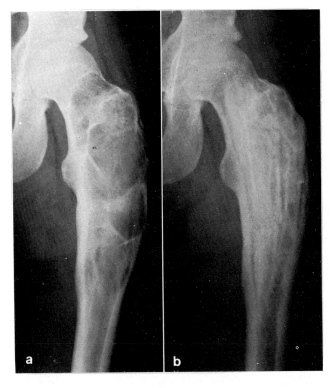

FIG. 348. - (a) Monostotic fibrous dysplasia in a male aged 18 years. The patient had previously been operated at 5 years of age, with no results. At 11 years of age there was pathologic fracture. (b) The patient was submitted to curettage and homoplastic corticocancellous grafting, obtaining excellent incorporation of the grafts after 4 years. In this case, as well, surgery was not necessary.

gical structure (very loose and much more hyperemic connective tissue, bone trabeculae with a lamellar structure bordered by osteoblasts, mosaic pattern).

On the contrary, in F.D. at an initial stage and in circumscribed monostotic cases, the radiographic diagnosis may be doubtful, suggesting numerous affections, from bone cyst to chondroma, from eosinophilic granuloma to chondromyxoid fibroma, from osteoblastoma to giant cell tumor. In some rare cases there may be problems of differential diagnosis even under microscopy.

Chondroma. Chondroma may be suggested not only because of the radiographic aspect (osteolytic area containing some nubecolae of radiopacity) but also because of the histological finding of cartilaginous tissue which, as previously observed, is not rare in F.D. It may be observed that the radiopacity of F.D. is more tenuous, diffused and faded than that of chondroma, and that the histological aspect of the cartilage of F.D. is different from that of chondroma. Above all, typical fibro-osseous tissue must be observed alongside the island of cartilage in F.D.

Bone cyst. When a very radiolucent lesion is observed, one localized in the proximal humerus, in the humeral diaphysis, in the proximal femur, in the iliac wing, radiograms may suggest a bone cyst. This impression may be confirmed by surgery if scarce fibrous tissue and cavities containing fluid are observed inside the lesion. Histologically, loose, edematous or myxoid fibrous tissue may be observed, with cystic spaces and few bone trabeculae. In this situation, which may be found in the adult, it is often difficult to establish whether we are dealing with a quiescent and cystic F.D. or an old bone cyst, partially filled with repair osteofibrosis.

Osteoblastoma. If a well-contained osteolytic area is observed radiographically, with some faded radiopacity; histologically, a very cellular connective tissue containing newly-formed bone trabeculae; theoretically, and exceptionally in a practical sense as well, some doubts may arise in deciding between F.D. and osteoblastoma. The histological differences are nearly always decisive. In osteoblastoma there is no fibrous stroma, the newly-formed bone is much more abundant, immature and, above all, surrounded by large osteoblasts, the tissue is much more vascularized.

Histiocytic fibroma. Apart from the radiographic differences, which are usually evident, histologically F.D. may appear in some fields to be the same as histiocytic fibroma (Fig. 343a). F.D. is diagnosed when, alongside these fields others with a histological aspect typical of F.D. are observed.

Osteofibrous dysplasia of the long bones (see next chapter).

COURSE

F.D. occur during childhood and then extend to a varying and unpredictable degree. It seems that the occurrence of lesions in the various bones takes place at approximately the same time, so that the initially monostotic or oligostotic forms generally remain as such. The extent of the dysplasia in the bone affected and the deformity tend to worsen, particularly during growth. After puberty, dysplastic areas rarely expand; the appearance of new foci is also a rare occurrence. In general, the progression of the skeletal lesions tends to be exhausted once adult age has been achieved.

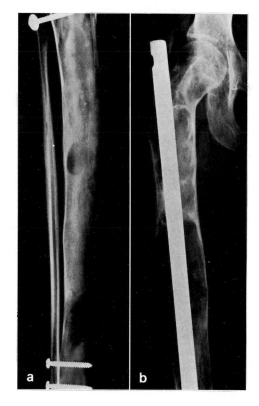

FIG. 349. - Female aged 24 years. Diffused fibrous dysplasia of the lower right limb. The patient had already had two pathologic fractures of the femur and leg. (a) Fibula-pro-tibia in the leg. (b) Closed Küntscher nailing in the femur. These operations, which aim at preventing fractures, may be more rational than the attempt to remove the dysplastic tissue. The patient was clinically healed after 15 years.

At times, particularly in the costal, pelvic, and metaphyseal sites (spongy bones) during adult age there may be some increase in a F.D. area, which is due more to hemorrhaging and to cystic transformations than to proliferative growth of the tissue. Similarly, a push in progression may be observed when the patient is pregnant, probably based on hyperemia-hemorrhage.

SARCOMATOUS TRANSFORMATION

The insurgence of a sarcoma on an area of F.D. is a rare occurrence: less than 1% of all cases (Figs. 345, 346). It is observed in both monostotic localized forms of the disease and in diffused polyostotic ones, and nearly always during adult age; at times, tens of years after the area of F.D. appeared to be stabilized and quiescent. The sarcoma which is most frequently observed is osteosarcoma, followed by fibrosarcoma and chondrosarcoma.

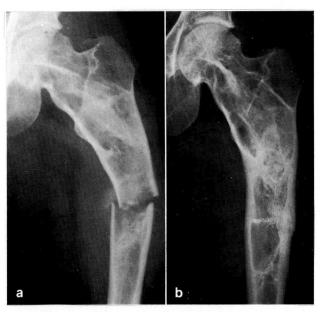

FIG. 350. - (a) Pathologic fracture in monostotic fibrous dysplasia in a female aged 21 years. (b) Treated nonsurgically, the fracture rapidly consolidated, and, after 10 years, the dysplasia appeared to be completely arrested and the cortex spontaneously reinforced so that no surgery was indicated.

TREATMENT

Treatment is exclusively surgical. Radiation therapy is absolutely contraindicated, because it is not very effective, and because of the risk of sarcomatous transformation.

Indications for surgery depend on three factors: symptoms and clinical-radiographic signs; age; extent of the dysplasia.

1) **Symptoms and signs**. F.D. does not deserve to be operated if there are no symptoms, or if there is no risk of impending fracture. The frequently occurring pathologic fracture usually does not constitute a problem, as it is easily consolidated (Fig. 350), and it generally does not change indications for therapy (conservative or surgical).

2) **Age**. There is a significant relationship between age and the results of curettage and bone grafting. In the child surgery is useless as the lesion does recur, often extending. Bone grafts placed inside the cavity are extensively

resorbed, even if they are large and made up of compact bone (Fig. 347). In the adolescent the probability of success or failure is approximately the same. In the adult success is nearly constant (Fig. 348).

3) **Extent of the dysplasia**. The probability of recurrence does not seem to depend on the extent of the dysplasia. When the dysplasia is very extensive, for example to an entire long bone, excision of the pathological tissue and its substitution with bone grafts become a problem due to the extension of surgery and the uncertainty of results (Fig. 347).

Therefore, curettage and bone grafting are rarely indicated and mainly in circumscribed and symptomatic F.D. in the adult. In the child it is best to limit treatment to corrective osteotomies of the deformities and internal fixation. The same may be said for extended forms, at any age. Resection of the skeletal segment may be used, but it is rarely necessary, in costal localizations.

In conclusion, in most cases of F.D., there are no indications for surgery (not even biopsy) with the exception of corrective osteotomy. Corrective osteotomies must be performed early (before deformities become too severe, particularly in the proximal femur), often they must be multiple, and associated with solid osteosynthesis.

PROGNOSIS

Prognosis may be accurately evaluated only after 10-12 years of age, as the progression of dysplasia during childhood may be unpredictable. Once adult age has been achieved, the lesions no longer progress, rather they tend to slowly improve. Prognosis is excellent in circumscribed lesions, except for the risk of sarcomatous progression, which however is a rare occurrence. Even some extensive forms achieve adult age with a relatively solid cortex, and very little deformity, so that symptoms are reduced to mild asymmetry of the limbs, sporadic pain, some risk of fracture. The most severe extensive and diffused forms of the disease may instead produce conspicuous deformity and shortening of the limbs, which is generally asymmetrical, deformity of the face, repeated fracture, severe disability.

REFERENCES

1937 ALBRIGHT F., BUTLER A. M., HAMPTON A. O., SMITH P.: Syndrome characterized by osteitis fibrosa disseminata, areas of pigmentation and endocrine dysfunction, with precocious puberty in females. Report of five cases. *New England Journal of Medicine*, **216**, 727-746.

1942 LICHTENSTEIN L., JAFFE H. L.: Fibrous dysplasia of bone. A condition affecting one, several or many bones, the graver cases of which may present abnormal pigmentation of skin, premature sexual development, hyperthyroidism or still other extraskeletal abnormalities. *Archiv of Pathology*, **33**, 777-816.

1961 DE PALMA A. F., DOOLD P. M.: Reconstructive surgery in fibrous dysplasia of bone. *Clinical Orthopaedics*, **19**, 132-147.

1962 HARRIS W. H., DUDLEY H. R. Jr., BARRY R. J.: The natural history of fibrous dysplasia. An orthopaedic, pathological, and roentgenographic study. *Journal of Bone and Joint Surgery*, **44-A**, 207-233.

1963 Van Horn P. E. Jr., Dahlin D. C., Bickel W. H.: Fibrous dysplasia. A clinical pathologic study of orthopedic surgical cases. *Mayo Clinic Proceedings*, **38**, 175-189.

1967 Chatterje S. K., Mazumder J. K.: Massive fibro-osseous dysplasia of the jaws in two generations. *British Journal of Surgery*, **54**, 335-340.

1969 Henry A.: Monostotic fibrous dysplasia. *Journal of Bone and Joint Surgery*, **51-B**, 300-306.

1970 Campanacci M., Leonessa C.: Displasia fibrosa dello scheletro. *Chirurgia degli Organi di Movimento*, **59**, 195-225.

1970 Schmaman A., Path MC., Smith I., Ackerman L. V.: Benign fibro-osseous lesions of the mandible and maxilla. A review of 35 cases. *Cancer*, **26**, 303-312.

1971 Keyl W.: Korrekturosteotomien an den unteren Extremitäten bei fibröser Knochendysplasie. *Zeitschrift für Orthopädie und ihre Grenzgebeite*, **109**, 73-81.

1972 Breck L. W.: Treatment of fibrous dysplasia of bone by total femoral plating and hip nailing. A case report. *Clinical Orthopaedics*, **82**, 82-83.

1972 Lejeune E., Bouvier M., Vanzelle J. L., Queneau P., Thomas J. D., Chandy J., Leung T. K., Deplante J. P.: Dysplasie fibreuse et myxomes des tissus mous. *Revue du Rhumatisme*, **39**, 281-288.

1972 Wirth W. A., Leavitt D., Enzinger F. M.: Multiple intramuscular myxomas. Another extraskeletal manifestation of fibrous dysplasia. *Cancer*, **27**, 1167-1173.

1973 De Palma A., Ahmad J.: Fibrous dysplasia associated with shepherd's crook deformity of the humerus. *Clinical Orthopaedics*, **97**, 38-39.

1973 Feintuch T. A.: Chondrosarcoma arising in a cartilaginous area of previously irradiated fibrous dyslplasia. *Cancer*, **31**, 877-881.

1974 Blauth W., Meves H.: Behandlungs Probleme bei der « aggressiven » Form der fibrösen Dysplasie. *Zeitschrift für Orthopädie und ihre Grenzgebiete*, **112**, 230-235.

1975 Abelanet R., Forest M., Meary R., Languepin A., Tomeno B.: Sarcome sur dysplasie fibreuse des os. A propos d'une forme complexe hémimelique et revue de la litérature. *Revue de Chirurgie Orthopedique*, **61**, 179-190.

1975 Campanacci M., Giunti A., Leonessa C., Pagani P. A., Trentani C.: Pathological fractures in osteopathies and bony dysplasias. *Italian Journal of Orthopaedics and Traumatology*, Supplementum I.

1975 Immenkamp M.: Die maligne Entartung bei fibröser Dysplasie. *Zeitschrift für Orthopadie und ihre Grenzgebeite*, **113**, 331-343.

1976 Logel J. R.: Recurrent intramuscular myxoma associated with Albright's syndrome. Case report and review of the literature. *Journal of Bone and Joint Surgery*, **58-A**, 565-568.

1979 Campanacci M., Bertoni F., Capanna R.: Degenerazione maligna in displasia fibrosa. Presentazione di 6 casi e revisione della letteratura. *Giornale Italiano di Ortopedia e Traumatologia*, **5**, 391-399.

1981 De Smet A.A., Travers H., Neff J.R.: Chondrosarcoma occurring in a patient with polyostotic fibrous dysplasia. *Skeletal Radiology*, **7**, 197-202.

1983 Derome P.J., Visot A.: La dysplasie fibreuse cranienne. *Neurochirurgie*, **29**, Suppl. 1.

1983 Lever E.G., Pettingale E.W.: Albright's syndrome associated with a soft-tissue myxoma and hypophosphatemic osteomalacia. *Journal of Bone and Joint Surgery*, **65-B**, 621-626.

1984 Helawa M., Ahmad A.: Chondrosarcoma in fibrous dysplasia in the pelvis. A case report and review of the literature. *Journal of Bone and Joint Surgery*, **66-B**, 760-764.

1986 Enneking W.F., Gearen P.F.: Fibrous dysplasia of the femoral neck. Treatment by cortical bone grafting. *Journal of Bone and Joint Surgery*, **68-A**, 1415-1422.

1987 Bi Hu L.: Case report 455. *Skeletal Radiology*, **16**, 679-684.

1987 Stephenson R.B., London M.D., Mankin F.M., Kaufer M.: Fibrous dysplasia An analysis of options for treatment. *Journal of Bone and Joint Surgery*, **69-A**, 400-409.

1988   TACONIS W.K.: Osteosarcoma in fibrous dysplasia. *Skeletal Radiology*, **17**, 163-170.

1988   YABUT S.M., KENAN S., SISSONS M.A., LEWIS M.M.: Malignant transformation of fibrous dysplasia. A case report and review of the literature. *Clinical Orthopaedics*, **228**, 281-289.

1989   SIMPSON A.M.R.W., CREASY T.S., WILLIAMSON D.M., WILDON D.J., SPIVEY J.S.: Cystic degeneration of fibrous dysplasia masquerading as sarcoma. *Journal of Bone and Joint Surgery*, **71-B**, 434-436.

OSTEOFIBROUS DYSPLASIA OF THE LONG BONES
(Synonyms: congenital fibrous defect of the tibia, ossifying fibroma)

DEFINITION

It is a congenital dysplasia, made up of fibrous and osseous tissue, the localization of which is nearly exclusively in the tibia and, at times, in the fibula; it is often associated with tibial anterior bowing, and its course is that of a more or less progressive hamartoma.

It is distinguished from fibrous dysplasia by age, site, radiographic aspect, histological picture and course (Table 6). We have delineated its essential features (Campanacci, 1976) and proposed calling it O.F.D.L.B.

FREQUENCY

It occurs more rarely than fibrous dysplasia, but it is not exceptional. Up until recently, most cases have gone unrecognized (Fig. 351).

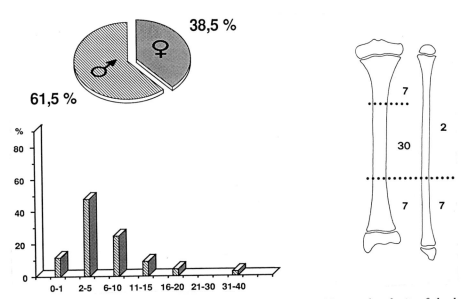

FIG. 351. - Sex, age and localization in 44 cases of osteofibrous dysplasia of the long bones (53 localizations). Only cases with histological confirmation are included.

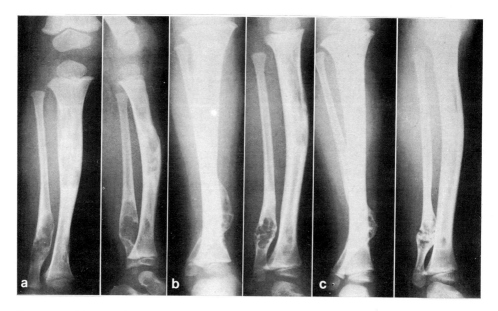

FIG. 352. - (a) Osteofibrous dysplasia of the right tibia and fibula in a boy aged 2 years. Similar milder lesions are also present in the left leg. (b) The lesions spontaneously healed after 1 year without treatment. (c) After 3 more years further spontaneous repair. The boy is clinically normal except for the protrusion due to severe curvation of the fibula. This may be dealt with when growth is more advanced. Similar spontaneous improvement is manifested in the contralateral limb.

SEX

There is predilection for the male sex (Fig. 351).

AGE

It is nearly always observed prior to 10 years of age, in most cases within the first 5 years of life (Fig. 351).

LOCALIZATION

O.F.D.L.B. typically and nearly exclusively occurs in the tibia. In some cases the homolateral fibula is also involved (Fig. 351). In exceptional cases it is bilateral (Fig. 352).

In the tibia, the most common localization is in the mid third of the diaphysis, from where the lesion may grow proximally and distally, followed by the distal third and the proximal third, in this order. In the fibula, it generally involves the distal third of the diaphysis. The lesion is typically diaphyseal, even if it rarely does extend to the metaphysis. In rare cases, the dysplastic areas are multiple in the same tibia.

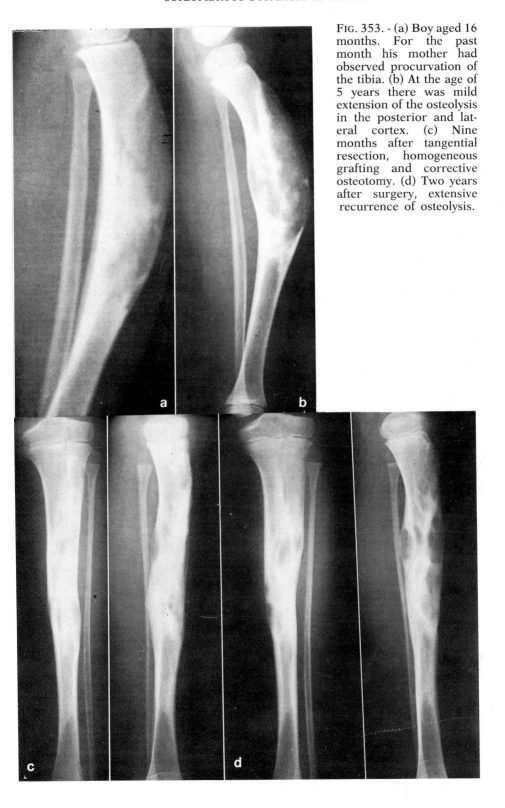

FIG. 353. - (a) Boy aged 16 months. For the past month his mother had observed procurvation of the tibia. (b) At the age of 5 years there was mild extension of the osteolysis in the posterior and lateral cortex. (c) Nine months after tangential resection, homogeneous grafting and corrective osteotomy. (d) Two years after surgery, extensive recurrence of osteolysis.

SYMPTOMS

O.F.D.L.B. is painless and generally revealed by cosmetic changes or palpation: bulging of the tibial bone profile, tibial anterior bowing. At times there is pathologic fracture, which is usually incomplete, characterized by pain and only a small amount of displacement. In rare cases there may be firm pseudarthrosis of the tibia and/or of the fibula.

RADIOGRAPHIC FEATURES

An eccentric intracortical osteolysis is generally observed. The subperiosteal surface of the cortex is more or less expanded, and it is very thin. To-

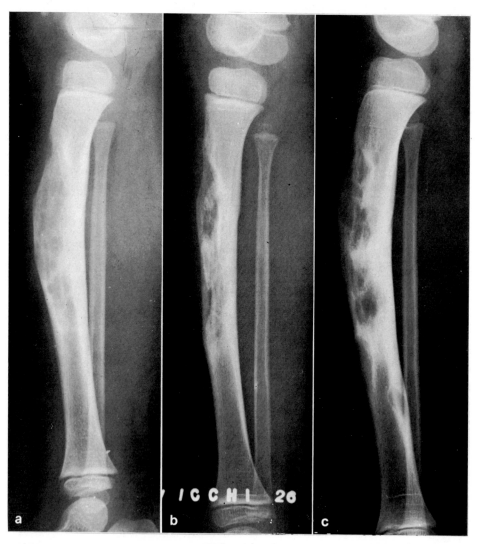

Fig. 354.

FIG. 354. - (a) Female aged 3 and 1/2 years. Deformity was observed at 1 year of age. (b) Ten months after a tangential resection and curettage. (c) After 2 years complete recurrence and occurrence of small new distal and posterior osteolysis. (d) One year later, new and wider tangential resection and homogeneous grafting. (e) After 18 years: despite limited recurrence of the osteolysis, the lesion is completely stabilized and does not cause any disturbances except mild procurvation.

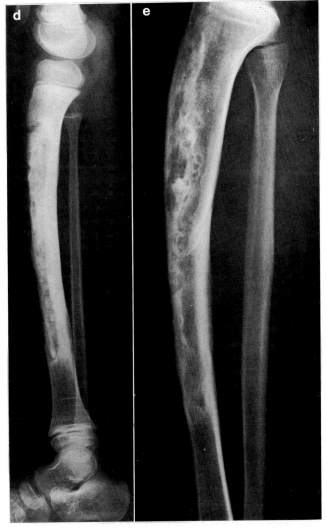

wards the inside of the bone and the medullary canal, on the contrary, the osteolysis is clearly delimited by a rim of sclerosis, with frequent narrowing of the medullary canal (Figs. 352-356). At times the osteolysis is single, at times it is made up of multiple bubbles. In the tibia it rarely involves the entire diaphyseal perimeter, while it commonly does so in the fibula. Rarely, as previously observed, tibial osteolyses are multiple and/or extended to most of the diaphysis (Fig. 357). At times inside the osteolysis a ground glass faded radiopacity is observed (Fig. 353). These radiographic aspects are so typical that usually the diagnosis may be made without biopsy.

GROSS PATHOLOGIC FEATURES

The periosteum is well-preserved. The underlying cortex is very thin. The tissue occupying the osteolytic area is compact, whitish, yellowish or reddish depending on the case, of soft to fibrous consistency; often it is slightly gritty.

HISTOPATHOLOGIC FEATURES

The histological picture is characterized by two essential aspects (Figs. 358-360).

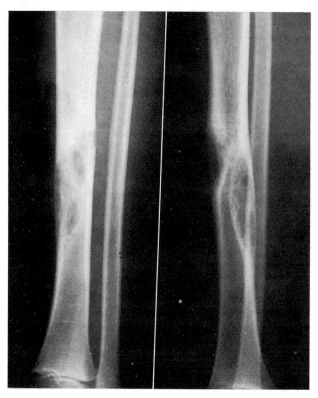

FIG. 355. - Boy aged 4 years. For the past 2 months mild swelling observed. The patient was submitted to curettage with typical histological finding.

1) Fibrous tissue embedding osseous trabeculae bordered by osteoblasts.

2) «Zonal» architecture.

The fibrous tissue is more or less cellular, generally less than is the case with fibrous dysplasia. It often has a whorled or storiform pattern, similar to that of histiocytic fibroma (Fig. 358b). Often it is rather loose, with delicate fibrillary texture; at times it is denser, with coarser closely-packed collagenous fibers. The fibroblasts are generally well-differeniated, they are rarely arge and plump. At times there are numerous multinucleate giant cells, probably related to microhemorrhage and resorption of bony substance.

The newly-formed bone trabeculae are sparse, slender and woven at the center of the lesion, more numerous, thick, anastomized amongst themselves, and lamellar towards the periphery. They are bordered by active osteoblasts (Fig. 359). This is the principal difference as compared to fibrous dysplasia.

In cases where biopsy included the entire lesion from periosteum to the depth of the lesion, we observed a zonal architecture (Figs. 359, 360). At the center of the osteolysis the fibrous tissue is exclusive or prevalent, with few, thin and immature woven bone trabeculae. If we proceed towards the peri-

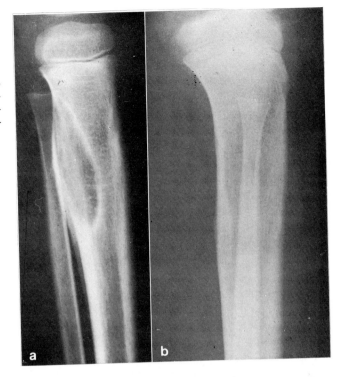

FIG. 356. - Boy aged 5 years. For the past month, after trauma, mild posterior swelling in the right tibia. (a) The patient was submitted to curettage with typical histological finding. (b) After 3 years repair is complete.

phery, that is, towards the periosteal surface and the medullary canal, the bone trabeculae become progressively more numerous, larger, more mature and lamellar, until they are anastomized and confused with the bone of the cortex. The fibrous tissue also gradually merges to that occupying the widened haversian spaces of the cortex, which is rather loose, not very cellular, with wide sinusoids.

HISTOGENESIS AND PATHOGENESIS

Doubtlessly, O.F.D.L.B. constitutes a hamartoma, made up of histio-fibroblasts and characterized by osteoblastic bone production. What is unique about this hamartoma is that its site is nearly exclusively the tibia, similar to adamantinoma.

DIAGNOSIS

As previously mentioned, diagnosis is easy and it may often be presumed from the clinical-radiographic picture alone, or by the isolated histological finding. The differences as compared to **fibrous dysplasia** are recalled in the various sections of this chapter and summarized in Table 6. At times, the radiographic image of O.F.D.L.B. may be similar to that of a **histiocytic fibroma**, particularly in localizations which are closer to the metaphysis. How-

Table 6

DIFFERENCES BETWEEN OSTEOFIBROUS DYSPLASIA
OF THE LONG BONES AND FIBROUS DYSPLASIA

	Osteo-fibrous dysplasia of the long bones	Fibrous dysplasia
Site	Exclusively (?) in the tibia and fibula	Practically any part of the skeleton
Distribution	Tibia and at times fibula	Often polyostotic
Age at onset of symptoms	0-10 years	Generally after 10 years of age in monostotic forms
Association with procurved tibia	Very frequent	Absent
Radiographic aspect	Expanding intracortical osteolysis	Generally intramedullary
Association with pseudarthrosis of the tibia	Very rare	Absent
Spontaneous regression	Rare but possible	No
Progression during childhood	Usually moderate	Variable. Often marked
Tendency towards recurrence prior to 10 years of age	High	High
Histological features	Connective tissue more mature Bone trabeculae bordered by osteoblasts Lamellar and woven bone Zonal architecture Continuous with the cortex	Connective tissue more cellular Bone trabeculae without osteoblasts Only woven bone No zonal architecture Separated from the cortex

ever, the histological picture is rather different, if considered in its entirety.

Above all, it is important to differentiate O.F.D.L.B. from **adamantinoma** of the tibia. Apart from the clinical (age), radiographic and progressive features, histologically adamantinoma, against a background which may be very similar to a fibrous dysplasia or to a O.F.D.L.B., will show the typical epitheliomorphous inclusions. Adamantinoma is generally observed during adult age, it causes pain, it has a different radiographic aspect, and it is progressive in the sense that the osteolysis slowly increases during adult age, and may expand in the soft tissues. Nonetheless, there are exceptional cases of adamantinoma which began during childhood, and are characterized by a radio-

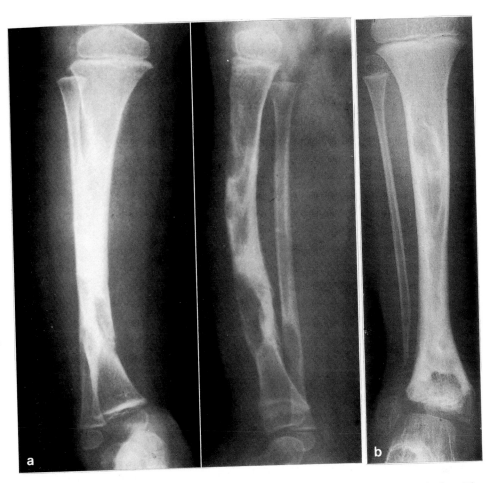

FIG. 357. - (a) Boy aged 2 years. Two months earlier, fracture of the distal tibia. The patient was submitted to curettage and homogeneous grafting. Surgery was followed by osteomyelitis and delayed union. (b) After 2 and 1/2 years union and spontaneous repair of the osteolysis.

graphic picture which is the same as that of a O.F.D.L.B. (Fig. 525). Thus, adamantinoma should be suspected, and ascertained by extensive biopsy, in cases of apparent O.F.D.L.B. showing unusual progression during childhood and, in particular, causing pain and continuing to evolve after puberty.

COURSE

The proliferative potential may be very moderate (hamartia), or more intense (hamartoma). Generally, it does not achieve the intensity and extent of some forms of fibrous dysplasia. Furthermore, it is more ephemeral, as it is completely exhausted prior to puberty. Some lesions remain small and cause no symptoms. Others, during the first years of life, tend to repair spontaneously. Others expand, even considerably, during the first years of life, to then

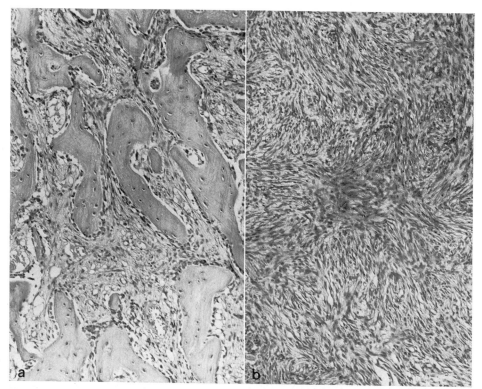

FIG. 358. - (a) Fibrous tissue with bone trabeculae bordered by osteoblasts. (b) Tissue is the same as that of histiocytic fibroma (*Hemat.-eos.*, 125, 125 x).

remain nearly stationary. Rather, after 10-12 years of age, it seems that the cortical bone is reinforced with slow hyperostotic thickening of the margins of the lesions, and slow narrowing of the osteolysis.

Such favorable evolution contrasts with the high tendency towards recurrence when the lesion is submitted to curettage or subperiosteal resection before 10 years of age. These recurrences are more frequent and repeated, the earlier the age at surgery. At times we are not dealing with recurrence, rather with a new lesion occurring in another site of the tibia.

Any pathologic fracture (like corrective osteotomies) nearly always heals by simple immobilization. Rare cases of pseudarthrosis of the tibia nearly always consolidate with osteosynthesis and/or bone grafting.

TREATMENT

During the first 5 years of life, O.F.D.L.B. should not be submitted to surgery, as it may tend towards spontaneous repair and because there is a high probability of recurrence. Even between 5 and 10 years of age surgical indication is influenced by the symptoms presented, and it should be delayed for as long as possible. When there is pathologic fracture, in most cases nonsurgical treatment may be used. Surgical treatment is indicated in the following

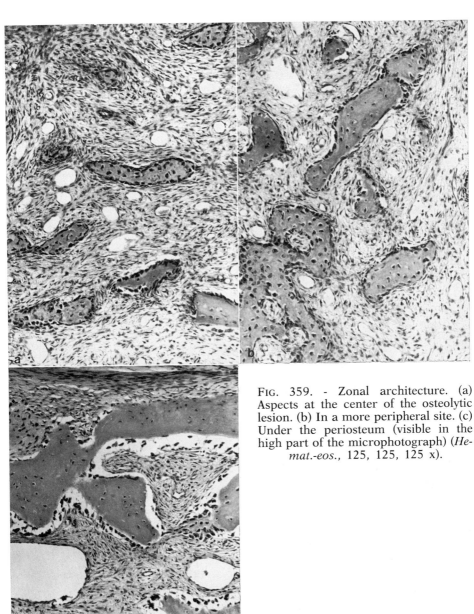

FIG. 359. - Zonal architecture. (a) Aspects at the center of the osteolytic lesion. (b) In a more peripheral site. (c) Under the periosteum (visible in the high part of the microphotograph) (*Hemat.-eos.*, 125, 125, 125 x).

conditions: 1) forms of the disease which are so extended that they considerably expand and/or weaken the bone. In cases such as these, it is best to use tangential resection by extraperiosteal approach, with bone grafting. 2) The presence of pseudarthrosis (solid osteosynthesis associated with strong bone grafting). 3) Accentuated tibial bowing, to be corrected by osteotomy after 10-12 years.

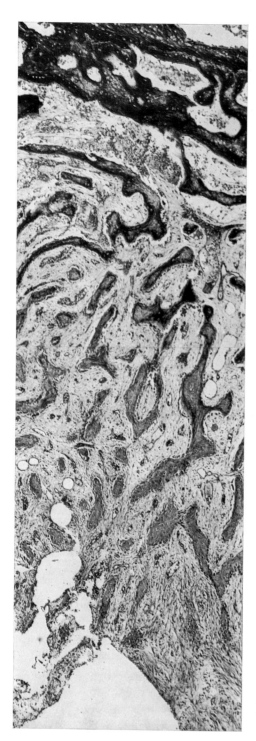

PROGNOSIS

Prognosis is generally excellent or good as the lesion, even if it is characterized by recurrence, and if it is complicated by pseudarthrosis, always ends up healing or in any case stabilizing and becoming asymptomatic. Rare more expansive forms of the disease, which were operated and which recurred several times during childhood, involve severe problems in surgical reconstruction.

In more extensive forms of the disease, during adult age, there often remains mild bowing of the tibial diaphysis clinically resembling Paget's disease.

FIG. 360. - Zonal archicture, with gradual transition from the fibrous area at the center of the osteolysis (below) to the cortex (above). Same case as Fig. 356 (Hemat.-eos., 40 x).

REFERENCES

1966 KEMPSON R.L.: Ossifying fibroma of the long bones. A light and electron microscopic study. *Archiv of Pathology*, **82**, 218-233.

1975 CAMPANACCI M., GIUNTI A., LEONESSA C., PAGANI P.A., TRENTANI C.: Pathological fractures in osteopathies and bony dysplasias. *Italian Journal of Orthopaedics and Traumatology*, Supplementum I.

1975 SEMIAN D.W., WILLIS J.B., BOVE K.E.: Congenital fibrous defect of the tibia mimicking fibrous dysplasia. A case report. *Journal of Bone and Joint Surgery*, **57-A**, 854-857.

1976 CAMPANACCI M.: Osteofibrous dysplasia of long bones. A new clinical entity. *Italian Journal of Orthopaedics and Traumatology*, **2**, 221-238.

1977 GEORGEN TH. G., DICKMAN P.S., RESNICK D., SALTZSTEIN S.L., O'DELL CH. W., AKESON W.H.: Long bone ossifying fibromas. *Cancer*, **39**, 2067-2072

1981 CAMPANACCI M., LAUS M.: Osteofibrous dysplasia of the tibia and fibula. *Journal of Bone and Joint Surgery*, **63-A**, 367-375.

1982 CAMPBELL C.J., HAWK TH.: A variant of fibrous dysplasia (Osteofibrous dysplasia). *Journal of Bone and Joint Surgery*, **64-A**, 231-236.

1983 NAKASHIMA Y., YAMAMURO T., FUJIWARA Y., KOJOURA J., MORI E., HAMASHIMA Y.: Osteofibrous dysplasia (ossifying fibroma of long bones). A study of 12 cases. *Cancer*, **52**, 909-914.

1983 SISSONS H., KANCHERLA P., WALLACE B.: Ossifying fibroma of bone. Report of two cases. *Bulletin of the Hospital for Joint Diseases*, **43**, 1-14.

1988 CASTELLOTE A., GARCIA-PEÑA P., LUCAYA J., LORENZO J.: Osteofibrous dysplasia. A report of two cases. *Skeletal Radiology*, **17**, 483- 486.

1990 RESNIK C.S., YOUNG J.W.R., LEVINE A.M., AISNER S.C.: Case report 604. *Skeletal Radiology*, **19**, 217-219.

PAROSTEAL OSTEOSARCOMA
(Synonyms: juxtacortical osteosarcoma; osteogenic juxtacortical or parosteal sarcoma; parosteal ossifying sarcoma)

DEFINITION

It is a bone-producing sarcoma (thus, an osteosarcoma) which derives from the periosteum and/or from parosteal tissue at the surface of the bone; it tends towards eburneous density, and it generally has a slow or very slow course. Its malignancy is overall much less than that of classic osteosarcoma; nonetheless, there are cases which from the beginning or in time (due to progression of the malignancy) become more aggressive.

FREQUENCY

P.O.S. occurs rarely (Fig. 361).

SEX

Unlike classic osteosarcoma, there is no predilection for sex (Fig. 361).

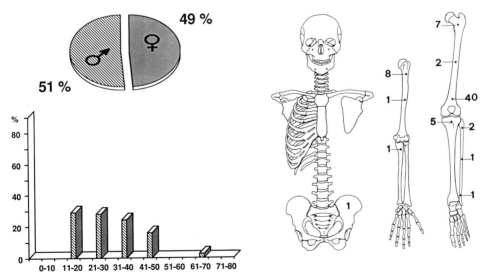

FIG. 361. - Sex, age and localization in 69 cases of parosteal osteosarcoma.

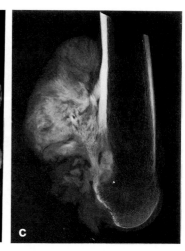

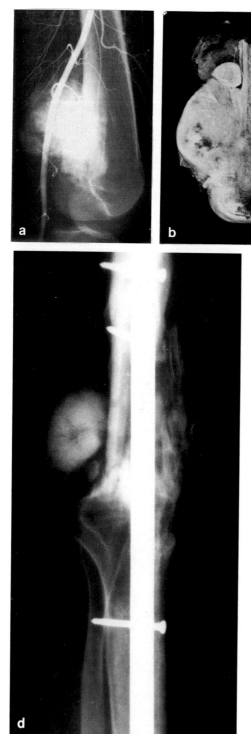

FIG. 362. - (a) Parosteal osteosarcoma in a girl aged 18 years. Onset of symptoms 4 years earlier. Arteriography. (b) and (c) Photo and radiogram of a thin slice of the resected segment. Histologically grade 1; observe initial penetration in the cortex and in the medullary spaces. In an area where the tumor adhered to the femoral vessels, resection was marginal. (d) After 5$\frac{1}{2}$ years, local recurrence, this time histological grade 2. Amputation, and N.E.D. after 8 years.

AGE

Age is generally above that of those affected with osteosarcoma. Most cases of P.O.S. begin to show symptoms between 15 and 40 years of age (Fig. 361). In exceptional cases P.O.S. may be observed prior to the end of skeletal growth. Nonetheless, the long latency of symptoms must be taken into account (see for example Figs. 362 and 363).

LOCALIZATION

The tumor is nearly exclusively observed in the long bones of the limbs, with evident predilection for the femur (2/3 of cases). This is followed, in this order, by the tibia, the humerus, the fibula, the bones of the forearm (Fig. 361). The neoplasm nearly always develops in the area of the metaphysis. Diaphyseal localizations are a rare occurrence. In agreement with its parosteal origin, it never originates from the epiphysis. But this tumor has an even more elective and typical site, which is the **posterior aspect of the distal femur**, from which it grows towards the popliteal space. Nearly half of all cases of P.O.S. are characterized by this localization (Fig. 361). This is followed, in this order, by the proximal femur, the proximal tibia, and the proximal humerus. It is hardly ever observed in the bones of the trunk, the hand or the foot.

SYMPTOMS

The main feature of P.O.S. is its slow growth. Nonetheless, cases with a relatively more rapid course are not rare.

As is the case in many tumoral forms characterized by indolent course, pain tends to be moderate and to occur late. In most cases the first symptom is swelling which, thereafter, may become painful. In deeper localizations, such as the popliteal and the proximal femur, the onset of symptoms may instead be constituted by mild discontinuous pain. When the neoplastic mass is located close to the joint, there may be joint function limitation.

Not rarely are patients observed who were previously operated conservatively, even several times, affected with local recurrence.

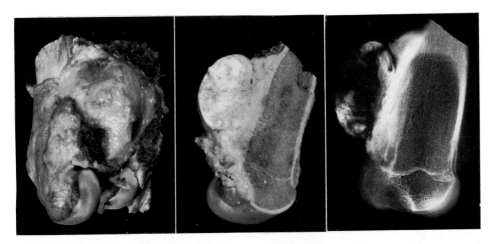

FIG. 363. - Parosteal osteosarcoma in a female aged 15 years, with onset of symptoms 6 months earlier. Photo and radiogram of a thin slice of the resected segment. Histological grade 1 with no penetration of the cortex. Resection was wide as the pseudocapsule of the tumor did not adhere to the vessels. N.E.D. after 13 years.

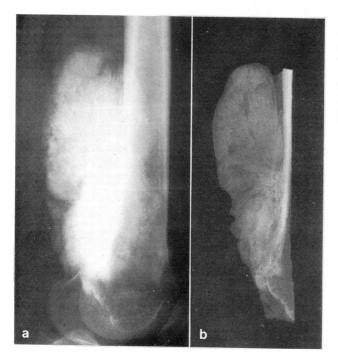

Fig. 364. - (a) Parosteal osteosarcoma in a female aged 30 years with symptoms for the past 6 months. (b) Thin slice of the anatomical specimen. Histological grade 1, with no invasion of the cortex. The patient is N.E.D. 29 years after amputation.

RADIOGRAPHIC FEATURES

The radiographic picture is very typical. It consists in an ossifying periosteal mass which, as it grows, tends to become more intensely radiopaque, to surround and even invade the implant bone (Figs. 362-367, 371-379).

In order to understand the radiographic details of P.O.S., it is best to follow the progression of the tumor, from the initial stages to the more advanced

Fig. 365. - (a) Parosteal osteosarcoma of enormous size surrounding the entire diaphysis of the humerus in a female aged 54 years. Symptoms date back 14 years. Forequarter amputation. Histological grade 2, with invasion of the medullary canal. (b) Metastasis in the cranial theca (see Fig. 370c, d). The pulmonary fields were radiographically unaffected.

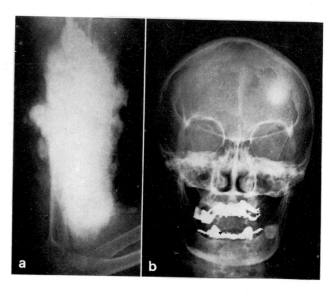

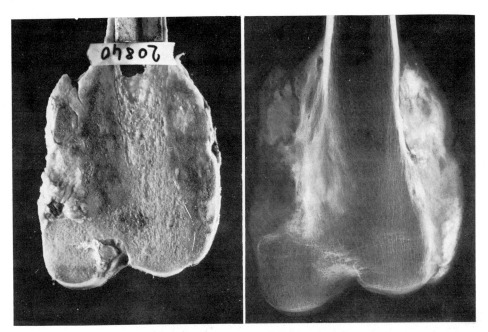

FIG. 366. - Parosteal osteosarcoma in a male aged 25 years. The patient had previously had three marginal/intralesional excisions in 6 years. Amputation. Photograph and X-ray of the anatomical specimen. Observe the penetration of the tumor within the cortex and the metaphyseal cancellous bone. Histological grade 2. N.E.D. 12 years after amputation.

ones. Furthermore, as the tumor tends to be intensely radiopaque, as it often becomes of considerable size and tends to surround the bone of origin, CAT and MRI should be obtained, and radiograms of thin slices of the anatomical specimen examined. These procedures will aid in revealing an aspect which is very important in terms of therapy and prognosis, such as any invasion of the tumor in the implant cortex and medullary spaces, and in exceptional cases, in the joint cavity.

At the onset of its growth the neoplasm may be characterized by moderate and faded radiopacity (Figs. 363c, 377, 379a, b). In more advanced stages, while it increases in volume, it reveals progressively more intense radiopacity until it becomes eburneous. The superficial layer of the tumor, which is that of more recent formation, tends to be less intensely radiopaque, so that the radiographic boundaries with the soft tissues may appear to be more or less faded (Figs. 362, 365, 372, 374). Instead, when the neoplastic mass is completely ossified and mature even at the surface, its external boundaries become more evident (Figs. 364, 367, 373, 375, 376). These radiographic aspects indicate that the newly-formed bone tissue of P.O.S. tends to mature, like that of hyperplastic lesions (bone callus, periosteal and muscular ossifications).

The surface of the neoplastic mass is roughly round-topped. In rare cases there may be multiple nodes originating from different areas of the metaphyseal perimeter (Fig. 376). If there is local recurrence after surgery, there

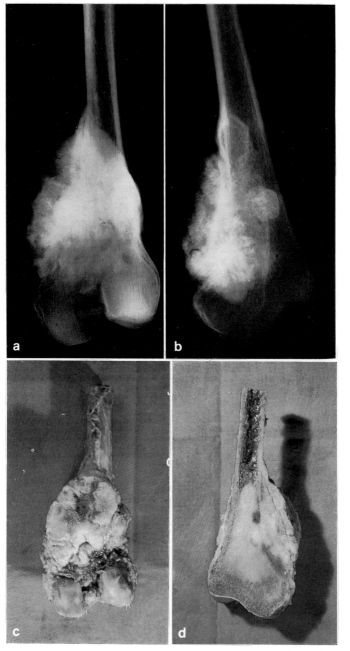

FIG. 367. - Parosteal osteosarcoma in a female aged 28 years. Onset of symptoms 15 years before. (a) and (b) Radiograms of anatomical specimen after amputation. The neoplasm which was intensely radiopaque originated from the posterior cortex of the femur, surrounding the posterior aspect of the bone and presenting very well-defined limits. (c) and (d) In the photograph of the segment transected longitudinally, there was neoplastic tissue which, in addition to surrounding the perimeter of the bone, pushed inwards, after interrupting the cortex. Histological grade 2. N.E.D. after 10 years.

may be radiopaque tumoral nodes in the soft tissues, which are completely separated from the skeletal surface (Fig. 378a).

The radiopacity of the tumor, analyzed on radiograms of the sliced anatomical specimens, is faded, cloudy, ground-glass in the initial, immature phases; as the tumor matures, convoluted bunches of thin and closely-packed

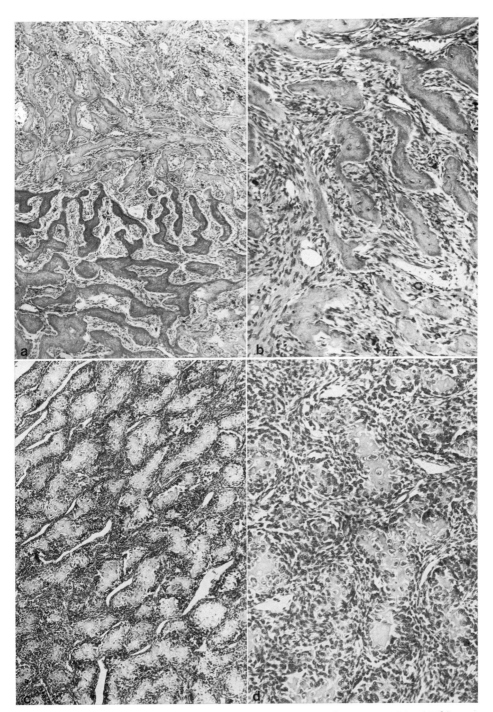

FIG. 368. - Different histological aspects of the same case (the same as Fig. 379b), corresponding to the recurrence of parosteal osteosarcoma. (a) and (b) Typical aspect of well-differentiated fibrosarcomatous stroma (grade 2) and relatively mature osteoid trabeculae. (c) and (d) Area with higher malignancy and poorly differentiated stroma (grade 3) and very immature osteoid tissue (*Hemat.-eos.*, 50, 125, 50, 125 x).

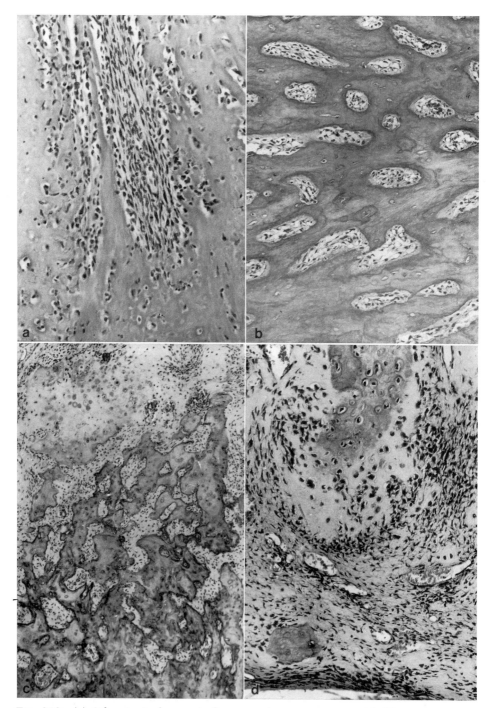

FIG. 369.- (a) Other typical aspect of parosteal osteosarcoma with fibrosarcomatous stroma (grade 2) and production of non-malignant osteoid tissue. (b) Area of more intense and mature ossification, where the stroma is scarcer and the aspects of malignancy less evident (same case as Fig. 379b). (c) and (d) Cartilaginous areas with aspects of malignancy (grade 2) (*Hemat.-eos.*, 125, 125, 50, 125 x).

bone trabeculae are observed (Figs. 362, 364, 374); finally, structures resembling adult bone characterized by thick trabecular structure or eburneous compactness are seen (Figs. 366, 367, 372, 373, 375, 376). These aspects cannot be visualized on standard radiograms, where the ossified mass appears to be amorphous. Within the tumoral radiopacity diaphanous spots may be observed, corresponding to areas which are not very osteogenetic or cartilaginous (Fig. 363c).

Of particular interest is the relationship between the tumor and the bone of origin. In less advanced forms, the cortex is nearly unmodified, and the tumor is intimately fused to it, but it may be distinguished by its radiopacity which is not as yet compact. More commonly, near its implant base, the sarcoma has an eburneous radiopacity which is completely confused with that of the thickened cortical bone (Figs. 362, 363, 364, 372, 373, 375). At times, in an area of the implant base of the neoplasm, the cortex appears to be excavated saucerlike and thickened (Figs. 377, 379); this aspect seems to announce the sarcomatous invasion of the medullary spaces of the host bone. In other cases still, or in other areas of the implant base, the cortical bone is spongy and its rarefied longitudinal trabeculae are confused with the neoplastic ones (Figs. 362, 364, 374, 376). In a successive phase, the cortex has disappeared and the tumor penetrates within the bone, with nodes which are to a greater or lesser extent radiopaque (Figs. 366, 367). Involvement of the cortex and the medullary spaces by the tumor is more frequent than has been postulated. It has to be searched for with the radiographic and histological study of multiple slices of the entire specimen, and, in vivo, by means of CAT and MRI. In our experience, this occurred in over half of the cases. It is directly correlated with the histological grade and the duration of symptoms.

From its implant base the neoplasm expands in two ways: 1) surrounding the metadiaphyseal perimeter; 2) towards the soft tissues and pushing, mushroom-like, towards the epiphysis and in particular towards the diaphysis. In the first case (where the tumor surrounds the meta-diaphysis), the single mass or the multiple nodes tend to be fused to the cortex (Figs. 366, 373, 374, 376). Instead, where the tumor mushrooms in the direction of the diaphysis, it often remains separated from the cortical bone of the diaphysis by means of a thin radiotransparent rima, which corresponds to a fibrous layer made up of the fusion between the pseudocapsule surrounding the tumor, and the periosteum (Figs. 362, 364, 366).

GROSS PATHOLOGIC FEATURES

The globose and round-topped surface of the tumor appears to be clearly delimited by a pseudocapsular layer, but, in some areas, it may be adherent to the soft tissues and to the joint capsule (Figs. 362, 363).

The general consistency of the tumor is rather hard. The superficial layer of the tumor is often less hard, as it is made up of fibrous, cartilaginous, or fibro-osteoid tissue. This is the part which most easily reveals the histological aspects of malignancy and thus must always be included in the biopsy specimen. Most of the tumor is ossified.

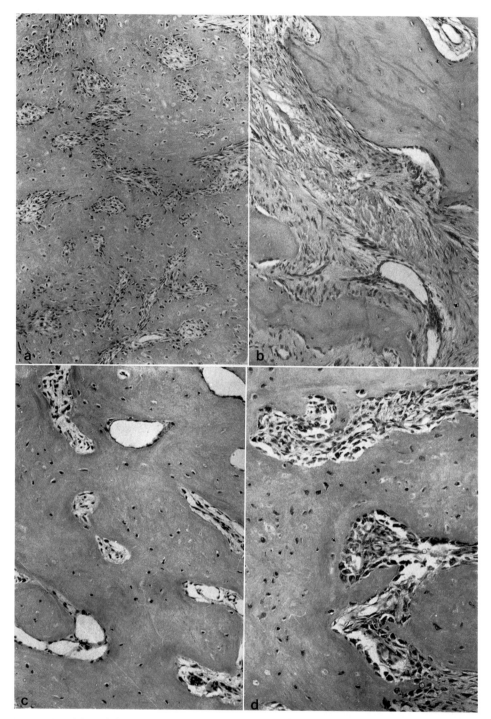

FIG. 370. - (a) and (b) Areas of parosteal osteosarcoma with very scarce or null cytological malignancy (grade 1). (c) and (d) In this eburneous tumor, as well, aspects of malignancy are minimal or absent: and yet this specimen corresponds to the metastasis illustrated in Fig. 365b (*Hemat.-eos.*, 125, 125, 125, 125 x).

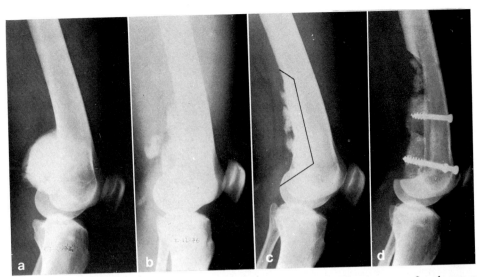

FIG. 371. - Female aged 25 years. Parosteal osteosarcoma with symptoms for the past year. (a) Radiographic aspect at diagnosis. The tumor was excised at the implant base (intralesional) with a posterior approach. (b) Extensive recurrence after 2 and 1/2 years; this was again excised marginally by the same popliteal access. (c) New recurrence after 3 years. (d) Wide resection of the posterior half of the distal femur, by means of two incisions, medial and lateral (see Fig. 26b). Homogeneous grafting. New recurrence in the soft tissues after 4 years. Wide excision including the femoro-popliteal vessels and repair with vascular by-pass. New recurrence in the soft tissues after 3 years; thigh amputation. In all of the recurrences and for 15 years the tumor always remained grade 1 and never penetrated the cortex.

On the cut surface, the non-ossified areas are whitish, juicy, of fibrous or cartilaginous aspect. The immature ossifying areas are more reddish, hyperemic, with a gritty surface (Fig. 366) or vaguely striated in the direction of the trabeculae. The mature and eburneous bony parts, finally, again appear to be whitish, and are characterized by an aspect which is not unlike that of normal almost compact bone (Fig. 373e).

The tumor is closely fused with the implant cortex. In the parts which, mushroomlike in growth, overflow towards the diaphysis, the tumoral mass may be separated from the cortex by means of a fibrous layer, which at times is musculoaponeurotic (Fig. 362). But where the tumor, surrounding the metaphyseal perimeter, grows within the periosteum, or remains compressed against the cortex, it is fused with it.

It is very important to use anatomical specimens to make an evaluation of any penetration of the tumor in the medullary spaces (Figs. 366, 367).

HISTOPATHOLOGIC FEATURES

P.O.S. is made up of a sarcomatous spindle cell and collagen stroma, containing osteoid and osseous trabeculae (with no features of malignancy) and, at times, malignant cartilage (Figs. 368-370).

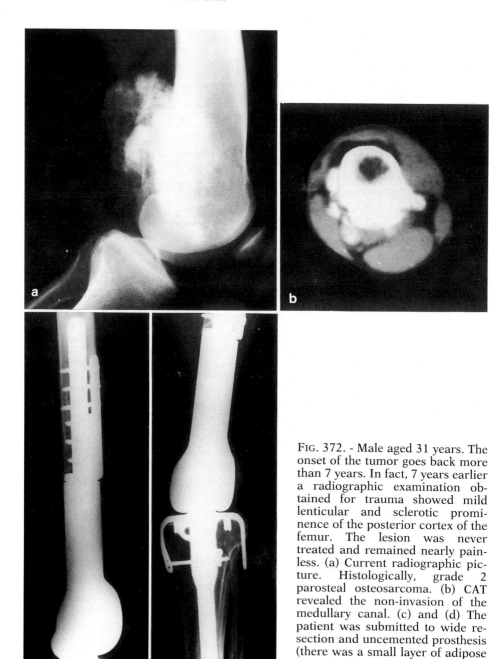

FIG. 372. - Male aged 31 years. The onset of the tumor goes back more than 7 years. In fact, 7 years earlier a radiographic examination obtained for trauma showed mild lenticular and sclerotic prominence of the posterior cortex of the femur. The lesion was never treated and remained nearly painless. (a) Current radiographic picture. Histologically, grade 2 parosteal osteosarcoma. (b) CAT revealed the non-invasion of the medullary canal. (c) and (d) The patient was submitted to wide resection and uncemented prosthesis (there was a small layer of adipose tissue between the surface of the tumor and the popliteal vessels). No signs of disease after 6 and 1/2 years.

In more typical areas of the tumor, the spindle cells are numerous and atypical, like those of a fibrosarcoma. The nuclei are large, oval, different in size, with some pleomorphism, abundant chromatin, some mitotic figures. The collagenous fibrillary component is more or less evident (Figs. 368a, b,

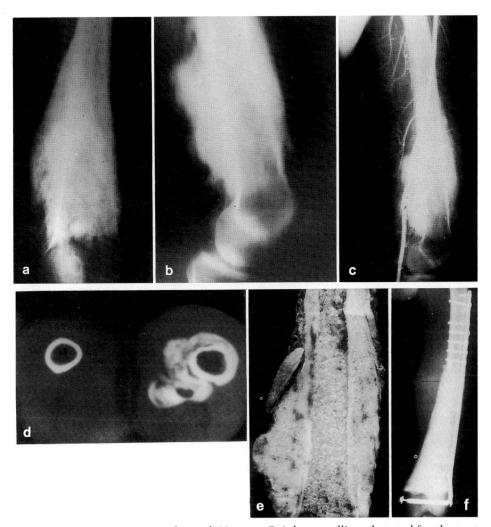

FIG. 373. - Osteosarcoma. Male aged 40 years. Painless swelling observed for the past year. Grade 2 parosteal osteosarcoma. (a) and (b) Typical radiographic aspect. (c) Arteriography (in two views) shows that the femoral artery is surrounded by the tumor. (d) CAT confirms that the femoral vessels are contained in an intratumoral tunnel. (e) and (f) Wide resection was performed, including the femoral vessels, and reconstruction with arterial bypass, acrylic cement and plate was carried out (because of deep infection, after several ineffective operations the limb was amputated 3 years after resection). No signs of disease 8 years after resection.

369a). At times the stroma takes on a myxoid aspect, with spindle-stellate cells.

The bone trabeculae are formed by direct metaplasia from the pseudo-fibrosarcomatous stroma, and thus, they are generally not bordered by osteoblasts. The osteocytes do not present aspects of malignancy (Figs. 368a, b, 369a, b). These trabeculae appear to be arranged rather regularly, and they tend to grow, become thicker and mature, from osteoid and woven bone, to

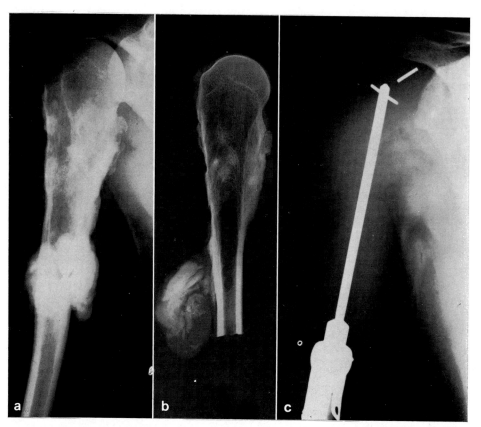

FIG. 374. - (a) Parosteal osteosarcoma in a male aged 29 years. Symptoms began 4 years earlier. The patient had already been submitted twice to marginal excision. (b) Thin slice of resected segment. Histological grade 2, invasion of the medullary canal. (c) Wide resection-endoprosthesis. The patient was N.E.D. after 19 years.

adult lamellar bone which is nearly normal. This maturation process progresses from the surface to the implant base. In more intensely ossified and mature areas the aspects of malignancy of the stroma decrease or totally regress (Fig. 370). Moreover, towards the implant base, reactive cortico-periosteal bone may be added to the neoplastic bone. It is very important to remember that the histological aspects of malignancy may be minimal or totally absent in vast areas of the tumor; and that histological malignancy may vary from area to area within the same tumor. That is why it is important to examine extensive histological specimens taken from different areas of the tumor and particularly from its surface.

Even where the aspects of malignancy are very subtle, one important feature suggesting P.O.S. is this: the tissue occupying the intertrabecular spaces is entirely composed by spindle cells and collagen fibers. In other words, one does not see the variety of elements (osteoblasts, osteoclasts, histiocytes, adipose cells, and fibrocytes) which characterize the non-neoplastic bone.

Often, the tumor contains cartilaginous areas, with evident aspects of malignancy. This neoplastic cartilage may calcify and be partially substituted by bone tissue (Fig. 369c, d).

The vascularity of the tumor is often abundant and the capillaries have their own continuous and clearly defined wall. Multinucleated giant cells in areas of hypervascularity, of interstitial hemorrhaging, or of intense bone resorption may be seen.

At the periphery of the tumor, there may be striated muscular cells and adipose cells embedded in the neoplasm, confirming its permeative growth.

P.O.S. is histologically graded from 1 to 3 based on the aspect of the spindle and cartilaginous cells, using the same criteria as those used to grade fibrosarcoma and condrosarcoma, respectively. The most frequent forms of the tumor are grade 1 and 2, grade 3 is observed in approximately 20% of all cases. Progression of malignancy may be observed. Thus, in the same tumor, there may be areas of differing grades, or the grade may increase in recurrences.

At times, grade 3 P.O.S. may have a structure which is similar to that of classic osteosarcoma (cells which are poorly differentiated, osteoid tissue ar-

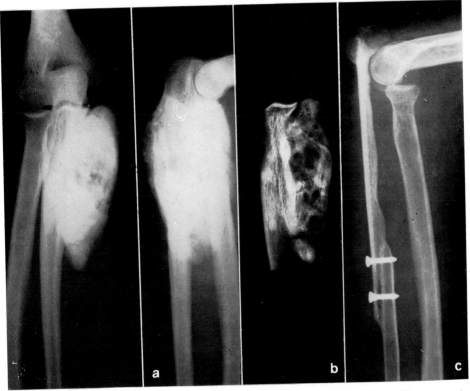

FIG. 375. - (a) Parosteal osteosarcoma in a female aged 19 years. Swelling was observed 5 years earlier. (b) Thin slice of the resected segment. Initial penetration in the medullary canal, histological grade 3. Note the perfectly well-defined outer boundaries of the tumor, in spite of its grade of malignancy. (c) Wide resection and autogenous tibial grafting. No signs of recurrence or metastasis 25 years after surgery.

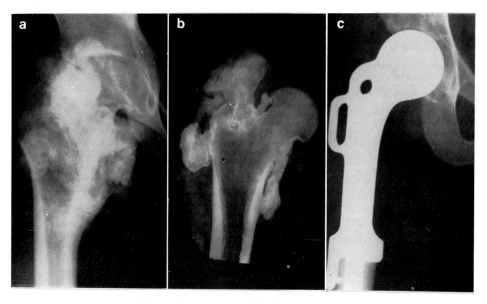

FIG. 376. - (a) Parosteal osteosarcoma in a female aged 27 years. Symptoms for the past 3 years. (b) Thin slice of resected segment. Note the multicentric implant of the tumor in the metaphyseal surface. Invasion of medullary spaces, histological grade 2. (c) Marginal resection and endoprosthesis. The patient died 6 months after surgery of pulmonary metastases.

ranged lacelike); but these aspects are only focal within a tumor which preserves the clinical-radiographic and histological features of P.O.S. A grade 4 P.O.S. is hardly ever observed (in a case such as this, on the other hand, the tumor is considered to be a classic osteosarcoma originating at the surface of the bone).

Pulmonary and skeletal metastases of P.O.S. are also intensely osteogenetic (Figs. 365, 370).

HISTOGENESIS AND PATHOGENESIS

P.O.S. seems to originate from the periosteum and/or from the capsulotendinous insertions at the bone. Its cells produce bone substance. Exceptional observations of P.O.S. after radiation therapy have been reported.

DIAGNOSIS

Diagnosis is easy, but it more than ever requires an overall evaluation of the clinical, radiographic and histological elements of the disease. Differential diagnosis may rarely be made with the forms listed below.

Periosteal and muscular ossifications (so called periostitis and myositis ossificans). Even when ossification is not isolated in the muscle but involves the periosteum and is adhered to the cortex, it is very difficult to mistake P.O.S. In fact, ossification was often preceded by trauma or repeated micro-trauma; the clinical progression and radiographic maturation of the tumor are rapidly achieved within a few months; localization is more often dia-physeal; the ossified mass is globose or pinnate and the bone trabeculae are less densely packed than those of P.O.S.; radiopacity, in globose forms of the

disease is greater at the periphery than at the center, and the bound-aries with the soft tis-sues are well-defined; the implant base at the bone is not as wide and as eburneous as it is in P.O.S. Anatomically, there is typical zonal architecture where the peripheral layers are more mature (bony) while the central core is made up of fibro-blasts and it may con-tain blood. Although the cells (fibroblasts, osteoblasts, and chon-droblasts) may reveal signs of lively growth (large deeply stained nuclei, slightly pleo-morphic, at times in mitosis) fibrosarcoma-tous stroma is never observed. Myositis os-sificans like P.O.S. may reveal groups of muscular cells entrapped in the newly-formed bone tissue.

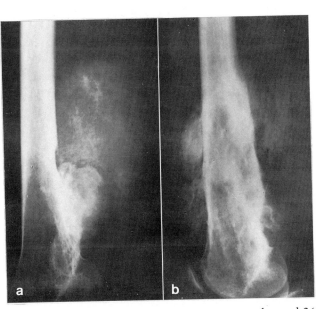

FIG. 377. - (a) Parosteal osteosarcoma in a male aged 26 years. Symptoms for the past 5 months. (b) Extensive re-currence, 5 years later, after two attempts at excision. The tumor did not penetrate the cortex and it was histo-logically grade 1 both in its primary form and in its re-currence. Amputation was performed and 31 years later there was no sign of disease.

Parosteal osteoma. In exceptional cases there may be diaphyseal or meta-physeal periosteal ossifications, which are rather dense and mature, nearly asymptomatic, which grow very slowly, and which are radiologically very si-milar or identical to P.O.S. If the histological examination does not reveal any aspect of malignancy, it is difficult to establish (Figs. 283b, c, 284) whe-ther it is a reactive periosteal ossification, a parosteal osteoma, or a very scler-osing P.O.S. characterized by a low grade of malignancy. In truth, only if the patient is monitored for many years can doubts be dispelled. In cases such as these the clinical-radiographic elements are just as important as the his-

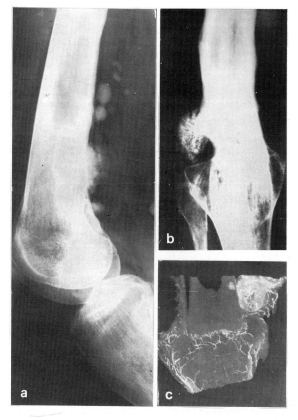

Fig. 378. - (a) Recurring parosteal osteosarcoma in a female aged 24 years. The patient was submitted to intralesional excision 1 year earlier. Histological grade 2, no invasion of the cortex. Amputation. The patient was N.E.D. after 13 years. (b) Recurring parosteal osteosarcoma on massive bone xenograft in a female aged 34 years. Onset of symptoms 17 years earlier, at the age of 17 years. At 19 years of age the patient was submitted to intralesional excision (grade 2, does not invade the cortex). At 20 years of age she was submitted to resection of the distal femur (due to recurrence) and arthrodesis (grade 2, invades the cortex). The radiogram shows recurrence on the graft occurring 14 years after resection (grade 2). Amputation. The patient died after 6 years (23 years after the onset of symptoms) due to pulmonary metastases. (c) Recurring parosteal osteosarcoma (grade 3) near a massive xenograft in a male aged 26 years. Onset of symptoms 11 years earlier. One year earlier submitted to resection of the distal femur and massive grafting (grade 3, invades the cortex). Amputation. Radiograph of the anatomical specimen, after arterial injection with minium. Recurrence in the form of a nodule is observed at the conjunction between the graft and the proximal tibial epiphysis. The patient died after 11 months (12 years after the onset of symptoms) of pulmonary metastases.

tological ones, and surgical treatment should be as conservative as possible, with careful monitoring of the patient. A similar problem, as previously observed, may occur in differential diagnosis between exostosis and peripheral chondrosarcoma.

Exostosis. We have recalled how some cases of P.O.S. present a radiographic structure of mature bone, which may seem to be not unlike that of certain exostoses characterized by a wide implant base. The basic radiographic difference is that the exostosis is made up of an evagination of the cortex and the metaphyseal cancellous bone, while P.O.S. is implanted on a thickened cortex. But macroscopically and microscopically the two forms are completely different. Let us recall, however, that P.O.S. may present a superficial cartilaginous layer (malignant).

Peripheral chondrosarcoma. Radiographically it has a finely bumpy surface, like a cauliflower, and radiopacity which is usually different, made up of a whole of many nodules, rings and amorphous granules, which are not structured (there is more calcification than ossification). The implant base is that of an exostosis, at least until the chondrosarcoma does not invade the host bone. Anatomically, there should be no doubt, as the two forms are completely different.

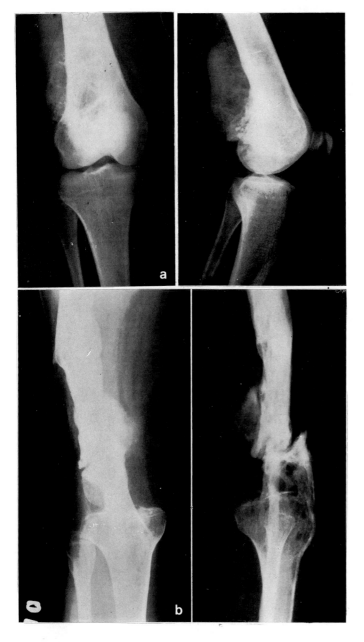

FIG. 379. - (a) Parosteal osteosarcoma in a female aged 36 years. Based on this picture, intralesional excision performed (grade 2, penetrates the cortex) with recurrence after 3 years. After 2 more years resection and allograft arthrodesis performed (grade 2, invades the canal). (b) Ten years after resection there was recurrence around the graft (see Figs. 368 and 369b) so that amputation was performed (grade 3). One year after amputation (17 years after onset of symptoms) pulmonary metastases occurred.

Periosteal chondrosarcoma. Usually, this tumor, of hemispherical shape, is radiolucent, or it contains a spray of calcar granules, and it lightly digs into the cortex dishlike. Differentiation is also entrusted to macroscopic and histological examination.

Osteosarcoma and fibrosarcoma. The speed of progression and the radiographic picture are generally sufficient to distinguish a classic osteosarcoma from P.O.S. Nonetheless, there are osteosarcomas characterized by a relatively slow course, and P.O.S. characterized by a relatively rapid one. There are osteosarcomas which develop abundantly, and in a sclerosing form outside the bone, and P.O.S. which destroy the cortex and penetrate within. Finally, there are rare cases of classic osteosarcoma which originates at the surface of the bone. These surface osteosarcomas have a course, and radiographic and histological aspects which are the same as classic osteosarcoma. Prognosis and treatment are also the same as for classic osteosarcoma. Histologically, osteosarcoma does not have a trabecular organoid structure, it never forms mature and lamellar bone, rather immature osteoid with a lacelike arrangement; it is characterized by greater atypia and scarce fibroblastic differentiation of its cells, as well as by a higher histological grade (4). However, there are osteosarcomas which are extensively fibroblastic, or primary fibrosarcomas of the bone, where the spindle cell sarcomatous tissue invades the spaces of the cancellous bone and surrounds the trabeculae. **This histological aspect may simulate a P.O.S.** Clinical-radiographic data will dispel any doubts. On the contrary, there are rare cases of P.O.S. which are histologically similar to a classic osteosarcoma (grade 3). In conclusion, in rare cases of osteogenetic and sclerosing tumor, at a very advanced stage and with aspects of high-grade malignancy, with partial destruction of the cortex and ample extension to the surrounding soft tissues, it may be difficult to distinguish between classic osteosarcoma and P.O.S. In cases such as these, the diagnostic decision would be facilitated by the possibility of having obtained radiograms during an earlier phase; however, the distinction is not of great importance, as treatment and prognosis are much the same.

Periosteal osteosarcoma. It is more often diaphyseal, it uplifts the periosteum in a lenticular form, it is more radiolucent and it contains thin radiopaque and faded spicules perpendicular to the cortex. Histologically, it is mostly chondroblastic and produces scarce and immature osteoid.

Osteosarcoma of the soft tissues. This very rare tumor may impress or erode the cortex from the outside. It is not by definition either periosteal or parosteal. Its radiopacity may be limited to a few nubecolae or nodules and be rather tenuous and faded, or absent. Its histological aspect and its malignancy are similar to those of classic osteosarcoma, not that of P.O.S.

COURSE

Usually, the course of the tumor is slow or very slow, on the average much slower than that of osteosarcoma. There are cases in which the tumor grows slowly for 5, 10, even 15 years, and, as the symptoms are absent or scarce, the patient is not operated for this entire period of time (Figs. 365, 372). In other cases, numerous attempts at excision of the tumor are followed by recurrence, within several years, without metastases occurring (Figs. 366, 371, 374, 377). Recurrence may be manifested even more than 10 years after excision, and metastases even more than 20 years after the onset of symptoms, and more than 5 years after surgery (Figs. 378b, c, 379).

Nonetheless, there are cases that show a more rapid course from the onset (Fig. 376) or in the course of time (Fig. 379) with a histological grade 3 malignancy. There may be **progression of malignancy** in time, which may be observed in cases of recurrence.

Metastases are generally pulmonary; at times other internal organs or the skeleton may be affected (Fig. 365).

TREATMENT

It is important not to be influenced by the slow course of the tumor. As the course of the tumor may become more rapid and aggressive at any time, treatment must be prompt and adequate.

Marginal excision of the tumor (following the pseudocapsular delimitation and detaching the implant base from the cortex) is not indicated because it is nearly always followed by local recurrence. Instead, wide resection of the tumor in healthy tissue is required (Figs. 25b, 371). If the tumor is very large, and/or it invades the medullary spaces, and/or it has a high grade of histological malignancy, resection of the entire skeletal segment affected is indicated (Figs. 362, 363, 372-376). When the tumor is adherent to the major vessels of the limb, these should be included in the resection, or amputation should be resorted to.

Finally, when the tumor is very large, when there is extensive local recurrence, when it has extensively invaded the implant bone, when it is histologically high grade, amputation will be required (Figs. 364-367, 377-379). Radiation treatment is not indicated. Chemotherapy, like that used to treat osteosarcoma, is advised in grade 3 cases where there is invasion of the medullary spaces.

PROGNOSIS

After surgery with wide margins, there is no local recurrence. Metastases are hardly ever observed in histological grade 1, whether or not there is penetration of the cortex. Metastases are also very unlikely in grades 2 and 3, when the tumor has not as yet penetrated the cortex and the medullary spaces. The highest histological grades (2 and, in particular, 3) and the penetration of the tumor in the medullary spaces are both clearly unfavorable prognostic factors.

If diagnosis is not made too late, and surgical treatment is adequate, this tumor should be healed, usually with conservative surgery, in more than 80% of cases.

REFERENCES

1951 GESCHICKTER C. F., COPELAND M. M.: Parosteal osteoma of bone: a new entity. *Annals of Surgery*, **133**, 790-807.

1954 DWINNEL L. A., DAHLIN D. C., GHORMLEY R. K.: Parosteal (Juxtacortical) osteogenic sarcoma. *Journal of Bone and Joint Surgery*, **36-A**, 732-744.

1958 JACOBSON S. A.: Early juxtacortical osteosarcoma (parosteal osteoma). *Journal of Bone and Joint Surgery*, **40-A**, 1310-1328.

1959 COPELAND M. M., GESCHICKTER C. F.: The treatment of parosteal osteoma of bone. *Surgery, Gynecology and Obstetrics*, **108**, 537-548.

1962 SCAGLIETTI O., CALANDRIELLO B.: Ossifying parosteal sarcoma. Parosteal osteoma or juxtacortical osteogenic sarcoma. *Journal of Bone and Joint Surgery*, **44-A**, 635-647.

1964 RANNIGER K.: The parosteal osteoid sarcoma. *Journal of Bone and Joint Surgery*, **46-A**, 1151-1151.

1967 VAN DER HEUL R. O., VON RONNEN J. R.: Juxtacortical osteosarcoma. Diagnosis, differential diagnosis, treatment, and an anlysis of eighteen cases. *Journal of Bone and Joint Surgery*, **49-A**, 415-439.

1968 CAMPANACCI M., GIUNTI A., GRANDESSO A.: Sarcoma periostale ossificante. 31 osservazioni. *Chirurgia degli Organi di Movimento*, **57**, 3-28.

1971 EDEIKEN J., FARRELL C., ACKERMAN L. V., SPJUT H. J.: Parosteal sarcoma. *American Journal of Röntgenology*, **11**, 579-583.

1972 FARR G. H., HUVOS A. G.: Juxtacortical osteogenic sarcoma. An analysis of fourteen cases. *Journal of Bone and Joint Surgery*, **54-A**, 1205-1216.

1976 CAMPANACCI M., GIUNTI A.: Periosteal osteosarcoma. *Italian Journal of Orthopaedics and Traumatology*, **2**, 23-36.

1976 UNNI K. K., DAHLIN D. C., BEABOUT J. W., IVINS J. C.: Parosteal osteogenic sarcoma. *Cancer*, **37**, 2466-2475.

1977 AHUDA S. C., VILLACIN A. B., SMITH J., BULLOUGH P. G., HUVOS A. G., MARCOVE R. C.: Juxtacortical (parosteal) osteogenic sarcoma. *Journal of Bone and Joint Surgery*, **59-A**, 632-647.

1980 LORENTZON R., LARSSON S. E., BOQUIST L.: Parosteal (juxtacortical) osteosarcoma. A clinical and histopathological study of 11 cases and a review of the literature. *Journal of Bone and Joint Sugery*, **62-B**, 86-92.

1984 CAMPANACCI M., PICCI P., GHERLINZONI F., GUERRA A., BERTONI F., NEFF J.R.: Parosteal osteosarcoma. *Journal of Bone and Joint Surgery*, **66-B**, 313-321.

1984 CAPANNA R., RUGGIERI P., BIAGINI R., CAMPANACCI M.: Emiresezione diafisometafisaria del femore. *Chirurgia degli Organi di Movimento*, **69**, 91-96.

1984 GREEN P., ILARDI C., BITTER J., DEE R.: Case report 260: parosteal osteosarcoma of the pubis. *Skeletal Radiology*, **11**, 141-143.

1984 WOLD L., UNNI K., BEABOUT J., SIM F., DAHLIN D.: Dedifferentiated parosteal osteosarcoma. *Journal of Bone and Joint Surgery*, **66-A**, 53-59.

1987 MARKS M., MARKS S., SEGALL H., SCHWINN C., FORRESTER D.: Case report 420: parosteal osteosarcoma of the sphenoid and orbit. *Skeletal Radiology*, **16**, 246-251.

1987 PICCI P., CAMPANACCI M., BACCI G., CAPANNA R., AYALA A.: Medullary involvement in parosteal osteosarcoma. A case report. *Journal of Bone and Joint Surgery*, **69-A**, 131-136.

1987 RITTS G.D., PRITCHARD D., UNNI K.K., BEABOUT J.W., ECKARDT J.J.: Parosteal osteosarcoma. *Clinical Orthopaedics*, **219**, 299-307.

1989 BAUM P.H., NELSON M.C., LACK E.E., BOGUMILL G.P.: Case report 560. *Skeletal Radiology*, **18**, 406-409.

1989 PINTADO S.O., LANE J., HUVOS A.G.: Parosteal osteogenic sarcoma of bone with coexistent low- and high-grade sarcomatous components. *Human Pathology*, **20**, 488-491.

CLASSIC OSTEOSARCOMA

DEFINITION

Classic osteosarcoma is a highly malignant tumor which nearly always originates within the bone[1] made up of mesenchymal cells which tend to produce bone substance, that is, to be differentiated in an osteoblastic sense.

Generally, the production of neoplastic bone is abundant and it may be observed on radiographic and macroscopic examination. Rarely, instead, it is so scarce and sporadic that it must be searched for in many histological specimens.

Often the sarcomatous tissue also shows aspects of fibroblastic and/or cartilaginous differentiation. Despite this, if the cells of the tumor form osteoid tissue, even if only in one site and in a small quantity, it is an O.S. Dahlin (1967) makes a prognostic distinction between prevalently osteoblastic O.S., prevalently chondroblastic O.S., and prevalently fibroblastic O.S. The prognostic value of this distinction, like that of the histological grade (3 or 4), is still to be demonstrated (see prognosis). The distinction made between osteolytic O.S. and sclerosing O.S. is also of little value, as in both cases the prognosis is the same.

FREQUENCY

After plasmacytoma, classic O.S. is the primary malignant tumor which most frequently occurs in the skeleton (Fig. 380). Nonetheless, in an absolute sense, it is an infrequent tumor. Among malignant neoplasms occurring in humans it constitutes a mere 0.2%. Its incidence is about 2-3 cases per 1,000,000 inhabitants per year (100-150 cases yearly in Italy).

SEX

There is predilection for the male sex at a ratio of 1.5-2:1 (Fig. 380).

---

[1] Periosteal osteosarcoma constitutes a distinct variety of osteosarcoma. Parosteal osteosarcoma may be considered to be a tumor in itself. In exceptional cases, classic O.S. originating at the surface of the bone may occur.

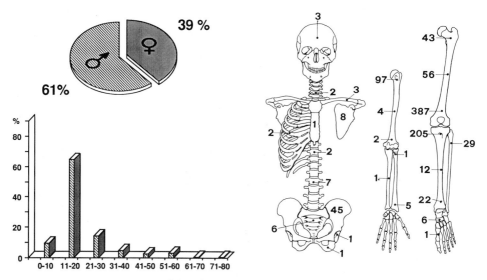

FIG. 380. - Sex, age, and localization in 952 cases of classic osteosarcoma.

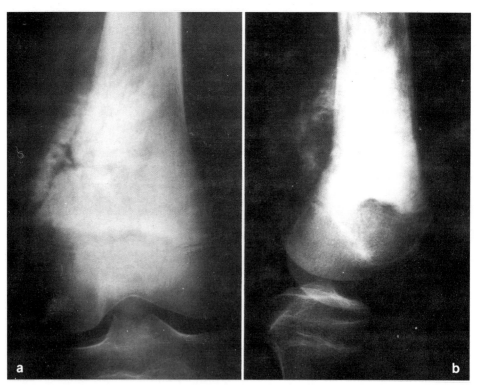

FIG. 381.

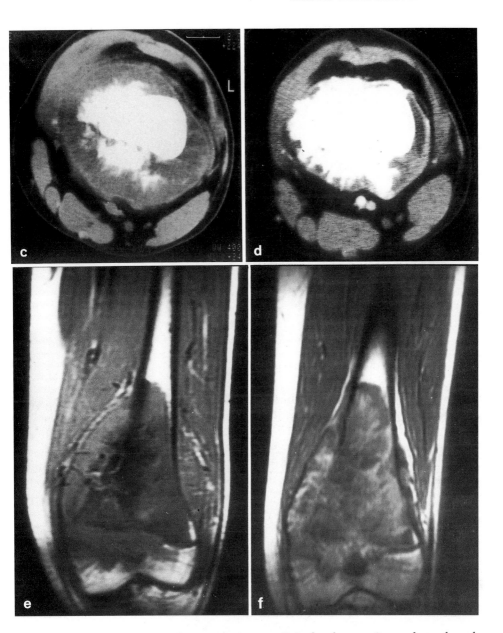

FIG. 381. - Osteosarcoma in a boy aged 12 years. Pain for the past 3 months and swelling for 2. (a), (b), (c), and (e) Typical radiographic picture, CAT and MRI at diagnosis. (d) and (f) CAT and MRI after preoperative chemotherapy: observe reduction in the volume of the tumor and better demarcation of the same in relation to the soft tissues and (in CAT) the popliteal vessels.

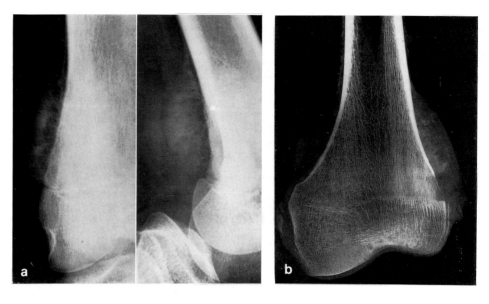

FIG. 382. - (a) Osteosarcoma of the distal femur in a female aged 12 years. (b) Osteosarcoma of the distal femur in a male aged 21 years.

AGE

In 75% of cases it is manifested between 10 and 30 years of age. It infrequently occurs prior to 10 years of age and after 30 (Fig. 380). Some cases of O.S. observed during advanced age are secondary (Pagetic bone, irradiated bone, dedifferentiated chondrosarcoma).

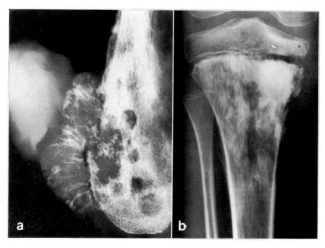

FIG. 383. - (a) Osteosarcoma of the scapula in a male aged 26 years. (b) Osteosarcoma in a boy aged 11 years.

LOCALIZATION

O.S. has no forbidden areas. Nonetheless, there are skeletal areas where there is very high predilection of the disease, others where the tumor is exceptionally rare (Fig. 380). The areas of predilection are, in this order, the distal femur and the proximal tibia, followed by the proximal humerus (the ratio for the frequency of these three sites is approximately 4:2:1). Approximately 3 out of 4 osteosarcomas are localized in the knee or in the shoulder. These are followed by the proximal femur, the diaphysis of the femur, and the pelvis. In other sites (proximal fibula, diaphysis and distal tibia) O.S. occurs rather rarely; it is decidedly rare in the vertebral column, scapula, clavicle, ribs, and sternum, in the distal humerus, the forearm and in the tarsus.

In the long bones there is predilection for O.S. in the metaphysis and the metadiaphysis. For as long as growth cartilage is present it constitutes an obstacle delaying invasion of the epiphysis. In the adult the tumor is easily extended to the epiphysis. O.S. rarely originates in a decidedly diaphyseal area. O.S. originating in an epiphysis is an exceptional observation.

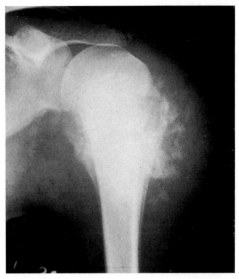

FIG. 384. - Osteosarcoma in a boy aged 16 years. Symptoms for the past 2 months.

SYMPTOMS

At the onset there are no typical symptoms. There is only pain, generally around the knee, which is mild and intermittent, worsened by function. As the patient is an adolescent or a young adult in perfectly good health, often devoted to physical activity, the pain may from the start be attributed to trauma, or explained and then treated as «rheumatic» pain. During this initial phase, radiographic examination is rarely considered to be necessary.

Within a few weeks, pain becomes more intense and continuous, while local swelling may already have occurred. Swelling increases, usually rapidly, at times relatively slowly. The skin above the tumor tends to be warm (due to the intense vascularity of the tumor); palpation is painful. During more advanced phases there is functional limitation of the nearby joint, infiltration and edema of the soft tissues, evidence of superficial venous net. In rare cases, prevalently osteolytic ones characterized by rapid progression, there may be pathologic fracture. Rarely, when the epiphysis is invaded by the tumor, as well, there is joint effusion.

The regional lymph nodes are not enlarged, except at a very advanced phase of the tumor; in this case, as well, it is usually a lymphadenitis due to resorption rather than metastasis.

The general conditions of the patient are nearly always good at diagnosis. When the patient begins to lose weight and become anemic, pulmonary metastases are generally already apparent or about to become so.

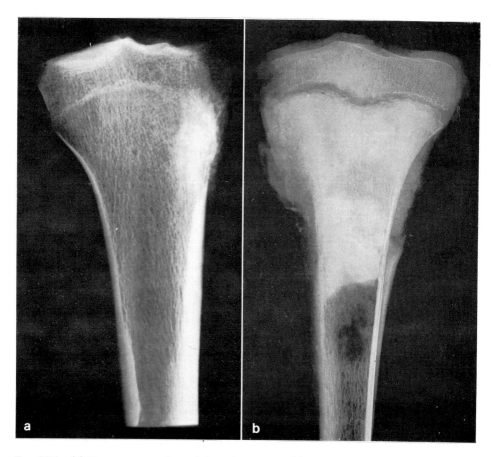

FIG. 385. - (a) Osteosarcoma in a girl aged 12 years. (b) In a boy aged 10 years (amputation specimens).

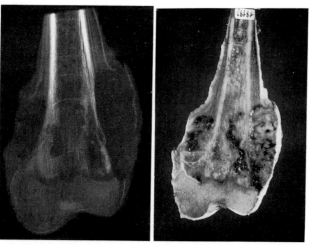

FIG. 386. - Osteosarcoma in a boy aged 15 years, with hemorrhagic areas. Amputation specimen.

The amount of time between the first symptoms and treatment is generally less than 6 months; rarely more than 1 year.

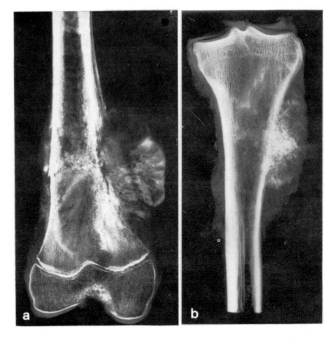

FIG. 387. - (a) Osteosarcoma in a boy aged 12 years. Symptoms for the past 3 months. (b) Osteosarcoma in a female aged 42 years. Amputation specimens.

HEMATOCHEMICAL FINDINGS

The only unconstant change consists in an increase in serum alkaline phosphatase [1]. The value of the phosphatase tends to decrease immediately after surgical removal of the tumor, to then increase if local recurrence or metastases occur.

RADIOGRAPHIC FEATURES

The radiographic picture is of essential importance, as it constitutes the only means of making an early diagnosis.

The radiographic picture of O.S. is that of a malignant tumor that originates within the bone, permeates and rapidly destroys the cancellous and cortical bones, uplifts and then surpasses the periosteum, produces neoplastic osteoid and bone in variable quantities. The radiographic picture may vary depending on the age of the patient, the site of the tumor, its speed of growth, phase of development, the amount of neoplastic bone production. Nonetheless, in many cases, which come to our observation when the tumor is already at an advanced stage, radiography provides rather typical elements, enough to allow for a nearly certain diagnosis, not only of malignancy but also of the nature of the neoplasm (Figs. 381-388).

---

[1] An increase in alkaline phosphatase, when there is no cholostasis, indicates an increase in the production of new bone tissue.

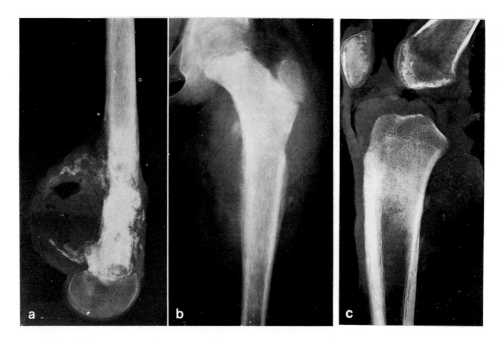

FIG. 388. - (a) Osteosarcoma in a boy aged 13 years (amputation specimen). (b) Diffused-ly chondroblastic osteosarcoma in a girl aged 10 years (the same as in Fig. 400); age, diffused radiopacity of the metaphysis, the type of periosteal reaction all suggest osteosarcoma rather than chondrosarcoma. Course was very rapid: death 4 months after the X-ray illustrated and after resection-endoprosthesis, with local recurrence and pulmonary metastases. (c) Diffusedly chondroblastic osteosarcoma in a male aged 19 years. In this case, as well as in the previous one, the histological examination was uncertain between chondroblastic osteosarcoma and grade 3 central chondrosar-coma. The patient presented recurrence on the amputation stump at the mid thigh: in the recurrence the neoplastic osteogenesis appeared to be histologically evident, con-firming the diagnosis of chondroblastic osteosarcoma (amputation specimen).

The classic radiographic picture of these advanced phases of the tumor includes an intraosseous area, which is **always characterized by faded bound-aries**, where normal trabeculation is substituted by radiolucency (prevalent-ly osteolytic forms) (Fig. 386), or by a combination of lucent and radiopaque areas (osteolytic and osteogenetic forms) (Figs. 384, 385) or by an intense and compact radiopacity (densely osteogenetic or sclerosing forms - Figs. 381, 391). The radiopacity of the tumor varies from tenuous and faded ground-glass type, to an eburneous one. The cortex may appear to be destroyed by the tumor. Often the cortex is perforated in several sites, which however can-not be seen on standard radiograms. But in this last case, as well, expansion of the tumor outside the cortex may be observed. Here, if the neoplasm is scarcely osteogenetic, a tumoral mass, deprived of radiopacity and expanded towards the soft tissues may be observed (Fig. 388); more often thin and fa-ded radiopaque bands perpendicular to the cortex may be observed. This toothcomb, brushlike or sun-ray image (Figs. 381, 382, 320a) is caused by the

FIG. 389. - (a) Diaphyseal osteosarcoma in a male aged 13 years. The radiographic aspect may suggest Ewing's sarcoma. (b) Diaphyseal osteosarcoma in a female aged 48 years. Age and the radiographic aspect had suggested lymphoma.

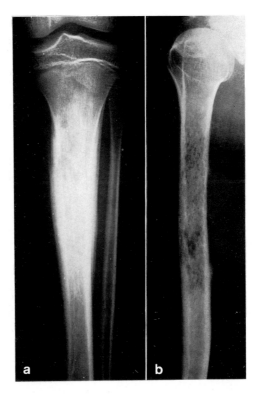

neoplastic osteogenesis, as well as by the reactive osteogenesis of the periosteum. In other intensely osteogenetic cases, very radiopaque bony nodes and bunches are observed outside the cortex (Figs. 384, 387, 390).

At the basal periphery of the neoplastic mass which has surpassed the cortex, the uplifted periosteum may react with lamellae of reactive ossification (non-neoplastic), producing the image known as Codman's triangle. Rarely, the lamellae of periosteal reaction are multiple and superimposed like onion peel (Figs. 388b, 389a), as in Ewing's sarcoma. This latter radiographic aspect may be observed in younger patients and in diaphyseal locations.

What always radiographically characterizes O.S. is the fact that the tumor, whether osteolytic or osteogenetic, has rather faded boundaries. Fine-detail radiograms show that the neoplastic bone is made up of thin trabeculae, which are anarchical in shape and distribution, and which confer diffused and faded radiopacity upon O.S.

When O.S. is observed during its initial stages, something which is becoming less and less rare, the radiographic picture is not so typical. All that may appear is a metaphyseal (rarely diaphyseal) eccentric spot of osteolysis (Figs. 393, 394, 395a) or of radiopacity (Figs. 385a, 391, 392, 396a) characterized by faded boundaries, while interruption of the cortex is hardly visible or totally absent. As a rule, in these cases, as well, CAT and MRI show a small interruption in the cortex and some neoplastic tissue invading the periosteal and parosteal soft tissues. More than 90% of all cases of classic O.S. are classified stage IIB.

In nearly exclusively osteolytic forms of the disease, which often pertain to the hemorrhagic variety of O.S. (see further on), radiograms do not show any aspect of neoplastic osteogenesis.

A preoperative study of O.S. includes bone scan, which reveals intense uptaking extended beyond the radiographic limits of the tumor, exceptionally skip metastasis, or other skeletal localizations. CAT is required to study the extent of the tumor in the soft tissues, its relationship with the large vessels or the internal organs, invasion of the articular tissues and joint cavity. MRI is the best method to evaluate and measure the extent of the tumor in the cancellous bone and along the medullary canal, to reveal skip metastasis, to study the peritumoral soft tissues. When the tumor displaces and compresses the large vessels angiography may be of use: this test (together with CAT with contrast medium and MRI) may reveal venous occlusion due to neoplastic thrombosis.

Pulmonary metastases are round in shape, often there is more than one, and they are characterized by the radiopacity of a compact tissue, but which is generally not ossifying. At times, instead, they show diffused ossification. To this may be added the image of pleural effusion. CAT may reveal pulmonary metastases in cases in which radiograms and tomograms are negative.

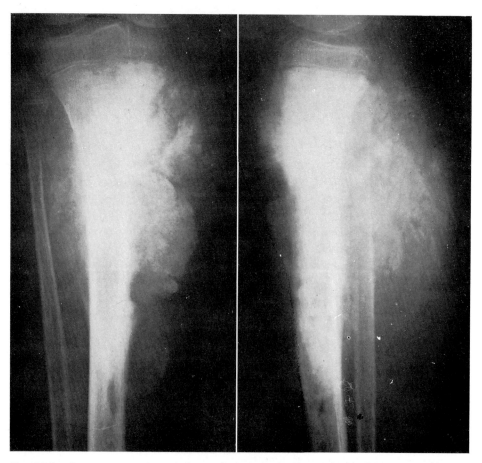

FIG. 390. - Osteosarcoma in a male aged 16 years, with nearly painless swelling for the past 8 months. The tumor was characterized by a rapid course, with death by metastases 1 year after radical amputation.

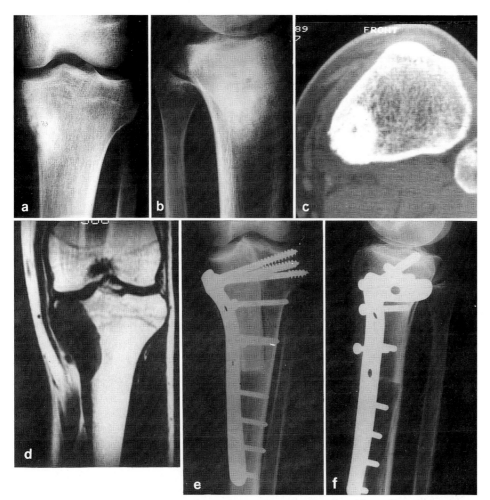

FIG. 391. - Osteosarcoma in a male aged 16 years. Pain and mild swelling for the past 15 days. Histologically, grade 3 osteoblastic osteosarcoma. (a), (b), (c) and (d) The tumor was staged IIA. (e) and (f) After preoperative chemotherapy, resection of half of the proximal tibia and substitution with an allograft were performed.

GROSS PATHOLOGIC FEATURES

In the past, when O.S. was treated by primary amputation, very frequently the entire tumor and its relationships with the surrounding tissues could be studied. The tumoral tissue, which is generally compact, tends to be whitish or rose-colored. The presence of neoplastic osteoid and bone gives it a harder consistency. The sclerosing areas are characterized by an eburneous hardness. As ossification increases vascularity decreases, so that the harder or more eburneous areas are also those which are whiter. Often, the naked eye can see the trabecular orientation of the neoplastic bone, in bands, bunches, or a very thick reticulum. But the picture is complicated by the fact

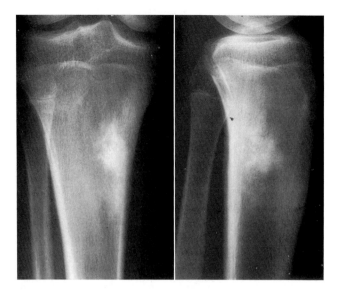

FIG. 392. - Osteosarcoma in a male aged 18 years, observed at its initial stage. The limited radiopaque area had suggested osteoid osteoma.

that often the osteogenetic neoplastic tissue permeates the structures of the host bone (cancellous and cortical) without completely destroying them, or it is intermingled with reactive bone tissue of endosteal and periosteal origin.

Nearly always the neoplastic tissue surpasses the cortex. At times, the

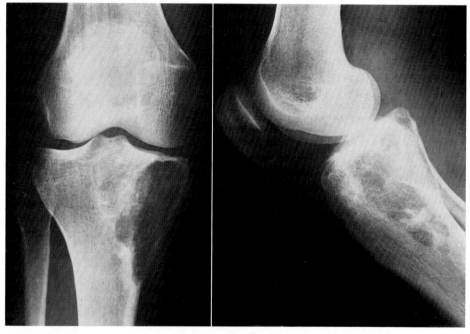

FIG. 393. - Osteosarcoma in a female aged 33 years. Pure osteolysis, with rather evident boundaries and an extremely attenuated but not clearly interrupted cortex had led to hypothesize a benign tumor.

Fig. 394. - (a) Osteosarcoma in a female aged 20 years. Considering the age of the patient, the radiographic picture could suggest chondroblastoma, clear-cell chondroblastoma, or even giant cell tumor. Nonetheless, it may be observed that the boundaries of the tumor are considerably faded. The patient died 16 months after radical amputation with pulmonary metastases. (b) Osteosarcoma in a male aged 14 years. The radiographic picture could have suggested chondrosarcoma. At surgery, instead, a cystic cavity with sero-hematic contents was observed, and with a small amount of tissue limited to the walls. This tissue also partially presented the features of an aneurysmal bone cyst, but it was also partially typical of osteosarcoma, hemorrhagic type.

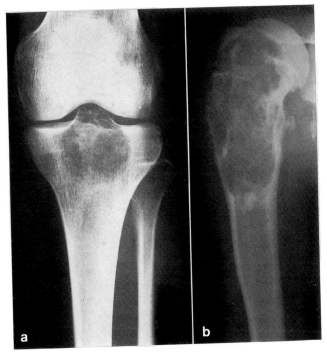

Fig. 395. - (a) Osteosarcoma in a female aged 46 years. Biopsy showed osteogenetic tissue with scarce aspects of malignancy. Influenced by the radiographic picture, which was apparently benign, osteoblastoma was diagnosed. (b) After 2 months the radiographic picture was obviously malignant. The new histological examination diagnosed osteosarcoma and even the previous specimens, a posteriori, were interpreted as osteosarcoma. The patient died with local recurrence and metastases 1 and 1/2 year after resection-endoprosthesis.

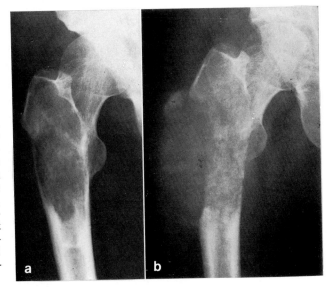

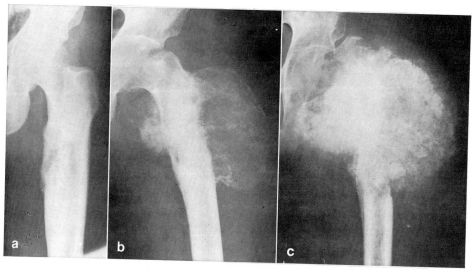

FIG. 396. - (a) Osteosarcoma in a male aged 26 years. Bioptic diagnosis was osteoblastoma, which was up to a certain point compatible with the radiographic picture. (b) Evidently malignant progression of the tumor after 11 months. (c) After 17 months. The patient refused amputation, and was treated with radiation therapy. The patient died 2 and 1/2 years later of pulmonary metastases. The biopsy specimens show that it was actually an osteosarcoma from the onset.

neoplastic tissue is fairly contained by the periosteum, other times, the periosteum, too, is invaded and the tumor infiltrates the muscles. The more external layers of the tumor are softer. Even in eburneous O.S., at the surface there is nearly always a small quantity of relatively soft tissue, which should be preferred for biopsy.

In O.S., hemorrhagic areas, yellowish dry areas of necrosis, cystic cavities are frequently observed. At times, whitish-translucent or mucoid areas may be observed due to a cartilaginous sarcomatous component, or white chalky foci of calcar precipitation (in chondroid areas or in areas of necrosis).

At times O.S. extends in the medullary canal of the diaphysis above that which seems to be its radiographic boundary. However, this extension rarely exceeds 1-2 cm and it is also rare to observe intramedullary neoplastic nodes which are separated from the main tumoral mass (skip metastases).

When growth cartilage is still present, often it is not surpassed by the tumor. In more aggressive and advanced forms of the tumor, nonetheless, the cartilage may appear to be destroyed, with neoplastic invasion of the epiphysis. In primarily (exceptional) or secondarily epiphyseal locations, similar resistance to the neoplastic invasion is provided by the articular cartilage.

HISTOPATHOLOGIC FEATURES

They consist of a sarcomatous tissue the cells of which produce osteoid and bone. The first element to be searched for in the specimen is thus its sar-

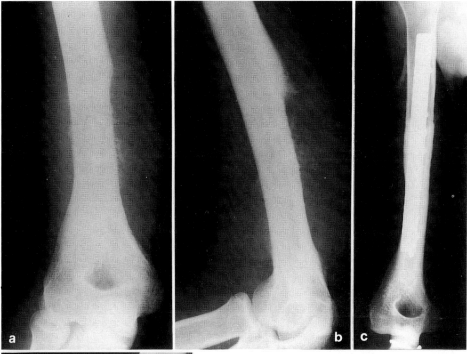

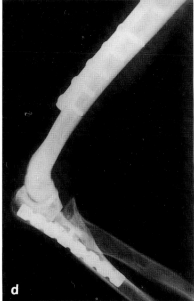

FIG. 397. - Chondroblastic osteosarcoma in a male aged 15 years with pain and swelling for the past 2 weeks. After preoperative chemotherapy the patient was submitted to wide extra-articular resection and substitution with whole articular allograft (distal humerus and proximal ulna).

comatous nature, immediately followed by the neoplastic osteogenesis defining O.S. (Fig. 398).

Usually, the more peripheral areas of the tumor are those which are less ossified, while the central areas are those which are more ossified. Scarcely osteogenetic areas are very cellular and the aspects of high-grade malignancy are fairly evident. Large cells, at times gigantic ones, considerable dysmetria and pleomorphism, atypia, hyperchromia, nuclear monstruosity, frequent and atypical mitotic figures are usually seen (Figs. 398, 399). Most cases of classic O.S. may be classified grade 4, some grade 3.

In this evidently sarcomatous tissue, the deposit of osteoid and osseous

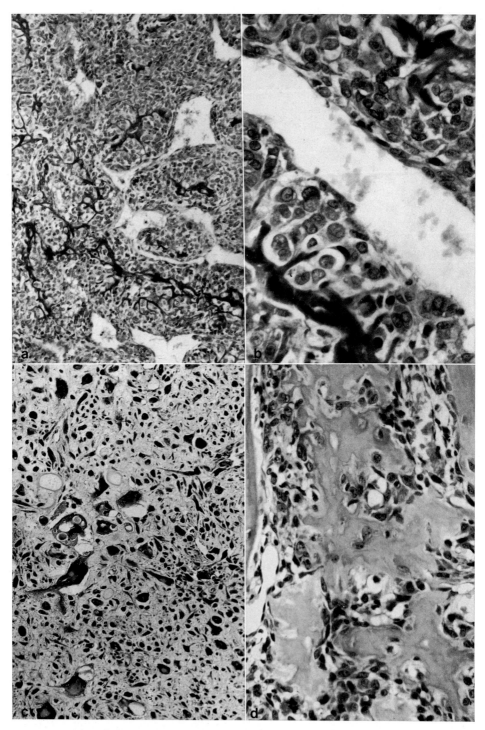

FIG. 398. - (a) and (b) Richly cellular osteosarcoma with production of a thin lace-like reticulum of osteoid. (c) Osteosarcoma with marked pleomorphism and cellular gigantism. (d) Osteosarcoma with abundant osteoid production. (*Mallory*, 125, 500, *Hemat.-eos.*, 125, 310 x).

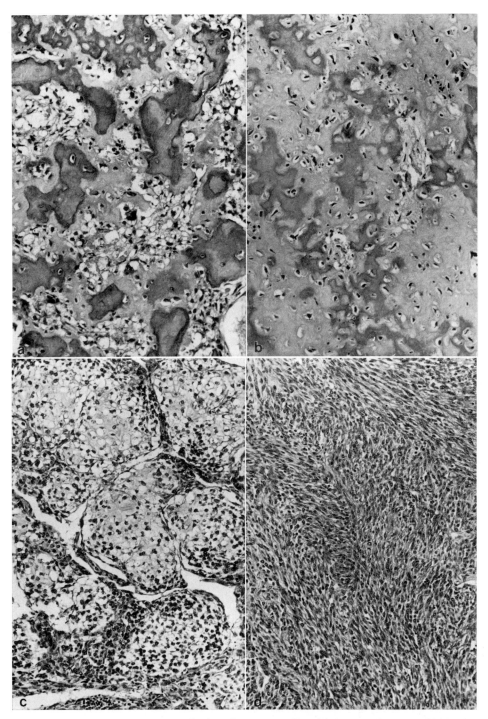

FIG. 399. - (a) Osteosarcoma with abundant osteoid and bone production. (b) In the same case, intensely osteogenetic area with scattering and decrease in volume of the cells. (c) Chondroblastic area in osteosarcoma. (d) In the same case, fibroblastic area (*Hemat.-eos.*, 125, 125, 125, 125 x).

material is observed. This material is shaped with an absolutely anarchical architecture. For example, it is nearly (Fig. 402) impossible to find trabeculae of neoplastic osteoid bordered by a regular row of osteoblasts. There are lace-like or distorted trabeculae, which never achieve structural maturation likening them to normal bone, not even when they are heavily calcified and closely-packed (Figs. 398, 399, 401).

In areas where the tumor is intensely osteogenetic, the cells, incarcerated in the abundant neoplastic bone substance, become scattered and scarce, their volume considerably decreases (Fig. 399b), their nuclei become small and with very dense chromatin up to pyknosis, the mitotic figures disappear (Fig. 401a, b). At times there is cellular necrosis (Fig. 401c, d). This rarefaction and wrinkling of the cells partially corresponds to the changes that physiologically transform the osteoblast into a mature osteocyte. This is what Jaffe (1958) calls the normalizing effect of the intense osteogenesis on sarcomatous cells. **In eburneous and/or devitalized areas of O.S., thus, more evident aspects of cellular malignancy may be searched for in vain**. But even in these unfavorable areas for a histological diagnosis, there are two important indications of O.S. The first is the **structural disorder** of the newly-formed bone (Figs. 399b, 401). The second is the fact that the neoplastic bone **permeates the medullary spaces** of the host bone. The bony trabeculae of the host, or what is left of them, are immerged in a bath of anomalous bone tissue, like relics of structures invaded by the flow of lava (Fig. 401a, b). This last finding is sufficient in itself for a diagnosis of O.S., even if the neoplastic tissue is totally eburneous, necrotic, and deprived of valid cytological elements for a sound evaluation (Fig. 401c).

The vessels of O.S. are more abundant in the scarcely and moderately osteogenetic areas, less so in the eburneous areas. These vessels are often ectatic sinusoid or actual cavernous cavities, and they do not have their own well-formed and continuous wall. In some areas they are directly walled by sarcomatous cells (Fig. 398a, b).

At times, the tissue of the O.S. has a limited or prevalent fibrosarcomatous aspect (Fig. 399d), or a chondrosarcomatous one (Figs. 399c, 400). Both the fibrosarcomatous and the chondrosarcomatous areas are characterized by high histological malignancy. (Often grade 4 for the cartilaginous component, a grade which is never observed in chondrosarcomas.) In some rare cases, osteogenesis is extremely scarce and it must be searched for on many histological specimens; or it is evident in the recurrence of the tumor[1].

Giant cells are frequently found in O.S. They may be gigantic neoplastic cells with one or more monstruous nuclei, that is, sarcomatous giant cells (Fig. 398c). In other cases, instead, there are multinucleate giant cells, with no nuclear atypia, identical to osteoclasts. The latter, of a reactive non-neoplastic nature, are particularly observed in areas of intense vascularity and

---

[1] In order to distinguish doubtful or minimum osteogenesis, it may be useful to use staining for alkaline phosphatase, or observation under phluorescent lighting after preoperative administration of tetracycline.

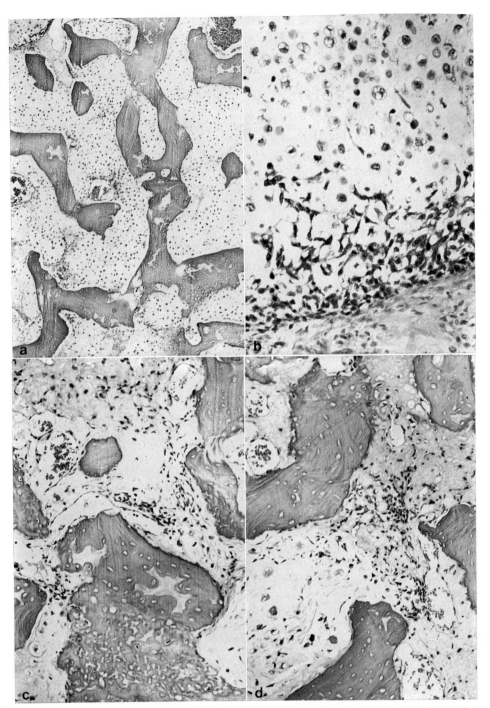

FIG. 400. - Diffusedly chondroblastic osteosarcoma (same case as in Fig. 388b). (a) The chondroblastic tissue diffusedly invades the medullary spaces of the host bone. (b) A cartilaginous lobule equal to that of a grade 3 central chondrosarcoma (see Fig. 227). (c) and (d) In the tissue submerging residues of host bone, there are rather uncertain aspects of neoplastic osteogenesis (*Hemat.-eos.*, 50, 310, 125, 125 x).

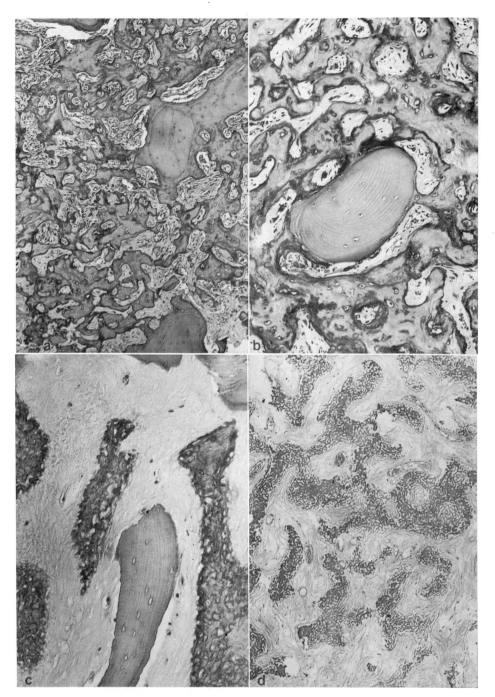

FIG. 401. - (a) and (b) Sclerosing osteosarcoma submerging the residues of host bone; in (b) there is a residue of the host bone at the center; furthermore, observe the absence of cellular malignancy. (c) Other sclerosing osteosarcoma. Above and at the center, residues of host bone. The remainder is osteosarcoma tissue which is nearly necrotic, with rare pyknotic nuclei. (d) Osteosarcoma after radiation therapy. The nuclei are nearly absent (*Hemat.-eos.*, 50, 125, 125, 50 x).

hemorrhage, surrounding dilated sinusoids or hematic cavities (cf. hemorrhagic O.S.).

Where O.S. is scarcely osteogenetic, the host bone tends to be rapidly resorbed. In very osteogenetic areas, instead, the neoplastic bone fills the medullary spaces, it fuses at the borders of the pre-existing trabeculae, and it substitutes them with a slower and more gradual process of resorption (Fig. 401a, b).

Where the neoplastic tissue surpasses the cortex, where it uplifts and then perforates the periosteum, a mixture of neoplastic osteogenesis and reactive periosteal osteogenesis is observed. Reactive periosteal osteogenesis prevalently contributes to the image of Codman's triangle; instead, and to a greater degree, neoplastic osteogenesis contributes to the tooth-comb image. Nonetheless, even the tooth-comb trabeculae may be to a considerable extent constituted by non-neoplastic reactive bone formed by periosteum.

Histochemical and biochemical studies have shown a high content of alkaline phosphatase in the cells of O.S. Electron microscopy indicates the production of collageneous fibrillae and of osteoid by the neoplastic cells.

HISTOGENESIS AND PATHOGENESIS

There is no doubt to the fact that O.S. originates from intraosseous mesenchymal cells which, once they have become sarcomatous, tend towards more or less diffused osteoblastic differentiation.

Some data suggest that O.S. is more likely to originate in areas of lively bone production and remodelling: the higher incidence of O.S. during the age of greatest skeletal growth and in areas where this growth is more intense (metaphyses of the knee and shoulder), the higher incidence of O.S. in youths who rapidly reach a high stature and, in animals, in large dogs; the insurgence of O.S. on pagetic bone (where bone turnover is elevated and persistent for many years). Furthermore, O.S. may develop on irradiated bone (see specific chapter). Recent studies in immunology and inoculation conducted in animals seem to indicate a viral etiology of O.S. Exceptional cases of heredity are described. O.S. may occur in patients who have survived retinoblastoma (tumor related to a congenital and hereditary change in the gene).

DIAGNOSIS

There are cases of **Ewing's sarcoma, lymphoma,** exceptionally **metastatic carcinoma** (particularly osteoplastic) which may radiographically simulate O.S., and, on the contrary, O.S. which are not at all radiographically typical. Particularly when the disease is located towards the diaphysis the radiographic picture may suggest Ewing's sarcoma (Fig. 389a), or lymphoma (Fig. 389b). In other cases, purely osteolytic ones, it may suggest any **malignant osteolytic neoplasm**. In exceptional cases, when the cortex is preserved, it may even resemble a **benign tumor** (Figs. 391, 392, 393, 394, 395a, 396a).

There are only three conditions, rare ones, in which diagnosis may remain uncertain even after histological examination.

1) A high-grade poorly-differentiated sarcoma where there is no neoplastic osteoid tissue, or where there are bands of material which could be osteoid just as they could be collagenous hyalin substance. In cases such as these, the diagnosis may remain uncertain between O.S., scarcely differentiated **fibrosarcoma** (Fig. 399) and **malignant fibrous histiocytoma**. 2) An extensively chondroblastic tissue, with grade 3 or 4 malignancy, and where it is not clear whether the scarce osteoid tissue is produced directly by the mesenchymal cells (O.S.) or by ossification of the cartilage (chondrosarcoma). In this case, the diagnosis may remain uncertain between O.S. and grade 3 **chondrosarcoma** (Fig. 400) (see also periosteal O.S.). 3) A sarcoma which radiographically causes doubts between **parosteal osteosarcoma** which has invaded the medullary canal, or a central O.S. which has extended to the outside of the cortex (Fig. 390); and which histologically shows intermediate features between those of the one and those of the other.

The main difficulty in making a histological diagnosis of O.S. was previously discussed in the section on histological findings. This is the normalizing effect that intense neoplastic osteogenesis may have on the tumor cells. If the examination were limited to a small specimen from an eburneous area of O.S., it could erroneously be considered an **osteoblastoma** or an **osteoid osteoma**. To this may be added that in exceptional cases the clinical-radiographic picture of O.S. may be rather atypical and deceiving, enough to vaguely mimic an osteoblastoma or another benign tumor (Figs. 391-396). As previously stated, essential elements for a diagnosis of O.S. — when there are no clear cytological features of malignancy — are the structural disorder of the tumoral tissue, and the fact that it infiltrates the medullary spaces of the host bone.

Much worse is the opposite error, that is, exchanging a benign form for O.S., such as **osteoblastoma**, **periosteal and muscular ossifications** (so-called periostitis and myositis ossificans). This error cannot be justified, but it is cited because it may be committed (see osteoblastoma and muscular and pseudotumoral periosteal ossifications).

Despite these possible difficulties, the diagnosis of classic O.S. is easy in most cases, and it may generally be ascertained by trocar biopsy.

COURSE

O.S. has a rapid course. At times the tumor may expand even in a few days. This instantaneous increase is in most cases caused by hemorrhaging in the tumor.

Nonetheless, there are cases of O.S. with slower growth: some-times the symptoms go back more than a year, and the tumor is still of relatively moderate size. These slow O.S. are more often of the sclerosing type.

O.S. metastasizes by hematic route, and thus to the lungs. Secondarily and during terminal phases it may metastasize in the skeleton. When skeletal metastases occur pulmonary metastases are nearly always present. It is rare to observe metastases in the internal organs in addition to pulmonary metastases, or metastases in the soft tissues.

Metastasis in the regional lymph nodes is quite rare.

TREATMENT

Treatment of O.S. remained nearly the same, limited to a usually ablative surgery, up until 1970. In the last 20 years, with the use of chemotherapy, it has changed radically, and this change is still underway.

Other forms of adjuvant therapy, such as the preoperative irradiation of the primary tumor, preventive irradiation of the pulmonary fields, various attempts at immunotherapy, have generally been abandoned.

The high incidence of pulmonary metastases (80-90%), after surgical ablation of the primary tumor, in historical cases shows that the colonization of neoplastic cells in the lungs has already begun, in most cases, at diagnosis. This affirmation is confirmed by calculating the doubling time for pulmonary metastases, based on which it may be assumed that the onset of metastases precedes the date of amputation or resection of the primary tumor. For this reason, we cannot solely rely on the surgical treatment of the primary tumor, however early it may have been performed. Therapeutic results could improve if we could destroy the pulmonary micrometastases already present at a first diagnosis of the primary tumor.

This consideration is at the basis of postoperative chemotherapy (begun in 1971). A successive step (1978) was taken with preoperative chemotherapy, which allowed us to drastically reduce amputation.

Chemotherapy

The drugs most used are methotrexate, cisplatin, adriamycin, a combination of bleomycin, cyclophosphamide, dactinomycin D (BCD) and iphosphamide. Methotrexate is used at high doses (8-12 gr/m2). Twelve to 24 hours after administration of the drug it is neutralized with folinic acid which is administered at intervals for 18-24 hours. The serum values of methotrexate must be monitored until they completely regress (which occurs in 48-72 hours) if necessary modifying the dosages of folinic acid and/or protracting administration of the same. The effectiveness of chemotherapy depends on the drugs used, on their dosage, and on their concentration in time.

All of the drugs listed are more or less myelotoxic. Furthermore, adriamycin is cardiotoxic, cisplatin potentially toxic for the kidney, for the acustic nerve and for the peripheral nerves.

We still are not aware of the extent of potential late damage that chemotherapy may cause: for example, the incidence of cardiopathy during advanced age in patients treated with adriamycin; the compromise of pulmonary and renal function after administration of bleomycin or cisplatin; its possible effects on reproduction; long-term carcinogenetic risk.

Chemotherapy is very costly (hospitalization and cost of drugs, particularly methotrexate).

Preoperative chemotherapy. This is carried out by intravenous or intra-arterial infusion (cisplatin). After a few cycles of chemotherapy (approximately 2 months), the clinical response is evaluated (decrease or regression of pain, reduction in mass, hardening), the laboratory response (decrease in serum alkaline phosphatase), the radiographic, CAT and MRI response (arrest of growth, ossification and capsulation of the tumor), the angiographic response (decreased tumoral and peritumoral vascularity), the bone scan response (reduced captation) (Figs. 24, 381).

Surgery is performed, more often it is conservative. It is performed when the platelets and neutrophiles have regained acceptable levels.

In rare cases preoperative chemotherapy may not be completed, because the tumor, which is very expanded and which grows rapidly, does not allow us to delay amputation.

After surgical ablation, at least one section of the entire tumor is examined histologically in order to evaluate the necrosis of neoplastic cells. This evaluation is considered to be a test of chemosensitivity in vivo. Indications for postoperative chemotherapy and prognosis are drawn from chemosensitivity.

There is good response to chemotherapy when tumoral necrosis exceeds 90%.

As these good responders have a much better prognosis than poor responders (necrosis less than 90%), the current tendency is that of using very aggressive preoperative chemotherapy (for example, associating methotrexate at high doses, cisdiaminoplatin and adriamycin) so that good responses may be obtained in as many patients as possible.

Postoperative chemotherapy. This is continued in cycles, after ablation of the primary tumor, for periods varying from 6 to 12 months. In protocols which include preoperative chemotherapy, if tumoral necrosis was good, the same drugs are continued to be administered. If instead necrosis and thus chemosensitivity in vivo was poor, the association of drugs is changed. Nonetheless, in poor responders, even when the drugs are changed prognosis does not seem to improve.

Surgical treatment

More than 90% of classic osteosarcomas erode the cortex and invade the soft tissues at diagnosis. That is, they are extracompartmental, stage IIB. If this invasion is limited, occurring in areas covered with muscular bellies and by other compartmental barriers (joint capsule, tendons and aponeuroses), wide and conservative surgery may be performed, with percentages of local recurrence not unlike those observed after amputation. Without preoperative chemotherapy, indications for conservative surgery were made in 25% of cases. With preoperative chemotherapy, the percentage of conservative operations has risen to 90%.

Based on the sites where osteosarcoma shows predilection, the most common types of operation are resection of the distal femur, of the proximal tibia, of the proximal humerus.

In resections of the distal femur, reconstruction may be carried out in arthrodesis or with an arthroprosthesis. An arthroprosthesis is more indicated when a good portion of the quadriceps muscle may be preserved, and when the patient adapts to a sedentary life. In patients aged less than 12 years, resection would cause subsequent severe leg length discrepancy. In cases such as these, arthrodesis may be performed, and lengthening of the tibia and femur may be postponed until chemotherapy has been completed. Often rotationplasty according to the Salzer method is indicated.

In resections of the proximal tibia, arthroprosthesis is indicated, with reinsertion of the patellar tendon on the fibula or on the gastrocnemius after they have been brought forward; otherwise, arthrodesis is indicated. In children amputation is preferred, or rarely rotationplasty may be performed.

A large portion of the capsule, the menisci and the cruciate ligaments are included in resections of the knee; at times, the patella with the entire extensor apparatus. In rare cases, totally extra-articular resection is required.

On the contrary, because of the shortness of the capsule, particularly the lower one, extra-articular resection is often performed in resections of the proximal humerus, removing the joint en bloc with the glenoid process, by means of osteotomy of the scapular neck. Resections of the proximal humerus are repaired by endoprosthesis. Arthrodesis may be performed in patients who wish to maintain more strength and some abductor function of the shoulder.

At times resections of the proximal femur must be extra-articular (with the acetabulum and without opening the joint); in cases such as these arthrodesis may be obtained by allograft (children) or a composite allograft-endoprosthesis can be used (adults). In intra-articular resections in the adult an endoprosthesis or an arthroprosthesis are used for reconstruction; in the child, arthrodesis is used.

At times diaphyseal resection is performed, leaving the epiphysis intact, and reconstructing by plates and grafts. If a bone bank is available, the best reconstruction system for diaphyseal resections and resections-arthrodeses is constituted by intercalary allografts; sometimes vascularized fibular autografts, or a combination of the two is preferred.

Articular allografts may also be used (shoulder, knee, elbow, wrist) in selected cases.

Surgical treatment of pulmonary metastases

If metastases occur in the lungs thoracotomy, which may be bilateral and repeated, and excision of all of the metastatic nodules is indicated. It is not known just how useful it is to associate metastasectomy with further chemotherapy, as is however done in many specialized centers. Prognosis is worse in metastases occurring early and rapidly increasing in extent and number. Five-year survival rate after thoracotomy is approximately 30%, as reported in selected case series.

PROGNOSIS

The percentage of survival after more than 10 years when surgical treatment alone is used is equal to 10-20%. Pulmonary metastases generally occur 1-2 years after amputation, with a maximum incidence during the first year. Nonetheless, they may occur (in 10-15% of cases) even after more than 2 years. In exceptional cases (2-5%) they occur after more than 5 years.

Nowadays, these figures have changed drastically. Survival after more than 5 years with no evidence of disease is approximately 60-70%. Metastases may also occur late and in anomalous sites, in addition to the lungs. These differences seem mainly to be attributed to adjuvant chemotherapy.

As the comparison made with historical case series is not scientifically correct, randomized prospective studies have been conducted, with a group of patients treated with surgery alone, and a group of patients treated with surgery and postoperative adjuvant chemotherapy. One of these studies, conducted at the Mayo Clinic on a limited number of cases, obtained results which are difficult to explain, and that is, there was no significant difference between the two groups, with survival after more than 2 years with no evidence of disease equal to approximately 45%. But the second study, conducted by several Institutes in collaboration and on a larger number of cases indicated that with surgery alone survival was as low as it was in past case series, while when adjuvant chemotherapy was used it was about 50%.

The use of preoperative chemotherapy, on the other hand, has histologically proved the effectiveness of drugs in causing necrosis of the cells of the primary tumor (as metastasectomy proved the same on metastases).

Some elements influence the prognosis of O.S. The first is expansion of the tumor at therapy. O.S. which are still small, which have just begun to attack or have not as yet reached the cortex, have a prognosis which is less severe than that of large O.S. which have extensively invaded the soft tissues. The second is the site of the tumor. The more proximal and the closer it is to the trunk, the worse the prognosis. Thus, O.S. of the tibia seem to have a higher possibility of survival; on the contrary, O.S. of the proximal humerus and of the proximal femur, and particularly those of the trunk, have the worst prognosis. Opinions differ as to whether age influences prognosis, in the sense that O.S. occurring prior to 15 years of age have a worse prognosis. Whether O.S. is osteolytic or sclerosing does not seem to have any reliable prognostic value.

With regard to prognosis, it still has not been proven just how important Dahlin's distinction between prevalently osteoblastic, chondroblastic, and fibroblastic forms is, nor the grade of histological malignancy (3 or 4). But the most important prognostic factor is constituted by **response to preoperative chemotherapy**. When necrosis exceeded 90%, prognosis is good in more than 80% of cases.

As metastases occur in most cases during the first 2 years, survival for 3 and, even more so, for 5 years is quite significant.

SECONDARY O.S.

In pagetic bone, in other benign lesions (fibrous dysplasia, benign cartilaginous tumors), in skeletal infarction, in chronic osteomyelitis, in radiated bone: see specific chapters. Furthermore, due to progression of malignancy, O.S. may occur from central chondrosarcoma (see dedifferentiated chondrosarcoma).

In the majority of cases metastases appear within the first 2 years after removal of the primary tumor. These cases of O.S. are often observed during adult age. Treatment is the same as that used for classic O.S., except for the fact that often chemotherapy cannot be carried out either totally or partially, due to the age of the patient. The prognosis of these secondary O.S. is particularly severe.

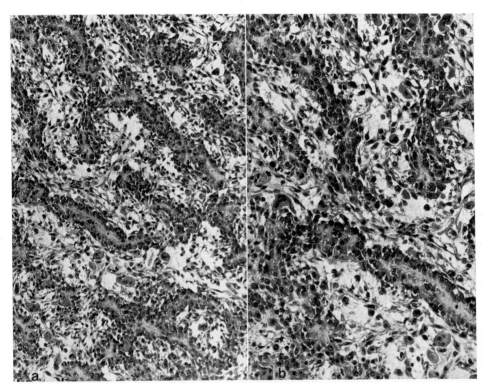

FIG. 402. - Osteosarcoma of the distal femur in a female aged 59 years. The bioptic finding throughout was that illustrated in the microphotography. The histological diagnosis was aggressive osteoblastoma, or characterized by possible malignant progression. The reason for this diagnosis depended on the considerable structural order, with thin bands of very immature osteoid tissue, bordered by regular strings of osteoblasts and with only a few cells in the interposed spaces. Actually, these osteoblasts are too large, hyperchromatic and too often in mitosis to be an osteoblastoma. The tumor was irradiated but after 5 months there was marked expansion and radiographic malignancy. A new histological examination carried out on the amputated limb revealed that alongside areas such as those illustrated there were other areas with more evident cytological malignancy and aspects of hemorrhagic osteosarcoma. The patient died after 2 years of pulmonary metastases (*Hemat.-eos.*, 125, 310 x).

O.S. OF THE MAXILLARY BONES

This tumor has a better prognosis as compared to what is generally the case with O.S., and despite the fact that the site evidently precludes very wide surgery. It is observed during middle age, more advanced than what is the case in other O.S. Histologically, there is often an extensive chondroblastic component.

HEMORRHAGIC (OR TELANGIECTATIC) O.S.

As observed, classic O.S. may contain hypervascular and hemorrhagic areas, with large sinusoids, hematic cavities and multinucleate giant cells reactive to hemorrhage. Thus, what may occur is that these aspects predominate and are diffused enough to change the entire anatomical-radiographic picture of O.S. These totally hemorrhagic O.S. are not different from classic type in terms of age and sex. Even the localization is similar, but perhaps there is greater predilection for the diaphysis (Fig. 403).

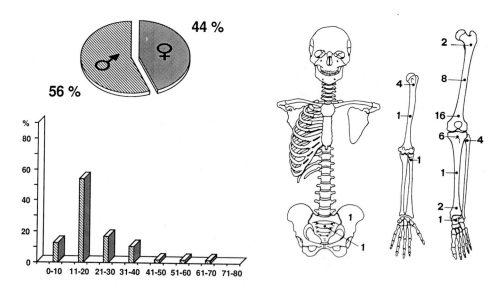

FIG. 403. - Sex, age and site in 48 cases of hemorrhagic osteosarcoma.

Radiographically, they are nearly exclusively osteolytic, with scarce osteogenetic reaction of the periosteum and usually (but not always: Fig. 394b) characterized by signs of considerable aggressiveness and rapid progression (Figs. 404-410).

Macroscopically, the tumor is rather soft and bleeding, as it is constituted by a sponge with large cavities filled with blood and clots (Fig. 404). The neoplastic tissue constitutes the septa and the walls, which are rather soft, at

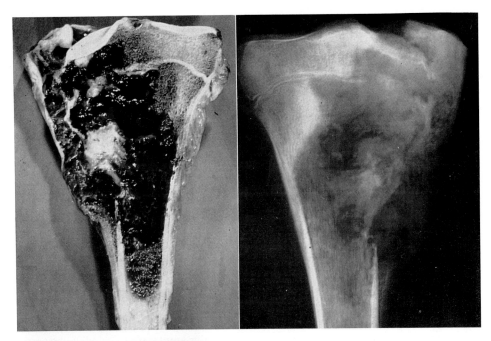

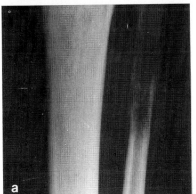

FIG. 404. - Hemorrhagic osteosarcoma in a boy aged 12 years. Observe the aggressive aspect with invasion of the epiphysis and the joint.

FIG. 405. - Hemorrhagic osteosarcoma in a male aged 23 years. Pain and swelling for the past 2 months. (a) Radiographic picture totally osteolytic and aggressive. (b) and (c) Angiography and CAT with contrast medium documented the hypervascularity of the tumor.

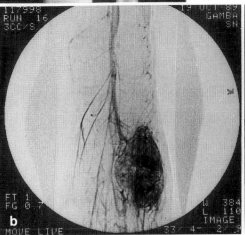

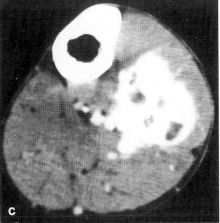

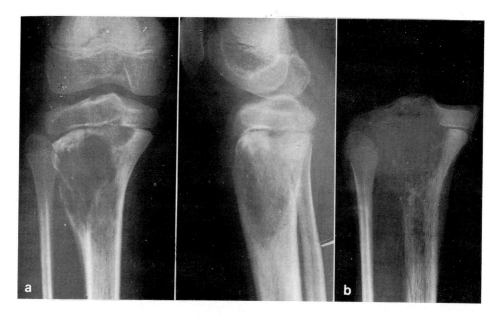

FIG. 406. - (a) Hemorrhagic osteosarcoma in a girl aged 10 years. Biopsy was interpreted as aneurysmal bone cyst. (b) Specimen from the amputation performed after 20 days as a result of severe expansion of the osteolysis. This time the histological finding was more clearly that of hemorrhagic osteosarcoma (see Fig. 411).

times thin. Generally, there is extensive destruction of the cortex and of the periosteum and invasion of the soft tissues. Exceptionally, however, the periosteum appears to be relatively intact, so that the macroscopic illusion of an aneurysmal bone cyst may be complete (Fig. 406).

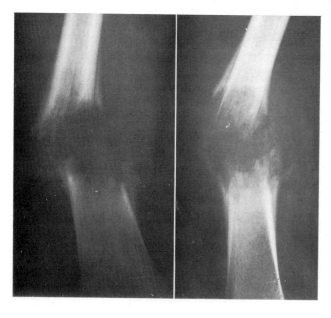

FIG. 407. - Hemorrhagic osteosarcoma in a girl aged 9 years.

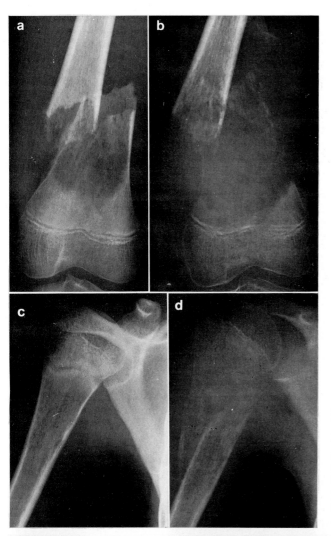

FIG. 408. - (a) Hemorrhagic osteosarcoma in a boy aged 12 years. (b) The same 40 days later. (c) Skeletal metastasis after 1 and 1/2 year. (d) The same 4 months later. At the same time pulmonary metastases occurred.

◀

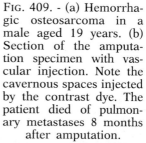

FIG. 409. - (a) Hemorrhagic osteosarcoma in a male aged 19 years. (b) Section of the amputation specimen with vascular injection. Note the cavernous spaces injected by the contrast dye. The patient died of pulmonary metastases 8 months after amputation.

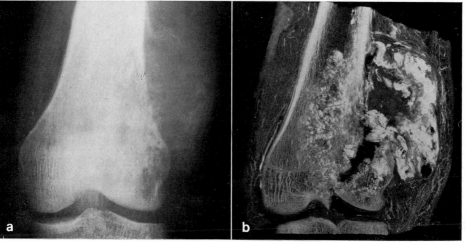

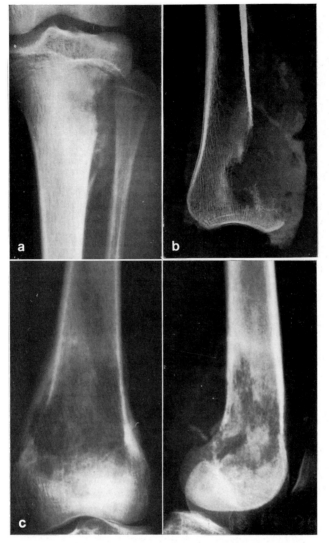

FIG. 410. - (a) Hemorrhagic osteosarcoma in a boy aged 12 years. (b) Hemorrhagic osteosarcoma of the distal tibia in a female aged 20 years. (c) Hemorrhagic osteosarcoma in a female aged 17 years. The patient was treated with wide resection and articular allograft; there were no signs of either recurrence or metastasis 21 years later (no chemotherapy).

Histologically, the tissue, under small enlargement, recalls or is the same as that of aneurysmal bone cyst: large hematic cavities alternated with septa and areas of tissue which, at times only under greater enlargement, reveals its sarcomatous nature (Figs. 411, 412). The cavities have no wall other than

▶

FIG. 411. - Hemorrhagic osteosarcoma (the same case as in Fig. 406). (a) Low power view recalls an aneurysmal bone cyst. (b) Under higher power the cytological malignancy is obvious.

▶

FIG. 412. - Another example of hemorrhagic osteosarcoma. Observe the numerous reactive multinucleate giant cells. Note the evident difference between the nuclei of these giant cells and those, decidedly larger, pleomorphic and hyperchromatic, of the sarcomatous cells (*Hemat.-eos.*, 150, 300, 125, 300 x).

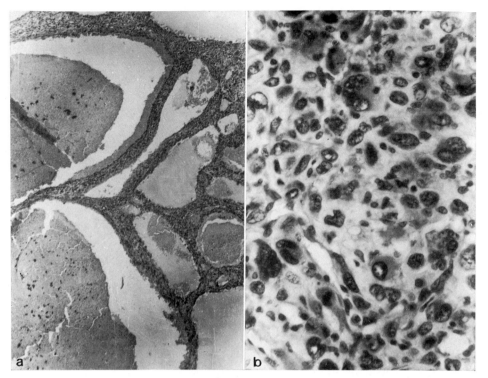

FIG. 411.

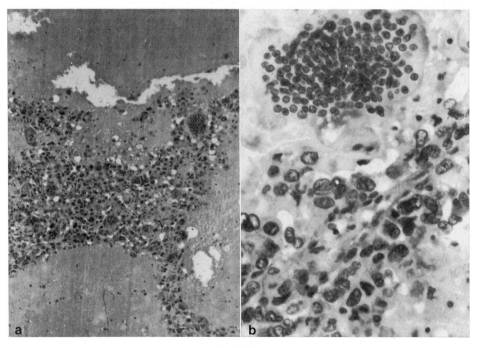

FIG. 412.

that constituted by the sarcomatous tissue itself. This shows elevated pleomorphism and cellular atypia. At times, mixed with the sarcomatous cells, there are numerous multinucleate giant cells identical to osteoclasts, deprived of any aspect of malignancy, because they are reactive to the hemorrhage. This aspect increases the possibility of confusing the tumor with aneurysmal bone cyst (Fig. 417b); in exceptional cases, when the tissue septa are thin and the sarcomatous cells scarce, if the specimen is not sufficiently extensive and representative, if the observer is not warned of this possibility, the error of underestimating O.S., exchanging it for aneurysmal bone cyst is truly possible. In other cases, instead, the sarcomatous tissue contains gigantic elements with one or more monstruous and hyperchromic nuclei, representing sarcomatous giant cells. Neoplastic osteogenesis is always rather scarce. Often, it must be searched for in numerous sections.

Hemorrhagic O.S. usually has a particularly aggressive and rapid **course**, and a high grade of histological malignancy (grade 4). Nonetheless, there are exceptional cases with reduced histological malignancy (grades 1-2) and a slow course, which must be included with low-grade central O.S. (see further on). The **treatment** and **prognosis** of hemorrhagic O.S. are the same as those for classic O.S.

LOW-GRADE CENTRAL O.S.

We mentioned the fact that some O.S., nearly always of the sclerosing type, have a relatively slow course. We also noted how the eburneous areas of O.S. histologically reveal the minor aspects of cellular malignancy. Nonetheless, these O.S. always contain some areas which are high-grade malignant, and do not show significant prognostic differences as compared to the average of classic O.S.

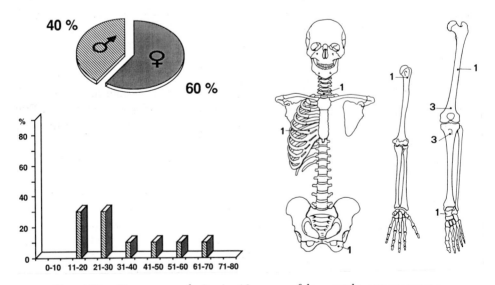

FIG. 413. - Sex, age and site in 12 cases of low-grade osteosarcoma.

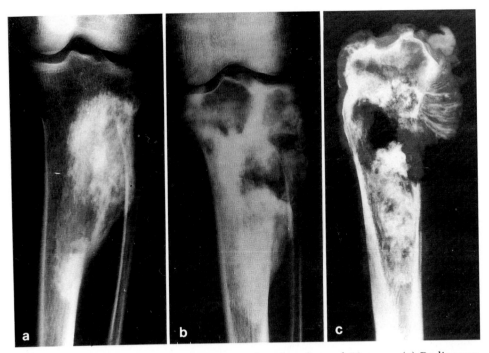

FIG. 414 - Low-grade central osteosarcoma in a female aged 53 years. (a) Radiogram obtained 7 years previously on which biopsy showed low-grade osteosarcoma. (b) Evolution of the tumor over 7 years with no treatment. The patient was then submitted to marginal resection and uncemented prosthesis. (c) Radiogram of the resected specimen. A histological examination of the entire tumor confirmed the diagnosis of grade 2 osteosarcoma with grade 3 peripheral areas. Local recurrence after 2 years and thigh amputation. No sign of disease after 2 more years.

However, there are exceptional cases (Fig. 413) where the tumor, whether osteolytic, sclerosing, or mixed, at the onset reveal a **radiographic** aspect which is not aggressive (Figs. 414-416) and which **histologically** appears to be similar to a fibrous dysplasia, or to a parosteal osteosarcoma, or to an osteoblastoma. In fact, there is somewhat of a histo-architectural order, with prevalently fibroblastic fields including osteoid and osseous trabeculae (Fig. 417a, b, c). The cells interposed with the osteoid trabeculae are prevalently spindle-shaped, with aspects of minimal or scarce and sporadic atypia. Furthermore, aspects of histological malignancy may be evident only in some areas of the tumor, and absent in others. Exceptionally, the tumor has a structure which is similar to that of an aneurysmal bone cyst (Fig. 417b). At times **diagnosis** is very difficult; the clinical-radiographic elements and the course of the tumor are of determining importance. The **course** of the tumor is slow or very slow, with local recurrence, even repeated, after intralesional or marginal surgery. At times, in recurrence, there may be progression of malignancy to a conventional O.S. (Fig. 417b, c, d). The **treatment** of choice is wide resection. Amputation is necessary in more expanded and recurring forms. **Prognosis** is relatively good. Nonetheless, some cases have metastasized.

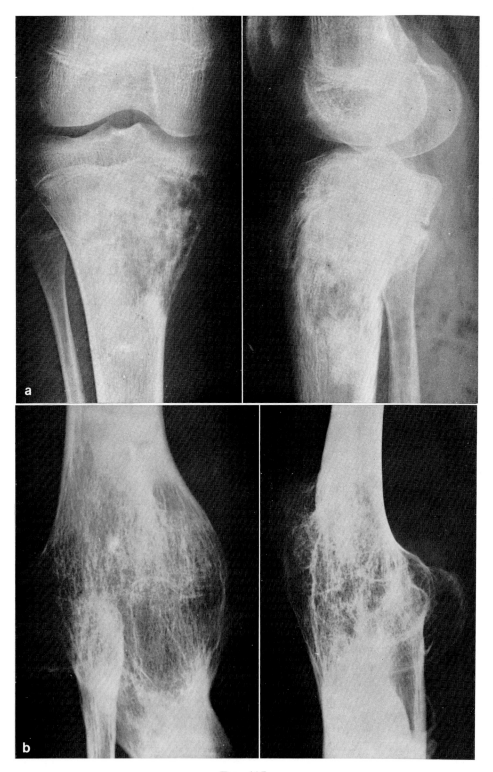

FIG. 415.

FIG. 415. - (a) Low-grade central osteosarcoma in a girl aged 12 years. Radiographically, too, the tumor appears to be well-contained. (b) The patient was submitted to resection and arthrodesis with autogenous grafts; there were no signs of recurrence or metastasis 30 years after surgery.

FIG. 416. - Male aged 12 years. Low-grade central osteosarcoma with localization in the epiphysis. Radiographically, too, the tumor is well-contained. The patient was submitted to resection and arthrodesis; there were no signs of recurrence or metastasis 22 years after surgery. Radiogram of a section of the anatomical specimen.

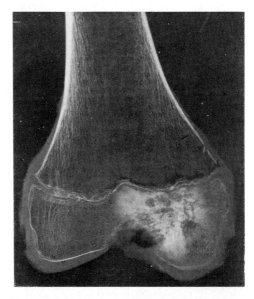

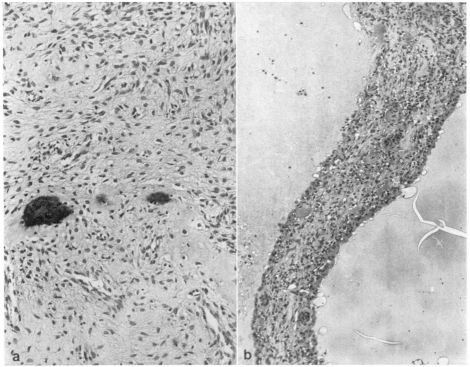

FIG. 417. (legend on the following page).

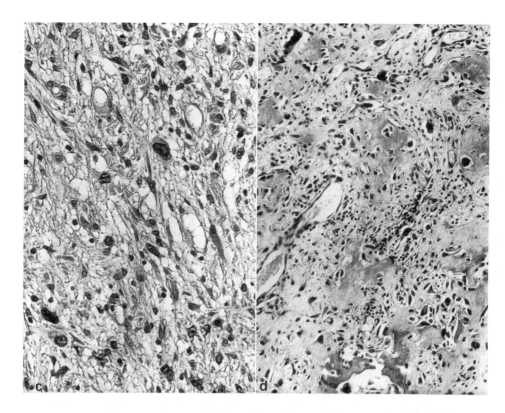

FIG. 417. - (a) Low-grade central osteosarcoma. The tissue of five extensive specimens had an aspect which was the same as this one throughout. It was a female aged 39 years whose symptoms dated back 2 and 1/2 years. (b) and (c) Hemorrhagic osteosarcoma, low grade of malignancy. The lesion was operated three times by curettage over 7 years and it was always diagnosed as aneurysmal bone cyst. Only in some areas (c) gigantism, pleomorphism, and hyperchromia of some of the cells could be observed. (d) The last biopsy after numerous recurrences and before amputation revealed high-grade malignancy of classic osteosarcoma (*Hemat.-eos.*, 125, 125, 310, 125 x).

SMALL-CELL O.S.

This is an interesting histological variety particularly because it may be exchanged for Ewing's sarcoma (Fig. 419). This error may be committed especially in extemporaneous frozen sections diagnosis. The small cells of the osteosarcoma, as compared to those of Ewing's sarcoma, have wider and deeply stained cytoplasms, nuclei which are more hyperchromatic, more pleomorphic, a nucleolus which is more evident, they are more often in mitosis; there is no cytoplasmatic glycogen. In other fields there is the typical osteogenesis of osteosarcoma. In terms of sex, age, localization (Fig. 418) and clinical-radiographic features, small-cell O.S. is not different from classic O.S. Its chemosensitivity seems to differ and prognosis to be more severe.

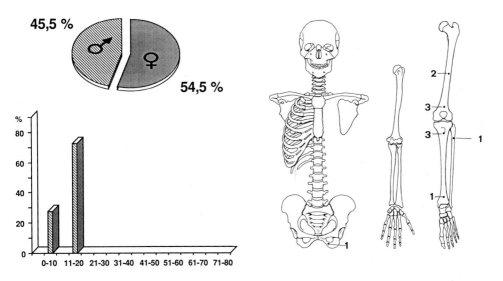

FIG. 418 - Sex, age and site in 11 cases of small-cell osteosarcoma.

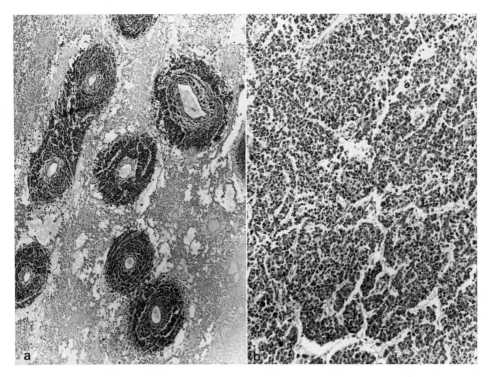

FIG. 419. - Small-cell osteosarcoma. (a) and (b) The presence of a mat of small cells, some with images of perivascular rings in the areas of necrosis, could confuse this osteosarcoma with Ewing's sarcoma. Under higher power (c) nonetheless, it was observed how the cells, unlike those of Ewing's sarcoma, had extensive and deeply stained cytoplasm, pleomorphic nuclei, with large chromatin blocks and numerous nucleoli. If specimens are extended, neoplastic osteogenesis is observed (d). (*Hemat.-eos.*, 50, 125, 300, 125 x).

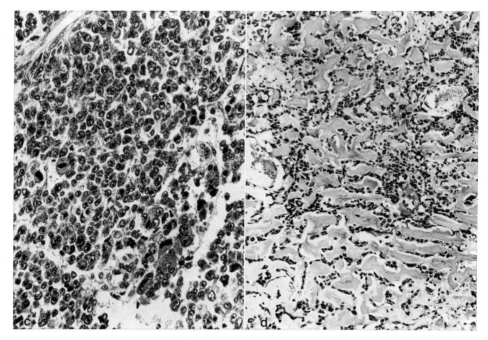

FIG. 419 c-d.

PERIOSTEAL O.S.

We are not referring here to the rare and previously mentioned conventional O.S. arising at the surface of the bone. Rather, we deal with an uncom-

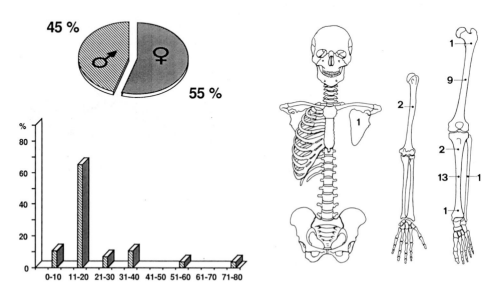

FIG. 420. - Sex, age, and localization in 30 cases of periosteal osteosarcoma.

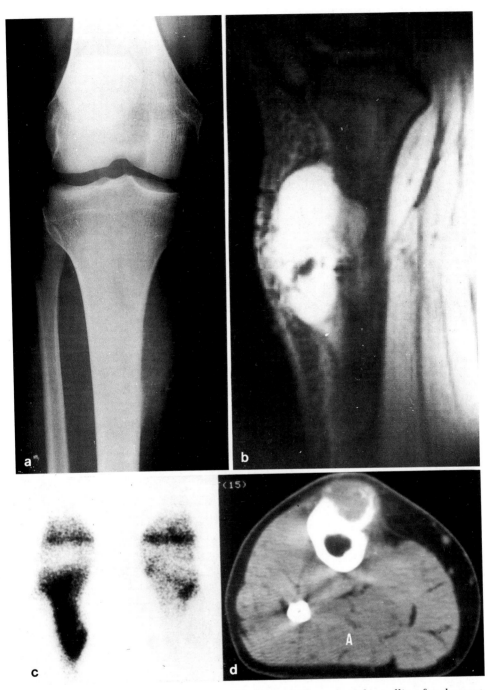

FIG. 421. - Periosteal osteosarcoma in a male aged 15 years with swelling for the past 3 months and little pain. Typical radiographic, MRI, bone scan and CAT aspects. The tumor did not invade the cortex and the medullary canal. Histologically, grade 3 chondroblastic osteosarcoma.

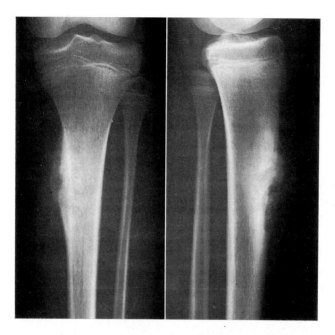

FIG. 422. - Periosteal osteosarcoma in a female aged 13 years. The patient was submitted to resection of the diaphyseal segment, no signs of recurrence or metastasis after 36 years.

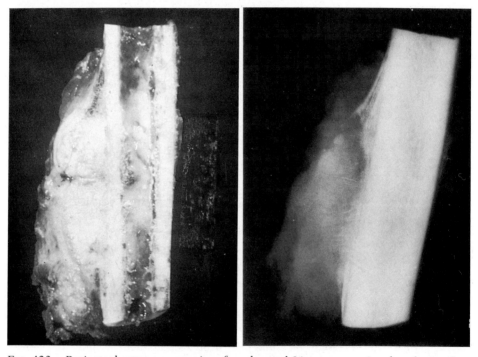

FIG. 423. - Periosteal osteosarcoma in a female aged 21 years, previously submitted to marginal excision, with recurrence after 6 months. Segment of wide resection. The tumor was not present in the medullary canal, the cortex was not invaded. New recurrence in the soft tissues after 1 year. This was excised and the patient had no evidence of disease after 16 years.

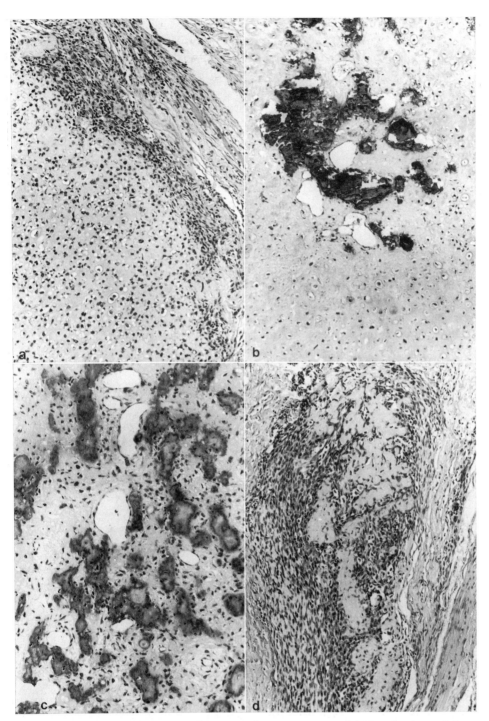

FIG. 424. - Histological aspects of periosteal osteosarcoma. (a) Neoplastic nodule at the surface, covered with its fibrous pseudocapsule (upper to the right). The aspect is that of a chondrosarcoma, with undifferentiated cells at the periphery of the lobule. (b) Calcification of the neoplastic cartilage. (c) Production of very immature osteoid tissue fading into the cartilaginous tissue. (d) Production of typical osteoid tissue by the neoplastic cells (*Hemat.-eos.*, 125, 125, 125, 125 x).

mon variety of O.S. which must be set apart as a distinct entity in its own (Fig. 420). Generally, it is located in the diaphysis of the long bones, particularly in the tibia and the femur, occurring during childhood-young age.

Radiographically, it appears to be a fusiform elevation of the periosteum, with erosion of the cortex from the outside but without any invasion, at least during its not too advanced phases, of the medullary canal (Figs. 421-423). Thin and faded ossification spiculae perpendicular to the cortex run through the radiolucent subperiosteal tumoral mass. This aspect helps to differentiate it from periosteal chondrosarcoma and from parosteal osteosarcoma (furthermore, these generally do not initiate from the diaphysis).

Histologically, periosteal O.S. is often and extensively chondroblastic but, alongside the cartilage, there is always neoplastic osteogenesis (Fig. 424). It has a mixed structure, with large mesenchymal spindle-stellate cells which are particularly crowded around the vessels and at the periphery of the large lobules; towards the center of the lobules the cells are rarefied due to chondroid differentiation which may be very immature, or more differentiated. In other fields, there is neoplastic production of osteoid tissue, which is nearly always immature, but which may usually be distinguished from neoplastic cartilage and from aspects of ossification of the cartilage and of reactive ossification. The chondroblastic aspects prevail over the osteoblastic ones. The neoplastic cartilage is not as well-differentiated as it is in periosteal chondrosarcoma. If observation were limited to chondroblastic fields alone, in most cases chondrosarcoma would be diagnosed. The bed and the borders of the tumor are often constituted by abundant reactive bone tissue, the intertrabecular spaces of which are partially infiltrated by the tumor. Finally, the picture is varied by necrosis, more frequently in the center of the lobules, and by calcification and ossification of the neoplastic cartilage. The histological grade is 3, less often 2. (There are also rare cases of O.S. which has developed at the surface of the bone and which is grade 4: these are classified together with classic O.S., for treatment and prognosis are the same).

The **prognosis** is much less severe than that of classic O.S. Here, too, the general rule that periosteal tumors are less malignant than their central equivalents is confirmed. The **treatment** of choice is wide resection of the skeletal segment affected. Generally, chemotherapy is not carried out. The incidence of metastases is rather low.

REFERENCES

1940   BRODERS A.C.: The microscopic grading of cancer. In: *Treatment of cancer and allied diseases*. G. P. Pack, E. M. Livingston, Paul B. Hoeber, New York.

1954   MAGNANI G.: Un caso di sarcoma osteogenico sclerosante a localizzazione multipla. *Archivio Putti di Chirurgia degli Organi di Movimento*, **4**, 454-454.

1955   CADE S.: Osteogenic sarcoma. A study based on 133 patients. *Journal of Royal College of Surgeons*, **1**, 79-111.

1957   CARROLL R. E.: Osteogenic sarcoma in the hand. *Journal of Bone and Joint Surgery*, **39-A**, 325-331.

1960 HAYLES A. B., DAHLIN D. C., COVENTRY M. B.: Osteogenic sarcoma in children. *Journal of the American Medical Association*, **174**, 1174-1177.

1961 DROMPP B. W.: Bilateral osteosarcoma in the phalanges of the hand. *Journal of Bone and Joint Surgery*, **43-A**, 199-204.

1961 PRICE C. H. G.: Osteogenic sarcoma. An analysis of survival and its relationship to histological grading and structure. *Journal of Bone and Joint Surgery*, **43-B**, 300-313.

1962 PRICE C. H. G.: The incidence of osteogenic sarcoma in South-West England and its relationship to Paget's disease of bone. *Journal of Bone and Joint Surgery*, **44-B**, 366-376.

1962 WEINFELD M. S., DUDLEY H. R. Jr.: Osteogenic sarcoma. A follow-up study of the ninety-four cases observed at the Massachusetts General Hospital from 1920 to 1960. *Journal of Bone and Joint Surgery*, **44-A**, 269-276.

1964 MIKI I., AZUMA H., TATEISHI A., ITO T., MITSUDA S., MIKAMI R., IWAKURA R., AZUMA A., ABE M.: Treatment of malignant tumors of the extremities by regional perfusion: a clinical report of twenty-one cases including nineteen osteogenic sarcomas. *Journal Japanensis of Orthopaedic Association*, **37**, 1-10.

1964 PHELAN J. T., CABRERA A.: Osteosarcoma of bone. *Surgery, Gynecology and Obstetrics*, **118**, 330-336.

1965 DAVIDSON J. W., CHACHA P. B., JAMES W.: Multiple osteosarcoma. Report of a case. *Journal of Bone and Joint Surgery*, **47-B**, 537-541.

1965 SPRATT J. S. Jr.: The rates of growth of skeletal sarcomas. *Cancer*, **18**, 14-24.

1966 GOIDINICH I. F., BATTAGLIA L., LENZI L., SILVA E.: Osteogenic sarcoma. Analysis of factors influencing prognosis in 100 cases. *Clinical Orthopedics*, **48**, 209-232.

1966 HARMON T. P., NORTON K. S.: Osteogenic sarcoma in four siblings. *Journal of Bone and Joint Surgery*, **48-B**, 493-498.

1966 MCKENNA R. J., SCHWINN C. P., SOONG K. Y., HIGINBOTHAM N. L.: Sarcomata of the osteogenic series (osteosarcoma, fibrosarcoma, chondrosarcoma, parosteal osteogenic sarcoma, and sarcomata arising in abnormal bone). An analysis of 552 cases. *Journal of Bone and Joint Surgery*, **48-A**, 1-26.

1966 NETHERLANDS COMMITTEE ON BONE TUMOUR: *Radiological atlas of bone tumours*. Volume I, Mouton e Co., The Hague, Parigi.

1966 TJALMA R. A.: Canine bone sarcoma: extimation of relative risk as a function of body size. *Journal National Cancer Institute*, **36**, 1137-1150.

1967 DAHLIN D. C., COVENTRY M. B.: Osteogenic sarcoma. A study of six hundred cases. *Journal of Bone and Joint Surgery*, **49-A**, 101-110.

1967 FRAUMENI J. F. Jr.: Stature and malignant tumors of bone in childood and adolescence. *Cancer*, **20**, 967-973.

1967 GARRINGTON G. E., SCOFIELD H. H., CORNYN J., POOKER S. P.: Osteosarcoma of the jaws. Analysis of 56 cases. *Cancer*, **20**, 377-391.

1967 TALERMAN A., GOLDING J. S. R., KIRKPATRICK D.: Bone tumours in Jamaica. *Journal of Bone and Joint Surgery*, **49-B**, 802-805.

1967 WOOD H. L. C.: Increased epiphyseal density in bone sarcoma. Report of two cases. *Journal of Bone and Joint Surgery*, **49-B**, 757-761.

1968 LAWBEER L.: Multifocal osteosarcomatosis. A rare entity. *Bulletin of Pathology*, **9**, 52-53.

1968 O'HARA J. M., HUTTER R. V. P., FOOTE F. W. Jr., MILLER T., WOODARD H. Q.: An analysis of thirty patients surviving longer than ten years after treatment for osteogenic sarcoma. *Journal of Bone and Joint Surgery*, **50-A**, 335-354.

1968 POPPE E., LIVERNOL K., EFSKIND J.: Osteosarcoma. *Acta Chirurgica Scandinavica*, **134**, 54%-556.

1969 AMSTUTZ H. C.: Multiple osteogenic sarcomata, metastatic or multicentric. Report of two cases and review of literature. *Cancer*, **24**, 923-931.

1969 NOSANCHUK J. S., WENTHERBEE L., BRODY G. L.: Osteogenic sarcoma. Prognosis related to epiphyseal closure. *Journal of the American Medical Association*, **208**, 2439-2441.

1970 CAMPANACCI M.: Manifestazioni atipiche dell'osteosarcoma. *Chirurgia degli Organi di Movimento*, **59**, 346-348.

1970   ENNEKING W. F.: Passive cellular immunity in the management of sarcoma. *Journal of Bone and Joint Surgery*, **52-B**, 779-779.

1970   EPSTEIN L. J., BIXLER D., BENET J. E.: An incidence of familial cancer. Including 3 cases of osteogenic sarcoma. *Cancer*, **25**, 889-891.

1970   GHADIALLY F. N., PRAN N. M.: Ultrastructure of osteogenic sarcoma. *Cancer*, **2/**, 1457-1467.

1970   MARCOVE R. S., MIKE V., HAJEK J. V., LEVIN A. G., HUTTER R. V. P.: Osteogenic sarcoma under the age of twentyone. A review of 145 operative cases. *Journal of Bone and Joint Surgery*, **52-A**, 411-423.

1970   MARSH H. O., CHOI C. B.: Primary osteogenic sarcoma of the cervical spine originally mistaken for benign osteoblastoma. A case report. *Journal of Bone and Joint Surgery*, **52-A**, 1467-1471.

1970   SWEETNAM R.: Osteosarcoma. *Journal of Bone and Joint Surgery*, **52-B**, 783-784.

1971   OHNO T.: Bronchial artery infusion with anticancer agents in the treatment of osteosarcoma. *Cancer*, **27**, 549-557.

1972   CACERES E., ZAHARIA M.: Massive preoperative radiation therapy in the treatment of osteogenic sarcoma. *Cancer*, **30**, 634-638.

1972   CAMPANACCI M., PIZZOFERRATO A.: Osteosarcoma emorragico. *Chirurgia degli Organi di Movimento*, **60**, 409-421.

1972   JENKIN R. D. T., ALLT W. E. C., FITZPATRICK P. J.: Osteosarcoma. *Cancer*, **30**, 393-400.

1972   MARSH B., FLYNN L., ENNEKING W.: Immunologic aspects of osteosarcoma and their application to therapy. *Journal of Bone and Joint Surgery*, **54-A**, 1367-1397.

1972   TRIFAUD A., MEARY R.: *Pronostic et traitment des sarcomes ostéogéniques.* Masson e Cie, Parigi.

1973   COHEN A. M.: Host immunity to growing sarcomas: tumor specific serum inhibition of a tumor specific cellular immunity. *Cancer*, **31**, 81-89.

1973   FITZGERALD R. H. Jr., DAHLIN D. C., SIM F. H.: Multiple metachronous osteogenic sarcoma: report of twelve cases with two long-term survivors. *Journal of Bone and Joint Surgery*, **55-A**, 595-605.

1973   MARCOVE R. C., MIKÈ V., HUVOS A. G., CHESTER M. S., LEVIN A. G.: Autogenous lysed cell vaccine in the treatment of osteogenic sarcoma - a preliminary report on fifteen cases. *Bone-Certain aspects of neoplasia*. Proceedings 24th Symposium Colston Research Society, Butterworths, London.

1974   ELLMAN H., GOLD R. H., MIRRA J. M.: Roentgenographically «benign» but rapidly lethal diaphyseal osteosarcoma. A case Report. *Journal of Bone and Joint Surgery*, **56-A**, 1267-1269.

1974   KREMENTZ E. T., MANSELL P. W. A., HORNUNG M. O., SAMUELS M. S., SUTHERLAND C. A., BENES E. N.: Immunotherapy of malignant disease; the use of viable sensitized lumphocites or transfer factor prepared from sensitized lymphocytes. *Cancer*, **33**, 394-401.

1974   LARSSON S. E., LORENTZON P.: The incidence of malignant primary bone tumours in relation to age, sex, and site. *Journal of Bone and Joint Surgery*, **56-B**, 534-540.

1974   LARSSON S. E., LORENTZON R.: The geographic variation of the incidence of malignant primary bone tumours in Sweden. *Journal of Bone and Joint Surgery*, **56-A**, 592-600.

1974   LEWIS R. J., LOTZ M. J.: Medullary extension of osteosarcoma. *Cancer*, **33**, 371-375.

1974   PRITCHARD D. J., REILLY C. A., FINKEL M. P., IVINS J. C.: Cytotoxicity of human osteosarcoma sera to hamster sarcoma cells. *Cancer*, **34**, 1935-1939.

1974   TWOMEY P. L., CATALONA W. J., CHRETIEN P. B.: Cellular immunity in cured cancer patients, *Cancer*, **33**, 435-440.

1975   BRAUN S. R., DOPICO G. A., OLSON C. E., CALDWELL W.: Low-dose radiation pneumonitis. *Cancer*, **35**, 1322-1324.

1975   CAMPANACCI M., CERVELLATI C.: Osteosarcoma. A review of 345 cases. *Italian Journal of Orthopaedics and Traumatology*, **1**, 5-22.

1975   DAHLIN D. C.: Pathology of osteosarcoma. *Clinical Orthopaedics*, **111**, 23-32.

1975   ENNEKING W. F., KAGAN A.: «Skip» metastases in osteosarcoma. *Cancer*, **36**, 2192-2205.

1975   FRIEDLAENDER G. E., MITSCHELL M. S.: A laboratory model for the study of the immunobiology of osteosarcoma. *Cancer*, **36**, 1631-1639.

1975   MARCOVE R. C., MARTINI N., ROSEN G.: The treatment of pulmonary metastasis in osteogenic sarcoma. *Clinical Orthopaedics*, **111**, 65-70.

1975   PASCHALL H. A., PASCHALL M. M.: Electron microscopic observations of 20 human osteosarcomas. *Clinical Orthopaedics*, **111**, 42-56.

1975   PRICE C. H. G., ZHUBER K., SALZER M. K., SALZER M., WILLERT H. G., IMMENKAMP M., GROH P., MATEJOVSKY Z., KEYL W.: Osteosarcoma in children. A study of 125 cases. *Journal of Bone and Joint Surgery*, **57-B**, 341-345.

1975   PRITCHARD D. J., FINKEL M. P., REILLY C. A.: The etiology of osteosarcoma. A review of current considerations. *Clinical Orthopaedics*, **111**, 14-22.

1975   ROSEN G., TAN C., SANMANEECHAL A., BEATTLE E., MARCOVE R, MURPHY M. L.: The rationale for multiple drug chemiotherapy in the treatment of osteogenic sarcoma. *Cancer*, **35**, 936-945.

1976   CZITROM A. A., PRITZKER K. P. H., LANGER F., GROSS A. E., LUK S. C.: Virus-induced osteosarcoma in rats. *Journal of Bone and Joint Surgery*, **58-A**, 303-308.

1976   FRIEDLAENDER G. E., MITCHELL M. S.: A virally induced osteosarcoma in rats. *Journal of Bone and Joint Surgery*, **58-A**, 295-302.

1976   MATSUNO T., UNNI K. K., MC LEOD R. A., DAHLIN D. C.: Telangiectatic osteogenic sarcoma. *Cancer*, **38**, 2538-2547.

1976   SPANOS P. K., PAYNE W. S., IVINS J. C., PRITCHARD D. J.: Pulmonary resection for metastatic osteogenic sarcoma. *Journal of Bone and Joint Surgery*, **58-A**, 624-628.

1976   SUTOW W. W., GEHAN E. A., VIETTI T. J., FRIAS A. E., DYMENT P. G.: Multidrug chemotherapy in primary treatment of osteosarcoma. *Jurnal of Bone and Joint Surgery*, **58-A**, 629-633.

1976   UNNI K. K., DAHLIN D. C., BEABOUT J. W.: Periosteal osteogenic sarcoma. *Cancer*, **37**, 2476-2485.

1976   WILLIAMS A. H., SCHWINN C. P., PARKER J. W.: The ultrastructure of osteosarcoma. *Cancer*, **37**, 1293-1301.

1977   DAHLIN D. C.: Case report 27. *Skeletal Radiology*, **1**, 249-252.

1977   DAHLIN D. C., UNNI K. K.: Osteosarcoma of bone and its important recognizable varietes. *American Journal of Surgical Pathology*, **1**, 61-72.

1977   JAFFE N., FREI E., TRAGGIN D., WATTS H.: Weekly high-dose methotrexate-citrovorum factor in osteogenic sarcoma. *Cancer*, **39**, 45-50.

1977   MILLER C. W., McLAUGHLIN R. E.: Osteosarcoma in siblings. *Journal of Bone and Joint Surgery*, **59-A**, 261-262.

1977   PRATT CH., SHANKS E., HUSTU O., RIVERA G., SMITH J., MAHESH K.: Adjuvant multiple drug chemotherapy for osteosarcoma of the extremity. *Cancer*, **39**, 51-57.

1977   SPJUT H. J., AYALA A. G., DE SANTOS L. A., MURRAY J. A.: Periosteal osteosarcoma, in *Management of primary bone and soft tissue tumours*, Year Book Medical Publishers, Chicago-London.

1977   UNNI K. K., DAHLIN D. C., McLEOD R. A., PRITCHARD D. J.: Intraosseous well-differentiated osteosarcoma. *Cancer*, **40**, 1337-1347.

1978   ENNEKING W. F., KAGAN A.: Transepiphyseal extension of osteosarcoma: incidence, mechanism, and implications. *Cancer*, **41**, 1526-1537.

1978   ROSEN G., HUVOS A. G., MOSENDE C., BEATTIE E. J., EXELBY P. R., CAPPAROS B., MARCOVE R. C.: Chemotherapy and thoracotomy for metastatic osteogenic sarcoma. A model for adjuvant chemotherapy and the rationale for the timing of thoracic surgery. *Cancer*, **41**, 841-849.

1979   MAHONEY J. P., SPANIER S. S., MORRIS J. L.: Multifocal osteosarcoma. A case report with review of the literature. *Cancer*, **44**, 1897-1907.

1979   ROSEN G., MARCOVE R.C., CAPARROS B., NIRENBERG A., KOSLOFF C., HUVOS A.G.: Primary osteogenic sarcoma. The rationale for preoperative chemotherapy and delayed surgery. *Cancer*, **43**, 2163-2177.

1979   SIM F. H., IVINS J. C., PRITCHARD D.: Osteosarcoma: new developments in diagnosis and treatment. *Journal of Bone and Joint Surgery*, **61-B**, 513-514.

1979   SIM F. H., UNNI K. K., BEABOUT J. W., DAHLIN D. C.: Osteosarcoma with small cells simulating Ewing's tumour. *Journal of Bone and Joint Surgery*, **61-A**, 207-215.

1979   THORPE W. P., REILLY J. J., ROSENBERG S. A.: Prognostic significance of alkaline phosphatase measurements in patients with osteogenic sarcoma receiving chemotherapy. *Cancer*, **43**, 2178-2181.

1980   CAMPANACCI M., BACCI G., PAGANI P., GIUNTI A.: Multiple drug chemotherapy for the primary treatment of osteosarcoma of the extremities. *Journal of Bone and Joint Surgery*, **62-B**, 93-101.

1980   CAMPANACCI M., LAUS M.: Local recurrence after amputation for osteosarcoma. *Journal of Bone and Joint Surgery*, **62-B**, 201, 207.

1980   DAHLIN D.C.: The problems in assessment of the new treatment regimens of osteosarcoma. *Clinical Orthopaedics*, **153**, 81-85.

1980   LAUS M.: Multicentric osteosarcoma. *Italian Journal of Orthopedics and Traumatology*, **6**, 249-254.

1980   REDDICK R., MICHLETICH H., LEVINE A., TRICHE T.: Osteogenic sarcoma. A study of ultrastructure. *Cancer*, **45**, 64-71.

1981   CAMPANACCI M., BACCI G., BERTONI F., PICCI P., MINUTILLO A., FRANCESCHI N.: The treatment of osteosarcoma of the extremities. Twenty year's experience at the Istituto Ortopedico Rizzoli. *Cancer*, **48**, 1569-1581.

1981   CAMPANACCI M., BERTONI F., CAPANNA R., CERVELLATI C.: Central osteosarcoma of low grade malignancy. *Italian Journal of Orthopedics and Traumatology*, **7**, 71-78.

1981   DAHLIN D. C.: The problems in assessment of new treatment regimens in osteosarcoma. *Clinical Orthopedics*, **153**, 81-85.

1981   LARSSON S. E., LORENZON R., WEDREN M., BOQUIST L.: The prognosis in osteosarcoma. *International Orthopedics* (SICOT), **5**, 305-310.

1981   LAWSON J.P., BARWICK K.W.: Case report 162: periosteal osteosarcoma of rib. *Skeletal Radiology*, **7**, 63-65.

1981   SUTOW W. W.: Multidrug chemotherapy in osteosarcoma. *Clinical Orthopedics*, **153**, 67-72.

1981   WEATHERBY R. P., DAHLIN D. C., IVINS J. C.: Postradiation sarcoma of bone. Review of 78 Mayo Clinic cases. *Mayo Clinic Proceedings*, **56**, 294-306.

1982   BACCI G., PICCI P., CALDERONI P., FIGUS E., BORGHI A.: Full lung tomograms and bone scanning in the initial work-up of patients with osteogenic sarcoma. *European Journal of Cancer*, **18**, 967-972.

1982   BERTONI F., BORIANI S., CAMPANACCI M.: Periosteal chondrosarcoma and periosteal osteosarcoma. Two distinct entities. *Journal of Bone and Joint Surgery*, **64-B**, 370-376.

1982   BLEYER W. A., HAAS J. E., PEIGL P., GREENLEE T. K., SCHALLER R. T. Jr.: Improved three-year disease-free survival in osteogenic sarcoma. Efficacy of adjunctive chemotherapy. *Journal of Bone and Joint Surgery*, **64-B**, 233-238.

1982   HUVOS A.G., ROSEN G., BRETSKY S., BUTLER A.: Teleangiectatic osteosarcoma. A clinico-pathologic study of 124 patients. *Cancer*, **49**, 1679-1689.

1982   MARTIN S.L., DWYER A., KISSANE J.M., COSTA J.: Small-cell osteosarcoma *Cancer*, **50**, 990-996.

1982   PICCI P., CALDERONI P., CAGNANO R., MINUTILLO A., GHERLINZONI F., BACCI: The hypotetical change in the natural history of osteosarcoma. The experience at the Bone Tumor Centre of the Istituto Ortopedico Rizzoli. *Chemioterapia*, **1**, 420-425.

1982   ROSEN G., CAPARROS B., HUVOS A. G., KOSLOFF C., NIRENBERG A., CACAVIO A., MARCOVE R. C., LANE J. M., MEHTA B., URBAN C.: Preoperative chemotherapy for osteogenic sarcoma: selection of postoperative adjuvant chemotherapy based on the response of the primary tumor to preoperative chemotherapy. *Cancer*, **49**, 1221-1230.

1982   TAUBER R., LANGUEPIN A.: Sarcomes osseux aprés radiotherapie. *Revue de Chirurgie Orthopedique*, **68**, 327-331.

1983   HUDSON T. M., SCHIEBLER M., SPRINGFIELD D. S., HAWKINS I. F. Jr., ENNEKING W. F., SPANIER S. S.: Radiologic imagin of osteosarcoma: role in planning surgical treatment. *Skel. Radiol.*, **10**, 137-146.

1983   PICCI P., BACCI G., BERTONI F., CALDERONI P., CAPANNA R., CERVELLATI C., GHERLINZONI F., GUERRA A., GIUNTI A., GUERNELLI N., MERCURI M., CAMPANACCI M.: Combined treatment in osteosarcoma. In «*Modern Trends in Orthopaedic surgery*», edited by M. Campanacci *et al.*. A. Gaggi Ed., Bologna.

1983   PICCI P., GHERLINZONI F., GUERRA A.: Intracortical osteosarcoma: rare entity or early manifestation of classical osteosarcoma? *Skeletal Radiology*, **9**, 255-258.

1984   CAMPANACCI M.: Terapia e prognosi dell'osteosarcoma: idee e numeri che cambiano. *Chirurgia Organi Movimento*, **69**, 7-9.

1984   GIULIANO A.E., FEIG S., EILBER F.R.: Changing metastatic patterns of osteosarcoma. *Cancer*, **54**, 2160-2164.

1984   JACOBS P. A.: Limb salvage and rotationplasty for osteosarcoma in children. *Clinical Orthopedics*, **188**, 217-222.

1985   BACCI G., CAMPANACCI M., PICCI P., GHERLINZONI F., CAPANNA R., JAFFE N., BETTELLI G.: Adjuvant chemotherapy with Adriamycin and high and moderate dose of Methotrexate for osteosarcoma of the extremities: an evaluation of results and comparison with a concurrent group treated with surgery alone. *Proceedings A.S.C.O.*, Huston, **495**, p. 127.

1985   BERTONI F., UNNI K., Mc LEOD R., DAHLIN D.: Osteosarcoma resembling osteoblastoma. *Cancer*, **55**, 416-426.

1985   DE SANTOS L. A., EDEIKEN B. S.: Subtle early osteosarcoma. *Skeletal Radiology*, **13**, 44-48.

1985   ESSELINCK W., HUAUX J. P., DEVOGELAER J. P., NOEL H., MALGHEM J., MALDAGUE B., GODISCAL H.: Transformation sarcomateuse dans la maladie osseuse del Paget. *Acta Orthopedica Belgica*, **51**, 5-17.

1985   GUERRA A., BACCI G., GHERLINZONI F.: Le traitement chirurgical conservateur dans les sarcomes osteogeniques des membres. *Revue de Chirurgie Orthopedique*, **71**, 463-471.

1985   HALL R., ROBINSON L., MALAWER M., DUHNAM W.: Periosteal osteosarcoma. *Cancer*, **55**, 165-171.

1985   HUVOS A.G., WOODARD H.Q., CAHAN W.G., HIGINBOTHAM N.L., STEWART F.W., BUTLER A., BRETSKY S.S.: Postirradiation osteogenic sarcoma of bone and soft tissue. A clinico-pathologic study of 66 patients. *Cancer*, **55**, 1244-1255.

1985   KALIFA C., VANDEL D., LEMERLE J.: La chemiothérapie des sarcomes ostéogéniques. *Revue de Chirurgie Orthopedique*, **71**, 429-434.

1985   LEVINE E., DE SMET A.A., HUNTRAKOON M.: Juxtacortical osteosarcoma: a radiologic and histologic spectrum. *Skeletal Radiology*, **14**, 38-46.

1985   PICCI P., BACCI G., CAMPANACCI M., GASPARINI M., PILOTTI S., CERASOLI S., BERTONI F., GUERRA A., CAPANNA R., ALBISINNI U., GALLETTI S., GHERLINZONI F., CALDERONI P., SUDANESE A., BALDINI N., BERNINI M., JAFFE N.: Histological evaluation of necrosis in osteosarcoma induced by chemotherapy. Regional mapping of viable and non viable tumor. *Cancer*, **56**, 1515-1521.

1985   ROSEN G.: Preoperative (neoadjuvant) chemotherapy for osteogenic sarcoma: a ten-year experience. *Orthopaedics*, **8**, 659-664.

1985   TAYLOR W. F., IVINS J. C., PRITCHARD D. J., DAHLIN D. C., GILCHRIST G. S., EDMONDSON J. H.: Trends and variability in survival among patients with osteosarcoma: a 7 year update. *Mayo Clinic Proceedings*, **60**, 91-104.

1985   XIPELL J.M., RUSH J.: Well-differentiated intraosseous osteosarcoma of the left femur. *Skeletal Radiology*, **14**, 312-316.

1986   HUVOS A.G.: Osteogenic sarcoma of bones and soft tissues in older persons. A clinicopathologic analysis of 117 patients older than 60. *Cancer*, **57**, 1442-1449.

1986   LANE J.M., HURSON B., BOLAND P.J., GLASSER D.B. : Osteogenic sarcoma. *Clinical Orthopaedics*, **204**, 93-110.

1986   LINK M., GOORIN A.M., MISER A.W., GREEN A., PRATT C.B., BELASCO J.B., PRIT-
       CHARD J., MALPAS J.S., BAKER A.R., KIRKPATRICK J.A., AYALA A.G., SHUSTER
       J.J., ABELSON H.T., SIMONE J.V., VIETTI T.J.: The effect of adjuvant chemo-
       therapy on relapse–free survival in patients with osteosarcoma of the extre-
       mity. *New England Journal of Medicine*, **314**, 1600-1606.

1986   ROSEN G., HUVOS A.G., MARCOVE R., NIRENBERG A.: Telangiectatic osteogenic
       sarcoma. Improved survival with combination chemotherapy. *Clinical Ortho-
       paedics*, **207**, 164-173.

1986   SUNDARAM M., HERBOLD D., MC GUIRE M.H.: Case report 370: low-grade intra-
       medullary osteosarcoma. *Skeletal Radiology*, **15**, 338-342.

1986   WEINER M., HARRIS M., LEWIS M., JONES R., SHERRY H., FEURER E., JOHNSON L.,
       LAHMAN E.: Neoadjuvant high-dose methotrexate, cisplatin and doxorubicin
       for management of patients with non-metastatic osteosarcoma. *Cancer
       Treatment Report*, **70**, 1431-1432.

1987   BACCI G., SPRINGFIELD D., CAPANNA R., PICCI P., GUERRA A., ALBISINNI U., RUG-
       GIERI P., BIAGINI R., CAMPANACCI M.: Neoadjuvant chemotherapy for osteo-
       sarcoma of the extremity. *Clinical Orthopaedics*, **224**, 268-276.

1987   EDEIKEN J., RAYMOND A.K., AYALA A.G., BENJAMIN R.S., MURRAY J.A., CARRASCO
       H.C.: Small-cell osteosarcoma. *Skeletal Radiology*, **16**, 621-628.

1987   HEATER K., COLLINS P.A.: Osteosarcoma in association with infarction of bone.
       Report of two cases. *Journal of Bone and Joint Surgery*, **69-A**, 300-302.

1987   JAFFE N., SPEARS R., EFTEKHARI F., ROBERTSON R., CANGIA A., TAKAVE Y., CARRA-
       SCO H., WALLACE S., AYALA A., RAIMOND K., WANG Y.M.: Pathologic fracture
       in osteosarcoma. Impact of chemotherapy on primary tumor and survival.
       Cancer, **59**, 701-709.

1987   PROVISOR A., NACHMAN J., KRAILO M., ETTINGER L., HAMMOND D.: Treatment
       of non-metastatic osteogenic sarcoma (os) of the extremities with pre and
       postoperative chemotherapy. In « *Proceedings twenty-third annual Meeting of
       ASCO* », Atlanta, USA.

1987   SUNDARAM M., MC GUIRE M.H., HERBOLD D.R.: Magnetic resonance imaging of
       osteosarcoma. *Skeletal Radiology*, **16**, 23-29.

1987   VANEL D., TCHENG S., CONTESSO G., ZAFRANI B., KALIFA C., DUBOUSSET J., KRON P.:
       The radiological appearances of telangiectatic osteosarcoma. A study of 14
       cases. *Skeletal Radiology*, **16**, 196-200.

1988   ALBISINNI U., GALLETTI S., MANFRINI M., PIGNATTI G., BIAGINI R., PICCI P.,
       BACCI G., CAPANNA R.: Valutazione angiografica della risposta dell'osteosar-
       coma alla chemioterapia neoadiuvante. *Radiologia Medica*, **75**, 381-385.

1988   BACCI G., AVELLA M., PICCI P., BRICCOLI A., DALLARI D., CAMPANACCI M.: Meta-
       static patterns in osteosarcoma. *Tumori*, **74**, 421-428.

1988   BENEDICT W.F., FUNG Y.T., MURPHREE A.L.: The gene responsible for the deve-
       lopment of retinoblastoma and osteosarcoma. *Cancer*, **62**, 1961-1964.

1988   BENJAMIN R.S., CHAWLA S.P., CARRASCO C., RAYMOND A.K., FANNING T., WALLACE
       S., AYALA A.G., MURRAY J.: Arterial infusion in the treatment of osteosarcoma.
       In « *Recent Concepts in Sarcoma Treatment* », edited by Rayan J.R. and
       Baker O., Academic Publishers, Kluwer.

1988   BENTZEN S.M., POUSEN M.S., KAAE S., JENSEN M., JOHANSEN M., MOURIDSEN H.T.,
       DAUGAARD S., ARNOLDI C.: Prognostic factors in osteosarcoma. A regression
       analysis. *Cancer*, **62**, 194-202.

1988   BURGERS J.M.V., VAN GLABBEKE M., BUSSON A., COHEN P. MAZABRAUD A.R., ABBA-
       TUCCI J.S., KALIFA C., TUBIANA M., LEMERLE J.S., VOUTE P.A., VAN OOSTEROM A.,
       WAGENER TH, VAN DER WERF-MESSING B., SOMERS R., DUEZ N.: Osteosarcoma
       of the limbs: report of the EORTC-SIOP 03 Trial 20781 investigating the
       value of adjuvant treatment with chemotherapy and/or prophylactic lung
       irradiation. *Cancer*, **61**, 1024-1031.

1988   FRENCH BONE TUMOR STUDY GROUP: Age and dose of chemotherapy as major
       prognostic factors in a trial of adjuvant therapy of osteosarcoma combining
       two alternating drug combinations and early prophylactic lung irradiation.
       Cancer, **61**, 1304-1311.

1988   SCHAJOWICZ F., MC GUIRE M.H., SANTIM ARAUJO E., MUSCOLO D.L., GITELIS S.:

Osteosarcomas arising on the surfaces of long bones. *Journal of Bone and Joint Surgery*, **70-A**, 555-564.

1988 SPRINGFIELD D.S., SCHMIDT R., GRAHAM POLE J., MARCUS R.B., SPANIER S.S., ENNEKING W.F.: Surgical treatment for osteosarcoma. *Journal of Bone and Joint Surgery*, **70-A**, 1124-1130.

1988 WHITE V.A., FANNING C.M., AYALA A.G., RAYMOND K., CARRASCO C.M., MURRAY J.A. Osteosarcoma and the role of fine-needle aspiration. A study of 51 cases. *Cancer*, **62**, 1238-1246.

1988 WINKLER K., BERON G., DELLING G., HEISE U., KABISCH H., PURFURST C., BERGER J., RITTER J., JURGENS H., GEREIN V., GRF N., RUSSE W., GRUEMAYER E.R., ERTELT W., KOTZ R., PREUSSER P., PRINDULL G., BRADEIS W., LANDBECK G.: Neoadjuvant chemotherapy of osteosarcoma: results of a randomized cooperative trial (COSS-82) with salvage chemotherapy based on histological tumor response. *Journal of Clinical Oncology*, **6**, 329-337.

1989 AYALA A.G., RO J.Y., RAYMOND A.K., JAFFE N., CHAWLA S., CARRASCO H., LINK M., JIMENEZ J., EDEIKEN J.. WALLACE S., MURRAY J.A., BENJAMIN R.: Small-cell osteosarcoma: a clinicopathologic study of 27 cases. *Cancer*, **64**, 2162-2173.

1989 BELLI L., SCHOLL S., LIVARTOWSKI A., ASHBY M., PALANGIE TH., LEVASSEUR PH., POUILLAT P.: Resection of pulmonary metastases in ostosarcoma. A retrospective analysis of 44 patients. *Cancer*, **63**, 2546-2550.

1989 BERTONI F., PRESENT D., BACCHINI P., PIGNATTI G., PICCI P., CAMPANACCI M.: The Istituto Rizzoli experience with small-cell osteosarcoma. *Cancer*, **64**, 2591-2599.

1989 KLEIN M.J., KENAN S., LEWIS M.M.: Osteosarcoma: clinical and pathological considerations. *Orthopaedic Clinics of North America*, **20**, 327-345.

1989 SIEGEL R.D., RYAN L.M., ANTMAN K.M.: Osteosarcoma in the adults. One Istitution's experience. *Clinical Orthopaedics*, **240**, 261-269.

1989 TAYLOR W.F., IVINS J.C., UNNI K.K., BEABOUT J., GOLENZER H., BLACK L.: Prognostic variable in osteosarcoma a multiinstitutional study. *Journal of National Cancer Institute*, **81**, 21-30.

1990 BACCI G., PICCI P., RUGGIERI P., MERCURI M., AVELLA M., CAPANNA R., BRACH DEL PREVER A., MANCINI A., GHERLINZONI F., PADOVANI G., LEONESSA C., BIAGINI R., FERRARO A., FERRUZZI A., CAZZOLA A., MANFRINI M., CAMPANACCI M.: Primary chemotherapy and delayed surgery (neoadjuvant chemotherapy) for osteosarcoma of the extremities. *Cancer*, **65**, 2539-2553.

1990 KURT A.M., UNNI K.K., MC LEOD R.A., PRITCHARD D.J.: Low-grade intraosseous osteosarcoma. *Cancer*, **65**, 1418-1428.

1990 SALEM R.A., GRAHAM-POLE J., CASSANO W., ABBOT F., VANDER GRIEND R.A., DICKSON N., METHA P., HEARE M., KEDAR A., HEARE T., GROSS S.: Response of osteogenic sarcoma to the combination of etoposide and cyclophosphamide as neoadjuvant chemotherapy. *Cancer*, **65**, 861-865.

1990 SPANIER S.S., SHUSTER J.J., VANDER GRIEND R.A.: The effect of local extent of the tumor on prognosis in osteosarcoma. *Journal of Bone and Joint Surgery*, **72-A**, 643-653.

1990 WUISMAN P., ENNEKING W.F.: Prognosis for patients who have osteosarcoma with skip metastasis. *Journal of Bone and Joint Surgery*, **72-A**, 60-68.

OSTEOSARCOMATOSIS
(Synonyms: multiple, multifocal or multicentric osteosarcoma, sclerosing osteosarcomatosis)

This is constituted by multiple foci of O.S. which occur in different areas of the skeleton, in an apparently simultaneous manner, or at brief intervals of time one from the other (Fig. 425).

It is an exceptionally rare form. It nearly always occurs prior to 15 years of age. The distribution of O.S. is very diffused. The foci may be very numerous, some very small. The **areas affected** are not limited to those preferred by

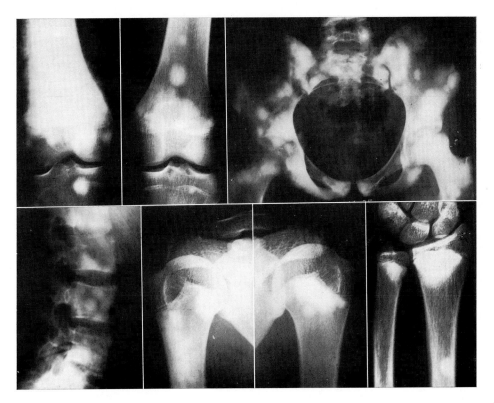

Fig. 425. - Osteosarcomatosis in a male aged 14 years. Pain in the right distal femur for the past 2 months. Good general health conditions. Very high alkaline phosphatase. No pulmonary metastases evident. Three months after the date of the radiograms and biopsy rapid decay in general state of the patient and pulmonary metastases. The patient died 9 months after the onset of symptoms. On autopsy, metastases of the mediastinum and diaphragm, as well as of the lungs (Case provided by Prof. G. Gherlinzoni).

O.S. In addition to the metaphyses of the knee and shoulder, other metaphyses may be affected, such as those of the ankle, and of the wrist; furthermore, the bones of the hand and foot (including the carpus and the tarsus), the epiphyses, the vertebral column, the flat bones.

The O.S. foci have the unique **radiographic** and anatomical feature of all being uniformly sclerosing or eburneous and, in most instances, of not surpassing the cortex.

Histologically, we are dealing with intensely and diffusedly osteogenetic O.S. The histological aspect, unlike that of classic O.S., seems to be considerably uniform in different areas of the tumor and in different tumors.

The **course** of the tumor is usually rapid and **prognosis** is fatal, generally within 1 year.

What is unique about the disease is that in some cases, despite the extensive diffusion of O.S., no pulmonary metastases were observed on autopsy.

All of these data suggest the following conclusions: a) that these multiple O.S. are of multicentric origin, rather than metastatic from a primary tumor; b) that this variety is clearly to be distinguished from classic O.S. Finally, these cases, which were not exposed to radiation or radioactive substances, are somewhat similar to multiple O.S. of the skeleton observed in subjects exposed to radium (radium dial painters) and to those obtained experimentally by administering radioactive substances.

EWING'S SARCOMA

DEFINITION

It is a malignant neoplasm composed of small round cells; it is undifferentiated and of uncertain histogenesis. At times the cells are characterized
by features of the neuro-epithelial type.

FREQUENCY

The tumor occurs relatively frequently. Among primary malignant tumors of the skeleton, it comes after plasmacytoma, osteosarcoma, and chondrosarcoma (Fig. 426).

SEX

There is predilection for the male sex, approximately at a ratio of 1.5:1
(Fig. 426).

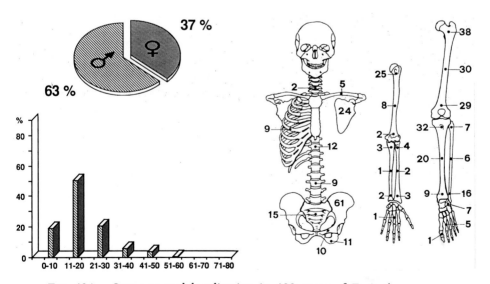

FIG. 426. - Sex, age and localization in 409 cases of Ewing's sarcoma.

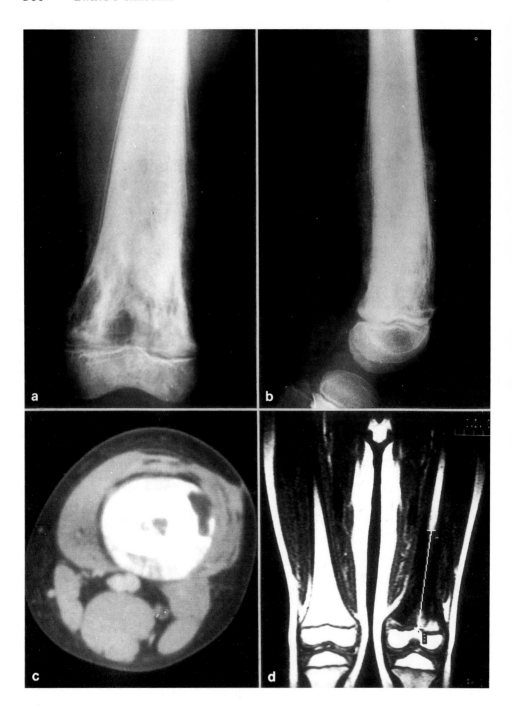

FIG. 427. - Ewing's sarcoma in a boy aged 6 years with pain for the past 2 months. (a) and (b) Radiograms show multiple areas of osteolysis and periosteal reaction of the onion-skin and brush-type. This brush-like reaction of the periosteum is also revealed by CAT (c). (d) MRI allows for accurate measurement of the extent of the tumor along the diaphysis.

Fig. 428. - (a) Ewing's sarcoma in a female aged 10 years. (b) Ewing's sarcoma during an advanced phase in a boy aged 13 years.

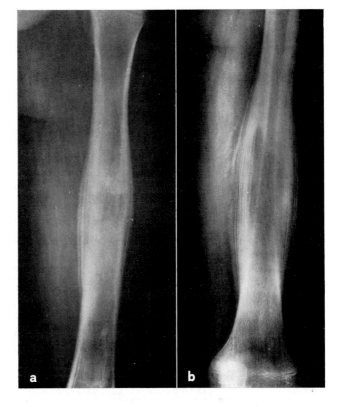

Fig. 428. - (a) Ewing's sarcoma in a female aged 10 years. (b) Ewing's sarcoma during an advanced phase in a boy aged 13 years.

AGE

Approximately 90% of all cases occur between 5 and 25 years of age, with a highest incidence of frequency between 10 and 20 years. E.S. is an exceptional occurrence before 5 and after 25 years of age (Fig. 426).

The age of the patient is of some diagnostic importance, as when the tumor is observed in a patient under 5 years of age differential diagnosis will involve skeletal metastasis due to neuroblastoma; if instead the patient is over 25 years of age, it will involve lymphoma and metastasis due to small-cell carcinoma.

LOCALIZATION

No site in the skeleton is immune from E.S.

Unlike other primary malignant tumors (except for lymphoma), E.S. shows evident predilection for the diaphyses and metadiaphyses of the long bones, and for the skeleton of the trunk (Fig. 426).

Among long bones, the most common localization of the tumor is in the femur, followed by, in this order, the tibia, humerus, fibula, bones of the forearm. In the long bones the neoplasm is prevalently localized in the metadiaphysis or in the diaphysis, rarely in the epiphysis. The epiphysis is hardly ever involved, as long as growth cartilage is present. Even if the tumor radiographically appears to be limited to one part of the bone, anatomically its extent may be greater, until almost the entire bone is involved (Fig. 433). In the skeleton of the trunk, the pelvis is clearly preferred (particularly the ilium), followed by the vertebral column, scapula, ribs, and clavicle. Finally, E.S. may be observed in the foot, and more rarely in the cranium, the maxillary bones, the hand.

In conclusion, it may be affirmed that more than 2/3 of all cases of E.S. are located in the lower limbs or in the pelvis.

SYMPTOMS

The earliest symptom is pain. At first pain is mild and discontinuous, then it may become intense, requiring the use of analgesic drugs. At times, particularly in vertebral or pelvic localizations, pain is irradiated.

Generally, swelling soon occurs; swelling is tense, elastic, tender, and increases rapidly. In fact, E.S. tends to quickly perforate the cortex and expand with a considerable or large neoplastic mass in the soft tissues (Figs. 430b, 433). Thus, the clinical finding of a large palpable mass, which may be visible, and the relative scarcity of radiographic bone lesions are disproportionate. This behavior is not the rule. There are cases in which E.S. left to itself even for several months extends in the cancellous bone or along the medul-

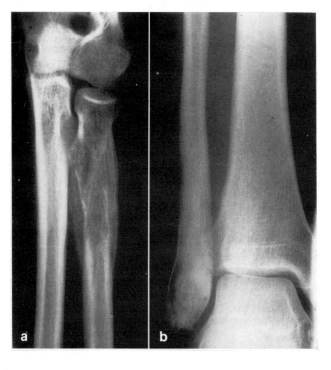

FIG. 429. - (a) Ewing's sarcoma in a female aged 13 years. The diagnosis was delayed by 4 months because ostemyelitis had initially been diagnosed (pain and fever appeared to have benefited from antibiotics). Resection of the proximal radius, radiation and chemotherapy were carried out. (b) Ewing's sarcoma in a male aged 19 years, at the distal end of the fibula. Observe the paucity of the radiographic signs of the tumor which involves the distal fourth of the fibula and extends to the epiphysis. There is some porosity of the cortex, a fair increase in diffused radiopacity, and a nearly null periosteal reaction.

lary canal of a long bone until a large portion of the latter is involved, without expanding outside the cortex (Figs. 434a, 437, 439, 440).

Other common symptoms are fever (remittent, about 38 degrees C.), anemia, increase in sedimentation rate, moderate leukocytosis, increase in serum L.D.H., weight loss. The more advanced the progression of the tumor, the more frequent and evident these symptoms. The prognostic value of the symptoms listed above is unfavorable.

In some cases, a varying amount of time after the onset of symptoms, the same symptoms may occur in another site in the skeleton. But only in exceptional cases do symptoms begin at the same time in two different skeletal sites.

RADIOGRAPHIC FEATURES

The radiographic picture varies considerably. It depends on the age of the patient, the site and degree of expansion of the tumor, on the reaction of the endosteum and of the periosteum. In order to understand the chang-

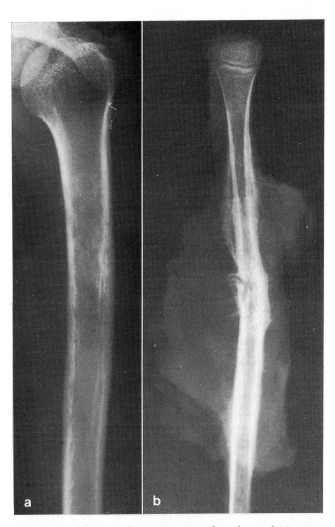

FIG. 430. - (a) Ewing's sarcoma in a female aged 20 years, with symptoms for the past 8 months. (b) Ewing's sarcoma of the fibula in a boy aged 10 years with symptoms for the past 2 months. Resection segment.

ing radiographic aspects of E.S. it must be recalled that this tumor usually grows by infiltrating the medullary spaces and the haversian canals, it rapidly reaches the periosteum, lifting it and then surpassing it. E.S. is prevalently osteolytic but it may cause reactive osteogenesis of the periosteum and — more rarely — of the endosteum. Nonetheless, the skeletal neo-osteogenesis

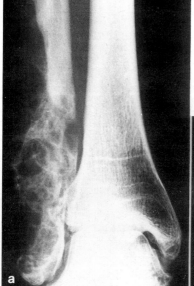

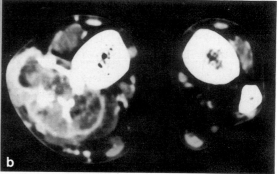

FIG. 431.- Ewing's sarcoma in a male aged 24 years. CAT (b) revealed expansion in the soft tissues which could not be suspected from the radiogram (a).

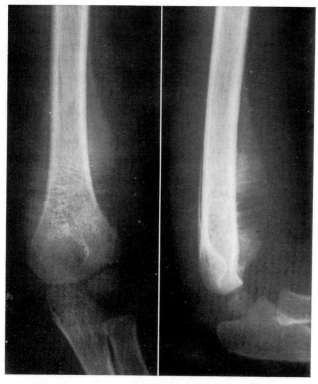

FIG. 432. - Ewing's sarcoma in a female aged 4 years. Brush-like periosteal reaction.

in E.S. always and exclusively derives from the host bone, never from tumor cells.

When bone infiltration is diffused, with focal formation of larger and confluent neoplastic nodules, very faded osteolytic spots are observed, characterized by small erosions of the cortex (spotted or moth-eaten aspect) (Figs. 429, 430a, 434b, 435a, 447a). Rarely, this diffused infiltration causes reactive hyperostosis with increase in skeletal opacity, which is faded and spotted as a result of the fact that it alternates with the osteolytic areas (Figs. 435b,

FIG. 433. - Ewing's sarcoma in a boy aged 12 years, submitted to disarticulation. Observe the discrepancy between the radiographic picture and the anatomical one: the latter shows how the tumor extends in the medullary canal as far as the proximal end of the diaphysis. This extension is not clearly seen in the radiograph, while it could have been visualized by CAT, bone scan, and especially MRI.

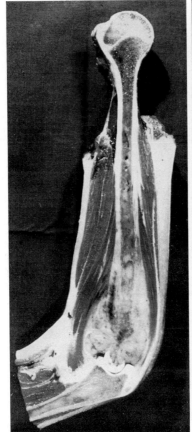
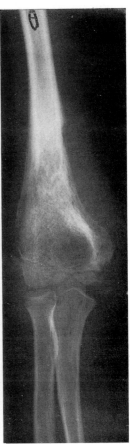

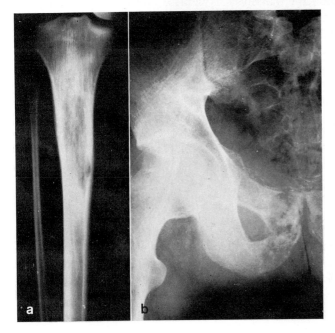

FIG. 434. - (a) Ewing's sarcoma in a female aged 20 years. (b) Ewing's sarcoma in a male aged 21 years with symptoms for the past year.

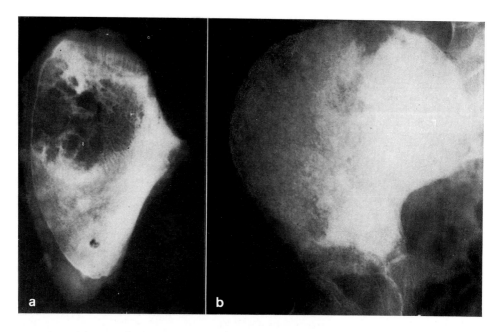

FIG. 435. - (a) Ewing's sarcoma in a boy aged 9 years submitted to subtotal resection of the scapula (anatomical specimen). (b) Ewing's sarcoma in a boy aged 12 years. Observe the prevalently sclerotic radiographic aspect.

447a). If the tumor forms a large compact mass, osteolysis is single, large, with extensive destruction of the cortex (Fig. 438a). Nonetheless, there are exceptional cases in which the osteolysis is central and the cortex does not appear to be clearly interrupted; rather it is thinned and at times slightly expanded by the tumor (Fig. 437, 440). In other cases, again exceptionally, the tumor seems to be periosteal, with a wide non-radiopaque mass expanding towards the soft tissues, superficial erosion of the cortex with triangular periosteal elevation at the two poles of the mass (saucer-like image) and very little radiographic compromise of the cortex and of the medullary canal (Fig. 438b).

In localizations of the tumor in the skeleton of the trunk, the metaphysis and, at times, in diaphyseal localizations, as well, there is little or no periosteal osteogenetic reaction (Figs. 429b, 430a, 434, 435, 439). Rather, in cases such as these, there is a neoplastic mass in the soft tissues, deprived of any radiopacity at all, or run through by some rare radiopaque streak of periosteal origin (Figs. 431, 433, 436). At times, strips of ossification perpendicular to the long bones may be observed, due to the reaction of the periosteum uplifted by the tumor, thinner and more regular than those of an osteosarcoma (brush-like) (Figs. 427, 430b, 432). Finally, there is the onion skin aspect to which value for a radiographic diagnosis of E.S. has been attributed (Figs. 428, 429a). This aspect is due to the fact that the tumor diffusedly and progressively infiltrates the subperiosteal cortical layers, without either lifting

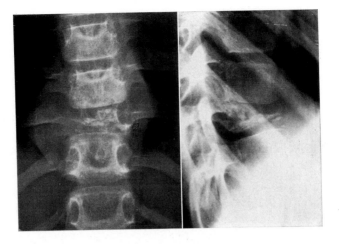

FIG. 436. - Ewing's sarcoma in a female aged 12 years. The radiographic picture could have suggested eosinophilic granuloma (which contrasts with the expanded mass in the soft tissues), or tubercular spondylitis (with which the integrity of the adjacent vertebrae contrasts).

or massively destroying the periosteum. In the site (diaphysis) and at the age (childhood-youth) in which the periosteum is particularly active, in response to this progressive neoplastic infiltration, the periosteum forms superimposed bone layers, either on one side, or on the entire diaphyseal circumference. As each layer or sheet is formed when the underlying sheet has been reached by the tumor, what follows is that the radiopaque sheets are often interrupted in some area. The latter is an important element for differential diagnosis with osteomyelitis. Nonetheless, it must be recalled that the radiographic onion skin aspect is not frequent in E.S., nor is it typical of this tumor. In fact, it may be caused by other neoplastic or inflammatory lesions which infiltrate the cortex and the periosteum of the diaphysis during childhood and youth in the same manner (osteomyelitis, eosinophilic granuloma, lymphoma, osteosarcoma).

Finally, it must be recalled that radiographic changes in the bone, when the first symptoms occur and even when there is considerable extra-skeletal swelling, may be truly minimal (Fig. 429b). Furthermore, there is always disproportion between the extent of the tumor which appears on radiograms and its actual anatomical extent (Fig. 433).

The extent in the bone, the expansion in the soft tissues, the details of the tumor as well as of the bone and the periosteal reaction, the relationships between the tumor and the vessels, nerves, internal organs, are best revealed by CAT and MRI (Figs. 427, 445, 446). Total body bone scan, as well, demonstrates the extent of the tumor in the bone and, in rare cases, it may indicate skeletal multiplicity from the first staging of the tumor.

GROSS PATHOLOGIC FEATURES

Tissue of the E.S. — like that of all sarcomas characterized by a very high cellular quota and very litte stroma — is soft, grayish-white, typically encephaloid. If it is incised and squeezed it often emits a milky fluid. In the areas modified by hemorrhage, which are commonly present, it becomes of gray-

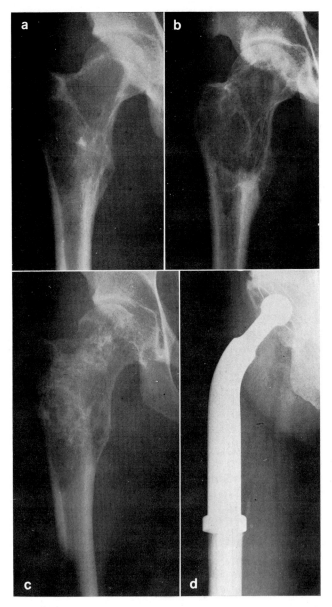

FIG. 437. - (a) Ewing's sarcoma in a male aged 19 years. Observe the relative preservation of the cortex. (b) Without any type of treatment, in 5 months the picture changed very little. In particular, the cortex remained well-preserved. At this point surgical curettage (in the false belief of a benign lesion), radiation and chemotherapy were carried out. (c) After 5 years of well-being pain occurred and the radiographic picture, illustrated here, showed signs of extensive local recurrence. (d) Thus, the patient was submitted to resection-arthroprosthesis. Macroscopic and histological examination of the resected segment confirmed the preservation of the cortex, and extensive intramedullary recurrence. The patient had no signs of metastases or recurrence 12 years after resection and 17 after diagnosis.

purple color or frankly hematic. Areas of necrosis are a frequent occurrence: the tissue is yellowish and sometimes fluid. The surgeon may mistake this semi-liquid tissue for pus and the tumor for osteomyelitis.

The neoplastic tissue may diffusedly infiltrate the medullary spaces without completely destroying the bone trabeculae, and grow along the haversian canals producing diffused porosity of the cortical bone. Furthermore, it forms scattered or confluent nodes, where the bone is completely resorbed, or disseminated in the medullary canal. Again, it may produce larger mas-

FIG. 438. - (a) Ewing's sarcoma of the fibula in a female aged 16 years. (b) Ewing's sarcoma of the femur in a male aged 12 years. Observe the prevalently periosteal location of the tumor, which produces hardly any osteogenetic reaction of the periosteum (saucer-like aspect of the cortex). The patient was well 19 years after radiation therapy.

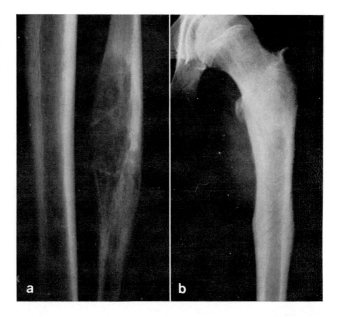

ses, with massive osteolysis and vast interruption of the cortex (Fig. 433b).

The neoplastic mass may extensively detach the periosteum and extend beyond it to the soft tissues. The onion skin periosteal reaction is usually observed in diaphyseal areas of diffused infiltration and porosity of the cortex. When biopsy is carried out, there is usually a good quantity of neoplastic tissue outside the cortex and the periosteum, even if radiographic changes are very scarce and initial. Nonetheless, there are cases, particularly those characterized by an onion skin image, in which the reactive periosteal layers only contain traces of neoplastic tissues or none at all. In cases such as these, the biopsy specimen should not be limited to the thickened periosteum, but include the whole thickness of the cortex and the contents of the medullary canal. In fact, the neoplastic tissue may only be present in the medullary canal and in the haversian canals, not among the periosteal sheets.

When obtaining the biopsy specimen, it is important to search for vital areas of the tumor, discarding necrotic, colliquative and hemorrhagic ones. It is a common autoptic finding to observe extensively diffused neoplastic nodules in the skeleton (particularly the vertebral column, cranium, ribs, sternum). Skeletal metastases occur more frequently than pulmonary metastases.

HISTOPATHOLOGIC FEATURES

In vital and unmodified areas of the tumor a uniform mat of small round nuclei, located close together and intensely stained is observed (Fig. 441). Cytoplasms are rather scarce, pale, vacuolated and characterized by faded boundaries. The nuclei, instead, are clearly visualized because of their intense color; as such, they constitute the diagnostic element of the tumor. They are twice as large as those of lymphocytes, round-oval in shape, with pulverulent chromatin and one or more very small nucleoli. Nearly all of the nuclei are of the same size, and characterized by a rather regular shape. Mitotic figures are rare, scarce, or numerous and not anomalous. Imprint specimens, or semi-fine sections may be of use for a study of these cellular details.

The behavior of the argyrophilous reticulum of E.S. is neither constant nor typical. In some cases it appears to be concentrated around the blood vessels and the neoplastic tissue contains none at all (Fig. 442b). In other cases the tumor is traversed by few sparse fibers (Fig. 441b); in others still, there is a thick reticulum surrounding nearly every cell such as in lymphoma.

Staining with P.A.S. and after alcoholic fixation, the cytoplasms reveal granules of glycogen (not stained after treatment with diasta-

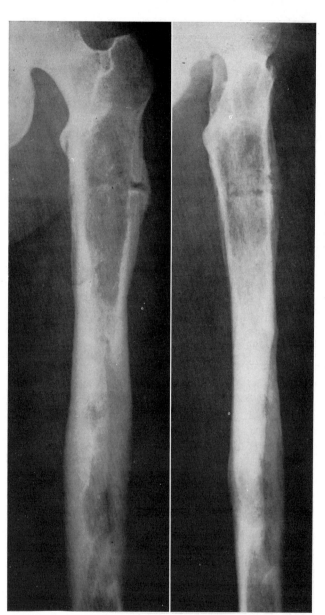

FIG. 439. - Ewing's sarcoma in a female aged 22 years. The patient had symptoms for 4 years. Biopsy performed 2 years earlier led first to a diagnosis of osteomyelitis. Observe the radiographic picture, after 4 years of symptoms, with a lesion which was apparently nearly totally contained within the medullary canal, but extended to most of the femur. A new biopsy showed the Ewing's sarcoma. Treated with radiation therapy, the patient died 2 years later of pulmonary metastases.

sis) (Fig. 441d). This abundant cellular glycogen is also evident under electron microscopy. Its presence is practically constant (glycogen is absent in lymphoma and in skeletal metastasis due to neuroblastoma; it is instead present in mesenchymal chondrosarcoma, in rhabdomyosarcoma, in hemangiopericytoma, in round-cell sarcoma of the soft tissues similar to Ewing's sarcoma).

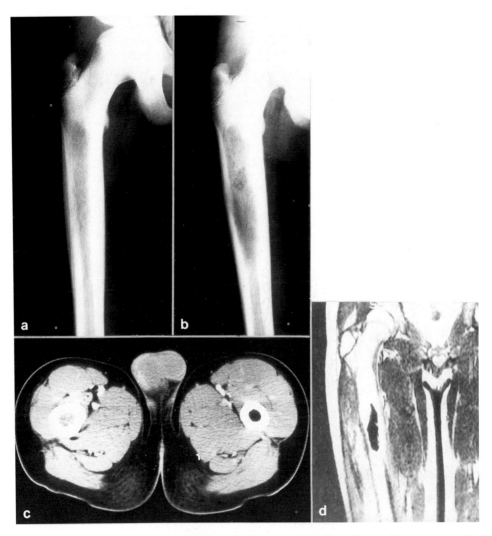

FIG. 440. - Ewing's sarcoma in boy aged 12 years. (a) When this radiogram was obtained the patient had had pain for only a few days with fever. There is periosteal reaction in regular and continuous sheets; the cortex appears to be mildly moth-eaten. ESR is moderately increased. As osteomyelitis is suspected (but, LDH dosage is not obtained), it is treated with antibiotics and there is complete regression of symptoms, which remain absent for 7 months. Then fever and mild pain recur. A radiogram obtained 1 year after the previous one (b) shows some increase in the osteolysis. Nonetheless, CAT and MRI (c, d) show that the tumor is totally intraperiosteal and that reaction of the periosteum is at a minimum. LDH is increased. Incisional biopsy reveals Ewing's sarcoma.

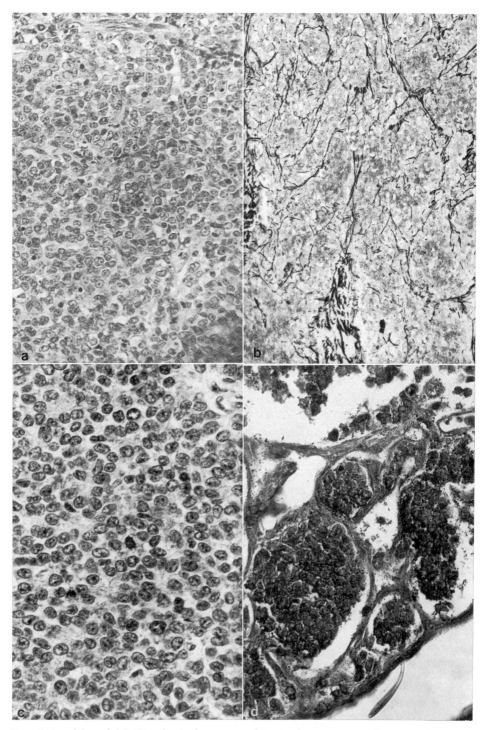

FIG. 441. - (a) and (c) Histological aspects of Ewing's sarcoma in *hematoxylin-eosin* specimens. (b) *Argentic impregnation*. (d) PAS for glycogen. (310, 200, 500, 310 x).

The blood vessels of E.S. are thin and provided with their own walls. They are usually scarce and located far apart, at times they are numerous.

In rare cases the cells are arranged in a rosette-like pattern. This aspect must be known of in order to avoid confusing the tumor with metastatic neuroblastoma. At the center of these pseudorosettes of E.S. there is a blood capillary or there may be a few necrotic cells (Fig. 442a).

At times, the neoplastic tissue forms perivascular rings (Fig. 442a). In specific cases, all of these rings have the same thickness throughout. At the center of the ring there is a blood vessel. At the periphery there is a thin layer of cells in degeneration, with pyknotic nuclei. Beyond this line there is total necrosis, where the cells can no longer be recognized. These morphological aspects indicate that the neoplastic tissue in these cases is nourished and survives only within a constant distance from the blood vessel. Beyond this distance cells die. This is another demonstration of the singular monomorphism and functional uniformity of the tumor cells. In necrotic areas there is considerable infiltration of polymorphonucleate leukocytes. This aspect, as we shall see, is important because of the possible diagnostic errors that may be made with osteomyelitis. Often, even in compact areas of the tumor, cells undergoing regression are abundantly scattered among vital cells. The former, as compared to the latter, have evident cytoplasmatic boundaries, acidophilic cytoplasm, smaller nuclei with

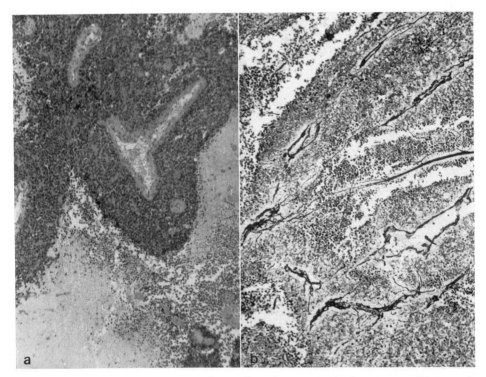

FIG. 442. - (a) Perivascular rings and pseudorosettes in Ewing's sarcoma. (b) *Argentic impregnation* for the reticulum. (*Hemat.-eos.*, 125x, *Arg.*, 125 x).

dense or pyknotic chromatin. Another regressive aspect is constituted by tumoral stripes where the cells are compressed together, and the nuclei are flattened, lengthened, filamentous, very dark and compactly massed together (Fig. 443a).

In areas where the tumor diffusedly infiltrates the bone, there are neoplastic nests and islands, at times surrounded by a fair amount of reactive fibrosis, at times by reactive osteogenesis. Faced with these cellular nests, surrounded by connective tissue, differential diagnosis may involve metastasis due to undifferentiated carcinoma (Fig. 441d).

HISTOGENESIS

In E.S. a characteristic chromosomal abnormality has been identified (reciprocal translocation in chromosomes 11 and 22).

As far as histogenesis is concerned, there is evidence that E.S. of bone is one, albeit undifferentiated, member of the family of neural tumors, distinct from neuroblastoma. These neural tumors, unlike neuroblastoma, occur in older patients, do not arise in the sympathetic nervous system, do not express catecholamines, nor the oncogene N-myc. However, they do present neural differentiation in vitro, and display certain neural features, such as the expression of neuron-specific enolase, S-100 protein, and electron microscopic structures (neurites, dense core granules).

The more differentiated forms of the spectrum of such neural tumors of bone have been referred to as peripheral neuroepithelioma. The E.S. would instead represent the less differentiated portion of such spectrum.

DIAGNOSIS

E.S. is characterized by numerous and delicate problems in differential diagnosis.

Based on clinical and radiographic elements alone, it is possible to make the reciprocal error of confusing the tumor with osteomyelitis, eosinophilic granuloma, osteoarticular tuberculosis, osteosarcoma, and other primary or secondary osteolytic tumors.

Based on the histological examination, instead, an error may be made involving metastasis due to neuroblastoma, lymphoma, metastasis due to undifferentiated carcinoma, small-cell osteosarcoma, mesenchymal chondrosarcoma, embryonal rhabdomyosarcoma.

Osteomyelitis

Age and, possibly, localization in the long bones are similar in hematogenous osteomyelitis and in E.S. The latter often causes fever, increase in sedimentation rate, anemia and leukocytosis (but also an increase in L.D.H.). Radiographically, small areas of central osteolysis and onion peel periosteal reaction may also typify osteomyelitis (Figs. 2-4). We have observed that in E.S. the radiopaque sheets of periosteal reaction are frequently interrupted,

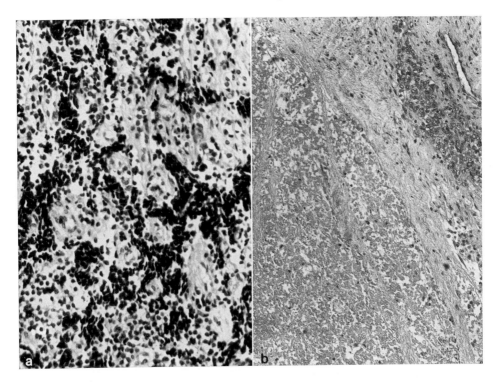

FIG. 443. - (a) Regressive aspects due to compression of the cells in Ewing's sarcoma. (b) Ewing's sarcoma after 4 sessions of radiation therapy; 80% of the cells are necrotic (*Hemat.-eos.*, 125, 125, x).

but they may also appear to be regular and continuous. There are rare cases of E.S. in which the tumor extends in the medullary canal, but it apparently interrupts neither the cortex nor the periosteum, even for several months. At biopsy, the surgeon may observe yellowish and semi-fluid tissue under the periosteum or in the medullary canal, and mistake it for pus. It has even occurred that the histopathologist to whom the material is submitted sees necrotic and hemorrhagic areas infiltrated by leukocytes, thus confirming an erroneous diagnosis of osteomyelitis.

It may also occur that, in a case of E.S. contained in the diaphysis and characterized by onion skin periosteal reaction, the surgeon is satisfied with taking a band of thickened periosteum and that the histopathologist, finding therein edema alone and mild inflammatory infiltration, makes a diagnosis of osteo-periostitis. Instead, the tumor would have been found if a sample of cortical bone and material from the medullary canal had been removed and examined.

Eosinophilic granuloma

There are cases of infantile eosinophilic granuloma which may radiographically suggest E.S. This happens in cases of spotted osteolysis or osteolysis

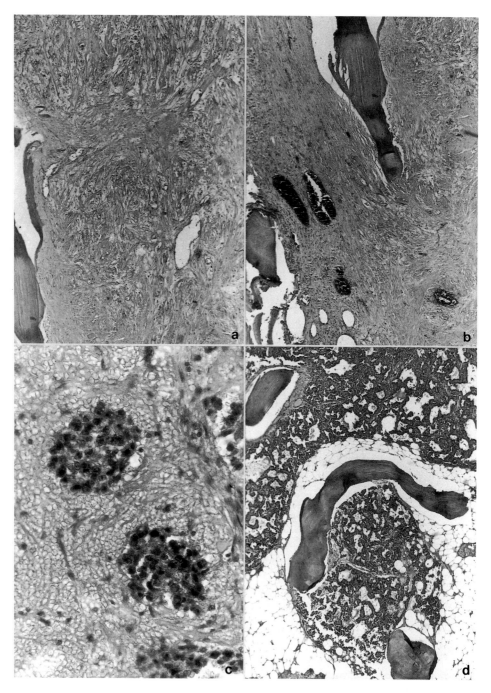

FIG. 444. - Effects of preoperative chemotherapy in Ewing's sarcoma. (a) Total necrosis. There is no trace of the tumor in the fibro-osseous scar tissue. (b) and (c) Microscopic tumoral residues in the form of small islands scattered in the scar tissue. (d) Macroscopic tumoral residues (*Hemat.-eos.*, 50, 50, 400 and 50x)

which is intense and rapidly progressive, with interruption of the cortex and (in the diaphysis of the long bones, in the clavicle) considerable periosteal reaction. On the other hand, there are rare cases of radiographically and well-contained osteolytic E.S., which may suggest eosinophilic granuloma. A histological examination will dispel any doubt.

Osteo-articular tuberculosis

In some exceptional cases vertebral E.S. is radiographically believed to be a tubercular spondylitis (Fig. 436). In fact, one or more vertebral bodies may appear to be sclerotic or spotted and, even if the intervertebral discs are usually not modified, the shadow of an extensive paravertebral neoplastic mass may simulate that of a cold abscess.

Osteosarcoma

We have observed how radiographically E.S. may be characterized by radiopaque periosteal strips perpendicular to the cortex (Figs. 427, 432). In

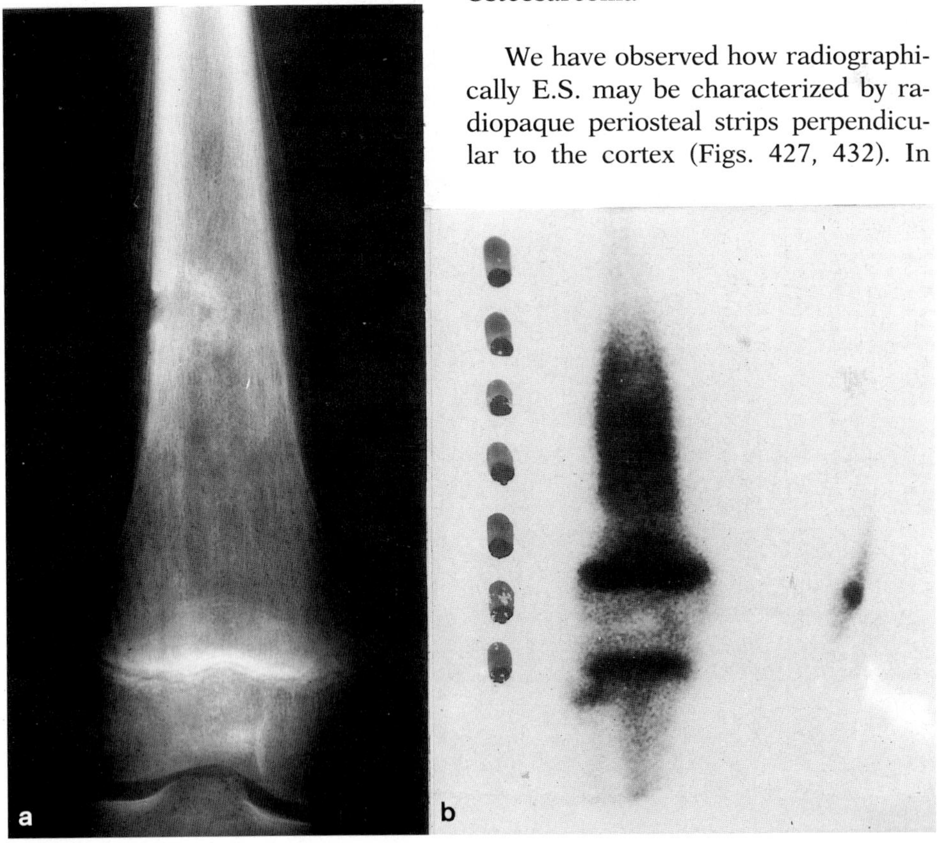

FIG. 445. - Ewing's sarcoma in a boy aged 13 years. (a), (b) and (c) Radiographic, scintigraphic and CAT pictures at diagnosis. (d) CAT after preoperative chemotherapy reveals regression of the tumor. (e) and (f) The patient was submitted to wide resection and reconstruction with an allograft and there were no signs of disease 6 months later.

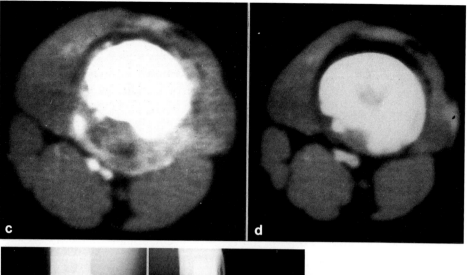

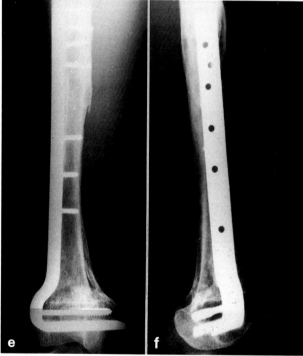

FIG. 445. (continued)

other cases, E.S. may produce a diffused, intense and faded increase in skeletal radiopacity (Fig. 435b). In both cases, the radiographic picture justifies the diagnostic hypothesis of osteosarcoma. On the contrary, there are rare cases of osteosarcoma which is extended towards the diaphysis, with a radiographic moth-eaten and/or onion skin image (Figs. 388b, 389a). Histologically, differential diagnosis may be made between E.S. and small-cell osteosarcoma (see specific chapter).

Metastasis due to neuroblastoma

If we are dealing with a child aged under 5 years, neuroblastoma is a more probable occurrence than E.S. Other diagnostic elements of neuroblastoma are the extent of the osteolytic lesions to different areas of the skeleton at the time of presentation, cranial lesions and exophthalmos, enlargement of the regional lymph nodes and CAT image of a retroperitoneal mass, at times containing small calcifications. Nonetheless, there are cases of initially solitary metastasis due to neuroblastoma which radiographically cannot be distinguished from E.S. Furthermore, neuroblastoma may also occur during late childhood, adolescence, and even during adult age. In neuroblastoma there is an increase in the metabolites of the catecholamines of the urine, which is absent in E.S. Histologically, neuroblastoma is made up of a mat of cells which are very similar to those of E.S. The most important differential feature is constituted by the fact that the cells of neuroblastoma tend to form actual rosettes, with nuclei at the periphery and cytoplasmatic elongations at the center (the rosettes which may be observed in E.S. are always pseudorosettes, with one blood capillary, or a few necrotic cells in the center). Nonetheless, although the rosettes are often observed in the primary neuroblastoma, they may be totally absent in skeletal metastases. Another histological differential element is constituted by the absence of glycogen in the cells of neuroblastoma. Finally, the cells of neuroblastoma may have more abundant cytoplasms and wider and more polydimensional nuclei as compared to E.S. Electron microscopy demonstrates granules of neurosecretion in the cytoplasms of neuroblastoma, glycogen in those of E.S.

Lymphoma

Despite the clinical, histological and prognostic differences (see diagnosis of lymphoma) fully justifying the separation of E.S. from lymphoma there are infrequent cases in which a definite distinction is not easy.

Metastasis due to undifferentiated carcinoma

In rare cases, an epithelial metastasis having small undifferentiated cells (for example, a pulmonary, thyroid, mammary, gastric, testicular carcinoma) may histologically simulate an E.S. Thus, if the skeletal lesion is observed in an adult or in an elderly person, the possibility of an epithelial metastasis must be taken into consideration, and clinical, radiographic and histological research conducted in-depth.

Mesenchymal chondrosarcoma

It may be histologically similar (the cells contain glycogen) in areas where it does not form chondroid islands.

Embryonal rhabdomyosarcoma

This tumor of the soft tissues may invade the skeleton by adjacency or

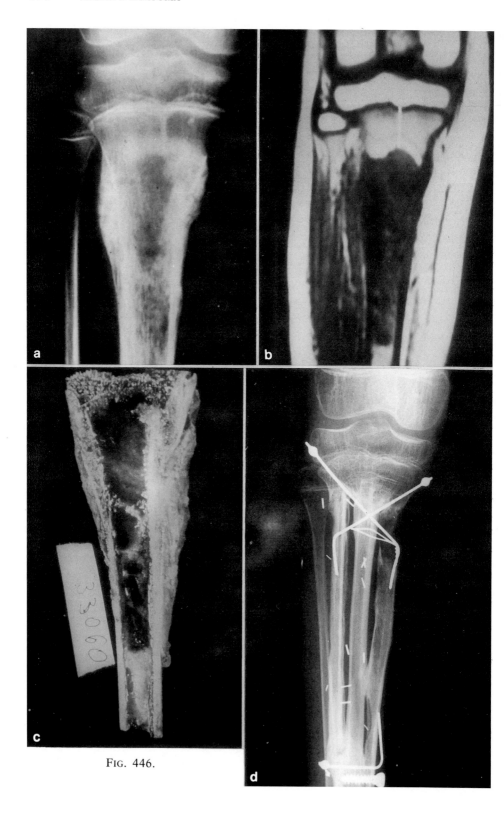

Fig. 446.

metastasis, and then be confused with E.S. Its cytoplasms are more abundant and intensely stained, they do contain glycogen and are positive for desmine, actine and myoglobine.

COURSE

Among primary tumors of the skeleton, the average course of E.S. is more rapid. In most cases, the amount of time between the first symptoms and diagnosis is considerably less than 6 months. The skeletal lesion may progress severely, and a large tumoral mass may form in the soft tissues within a few weeks. Nonetheless, as previously observed, there are exceptions to the rule. At times, expansion of the tumor is slower and it remains rather contained in the bone, so that the interval between the first symptoms and diagnosis may be 1 year or even more (Figs. 439, 440).

E.S. which is left untreated ends up being disseminated to different areas of the skeleton. Exceptionally, there is more than one skeletal lesion at the onset of symptoms. On autopsy, instead, there is nearly always skeletal dissemination of neoplastic nodes, mostly or all asymptomatic and not visible on radiograms. This skeletal diffusion may also occur in the absence of pulmonary metastases. It cannot be established whether we are dealing with multicentric and primary skeletal localizations, or skeletal metastases secondary to the primary tumor. In this second case, which seems to be the most probable one, it must be admitted that the cells have skipped over the pulmonary filter.

Pulmonary metastases are a frequent occurrence. Metastases of different internal organs are also frequent. Metastases to the regional lymph nodes are not rare, particularly in paravertebral and pelvic lymph nodes.

TREATMENT

Treatment is **antiblastic, surgical and radiation**.

Radiation treatment is the most traditional type of therapy, at one time it was the only one used. The tumor is very sensitive to radiation (Fig. 443b). After just a few applications pain and fever regress. The palpable tumoral mass is reduced more slowly (because the necrotic cells must be resorbed) but this, too, tends to regress completely within a few months. Even slower is reconstruction of the bone, which is nonetheless manifested, at times in a

◀

FIG. 446. - Ewing's sarcoma in a girl aged 7 years with pain for the past 6 months and swelling for the past 2. (a) and (b) Radiographic picture and MRI after preoperative chemotherapy. (c) The patient was submitted to wide resection. (d) Reconstruction involved a vascularized autogenous fibula (at center) and two fibular allografts (on the sides). Observe the partial resorption of the latter, while the vascularized graft is hypertrophic (compare it with the fibula in the same limb). There were no signs of disease after 2 years.

surprising manner. Radiograms show the tendency of osteolytic areas and of the periosteal layer invaded by the tumor to ossify, so that generally there is skeletal thickening in the area of the tumor.

About 5000-6000 r are required. Irradiation must be extended at least 5 cm beyond the radiographic (bone scan, CAT, MRI) boundaries of the tumor, but it does not seem necessary to always include the entire bone affected.

Chemotherapy was introduced over the last 30 years, and has radically changed things. The most frequent association of drugs is vincristine, adriablastin, cyclophosphamide, and actinomycin D. For many years this poly-chemotherapy was used at the same time as radiation treatment, limiting the use of surgery to few indications.

Since chemotherapy has drastically increased the survival rate, numerous (about 20%) cases of local recurrence of the irradiated sarcoma have been observed. This shows that radiation therapy, although associated with chemotherapy, does not always destroy the entire tumor. Probably, the center of the tumoral mass, which is poorly vascularized and hypoxic, is radio- and chemo-resistant.

Local recurrence is observed more rarely and prognosis is thus better in cases in which the primary tumor was removed surgically. Furthermore, ra-

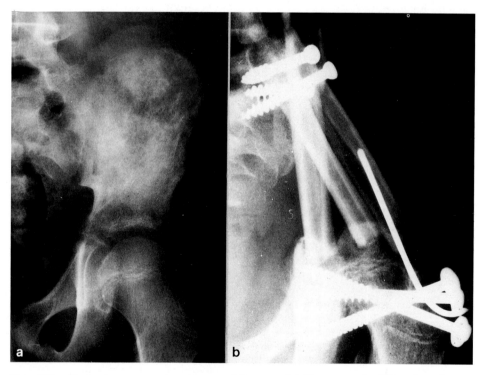

Fig. 447. - Ewing's sarcoma in a boy aged 9 years. (a) The tumor is diffused to the entire iliac bone and the reactive hyperostosis causes an increase in skeletal radiopacity. (b) After preoperative chemotherapy wide resection of the ilium and reconstruction with arthrodesis and bridge grafting (fibular allograft) were performed.

diation treatment causes different complications: fibrosis of the soft tissues, shortening of the limb in subjects who are still growing, joint stiffness and deformity, fractures which are difficult to heal, osteonecrosis and, worst of all, late radio-induced sarcoma. The latter, which occurs more than 5 years after irradiation and is generally osteosarcoma or malignant fibrous histiocytoma, is observed more and more often, as the number of cases of long surviving E.S. increases.

These observations have led to a re-evaluation of **surgical treatment**, and the use of **preoperative chemotherapy**, similar to what is done to treat osteosarcoma. Chemotherapy obtains nearly complete clinical-radiographic regression of the primary tumor. This remission often makes surgical resection possible. If resection has been marginal or intralesional, radiation therapy follows; if resection has been wide or compartmental, radiation therapy may be omitted (Figs. 445, 446, 447).

In cases which are not operated after induction chemotherapy (very extensive tumors, vertebral localizations, multicentric skeletal forms, or metastases at the onset) radiation therapy alone is used. After ablation (surgical or radiation) of the primary tumor, chemotherapy is continued for 12 months.

Preoperative chemotherapy allows for a histological verification of its effect on the tumor. In most cases, it causes the regression of most or all of the neoplastic tissue. This often remains constituted by some micronodules or more extensive areas of vital cells, scattered within scarring fibro-osseous tissue (Fig. 444).

Surgical treatment of E.S., like and more than that of osteosarcoma, involves problems related to the age of the patient. An arthroprosthesis or an arthrodesis are not very acceptable, in a hip or in a knee, during childhood. Another problem involves the frequent extent of E.S. to much of the bone affected. Another still involves the fact that the use of bone grafting is not advised if radiation therapy must follow surgery. At times, particularly in smaller children and in sites distal to the knee, or when there is pathologic fracture, or when the tumoral mass is very large, the best type of surgery is amputation. Surgical indications and methods are currently progressing. Doubtless, thanks to chemotherapy, E.S. has partially become a surgical affection; and indications must be personalized for each individual patient.

Surgical resection may still be performed after the bone has been irradiated and at the end of chemotherapy, with the aim of reducing the risk of local recurrence and radiation-induced sarcoma.

Pulmonary metastases are treated either with radiation therapy or with thoracotomy. Skeletal metastases are treated with radiation therapy, as well as with chemotherapy.

PROGNOSIS

Before chemotherapy was used prognosis was very poor, with a 10-year survival-rate less than 5%. In rare cases, death occurred several years after therapy, so that the 5-year term is not totally significant.

Since chemotherapy has been in use, the percentage of survival has increased, during the first 5 years, to 50%. Local recurrence and metastases may be observed, however, even after several years, more than is the case in osteosarcoma. Thus, more than in osteosarcoma, survival should be evaluated after 10 years. Local recurrence in E.S. is a particularly dreadful event, as in most cases it is associated with or soon followed by metastatic diffusion.

One complication is brain metastasis (antiblastics do not go beyond the hemato-liquoral barrier). This observation, which has caused some to recommend preventive irradiation of the encephalus or the use of antiblastics in the liquor, is not, however, at least in our experience, frequent enough to recommend the use of these measures.

Unfavorable prognostic factors are male sex, the presence of general signs such as fever, anemia, weight loss, increase in sedimetation rate, increase in serum L.D.H., localization of the tumor in the pelvis and sacrum. Chemotherapy with four drugs has obtained better results than that with three. The association of surgery obtains evidently better results than radio- and chemotherapy alone.

REFERENCES

1959 SCHAJOWICZ F.: Ewing's sarcoma and reticulum-cell sarcoma of bone. With special reference to the histochemical demonstration of glycogen as an aid to differential diagnosis. *Journal of Bone and Joint Surgical*, **41-A**, 349-356.

1963 BHANSALI S. K., DESAI P. B.: Ewing's sarcoma. Osbervations on 107 cases. *Journal of Bone and Joint Surgery*, **45-A**, 541-553.

1966 JENKIN R. D. T.: Ewing's sarcoma. A study of treatement methods. *Clinical Radiology*, **17**, 97-106.

1967 BOYER C. W. Jr., PERRY R. H.: Ewing's sarcoma. Case against surgery. *Cancer*, **20**, 1602-1606.

1967 FALK S., ALPERT M.: Five years survival of patients with Ewing's sarcoma. *Surgery, Gynecology and Obstetrics*, **124**, 319-324.

1967 PHILIPS R. F., HIGINBOTHAM N. L.: The curability of Ewing's endotelioma of bone in children. *Journal of Pediatry*, **70**, 391-397.

1967 VOHRA V. G.: Roentgen manifestations in Ewing's sarcoma. A study of 156 cases. *Cancer*, **20**, 727-733.

1968 FRIEDMAN P., GOLD H.: Ultrastructure of Ewing's sarcoma of bone. *Cancer*, **22**, 307-322.

1968 HUSTU H. P., HOLTON C., JAMES D. Jr., PINKEL D.: Treatment of Ewing's sarcoma with concurrent radiotherapy and chemotherapy. *Journal of Pediatry*, **73**, 249-251.

1969 MATHEWS R. S., LINCOLN C. R., GOLDNER L., BRADFORD W. D., CAVANAUGH P. J.: Ewing's tumor treatment with supervoltage radiation and chemotherapy. *Journal of Bone and Joint Surgery*, **51-A**, 1038-1038.

1971 DICK H. M., FRANCIS K. C., JOHNSTON A. D.: Ewing's sarcoma of the hand. *Journal of Bone and Joint Surgery*, **53-A**, 345-348.

1971 FRIEDMAN B., HANAOKA H.: Round-cell sarcomas of bone. A light and electron microscopic study. *Journal of Bone and Joint Surgery*, **53-A**, 1118-1136.

1971 MARSA W. G., JOHNSON R. E.: Altered pattern of metastasis following treatment of Ewing's sarcoma with radiotherapy and adjuvant chemotherapy. *Cancer*, **27**, 1051-1054.

1971 MARSHALL E. K., BENSCH K. G.: On the origin of Ewing's tumor. *Cancer*, **27**, 257-273.

1972 Freeman A. J., Sachatello C., Gaeta J., Shah N. K., Wang J. J., Sinks L. F.: An analysis of Ewing's tumor in children at Roswell Park Memorial Institute. *Cancer*, **29**, 1563-1569.

1972 Hou-Jensen K., Priori E., Dmochowski L.: Studies on ultrastructure of Ewing's sarcoma of bone. *Cancer*, **29**, 280-286.

1972 Hustu U. H., Pinkel D., Pratt C. B.: Treatment of clinically localized Ewing's sarcoma with radiotherapy and combination chemoterapy. *Cancer*, **30**, 1522-1527.

1973 Kofman S., Perlia C. P., Economou S. G.: Mithramycin in the treatment of metastatic Ewing's sarcoma. *Cancer*, **31**, 889-893.

1973 Price C. H. G.: A critique of Ewing's tumour of bone, in «*Bone - Certain aspects of neoplasia*», Butterworths, London.

1973 Schajowicz F.: Differential diagnosis of Ewing's sarcoma, in «*Bone - Certain aspects of neoplasia*», Butterworths, London.

1973 Suit H. D., Fernandez C., Sutow W., Samuels M., Wilbur J.: Radiation therapy and multi-drug chemotherapy in management of patients with Ewing's sarcoma, in «*Bone - Certain aspects of neoplasia*», Butterworths, London.

1974 Fernandez C. H., Lindberg R. D., Sutow W. W., Samuels M. L.: Localized Ewing's sarcoma. Treatment and results. *Cancer*, **34**, 143-148.

1974 Mehta Y., Hendrickson F. R.: Central nervous system involvement in Ewing's sarcoma. *Cancer*, **33**, 859-862.

1974 Rosen G., Wollner N., Tan C., Wu S. J., Hajdu S. I., Cham W., D'Angio G. J., Murphy M. L.: Disease-free survival in children with Ewing's sarcoma treated with radiation therapy and adjuvant four-drug sequantial chemotheraphy. *Cancer*, **33**, 384-393.

1975 Macintosh D. J., Price C. H. G., Jeffree G. M.: Ewing's tumor. A study of behaviour and treatment in forty-seven cases. *Journal of Bone and Joint surgery*, **57-B**, 331-340.

1975 Pomeroy T. C., Johnson R. E.: Combined modality therapy of Ewing's sarcoma. *Cancer*, **35**, 36-47.

1975 Pritchard D. J., Dahlin D. C., Dauphine R. T., Taylor W. F., Beabout J. W.: Ewing's sarcoma. A clinico-pathological and statistical analysis of patients surviving five years or longer. *Journal of Bone and Joint Surgery*, **57-A**, 10-16.

1975 Suit H. D.: Role of therapeutic radiology in cancer of bone. *Cancer*, **35**, 930-936.

1977 Lewis R. J., Marcove R. C., Rosen G.: Ewing's sarcoma. Functional effects of radiation therapy. *Journal of Bone and Joint Surgery*, **59-A**, 325-331.

1977 Perez C. A., Razek A., Tefft M., Nesbit M., Burgert E. O., Kissane J., Vietti T., Gehan E. A.: Analysis of local tumor control in Ewing's sarcoma. Preliminary results of a cooperative intergroup study. *Cancer*, **40**, 2864-2873.

1977 Tefft M., Mc Chabora B., Rosen G.: Radiation in bone sarcoma. A re-evaluation in the era of intensive systemic chematherapy. *Cancer*, **39**,806-816.

1978 Bacci G., Campanacci M., Pagani P. A.: Adjuvant chemotherapy in the treatment of clinically localized Ewing's sarcoma. *Journal of Bone and Joint Surgery*, **60-B**, 567-574.

1978 Lambart-Bosch A., Blache R., Peydro-Olaya A.: Ultrastructural study of 28 cases of Ewing's sarcoma: typical and atypical forms. *Cancer*, **41**, 1362-1373.

1978 Rosen G., Caparros B., Mosende C., Mccormick B., Huvos A. G., Marcove R. C.: Curability of Ewing's sarcoma and considerations for future therapeutic trials. *Cancer*, **41**, 888-899.

1978 Telles N. C., Rabson A. S., Pomeroy T. C.: Ewing's sarcoma: an autopsy study. *Cancer*, **41**, 2321-2329.

1979 Campanacci M., Bacci G., Boriani S., Laus M.: Sarcoma di Ewing. Studio di 195 osservazioni. *Giornale Italiano di Ortopedia e Traumatologia*, **5**, 307-315.

1979 Chan R. C., Sutow W. W., Lindberg R. D., Samuels M. L., Murray J. A., Johnston D. A.: Management and results of localized Ewing's sarcoma. *Cancer*, **43**, 1001-1006.

1980 Glaubiger D. L., Makugh R., Schwarz J., Levine A. S., Johnson R. E.: Determination of prognostic factors and their influence on therapeutic results in patients with Ewing's sarcoma. *Cancer*, **45**, 2213-2219.

1980   Razek A., Perez C. A., Tefft M., Nesbit M., Vietti T., Burgert E. O. Jr., Kissane J., Pritchard D. J., Gehan E. A.: Integroup Ewing's sarcoma study. Local control related to radiation dose, volume, and site of primary lesion in Ewing's sarcoma. *Cancer*, **46**, 516-521.

1980   Tepper J., Glaubiger R. D., Lichter A., Wackenhut J., Glatstein E.: Local control of Ewing's sarcoma of bone with radiotherapy and combination chemotherapy. *Cancer*, **46**, 1969-1975.

1981   Marcove R. C., Rosen G.: Radical en bloc excision of Ewing's sarcoma. *Clinical Orthopedics*, **153**, 86-91.

1981   Pritchard D. J.: Indications for surgical treatment of localized Ewing's sarcoma of bone. *Clinical Orthopedics*, **153**, 39-43.

1981   Rosen G., Caparros B., Nirenberg A., Marcove R. C., Huvos A. G., Kosloff C., Lane J., Murphy M. L.: Ewing's sarcoma: ten-year experience with adjuvant chemotherapy. *Cancer*, **47**, 2204-2213.

1982   Bacci G., Picci P., Gitelis S., Borghi A., Campanacci M.: The treatment of localized Ewing's sarcoma: the experience at the Istituto Ortopedico Rizzoli in 163 cases treated with and without adjuvant chemotherapy. *Cancer*, **49**, 1561-1578.

1982   Gherlinzoni F., Calderoni P., Guerra A., Bertoni F., Picci P., Bacci G.: Il ruolo della chirurgia nel trattamento del sarcoma di Ewing non metastatico. Esperienza dell'Istituto Ortopedico Rizzoli relativa a 163 casi. *Chirurgia Organi Movimento*, **67**, 1-13.

1982   Kliman M., Harwood A. R., Jenkin R. D., Cummings B. J., Langer F., Quirt J., Fornasier U. L.: Radical radiotherapy as primary treatment for Ewing's sarcoma distal to the elbow and knee. *Clinical Orthopedics*, **165**, 233-238.

1983   Bacci G., Bertoni F., Borghi A., Calderoni P., Capanna R., Cervellati C., Gherlinzoni F., Giunti A., Guerra A., Guernelli N., Mercuri M., Picci P., Putti C., Campanacci M.: Combined treatment in Ewing's sarcoma. In «*Modern trends in orthopaedic surgery*» edited by M. Campanacci et al., A. Gaggi Bologna.

1983   Hayes F. A., Thompson E. I., Hustu H. O., Kumar M., Coburn T., Webber B.: The response of Ewing's sarcoma to sequential cyclophosphamide and adriamycin induction therapy. *Journal of Clinical Oncology*, **1** (1), 45-51.

1983   Kissane J. M., Askin F. B., Foulkes M., Stratton L. B., Shirley S. F.: Ewing's sarcoma of bone: clinicopathologic aspects of 303 cases from the Intergroup Ewing'Sarcoma Study. *Human Pathology*, **14** (9), 773-9.

1983   Jurgens H., Cserhati M., Gobel U., Gutjahr P., Jobke A., Kaatsch P., Kuhl J., Sekera J., Winlker K.: The CESS 81 cooperative Ewing sarcoma study of the Society for Pediatric Oncology, an interim report. *Clinical Pediatrics*, **195**, 207-13.

1983   Li W. K., Lane J. M., Rosen G., Marcove R. C., Caparros B., Huvos A., Groshen S.: Pelvic Ewing's sarcoma. Advances in treatment. *Journal of Bone and Joint Surgery*, **65**, 738-47.

1983   Picci P., Bacci G., Gherlinzoni F., Laudati M., Manduchi R.: The value of serum lactic acid dehydrogenase (LDH) level as a prognostic factor in localized Ewing's sarcoma. *Chemioterapia*, **6**, 372-375.

1983   Schifter S., Vendelbo L., Jensen O., Kaae S.: Ewing's tumor following bilateral retinoblastoma: a case report. *Cancer*, **51**, 1746-1749.

1983   Spaziante R., De Divitiis E., Giamundo A., Gambardella A., Di Prisco G.: Ewing's sarcoma arising primarily in the spinal epidural space, fifth case report. *Neurosurgery*, **12**, 337-41.

1983   Zucker J. M., Henry-Amar M., Sarrazin D., Blache R., Patte C., Schweisguth O.: Intensive systemic chemotherapy in localized Ewing's sarcoma in childhood. A historical trial. *Cancer*, **52**, 415-23.

1984   Demeocq F., Carton P., Patte C., Oberlin O., Sarrazin D., Lemerle J.: Treatment of Ewing's sarcoma with intensive initial chemotherapy. 1st evaluation of a French pediatric multicenter protocol. *Presse Médicale*, **13**, 717-21.

1984   Evans R. G., Burgert E. O., Gilchrist G. S., Smithson W. A., Pritchard D. J., Bruckman J. E.: Sequential half-body irradiation (SHBI) and combination chemotherapy as salvage treatment for failed Ewing's sarcoma, a pilot study. *Int. J. Radiat. Oncol. Biol. Phys.*, **10**, 2363-8.

1984 JOYCE M., HARMON D., MANKIN H., SUIT H., SCHILLER A.L., TRUMAN J.T.: Ewing's sarcoma in female siblings: a clinical report and review of the literature. *Cancer*, **53**, 1959-1962.

1984 KOSLOWSKI K., BELUFFI G., MASEL J., DIARD F., FERRARI-GIBOLDI F., LE DOSSEUR P., LABATUT J.: Primary vertebral tumours in children. Report of 20 cases with brief literature review. *Pediatric Radiology*, **14**, 129-39.

1984 LINK M. P., DONALDSON S. S., KEMPSON R. L., WILBUR J. R., GLADER B. E.: Acute nonlymphocytic leukemia developing during the course of Ewing's sarcoma. *Medical Pediatric Oncology*, **12**, 194-200.

1984 NAVAS-PALACIOS J.J., APPARICIO-DUQUE R., VALDES M.: On the histogenesis of Ewing's sarcoma: an ultrastructural, immunohistochemical and cytochemical study. *Cancer*, **53**, 1882-1901.

1984 SHIRLEY S. K., GILULA L. A., SIEGAL G. P., FOULKES M. A., KISSANE J. M., ASKIN F. B.: Roentgenographic-pathologic correlation of diffuse sclerosis in Ewing sarcoma of bone. *Skeletal Radiology*, **12**, 69-78.

1984 THOMAS P. R., PEREZ C. A., NEFF J. R., NESBIT M. E., EVANS R. G.: The management of Ewing's sarcoma, role of radiotherapy in local tumor control. *Cancer Treatment Report*, **68**, 703-10.

1984 TURC-CAREL C., PHILIP I., BERGER M. P., PHILIP T., LENOIR G. M.: Chromosome study of Ewing's sarcoma (ES) cell lines. Consistency of a reciprocal translocation. *Cancer Genet. Cytogenet.*, **12**, 1-19.

1984 WALD S. L., ROLAND T. A.: Intradural spinal metastasis in Ewing's sarcoma: case report and review of the literature. *Neurosurgery*, **15**, 873-7.

1984 WEINSTEIN J. B., SIEGEL M. J., GRIFFITH R. C.: Spinal Ewing sarcoma misleading appearances. *Skeletal Radiology*, **11**, 262-5.

1985 AKHTAR M., ASHRAF M., SABBAH R.: Aspiration cytology of Ewing's sarcoma: light and electron microscopic correlations. *Cancer*, **56**, 2051-2060.

1985 BACCI G., CAPANNA R., ORLANDI M., MANCINI I., BETTELLI G., DALLARI D., CAMPANACCI M.: Prognostic significance of serum lactic acide dehydrogenase in Ewing's tumor of bone. *Ric. Clin. Lab.*, **15**, 89-96.

1985 BACCI G., PICCI P., GHERLINZONI F., CAPANNA R., CALDERONI P., PUTTI C., MANCINI A., CAMPANACCI M.: Localized Ewing's sarcoma of bone: ten years experience at the Istituto Ortopedico Rizzoli in 124 cases treated with multimodal therapy. *European Journal of Cancer*, **21**, 163-173.

1985 SPRINGFIELD D. S., PAGLIARULO C.: Fractures of long bones previously treated for Ewing's sarcoma. *Journal of Bone and Joint Surgery.*, **67**-A, 477-481.

1986 ADVANY S.H., RAO D.N., DINSHAW K.A., NAIR C.N., GOPAL R., VYAS J.J., DESAY P.B.: Adjuvant chemotherapy in Ewing's sarcoma. *Journal of Surgical Oncology*, **32**, 76-78.

1986 KIM T.E., GHAZI G., ATKINSON G., McLAREN J.R., RAGAB A.H.: Ewing's sarcoma of a lower extremity in an infant: a therapeutic dilemma. *Cancer*, **58**, 187-189.

1986 NEFF J.R.: Non-metastatic Ewing's sarcoma of bone: the role of surgical therapy. *Clinical Orthopaedics*, **204**, 111-118.

1986 WILKINS R., PRITCHARD D., BURGERT O., UNNI K.: Ewing's sarcoma of bone: experience with 140 patients. *Cancer*, **58**, 2551-2555.

1987 LLOMBART-BOSCH A., LACOMBE M., CONTESSO G., PEYDRO-OLAYA A.: Small round blue cell sarcoma of bone mimicking atypical Ewing's sarcoma with neuroectodermal features. An analysis of five cases with immunohistochemical and electron microscopic support. *Cancer*, **60**, 1570-1582.

1988 BORIANI S., PICCI P., SUDANESE A., TONI A., MANCINI A., FREZZA G., BARBIERI E., BALDINI N., MONESI M., CIARONI D., BACCI G.: Radioinduced sarcomas in survivors of Ewing's sarcoma. *Tumori*, **74**, 543-551.

1988 FROUGE C., VANEL D., COFFRE C., COVANER D., CONTESSO G., SARRAZIN D.: The role of magnetic resonance in the evaluation of Ewing's sarcoma. A report of 27 cases. *Skeletal Radiology*, **17**, 387-392.

1988 JURGENS M., EXNER V., GADNER H., HARMS D., MICHAELIS J., SAUER R., TREUNER J., VOUTE T., WINKELMANN W., WINKLER K., GOBEL U.: Multidisciplinary treatment of primary Ewing's sarcoma of bone: a 6-year experience of a European cooperative trial. *Cancer*, **61**, 23-32.

1989 LLOMBART-BOSCH A., TERRIER-LACOMBE J., PEYDRO-OLAYA A., CONTESSO G.: Peripheral neuroectodermal sarcoma of soft tissue (peripheral neuroepithelioma): a pathologic study of ten cases with differential diagnosis regarding other small round-cell sarcomas. *Human Pathology*, **20**, 273-280.

1989 PINTO A., GRANT L.M., HAYES F.A., SCHELL M.J., PARHAM D.M.: Immunohistochemical expression of neuron-specific enolase and leu 7 in Ewing's sarcoma of bone. *Cancer*, **64**, 1266-1273.

1989 PRITCHARD D.J.: Small round-cell tumors. *Orthopaedic Clinics of North America*, **20**, 367-375.

1990 CAPANNA R., TONI A., SUDANESE A., MCDONALD D., BACCI G., CAMPANACCI M.: Ewing's sarcoma of the pelvis. *International Orthopaedics*, **14**, 57-61.

1990 ISAYAMA T., IWASAKI H., KIKUCHI M., YOH S., TAKAGISHI N.: Neuroectodermal tumor of bone. Evidence for neural differentiation in a cultured cell line. *Cancer*, **65**, 1771-1781.

1990 STREGE D.W., MANEL D.P. VOGLER C., SCHAJOWICZ F.: Ewing's sarcoma in a phalanx of an infant's finger. *Journal of Bone and Joint Surgery*, **71-A**, 1262-1265.

1990 SUNDARAM M., MERENDA G., MCGUIRE M.M.: A skip lesion in association with Ewing's sarcoma. Report of a case. *Journal of Bone and Joint Surgery*, **71-A**, 764-768.

SKELETAL LESIONS IN SYSTEMIC MALIGNANT LYMPHOMAS AND PRIMARY LYMPHOMA OF BONE

By malignant lymphomas we mean a group of systemic neoplasms of the lymphoblastic tissue, and particularly two, involving skeletal pathology: **Hodgkin's disease**, and **non-Hodgkin lymphomas**.

The skeletal localization of systemic malignant lymphoma may occur in three ways: a) by invasion of the bone by adjacent lymph nodes; this explains the frequent localization of the disease in the vertebral column, the pelvis, the ribs, and the sternum; b) by hematogenous or lymphatic metastases; c) by autochthonous development from the bone marrow.

When the skeleton is examined on autopsy in a case of malignant lymphoma which has followed its course, there is nearly always a fair amount of medullary neoplastic dissemination characterized by small nodes. This dissemination is clinically and radiographically silent. At times it may be visualized by bone scan. Skeletal lesions due to malignant lymphoma, which we deal with, are instead the more massive and rarer ones causing clinical and radiographic signs.

Hodgkin's disease may be manifested by skeletal lesions constituting the first symptom of the disease, when changes in the lymph nodes are still not very apparent, or totally latent. Nonetheless, the latter always end up being manifested, and skeletal localizations are classified as the systemic extent of the disease.

Non-Hodgkin lymphomas may produce skeletal lesions which are sooner or later associated with systemic diffusion in the lymph nodes and the internal organs, but they may also remain indefinitely localized in the skeleton. Thus, lymphoma includes two varieties. One with involvement of the lymph nodes, of the internal organs, and frequently of the skeleton, which is classified among systemic malignant lymphomas. The other, instead, constitutes a non-systemic primary tumor of bone. These two varieties cannot be distinguished on a histological level, and on a clinical level they are characterized by phases of passage and intermediate forms between one and the other. This is why primary lymphoma must be considered together with systemic malignant lymphomas. Of these, it constitutes the most frequent form and the most important one for anyone interested in skeletal pathology. Let us not overlook the fact that lymphoma of bone cannot be considered primary and non-systemic unless it is followed in its course for several years. In cases of apparently primary lymphoma of bone, an accurate study of the lymph nodes, of the remainder of the skeleton, of the internal organs, of the bone marrow and of the peripheral blood is required.

HODGKIN'S DISEASE

There is predilection for the male sex and for those aged from 20 to 40 years. In comparison with primary lymphomas of bone it is observed at a younger age.

On autopsy, tumoral nodes scattered throughout the skeleton are frequently observed. This moderate, late or terminal skeletal dissemination is not of clinical importance, and cannot be visualized on radiograms. We instead wish to deal with skeletal localizations which are clinically, radiographically, or scintigraphically manifested. These are observed in 10-20% of all cases (Jaffe, 1958) and they may rarely constitute the onset of the disease, so that skeletal biopsy becomes the key to diagnosis.

The most frequent skeletal **localization** is the vertebral column (vertebral body), particularly the thoracolumbar region. This is followed by the iliac bone, the ribs and sternum, the proximal femur, the proximal humerus. The skeletal localizations are often multiple.

Clinically, the skeletal lesion is manifested by pain; in vertebral localizations this may be irradiated and associated with neurological disorders. Involvement of the skeleton is more probable in cases characterized by anemia, leukopenia and/or thrombocytopenia, and during advanced stages of the disease.

Radiograms may remain silent for weeks or months after the onset of symptoms. Radiographic modification mainly consists in osteolysis with faded boundaries, at times multiple spots (Fig. 448). Nonetheless, the hodgkinian tissue often causes reactive hyperostosis. Thus, there may be an increase in skeletal opacity, which is generally alternated with spots of osteolysis (Fig. 449). Exceptionally, there have been reports of an «ivory vertebra» in

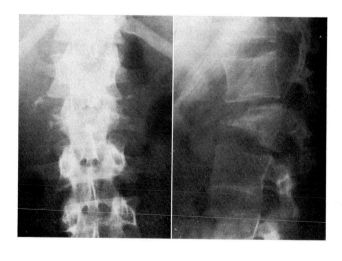

Fig. 448. - Vertebral localization of Hodgkin's disease in a female aged 32 years.

FIG. 449. - Multiple vertebral localizations due to
Hodgkin's disease in a female aged 36 years. Ob-
serve the extent of the lesion to several vertebrae,
the association of osteo-
lysis with osteosclerosis,
and anterior marginal
erosion of two vertebral
bodies.

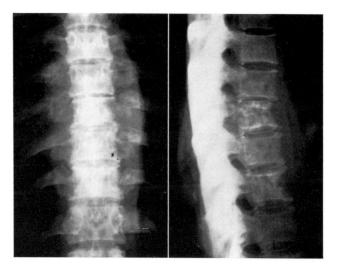

Hodgkin's disease. When the tumoral tissue invades the bone from adjacent
lymph nodes, there is erosion of the cortex from the outside (marginal erosions of the vertebral bodies) (Fig. 449), and CAT shows tumoral masses in
the parosteal soft tissues in continuity with the osteolytic areas. The intervertebral disc remains preserved for a long time. If the entire skeleton is examined radiographically and scintigraphically, other less evident lesions may
be observed.

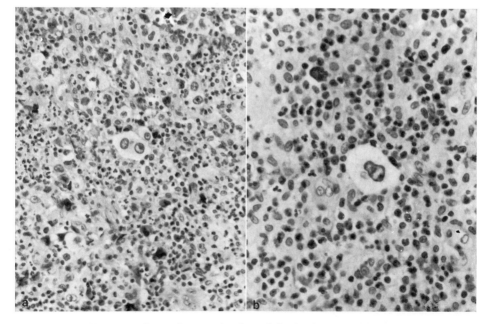

FIG. 450. - Histological aspects of Hodgkin's disease in the skeleton.

Macroscopic examination often shows that the skeletal invasion derives from large adjacent lymph node masses. In other cases or in other areas of the skeleton, instead, there are multiple neoplastic nodules within the medullary canal or the cancellous bone, which are clearly metastatic or autochthonous.

Histologically, the tumoral tissue is the same as that of lymph node localizations (Fig. 450): it has a pseudogranuloma aspect, histio-fibroblasts, lymphocytes, plasmacells, neutrophiles, eosinophiles, Hodgkin cells and Reed-Sternberg cells; areas of necrosis and reactive fibrosis. The tissue may be rich in eosinophiles. In fact, there might be a problem of reciprocal differential diagnosis between Hodgkin's lymphoma and **eosinophilic granuloma**. In eosinophilic granuloma there is a pattern of histiocytes at the background. Even if their nuclei are swollen or rather large, they are never characterized by pleomorphism or hyperchromia, and Reed-Sternberg cells are absent. Moreover, there is no reactive fibrosis, which is frequently observed in Hodgkin's disease.

Even when hodgkinian lesion initially appears to be localized in the bone, during the **course** of the disease, sooner or later, typical systemic changes and ones involving the lymph nodes occur.

PRIMARY LYMPHOMA OF BONE

It is a L. which primarily originates in the bone. If it is not treated, it remains localized and at least apparently exclusive of one (or more) skeletal segments even for several years. If it is treated, it has a high probability of cure [1].

DEFINITION

Primary L. of bone is a round-cell sarcoma which originated from the lymphoid cells of the bone marrow, with histological and clinical features and a course and prognosis which are distinct from those of Ewing's sarcoma. Nonetheless, this distinction is not always evident; even less evident is the separation between primary L. of bone and systemic L. In primary L. of bone a morphological and immunological classification, such as that adopted for systemic L., is not available.

FREQUENCY

It occurs much less frequently than Ewing's sarcoma (Fig. 451).

---

[1] Parker and Jackson 1939 isolated primary «reticulosarcoma» of bone from Ewing's sarcoma, for which it had been mistaken up until that time, based on the observation that some cases were not characterized by a rapid course and the death rate typical of that sarcoma.

SEX

There is predilection for the male sex (Fig. 451).

AGE

In contrast with Ewing's sarcoma, L. is a tumor which occurs during adult and advanced age. Most cases are observed after 25-30 years. It is rarely observed prior to 20 years, and exceptionally prior to 15 (Fig. 451).

LOCALIZATION

Even more than is the case with Ewing's sarcoma, there is predilection for the skeleton of the trunk and the cranio-facial bones (approximately half of all cases). The other half is localized in the long bones, nearly exclusively in the femur, the tibia and the humerus (Fig. 451).

In the long bones it may equally be observed in the meta-epiphysis and in the diaphysis. The epiphysis is involved more frequently than is the case in Ewing's sarcoma, as L. is mostly manifested when the growth cartilage has disappeared.

Not rarely does L. involve two or more adjacent or distant bones.

In some localizations in the spinal epidural space it may be difficult or impossible to establish whether the tumor derives from the bone, on the basis of imaging techniques and findings at laminectomy.

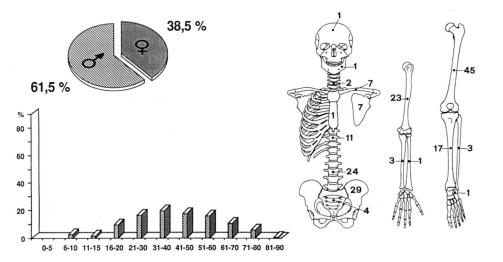

FIG. 451. - Sex, age and localization in 176 cases of lymphoma of bone (apparently primary).

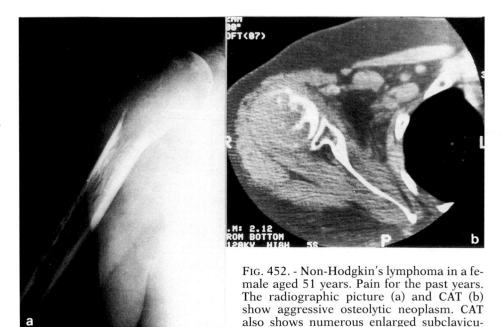

FIG. 452. - Non-Hodgkin's lymphoma in a female aged 51 years. Pain for the past years. The radiographic picture (a) and CAT (b) show aggressive osteolytic neoplasm. CAT also shows numerous enlarged subclavicular lymph nodes.

SYMPTOMS

A first striking feature, in contrast with Ewing's sarcoma, is the perfect integrity of the general conditions of the patient, at least for a long period of time. There is no fever, no anemia, no weight loss, no increase in sedimentation rate, no leukocytosis.

The main symptom is pain, which may remain mild and discontinuous for a long time. Other possible symptoms are local swelling, pathologic fracture, irradiated pain and neurological deficit if there is myeloradicular compression. In L., as compared to Ewing's sarcoma, enlargement of the regional lymph nodes is less rare.

When L. is suspected or actually diagnosed, it is important to explore the entire skeleton (bone scan), the lymph node stations, the liver and the spleen, and study the medullary smears and the peripheral blood.

RADIOGRAPHIC FEATURES

The radiographic picture is not very different from that of Ewing's sarcoma and, similarly, it has few typical elements. Some differences, in relation to Ewing's sarcoma, are due to the fact that L. grows more slowly and, as it is nearly always manifested during adult age, it causes a scarcer osteogenetic reaction of the periosteum.

The radiographic picture is dominated by osteolysis, which is generally spotted and very faded. Often, the bone appears to be moth-eaten; more rare-

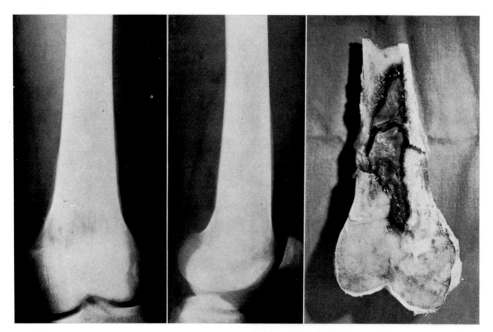

FIG. 453. - Primary lymphoma of bone in a male aged 21 years. Pain for the past 2 months. The radiographic alteration was relatively moderate, with small spots of central osteosclerosis and mild onion peel periosteal reaction. The patient was submitted to en bloc resection: anatomical section of the segment revealed much greater extent of the tumor than was visible on X-ray.

ly, the osteolysis is confluent in a homogeneous area (Figs. 452, 454a, 455, 456, 459).

Alongside osteolysis, there may be areas of increased opacity, due to reactive hyperostosis of the bone which is diffusedly permeated and not resorbed (Figs. 454b, 458b). Rarely, hyperopaque sclerosis dominates the radiographic picture.

The cortex is generally interrupted, but at times it appears to be relatively preserved (Figs. 455, 457a, 462a). In more advanced forms of the tumor, it expands in the soft tissues with masses which are deprived of radiopacity and faded, or run through by some streaks of reactive ossification (Figs. 457b, 461a). The osteogenetic reaction of the periosteum is absent (Fig. 458b) or rather scarce. It may be more lively in the diaphysis and during youth, but it rarely achieves an onion skin aspect (Figs. 453, 458a). Pathologic fractures occur quite frequently (Figs. 456, 458b, 461, 462).

As is the case in Ewing's sarcoma, the anatomical lesion tends to be rather more extensive than is visualized in the radiogram (Fig. 453). In this sense **bone scan** and **MRI** are very demonstrative. Nonetheless, in some cases because of the slow course and scarcity of symptoms, the lesion (of long duration and rather advanced on diagnosis) appears to be very extended even in radiograms. At times the radiographic alteration is extended to nearly half of the entire bone, or even to the entire diaphysis.

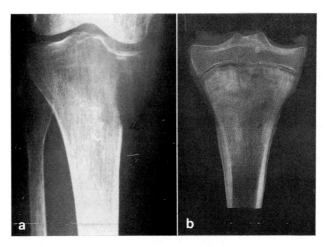

FIG. 454. - (a) Primary lymphoma of bone in a female aged 60 years. For the past 3 months pain and swelling. Laterocervical adenopathy. Completely osteolytic form: the patient died after 4 months due to diffusion of the neoplasm. (b) Primary skeletal lymphoma in a female aged 15 years. For the past year pain and swelling after trauma. The patient was submitted to en bloc resection. Radiogram of the anatomical specimen. Prevalently sclerosing form of the disease. The patient was well 13 years after resection.

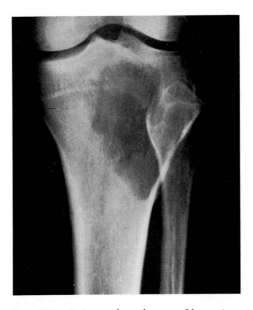

FIG. 455. - Primary lymphoma of bone in a female aged 34 years. The radiographic aspect could suggest giant cell tumor.

Lymphography is indicated for a study of the regional lymph nodes, and **total body bone scan** in order to exclude other skeletal localizations, as well as **hepatic and splenic isotope scan**.

GROSS PATHOLOGIC FEATURES

The tumoral tissue which is vital and not altered is grayish-white, soft, juicy, encephaloid. It is not differentiated from the tissue of all malignant lymphomas, of Ewing's sarcoma, and of any very cellular sarcoma.

Like Ewing's sarcoma, it frequently expands outside the cortex and tends to extend in the bone, considerably far from the main lesion, with multiple nodes and/or diffused infiltration.

Like Ewing's sarcoma, it often presents areas of hemorrhaging, necrosis and liquefaction. The latter may cause the false impression during surgical exploration of an osteomyelitis.

At times, the regional lymph nodes are enlarged, of firm-elastic consistency, at times fused in a packet. On the cut surface, the lymph node pulp is totally or partially substituted by whitish bulging, encephaloid tissue.

HISTOPATHOLOGIC FEATURES

It is a richly cellular tissue. The cells have pale and scarce cytoplasm, but in some it is more abundant and clearly delimited. There may be a delicate intercellular reticulum formed by the union between the cytoplasmatic processes.

The nuclei are generally larger than those of Ewing's sarcoma, with considerable polydimensionality and pleomorphism. Some are roundish or oval; others are kidney-shaped, pearhaped, indented or lobulated. Some cells may have a rather large nucleus or double nucleus, but there are no giant cells. At times the chromatin is pulverulent, other times it is in rougher blocks. The nucleus may tend to be vesicular and often one or more nucleoli, even

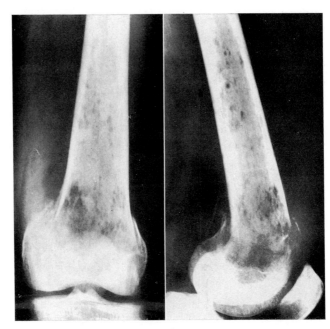

FIG. 456. - Primary lymphoma of bone in a male aged 38 years. Extensive moth-eaten image with pathologic fracture.

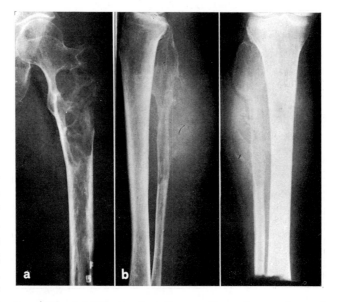

FIG. 457. - (a) Primary lymphoma of bone in a male aged 40 years. Extensive osteolytic bubbly lesion with relatively well-defined margins. (b) Female aged 35 years. Large lesion, completely osteolytic, with faded boundaries and extensive invasion of the soft tissues. In both cases there was no periosteal reaction.

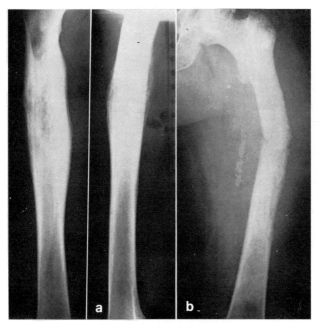

FIG. 458. - (a) Primary lymphoma of bone in a male aged 19 years. The symptoms had been interpreted as osteomyelitis. The patient was treated with radiation therapy alone, and was well after 17 years. (b) Primary lymphoma of bone in a female aged 52 years. For the past year pain and 2 months earlier pathologic fracture. The lesion was diffused to approximately 2/3 of the femur, with an extensive mass in the soft tissues. Hip disarticulation, the patient died after 1 year due to diffusion of the tumor.

large ones, are evident. Mitotic figures are frequent (Fig. 460a, b). Among these reticular cells numerous lymphoblasts and lymphocytes are often disseminated (Fig. 460c).

There are collagenous bands, which may be delicate or rougher, and which may divide the tissue into irregular alveoli. Argentic impregnation often but not always reveals a thick reticulum surrounding small groups of cells and even single cells (Fig. 460d). P.A.S. does not reveal cellular glycogen. Immunohistochemistry (in undecalcified specimens) may reveal positive for lymphocytic markers.

In better differentiated L., the cells are diffusedly small, of lymphoid appearance. The nuclei are smaller and darker, as compared with Ewing's sarcoma, but the cytoplasmatic borders are more distinct.

FIG. 459. - Lymphoma of bone in a male aged 41 years. For 9 years the patient was treated for myeloid chronic leukemia. (a) Radiogram obtained 2 months after the onset of right lumbar sciatic pain at L5. There was mild erosion of the lateral right somatic border at L4. (a) Progression of osteolysis after 1 month. The patient died a few weeks later with neoplastic diffusion.

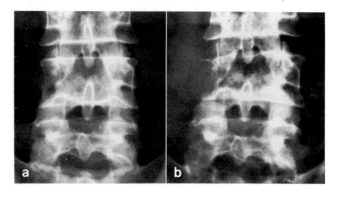

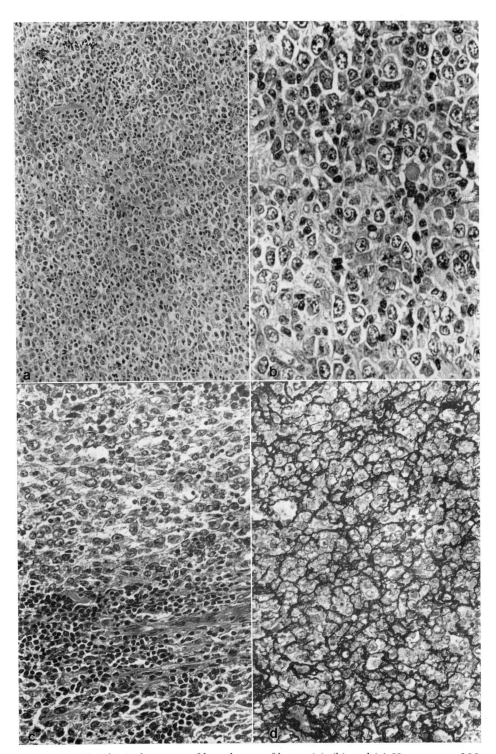

FIG. 460. - Histological aspects of lymphoma of bone. (a), (b) and (c) *Hemat.-eos.*, 200, 500, 300 x; (d) *argentic impregnation* 300 x.

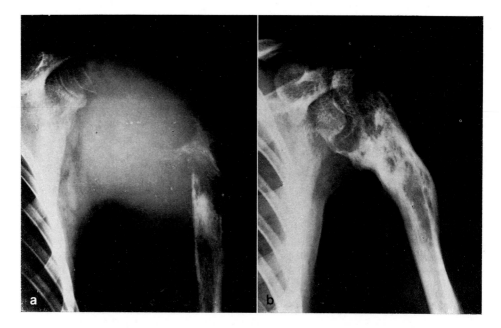

FIG. 461. - Primary lymphoma of bone in a male aged 17 years. (a) Severely destructive and expanded lesion of the proximal humerus. (b) Reconstruction of the humerus 2 years after radiation therapy. The patient had several other skeletal localizations, all irradiated, and was well 6 years after diagnosis.

HISTOGENESIS AND PATHOGENESIS

It originates from the medullary lymphoid cells. It occurs more frequently in association with immunological disorders, such as A.I.D.S.

DIAGNOSIS

Based on clinical and radiographic data, some L. may mimic a non-neoplastic lesion, such as **osteomyelitis** or **eosinophilic granuloma**. More often, the radiographic alteration is evidently neoplastic but, depending on the individual case, it cannot be distinguished from a **metastasis** due to a carcinoma, a **fibrosarcoma**, a **malignant fibrous histiocytoma**, an **Ewing's sarcoma**, an **osteosarcoma** (Fig. 389b).

The surgical macroscopic finding, in rare cases of tumor which is contained and extensively liquefied, may suggest **osteomyelitis**.

Diagnosis is above all histological. But it is not always easy. If a tissue with the histological features described above derives from a lymph node, then diagnosis is certain, at most with some superimposition in relation to that of Hodgkin's sarcoma. When, instead, the tissue originates from the bone, histological differential diagnosis with **Ewing's sarcoma** is not always convincing. The histological aspects differentiating L. from Ewing's sarcoma are as follows. More extensive and distinct cytoplasms, larger pleomorphic nuclei, tending to be vesicular and at times having indentations in their profile, a rougher chromatin pattern, and more evident nucleoli, more frequent mitotic figures, more abundant collagenous fibers, a more regular and thicker argyrophilous reticulum (but not always), absence of cellular glycogen, positivity for immunological markers. Numerous lymphoblasts and lymphocytes are often observed in L. However, there are cases of Ewing's sarcoma where the nuclei are larger and slightly pleomorphic, or with scarce or doubtful evidence of the glycogen, or with a more abundant reticulum. The clinical features which differentiate L. from Ewing's sarcoma are as follows. Adult or advanced age, absence of fever, anemia, weight loss, tendency to remain for a longer period of time circumscribed to a single area of the skeleton, at times lymph node metastases or systemic manifestations in the lymph nodes, a slower course and a better prognosis.

Finally, L. may, although rarely, cause problems in histological differentiation with an undifferentiated **epithelial metastasis** (cf. diagnosis of Ewing's sarcoma), or with a skeletal lesion of **histiocytosis X** (cf. diagnosis of histiocytosis X). This last problem in diagnosis may occur if a marginal area of L. is examined, where peritumoral inflammatory reaction prevails.

COURSE

Although there may be considerable variations, L. often grows slowly. In general, the duration of symptoms prior to diagnosis is greater than 6 months-1 year, but it may even be a few years. The course of the disease is always varied and unpredictable. There are cases in which the tumor remains localized in a skeletal segment and, if it is treated, it does heal. In other cases, there may be metastases in the regional lymph nodes. These, too, may heal. In other cases still, a second localization, or localizations, in the skeleton may occur early or after several years. In these cases, as well, the neoplasm remains concentrated in the skeleton and it may extend to the regional lymph nodes alone. Finally, there are cases in which primary and apparently single L. of bone is followed by systemic diffusion to the lymph nodes, the liver, the spleen, and other internal organs, even after many years. The latter constitute systemic L. which began in the bone. Pulmonary metastases occur rarely.

TREATMENT

L. is very sensitive to radiation therapy (Fig. 461), which constitutes the treatment of choice for primary localizations, metastases, and multicentric skeletal localizations. The dose generally varies from 5000 to 8000 r. Irradiation must be extended to a wider volume than that occupied by the radiographic lesion, generally to the entire bone affected.

Radiation therapy must be associated with cyclical and long-lasting poly-chemotherapy.

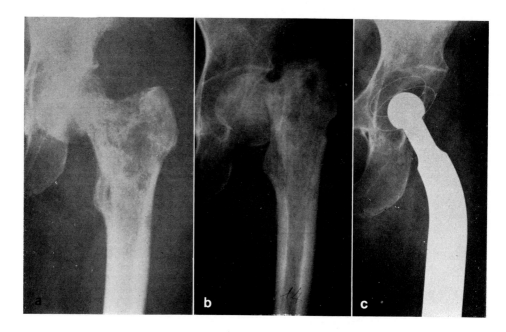

Fig. 462. - Primary lymphoma of bone in a female aged 37 years. After radiation therapy there was pathologic fracture (a), which worsened (b). The patient was thus submitted to resection and arthroprosthesis (c).

If there should be myeloradicular compression, decompressive laminectomy with biopsy is indicated, followed by radiation therapy; or immediate radiation therapy after needle-biopsy. When dealing with very destructive lesions of the long bones with pathologic fracture or impending fracture, resection, the application of endo- or arthroprosthesis (Fig. 462), osteosynthesis possibly associated with the use of acrylic cement are all indicated. Radiation and chemotherapy must be carried out after surgery, as stated above. Resection may also be indicated in lesions of the scapula, ribs, anterior pelvic arch, in association with the chemo- and radiation therapy.

Amputation is restricted to rare cases where expansion of the tumor contraindicates conservative surgical treatment and radiation therapy, or when the latter proves to be insufficient to manage the tumor, or in cases of extensive local recurrence after radiation therapy.

PROGNOSIS

The variable, slow and insidious course of the disease will not allow us to speak of certain healing, not even 10 years after treatment. Obviously, five-year survival rate is of little importance. It was rather high, even prior to the use of chemotherapy, with approximately 40-50% of all cases. But survival after 10 years was approximately 30%. The association of chemotherapy has increased the percentage of survival to 60-80%. As may be observed, the prognosis is better than that of Ewing's sarcoma.

Elements indicating a worse prognosis are the wide extent of the neoplasm to the bone and localizations in the pelvis and skeleton of the trunk. At times, L. recurs in irradiated skeletal areas. In exceptional cases, after several years, radiation sarcoma is manifested in the same site.

REFERENCES

1939 PARKER F. Jr., JACKSON H. Jr.: Primary reticulum cell sarcoma of bone. *Surgery, Gynecology and Obstetrics*, **68**, 45-53.

1954 FRANCIS K. C., HIGINBOTHAM N. L., COLEY B. L.: Primary reticulum cell sercoma of bone. Report of 44 cases. *Surgery, Gynecology and Obstetrics*, **99**, 142-146.

1958 JAFFE H. L.: *Tumors and tumorous conditions of the bones and joints*. Lea & Febiger, Philadelphia.

1960 HARDER J.: Über Knochenlymphogranulomatose. *Fortschritte auf dem Gebiete der Röntgenstrahlen und Nuklearmedizin*, **93**, 445-455.

1963 IVINS J. C., DAHLIN D. C.: Malignant lymphoma (reticulum cell sarcoma) of bone. *Mayo Clinic Proceedings*, **38**, 375-385.

1963 MOSELEY J. E.: *Bone changes in hematologic disorders*. Grune & Stratton, New York and London.

1967 EDEIKEN J., HODES P. J.: Reticulum cell sarcoma (primary of bone), in « *Röntgen diagnosis of disease of bone* », Williams & Wilkins Company, Baltimora.

1967 FRANSSILA K. O., KALIMA T. V., VOUTILAINEN A.: Histologic classification of Hodgkin's disease. *Cancer*, **20**, 1594-1601.

1967 GRANGER W., WHITAKER R.: Hodgkin's disease in bone, with special reference to periosteal reaction. *British Journal of Radiology*, **40**, 939-948.

1967 HUSTU H. O., PINKEL D.: Lymphosarcoma, Hodgkin's disease and leukemia in bone. *Clinical Orthopaedics*, **52**, 83-93.

1968 HARBERT J. C., ASHBURN W. L.: Radiostrontium bone scanning in Hodgkin's disease. *Cancer*, **22**, 58-63.

1968 WANG C. C., FLEISCHLI D. J.: Primary reticulum cell sarcoma of bone. With emphasis on radiation therapy. *Cancer*, **22**, 994-998.

1969 HORAN F. T.: Bone involvement in Hodgkin's disease. A survey of 201 cases. *British Journal of Surgery*, **56**, 277-281.

1970 GROSSMAN M.: Roentgenographic changes in childhood Hodgkin's disease. *American Journal of Roentgenology*, **108**, 354-364.

1971 DUHAMEL G., NAJMAN A., ANDRÈ R.: Les localisations a la moelle osseuse de la maladie de Hodgkin. *Presse Medicale*, **79**, 2305-2308.

1971 MILLER T. R., NICHOLSON J. T.: End results in reticulum cell sarcoma of bone treated by bacterial toxin therapy alone or combined with surgery and/or radiotherapy (47 cases) or with concurrent infection (5 cases). *Cancer*, **27**, 524-548.

1971 SHOJI H., MILLER T. R.: Primary reticulum cell sarcoma of bone. *Cancer*, **28**, 1234-1244.

1971 SILVERBERGER I. J., JACOBS E. M.: Treatment of spinal cord compression in Hodgkin's disease. *Cancer*, **27**, 308-313.

1972 BEACHLEY M. C., LAV B. P., KING E. R.: Bone involvement in Hcdgkin's disease. *American Journal of Roentgenology*, **114**, 559-563.

1972 JONES S. E., ROSENBERG S. A., KAPLAN S. H.: Non-Hodgkin's lymphomas. *Cancer*, **29**, 954-960.

1972 LEVITT M., MARSH J. C., DE CONTI R. C.,. MITCHELL M. S., SKEEL R. T., FARBER L. R., BERTINO J. R.: Combination sequential chemotherapy in advanced reticulum cell sarcoma. *Cancer*, **29**, 630-636.

1973 DAHLIN D. C.: Primary malignant lynphoma (reticulum cell sarcoma) of bone, in « *Bone - Certain aspects of neoplasia* », Butterworths, London.

1974 BOSTON H. C. Jr., DAHLIN D. C., IVINS J. C., CUPPS R. E.: Malignant lymphoma (so-called reticulum cell sarcoma) of bone. *Cancer*, **34**, 1131-1137.

1975 FERRANT A., RODHAIN J., MICHAUX J. L., PIRET L., MALDAGUE D., SOKAL G.: Detection of skeletal involvement in Hodgkin's disease: a comparison of radiography, bone scanning, and bone marrow biopsy in 38 patients. *Cancer*, **35**, 1346-1353.

1975 WEISS R. B., BRUNNING R. D., KENNEDY B. J.: Hodgkin's disease in the bone marrow. *Cancer*, **36**, 2077-2085.

1976 FRIEDMAN M., KIM T. H., PANAHON A. M.: Spinal cord compression in malignant lymphoma. Treatment and results. *Cancer*, **37**, 1485-1491.

1976 SCHECHTER J. P., JONES S. E., WOOLFENDEN J. M., LILIEN D. L., O'MARA R. E.: Bone scanning in lymphoma. *Cancer*, **38**, 1142-1148.

1976 STEIN R. S., ULTMANN J. E., BYRNE G. E., MORAN E. M., GOLOMB H. M., OETZEL N.: Bone marrow involvement in non-Hodgkin's lymphoma. Implications for staging and therapy. *Cancer*, **37**, 629-636.

1982 BACCI G., PICCI P., BERTONI F., GHERLINZONI F., CALDERONI P., CAMPANACCI M.: Primary non-Hodgkin's lymphoma of bone: results in 15 patients treated by radiotherapy combined with systemic chemotherapy. *Cancer Treatment Report*, **66**, 1859-1862.

1982 DOSORETZ D., RAYMOND K., MURPHY G., DOPPKE K.P., SCHILLER A.L., WANG C.C., SUIT H.D.: Primary lymphoma of bone: the relationship of morphological diversity to clinical behaviour. *Cancer*, **50**, 1009-1014.

1985 BACCI G., JAFFE N., EMILIANI E., CAPANNA R., CALDERONI P., PICCI P., BERTONI F., GHERLINZONI F., CAMPANACCI M.: Staging, therapy and prognosis of primary non-Hodgin's lymphoma of bone and comparison of results with localized Ewing's sarcoma: ten years' experience at the Istituto Ortopedico Rizzoli. *Tumori*, **71**, 345-354.

1986 OSTROWSKI M.L., UNNI K.K., BANKS P.M., SHIVES T.C., EVANS R.G., O'CONNEL M.J., TAYLOR W.F.: Malignant lymphoma of bone. *Cancer*, **58**, 2646-2655.

1987 AHMED T., WORMSER G.P., STAHL R.E., RAVINDER M., CIMINO J., GLASSER M., MITTELMAN A., FRIEDLAND M., ARLIN Z.: Malignant lymphomas in a population at risk for acquired immunodeficiency syndrome. *Cancer*, **60**, 719-723.

1987 CLAYTON F., BUTLER J.J., AYALA A.G., RO J.V., ZORNOZA J.: Non Hodgkin's lymphoma in bone: pathologic and radiologic features with clinical correlates. *Cancer*, **60**, 2494-2501.

1987 HOWART A.T., THOMAS H., WATERS K.T., CAMPBELL P.E.: Malignant lymphoma of bone in children. *Cancer*, **59**, 335-339.

1987 SAMUELS T.S., HOWARD B.A., RUBENSTEIN J.D., SRIGLEY J.: Case report 409. *Skeletal Radiology*, **16**, 78-81.

1989 UEDA T., AOZASA K., OHSAWA M., YOSHIKAWA H., UCHIDA A., ONO K., MATSUMOTO K.: Malignant lymphomas of bone in Japan.*Cancer*, **64**, 2387-2392.

1990 PETTIT C.K., ZUKERBERG L.R., GRAY M.H., FERRY J.A., ROSENBERG A.E., HARMON D.C., HARRIS N.L.: Primary lymphoma of bone. A B-cell neoplasm with a high frequency of multilobulated cells. *American Journal of Surgical Pathology*, **14**, 329-334.

1990 PORTLOCK C.S.: Non-Hodgkin lymphomas. Advances in diagnosis, staging and management. *Cancer*, **65**, 718-722.

1990 SANTOS G.W.: Bone marrow transplantation in hematologic malignancies. Current status. *Cancer*, **65**, 786-791.

SKELETAL LESIONS IN LEUKEMIA

We particularly intend to discuss skeletal manifestations of **acute leukemia in the child**. This type of leukemia, which is more often lymphatic, causes radiographic skeletal alterations in nearly half of all cases and osteoarticular symptoms in a smaller but still significant number of patients. The skeletal manifestations of infantile leukemia are very important because they often represent the only symptom at onset.

When dealing with a child who complains of osteoarticular pain, at times characterized by mild joint swelling and fever, with a normal picture of peripheral blood (infantile leukemia often remains aleukemic) it is easy to imagine rheumatic disease or Still's disease, unless the behavior of leukemia is not known, and the radiographic picture is not interpreted correctly. The presence of moderate enlargement of the spleen and/or the lymph nodes may be interpreted as a component of Still's disease. Radiograms reveal peculiar leukemic alterations of the skeleton, and direct us towards a correct diagnosis, which will be confirmed by the marrow aspiration smear.

The **initial radiographic aspect**, the most frequent and typical one, consists in a metaphyseal band of faded radiotransparence. This is immediately adjacent to the growth cartilage and it is initially thin. There may be a first radiotransparent line (cartilage) in the metaphysis, followed by a thin radiopaque line (the layer of calcified cartilage) and then by a second transparent line (Fig. 463a). This osteoporosis or osteolysis is particularly intense (and thus it achieves the threshold of radiographic evidence) in the region of newly-formed bony trabeculae of the metaphysis, because in this location the compression on the part of the leukemic tissue filling the medullary spaces acts on a very delicate bone or rather it obstructs its neoformation. For the same reason, radiotransparent bands are observed particularly in those metaphyses where skeletal growth is livelier, that is, the knee, the shoulder, the wrist.

In a more advanced phase, the development of leukemic tissue causes a widening of the metaphyseal osteolytic bands, which furthermore occur in all of the metaphyses and is associated with dotting, and faded osteolytic spots. This fine moth-eaten aspect or diffused osteoporosis or spotted osteolysis prevails in the spongy bone: metaphyses, epiphyses, bones of the hand and foot, vertebral column, cranium, pelvis.

More massive areas of osteolysis, which may lead to pathologic fracture, are rarely manifested. The latter aspects are similar to those of metastases

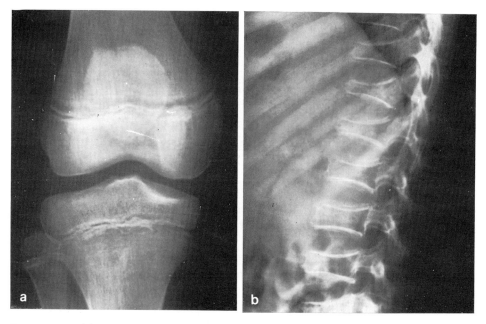

FIG. 463. - (a) and (b) Acute lymphatic leukemia in a child aged 9. (b) Fish vertebrae.

due to neuroblastoma. It must be recalled, however, that these hardly ever involve the limbs distal to the knee, where leukemic lesions may be evident in the hand and foot, as well.

In the vertebral column diffused osteoporosis may be observed, with a reduction in height and biconcave deformity of the vertebrae, and relative increase in thickness and in convexity of the intervertebral disks (fish vertebrae, Fig. 463b).

Finally, one common radiographic finding is diffused osteogenetic periosteal reaction of the diaphyses, in faded laminar and/or wrinkled form. This is secondary to the leukemic infiltration which occurs in the haversian canals uplifting the periosteum. This radiographic aspect must not be confused with that of osteomyelitis or Ewing's sarcoma (particularly if there is fever).

All radiographic alterations of the skeleton tend to completely regress if therapy produces remission of the leukemia. In particular, radiotransparent metaphyseal bands regress, and are often substituted by bands of increased radiopacity, similar to those due to intoxication with heavy metal.

In **chronic leukemia in the adult**, clinical manifestations and radiographic alterations of the skeleton are quite rare, and they hardly ever initiate the symptomatological picture. In the adult, unlike what occurs in the child, skeletal alterations, when they do in fact exist, are above all observed in the skeleton of the trunk, where the hemopoietic marrow is concentrated.

At most, diffused osteoporosis may be observed, particularly vertebral, and possibly some collapsed vertebrae; or fine moth-eaten aspect in the cranium; or confluent moth-eaten aspect in some other skeletal segment. It is interesting to recall that anatomically, in addition to the osteoporosis induced by the pressure of the medullary leukemic tissue, necrosis of the bone trabeculae (and of the leukemic tissue) due to obliteration of the medullary vessels may be observed, at times favored by cortisone therapy. This necrosis may facilitate collapse and pathological fracture, particularly in the femoral head.

REFERENCES

1961 THOMAS L. B., FORKNER C. E. Jr. Frei, BRESSE B. E. Jr., STABENAU J. R.: The skeletal lesions of acute leukemia. *Cancer*, **14**, 608-621.

1963 MOSELEY J. E.: *Bone changes in hematologic disorders (roentgen aspects)*. Grune & Stratton, New York and London.

1969 CHABNER B. A., HOSKELL C. M., CANELLOS G. P.: Destructive bone lesions in chronic granulocityc leukemia. *Medicine*, **48**, 401-410.

1975 CAMPBELL E., MALDONADO W., SUHRLAND G.: Painful lytic bone lesion in an adult with chronic myelogenous leukemia. *Cancer*, **35**, 1354-1356.

1981 TOOLIS F., POTTER B., ALLAN N.C., LANGLANDS A.O.: Radiation induced leukemias in ankylosing spondylitis. *Cancer*, **48**, 1582-1585.

1982 DEMANES D.J., LANE N., BECKSTEAD J.H.: Bone involvement in hairy-cell leukemia. *Cancer*, **49**, 1697-1701.

1986 DHARMASENA F., WICKHAM N., McHUGH P.J., CATOVSKY D., GALTON D.A.G.: Osteolytic tumors in acute megacaryoblastic leukemia. *Cancer*, **58**, 2273-2277.

1986 ROGALKY R.J., BLACK G.B., KEED M.H.: Orthopaedic manifestations of leukemia in children. *Journal of Bone and Joint Surgery*, **68-A**, 494-501.

1987 CAUDLE R.J., CRAWFORD A.H., GELFAND M.J., GRUPPO R.A.: Childhood acute lymphoblastic leukemia presenting as « cold » lesions on bone scan: a report of two cases. *Journal of Pediatric Orthopaedics*, **7**, 93-95.

1987 COHN S.L., MORGAN E.R., MALLETTE L.E.: The spectrum of metabolic bone disease in lymphoblastic leukemia. *Cancer*, **59**, 346-350.

1987 SAMUDA G.M., CHENG M.Y., YEUNG C.Y.: Back pain in vertebral compression: an uncommon presentation of childhood acute lymphoblastic leukemia. *Journal of Pediatric Orthopaedics*, **7**, 175-178.

1988 HEALEY J.H., LANE J.M., ERLANDSON R.A., BULLOUGH P.G.: Solid leukemic tumor. An uncommon presentation of a common disease. *Clinical Orthopaedics*, **194**, 248-251.

1988 HEROLD C.J., WITTICH G.R., SCHWARZINGER I., HALLER J., CHOTT A., MOSTBECK G., HAJEK P.G.: Skeletal involvement in hair-cell leukemia. *Skeletal Radiology*, **17**, 171-175.

1988 RIBEIRO R.C., PUI C.H., SCHELL M.J.: Vertebral compression fracture as a presenting feature of acute lymphocytic leukemia in children. *Cancer*, **61**, 589-592.

1988 SALIMI Z., SUNDARAM M.: Avascular bone necrosis in an untreated case of chronic myelogenous leukemia. *Skeletal Radiology*, **17**, 353-355.

1989 GOERG C., GOERG K., PFLUEGER K.H., HAVEMANN K.: Neurofibromatosis and acute monocytic leukemia in adults. *Cancer*, **64**, 1717-1719.

PLASMACYTOMA
(Synonyms: myeloma, multiple myeloma, myelomatosis, plasmacellular myeloma)

DEFINITION

It is a primary and systemic malignant neoplasm of the bone marrow, which originates from the B lymphoid cells, and is characterized by plasmacellular differentiation. The occurrence of a skeletal P. which is truly solitary and thus curable is doubtless and certainly exceptional [1].

FREQUENCY

The tumor occurs frequently, much moreso than osteosarcoma, even if our series does not include as many cases as those of the latter (Fig. 464).

SEX

There is predilection for the male sex, at a ratio of 1.5:1 (Fig. 464).

AGE

P. is a tumor which affects mature or advanced age. It is nearly always observed after 40-50 years of age. It is very rarely observed prior to 30 years of age, and it is practically unknown prior to puberty.

---

[1] There is also a type of P. which initiates in the soft tissues, particularly the nose-pharynx, conjunctiva, or lymph nodes. This often remains localized, without skeletal diffusion, and it may heal: extraosseous plasmacytoma, which is for the most part benign or, better yet, characterized by local malignancy.

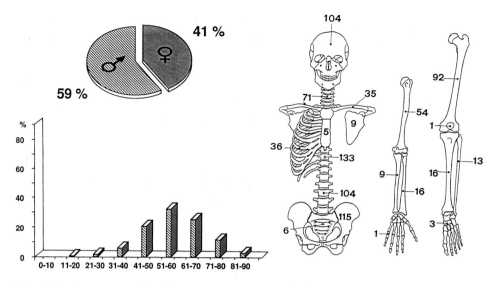

F<small>IG</small>. 464. - Age, sex and localization in 344 cases of plasmacytoma. Only radiographically evident and prevalent localizations are indicated.

LOCALIZATION

As we are dealing with a systemic neoplasm of the bone marrow, P. will
sooner or later extend to most of the skeleton, particularly to those areas
which contain red marrow in the adult. These are the areas of the cancellous
bone in the trunk, the cranium and the metaepiphyses, particularly those of
the hip and shoulder.

Diffusion to the skeleton is neither simultaneous nor uniform. Generally,
in a specific stage of the disease, some bones are affected more (Fig. 464),
while in others the alteration is not as yet present, or rather, it may only be
visualized microscopically.

Not rarely, P. is revealed at the onset by a single tumoral mass circumscribed to a single skeletal segment: **solitary P.** However, only exceptionally
does solitary P. remain as such. Nearly always it is followed by skeletal diffusion and death, even after several years. The most common localization of solitary P. is the vertebral column (one or two vertebrae). This is followed by
the bones of the trunk and the upper end of the femur.

SYMPTOMS

The first symptoms, often for weeks or months, remain vague or not localized. They may consist in mild skeletal pain, asthenia, weight loss, moderate
anemia. Often, the patient complains of low back pain, which may be extended to the thoracic region. When the rachialgia — more often low back pain
— is considerable, pain may be exacerbated by movement, and the paravertebral musculature is contracted. Percussion of the spinous apophyses may

awaken pain. In some cases the low back pain is associated with sciatic or crural pain, due to nerve root compression by the myelomatous tissue. At times, vertebral pain becomes intense. When this occurs suddenly (after stress, mild trauma, or even without apparent cause), it is a sign that pathologic vertebral fracture has occurred. In more expanded vertebral localizations, paralysis due to gradual or sudden medullary compression with or without vertebral collapse may occur.

More infrequently the onset of symptoms includes pain and, at times, pathologic fracture in a long bone. These symptoms occur more often during the course of the disease which is already evident.

In advanced stages of the disease, there may be swelling of the superficial bones (ribs, sternum, clavicle), progressive weight loss and anemia, fever, hyperazotemia, hemorrhagic diathesis, hypercalcemic and hyperuricemic syndrome, extraskeletal myelomatous masses, macrogloxia due to amyloidosis. In rare cases, there is severe and uremic renal insufficiency.

LABORATORY FINDINGS

The **bone marrow smear** often reveals P. even when the symptoms are just initiating or uncertain. Obviously, a negative smear does not exclude the existence of the disease. If the smear contains more than 3% of plasmacells it may be suspected. If it contains 10% the disease is very likely, but other conditions, such as hepatic affections and bone metastases due to carcinoma, may cause a diffused or perimetastatic increase in medullary plasmacells. If the plasmacellular percentage is even more elevated (it may go as far as 70%) and if alongside typical plasmacells ones with a large or double nucleus and even more immature and atypical elements are observed, diagnosis is certain. Naturally, the more advanced the disease, the more frequent the positiveness of the cytological finding.

Serum proteins. In a high percentage of cases there is an increase in globulins, with inversion of the albumin/globulin ratio. Electrophoresis and, in particular, immuno-electrophoresis shows, even when the total globulins are not very increased, a narrow and sharp peak located in the area of the α or the γ globulin bands of the electrophoresis. This is due to the excess presence of a monoclonal immunoglobulin. The electrophoretic alteration is present in nearly all cases with disseminated lesions [1]. It may be absent at the onset, particularly in cases of solitary P. Rarely, serum electrophoresis is not demonstrative, while urinary electrophoresis is.

Bence-Jones proteinuria. More sensitive than the traditional research which involves heating the urine, are urinary electrophoresis and immuno-

[1] Moreover, it must be recalled that there are exceptional observations of monoclonal macroglobulinemia (similar to the Waldenstrom form) with diffused and multiple osteolyses resembling those of P., without there being any P.

electrophoresis. It is rarely positive, and observed in P. secreting light chains globulins (k or l).

Calcemia. It is often elevated due to diffused bone resorption induced by myelomatous proliferation.

Uricemia and azotemia. They are both frequently increased. The hyperuricemia is due to the excessive catabolism of the nucleic acids, as occurs in all severe medullary proliferations. The hyperazotemia is due to myelomatous renal modifications.

Peripheral blood. It reveals anemia. The white blood cells are generally not modified. In rare cases, nonetheless, there may be considerable leukocytosis, and even a good number of plasmacells. Cases such as these have been referred to as plasmacellular leukemia.

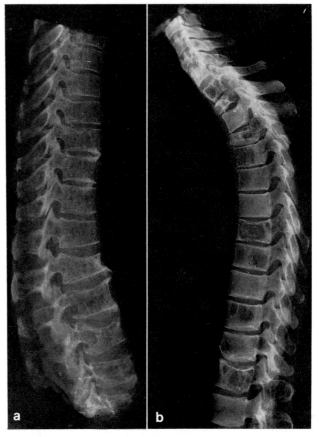

FIG. 465. - Two radiographic images of plasmacytoma, diffused (a) and respectively in multiple nodes (b), in the vertebral column. Anatomical specimens.

RADIOGRAPHIC FEATURES

There is a radiographic latency phase and a disproportion between anatomical and radiographic extent of P. Even when the medullary spaces are diffusedly infiltrated by the pathologic tissue, but there is still no important resorption of the trabeculae and cortex, radiograms remain negative.

When the myelomatous tissue makes the skeletal structures considerably porous, radiographically there may be diffused osteoporosis, with thinning of the cortex (Fig. 467). This finding is particularly frequent in initial phases of the disease and in the vertebral column.

In an even more advanced phase, the myelomatous tissue not only diffusedly infiltrates the medullary spaces, it also forms disseminated nodules, which are at first minute and then larger and confluent. This anatomical phase determines the most typical radiographic aspects of P. which consist in a minute moth-eaten aspect, in rounded osteolytic spots, in confluent bubbly images, and, finally, in rather expanded osteolytic lesions. What is typical is the fact that there is no rim of opacity around the osteolytic lacunae. At the same time, the cortical bones are thinned as a result of internal erosion and in some areas they may be cancelled (Fig. 465).

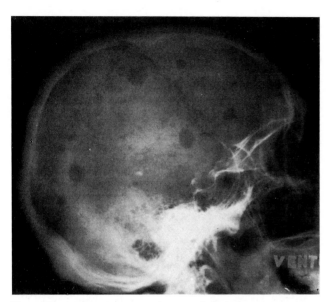

FIG. 466. - Plasmacytoma in a male aged 52 years. Lesions of the cranium.

Very fine porosity may be observed in the cranium, like very close pin points, having a ground glass image. In a more advanced phase of the disease, furthermore, round, unequal, diffused, ever-growing and possibly confluent osteolytic lacunae occur. The osteolytic lacunae have a typical punched-out aspect, and the cranium seems to be sprayed (Fig. 466).

In the vertebral column, osteoporosis becomes more intense, until there is a reduction in height and biconcave deformity of the vertebrae, with a relative increase in thickness and convexity of the disc spaces. Within this severe osteoporosis there may be osteolytic lacunae. What is typical is the fact that the osteolytic lacunae are also located in the posterior vertebral arch and in the ribs. The cortices, both vertebral and costal, are very attenuated, here and there mildly expanded in bubbly form, or interrupted in some areas. Often there is multiple vertebral collapse (Figs. 465, 467). Similar modifications may be observed in the pelvis (Figs. 468, 469, 470).

In the long bones, osteoporosis, a moth-eaten

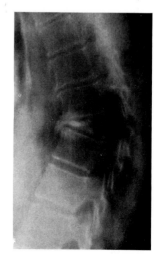

FIG. 467. - Plasmacytoma in a female aged 52 years. Osteolysis and collapse of the 9th thoracic vertebra. Tomography.

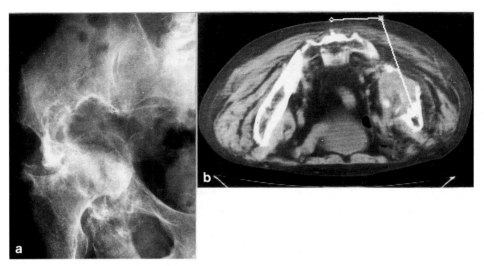

FIG. 468. - Plasmacytoma in a male aged 75 years. Pain in the hip for the past 2 years. (a) and (b) Pelvic osteolysis with intrapelvic protrusion of the femoral head. In (b) observe the trace for needle biopsy under CAT monitoring.

image, honey-combed and bubbly osteolysis with thinning of the cortex from the inside, confluent and massive osteolyses with destruction of the cortex and possibly pathologic fracture prevail in the meta-epiphysis, particularly at the proximal parts of the limbs. Nonetheless, in advanced forms of the disease, the diaphyses may also appear to be more or less roughly involved (Figs. 471, 472).

In exceptional cases, there may be P. which causes reactive hyperostosis and radiographic sclerosis. The hyperostosis may be diffused, even very intense, and contain some osteolytic lacunae or moth-eaten images.

In **solitary skeletal P.** there is localized and massive osteolysis (Fig. 473).

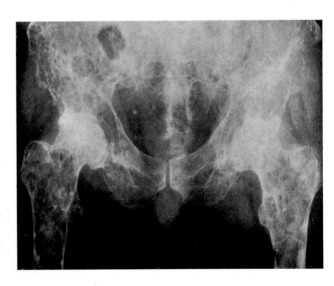

FIG. 469. - Plasmacytoma in a male aged 63 years. Severe and generalized lesions to the pelvis and proximal femurs.

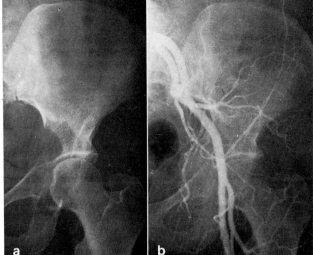

FIG. 470. - Plasmacytoma in a female aged 45 years. (a) Severe osteolysis of the acetabulum cancelling the cortex. (b) Angiography reveals moderate vascularization of the tumor.

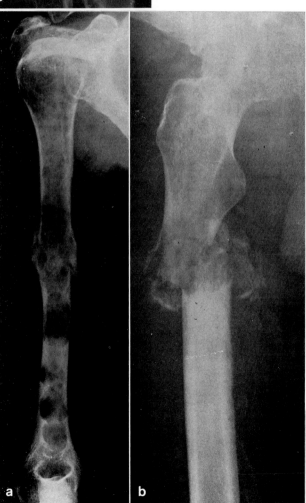

FIG. 471. - (a) Plasmacytoma in a female aged 50 years. (b) Male aged 74 years. In both cases pathologic fracture.

At times it is homogeneous, with or without erosion of the cortex; at times it is formed by the confluence of multiple spots; other times it swells the bone and is run through by thin soap-bubble-like trabeculae (Fig. 474).

Bone scan of the skeleton may be negative, even in areas corresponding to massive and radiographically evident lesions.

GROSS PATHOLOGIC FEATURES

The myelomatous tissue is similar to that of all neoplastic forms exclusively or nearly exclusively made up of cells: grayish or reddish, soft, encephaloid, at times almost fluid. As previously observed, it diffusedly permeates the medullary spaces and forms rounded nodules, which are increasingly large and confluent. At times in diffused forms and always in solitary ones, it constitutes larger tumoral masses, where hemorrhagic, cystic, necrotic changes are a frequent occurrence. The tissue, which has worn down the cortex, may expand externally. This expansion, in the vertebral column, may cause compression on the cord and the spinal roots.

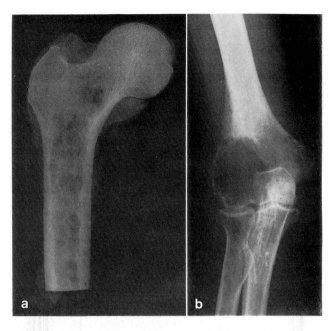

FIG. 472. - (a) Plasmacytoma in a male aged 72 years. Section of the anatomical specimen. (b) Male aged 53 years.

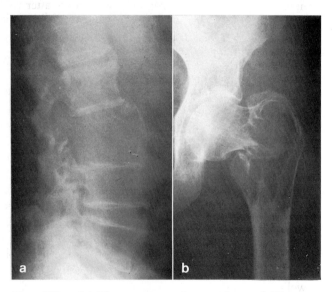

FIG. 473. - (a) Plasmacytoma in a male aged 72 years. Complete osteolysis with no collapse of the body at L3. (b) Female aged 66 years. Pathologic fracture.

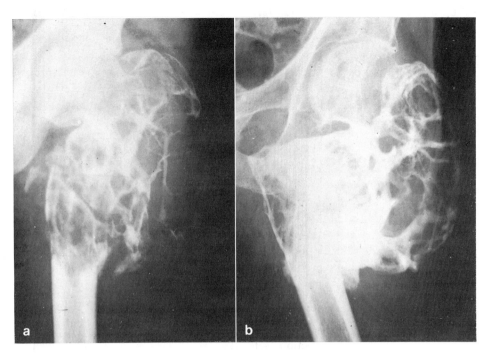

FIG. 474. - Male aged 61 years. (a) Enormous «solitary» plasmacytoma with onset of symptoms two years previously. (b) Three years after radiation therapy. The patient survived 9 years after diagnosis.

HISTOPATHOLOGIC FEATURES

The tissue is exclusively made up of a very thick mat of cells. There is hardly any intercellular stroma (Fig. 475).

These cells, at least partially, may be recognized as plasmacells. They have a rather extensive cytoplasm, which is deeply stained and basophile[1], with evident boundaries. The round nucleus is eccentric, and there is a clear perinuclear halo (corresponding to a very developed Golgi apparatus). The chromatin is in distinct blocks, which are often oriented towards the nuclear membrane («cart-wheel or leopard skin» nucleus). At times, external or internal to the cytoplasm, square or triangular crystals are observed, which are perfectly revealed under electron microscopy. Alongside these more or less typical plasmacells are other larger ones, at times having a double nucleus. Here and there mitotic figures are observed. When the tissue is characterized by this aspect, it is a well-differentiated P.

---

[1] When hematoxylin-eosin is used, depending on the case, it may be purplish in color (basophile) or reddish (ossiphile). Thus, staining with methyl green-pironine which colors the RNA is useful. Imprint specimens stained with May-Grunwald-Giemsa (basophile cytoplasms) are useful. The plasmacells are clearly distinguished under electron microscopy, as well.

In other cases, instead, cytology is much more anaplastic and atypical. Large cells, at times gigantic ones, prevail; the cytoplasms are deeply stained, at times containing extensive vacuoles; there is considerable or extreme nuclear pleomorphism, with hyperchromia, large nucleoli, atypical mitoses. Not rarely giant cells with several nuclei or a bizzarre nucleus are observed. Nonetheless, it is nearly always possible to observe scattered cells which are more differentiated, and which may be recognized as plasmacells.

LESIONS OF THE KIDNEYS

These above all consist in abundant protein cylinders obstructing the tubules, particularly the Henle loops and the collector canals. The tubular epithelium undergoes regressive and atrophic phenomena. Tubular dilations and paramyloid deposits, phlogosis and interstitial fibrosis may be associated. Glomerular changes are scarce or absent. Impairment of renal function rarely achieves severe uremic insufficiency.

EXTRASKELETAL CALCIFICATIONS

Hypercalcemia, which may be intense, may lead to extensive calcification, in the kidneys, lungs, or other soft tissues, rarely in the paramyloid masses.

PARAMYLOIDOSIS

Microscopic deposits of protein (paramyloid) are frequently observed in myelomatous tissue (Fig. 475c, d). Rarely, this paramyloid substance fills the cytoplasms of myelomatous cells, making them vitreous. At times, the paramyloid substance forms macroscopic masses, which may even be large, either in the myelomatous tissue or outside the skeleton, exceptionally in the skin and mucosae, lymph nodes, internal organs. Macroscopically, the paramyloid masses have a compact aspect which is yellowish-gray or pink in color, and gelatinous. The specific metachromatic reactions of amyloid (crystal-violet) are not always positive. Histologically, they are globules or masses with a polycyclical contour of an amorphous, homogeneous, eosinophilic material, which may be partially calcified. At its borders multinucleated giant cells (macrophages) may be observed.

DIAGNOSIS

Although diagnosis is easy in the patent and advanced forms, this is not so during the early stages of the disease, which may remain indolent, with mild and faded signs, even for several months or years.

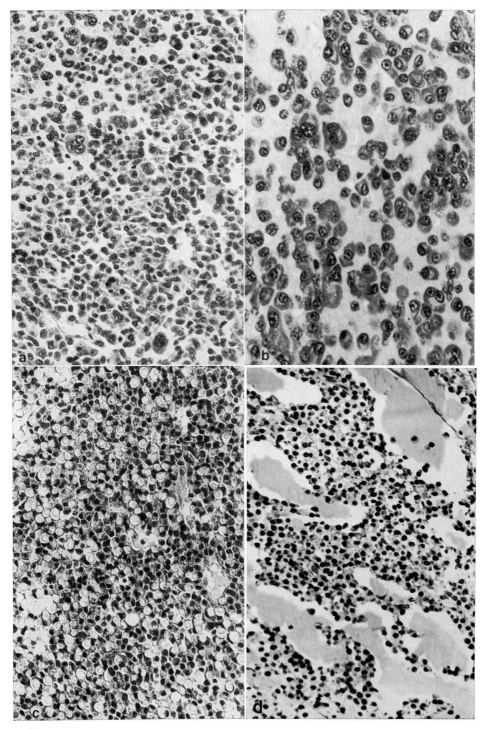

FIG. 475. - Histological aspects of plasmacytoma. In (c) observe small drops of para-myloid and in (d) more extensive deposits of the same material. (*Hemat.-eos.*, 300, 500, 300, 200 x).

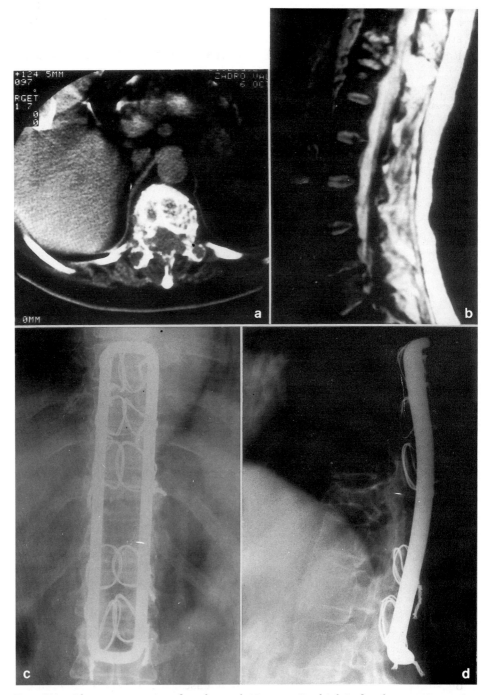

FIG. 476. - Plasmacytoma in a female aged 60 years. Rachialgia for the past 8 months, paraparesis for 2. (a) CAT reveals beehive-like osteolysis at D11 extended to the posterior vertebral arch. (b) MRI shows medullary compression. (c) and (d) The patient was submitted to decompressive laminectomy, biopsy and stabilization with a Hartshill rectangle, then to radiation and chemotherapy. Complete recovery of neurologic lesion in 3 months.

Clinically, if a patient aged over 40 years presents with vague skeletal pain and/or diffused low back pain, asthenia, pallor, mild weight loss, P. may be suspected.

Radiographically, if there is diffused vertebral osteoporosis, the origin of which is not clear, particularly if it is associated with the aforementioned symptoms and/or accompanied by moth-eaten images of the cancellous bone (including that of the vertebral pedicles and the ribs) and considerable thinning of the cortical bones, the diagnosis of P. may be even more strongly suspected. In some advanced osteolytic forms radiographic differential diagnosis may include **diffused epithelial metastases**. But usually the general radiographic picture of the skeleton is rather indicative of P. In exceptional sclerosing forms of the disease, instead, differential diagnosis with **diffused metastases due to prostatic carcinoma** may be impossible if solely based on radiographs. Theoretically, a radiographic differential diagnosis may be made between diffused osteolytic P. and **primary hyperparathyroidism** with severe bone resorption and cystic images due to brown tumors (P., too, causes hypercalcemia). Apart from the numerous differences in clinical and laboratory data, there are important differential radiographic aspects. Hyperparathyroid osteoporosis (even if it associates with large osteolyses due to brown tumors) is due to a uniform enlargement of the haversian canals and of the medullary spaces of the cancellous bone. Thus, it is made up of regular and diffused micro-pores, characterized by slow progression, which never interrupt the cortex. Myelomatous osteolysis is instead produced by the dissemination and confluence of malignant neoplastic nodes, and it is thus irregular, spotted, aggressive and destructive. In hyperparathyroid osteosis, furthermore, the cranium may show fine ground glass porosity, not the osteolytic spots of P.; the vertebral column is scarcely involved; there is typical faded subperiosteal resorption of many metaphyseal regions and in particular of the phalanges of the hand, resorption of the dental alveoli, and of the acromial end of the clavicle.

In cases of **solitary P.** diagnosis cannot be based on imaging techniques only. In the long bones it may be suspected based on the finely trabeculated and bubbly osteolysis, which at times swells the meta-epiphysis.

The **tests which are usually requested** in order to ascertain diagnosis of P. are as follows. Radiograms of the cranium, spine, pelvis and proximal limbs. Bone scan. Serum electrophoresis and immuno-electrophoresis (calcemia, uricemia). Search for Bence-Jones proteins and urinary electrophoresis on the urine of 24 hours (renal clearances). Sternal or iliac bone marrow smear. Open or needle biopsy in some cases of evident osteolytic lesions, of spinal medullary compression and of solitary P.

Serum immunoelectrophoresis is the most important diagnostic examination. It reveals globulin anomalies in most cases. It is rarely negative in cases of solitary or even diffused P. Urinary electrophoresis is particularly interesting as, rarely, it may be positive in cases where serum electrophoresis is not.

The marrow smear can be negative in initial or solitary cases. When the smear nearly exclusively reveals undifferentiated anaplastic elements, considered by itself, it may raise some uncertainty with regard to lymphoma.

Biopsy: it is important that the sample may be taken from vital neoplastic tissue, that the histological section is very thin, and that the specimen is fixed and stained perfectly. In fact, a specimen which is not suitable may reveal a small-cell «blue» tumor, which is not much unlike a **lymphoma**, or an **Ewing's sarcoma**. If large and pleomorphic anaplastic elements prevail, we must be careful to search for and evaluate the aspects of plasmacytary differentiation and take into account the clinical, radiographic and laboratory data, in order to avoid the erroneous diagnosis of lymphoma. Furthermore, as compared to lymphoma, there are giant cells which may be multinucleate and there are no argyrophilous fibers. At times, doubts may arise with regard to an **inflammatory lesion** having a high or exclusive plasmacellular quota. The differences lie in the histo-structure as well as in the cytology. In the inflammatory process, in fact, there is always a fibrosis surrounding groups of cells, while in P. there are cellular fields which are totally deprived of any stroma, except for a few blood capillaries. Furthermore, in the inflammatory process the plasmacells are all well-differentiated and mature and are associated with lymphocytes and granulocytes. Nonetheless, if the P. specimen consists in a fibrous or fibrotized area, where the neoplastic cells are scattered and surrounded by collagenous fields, the doubt may be difficult to dispel.

COURSE AND PROGNOSIS

The course of the disease may vary. Often only a few months pass from the onset of symptoms and the diagnosis, and death occurs within 2-5 years. However, there are cases, particularly of solitary P., in which the symptoms are mild even for 5-10 years.

The course of the disease is not very predictable. There does not seem to be a significant relationship beween the histological aspect of the neoplasm and its course. It is instead certain that P. which is initially solitary in the skeleton generally has a slower course. At times the tumor remains single for many years. Only exceptional cases may be considered to be truly solitary, and thus able to be healed more than 10-15 years after treatment. Nearly always systemic diffusion is manifested, but it may even occur 8-12 years after the occurrence and treatment of initial P.

With these very rare exceptions, prognosis is almost always fatal and not long-term. Unfavorable prognostic elements are: extent of the area of osteolysis, intensity of the anemia, hypercalcemia, and of the increase in monoclonal protein in the serum.

As previously observed, extraskeletal solitary P. (nearly all of the nosepharynx) instead heal frequently.

Death occurs due to complications, usually pneumonia, more rarely cysto-pielitis due to paraplegia, or hemorrhagic phenomena. Or due to cachexia, cardio-circulatory insufficiency, uremia.

As for metastatic diffusion, extraskeletal neoplastic macroscopic nodules are an infrequent finding on autopsy: mostly in the liver, the spleen, the lymph nodes and kidneys. A more frequent finding is microscopic myelomatous infiltration in these same sites.

TREATMENT

Treatment is based on antiblastic drugs, among which the most effective are cyclophosphamide (Endoxan) and melphalan (Alkeran), associated with corticosteroids (Prednisone). Vincristine, adriamycin and others are also used.

Radiation treatment is often used, to relieve pain, decrease spinal cord compressive phenomena, or prevent pathologic fracture, when there are major and circumscribed osteolyses. In younger patients allogenic bone marrow transplant may be used.

Surgery may be indicated in order to decompress the spinal cord in cases of initial paraplegia, or in order to treat and prevent pathologic fractures (osteosynthesis, osteosynthesis with acrylic cement, resection-endo or arthroprosthesis).

Depending on the case, solitary P. is usually treated by irradiation, by surgical ablation (wide resection), or by combined radiotherapy and surgery.

REFERENCES

1943 HELLWIG C. A.: Extramedullary plasma-cell tumors as observed in various locations. *Archives of Pathology*, **36**, 95-111.

1955 CARSON C. P., ACKERMAN L. V., MALTBY J. D.: Plasma-cell myeloma. A clinical, pathologic and roentgenologic review of 90 cases. *American Journal of Clinical Pathology*, **25**, 849-888.

1963 PORTER F. S. Jr.: Multiple myeloma in a child. *Journal of Pediatry*, **62**, 602-604.

1964 COHEN D. M., SVIEN H. J., DAHLIN D. C.: Long-term survival of patients with myeloma of the vertebral column. *Journal of the American Medical Association*, **187**, 914-917.

1964 MIDWEST COOPERATIVE CHEMOTHERAPY GROUP: Multiple myeloma. General aspects of diagnosis, course, and survival. *Journal of the American Medical Association*, **188**, 741-745.

1966 DRIVSHOLM A., VIDEBOEK A.: Alkeran (Melphalan) in the treatment of myelomatosis. *Acta Medica Scandinavica*, Suppl. **445**, 187-193.

1966 GRIFFITHS D. L.: Orthopaedic aspects of myelomatosis. *Journal of Bone and Joint Surgery*, **48-B**, 709-728.

1966 MALDONADO J. E., BROWN A. L. Jr., BAYRD E. D., PEASE G. L.: Ultrastructure of the myeloma cell. *Cancer*, **19**, 1613-1627.

1966 NORDENSON N. G.: Myelomatosis. A clinical review of 310 cases. *Acta Medica Scandinavica*, Suppl. **445**, 179-183.

1967 BERGSAGEL D. E., GRIFFITH K. M., HAUT A., STUCKEY W. J. Jr.: The treatment of plasma-cell myeloma. *Advances Cancer Research*, **10**, 311-359.

1968 VALDERRAMA J. A. F., BULLOUGH P. G.: Solitary myeloma of the spine. *Journal of Bone and Joint Surgery*, **50-B**, 82-90.

1969 PASMONTIER M. W., AXAR H. A.: Extraskeletal spread in multiple plasma-cell myeloma. A review of 57 autopsied cases. *Cancer*, **23**, 167-174.

1971 MANGALIK A., VELIATH A. J.: Osteosclerotic myeloma and peripheral neuropathy. *Cancer*, **28**, 1040-1045.

1971 VELEZ GARCIA E., MALDONADO N.: Long-term follow-up and therapy in multiple myeloma. *Cancer*, **27**, 44-50.

1972 ALEXANIAN R., BONNET J., GEHAN E., HAUT A., HEWLETT J., LANE M., MONTO R., WILSON H.: Combination chemotherapy for multiple myeloma. *Cancer*, **30**, 382-389.

1973 MC LAUCHLAN J.: Solitary myeloma of the clavicle with long survival after total excision. *Journal of Bone and Joint Surgery*, **55-B**, 357-358.

1974 HIMMELFARB E., SEBES J., RABINOWITZ J.: Unusual roentgenographic presentations of multiple myeloma. *Journal of Bone and Joint Surgery*, **56-A**, 1723-1728.

1974 LEE B. J., SAHAKIAN G., CLARKSON B. D., KRANKOFF I. H.: Combination chemotherapy of multiple myeloma with Alkeran, Cytoxan, Vincristine, Prednisone, and BCNU. *Cancer*, **33**, 533-538.

1975 ALAXANIAN R., BALCERZAK S., BONNET D. J., GEHAN E. A., HAUT A., HEWLETT J. S., MONTO R. W.: Prognostic factors in multiple myeloma. *Cancer*, **36**, 1192-1201.

1975 DURIE B. G., SALMON S. E.: A clinical staging system for multiple myeloma. *Cancer*, **36**, 842-854.

1975 KYLE R. A.: Multiple myeloma: review of 869 cases. *Mayo Clinic Proceedings*, **50**, 29-40.

1976 AHMED N., RAMOS S., SIKA J., LEEVEN H. H., PICCONE V. A.: Primary extramedullary esophageal plasmacytoma. First case report. *Cancer*, **38**, 943-947.

1976 MANCILLA-JIMENEZ R., TAVASSOLI F. A.: Solitary meningeal plasmacytoma. Report of a case with electron microscopic and immunohistologic observations. *Cancer*, **38**, 798-806.

1977 ALEXANIAN R., SALMON S., BONNET J., GEHAN E., HAUT A., WEICK J.: Combination therapy for multiple myeloma. *Cancer*, **40**, 2765-2771.

1977 HOKANSON J. A., BROWN B. W., THOMPSON J. R., DREWINKO B., ALEXANIAN R.: Tumor growth patterns in multiple myeloma. *Cancer*, **39**, 1077-1084.

1979 CORWIN J., LINDBERG R. D.: Solitary plasmacytoma of bone vs. extramedullary plasmacytoma and their relationship to multiple myeloma. *Cancer*, **43**, 1007-1013.

1979 WOODRUFF R. K., WHITTLE J. M., MALPAS J. S.: Solitary plasmacytoma: I: Extramedullary soft tissue plasmacytoma. *Cancer*, **43**, 2340-2343.

1979 WOODRUFF R. K., MALPAS J. S., WHITE F. E.: Solitary plasmacytoma: II: Solitary plasmacytoma of bone. *Cancer*, **43**, 2344-2347.

1981 BLATTUER W., BLAIR A., MASON T.: Multiple myeloma in the United States 1950-1970. *Cancer*, **48**, 2547-2554.

1981 DAVIS B.W., COUSAR J.B., COLLINS R.D.: Dysplastic myeloma: an aggressive variant of multiple myeloma. *Laboratory Investigation*, **44**, 14A.

1982 BATAILLE R.: Localized plasmocytoma. *Clinical Haematology*, **11**, 113-121.

1983 FOUCAR K., RABER M., FOUCAR E., BARLOGIE B., SANDLER C.M., ALEXANIAN R.: Anaplastic myeloma with massive extramedullary involvement. Report of two cases. *Cancer*, **51**, 166-174.

1986 GOODMAN M.A.: Plasma cell tumors. *Clinical Orthopaedics*, **204**, 86-92.

1987 CARTER A., HOCHERMAN I., LINN S., COHEN Y., TATARSKY I.: Prognostic significance of plasma cell morphology in multiple myeloma. *Cancer*, **60**, 1060-1065.

1987 MEIS J., BUTLER J., OSBORNE B., ORDONEZ N.: Solitary plasmacytomas of bone and extramedullary plasmacytomas. *Cancer*, **59**, 1475-1485.

1988 DELAUCHE-CAVALLIER M., LAREDO J.D., WYBIER M., BARD M., MAZABRAUD A., DARNE J.L.L., KUNTZ D., RYCKEWAERT A:. Solitary plasmacytoma of the spine. *Cancer*, **61**, 1707-1714.

1988 HALL F.M., GORE S.M.: Osteosclerotic myeloma variants. *Skeletal Radiology*, **17**, 101-105.

1988 TORDEUR F., CZERNICHOW P., LE LOET X., DESHAYES P.: Contribution à l'étude épidemiologique du myélome multiple en France. *Revue du Rhumatisme*, **55**, 87-94.

HEMANGIOMA

DEFINITION

In many cases H. seems to be a blood vascular hamartoma, that is, a proliferation of anomalous vessels originating from an area of excluded embryonary angioblastic tissue.

Before describing actual H. of the skeleton, it is important to clear the field of those **senile angectatic vertebral foci** that traditionally and erroneously have been called angiomas (Figs. 477, 478).

SENILE ANGIECTATIC VERTEBRAL FOCI

These are spots of osteolysis of one or more vertebral bodies, central, small and round, occupied by adipose tissue rich in dilated sinusoids. These spots of rarefaction of the cancellous bone with angiectasia are rather frequent, particularly during advanced age. They are totally asymptomatic and little or not at all apparent in radiograms. Thus, they constitute an autoptic finding of no clinical significance.

On thousands of autopsies, vertebral angiectatic foci are observed in approximately 12% of the vertebral columns examined. There is a fair predilection for the female sex. The lesion is nearly exclusively observed after 40 years of age and it becomes more frequent with age.

Angiectatic foci are completely asymptomatic. In most cases, even radiographic examination does not reveal any change, either in vivo, or x-raying the isolated column (Fig. 477b). Only radiograms of thin slices of the vertebral body may reveal a central and round area of trabecular rarefaction, which may be run through by few rough vertical trabeculae.

The angectatic areas are mostly localized in the lower thoracic and lumbar regions, and always in the vertebral body. Often, they are present in more than one vertebral body, but each vertebra contains only one.

Macroscopically, once the vertebra is transected, a small round spot (from a few millimeters to 1-2 centimeters in diameter), which is either central or moderately eccentric, wine-red in color, soft due to the nearly complete absence of bone trabeculae, with clear boundaries with the surrounding bone may be observed (Fig. 477a). The cortex is never either thinned or expanded. The spots of trabecular rarefaction may be yellowish in color, as

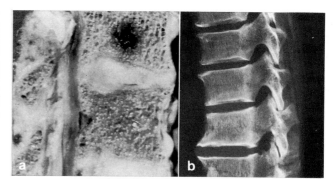

they are occupied by adipose tissue which is hardly angiectatic. Red and yellow spots may be associated in the same case.

Histologically, the bone trabeculae and the hemopoietic marrow have disappeared. In their place is edematous adipose tissue run through by numerous small blood vessels (sinusoids and venules) which are ectatic and filled
with blood, at times thrombized. Here and there minor blood effusion may
be observed in the adipose tissue. The boundaries of the angectatic area are
regularly circular and rather clear, but with no capsular delimitation (Fig.
478).

The frequency of the finding, its constant site, multiplicity, predilection
for more advanced age, anatomical features, clearly show that it is a circum-

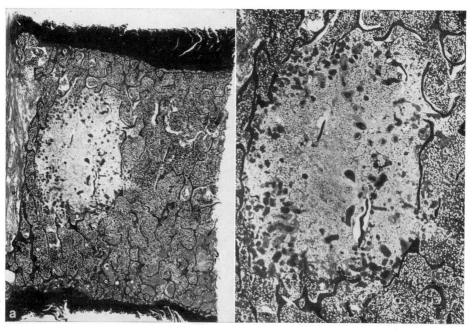

FIG. 478. - Senile angiectatic vertebral area. Histological aspect. Female aged 67
years. Occasional finding on autopsy (*Hemat.-eos.*, 3, 15 x).

scribed osteomedullary area of atrophy: of regressive origin, not hamartomatous, much less neoplastic. The capillary and venular varicosities are probably secondary to local hemodynamic modifications.

Senile angiectagic vertebral foci are of no clinical importance, as they
cause no symptoms. They are probably also irrelevant from a radiological
point of view, as generally they are not visualized on radiograms in vivo (Fig.
477b).

* * *

True H. of the skeleton are an infrequent occurrence and are manifested
in three localizations: the vertebral column, the flat bones (particularly of
the cranium), the skeleton of the limbs (Fig. 479).

FREQUENCY

Vertebral H. occur most frequently. They are followed by those of the flat
bones, which are nearly always localized in the cranium. H. of the skeleton of
the limbs are an exceptional occurrence.

SEX

Like all H., those of the skeleton show predilection for the female sex (Fig.
479).

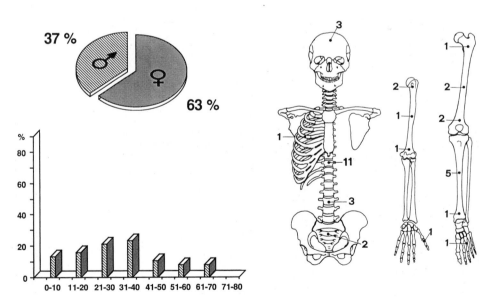

FIG. 479. - Sex, age and localization in 37 cases of angioma of the skeleton (only those
cases submitted to surgery and confirmed histologically).

AGE

It is impossible to establish the age at which the lesion initiates, because the H. may remain asymptomatic for a long time, even a life-time. H. which cause symptoms or are observed on radiograms obtained for other reasons are more often observed during adult age, rarely during childhood (Fig. 479).

LOCALIZATION

Vertebral H. are prevalently observed in the thoracic and lumbar regions, in this order. H. always involves the vertebral body, but it may extend to the posterior arch as well. In rare cases it involves more than one vertebra.

In the **cranium** the most frequent localization is the frontal and parietal bone. It is not an exceptional occurrence in the facial bones, such as the maxillary bones. In the other flat bones, it is observed only exceptionally in the ribs, scapula, pelvis.

In the **skeleton of the limbs** H. has been observed in the long bones — where it seems to prefer the meta-diaphyseal region — and in the hand and foot. In exceptional cases H. is circumscribed to the periosteum in the form of a lenticular, purplish and painful spot.

Exceptional cases of multiple H., located in different parts of the skeleton (**angiomatosis**), may occur in children. H. of the skeleton are rarely associated (Fig. 493) with angiomas of the soft tissues or of other tissues. Even in diffused angiomatosis of the soft tissues of the limbs, the bone is usually singularly left intact.

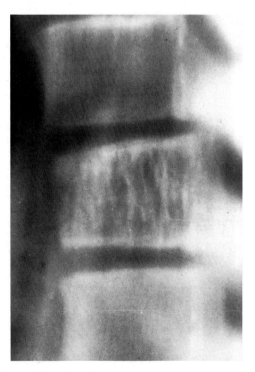

FIG. 480. - Vertebral angioma in a male aged 23 years. Chance radiographic finding. Diagnosis only radiographic.

SYMPTOMS

In the case of **vertebral H**. it is possible to distinguish between three possibilities: a) asymptomatic vertebral H. This is the most frequent occurrence. At times low back pain is associated with the radiographic picture of a striated vertebra (Figs. 480, 481, 482). An accurate clinical

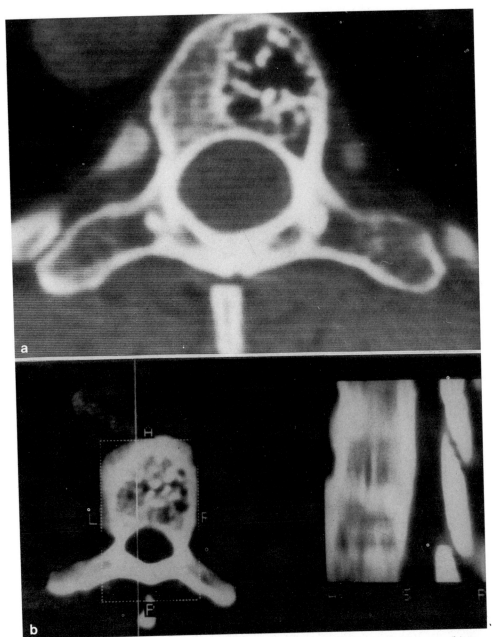

FIG. 481. - (a) Angioma of the sixth thoracic vertebra in a female aged 43 years. (b) Angioma of the fifth thoracic vertebra in a female aged 50 years. Polka-dot CAT images.

examination instead shows that the low back pain is of discal origin, and that it is unrelated to the presence of the angioma. (b) Vertebral H. causing local pain, with no signs of myelo-radicular compression (Fig. 482a). c) Vertebral H. associated with signs of myelo-radicular compression (Fig. 483).

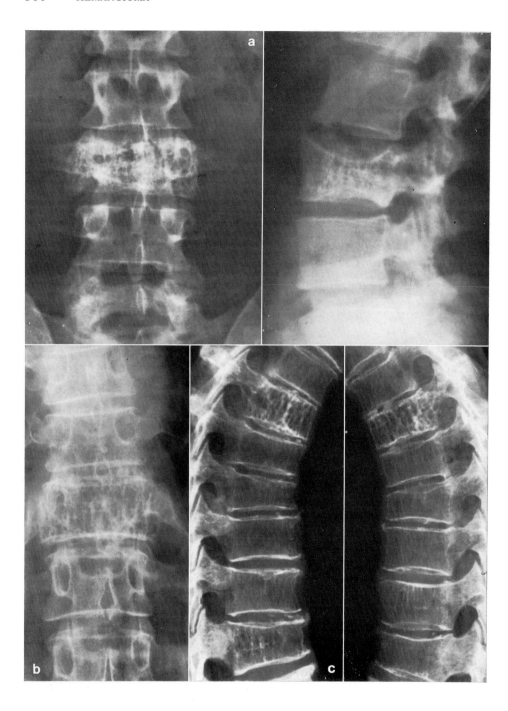

Fig. 482. - Vertebral hemangiomas. (a) Female aged 37 years. Angioma of the 3rd lumbar vertebra. Diagnosis ascertained histologically. (b) Male aged 43 years. Angioma of the 12th thoracic vertebra. Diagnosis only radiographic. (c) Female aged 63 years. Angioma of the 5th thoracic vertebra. Occasional finding on autopsy. Diagnosis ascertained histologically.

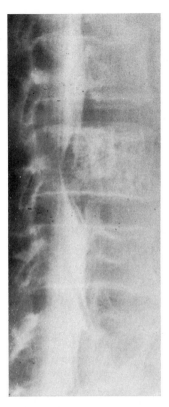

FIG. 483. - Female aged 35 years. For the past 3 months lumbar crural pain with signs of compression of the 3rd lumbar root. «Striated» vertebra and saccoradiculography revealing compression of the sac by posterior ballooning of the vertebral body. Diagnosis ascertained by biopsy. Laminectomy and radiation therapy achieved a cure lasting 12 years.

These in particular include H. of the thoracic region and mostly reveal expansion of the vertebral body and extent to the posterior arch. H. as described in a) and b) are usually not submitted to biopsy, thus, diagnosis remains radiological and presumed.

In the **cranium** H. is clinical manifested — when it is manifested — with slow-growing swelling and, rarely, mild pain. In exceptional cases it may compress the brain.

In the **bones of the limbs** the main symptom is pain.

RADIOGRAPHIC FEATURES

The most common radiographic picture of **vertebral H**. is that of «striated vertebrae». This is a bone rarefaction characterized by the presence of rough and scarce vertical trabeculae. CAT reveals a typical «polka dot» aspect (Figs. 480, 481, 482). This aspect is so typical that it is considered to be pathognomic and sufficient for diagnosis. In truth, all cases of striated vertebra operated on and biopsied were clearly angiomas from a histological point of view. These cases, however, constitute a small minority, because most times striated vertebra does not cause symptoms sufficient to justify laminectomy and biopsy. At times, instead, there is a «moth-eaten» or «honey-comb» aspect of the vertebral body, with no evident striation. This aspect is the most frequent one in vertebral H. with neurological symptoms, and thus ascertained histologically (Fig. 483). In other cases, there is wedge-shaped collapse of the vertebral body; this obscures the pre-existing honey-comb or striated image. When H. causes symptoms of myelo-radicular compression, there is often expansion of the vertebral body and/or diffusion of the osteolysis to the posterior vertebral arch. Nonetheless, diffusion to the posterior arch may be observed in cases of asymptomatic H., as well (Fig. 482). In conclusion, the striated aspect seems to correspond to most of the H. which have by now exhausted growth. The honey-comb aspect, with vertebral expansion and/or collapse, corresponds to H. which proliferate and expand. Between the «honey-comb» vertebrae and the «striated» ones all of the degrees of passage may be observed.

H. of the **cranium** have a typical «sun-ray» or «rosette» aspect. It is a rounded area, with clear boundaries, and bone trabeculae forming a thick reticulum irradiated from the center to the periphery. In tangential view, the external cortex is substituted by lenticular swelling formed by bone trabeculae perpendicular to the surface («like sun-rays»). The internal cortex is usually not deformed. Nonetheless, there are cases with expansion of both cortices (Fig. 486a, b). Similar aspects are observed in rare cases of H. of the other flat bones (Figs. 488b, 492).

In the **skeleton of the limbs** the radiographic aspect is not so typical. At times there is a single spot of osteolysis, other times small spots close together with mildly faded boundaries. The cortex is often thinned and swollen (Fig. 490), while it is never interrupted. In some cases, within the radiolucent area there is a bone trabeculation with «honey-comb», «bubbly», «sun ray» (Figs. 487, 488a, 493), or «striated» aspects.

Exceptional cases of multiple skeletal H. are observed (**skeletal angiomatosis**) with a radiographic image of multiple lytic lacunae of the cancellous bone, with no involvement of the cortex.

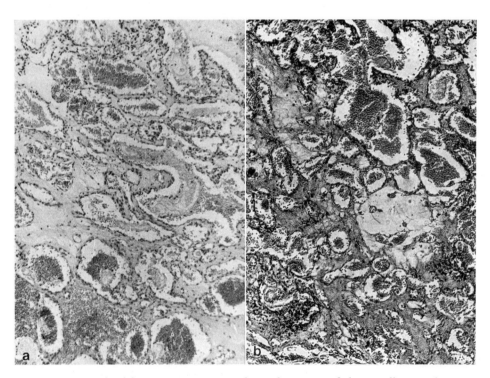

FIG. 484. - Vertebral hemangiomas. Histological aspects of the capillary and cavernous type (*Hemat.-eos.*, 125, 125 x).

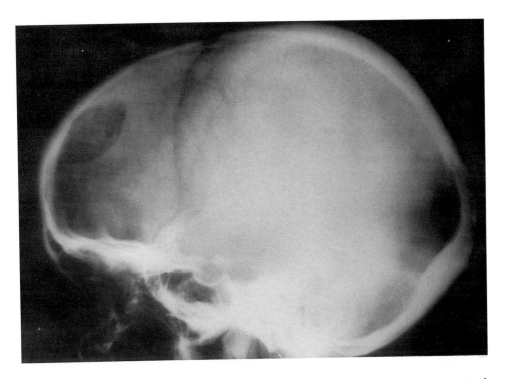

FIG. 485. - Cranial angioma in a female aged 30 years Diagnosis ascertained histologically.

GROSS PATHOLOGIC FEATURES

In the areas of osteolysis and in the spaces alternating with rarefied bone septa there is a typical bright red or bluish-red tissue, which is soft and very bloody. In the vertebral column, when surgery is performed for neurological disorders, involvement of the posterior arch is often observed; the arch is honey-combed by intensely bleeding vascular spaces; the posterior cortex of the vertebral body, is bulging, very thin or lacking, showing a soft bluish-red tissue which, deriving from the vertebral body, compresses the dural sac. In cranial localizations and in those of the bones of the limbs, as well, the same type of tissue is observed (Fig. 486b). Hemorrhage which is provoked during surgery, when an angioma is incised or pricked with a needle, may be so abundant that even biopsy may be obstructed, and very prolonged compression is necessary in order to ensure hemostasis.

HISTOPATHOLOGIC FEATURES

A thick ensemble of clearly neoformed and anomalous vascular spaces is observed (Figs. 489, 494c, 495, 496a). These may be capillaries, more or less dilated until cavernous bunches (Figs. 484, 486c, d, 494a, b, 496b), or wide in-

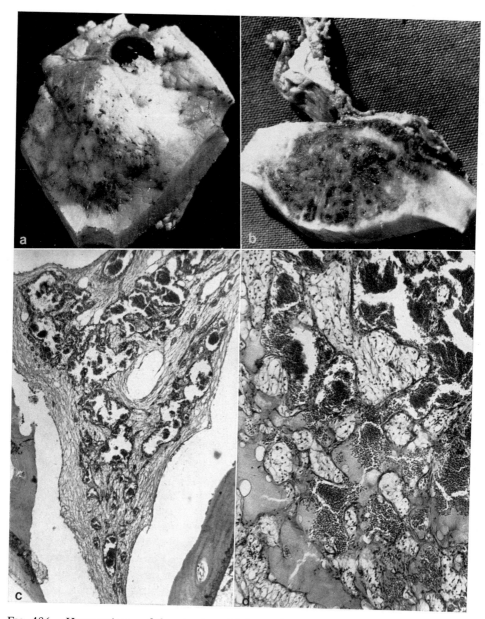

FIG. 486. - Hemangioma of the cranium. Male aged 29 years. (a) and (b) Macroscopic aspect of the internal aspect and on the cut surface. (c) and (d) Histological aspect of mature cavernous angioma (*Hemat.-eos.*, 50, 125 x).

tercommunicating labyrinthic spaces are formed. The coating endothelium in a single layer is mostly well-differentiated and relatively mature. The vascular wall is made up of a thin collagenous layer. The vascular lumi are generally filled with blood. The aspect is that usual to capillary and cavernous angiomas.

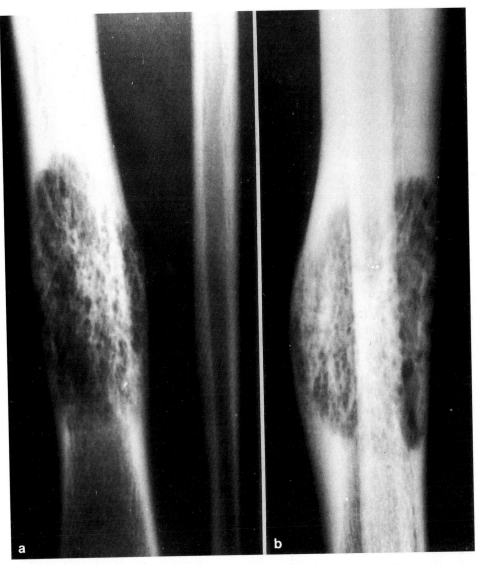

FIG. 487. - Angioma in a male aged 31 years. Pain for the past year. The patient was submitted to curettage. The lesion was repaired after 5 years.

Some interesting details may be observed. Pseudoarterioles and pseudo-veins having a thick collagenous, muscular and elastic wall are never ob-served, which are instead typical of angiomas of the soft tissues. As cavernous H. constitutes a stage of maturation and quiescence, the capillary one an ini-tial and proliferative stage, in expansive vertebral H. submitted to surgery for the treatment of medullary compression, and in symptomatic ones, in gen-eral, the capillary and microcavernous structures prevail, with aspects of live-ly proliferation (Figs. 494c, 495, 496a). In asymptomatic H., in those which go back a long time and which are not very expanded (as is commonly the

FIG. 488. - (a) Hemangioma in a male aged 22 years. The lesion had been biopsied 6 years earlier and had thus remained asymptomatic for 6 years. Suddenly, for the past 2 months, it had begun to expand with evident swelling in the soft tissues. Radiograms of the resected segment. (b) Male aged 30 years. Swelling angioma of a rib. Radiogram of the resected segment.

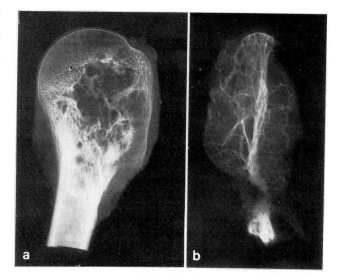

case in striated vertebrae and in cranial H.) large mature caverns are observed, instead, with residual and/or newly-formed bone trabeculae alternating with the cavernous bunches (Figs. 484b, 486c, d).

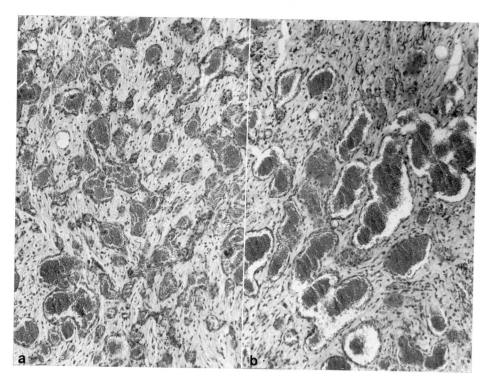

FIG. 489. - Hemangioma of the tibial diaphysis. Female aged 29 years. Capillary histological aspect (*Hemat.-eos.*, 125, 125 x).

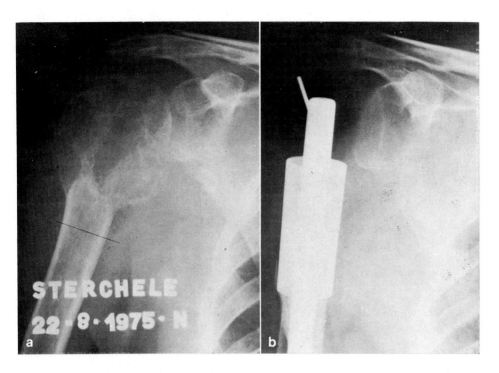

FIG. 490. - Hemangioma in a female aged 35 years. (a) The lesion could radiographically have suggested a giant cell tumor. On biopsy rather intense hemorrhaging was produced from the tumor. (b) Marginal resection and endoprosthesis. No recurrence after 15 years.

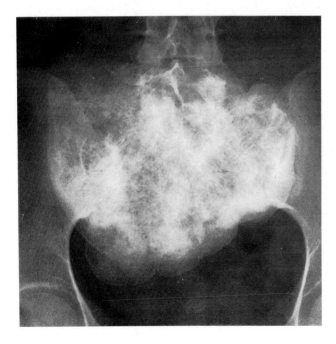

FIG. 491. - Hemangioma in a female aged 22 years. The lesion was biopsied 8 years earlier and since then radiographically it has no longer expanded, rather it has gradually become sclerotic (radiation therapy was carried out).

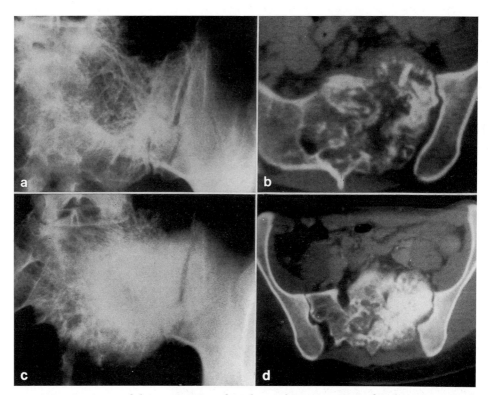

FIG. 492. - Angioma of the sacrum in a female aged 21 years. Pain for the past year after trauma. Diagnosis ascertained with biopsy. (a) and (b) Radiographic picture and CAT. (c) and (d) Ossification of the angioma after two successive embolizations, after 14 months.

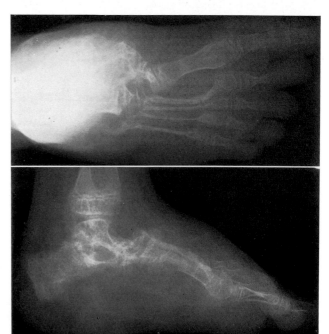

FIG. 493. - Diffused intra and extraskeletal angiomatosis of the foot in a girl aged 7 years. Observe intense skeletal atrophy associated with shortening, joint stiffness and pain. These symptoms led to amputation.

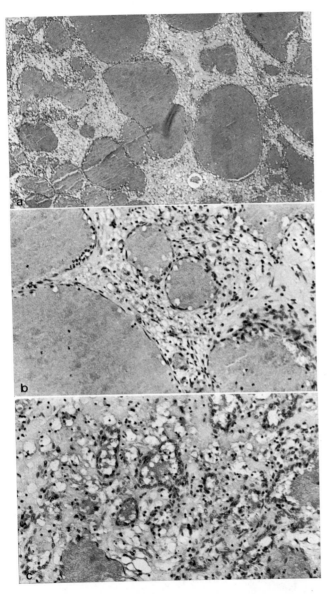

HISTOGENESIS AND PATHOGENESIS

Skeletal H. is a vascular hamartoma. This is demonstrated by its anatomical identity with H. of other tissues (of which the hamartomatous nature is generally unquestionable) and the existence of exceptional skeletal angiomatoses initiating during childhood. The lively proliferation of some cases of H. in adult or advanced age may be ascribed to the resumption of hamartomatous activity which has remained latent for a long time, perhaps even stimulated by hemodynamic modifications. Or it could, in these cases, be a benign neoplasm similar to hemangioendothelioma.

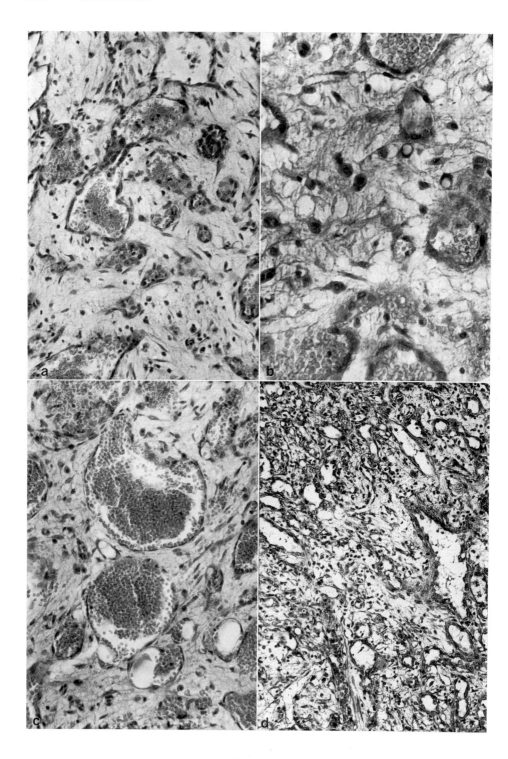

FIG. 495. - Histological aspects of capillary hemangioma of the bone. In (b) observe two angioblasts in the cytoplasm of which the primary vascular cavity is formed. (*He-*

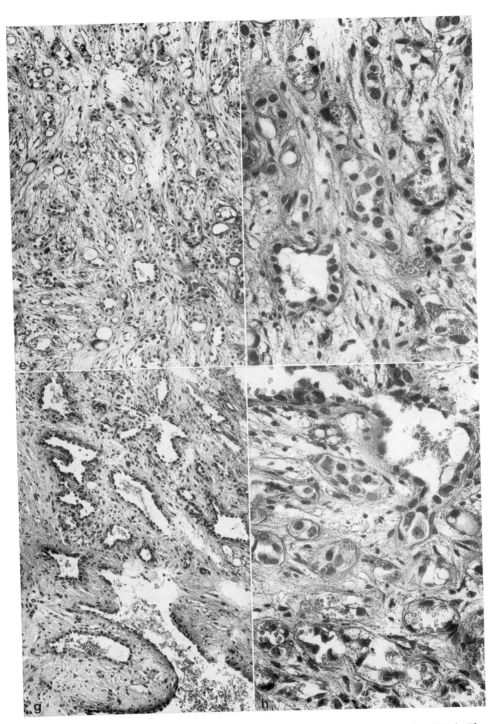

FIG. 495. (continued) - *mat.-eos.*, 200, 300, 200, 125 x). (e-h) (Case in Fig. 488a). The walls of the capillaries are at times matted by plump endothelial cells. This aspect may liken capillary angioma to hemangioendothelioma (*Hemat.-eos.*, 125, 300, 125, 300 x).

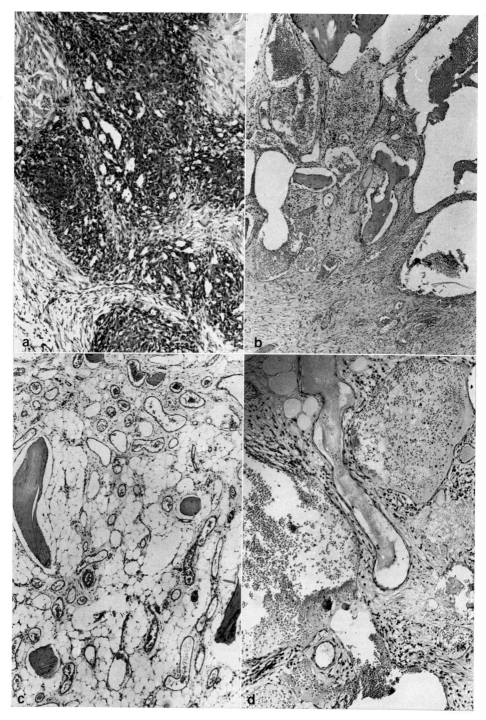

FIG. 496. - Histological aspects in the case of Fig. 493. (a) Capillary hemangioma. (b) Cavernous hemangioma. (c) There is dilatation and hyperplasia of the small vessels probably on a hemodynamic basis. (d) Dilatation of the sinusoids and cavernous spaces (*Hemat.-eos.*, 125, 50, 50, 125 x).

DIAGNOSIS

We have already observed how the striated radiographic aspect is typical of vertebral H. So much so that diagnosis may be founded on the basis of radiograms alone. Nonetheless, a striated vertebra is prevalently observed in quiescent and asymptomatic H. In more actively proliferating forms, causing myelo-radicular symptoms, a «honey-comb» aspect, or vertebral collapse is more easily observed. The radiographic aspect of cranial H. is also often typical. Radiological differential diagnosis is rarely made with cranial metastasis due to carcinoma. In H. localized in other skeletal sites, instead, diagnosis is above all histological. From a histological point of view, diagnosis is easy, and errors involving other types of diseases cannot be made.

COURSE

H. probably develops during childhood-youth achieving maturity and quiescence during adult age (Fig. 491). These are the asymptomatic and stationary H. which often do not modify further for the entire life of the patient. At times, instead, H. expands during adult age, even after many years of quiescence. At times, a H. may begin to grow again during pregnancy.

TREATMENT

Asymptomatic H. (like «striated vertebra») do not require any type of treatment. H. which cause pain may be treated by surgical ablation or (vertebral H.) selective arterial embolization and/or radiation therapy. Vertebral H. with medullary symptoms must be submitted to laminectomy, decompression of the spinal cord, and then radiation therapy. Curettage and, at times, biopsy may be difficult or impossible due to profuse hemorrhaging. This, instead, does not disturb the extraperiosteal resection which may instead be indicated in more extensive forms of the skeleton of the trunk and limbs (Figs. 488, 490). Selective arterial embolization is important as a therapeutic measure by itself (Fig. 492), or immediately prior to surgery, especially in vertebral localizations of the disease.

PROGNOSIS

Surgical removal is followed by healing. If removal is incomplete, there may be recurrence (Fig. 488a). Radiation therapy and embolization may obtain good results, obstructing progression of the H. (Figs. 491, 492). If laminectomy is performed early, it may allow for regression of symptoms due to medullary compression.

REFERENCES

1927 MAKRYCOSTAS K.: Über das Wirbelangiom, Lipom und Osteom, *Wirchows Archiv Pathologishe Anatomie*, **265**, 259-303.

1928 TÖPFER D.: Über ein infiltrierend wacksends Hämangiom der Haut und inneren Organe. Zur Kenntnis der Wirbelangiome. *Frankfurter Zeitschrift für Pathologie*, **36**, 337-345.

1941 GHORMLEY R. K., ADSON A. W.: Hemangioma of vertebral column. *Journal of Bone and Joint Surgery*, **23**, 887-895.

1942 THOMAS A.: Vascular tumors of bone. A pathological and clinical study of twenty seven cases. *Surgery Gynecology and Obstretrics*, **74**, 777-795.

1953 ZAKOV S. B.: Vertebral Hemangioma. *Vestnik Rentghenologhii i Radiologhii*, **6**, 54-59.

1957 KLEINSASSER O., ALBRECHT H.: Bei Hämangiome der Schadelknochen. *Langenbeck Archiv für Chirurgie*, **285**, 115-133.

1958 ARSENI C., SIMIONESCU M. D.: Vertebral hemangiomata. Report on 15 cases. *Acta Psychiatrica et Neurologica Scandinavica*, **34**, 1.

1962 SPIJUT H. I., LINDHOM A.: Skeletal angiomatosis. Report of two cases. *Acta Pathologica Microbiologica Scandinavica*, **55**, 49-58.

1966 NEHRKORN O., WOLFERT E.: Generalisierte Knochenhämangiomatose mit Lungenbeteiligung. *Fortschritte auf dem Gebiete der Röntgenstrahlen und Nuklearmedizin*, **104**, 107-112.

1968 CAMPANACCI M., CENNI F., GIUNTI A.: Angectasie, amartomi e neoplasmi vascolari dello scheletro. *Chirurgia degli Organi di Movimento*, **58**, 472-498.

1968 GOIDANICH I. F., CAMPANACCI M.: *Vascular hamartomas and angiodysplasias of the extremities.* Charles C. Thomas, Springfield, Illinois.

1971 SCHMORL G., JUNGHANNS H.: *The human spine in health and diseases.* Grune & Stratton, New York and London.

1972 BOYLE W. J.: Cystic angiomatosis of bone. A report of three cases and review of the literature. *Journal of Bone and Joint Surgery*, **54-B**, 626-636.

1978 SCHAJOWICZ F., AIELLO C. L., FRANCONE M. V., GIANNINI R. E.: Cystic angiomatosis (hamartous haemolymphangiomatosis) of bone. A clinicopathological study of three cases. *Journal of Bone and Joint Surgery*, **60-B**, 100-106.

1984 GUERM C., CYWINER-GOLENZER C., AMOUROUX J.: Angiome et angiomatose des os. *L'Actualité Rhumatologique*, **21**, 55-66.

1986 BAKER N.D., GREENSPAN A., NEUWIRTH M.: Symptomatic vertebral hemangiomas: a report of four cases. *Cancer*, **15**, 458-463.

1986 PALEY D., EVANS D.C.: Angiomatous involvement of an extremity. A spectrum of syndromes. *Clinical Orthopaedics*, **206**, 215-218.

1986 SCHNYDER P., FANKHAUSER H., MANSOURI B.: Computed tomography in spinal hemangioma with cord compression. Report of two cases. *Skeletal Radiology*, **15**, 372-376.

1988 KENAN S., BONAR S., JONES C., LEWIS M.M.: Subperiosteal hemangioma. A case report and review of the literature. *Clinical Orthopaedics*, **232**, 279-283.

1989 REID A.B., REID I.L., JOHNSON G., HAMONIC M., MAJOR P.: Familial diffuse cystic angiomatosis of bone. *Clinical Orthopaedics*, **238**, 211-218.

1990 HAWNAUR J.M., WHITEHOUSE R.W., JENKINS J.P.R., ISHERWOOD I.: Musculoskeletal haemangiomas: comparison of MRI and CT. *Skeletal Radiology*, **19**, 251-258.

LYMPHANGIOMA

This tumor occurs only exceptionally. The few cases described in the literature concern infancy or early childhood. At times, chronic lymphedema of a limb or lymphangioma of the soft tissues are associated. The skeletal lesions are disseminated, in the form of small or extensive areolar osteolyses. Histologically, the lymphatic vessels are observed to be dilated and at times cavernous, in the periosteum and in the bone. It probably is a hamartoma. When indicated, treatment is surgical, sometimes either partial or palliative.

REFERENCES

1947 BICKEL W. H., BRODERS A. C.: Primary lynphangioma of the ilium. Report of a case. *Journal of Bone and Joint Surgery*, **29**, 517-522.
1950 HARRIS R., PRANDONI A. G.: Generalized primary lymphangiomas of bone; report of a case associated with congenital lymphedema of forearm. *Annals Internal Medicine*, **33**, 1302-1313.
1955 COHEN J., CRAIG J. M.: Multiple lymphangiectases of bone. *Journal of Bone and Joint Surgery*, **37-A**, 585-596.
1956 FALKAMER S., TILLING G.: Primary lymphangioma of bone. *Acta Orthopedica Scandinavica*, **26**, 99-110.
1961 SCHOPFNER C. E., PARKER A. R.: Lymphangioma of bone. *Radiology*, **76**, 449.
1968 ROSENQUIST C. J., WOLFE D. C.: Lymphangioma of bone. *Journal of Bone and Joint Surgery*, **50-A**, 158-162.
1976 BULLOUGH P. G., GOODFELLOW J. W.: Solitary lymphangioma of bone. *Journal of Bone and Joint Surgery*, **58-A**, 418-419.
1983 EDWARDS W.H., THOMPSON R.C., VARSA E.W.: Lymphangiomatosis and massive osteolysis of the cervical spine. A case report and review of the literature. *Clinical Orthopaedics*, **177**, 222-229.
1984 JUMBELIC M., FEUERSTEIN I.M., DORFMAN H.D.: Solitary intraosseous lymphangioma. A case report. *Journal of Bone and Joint Surgery*, **66-A**, 1478-1481.
1987 PAZZAGLIA U.E., MORA R., CECILIANI L.: Lymphangiomatosis of the arm with massive osteolysis. A case report. *International Orthopaedics*, **11**, 367-369.

HEMANGIOENDOTHELIOMA AND ANGIOSARCOMA

DEFINITION

These neoplasms are formed by mesenchymal cells which tend to differentiate in an angioblastic sense, and to form blood vessels. H.H. occurs with different grades of malignancy. Grade 1 H.H. is very low-grade malignant. (Maybe even a benign H.H. exists: grade 0). Grades 3 and 4 H.H. are very aggressively malignant tumors. Grade 2 H.H. is in between the two ends of the spectrum, and, due to the rarity of this tumor, we still do not precisely know the biological behavior and prognosis of these intermediate forms. Moreover, the distinction between grades 2 and 3 is somehow subjective and controversial. There is also the possibility that H.H. may undergo a progression in malignancy, thus showing a different grade in different areas of the same tumor, or in subsequent periods of time in the same patient. For all these reasons, H.H. of bone represents a difficult problem and awaits further experience and study.

FREQUENCY

The tumor occurs rarely.

SEX, AGE

There is predilection for the male sex, at a ratio of 2:1. It is observed at every age between 10 and 70 years (Fig. 497).

LOCALIZATION

The most frequent sites are the bones of the lower limb (particularly the femur), where the tumor may be localized in either the metaphysis or the diaphysis. When localization is metaphyseal, as adults are generally involved, the disease easily expands to the epiphysis. These sites are followed by localizations in the pelvis, the vertebral column, where it is generally found in the body of a thoracic or lumbar vertebra, and in the upper limb. More rarely, it affects other flat bones (scapula, sternum, ribs, clavicle, cranium) (Fig. 497).

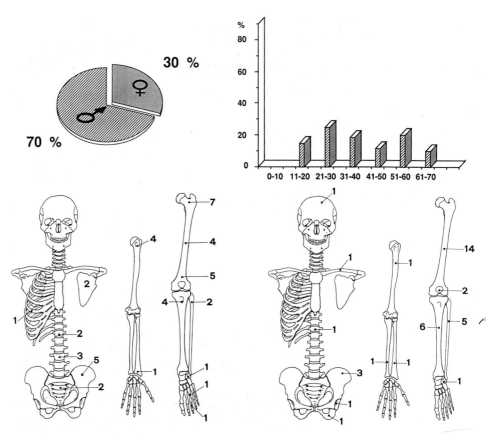

FIG. 497. - Sex, age and localization in 60 cases of hemangioendothelioma of the skeleton. On the left the localizations in solitary lesions. On the right, in 15 multicentric tumors (39 localizations).

In approximately 1/4 of all cases H.H. is **multicentric**, either in the same bone or in different nearby bones. Generally, multicentric lesions remain limited to a single limb (Fig. 497), but in exceptional cases they may be extended to several limbs and/or to the skeleton of the trunk. When, instead, H.H. is characterized by several skeletal localizations, which are not synchronous, and are distant from one another, they must be considered to be metastatic.

SYMPTOMS

The main symptom is pain. Swelling occurs rarely, and only in the more superficial bones and/or in more expanded tumors. Occasionally, symptoms may initiate suddenly with a pathologic fracture. Vertebral localizations may cause signs of myelo-radicular compression.

FIG. 498. - (a) Male aged 27 years. Grade 1 hemangioendothelioma. Curettage was performed, bone grafting and then irradiation. The lesion is repaired at 37 year follow-up. (b) Male aged 18 years. Grade 1 hemangioendothelioma. The patient was submitted to marginal resection and grafting with an autoplastic fibula. There were no signs of recurrence after 46 years. (c) Male aged 34 years. Grade 1 hemangioendothelioma. Marginal resection of the distal portion of the third metatarsal. Healed after 34 years.

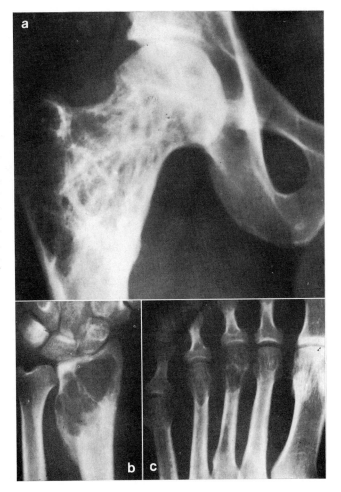

RADIOGRAPHIC FEATURES

H.H. are intensely and exclusively osteolytic tumors. In multicentric forms, rounded, central or intracortical osteolytic images are observed. As they expand, they tend to flow together in more extensive radiolucent areas, ones which are polycyclical, of «bubbly or honey-comb» aspect. Even when the tumoral image is a single one, it may appear to be «bubbly», due to its polycyclical boundaries and the existence of thin septa, enough to give the impression of originating from the confluence of different neoplastic nodes (Figs. 498-501).

In low-grade forms of the disease, the boundaries of the osteolytic images are rather well-defined and sometimes marked by a rim of osteosclerosis. The cortex may be thinned and/or expanded, but it is usually continuous (Figs. 498-500). In other cases, the cortex may appear to be very thinned and in some areas absent (Fig. 501). High-grade H.H. is manifested by an osteo-

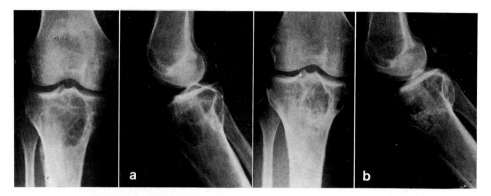

FIG. 499. - Male aged 40 years. (a) Grade 1 multicentric hemangioendothelioma in the proximal tibia, in the patella (a third lesion in the diaphysis of the femur), all in the same limb. (b) Lesions were for the most part repaired, and no signs of activity were apparent after 20 years. The patient was treated by patellectomy and irradiation of the other lesions.

lysis which is similar to that described, but its boundaries are usually more faded. At times, it is single osteolysis, other times it is a group of small «moth-eaten» images. The cortex is often cancelled (Figs. 502-505).

Both in low and high-grade forms of the disease there is very little or no periosteal reactive osteogenesis.

GROSS PATHOLOGIC FEATURES

In low-grade H.H. the cortex and the periosteum may be continuous. The neoplastic tissue is soft, wine or dark red, considerably bloody. At times it is a homogeneous tissue, other times it includes large cavities filled with blood

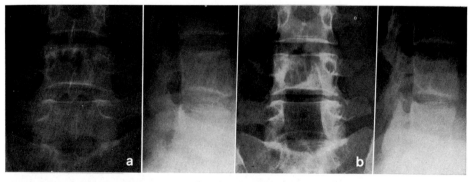

FIG. 500. - Female aged 23 years. (a) Grade 2 hemangioendothelioma of the body at L4. (b) Treated by laminectomy and radiation therapy, the lesion is repaired after 17 years.

FIG. 501. - Male aged 29 years. Grade 2 multicentric hemangioendothelioma in all of the bones of a lower limb. The patient was submitted to curettage of some tibial lesions, and was almost stationary after 6 years.

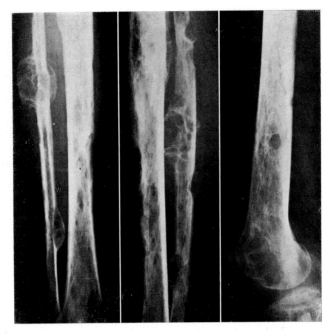

and/or coagula. In high-grade H.H. the tissue has approximately the same macroscopic features, but the cortex and the periosteum are permeated and often there is invasion of the soft tissues. H.H. may even appear to be pale, even whitish, when the collagenous stroma of the tumor is very abundant or angioblasts form solid fields without vascular cavitation.

HISTOPATHOLOGIC FEATURES

In order to understand the histologic picture of these tumors, it is important

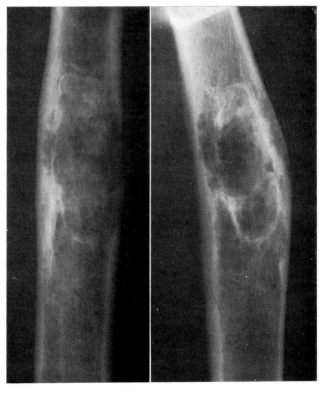

FIG. 502. - Male aed 52 years. Grade 3 hemangioendothelioma. Hip disarticulation. The patient died after 1 year of pulmonary metastases.

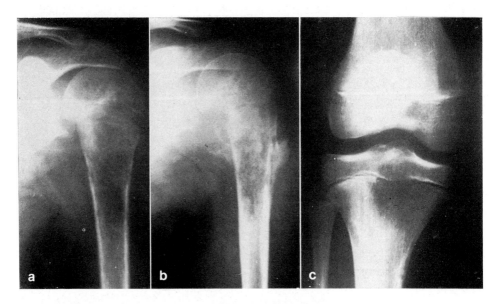

FIG. 503. - Girl aged 12 years. (a) Grade 4 hemangioendothelioma treated with radiation therapy. (b) The same lesion after 4 months. (c) Metastasis in the proximal tibia. The patient died after 1 year of pulmonary and bone metastases.

to recall the morphology and the differentiation of the angioblast. Angioblasts are mesenchymal cells which at first form solid cords having a unicellular section. The cell has extensive cytoplasm which is intensely colored and P.A.S. positive, and which tends to join those of the nearby cells in syncytia. In the cytoplasm a fissure is formed and dilates pushing the nucleus towards the periphery. The lumen of the primary capillary is thus derived within the cytoplasm by vacuolization. The angioblastic growth is associated with some histio-fibroblasts and monocytes.

H.H. are constituted by elements demonstrating an angioblastic differentiation. Immunohistochemistry shows that the cytoplasms are positive for factor VIII. The tumor at times presents a microscopic distribution in isolated or confluent multiple foci. This observation agrees with the radiographic features.

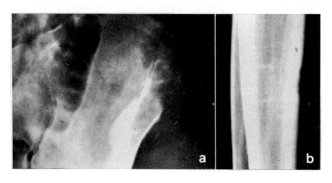

FIG. 504. - Male aged 40 years. Grade 3 hemangioendothelioma. (a) Radiographic aspect of the first iliac localization. (b) Subperiosteal metastases of the homolateral tibia, which occurred after 4 months. Treated with radiation therapy the patient died due to neoplastic dissemination after 1 year.

FIG. 505. - Female aged 74 years. (a) Right femur with bone infarct. (b) Left femur with similar infarct and, at the distal end, osteolytic lesions due to grade 3 hemangioendothelioma. Treated with radiation therapy, the patient died after 6 months of pulmonary metastases.

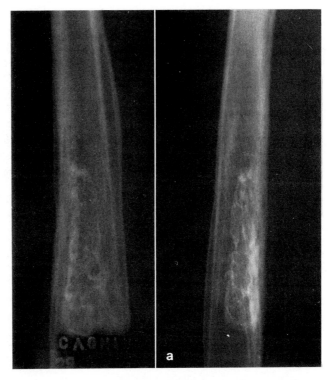

The features of the supporting stroma, including the singular frequency of a considerable or intense amount of leukocyte infiltration, and particularly of **eosinophilic leukocytes**, are substantially the same in low-grade and in high-grade tumors.

1) **Grade 1 H.H.** (Figs. 506a, 507).

It is made up of cords and thin vascular canals. The angioblastic cells are of average size, they have extensive and colorful cytoplasms, basophiles. The nuclei are globose, oval or elongated, with finely pulverulent chromatin and a clear nuclear membrane. Only some of the nuclei reveal a small nucleolus. The nuclei are not very large, even if moderate pleomorphism may be observed.

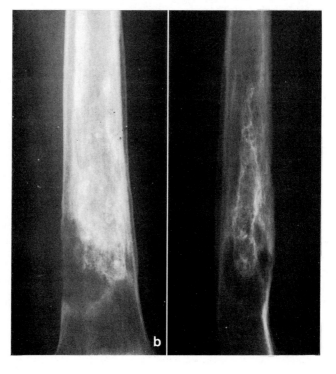

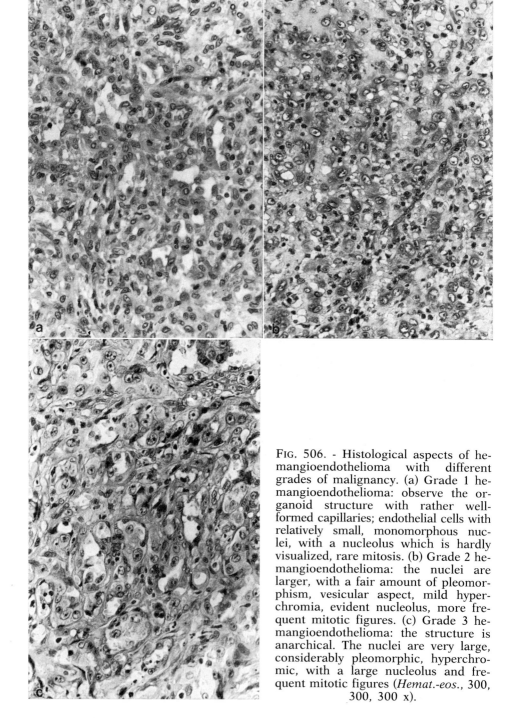

Fig. 506. - Histological aspects of hemangioendothelioma with different grades of malignancy. (a) Grade 1 hemangioendothelioma: observe the organoid structure with rather well-formed capillaries; endothelial cells with relatively small, monomorphous nuclei, with a nucleolus which is hardly visualized, rare mitosis. (b) Grade 2 hemangioendothelioma: the nuclei are larger, with a fair amount of pleomorphism, vesicular aspect, mild hyperchromia, evident nucleolus, more frequent mitotic figures. (c) Grade 3 hemangioendothelioma: the structure is anarchical. The nuclei are very large, considerably pleomorphic, hyperchromic, with a large nucleolus and frequent mitotic figures (Hemat.-eos., 300, 300, 300 x).

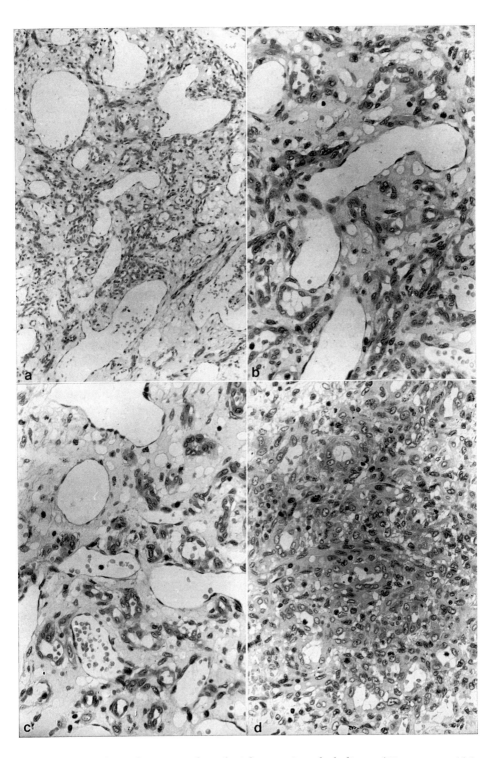

FIG. 507. - Histological aspects of grade 1 hemangioendothelioma (*Hemat.-eos.*, 125, 300, 300, 300 x).

There are neither hyperchromia nor vesicular nuclei. There are no or exceptional mitotic figures. At times the cells are joined in syncytia, so that they may appear to be binucleate and even form multinucleate giant cells. The cytoplasms, even in the most solid areas, tend to vacuolate. Trichromic staining for the connective tissue distinguishes cords and cellular nests rather well, with a hint at the formation of cavities for the vacuolization of the cytoplasms. Some of the cells are characterized by a nucleus at the periphery. In other cases, and this is the most differentiated and typical aspect, the endothelial cells form a net of thin cord and canals; they are flatter, generally in a single layer, with nuclei protruding towards the lumen. This may contain some red blood cells. Generally, the angioblastic neoformation is limited to thin capillaries. In some cases, instead, there are aspects of transition between these capillaries and wider cavities, where the parietal endothelium appears to be more flattened and mature. These are cases in which differentiation between grade 1 H.H. and capillary hemangioma may be more difficult.

Connective support stroma surrounds the more differentiated cords and tubules: the stroma may be loose, or denser collagenous. In general, there is stromal infiltration of monocytes and granulocytes, with unconstant prevalence of eosinophilic ones. At times the infiltration of eosinophiles is very intense.

In some fields interstitial hemorrhage is observed, with red blood cells scattered in the stroma, accumulations of hemosiderin pigment and multinucleate giant cells (macrophages) reactive to the hemorrhage. In the stroma there are capillaries and sinusoids, which are not neoplastic, and which are completely different from angioendotheliomatous capillaries.

2) Grade 2 H.H. (Figs. 506b, 508).

In this case, as well, the angioblastic tissue may appear to be cellular, nearly compact, or it may form cords and vascular canals. At times, rather large vascular cavities are observed, ones which are cavernous and filled with blood, recalling those of aneurysmal bone cysts. But, unlike aneurysmal bone cysts, the cavities are matted with neoplastic endothelial cells. In these larger cavities small globose parietal «villi» may be observed, constituted by a fibro-hyalin support and by the coating of swollen endothelial cells.

As compared to grade 1 H.H. the nuclei are larger, with evident pleomorphism. Some of the nuclei are very large. As compared to the grade 1 form, there is also mild hyperchromia, often camouflaged by the fact that the nuclei tend to be vesicular. The nucleoli are more evident, but they are rarely large. Mitotic figures are more frequently observed.

3) Grades 3-4 H.H. (or angiosarcoma) (Figs. 506c, 509).

The aspect becomes frankly malignant, its structure is anarchical. There are more frequently solid cellular fields, with globose or spindle-shaped mesenchymal cells; in other sites there are nests, cords, and cellular tubules; in

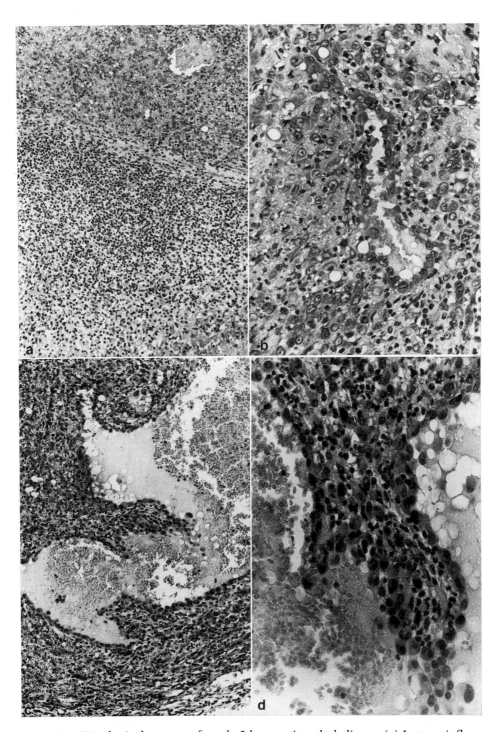

FIG. 508. - Histological aspects of grade 2 hemangioendothelioma. (a) Intense inflammatory infiltration in which eosinophilic granulocytes predominate. (c) and (d) Cavities filled with blood may recall those of aneurysmal bone cyst: these cavities are coated by endothelial cells (*Hemat.-eos.*, 50, 300, 125, 300 x).

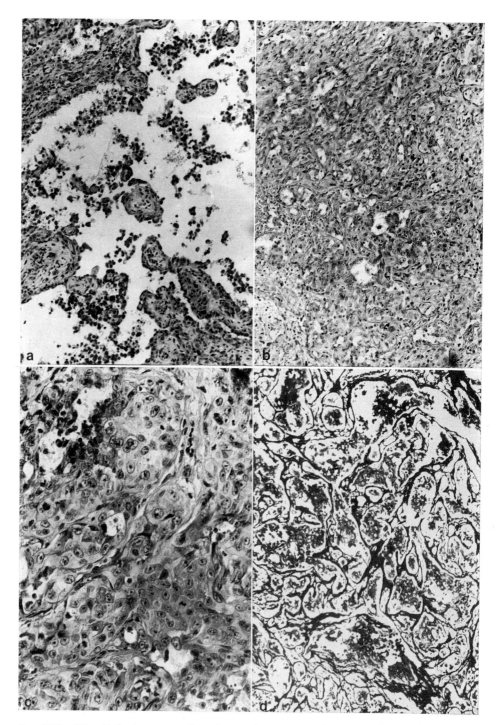

Fig. 509. - Histological aspects of grades 3-4 hemangioendothelioma. (a) Large vascular cavities with small papillary vegetations in the lumen. (b) and (c) Nearly solid angioblastic production. (d) The endothelial cells form tubes and cords surrounded by reticular membranes (*Hemat.-eos.*, 125, 125, 300 x; *argentic impregnation*, 125 x).

still other areas there are wide cavities matted with neoplastic endothelial cells in one or more layers. Endocavitary globose villi are frequently observed, with fibro-hyaline support and endothelio-sarcomatous coating.

The cells are large or very large, with dark basophile cytoplasms, joined in sincitia, often vacuolated. The nuclei are large or very large, evidently vesicular, hyperchromatic, pleomorphic. A frequent finding is the presence of one or more large nucleoli. Mitotic figures abound, they are often atypical. Cells having two, three or more nuclei are a frequent finding.

HISTOGENESIS AND PATHOGENESIS

These are neoplasms which originated from angioblasts, of which they preserve the morpho-functional attitude. In angiomas (vascular hamartomas) there is proliferation of capillaries which are identical to embryonal vessels, and generally achieve complete maturation. Here, on the contrary, angioblastic cells, even those of low-grade H.H., are larger and more pleomorphic than normal, and they never completely mature. As previously observed, nonetheless, there are cases in which it may be difficult to distinguish between grade 1 H.H. and capillary angioma.

In three of our observations high-grade H.H. occurred on an old osteomyelitis. In one of Lichtenstein's cases and in one of Dube and Fisher's (1972), a high-grade H.H. developed near a metallic internal fixation. In two other cases of ours, a high-grade H.H. developed in the area of an old chondroma and respectively in a diaphyseal bone infarct.

DIAGNOSIS

Diagnosis is histological. Nonetheless, low-grade H.H. may be suspected based on radiographs because of the osteolysis with polycyclical boundaries, and above all, in the case of multicentric osteolyses. In truth, the radiographic observation of multiple osteolytic lesions (usually in the same lower limb), with no diffused osteoporosis (thus, excluding **hyperparathyroidism**) and having no features of **metastatic** lesions or those of **plasmacytoma** is very indicative of H.H.

The more aggressive osteolytic lesion of a high-grade H.H., instead, cannot be radiographically differentiated from that of any **osteolytic sarcoma or skeletal metastasis**.

The histological picture is very typical and it is rarely interpreted erroneously. There are two diagnostic elements: structure in cords, canals, vascular lacunae; cellular features. As for the first element, trichromic and silver staining for the reticular and collagenous fibers may be of considerable aid. These stainings reveal the structure in cords and tubules, which may not be as evident when hematoxylin-eosin is used, and it is observed that the cells are inside the reticular membrane (while in hemangiopericytoma they are outside). The cellular features are very important because they are constant.

In truth, if a tumor does not have these features (large cytoplasms which are well-stained and basophile, cytoplasmatic vacuoles, the formation of syncytia, globose-oval nuclei with pulverulent chromatin and evident nuclear membrane; in more malignant forms of the disease, large vesicular nuclei, with a large nucleolus) it is not an angioblastic tumor. The cytoplasms are positive for factor VIII.

The histological differential diagnosis of high-grade H.H. is above all made with **epithelial metastasis (particularly renal)**, which may reveal cellular cords with well-stained or vacuolated cytoplasms (clear cells), spindle-shaped epithelial cells, intense vascularization and hemorrhagic areas.

Low-grade H.H., as mentioned, present transition phases and similarities with **capillary angiomas**, compared to which differential diagnosis may be difficult (Fig. 495 e-h).

The most important and delicate histodiagnostic problem concerns the **grading of malignancy**. Such grading is evident and clear in grade 1 and grade 4 tumors. It may be more difficult to distinguish between grades 2 and 3. Rarely, an H.H. graded 2 may prove to be locally aggressive and metastatic. This could also depend on the fact that areas of more or less malignant aspect coexist in the same tumor (thus it is important to examine numerous and large sections, or the entire tumor).

COURSE

In **low-grade H.H.** neoplastic growth is slow or very slow. Often, the duration of symptoms achieves or exceeds 1 year at diagnosis, but in some cases it is evident that the tumor existed prior to the occurrence of the first symptoms. If it is not treated, the tumor may remain stationary or progress slowly, even for several years. When it is multicentric, the different lesions are generally present at diagnosis. Nonetheless, others may occur successively.

It is still not known whether H.H. may reveal **progression in malignancy**.

The course of **high-grade H.H.** is often very rapid. The duration of symptoms is usually less than 6 months, often less than 3. Metastases occur nearly always in the lungs within 1 year. Recurrence on the amputation stump may be observed, and there may be visceral and skeletal metastases, as well. Metastases in the lymph nodes are rarely observed.

TREATMENT

In **grade 1 H.H.** marginal resection or even thorough curettage with local adjuvants is indicated. In **grade 2 H.H.** wide resection should be used. In **high-grade (3-4) H.H.** surgical treatment should be very aggressive, either wide or radical and often (stage II-B lesions) it implies amputation.

It is not known, yet, if preoperative chemotherapy could permit, in good responders, extending the indication for conservative wide surgery.

In multicentric tumors and in vertebral locations of low-grade malignancy, curettage and radiation therapy can be used. In multicentric and vertebral locations of high-grade malignancy, when wide surgical ablation is either impractical or unfeasible, treatment is limited to radiation and chemotherapy.

Provisionally, chemotherapy similar to that use for osteosarcoma is used in high-grade H.H.

The treatment program must always be based on an accurate histological study, and thus preceded by biopsy, preferably incisional.

PROGNOSIS

Grade 1 H.H. heals constantly with conservative surgical treatment and with radiation treatment, or with the association of both. We do not fully know the course of **grade 2 H.H.** Usually it is cured by wide surgical removal and, at times, even by marginal or intralesional surgery plus radiation therapy. We do not know whether grade 2 H.H. is capable of progressing in malignancy and whether this is favored by radiation therapy. Recurrence may occur in other sites of the skeleton (usually in the same limb). Rare cases have given metastases. The prognosis of **grades 3 and 4 H.H.** is poor. With surgical or radiation treatment only, survival for more than 5 years is rare. Prognosis with the use of adjuvant and neoadjuvant chemotherapy is not yet known.

REFERENCES

1962 HARTMANN W. H., STEWART F. W.: Hemangioendothelioma of bone. Unusual tumor characterized by indolent course. *Cancer*, **15**, 846-854.

1964 ZANASI R.: Endotelioma benigno dello scheletro. *Archivio di Ortopedia*, **77**, 41-47.

1965 BUNDENS W. D., BRIGHTON C. T.: Malignant hemangioendothelioma of bone. Report of two cases and review of the literature. *Journal of Bone and Joint Surgery*, **47-A**, 762-772.

1968 OTIS J., HUTTER R. V. P., FOOTE F. W. Jr., MARCOVE R. C., STEWART F. W.: Hemangioendothelioma of bone. *Surgery Gynecology and Obstetrics*, **127**, 295-305.

1969 CAMPANACCI M., CENNI F., GIUNTI A.: Angectasie, amartomi e neoplasie vascolari dello scheletro. *Chirurgia degli Organi di Movimento*, **58**, 472-498.

1971 DORFMAN H. D., STEINER G. C., JAFFE H. L.: Vascular tumours of bone. *Human Pathology*, **2**, 349-376.

1971 UNNI K. K., IVINS J. C., BEABOUT J. W., DAHLIN D. C.: Hemangioma, hemangiopericytoma and hemangioendothelioma (angiosarcoma) of bone. *Cancer*, **27**, 1403-1414.

1972 DUBE V. E., FISHER D. E.: Hemangioendothelioma of the leg following metallic fixation of the tibia. *Cancer*, **30**, 1260-1266.

1972 STEINER G. C., DORFMAN H. D.: Ultrastructure of hemangioendothelial sarcoma of bone. *Cancer*, **29**, 122-135.

1975 LARSSON S. E., LORENTZON R., BOQUIST L.: Malignant hemangioendothelioma of bone. *Journal of Bone and Joint Surgery*, **57-A**, 84-89.

1979 CRAVER W. L., BROWN B. S.: Hemangioendothelioma of bone with pulmonary metastases: a 25-year course. Report of a case. *Cancer*, **43**, 1917-1923.

1980 CAMPANACCI M., BORIANI S., GIUNTI A.: Hemangioendothelioma of bone. A study of 29 cases. *Cancer*, **46**, 804-814.

1982 VOLPE R., MAZABRAUD A.: Hemangioendothelioma (angiosarcoma) of bone: a distinct pathologic entity with an unpredictable course? *Cancer*, **49**, 727-736.

1988 LYE D.J., WEPFER J.F., HASKEL D.S.: Case report 458. *Skeletal Radiology*, **17**, 57-59.

HEMANGIOPERICYTOMA

This tumor is extremely rare in the bone. Only a few cases have been described up to now in the literature. It seems to particularly occur in the long bones. It causes osteolysis with faded boundaries, with possible erosion of the cortex (Fig. 510). Histologically, it is constituted by a thick proliferation of cells, with round-oval nuclei, arranged around numerous small vessels. In order to obtain a diagnosis staining for the reticular and collagen fibers is required (trichromic, P.A.S., argentic impregnation, Fig. 511). These show that the cells (surrounded by a dense argyrophylous reticulum) are arranged out-

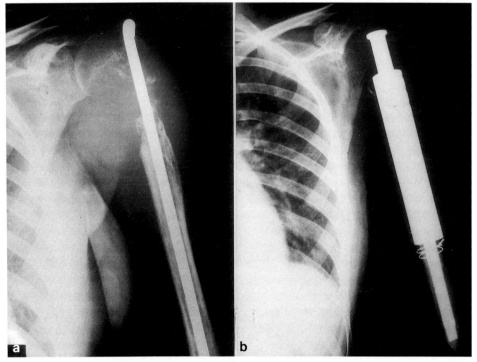

FIG. 510. - Female aged 21 years. Grade 3 hemangiopericytoma. (a) The patient was operated elsewhere by biopsy and Rush nailing. (b) Extra articular resection of the proximal humerus, wide but contaminated by the presence of the nail. Reconstruction with cemented modular prosthesis. Post-operative radiotherapy. No signs of disease after 1 year.

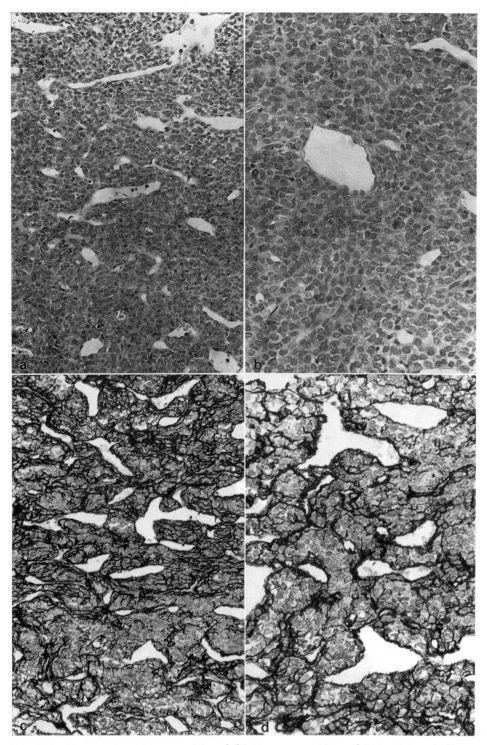

FIG. 511. - Hemangiopericytoma. (a) and (b) *Hemat.-eos.* 200 and 300 x. (c) and (d) *Argentic impregnation* 200 and 300 x.

side the basal membrane of the vessels, instead of inside, as is the case in he-mangioendothelioma. Histological differential diagnosis involves Ewing's sarcoma (the cytoplasms are P.A.S. positive even in hemangiopericytoma) and particularly mesenchymal chondrosarcoma. The course and prognosis of the disease are to a great extent unpredictable: some cases have metasta-sized, even many years after treatment. This must be based on decidedly wide surgical removal.

REFERENCES

1960 MARCIAL-ROJAS R. A.: Primary haemangiopericytoma of bone. Review of the literature and report of the first case with metastases. *Cancer*, **13**, 308-311.

1971 UNNI K. K., IVINS J. C., BEABOUT J. W., DAHLIN D. C.: Haemangioma, haeman-giopericytoma and haemangioendothelioma (angiosarcoma) of bone. *Cancer*, **27**, 1403-1414.

1973 DUNLOP J.: Primary haemangiopericytoma of bone. Report of two cases. *Journal of Bone and Joint Surgery*, **55-B**, 854-857.

1973 HAHN M. J., DAWSON P., ESTERLY J. A.: Haemangiopericytoma. An ultrastruc-tural study. *Cancer*, **31**, 255-261.

1980 VANG P.S., FALK E.: Hemangiopericytoma of bone. Review of the literature and report of a case. *Acta Orthopaedica Scandinavica*, **51**, 903-907.

1981 McGAHAN J.P., HAUSEN S.K., PALMER P.E.S.: Case report 163. *Skeletal Radio-logy*, **7**, 66-96.

1982 GIUNTI A., CALDERONI P., MARTUCCI E.: Haemangiopericytoma of bone. *Italian Journal of Orthopaedics and Traumatology*, **8**, 347-350.

1986 CHEN K.T.K., KASSEL S.H.: Congenital hemangiopericytoma. *Journal of Surgi-cal Oncology*, **31**, 127-129.

1988 TANG J.S.M., GOLD R.M., MIRRA J.M., ECKARDT J.: Hemangiopericytoma of bone. *Cancer*, **62**, 848-859.

NEURINOMA. MODIFICATIONS
OF THE SKELETON ASSOCIATED
WITH NEUROFIBROMATOSIS

NEURINOMA
(Synonyms: neurilemmoma, schwannoma)

N. is a benign tumor originating from Schwann cells. In the bones it originates from the small nervous branches of the periosteum (periosteal N.) or from those which accompany the nutrient vessels of the bone. Skeletal N. occurs very rarely, but a small number of undebatable cases are reported in the literature. The tumor may be manifested at any age, prevalently during adult **age**. The **sites** observed are the long bones (diaphysis, metaphysis, rarely the meta-epiphysis), a rib, the scapula, the patella, the tubular bones of the hand. The tumor grows slowly and causes mild and late **symptoms** (symptoms may date back 15-20 years). Periosteal N. are less rare, which **radiographically** resemble a lenticular excavation of the cortex, with a sclerotic border, or like an intracortical vesicular osteolysis covered by a thin and somewhat bulging shell of bone, sometimes multiloculated. Central N. of the

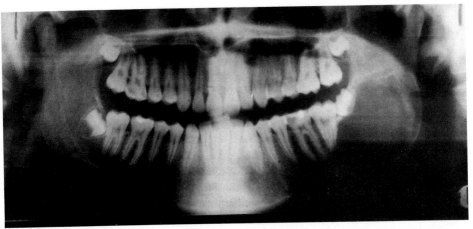

FIG. 512. - Neurinoma of the mandible in a boy aged 14 years. Observe the osteolytic lesion of the left angle of the mandible, slightly swollen and well delimited.

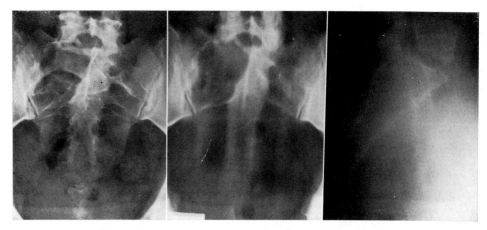

FIG. 513. - Female aged 32 years. Neurinoma (originating from a sacral root) excavating the sacrum and simulating a skeletal tumor.

bone radiographically reveal a globose area of osteolysis, with well-defined margins marked by a thin line of hyperostosis (Fig. 515). In any case, the tumor tends to be small or moderate in size. **Macroscopically**, it is clearly delimited, rather soft, grayish, with frequent hemorrhagic and cystic areas. **Histologically**, it has the typical spindle-cell structure with currents of wavy fi-

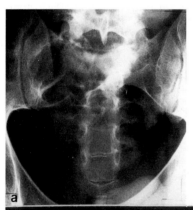

FIG. 514. - Neurinoma of the sacrum in a male aged 24 years. Recurring lumbar-sciatic pain for the past 9 years, which worsened in the last 2. Signs of nerve root deficit at S1. (a) The radiogram shows osteolysis having well defined limits of the wing and of the first sacral foramen to the right. (b) and (d) CAT shows osteolysis having sharp borders and the tumor which protrudes forwards outside of the sacrum, probably through the anterior sacral foramen. The patient was treated with three selective arterial embolizations, and then curettage by anterior approach. Symptoms regressed and CAT is stationary after 4 years.

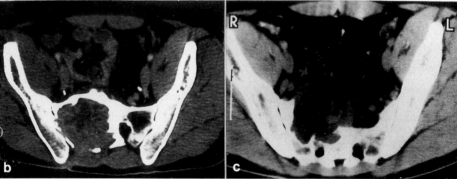

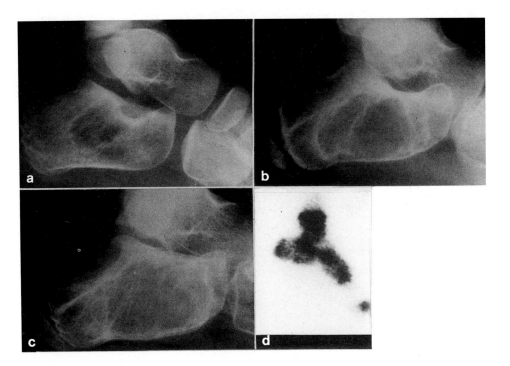

FIG. 515. - Neurinoma in a girl aged 6 years. Pain for the past 2 months after trauma. (a) Radiogram shows central osteolysis with sharp borders. Expansion of the osteolysis after 13 months (b) and after 6 further months (c). Bone scan (d) shows scarse uptaking of the lesion. The patient was submitted to curettage following frozen section biopsy. There were no signs of recurrence after 2 years.

bers (Antoni type A). The nuclei are oval, at times palisading. Fibers and nuclei may be arranged in whorls (Verocay bodies) (Fig. 517). The structure characterized by dissociated fibers and cells having abundant intercellular fluid and the formation of cystic cavities (Antoni type B) is less frequent than is observed in extraskeletal N. The blood vessels are numerous, with a thick collagen wall.

It is important to recall that sparse large nuclei are commonly observed in N., with considerable polydimensionality and pleomorphism, and with a fair amount of hyperchromia, without this implying malignancy. There does not seem to be any demonstrative case of malignant N. in the bone.

There are cases of N. which impress and excavate the bone from the outside or starting from a skeletal foramen, particularly in the vertebral column, the sacrum and the mandible (where they mostly originate from the spinal roots and nerves and respectively from the mandibular nerve) (Figs. 512, 513). Some N. of the sacrum achieve very large size. Radiographically they may be suspected, as the osteolysis has rather clear boundaries and the tumor expands with lobulations that follow the sacral foramina (Fig. 514).

FIG. 516. - Female aged 40 years. Neurofibromatosis. (a) Enlargement of the interpedicular distance, considerable narrowing of the laminae, vast osteolysis of the sacrum, with clear boundaries. (b) Typical dishlike erosion of the posterior aspect of the vertebral bodies.

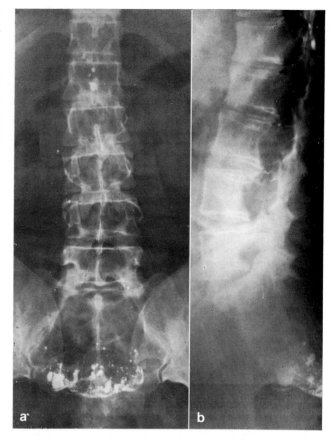

MODIFICATIONS IN THE SKELETON
ASSOCIATED WITH NEUROFIBROMATOSIS

In N.F., too, periosteal or intraosseous neurofibromas may be observed in exceptional cases; nonetheless, most skeletal modifications observed in this disease are of another nature, not tumoral.

N.F., or Von Recklinghausen disease, is a complex congenital dysplasia involving both the neuroectodermic derivates (particularly the peripheral nerves and skin) and the mesodermic derivates (skeleton and soft tissues). The pre-eminent modification, which gives its name to the disease, is the proliferation of Schwann cells and of peripheral nerve fibers, probably of the hamartomatous type. This proliferation involves the nerve trunks in a very irregular manner, causing nodular enlargement or diffused enlargement and elongation (plexiform); and the nerve endings, where nodular (circumscribed cutaneous) or diffused (cutaneous and subcutaneous thickening) lesions may appear. A second component is constituted by skin café au lait spots. N.F. is a hereditary disease, and is generally manifested during early childhood. Its severity varies considerably, from mild forms where only skin

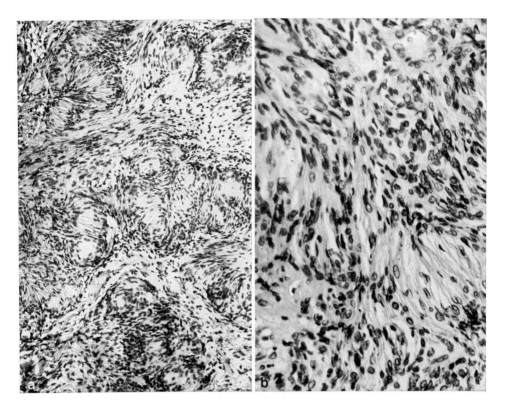

FIG. 517. - Histological aspects of neurinoma (*Hemat.-eos.*, 125 and 300 x).

spots and at most some small nodules are present, to severe forms, which in the words of Jaffe constitute a museum of anomalies.

Skeletal modifications in N.F. may be radiographically revealed in more than 1/3 of all cases. These modifications may be numbered as follows.

1) Periosteal and intraosseous neurofibromas.

These are rare and of moderate size, at times they are multiple. Periosteal ones are those most documented, in the form of little nodules or rather diffused thickening of the periosteum. Radiographically, they may resemble small dish-like erosions of the cortex, or oblique and faded bands of relative radiolucency (caused by depressions or furrows of the outer surface of the cortex in the cases of diffused periosteal thickening).

2) Scoliosis.

These scolioses tend to be early and to progress rapidly even during childhood. Etiology and the relationship with other anomalies of N.F. are not well-known.

3) Modifications — in defect or in excess — in the growth of one or more limbs.

These are associated with diffused hypertrophy and pseudo-elephantiasis of the soft tissues and osteo-articular deformities. These modifications, too, are of varying severity and extent ranges from a minimum (a part of the hand or of the foot) to a maximum (all of the limb). In these pseudo-elephantiasic limbs, vast ossifying periosteal hematomas of the long bones have been observed.

4) Slendering, hypoplasia, aplasia of the bones of the limbs, and, in particular, congenital bowed tibia and congenital or infantile pseudarthrosis of the tibia.

In the site of these pseudarthroses no neurofibromatous tissue is found. When osteolytic areas of the tibial diaphysis are associated with the bowed tibia, which is rarely pseudarthrosic, it is not a neurofibroma, rather osteo-fibrous dysplasia of the tibia (see specific chapter).

5) Multicentric histiocytic fibromas of the skeleton, with typical radiographic aspect (see specific chapter).

6) Excavations of the surfaces of the vertebrae.

Due to compression by the neurofibromas and/or spinal meningoceles, lar and multiple excavations may be observed, which may even be rather deep, of the posterior aspect of the vertebral bodies and/or enlargement of the intervertebral foramina (Fig. 516).

7) Rare associations.

These include spina bifida, congenital dislocation of the hip, congenital club foot.

REFERENCES

1940 DE SANTO D. A., BURGESS E.: Primary and secondary neurilemmoma of bone. *Surgery, Gynecology and Obstetrics*, **71**, 454-461.

1940 UHLMANN E., GROSSMAN A.: Von Recklinghausen's neurofibromatosis with bone manifestations. *Annals of Internal Medicine*, **14**, 225-241.

1948 HOLT J. F., WRIGHT E. M.: The radiologic features of nerofibromatosis. *Radiology*, **51**, 647-664.

1950 MC CARROL H. R.: Clinical manifestations of congenital neurofibromatosis. *Journal of Bone and Joint Surgery*, **32-A**, 601-617.

1953 DIVERTIE M. B., DAHLIN D. C.: Neurilemmoma of rib. Report of a case. *Disease of Chest*, **44**, 635-637.

1953 HENSLEY C. D. Jr.: Rapid development of a « subperiosteal bone cyst » in multiple neurofibromatosis. A case report. *Journal of Bone and Joint Surgery*, **35-A**, 197-203.

1958 HART M. S., BASOM W. C.: Neurilemmoma involving bone. *Journal of Bone and Joint Surgery*, **40-A**, 465-468.

1960 SANTER T. G., VELIOS F., SHAFER W. G.: Neurilemmoma of bone. Report of 3 cases with a review of the literature. *Radiology*, **75**, 215-222.

1961 CALDWELL J. B., HUGHES K. W., COX R. S. Jr.: Neurofibroma of the mandible. Report of a case. *Journal of Oral Surgery*, **19**, 166-171.

1961 FRIEDMAN M.: Intraosseous schwannoma. Report of a case. *Oral Surgery*, **18**, 90-96.

1961 HUNT J. C., PUGH D. G.: Skeletal lesions in neurofibromatosis. *Radiology*, **76**, 1-20.

1964 MORTON M. S., VASSAR P. D.: Neurilemmoma in bone. Report of a case. *Canadian Journal of Surgery*, **7**, 187-189.

1967 FAWCETT K. J., DAHLIN D. C.: Neurilemmoma of bone. *American Journal of Clinical Pathology*, **47**, 759-766.

1969 CURTISS B. H., FISHER R. L., BUTTERFIELD F., SAUNDERS P.: Neurofibromatosis with paraplegia. *Journal of Bone and Joint Surgery*, **51-A**, 843-861.

1971 DICKSON J. H., WALTZ T. A., FECHRER R. E.: Intraosseous neurilemmoma of the third lumbar vertebra. *Journal of Bone and Joint Surgery*, **53-A**, 349-355.

1971 SANE S., YUNIS E., GREER R.: Subperiosteal or cortical cyst and intramedullary neurofibromatosis. Uncommon manifestations of neurofibromatosis. A case report. *Journal of Bone and Joint Surgery*, **53-A**, 1194-1200.

1972 KULLMANN L., WONTERS H. W.: Neurofibromatosis; gigantism and subperiosteal haematoma. Report of two children with extensive subperiosteal bone formation. *Journal of Bone and Joint Surgery*, **54-B**, 130-138.

1976 CHAGLASSIAN J. H., RISEBOROUGH E. J., HALL J. E.: Neurofibromatous scoliosis. Natural history and results of treatment in thirty-seven cases. *Journal of Bone and Joint Surgery*, **58-A**, 695-702.

1976 GORDON E. J.: Solitary intraosseous neurilemmoma of the tibia. Review of intraosseous neurilemmoma and neurofibroma. *Clinical Orthopaedics*, **117**, 271-282.

1978 MORRISON M. J., IVINS J. C.: Case report 47. *Skeletal Radiology*, **2**, 177-178.

1981 SCHAJOWICZ F.: *Tumors and tumor-like lesions of bone and joints.* Springer Verlag, New York.

1982 WILNER D.: *Radiology of bone tumors and allied disorders.* Vol. 1. W.B. Saunders, Philadelphia.

LIPOMA AND LIPOSARCOMA.
MALIGNANT MESENCHYMOMA

Despite the abundance of adipose tissue in the bone marrow, the occurrence of intraosseous L. and L.S. is extremely rare. We have never observed a case of undebatable skeletal L. and our experience with L.S. is limited to one case.

Probably, some cases referred to as skeletal lipoma are not actually skeletal **lipoma**, rather they represent areas of skeletal atrophy with adipose substitution (see senile angiectatic vertebral areas). Among the very rare cases of skeletal L. reported in the literature, those which are less rare and more convincing seem to be periosteal and parosteal ones, which may cause epicortical osteolysis with well-defined boundaries, marked by a thin line of hyperostosis. Skeletal L. has been described in the cranio-facial bones, ribs, ulna, tibia, fibula, sacrum and calcaneus. Its anatomical features are the same as those of common L. of the soft tissues. That is, it is a globose or plurilobulated small mass, well-circumscribed, compact, pale yellow in color and of firm and pasty consistency. The histological aspect is that of mature fat, in closely packed lobules, at times including some small groups of cells resembling immature fat or «brown fat».

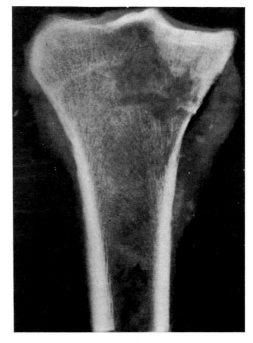

Even the diagnosis of **liposarcoma**, in some cases reported in the literature, must be accepted with caution, as it could in truth be a malignant mesenchymoma (see further on) and because foam cells may be observed in malignant fibrous histiocytomas. The exceptional examples

Fig. 518. - Male aged 15 years. Malignant mesenchymoma. X-ray of the anatomical specimen.

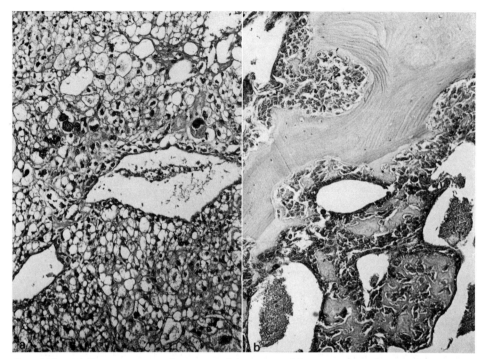

FIG. 519. - Malignant mesenchymoma. (a) Aspect of liposarcoma. (b) Aspect of osteosarcoma (*Hemat.-eos.*, 125, 125 x).

of skeletal L.S. have been observed during adult age and in the diaphyses or
meta-diaphyses of the long bones. Radiographically, osteolysis is observed
which tends to destroy the cortex. Histologically, the tumor is the same as
poorly differentiated high-grade L.S. of the soft tissues. Alongside areas of fibroblastic differentiation and/or myxoid areas, are aspects of lipoblastic differentiation, with cells having vacuolated cytoplasm and filled with lipoids.
Cellular atypia is generally very high.

Malignant mesenchymoma is a primary sarcoma of bone with aspects of
differentiation in two or more tissue types, besides the fibroblastic. In the
few reported cases, associated liposarcomatous and osteosarcomatous differentiation have been described. It occurs exceptionally rarely, and its clinical,
radiographic, prognostic and therapeutic features resemble those of osteosarcoma (Figs. 518, 519).

REFERENCES

1953 CATTO V., STEVENS J.: Liposarcoma of bone. *Journal of Pathology and Bacteriology*, **86**, 248-253.
1954 GOLDMAN R. L.: Primary liposarcoma of bone. Report of a case. *American
Journal of Clinical Pathology*, **42**, 503-508.
1955 CHILD P. L.: Lipoma of the os calcis. Report of a case. *American Journal of
Clinical Pathology*, **25**, 1050-1052.

1955 DAWSON E. K.: Liposarcoma of bone. *Journal of Pathology and Bacteriology*, **70**, 513-520.

1957 GOIDANICH I. F.: *I tumori primitivi dell'osso*. S.p.A. Poligrafici « Il Resto del Carlino », Bologna.

1965 PELOUX Y., THEVENOL P., BOUFFARD A.: Le lipome intramédullaire osseous. Etude d'un nouveau cas observé au Dahomay. *Presse Médicale*, **73**, 2057-2058.

1966 SCHAJOWICZ F., CUEVILLAS A. R., SILBERMAN F. S.: Primary malignant mesenchymoma of bone. A new tumor entity. *Cancer*, **19**, 1423-1428.

1969 ROSS F. C., DADFIELD: Primary osteo-liposarcoma of bone (malignant mesenchymoma). Report of a case. *Journal of Bone and Joint Surgery*, **50-B**, 639-643.

1970 SCHWARTZ A., BECKER S. M.: Liposarcoma of bone. Report of a case and review of the literature. *Journal of Bone and Joint Surgery*, **52-A**, 171-177.

1971 ZORN D. T., CORDRAY D. P., RANDELS P. H.: Intraosseous lipoma of bone involving the sacrum. *Journal of Bone and Joint Surgery*, **53-A**, 1201-1204.

1975 LARSSON S. E., LORENTZON R., BOQUIST L.: Primary liposarcoma of bone. *Acta Orthopedica Scandinavica*, **46**, 869-876.

1978 BERTONI F., LAUS M.: Mesenchimoma maligno primitivo dell'osso. Segnalazione di un caso. *Giornale Italiano di Ortopedia e Traumatologia*, **4**, 105-108.

1978 DE LEE J.C.: Intraosseous lipoma of the proximal part of the femur. Case report. *Journal of Bone and Joint Surgery*, **61-A**, 601-603.

1980 SCHNEIDER H.M., WUNDERLICH T., PULS P.: The primary liposarcoma of bone. *Archives of Orthopaedic and Trauma Surgery*, **96**, 235-239.

1981 PARDO-MINDAN F.J., AYALA H., JOLY M., GIMENO E., VAZQUEZ J.: Primary liposarcoma of bone: light and electron microscopic surgery. *Cancer*, **48**, 274-280.

1981 SCHAJOWICZ F.: *Tumors and tumor-like lesions*. Springer Verlag, New York.

1982 WILNER D.: *Radiology of bone tumors and allied disorders*. Vol. 1. W.B. Saunders, Philadelphia.

1983 LEESON M., KAY D., SMITH B.: Intraosseous lipoma. *Clinical Orthopaedics*, **181**, 186-190.

1983 TOROK G., MELLER Y., MAOR E.: Primary liposarcoma of bone. Case report and review of the literature. *Bulletin of Hospital of Joint Diseases*, **43**, 28-37.

1984 BOGUMILL G.P., SCHWAMM H.A.: *Orthopaedic pathology*. W.B. Saunders, Philadephia.

1984 GOLDMAN A.B., MARCOVE R.C., HUVOS A.G.: Intraosseous lipoma of the tibia. *Skeletal Radiology*, **12**, 209-212.

1988 MILGRAM J.W.: Intraosseous lipoma. A clinicopathologic study of 66 cases. *Clinical Orthopaedics*, **231**, 277-302.

ADAMANTINOMA OF THE LONG BONES

DEFINITION

It is a low-grade malignant tumor probably of mixed mesenchymal and epithelial nature, which develops in the diaphyses and metaphyses of the long bones, prevalently of the tibia. It has incorrectly been defined «adamantinoma» because its histological aspect may recall that of ameloblastoma of the maxillary bones.

FREQUENCY

A. is the rarest primary bone tumor after neurogegenous and lipogenous tumors.

AGE

It is observed between 10 and 70 years of age, prevalently between 20 and 40 years. It is an exceptional occurrence before 10 years of age (Fig. 520).

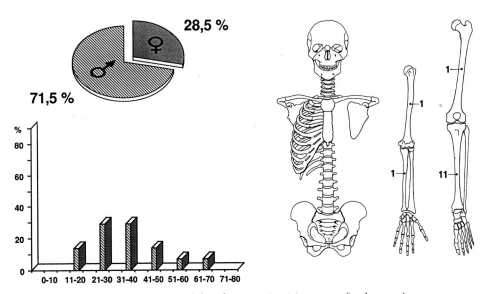

Fig. 520. - Sex, age and localization in 14 cases of adamantinoma.

SEX

There is predilection for the male sex.

LOCALIZATION

The site which is most preferred (in almost 90% of all cases) is the tibia. Localizations in the ulna, fibula, femur, radius, humerus, exceptionally elsewhere, have been observed.

The tumor generally develops in the diaphyses, at times in the metaphyses, never in the epiphyses.

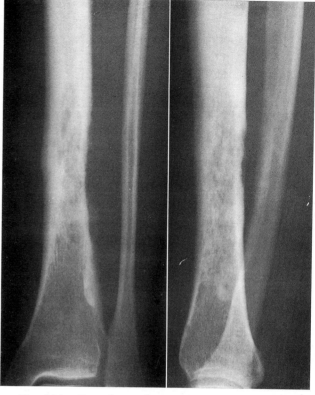

Fig. 521. - Female aged 48 years. Recurrence of adamantinoma after three attempts at intralesional excision over 3 years.

SYMPTOMS

Symptoms are those of a tumor characterized by torpid growth and which develops in a very superficial bone such as the tibia. At times, the patient becomes aware of slow-growing swelling. At times the main symptom is pain, which is never very intense. The neoplasm rarely has achieved a large size at surgery. It may cause a pathologic fracture.

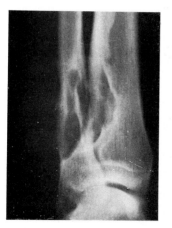

Fig. 522. - Male aged 24 years. Adamantinoma involving the tibia and the fibula and expanding in the soft tissues. Onset of symptoms 3 years earlier.

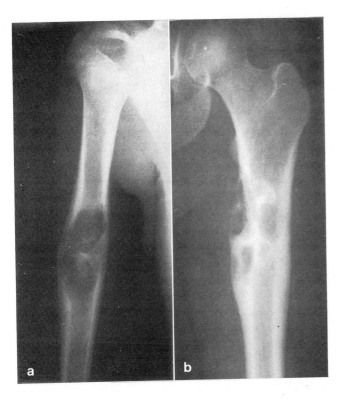

FIG. 523. - (a) Boy aged 12 years. Pain for the past 4 months. (b) Female aged 22 years. The lesion had been intralesionally excised and then irradiated 3 years earlier. The recurrence visible on radiogram was treated by wide resection. No sign of recurrence after 16 years.

RADIOGRAPHIC FEATURES

There is a rather lucent area of osteolysis, with faded (but sometimes well-defined) boundaries, uniform or honeycombed or bubbly. When osteolysis is central, as is more often the case, the cortex may appear to be moderately expanded and attenuated. It is rarely interrupted, with invasion of the soft tissues (Figs. 521, 523).

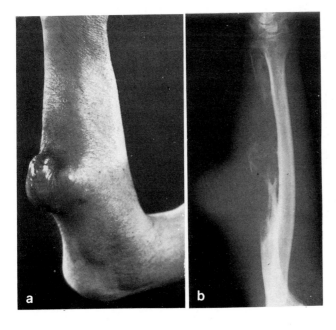

FIG. 524. - Male aged 63 years. Eight years earlier, progressive swelling on the diaphysis of the ulna. (After 2 years intralesional excision. After 4 more years local recurrence. After 2 more years the recurring mass was seen to be progressively expanding). (a) Clinical picture; (b) radiographic picture. Amputation was carried out. Died after 3 years with pulmonary metastases.

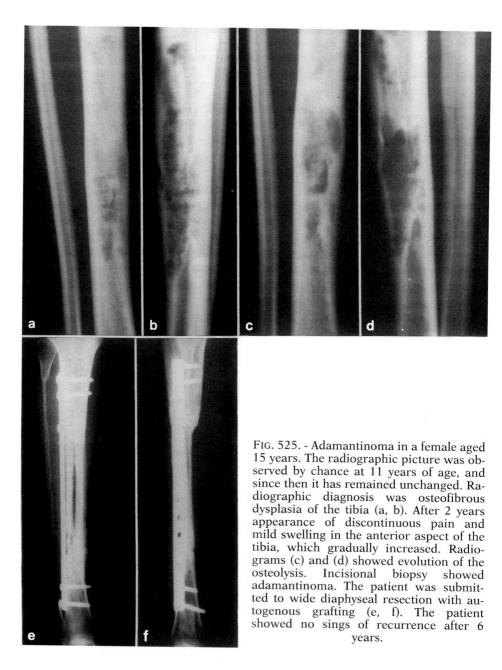

FIG. 525. - Adamantinoma in a female aged 15 years. The radiographic picture was observed by chance at 11 years of age, and since then it has remained unchanged. Radiographic diagnosis was osteofibrous dysplasia of the tibia (a, b). After 2 years appearance of discontinuous pain and mild swelling in the anterior aspect of the tibia, which gradually increased. Radiograms (c) and (d) showed evolution of the osteolysis. Incisional biopsy showed adamantinoma. The patient was submitted to wide diaphyseal resection with autogenous grafting (e, f). The patient showed no sings of recurrence after 6 years.

In some cases the osteolysis is eccentric, with the cortex cancelled on one side alone; or the cortex appears to be scooped out by the tumoral mass which seems to be of periosteal origin (Fig. 522).

In central and eccentric or periosteal forms of the disease, the osteogenetic reaction of the periosteum is very scarce or absent. At times A. has a radiographic aspect which is similar to or the same as that of osteofibrous dysplasia of the tibia (see specific chapter)(Fig. 525).

GROSS PATHOLOGIC FEATURES

Generally contained by the cortex or the periosteum, the tumor appears to be whitish, compact, with a vaguely nodular structure, of firm consistency, and chracterized by little bleeding. At times there are cystic or hemorrhagic areas. In some cases the neoplasm invades the soft tissues.

HISTOPATHOLOGIC FEATURES

The histological picture varies from case to case, even within the same specimen. The main histological aspects may be classified as follows (Weiss and Dorfman, 1977). 1) **Basalioid aspect**: cords and islands of cells similar to basal cell carcinoma. These cells may be spindling in the center of the islands, while at the periphery a layer of cubic or cylindrical palisading cells may be seen. The reticulin fibers surround cellular fields, not single cells. This aspect recalls that of basaliomas and ameloblastoma of jaw. 2) **Spindlecellular aspect**. Similar to the previous one, but with no peripheral palisading layer. At times the cells are arranged in whorls. The reticulin fibers surround single cells (typical of mesenchymal tumor). This aspect may resemble a fibrosarcoma. 3) **Tubular aspect**. Small ramified tubules or alveolar cavities, matted by cubic-cylindrical cells, in one or more layers. This aspect may resemble that of an adenocarcinoma or a hemangioendothelioma. 4) **Squamocellular** aspect. At times, but not frequently, there are nodules of squamous cells, even with evidence of prickle cells and epithelial pearls. The cells stain positively with keratin antibodies and, at E.M., show desmosomes, tonofibrils and microfilaments.

Deposits of immature osteoid similar to that of osteosarcoma around the neoplastic cells have been described.

All of the aforementioned cellular aggregates are surrounded by a bland fibrous stroma, in relation to which they may be clearly distinguished. This collagenous connective tissue is usually abundant and dense. This explains the sustained consistency, and the whitish color of A. At the periphery and alongside A. there may be fibrous tissue which is nearly or totally the same as that of fibrous dysplasia, and like this, it contains trabeculae of reticular bone. At times these trabeculae are bordered by osteoblasts so that the aspect is that of an osteofibrous dysplasia of the tibia. This mesenchymal tissue is benign and contains small nidi of epithelioid aspect or penetrates the tissue typical of A. Thus, it seems that this tissue is part of the tumor.

HISTOGENESIS AND PATHOGENESIS

The histogenesis of A. is still hypothetical and controversial. The epithelial origin is sustained by several givens. a) The presence of squamous cells and epithelial pearls. b) The demonstration under electron microscopy of tonofibrils and desmosomes in the cytoplasm and forming a bridge among the

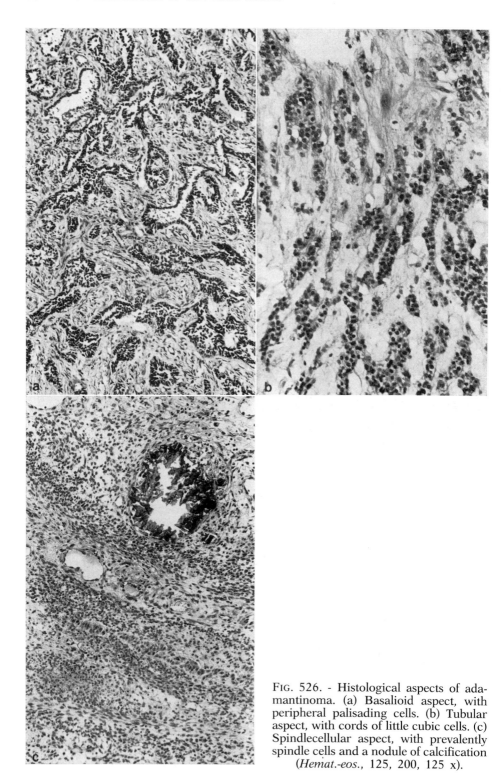

Fig. 526. - Histological aspects of adamantinoma. (a) Basalioid aspect, with
peripheral palisading cells. (b) Tubular
aspect, with cords of little cubic cells. (c)
Spindlecellular aspect, with prevalently
spindle cells and a nodule of calcification
(*Hemat.-eos.*, 125, 200, 125 x).

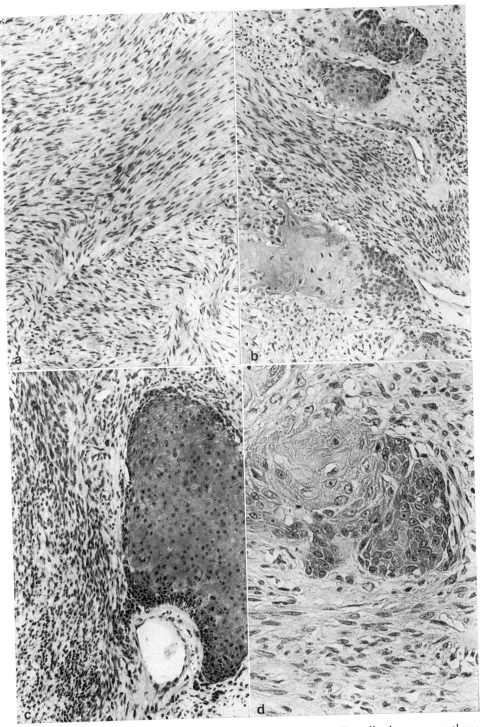

FIG. 527. - Histological aspects of adamantinoma. (a) Spindle cells the same as those of fibrosarcoma. (b), (c), (d) Squamous cells, prickle cells and epithelial pearls. (*Hemat.-eos.*, 125, 125 x, Van Gieson, 125, 300 x).

cells. c) The presence of tubules or alveoli matted by cubic-cylindrical cells; of solid areas similar to those of basaliomas; of cylindrical palisading cells surrounding spindle-stellate fields, as occurs in ameloblastoma. What instead contrasts with epithelial histogenesis is the presence of reticulin and collagen fibers and, in exceptional cases, of osteoid material between tumoral cells, as well as the fact that some areas of the tumor and some pulmonary metastases have an exclusively spindle cellular and sarcomatous structure; finally, tumoral areas may appear identical to a fibrous or osteofibrous dysplasia.

It may be affirmed that so-called A. of the long bones is a tumor constituted by cells capable of different differentiation, epithelial and mesenchymal. It seems that A. may originate in association with an osteofibrous dysplasia of the tibia.

DIAGNOSIS

Diagnosis of A. is not easy because of its rarity, its changeable and differing histological aspects, because of the possibility of its histologically resembling **epithelial metastasis, hemangioendothelioma, fibrous or osteofibrous dysplasia**. A valid aid to diagnosis is the history of the patient, age, and, in particular, the site (in the diaphysis of the tibia).

We are aware of the fact that there do exist exceptional cases of osteofibrous dysplasia of the tibia, having a typical clinical-radiographic and histological picture, which, after puberty (hardly ever before) prove to be A. (Fig. 525). This does not justify performing biopsy of all osteofibrous dysplasias of the tibia, first of all because A. in such cases is a very rare occurrence, and secondly because biopsy, if negative, would not exclude A. On the other hand, the malignancy of A. is so low that a very early diagnosis is not so important. A. must instead be suspected when a tibial lesion, whether or not characterized by the aspect of an osteofibrous dysplasia, becomes painful and/or it grows after puberty. In cases such as these, biopsy must be taken from the most radiolucent area, and that which expanded most on subsequent radiograms.

COURSE

A. grows slowly or very slowly. Cases have been described in which the interval between the first symptoms and surgical treatment was almost 20 years, without the occurrence of any metastasis. Metastases may be manifested even more than 10 years after surgery. Metastases are rare and mostly localized in the lungs, but they may also occur in the lymph nodes and skeleton.

TREATMENT

If the tumor is still contained in the cortex, it must be widely resected with the affected bone segment and the periosteum. The tibia may be reconstructed by means of auto- or allografts and solid osteosynthesis (Fig. 525).

If the tumor has extensively interrupted the cortex and is very expanded in the soft tissues, or if it has locally and widely recurred after conservative surgery, amputation is indicated. An attempt at resection in cases such as these would expose the patient to a high risk of recurrence.

If the inguinal lymph nodes show possible or certain signs of metastatic invasion, they must be removed en bloc. Because of the slow growth of the tumor, excision of the pulmonary metastases is indicated.

PROGNOSIS

If the tumor is not widely removed it recurs. Depending on the specific case series, death by metastasis has occurred in 10-30% of cases followed-up in time. Thus, metastases occur infrequently and usually late. If treatment is prompt and adequate, prognosis is favorable in most cases.

REFERENCES

1954 BAKER P. L., DOCKERTY M. B., COVENTRY M. B.: Adamantinoma (so-called) of the long bones. Review of the literature and a report of three new cases. *Journal of Bone and Joint Surgery*, **36-A**, 704-720.

1954 CHANGUS G. W., SPEED J. S., STEWART F. W.: Malignant angioblastoma of bone. A reappraisal of adamantinoma of long bone. *Cancer*, **10**, 540-549.

1954 HICKS J. D.: Synovial sarcoma of the tibia. *Journal of Pathology and Bacteriology*, **67**, 151-161.

1954 LEDERER H., SINCLAIR A. J.: Malignant synovioma simulating adamantinoma of the tibia. *Journal of Pathology and Bacteriology*, **67**, 163-168.

1962 COLHEN D. M., DAHLIN D. C., PUGH D. G.: Fibrous dysplasia associated with adamantinoma of the long bones. *Cancer*, **15**, 515-521.

1964 NAIY A. F., MURPHY Y. A., STASNEY R. J., NEVILLE W. E., CHRENKA P.: So-Called adamantinoma of long bones. Report of a case with massive pulmonary metastasis. *Journal of Bone and Joint Surgery*, **46-A**, 151-158.

1965 MOON N. F.: Adamantinoma of the appendicular skeleton. A statistical review of reported cases and inclusion of 10 new cases. *Clinical Orthopaedics* **43**, 189-213.

1966 DONNER R., DIKLAND R.: Adamantinoma of the tibia. A long-standing case with unusual histological features. *Journal of Bone and Joint Surgery*, **48-B**, 138-144.

1967 SCHAJOWICZ F., GALLARDO H.: Adamantinoma de tibia. Revision bibliografica y consideracion de un nuevo caso. *Revista de Ortopedia y Traumatologia*, **12/L.A.**, 105-118.

1968 ALBORES-SAAVEDRA J., DIAN-GUTIERREZ D., ALTAMIRANO-DIMAS M.: Adamantinoma de la tibia. Observaciones ultrastructurales. *Revista de Medicina del Hospital General de Mexico*, **31**, 241-252.

1969 ROSAI J.: Adamantinoma of the tibia. Electron microscopic evidence of its epithelial origin. *American Journal of Clinical Pathology*, **51**, 786-792.

1971 SCHAJOWICZ F., CABRINI R.L., SIMES R.J.: Microscopia electronica del « adamantinoma » de los huesos largos. *Revista de Ortopedia y Traumatologia*, **16/L.A.**, 185-194.

1973 SCHAJOWICZ F., DE PAOLI J.M.: Adamantinoma de los huesos largos a focos multiples. *Societad Argentina de Ortopedia y Traumatologia*, **38**, 423-435.

1974 UNNI K.K., DAHLIN D.C., BEABOUT J.W., IVINS J.C.: Adamantinomas of long bones. *Cancer*, **34**, 1796-1805.

1975 HUVOS A.G., MARCOVE R.C.: Adamantinoma of long bones. A clinicopathological study of fourteen cases with vascular origin suggested. *Journal of Bone and Joint Surgery*, **57-A**, 148-154.

1977 YONEYAMA T., WINTER W.G., MILSOW L.: Tibial adamantinoma: its histogenesis from ultrastructural studies. *Cancer*, **40**, 1138-1142.

1977 WEISS S.W., DORFMAN H.D.: Adamantinoma of long bone. *Human Pathology*, **8**, 141-153.

1981 CAMPANACCI M., GIUNTI A., BERTONI F., LAUS M., GITELIS S.: Adamantinoma of the long bones. The experience at the Istituto Ortopedico Rizzoli. *American Journal of Surgical Pathology*, **5**, 533-542.

1983 MORI H., YAMAMOTO S., HIRAMATSU K., MIURA T., MOON N.F.: Adamantinoma of the tibia. Ultrastructural and immunohistochemical study with reference to histogenesis. *Clinical Orthopaedics*, **190**, 299-310.

1983 ROCK M.G., BEABOUT J.W., UNNI K.K., SIM F.H.: Adamantinoma. *Orthopaedics*, **6**, 472-483.

1985 PEREZ-ADAYDE A.R., KOZAKEWICH P.W., VAWTER G.F.: Adamantinoma of the tibia. An ultrastructural and immunohistochemical study. *Cancer*, **55**, 1015-1023.

1986 MOON N.F., MORI H.: Adamantinoma of the appendicular skeleton updated. *Clinical Orthopaedics*, **204**, 214-237.

1987 BRAUD P., TOMENO B., COURPIED J.P., RAMADIER J.O., FAGOT J., FOREST M., MERLE D'AUBIGNÉ R.: Une tumeur singulière. L'adamantinome des os longs. *Revue de Chirurgie Orthopedique*, **73**, 3-13.

1988 BOURNE M.H., WOOD M.B., SHIVES T.C.: Adamantinoma of the radius. A case report. *Orthopaedics*, **11**, 1565-1566.

1989 CZERNIAK B., ROJAS-CORONA R.R., DORFMAN D.: Morphologic diversity of long-bone adamantinoma. The concept of differentiated (regressing) adamantinoma and its relationship to osteofibrous dysplasia. *Cancer*, **64**, 2319-2334.

1989 KEENEY G.L., UNNI K.K., BEABOUT J.W., PRITCHARD D.J.: Adamantinoma of long bones: a clinicopathologic study of 85 cases. *Cancer*, **64**, 730-737.

1990 ADLER C.P.: Case report 587. *Skeletal Radiology*, **19**, 55-58.

CHORDOMA

DEFINITION

It is a malignant tumor originating from the residues of the notochord in the cranial base and the vertebral column. Although it may initiate at the surface of the bone and originate from a tissue which does not belong to the bone, it always invades a part of the skeleton and may thus be classified among tumors of the skeleton.

FREQUENCY

CD. occurs rarely.

SEX

There is predilection for the male sex at a ratio of 2-3:1 (Fig. 528).

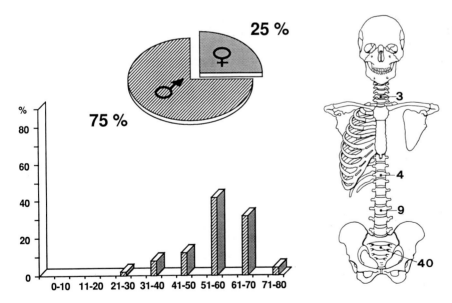

FIG. 528. - Sex, age and localization in 50 cases of chordoma of the vertebral column and sacrum.

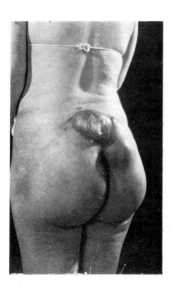

FIG. 529. - Female aged 43 years. For the past 10 years mild sacral pain. Five years earlier the patient had been submitted to intralesional resection and then irradiated. An enormous local recurrence is observed 5 years after surgery. The patient died 1 year later of pulmonary metastasis.

AGE

It is a tumor of adult and advanced age, with a maximum incidence after 50 years. CD. of the cranial base are generally manifested before those of the sacro-coccyx because they cause symptoms even when they are of small size, and because CD. grows slowly. In any case, CD. is exceptionally observed prior to 25 years of age (Fig. 528).

LOCALIZATION

The site of CD. is so exclusive that it constitutes an important element for diagnosis. Approximately 85% of all cases of CD. are observed in the sacro-coccyx or in the cranial base (spheno-occipital region). The remaining cases are observed in the spine (vertebral body) (Fig. 528).

SYMPTOMS

CD. of the spheno-occipital region cause earlier symptoms, due to the compression that they exert even during the earliest phases of their expansion. Symptoms may be manifested as a result of lesions of the hypophysis or of the cranial nerves (particularly the optic and oculomotor nerves); due to obstruction of the nose-pharynx; due to expansion in the ponto-cerebellar angle; due to increase in intracranial pressure.

CD. of the sacro-coccyx cause symptoms which occur late or very late, at times when the tumor has become of considerable size. Symptoms include insidious pain, constipation, hemorrhoids, dysuria, in exceptional cases limping (if the sacroiliac joint is involved) and deficit due to compression of the sacral nerve roots (hypoesthesia, sphincteric paresis). The tumoral mass may

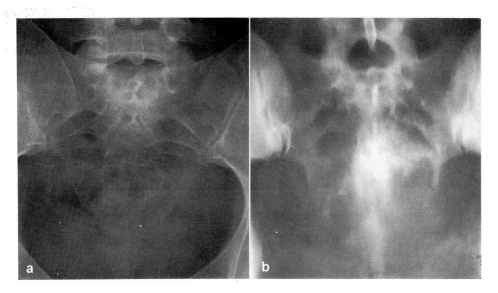

FIG. 530. - (a) Same case as the previous one. Radiogram obtained prior to surgery. (b) Female aged 28 years. Pain for the past year.

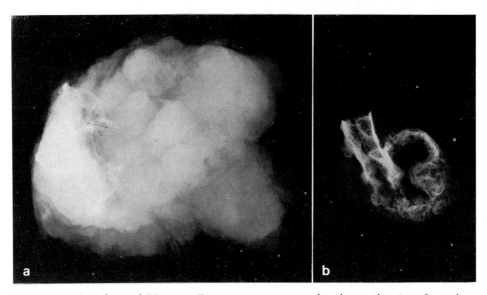

FIG. 531. - (a) Male aged 50 years. Enormous recurrent chordoma, the size of a melon, which expanded anteriorly. (b) Male aged 57 years. Recurrent chordoma. Both of the radiograms were obtained from the resection specimen. These wide resections are possible and the probability of success considerable when the tumor does not proximally surpass the second sacral metamere and particularly if it does not invade the sacro-iliac joint, and if it has not been disseminated by previous surgery.

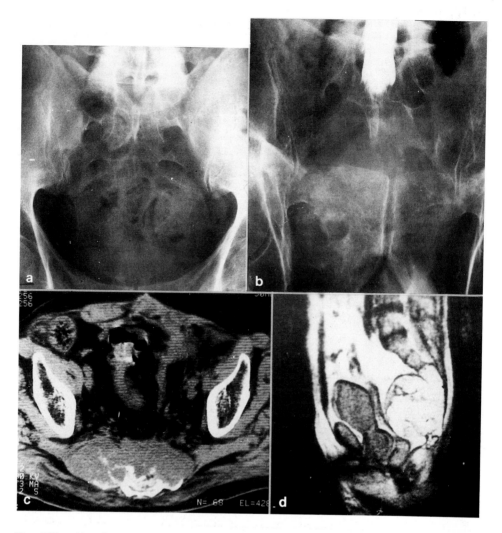

FIG. 532. - Chordoma of the sacrum in a male aged 62 years. Pain for the past 5 years. Faded osteolysis of the caudal part of the sacrum (a). Compression on the dural sac and at the level of the first sacral foramen: myelography (b). CAT shows infiltration along the piriformis muscle to the right (c). MRI shows the tumor mass protruding behind the rectum and rising in the sacral canal slightly above S2.

be palpated on rectal examination. In more advanced forms of the disease the neoplastic mass may be palpated in the sacral or sacro-coccygeal region, at times in the gluteal region (Figs. 529, 534).

In vertebral locations CD. may be manifested by signs of myelo-radicular compression. In forms characterized by anterior expansion, it may simulate a tubercular abscess.

RADIOGRAPHIC FEATURES

In most cases of CD., when the first symptoms occur it is already producing osteolysis which is radiographically visible.

In the cranial base, osteolysis particularly involves the clivus and the sella turcica. CAT and MRI reveal the tumoral mass.

Osteolysis is observed in the sacro-coccyx cancelling the outlines of the bone and the lines of the sacral foramina (Fig. 530). This osteolysis generally has faded boundaries on radiogram, and continues with an extraosseous tumoral mass (CAT, MRI) which generally protrudes more anteriorly than posteriorly (Fig. 531). Typical of CD. is its central origin in the sacrum, its globose even somewhat lobulated form, its relatively well-defined borders in CAT and MRI. The tumor may contain non-structured and faded radiopaque spots, corresponding to intratumoral calcifications (Fig. 531b). This finding is important because it makes the radiographic distinction between CD. and chondrosarcoma impossible. **CAT, MRI** and at times **saccoradiculography** and **angiography** are of essential importance, particularly when planning surgery (Figs. 532, 534).

In localizations of the tumor in the cervical or thoracolumbar vertebrae, osteolysis of a vertebral body is observed, often having relatively well-defined limits marked by a rim of osteosclerosis; at times, it is associated with increased radiopacity due to calcification, due to reactive hyperostosis, or due to bone necrosis. In these cases, as well, an extraosseous mass may be observed, which may suggest a tubercular abscess. In some cases there is destruction of the disc with extent to the vertebra and/or vertebral collapse.

GROSS PATHOLOGIC FEATURES

When localized in the base of the cranium CD. does not usually achieve a large size, as death occurs first. It erodes the bone from the spheno-occipital junction, extending to the sella turcica, to the sphenoidal sinuses, at times in the orbit. It may protrude in the nose-pharynx and it may perforate the dura mater.

When localized in the sacro-coccyx, on the contrary, large or very large tumors are frequently observed, destroying the bone and expanded in large extraosseous masses. On the cut surface, CD. is of lobular structure, divided by thin fibrous septa. The tissue of the lobules, which are irregular and confluent, is grayish, soft, with a typical translucid, gelatinous and **mucoid** aspect. This aspect recalls that of some chondrosarcomas. Hemorrhagic, necrotic and cystic areas are commonly observed. The tumor expands in the sacral foramina and plugs proximally in the sacral vertebral canal (Fig. 532d). Even if its boundaries may appear to be evident, it has no capsular coating. Posteriorly and laterally it invades the gluteal and piriformis muscles, the subcutaneous fat, the sacroischiatic ligaments. Anteriorly, instead, it is contained by the presacral fascia and it generally does not adhere to the rectal wall.

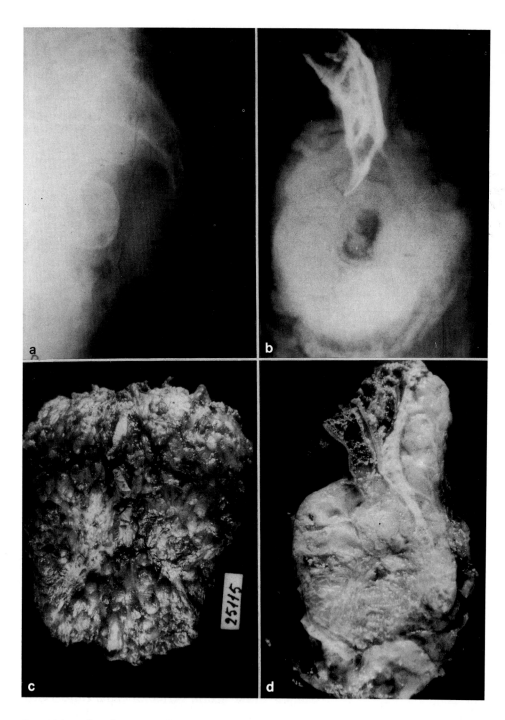

FIG. 533. - Chordoma in a female aged 73 years. Pain for the past 3 years. (a) and (b) Radiogram of the patient and of the resected segment (through the third sacral foramen). (c) and (d) Posterior aspect and surface of sagittal section of the segment. Resection was wide/contaminated. There were no signs of recurrence or metastasis after 6 years.

HISTOPATHOLOGIC FEATURES

The histological picture of CD. varies from case to case, and even from field to field within the same tumor. This variability depends on the various stages of differentiation of the cells of notochordal origin, and also on the differing grade of cellular malignancy.

The histological structure of the tumor is roughly lobular, with fibrovascular shoots separating the neoplastic lobules. These are not totally deprived of vessels (Fig. 536) (unlike chondrosarcoma) but, in more mature and mucoid areas, the vessels are scarce or absent. In some tumors or in some fields, where the tissue is scarcely differentiated, this appears to be more cellular and constituted by small, roundish elements, having evident cytoplasmatic boundaries and little or no vacuolization of the cytoplasm. It would be difficult or impossible to make a diagnosis based solely on the examination of an area of this type. In other, more differentiated areas, the cells are characterized by large cytoplasmatic vacuoles, with the nucleus at the center or shifted to the periphery (signet ring-cell). The vacuoles may also be gigantic and stain with mucin specific dyes. These cells are known as physaliphorous, from the Greek fisaein = to swell (Figs. 535, 536). The mucin produced by the cells tends to collect outside them, in a large quantity. Thus, small groups of physaliphorous cells scattered in the mucoid substance may be observed. This groups may be of spheric shape, formed by concentric cells. Another very common and typical aspect is that of cellular cords, isolated and anastomized, and contained in the mucoid substance. These cells have deep pink cytoplasms, colored by eosin (ossiphiles) and fused in syncytia (Fig. 535). At times they have the aspect of physaliphorous cells, but in other cases they are rather spindling, with oval nuclei and stretched cytoplasms.

The nuclei are always deeply stained; at times they are rather small and monomorphous, at times large, hyperchromic and very pleomorphic. In this last case double nuclei and bizarre nuclei may be observed with mitotic figures. In other words, the aspects of cellular malignancy may either be minimal or very striking. Moreover, this is not believed to have much of an influence on the clinical course of the tumor or on its prognosis.

In exceptional cases of sacro-coccygeal and vertebral CD., aspects of cartilaginous differentiation are observed. These are rather frequent in tumors of the base of the cranium. Dahlin (Heffelfinger et. al., 1973) uses the term «chondroid chordomas» for tumors such as these, and affirms that many of the tumors described as chondrosarcomas of the base of the cranium are actually CD.

Rarely a CD. may transform into a high-grade sarcoma, such as malignant fibrous histiocytoma («dedifferentiated chordoma»). In such a case, the course and prognosis become those of the more malignant sarcoma.

HISTOGENESIS AND PATHOGENESIS

In the adult, traces of notochordal tissue remain in the center of the intervertebral disks. Furthermore, residues of the same tissue may be observed at

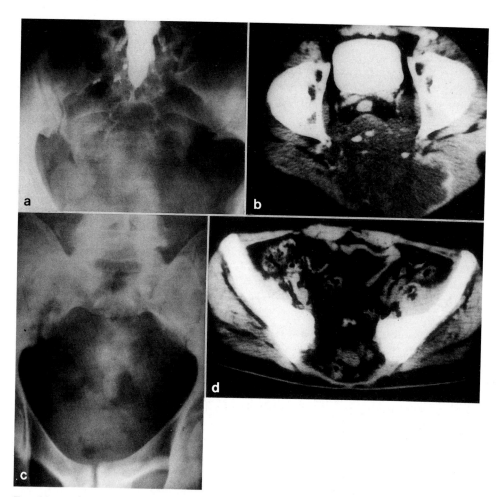

FIG. 534. - Chordoma in a male aged 38 years. Pain for the past 5 years. Sacral and gluteal swelling for 1 year. Radiographic picture and CAT (a,b) show osteolysis extended
as far as the second sacral foramen (a). The tumor mass totally destroys the sacrum,
shifts the rectum forward, reaches both sides of the ischiatic spines and widely invades the gluteus maximus, particularly on the left (b). (c) and (d) The patient was submitted to sacral resection between S1 and S2. Resection was mostly wide, marginal
in some areas corresponding to the wall of the rectum. There were no signs of local recurrence after 3 years. Instead, there was metastasis in the brachial biceps and in the
fourth thoracic vertebra.

the base of the cranium, in proximity of the spheno-occipital synchondrosis.
Similar residues may persist in the vertebrae and sacro-coccyx. These notochordal residues are particularly known in the base of the cranium (not so
much in the sacro-coccyx) due to the fact that on autopsy they are easily visualized, on the surface of the clivus, under the dura mater. They are present
in 1-2% of all autopsies (Jaffe, 1958). Their appearance is that of a nodule not
larger than a peppercorn, which is trasparent and gelatinous. Histologically,
it is made up of vacuolated cells (containing mucin) and abundant extracel-

lular mucin. These are hamartiae of the notochord, the proliferative potential of which is so scarce that they do not deserve the name of hamartoma. These nodules are known as **spheno-occipital ecchordosis physaliphora** and their interest is solely related to the pathogenesis of CD. In fact, although it cannot be demonstrated, the fact that CD. prevalently originate where there are no intervertebral disks, while instead these hamartiae of the notochord do exist (which go unused and «excluded» unlike the notochordal remains that participate in the formation of the disks), probably indicates that CD. originates from these ecchordoses physaliphorae.

It is not surprising that CD. are associated with areas of cartilaginous differentiation, considering the embryogenetic similarity of notochord and primitive cartilage.

DIAGNOSIS

The diagnosis of CD. cannot be ascertained radiographically. In the cranial site it may be confused with different intracranial or pharyngeal tumors. In sacro-coccygeal localizations, it may even suggest **chondrosarcoma** (intratumoral calcifications are possible in both), **giant cell tumor, epithelial metastasis**, or **neurinoma**. Central chondrosarcoma is a rare occurrence in the sacrum and, at any rate, treatment is the same as that of CD. Giant cell tumor occurs rarely after 50 years of age, but its radiographic aspect may be quite similar to that of CD. Metastasis due to carcinoma tends to produce a more eccentric and irregular osteolysis, with margins which are more faded than those of CD. Sacral neurinoma is observed at a younger age and its radiographic margins are more clearly defined. In rare vertebral sites of the tumor, diagnosis is even more uncertain, and it may go from eosinophilic granuloma to tubercular spondylitis, from primary bone tumor to metastatic tumor. Even the gross aspect of CD. may suggest chondrosarcoma or mucin-secreting epithelial metastasis.

Thus, diagnosis is always based on histology. The histological aspect may suggest **chondrosarcoma**: it may be recalled that true chondroid and chondrosarcomatous areas may exceptionally be observed in extracranial CD. and frequently in those of the cranial base.

If the histopathologist does not take the clinical radiographic picture into consideration, he or she could even mistake CD. for a **mucin-secreting adenocarcinoma** (for example, of the rectum). Nonetheless, even a correct evaluation of the structure and the cytology of the tumor is sufficient to avoid this error.

COURSE

CD. grows slowly. The tumor shows prevalently local malignancy, as it is invasive and recurs if removal is not wide, but its tendency to metastasize is

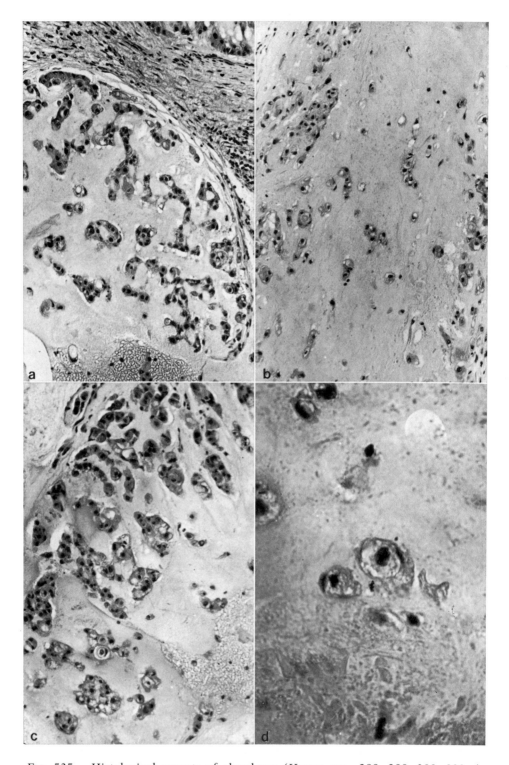

FIG. 535. - Histological aspects of chordoma (*Hemat.-eos.*, 200, 200, 200, 800 x).

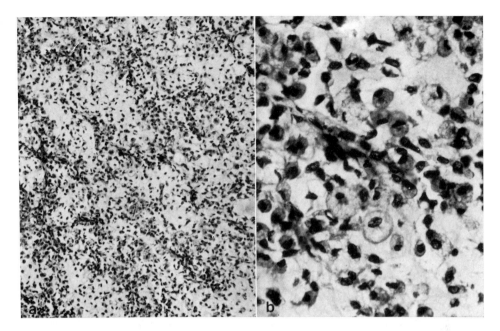

FIG. 536. - Chordoma (*Hemat.-eos.*, 125 and 500 x).

scarce and occurs late. CD. located at the base of the cranium hardly ever metastasize, also because the patient dies before. CD. at the base of the cranium characterized by cartilaginous histological aspects have a slower and less malignant course (Heffelfinger *et. al.*, 1973). In sacro-coccygeal CD. metastases probably occur in 10% of all cases. The tumor may erode the wall of the veins (similar to some chondrosarcomas) and metastasize in the liver or in the lungs. At times metastases occur in the lymph nodes; rarely, metastases by hematogenous route are more diffused. In most cases death occurs due to local neoplastic invasion (particularly in the interior of the pelvis).

TREATMENT

The treatment of choice is wide resection of the entire tumor with a layer of healthy surrounding tissue. Localization of the tumor and its considerable size at diagnosis may make this type of surgery very difficult or impossible.

In CD. localized in the sacro-coccyx, nonetheless, particularly of the tumor occupies the caudal part of the sacrum (from the second metamere downwards) wide resection may be performed, even if this means sacrificing some of the nerve roots (Figs. 532, 533, 534). When the tumor adheres to the rectal wall (which is rarely the case) or when biopsy has been performed by rectal route (which is absolutely forbidden) the rectum should be included in the resection block and abdominal colostomy performed. In more expanded and infiltrative forms of the disease, removal of the tumor is as complete as possible, but there is little hope of avoiding recurrence.

Some CD. demonstrate a fair amount of radiosensitivity. Radiation therapy at strong doses may thus be applied in unoperable forms of the tumor, and it may even allow for rather prolonged remission of the disease.

PROGNOSIS

Despite its slow growth, and the scarce tendency of the tumor to metastasize, CD. may be fatal. Many CD. of the base of the cranium cause death within 2-3 years. The best prognosis is observed in «chondroid chordoma», some of which, when operated, may result in a long survival rate and even healing (Heffelfinger *et al.*, 1973). Sacro-coccygeal tumors, treated in an inadequate surgical manner and/or by radiation therapy, may have a longer survival rate, even 5-15 years; or they may be cured when surgical resection was wide. Local recurrence and metastases may occur even after many years. They may be successfully treated by further surgery. Survival with no evidence of disease after more than 10 years reported in the literature for CD. of the sacro-coccyx is usually low. This is due to the fact that in many cases surgical treatment was late and/or inadequate.

REFERENCES

1958 JAFFE H. L.: *Tumors and tumorous conditions of the bones and joints.* Lea & Febiger, Philadelphia.

1964 PONTE A., FRANCIS K. C.: Il cordoma. *Archivio Putti*, **19**, 76-95.

1967 HIGINBOTHAM N. L., PHILLIPS R. F., FARR H. W., HUSTU H. O.: Chordoma. Thirty-five years study at Memorial Hospital. *Cancer*, **20**, 1841-1850.

1967 LOCALIO S. A., FRANCIS K. C., ROSSANO P. Q.: Abdominosacral resection of sacrococcygeal chordoma. *Annals of Surgery*, **166**, 394-402.

1968 ANDERSON W. B., MEYERS H. I.: Multicentric chordoma. Report of a case. *Cancer*, **21**, 126-128.

1970 MURAD M. T., MURTHY NARASIMHA M. S.: Ultrastructure of chordoma. *Cancer*, **25**, 1204-1215.

1973 HEFFELFINGER J. M., DAHLIN D. C., MC CARTY C. S., BEABOUT J. W.: Chordomas and cartilaginous tumors at the skull base. *Cancer*, **32**, 410-420.

1975 GRAY S. W., SINGHABHANDU B., SMITH R. A., SKANDALAKIS J. E.: Sacrococcygeal chordoma: report of a case and review of the literature. *Surgery*, **78**, 573-582.

1975 WELLINGER CL.: Le chordome rachidien. I. Revue de la littérature depuis 1960. *Revue du Rhumatisme*, **42**, 109-116.

1978 STENER B., GUNTERBERG B.: High amputation of the sacrum for extirpation of tumors. Principles and technique. *Spine*, **3**, 351-366.

1979 SUNDARESAN N., GALICICH J.H., CHU F.C.H., HUVOS A.G.: Spinal chordomas. *Journal of Neurosurgery*, **50**, 312-319.

1981 GENNARI L., AZZARELLI A., QUAGLIUOLO V.: A posterior approach for the excision of sacral chordoma. *Journal of Bone and Joint Surgery*, **69-B**, 565-568.

1981 MEIS J.M., RAYMOND A.K., EVANS H.L., CHARLES R.E., GIRALDO A.A.: «Dedifferentiated» chordoma. A clinicopathologic and immunohistochemical study of three cases. *American Journal of Surgical Pathology*, **11**, 516-525.

1981 MINDELL E.R.: Current concepts review: chordoma. *Journal of Bone and Joint Surgery*, **63-A**, 501-505.

1981 PARDO-MINDAN F.J., GUILEN F.J., VILLAS C., VAZQUES J.J.: A comparative ultra-structural study of chondrosarcoma, chondroid sarcoma and chordoma. *Cancer*, **47**, 2611-2619.

1982 STOKER D.J., PRINGLE J.: Case report 205-chordoma of mid-cervical spine. *Skeletal Radiology*, **8**, 306-310.

1982 ULICH T.R., MIRRA J.M.: Ecchordosis phisaliphora vertebralis. *Clinical Orthopaedics*, **163**, 282-289.

1982 WILNER D.: *Radiology of bone tumors and allied disorders*. Vol. 4. W.B. Saunders, Philadelphia.

1983 WORLD L.E., LAWS E.R.: Cranial chordoma in children and young adults. *Journal of Neurosurgery*, **59**, 1043-1047.

1984 MEYER J.E., LEPKE R.A., LINDFORS K.K., PAGANI J.J.: Chordomas: their CT appearance in the cervical, thoracic, and lumbar spine. *Radiology*, **153**, 693-696.

1985 DAVIDSON J.K., MUCCI B.: Case report 322. *Skeletal Radiology*, **14**, 76-80.

1985 RICH T.A., SCHILLER A., SUIT H.D., MANKIN H.J.: Clinical and pathologic review of 48 cases of chordoma. *Cancer*, **56**, 182-187.

1985 ROSENTHAL D., SCOTT J.A., MANKIN H.J., WISMER G.L., BRADY T.J.: Sacrococcygeal chordoma: magnetic resonance imaging and computed tomography. *American Journal of Radiology*, **145**, 143-147.

1985 SALISBURY J., ISAACSON P.: Demonstration of cytokeratins and an epithelial membrane antigen in chordomas and human fetal notochord. *American Journal of Surgical Pathology*, **9**, 791-797.

1986 SUNDARESAN N.: Chordomas. *Clinical Orthopaedics*, **204**, 135-142.

1987 CHIRAS J., GAGNA G., ROSE M., SAILLANT G., BORIES J., ROY-CAMILLE R.: Artériographie et embolisation des tumeurs du sacrum. *Revue de Chirurgie Orthopedique*, **73**, 99-103.

1987 GENIN J., MISSENARD G.: Les chordomes sacro-coccygiens. *Revue de Chirurgie Orthopedique*, **73**, 79-81.

1987 SMITH J., LUDWIG R.L., MARCOVE R.C.: Sacrococcygeal chordoma. A clinico-radiological study of 60 patients. *Skeletal Radiology*, **16**, 37-44.

1987 STENER B.: Traitement chirurgical des tumeurs du sacrum. *Revue de Chirurgie Orthopedique*, **73**, 114-121.

1987 SUNG H.W., SHU W.P., WANG M.M., YUAI S.Y., TSAI Y.B.: Surgical treatment of primary tumors of the sacrum. *Clinical Orthopaedics*, **215**, 91-98.

1989 HEALEY J.H., LANE J.M.: Chordoma: a critical review of diagnosis and treatment. *Orthopaedic Clinics of North America*, **20**, 417-426.

1989 RESNIK C.S., YOUNK J.W.R., LEVINE A.M., AISNER S.C.: Case report 544. *Skeletal Radiology*, **18**, 303-305.

1990 SMITH J., REUTER V., DEMAS B.: Case report 576. *Skeletal Radiology*, **18**, 561-564.

SARCOMA ON PAGETIC BONE

It is a rare but not exceptional occurrence to observe a sarcoma developing on pagetic bone: a 0.2% incidence, that is 1 case out of 600 of Paget's disease, has been suggested. Nonetheless, it is impossible to figure out the incidence of this complication as most of Paget's cases are asymptomatic and thus remain unrecognized. We do know that the occurrence of sarcoma is less rare in severe polyostotic forms of Paget's disease.

Sarcoma in Paget's disease is nearly always manifested after **50 years of age** and it is much more frequent in **males**. There is predilection for the following **localizations** in this order: the femur, humerus, pelvis, tibia, and cranium (Fig. 537). This distribution does not correspond to that of Paget's disease, which, for example, is frequent in the vertebrae, whereas sarcoma is instead rare. As compared to primary osteosarcoma, sarcoma in Paget in the long bones is more often diaphyseal; in the humerus, it may be localized in the distal portion, while primary osteosarcoma is nearly exclusively local-

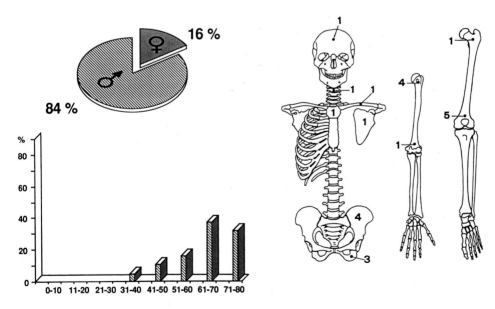

FIG. 537. - Sex, age and localization in 19 cases of sarcoma in pagetic bone (23 localizations).

FIG. 538. - Grade 4 malignant fibrous histiocytoma in Paget's disease. Male
aged 66 years. For the past 5 months
pain and for 3 swelling. The radiogram
shows typical pagetic osteopathy plus
aggressive osteolysis at the upper end
of the humerus. At diagnosis there were
disseminated pulmonary metastases.

▶

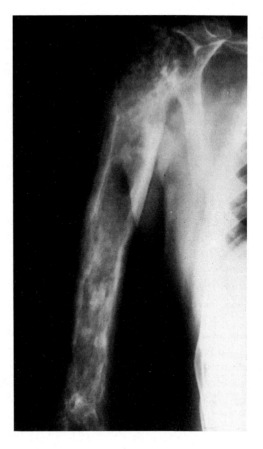

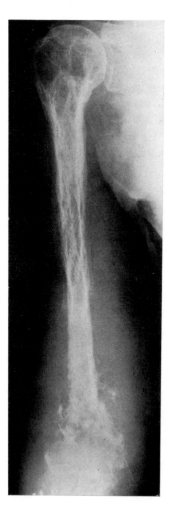

◀

FIG. 539. - Male aged 76 years. Four months earlier
pathologic fracture. There were bilateral pulmonary metastases. The patient died after 7 months.
The radiogram reveals typical sarcomatous transformation. Histologically, osteosarcoma of the distal half of the humerus; typical pagetic alteration
of the proximal half.

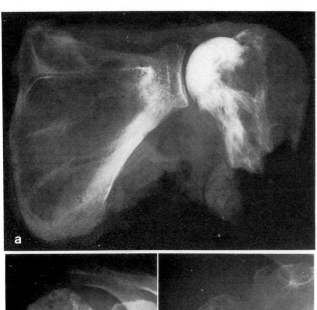

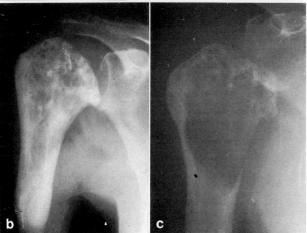

FIG. 540. - (a) Male aged 47 years. Sarcoma in Peget's disease of the proximal humerus (histologically osteosarcoma). X-ray of the anatomical specimen after interscapulothoracic amputation. The segment only includes the proximal part of the humerus, above a pathologic fracture. The patient died 8 months later of pulmonary metastases. (b) and (c): male aged 76 years. Sarcoma in Paget's disease (histiologically malignant fibrous histiocytoma), at the onset of the painful stage (b) and after 6 months (c).

ized in the proximal humerus. At times, multicentric sarcomas occur (non-metastatic) in the same bone or in different bones, but all on pagetic terrain.

Clinically, the symptoms due to the sarcoma may reveal Paget's disease which has until that moment been asymptomatic and gone unrecognized. In other cases, mild and chronic symptoms of pagetic osteopathy suddenly result in more intense pain and swelling, which should cause suspicion of malignant transformation. At times, there is spontaneous fracture.

Radiographically, Paget's sarcomas are mostly osteolytic (Figs. 538, 539, 540). First, there is intracortical osteolysis with fuzzy limits. Rapidly the osteolysis extends, dissolving the radiographic image of the pagetic bone and cancelling the cortex. Sarcoma rarely appears to be intensely osteogenetic and sclerosing. Even the osteogenetic reaction of the periosteum tends to be scarce. The radiographic stigmata of Paget's disease are recognized in the skeletal segment which is the site of the sarcoma, and often in other parts of the skeleton. When an osteosarcoma is observed in an elderly patient, it is best to examine the skeleton in order to avoid any associated pagetic modifications (total body bone scan, specific X-rays).

Macroscopically, there is a strongly invasive mass, of parenchymatous aspect, with frequent hemorrhagic and cystic areas. At times the tissue contains granulosity due to an immature osteogenesis; it rarely contains hard or eburneous bony areas.

Histologically, sarcomas in Paget's disease are mostly categorized as osteosarcomas. These are scarcely osteogenetic osteosarcomas, rarely sclerosing. The cellular component is scarcely differentiated and very pleomorphic, with large atypical nuclei and frequent multinucleate giant cells, which may or may not be malignant. At times there is no evidence of osteogenesis and the tumor is classified as a malignant fibrous histiocytoma, or as a poorly differentiated fibrosarcoma. Finally, in exceptional cases the diagnosis is scarcely differentiated chondrosarcoma. The sarcoma always has a high grade of histological malignancy.

The **occurrence of sarcoma** is certainly favored by bone turnover and cellular renewal which, in pagetic areas, are intense, continuous and prolonged for many years (cf. pathogenesis of osteosarcoma).

The **course of the tumor** is always rapid. Pulmonary metastases are manifested early. We have already observed how multiple skeletal sarcomas in the pagetic skeleton are more often multicentric than metastatic.

In theory, **treatment** is the same as that for osteosarcoma. Nonetheless, as we are mostly dealing with elderly patients, chemotherapy is rarely used, and the type of surgical treatment which is most often indicated is amputation.

Prognosis is generally severe. Survival rate for more than 5 years is very low. Death generally occurs within 2-3 years.

REFERENCES

1927   BIRD C. E.: Sarcoma complicating Paget's disease of bone. Report of nine cases, five with pathologic verification. *Archives of Surgery*, **14**, 1187-1208.

1950   MINER I. E.: Sarcoma in Paget's disease of bone. *Bulletin of the Hospital for Joint Diseases*, **2**, 26-42.

1957   PORRETTA C. A., DAHLIN D. C., JANES J. M.: Sarcoma in Paget's disease of bone. *Journal of Bone and Joint Surgery*, **39-A**, 1314-29.

1958   STEVENS J., LENNOX B.: Long survival after amputation for Paget's sarcoma of bone. *Journal of Bone and Joint Surgery*, **40-B**, 735-741.

1964   MC KENNA R. J., SCHWINN C. P., SOONG K. Y., HIGINBOTHAM N. L.: Osteogenic sarcoma arising in Paget's disease. *Cancer*, **17**, 42-66.

1969   PRICE C. H. G., GOLDE W.: Paget's sarcoma of bone. A study of eighty cases from the Bristol and the Leeds Bone Tumour Registries. *Journal of Bone and Joint Surgery*, **51-B**, 205-224.

1973   ROSS F. G. M., MIDDLEMISS J. H., FITTON J. M.: Paget's sarcoma in bone. A radiological study, in « *Bone - Certain aspects of neoplasia* », Butterworths, London.

1979   GIUNTI A., LAUS M.: Sarcomi in morbo di Paget. Presentazione di 11 casi. *Giornale Italiano di Ortopedia e Traumatologia*, **5**, 325-335.

GIANT CELL TUMOR ON PAGETIC BONE

It is an exceptional occurrence. It above all occurs in the male **sex** and always after 50 years of **age**. These tumors evidently prefer the cranio-facial bones and the pelvis, but they have been observed in the vertebral column (Figs. 541, 542), humerus and tibia, as well. They are manifested by nearly painless swelling, characterized by a slow course. At times they are multiple, occurring at the same time or subsequently. **Radiographically**, they produce

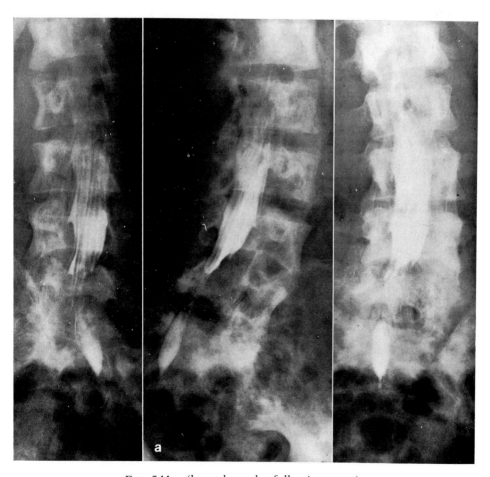

FIG. 541a. (legend on the following page).

FIG. 541. - (a) Male aged 54 years affected with Paget's osteopathy in the pelvis and lumbar spine. For the past year intense lumbar and sciatic pain with signs of compression of right L5 and S1 roots. Sacco-radiculography reveals severe narrowing of the sac at the level of L5. Hemilaminectomy revealed soft tissue protruding from the body of L5 and compressing the sac and the nerve roots. On histological examination the aspect was that of a giant cell tumor (Fig. 543). (b) The patient was alive after 18 years, with the presence of an enormous lumbar and pelvic tumoral mass.

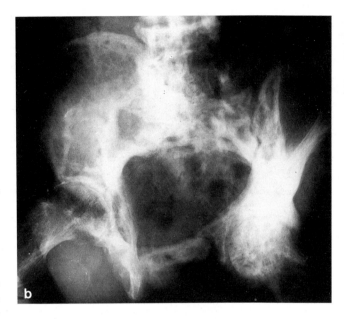

an image of osteolysis with rather faded boundaries. **Histologically**, they seem to be the same as primary, conventional giant cell tumor (Fig. 543).

No examples of malignant transformation have been reported. **Treatment** should be surgical and conservative as much as possible, limiting radiation

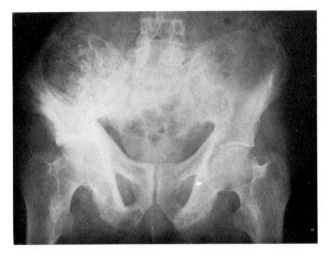

FIG. 542. - Giant cell tumor of the pelvis in Paget's disease in a male aged 55 years. The Paget's disease was apparent only in the pelvis. The iliac tumors had been discovered 6 years previously and were repeatedly irradiated. For the past year they seemed to be stationary. Both of the lesions were ascertained histologically (aspect the same as that of a giant cell tumor alongside typical pagetic bone). After 14 years the tumor lesions were extended to an enormous size, but no metastases had appeared.

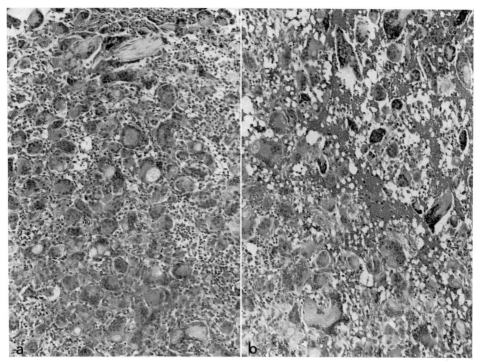

FIG. 543. - Histological features of a giant cell on pagetic bone (*Hemat.-eos.*, 125, 125x).

treatment solely to forms which cannot be managed surgically. In fact, radiation treatment is not recommended as it may favor the occurrence of a sarcoma (in pagetic bone and/or in giant cell tumor).

REFERENCES

1963 HUTTER R. V. P., FOOTE F. W. Jr., FRAZELL E. L., FRANCIS K. C.: Giant cell tumors complicating Paget's disease of bone. *Cancer*, **16**, 1044-1056.
1966 SCHAJOWICZ F., SLULLITEL I.: Giant-cell tumor associated with Paget's disease of bone. A case report. *Journal of Bone and Joint Surgery*, **48-A**, 1340-1349.
1971 LEVINE H. A., ENRILE F.: Giant-cell tumor of patellar tendon coincident with Paget's disease. *Journal of Bone and Joint Surgery*, **53-A**, 335-340.
1977 BONAKDARPOUR A., HARWICK R., PICKERING J.: Case report 34. *Skeletal Radiology*, **2**, 52-55.
1979 DONATI U., MARTUCCI E.: Così detto tumore a cellule giganti su osso pagetico. Presentazione di un caso in sede vertebrale. *Giornale Italiano di Ortopedia e Traumatologia*, **5**, 265-269.
1979 JACOBS T. P., MICHELSEN J., POLAY J. S., D'ADAMO A. C., CANFIELD R. E.: Giant cell tumor in Paget's disease of bone. Familial and geographic clustering. *Cancer*, **44**, 742-747.
1981 MIRRA J.M., BAUER F., GRANT T.: Giant-cell tumor with viral-like inclusions associated with Paget's disease. *Clinical Orthopaedics*, **158**, 243-251.
1982 MIRRA J.M., GOLD R.H.: Case report 186. *Skeletal Radiology*, **8**, 67-70.
1988 PAZZAGLIA U.E., BARBIERI D., CECILIANI L.: An epiphyseal giant-cell tumor associated with early Paget's disease. *Clinical Orthopaedics*, **26**, 217-220.

CARCINOMAS AND SARCOMAS
ON CHRONIC OSTEOMYELITIS

A squamous cell carcinoma, exceptionally a sarcoma, may develop from the outer rim or the walls of a draining sinus tract of a chronic osteomyelitis lasting many years; generally, more than 20 years. When a fistulized osteomyelitis has achieved these extreme degrees of chronicity, the risk of malignant transformation, together with the poor conditions of the skin, the deformity, and the joint stiffness, constitute one more reason for suggesting amputation without further delay.

Due to the prevailing incidence of traumatic osteomyelitis, there is predilection for the male **sex**, **age** is adult to advanced, the most frequent **site** is the tibia; this is followed by the femur, the bones of the foot, exceptionally the upper limb (Fig. 544).

Nearly always we are dealing with a **squamous cell carcinoma**. This usually develops from the outer rim of the sinus which becomes raised and

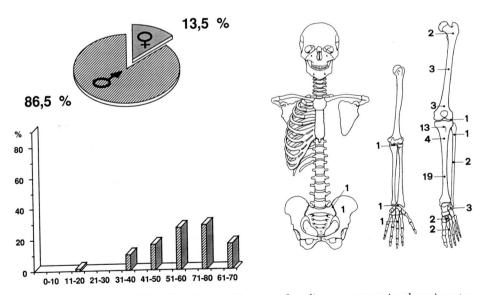

FIG. 544. - Sex, age and localization in 60 cases of malignant tumor in chronic osteomyelitis (53 squamous cell carcinomas and 7 sarcomas: fibrosarcoma, malignant fibrous histiocytoma, osteosarcoma, angiosarcoma, chondrosarcoma).

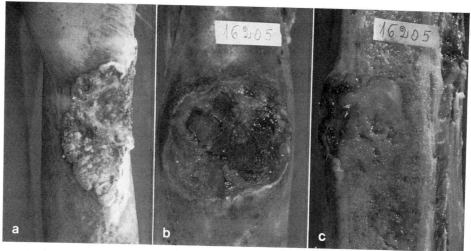

Fig. 545. - (a) Male aged 60 years. Squamous cell carcinoma occurring on torpid ulcer in osteomyelitis of the proximal tibia. (b) and (c) Male aged 45 years. Angiosarcoma in chronic osteomyelitis of the tibia: (c: section of the anatomical specimen).

bumpy, hard, frequently ulcerated, and slowly progressing (Fig. 545a). Rarely, the carcinoma originates more deeply, from the epithelium covering the sinus tract and which may coat some bone cavities. In this case the first symp-

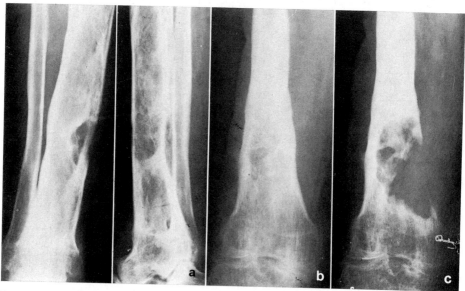

Fig. 546. - (a) Male aged 38 years. Chronic osteomyelitis lasting 30 years. Angiosarcoma. Thigh amputation. The patient was well after 5 years. (b) Male aged 64 years. Chronic osteomyelitis lasting 49 years. (c) After 8 months, severe osteolysis. Squamous cell carcinoma. Thigh amputation. The patient died after 16 years for unrelated causes.

toms are constituted by the occurrence or accentuation of pain, by putrid secretion and by bleeding. In more advanced phases a fleshy mass fills the sinus and expands mushroomlike in the surface.

Exceptionally a **sarcoma** originates from the sinus tract or the osteomyelitic bone, and similarly may vegetate at the skin surface (Fig. 545b, c).

When the neoplasm — carcinoma or sarcoma — invades the bone, osteolytic progressive erosion is observed on **radiograms** (Fig. 546) and pathologic fracture may occur.

Histologically, we are dealing with well-differentiated squamous cell carcinomas, with the formation of epithelial pearls (Fig. 547). Rarely, the cells are less differentiated, and at times they are elongated or spindle-shaped, so that sarcoma may be suggested. When it truly is a sarcoma, it is generally a scarcely differentiated fibrosarcoma, or a malignant fibrous histiocytoma, exceptionally an angiosarcoma, an osteosarcoma, a chondrosarcoma.

The only **diagnostic** problem (clinical and histological) involves distinguishing between a carcinoma and a chronic epithelial hyperplasia. The latter is characterized by a less vegetating and invasive gross aspect, prevalently cheratinized; and histologically, by wide epithelial digitations, which are long and ramified, having intense acanthosis and cheratopoiesis at the surface,

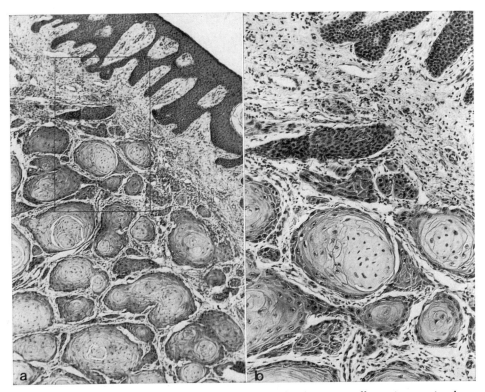

FIG. 547. - Histological aspect of well-differentiated squamous cell carcinoma, in chronic osteomyelitis (*Hemat.-eos.*, 50, 125 x).

with no nuclear atypia, and evident basal delimitation with the underlying connective chorion. Nonetheless, these pseudoepitheliomatous hyperplasias, as well, must be observed carefully and monitored in time for progression in carcinoma.

Often the regional lymph nodes are enlarged, but we are generally dealing with chronic lymphadenitis, infrequently with metastases.

Treatment consists in amputation, associated with excision of the regional lymph nodes if these are enlarged. If there are no lymph node metastases at amputation, prognosis is rather good. Contrarily, there is a considerable possibility of ascendent lymph node and visceral metastases. Overall, approximately 30% of all cases of these carcinomas have metastasized. The **prognosis** is generally more severe in the case of sarcoma (metastases in more than half of the cases).

REFERENCES

1963 SEDLIN E. D., FLEMING J. L.: Epidermoid carcinoma arising in chronic osteomyelitic foci. *Journal of Bone and Joint Surgery*, **45-A**, 827-838.

1964 MORRIS J. M., LUCAS D. B.: Fibrosarcoma within a sinus tract of chronic draining osteomyelitis. Case report and review of literature. *Journal of Bone and Joint Surgery*, **46-A**, 853-857.

1965 HEJNA W. F.: Epidermoid carcinoma in chronic osteomyelitis: diagnostic problems and management. Report of ten cases. *Journal of Bone and Joint Surgery*, **47-A**, 133-145.

1976 BEHROOZ A. A., WIRTH C., COLMAN N.: Fibrosarcoma arising from chronic osteomyelitis. *Journal of Bone and Joint Surgery*, **58-A**, 123-125.

1976 DRÄNERT K., RÜTER A., BURRI C., WILLENEGER H.: Fistelmalignome bei chronischer Osteomyelitis. *Archiv für Orthopädische und Unfall-Chirurgie*, **84**, 199-210.

1976 FITZGERALD R. H., BREWER N. S., DAHLIN D. C.: Squamous-cell carcinoma complicating chronic osteomyelitis. *Journal of Bone and Joint Surgery*, **58-A**, 1146-1148.

1978 GIUNTI A., LAUS M.: Tumori maligni in osteomielite cronica. Presentazione di 39 casi, 26 controllati a distanza. *Giornale Italiano di Ortopedia e Traumatologia*, **4**, 167-177.

THE EFFECTS OF RADIATION ON THE SKELETON AND RADIATION INDUCED SARCOMAS OF BONE

Internal radiation as well as external radiation produce similar effects on the skeleton. These effects consist in necrotic changes, which are constant if a certain radiation dose is exceeded and, very rarely, in the development of a sarcoma.

The effects of **internal radiation** were studied in the United States in a group of more than 5000 persons, particularly young women who in the twenties, painting the luminous dials of clocks inhaled or ingested (due to the habit of sharpening their paintbrush points with their lips) radium and mesotorium contained in the phosphorescent paint. Another source of internal radiation were radium or torium salts used in the treatment of tuberculosis and ankylosing spondylarthritis. Today, this pathogenous cause has returned up-to-date with the use of atomic energy and «fall out» products containing Sr89 and Sr90. The effects of internal radiation on the skeleton were experimetally studied by using Sr89 and Ca45 in particular. Practically every radioactive element which is not excreted is accumulated in the bone tissue where it continues to exert its action for many years. It seems that most of the substance is fixed where bone exchange is more active, thus in the growth areas and, in the adult, in the cancellous bone of the epiphyses. The ffects of internal radiation include disseminated bone necrosis and even multiple bone sarcomas, anemia, osteomyelitis of the jaws, leukemia.

On the contrary, the action of **external radiation** is circumscribed and thus includes necrosis and sarcoma (single). Another difference seems to be the latency time between the exposure and the occurrence of skeletal sarcoma, which is greater for internal radiation (where the radiation effect is more tenuous but continues for many years after exposure) than for external radiation (the effect of which is limited to the period of exposure but is more intense). Apart from these, there are no other significant differences in the effects that the two types of radiation have on the skeleton.

It is difficult to provide figures for risk doses, as they depend on the modalities and the times of assumption or application. Nonetheless, it seems that for internal radiation the risk dose is an overall uptake exceeding 0.5 micrograms of radium salts. For external radiation, instead, a dose exceeding 2000 r causes modifications in enchondral growth and more than 3-4000 r may cause sarcoma. Low-voltage radiation is more dangerous, in terms of the occurence of sarcomas, than high-voltage radiation.

THE EFFECTS OF RADIATION ON THE SKELETON

These consist in the arrest of cellular proliferation, particularly evident in the fertile cartilage and in the hemopoietic marrow. At higher doses necrosis of all of the cells is manifested, those of the bone marrow, of the endosteum, of the periosteum and the osteocytes. In the case of internal radiation, these phenomena occur many years after exposure, which, in turn, may be protracted over years. In the case of external radiation, the same phenomena are generally revealed 1-2 years after irradiation. Furthermore, in the first case, they are diffused to the entire skeleton, particularly involving the meta-epiphyses but also the diaphyses; in the second, they are circumscribed to the irradiated area.

Lesion of the fertile cartilage is manifested clinically by shortening, which occurs in a long bone, and at times by deformity by asymmetrical arrest in growth. The deformity may involve a limb (for example varus or valgus knee) or the vertebral column (scoliosis). Radiographically and macroscopically the growth cartilage at first appears to be increased in thickness, as in addition to the proliferation of the chondrocytes, that of the osteoblasts and thus ossification of the calcified cartilage is arrested. Then, the physis appears to be irregular, here and there narrowed and finally precociously

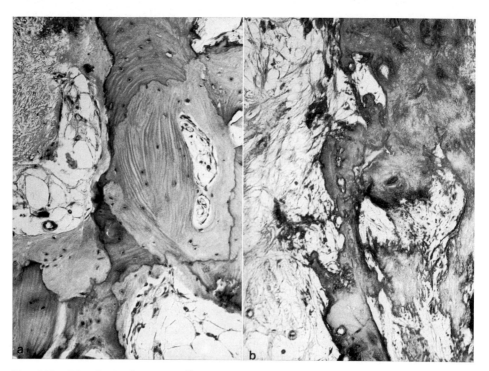

FIG. 548. - Histological aspects of bone necrosis due to radiation. (a) Incomplete necrosis with necrotic bone partially substituted by vital bone. (b) Complete necrosis with bone disgregation (*Hemat.-eos.*, 125, 125 x).

fused. The metaphysis may be widened (as in achondroplasia). Rarely, **exostoses** occur, the same as primary exostoses (see specific chapter). Histologically, at first an increase in cartilaginous thickness, disorganization of the co-
lumnated layer, increase in the hypertrophic layer are observed. Then, the
thickness of the growth cartilage decreases more and more, the proli-ferative and column layers regress, few hypertrophic cells remain, dis-tributed in a disorderly manner. On the metaphyseal aspect of the cartilage the osteoblasts and other proliferating cells decrease, and medullary fibrosis is observed. The vertical fringe of thin, newly-formed bone trabeculae has disappeared. In its place is a horizontal and irregular layer of mature bone limit-ing the cartilage. In short, these are the classic aspects of the growth arrest however produced.

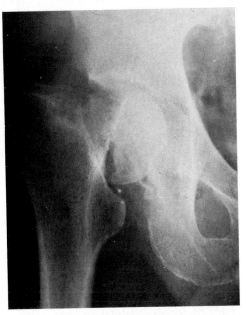

FIG. 549. - Male aged 47 years. Radiation treatment in the inguinal regions for Hodgkin's disease performed 2 years earlier. Spontaneous fracture of the femoral neck.

Bone lesions consist in necrosis of the bone and medullary tissue, precipitation of calcium salts in the medullary fibrous tissue, disgrega-tion of the necrotic bone, attempts at repair on the part of the vital connective tissue left intact (Fig. 548). These phenomena are similar to those of ischemic bone necrosis. The bone which is thus altered is more fragile and (as always occurs in devitalized and poorly vascularized bone) more subject to infection, which is particularly possible in the jaws by dental or parodontal propagation.

Clinically, **pathologic fracture** may be manifested, particularly in the epi-physes and metaphyses of the lower limbs. Generally, these are stress frac-tures. In the epiphyses we generally observe gradual collapse of the cancellous bone and of the joint surface. In cases such as these, pain may be less import-ant than occurs in ischemic epiphyseal necrosis, because the synovial mem-brane and joint capsule are devitalized by the radiation. In the metaphyses the most frequent fracture is that of the femoral neck (Fig. 549), which is above all observed in females irradiated for pelvic carcinoma, more rarely in males irradiated for cancer of the prostate, the bladder, or seminoma. Frac-tures in irradiated bone consolidate with difficulty or do not consolidate at all (Fig. 551).

Radiographically, bands, spots or vast areas of intense radiopacity char-acterized by faded boundaries may be observed, often alternated with areas

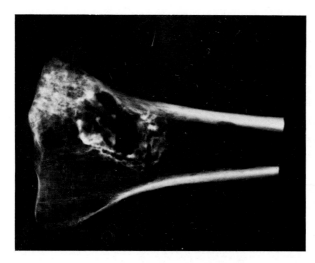

FIG. 550. - Female aged 23 years. Seven years earlier irradiated in the knee (7000 r) for an undetermined tumor in the tibia. After 6 years fibrosarcoma of the soft tissues developed in the popliteal fossa, probably secondary to radiations. After two attempts at local excision followed by local recurrence, amputation was performed. Radiogram of the anatomical transected specimen shows necrosis due to radiation of the tibia (histologically there were no traces of tumor in the tibia).

of hypertransparence of the cancellous and the cortical bone, these too having faded boundaries (Fig. 550) These radiographic aspects are rather typical and must not be exchanged for a neoplastic lesion. It is not necessary to perform biopsy, osteopathy due to radiation being confirmed by the history of the patient (irradiation at least 1 year previously and at a necrotizing dose), by CAT-MRI (no mass of newly-formed extraosseous tissue), by radiograms repeated in time (no progression of skeletal changes) (Fig. 551).

A **microscopic** study of these skeletal necroses caused by irradiation, in man and in the experimental animal, clearly illustrates the nature and the progression of lesions and at times allows us to visualize cellular modifications which might be considered to be presarcomatous. The bone tissue of the trabeculae and of the cortex is necrotic. The bone lacunae are empty due to the disappearance of osteocytes. The tissue filling the medullary spaces and the haversian canals is necrotic as well; it is made up of compact fibrohyaline material, or disgregated in fibrillary tufts having no order, or amorphous. The cells are totally absent or represented by sparse fibrocytes having a shrunken, dark nucleus. This medullary tissue is frequently impregnated with calcium salts, particularly at the borders of the necrotic bone. As cellular life does not exist, the latter cannot be resorbed; its surfaces are lacking images of lacunary erosion. These areas of total necrosis correspond to radiographically sclerotic areas, as the radiopacity of the bone which is not resorbed, is added to that due to calcification of the necrotic medullary connective tissue. In time, the necrotic bone tissue tends to disgregate and fracture. In areas where the necrosis is not complete and at the boundaries of the necrotic tissue, there is more or less cellular repair tissue, with aspects of osteoclastic bone resorption, of medullary fibrosis, of scarce osteogenesis. Due to the prevalent bone resorption, these areas correspond to radiographic hyper-

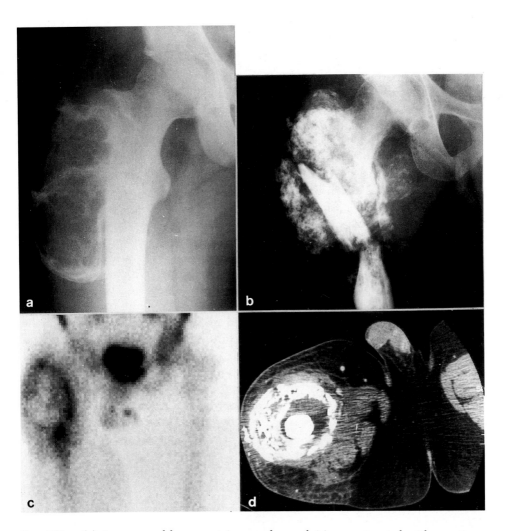

FIG. 551. - (a) Aneurysmal bone cyst in a male aged 14 years treated with curettage and radiation (6000 Rad). (b), (c) and (d) Radiation-induced bone necrosis with multiple fractures after 17 years. Observe the calcifications and ossifications in the scarring soft tissues; bone scan in positive in these reactive ossifications and negative in the necrotic bone.

transparent areas of the cancellous and cortical bone. The different aspects listed (total necrosis, partial necrosis and repair phenomena) are varyingly associated (Fig. 548). In the fibrous and fibro-osseous tissue of the irradiated areas cells with a fair amount of pleomorphism and hyperchromia of the nuclei may be observed, which could constitute a presarcomatous stage.

RADIATION INDUCED SARCOMAS

The incidence of sarcoma in healthy bone exposed to external radiation is very low: it has been evaluated at around 0.1% out of 2300 patients irradiated and followed-up for at least 5 years (Phillips and Seline, 1963). The frequency of skeletal sarcoma seems to be very high in certain cases of internal radiation (occupational or therapeutic) where it comes close to 10% (Evans, 1966; Spiess *et al.*, 1962). Then, there are cases of sarcoma occuring on preexisting irradiated benign skeletal tumors, where the problem of the real effect due to rays arises (Fig. 552). This problem particularly exists in the case of giant cell tumor which we know may spontaneously progress in sarcoma (see specific chapter). Similarly, the effect of radiation may be discussed when a sarcoma occurs in the irradiated area of a pre-existing skeletal lesion capable of spontaneous progression in sarcoma (for example, exostosis, chondroma, fibrous dysplasia, Paget's disease). In general, the most certain examples of sarcoma induced by radiation are those which respond to the following features. (Fig. 553) 1) The sarcoma develops on a healthy bone, or on a skeletal lesion incapable of spontaneous malignant progression (for example, tuberculosis, bone cyst), or again in the site of a pre-existing malignant tumor but one with completely different histological features (for

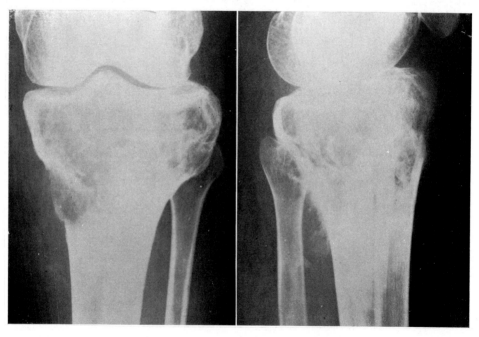

FIG. 552. - Female aged 21 years. Six years earlier irradiated (5000 r) for chondromyxoid fibroma of the tibia. The radiogram shows radiation-induced osteosarcoma (ascertained histologically). The patient refused amputation and died 1 year later of pulmonary metastases.

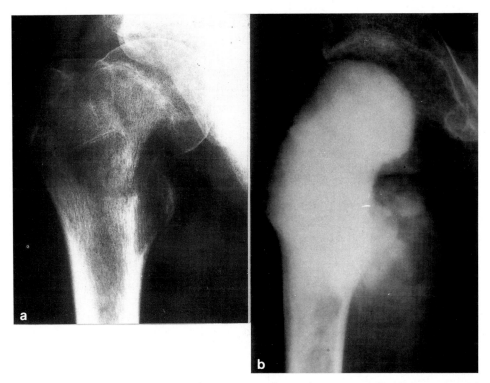

FIG. 553. - (a) Eosinophilic granuloma in a male aged 14 years. After biopsy, treated with radiation (4000 Rad). (b) After 10 years radio-induced sclerosing osteosarcoma. At diagnosis there were multiple pulmonary metastases.

example, osteosarcoma or malignant fibrous histiocytoma on irradiated Ewing's sarcoma). 2) The sarcoma occurs several years after irradiation. 3) In the period of time between irradiation and the occurrence of sarcoma, the primary tumor has appeared to be completely inactive.

However, the copious clinical data and the experimental data show with certainty that the possibility of radiation-induced sarcoma exists. In the human being, the **doses of external radiation** used are generally greater than 3-4000 r. The **interval** of time between irradiation and the sarcomatous mani-

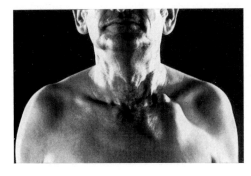

FIG. 554. - Male aged 51 years. Twenty-two years earlier irradiated on the thyroid region (5000 r) for a hyperfunctioning goiter. Eighteen months earlier pathologic fracture of the clavicle. Radiodermitis was observed as well as vast clavear and subclavear swelling. It was a grade 3 radiation-induced fibrosarcoma. N.E.D. 15 years after resection of the clavicle.

festation varies from 3 to more than 40 years, but generally it is between 5 and 10 years. Sarcomas induced by internal radiation have a longer latency, on the average around 20 years.

Radiation-induced sarcoma may be observed in healthy bone included in the field of irradiation used for extraosseous affections, among which carcinoma of the breast, carcinomas of the pelvic organs, lymphomas, retinoblastoma, skin tumors, thyroid tumors (Fig. 554). Furthermore, in the skeletal site irradiated for tubercular osteoarthritis, osteomyelitis, ankylosing spondylarthritis, histiocytosis X, bone cyst, aneurysmal bone cyst, chondroblastoma, osteoblastoma, fibrous dysplasia. There are cases in which irradiation fully eradicated a primary sarcoma such as Ewing's sarcoma and, after many years, a different sarcoma occurred in the irradiated bone. We have already discussed the occurrence of sarcoma on irradiated giant cell tumor.

Finally, it must be observed that radiations may also cause sarcoma of the soft tissues (Fig. 550).

Radiographically, we are usually dealing with osteolytic or prevalently osteolytic sarcomas (rarely osteogenetic ones) which are very invasive.

Histologically, they are mostly not very differentiated high-grade malignant tumors. Often evidence of osteogenesis classifies them among osteosarcomas. Less frequently we are dealing with malignant fibrous histiocytomas, or scarcely differentiated fibrosarcomas. Exceptionally, with other sarcomas. Internal radiation generally produces osteosarcoma, which is often multicentric, particularly localized around the hip and knee. Some of these osteosarcomas occur in atypical sites for primary osteosarcoma, such as the cranium, the sternum, the hand.

At any rate, as shown by the histological aspect as well, these are very malignant sarcomas, with a rapid **course**. **Prognosis** seems to allow less than a 20% survival rate 10 years after wide or radical surgery. The effectiveness of chemotherapy is still unknown.

REFERENCES

1931 MARTLAND H. S.: The occurrence of malignancy in radioactive persons. A general review of data gathered in the study of the radium dial painters, with special reference to the occurrence of osteogenic sarcoma and the interrelationship of certain blood diseases. *Cancer*, **15**, 2435-2516.

1945 HATCHER C. H.: Development of sarcoma in bone subjected to roentgen or radium irradiation. *Journal of Bone and Joint Surgery*, **27**, 179-195.

1952 AUB J. C., EVANS R. D., HEMPELMANN L. H., MARTLAND H. S.: The late effects of internally deposited radioactive materials in man. *Medicine*, **31**, 221-329.

1953 LOONEY W. B., WOODRUFF I. A.: Investigation of radium deposition in human skeleton by gross and detailed autoradiography. *Archives of Pathology*, **56**, 1-12.

1955 LOONEY W. B., HASTELIK R. J., BRUES A. M., SKIRMANT E.: A clinical investigation of the chronic effects of radium salts administered therapeutically (1915-1931). *American Journal of Roentgenology*, **73**, 1006-1037.

1955 LOONEY W. B.: Late effects (twenty-five to forty years) of the early medical and industrial use of radioactive materials. Their relation to the more accurate establishment of maximum permissible amounts of radioactive elements in the body. *Journal of Bone and Joint Surgery*, **37**-A, Part I, 1169-1187. **38**-A, Part II, 175-218.

1957   CRUZ M., COLEY B. L., STEWART F. W.: Post-radiation bone sarcoma. Report of eleven cases. *Cancer*, **10**, 72-88.

1962   SPIESS H., POPPE H., SCHOEN H.: Strahleninduzierte Knochentumoren nach Thorium X-Behandlung. *Monatschrift für Unfallheilkunde*, **110**, 198-201.

1962   WOODARD H. R., HIGINBOTHAM N. L.: Development of osteogenic sarcoma in a radium dial painter thirty-seven years after the end of exposure. *American Journal of Medicine*, **32**, 96-102.

1963   PHILIPS T. L., SHELINE G. E.: Bone sarcomas following radiation therapy. *Radiology*, **81**, 992-996.

1965   POZNANSKI S. W., FRANKEL S.: The roentgenographic develompent of radiostrontium (Sr90) induced osteogenic sarcoma in the rat. *Journal of Bone and Joint Surgery*, **47**-A, 349-358.

1965   STEINER G. C.: Post-radiation sarcoma of bone. *Cancer*, **18**, 603-612.

1966   EVANS R. D.: The effect of skeletally deposited alpharay emitters in man. *British Journal of Radiology*, **39**, 881-895.

1967   SOLOWAY H. B.: Radiation induced neoplasms following curative therapy for retinoblastoma. *Cancer*, **19**, 1984-1988.

1967   BONARIGO B. C., RUBIN P.: Non union of pathologic fractures after radiation therapy. *Radiology*, **88**, 889-898.

1967   CASTRO L., CHOI S. H., SHEENAN F. R.: Radiation induced bone sarcomas. Report of five cases. *American Journal of Roentgenology*, **100**, 924-930.

1967   SEARS W. P., TEFT M., COHEN J.: Post-irradiation mesenchymal chondrosarcoma. A case report. *Pediatrics*, **41**, 254-258.

1968   WAUGHAN J.: The effects of skeletal irradiation. *Clinical Orthopaedics*, **56**, 283-303.

1969   KATZMAN H., WAUGH J., BERDON W.: Skeletal changes following irradiation of childhood tumors. *Journal of Bone and Joint Surgery*, **51**-A, 825-842.

1971   ARLEN M., HIGINBOTHAM N., HUVOS A. G., MARCOVE R. C., MILLER T., SHAH I. C.: Radiation induced sarcoma of bone. *Cancer*, **28**, 1087-1099.

1971   DUPARC L., PRAT B.: Fracture du col fémoral aprés irradiation pelvienne. *Revue de Chirurgie Orthopedique*, **57**, 227-241.

1972   EDGAR M. A.: Fibrosarcoma complicating ankylosing spondylitis. *Journal of Bone and Joint Surgery*, **54**-B, 199-199.

1972   SIM H. F., CUPPS R. E., DAHLIN D. C., IVINS J. C.: Post-radiation sarcoma of bone. *Journal of Bone and Joint Surgery*, **54**-A, 1479-1489.

1976   RISENBOROUGH E., STANLEY L. G., BURTON R., JAFFE N.: Skeletal alterations following irradiation for Wilms' tumor. *Journal of Bone and Joint Surgery*, **58**-A, 526-536.

1978   SINDELAR W. F., COSTA J., KETCHAM A. S.: Osteosarcoma associated with thorotrast administration. Report of two cases and literature review. *Cancer*, **42**, 2604-2609.

1979   TOUNTAS A. A., FORNASIER V. L., HARWOOD A. R., LEUNG P. M. K.: Postirradiation sarcoma of bone. A perspective. *Cancer*, **43**, 182-187.

1980   MEADOWS A., STRONG L.C., LI F., D'ANGIÒ G.J., SCHWEIGSGUTH O., FREEMAN A.I., JENKIN R.D., MORRIS-JONES P., NESBIT M.E.: Bone sarcoma as a second malignant neoplasm in children. Influence of radiation and genetic predisposition. *Cancer*, **46**, 2603-2606.

1984   MASUDA S., MURAKAWA Y.: Postirradiation parosteal osteosarcoma: a case report. *Clinical Orthopaedics*, **184**, 204-207.

1984   ROY-CAMILLE R., SAILLANT G., CHIRAS J., ARLET J., FICAT P., HENRY P., LEONARD PH.: Ostéosarcome de C4-C5 radio-induit. *Revue de Chirurgie Orthopedique*, **70**, Suppl., 99-100.

1985   HUVOS A.G., WOODARD H.Q., CAHAN W.G., HIGINBOTHAM N.L., STEWART F.W., BUTLER A., BRETSKY S.S.: Postirradiation osteogenic sarcoma of bone and soft tissues. *Cancer*, **55**, 1244-1255.

1987   SMITH J.: Postirradiation sarcoma of bone in Hodgkin disease. *Skeletal Radiology*, **16**, 524-532.

1988 BORIANI S., PICCI P., SUDANESE A., TONI A., MANCINI A., FREZZA G., BARBIE-
      RI E., BALDINI N., MONESI M., CIARONI D., BACCI G.: Radioinduced sarcomas
      in survivors of Ewing's sarcoma. *Tumori*, **74**, 543-551.

SARCOMAS ON BONE INFARCTS OR NECROSIS

There are rare cases in which sarcoma — malignant fibrous histiocytoma, fibrosarcoma, osteosarcoma, angiosarcoma (Fig. 505) — develops in the area of an old bone infarct, due to decompression air emboli or of unknown origin. These sarcomas have been observed only in the femur and in the tibia (see chapters on tumors listed above). Exceptionally, there may be a sarcoma occurring on a benign tumor, for example a giant cell tumor, submitted many years earlier to curettage and bone grafting, or on an old calcified chondroma. These sarcomas may have originated from the reactive cells around a necrotic calcified material, present for many years.

BONE METASTASES FROM CARCINOMAS

DEFINITION

By M. to the skeleton, we usually mean M. due to carcinomas. M. from sarcomas, including sarcomas of bone, are rare and terminal, and thus of little clinical interest. M. from carcinoma, instead, are of considerable clinical importance, not only because of their frequency, but also because they often constitute a problem in diagnosis (when they are manifested prior to the primary tumor) and often constitute a therapeutic problem.

FREQUENCY

Carcinomatous M. constitute the most frequent malignant tumor of the skeleton. If the clinical and radiographic material available is evaluated, about 15% of all carcinomas manifest skeletal M. But if autoptic material is examined, the percentage probably increases to 30%.

Most cases of bone M. derive from carcinomas of four organs: breast, prostate, lung, kidney. These are followed by the thyroid, stomach, colon and rectum, pancreas, and all the others. Carcinomas of the first five organs listed (breast, prostate, lung, kidney and thyroid) are also those which metastasize with a maximum frequency to the bone (cf. pathogenesis).

SEX, AGE

Sex and age are those of the primary carcinoma involved (Fig. 555). It must however be recalled, and particularly in the case of M. from pulmonary carcinoma and hypernephroma, that it is not an exceptional occurrence in young patients, aged from 30 to 40 years; M. of thyroid carcinoma may even be observed between 20 and 30 years of age.

LOCALIZATION

There is evident predilection for the skeleton of the trunk and the limb girdles. The first localization is the vertebral column, particularly the thoracic and lumbar regions. These are followed by the pelvis, the proximal end of

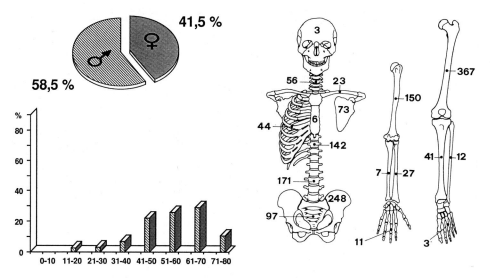

FIG. 555. - Sex and age in 1877 cases of bone metastases from carcinoma. Localization in 1481 apparently solitary metastases (as there was no systematic study of the entire skeleton).

the femur, the proximal end of the humerus. M. rarely occur distal to the knee and elbow, nonetheless, they may occur anywhere, even in the hand (Fig. 555).

In the spine they prevalently involve the vertebral body; the posterior arch is usually in the involved advanced form of the disease, by invasion from the body and the pedicles. In the pelvis M. is more frequent in the iliac bone. In the cranium it affects the skull, hardly ever the facial bones. In the long bones of the limbs it may occur in the metaphyses or in the diaphyses, less often in the epiphyses.

By nature, M. tends to be multiple. Nonetheless, it frequently occurs that at the onset bone M. is the only one visible. Thereafter, others may occur, which may be skeletal and/or extraskeletal.

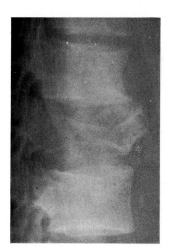

FIG. 556. - Male aged 58 years. Metastasis of hypernephroma.

Furthermore, there is a tendency to prefer certain sites depending on the primary tumor. M. of prostatic and uterine carcinoma occurs more frequently in the lumbar column, sacrum, and pelvis. M. of breast and thyroid cancer are preferably localized in the skeleton of the trunk and in the cranium. M. of pulmonary carcinoma may even reach as far as the ends of the limbs and may be periosteal or intracortical (Fig. 560). M. of prostate and breast carcinoma (but at times also of other epithelial organs) may be very disseminated, nearly diffused to the entire skeleton. Those of hypernephroma and of

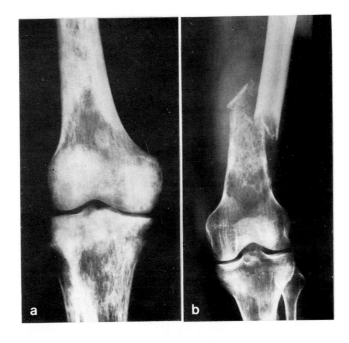

FIG. 557. - (a) Male aged 170 years. Diffused metastases of prostatic carcinoma. (b) Male aged 66 years. Metastasis of hypernephroma with pathologic fracture.

thyroid follicular carcinoma may be solitary and remain so for a long period of time.

SYMPTOMS

Anatomical evidence of M. does not signify radiographic evidence of M., nor does the latter always signify clinical evidence of M. In other words, many skeletal M. observed on autopsy cannot be visualized on radiograms, and some M. which may be visualized radiographically do not cause any symptoms. Absence or mildness of symptoms in radiographically visible M. frequently occurs in blastic and mixed lytic-blastic M. (prostate, breast), which may even be multiple, and considerably extended without causing symptoms.

On the contrary, in many cases pain may precede radiographic manifestation of osteolytic M. (particularly in the cancellous bone of the spine, pelvis, ribs, femoral neck). Some cases of lumbar M. with a negative radiographic report may simulate herniated disc syndrome. At times the patient (in most cases elderly females) is hospitalized for a fracture of the upper end of the femur, occurring during good health and which is apparently traumatic. Radiograms of the fracture may not be very revealing, or they are easily underevaluated, and M. may be discovered during endoprosthetic surgery. Similarly, insistent coxo-pelvic and costo-sternal pain during advanced adult age, and even moreso if in the presence of some associated clinical data or element in the patient's history, should lead to suspicion of M. even if the radiographic picture is negative at that time.

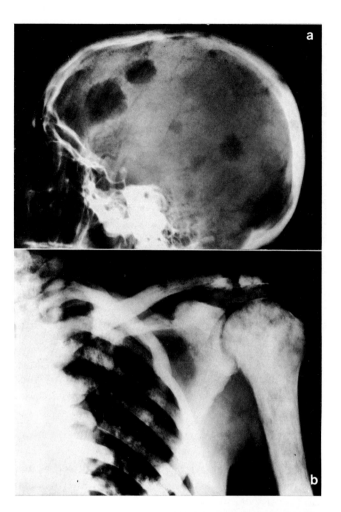

Symptoms do not differ from those of a primary malignant bone tumor, and include pain, functional deficit, swelling, pathologic fracture and — in the vertebral column — signs of nerve root-spinal cord compression. Based on their nature, site, multiplicity, relative radio-resistance, M. are

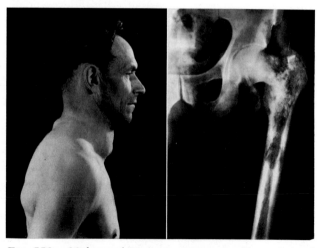

FIG. 559. - Male aged 51 years. Metastases from thyroid carcinoma with pathologic fracture.

not treated with the same radicality used to treat primary bone tumors; as a result, these symptoms often become of an intensity which considerably exceeds that of most skeletal sarcomas. In particular, pathologic fracture is a very frequent occurrence (Figs. 556, 557b, 559b, 568a).

Because of their rich vascularization, M. due to hypernephroma occurring in superficial bone may pulsate on palpation (Fig. 565).

When metastatic lesion is suspected, clinical examination of the breast, prostate, thyroid, chest and abdomen is essential.

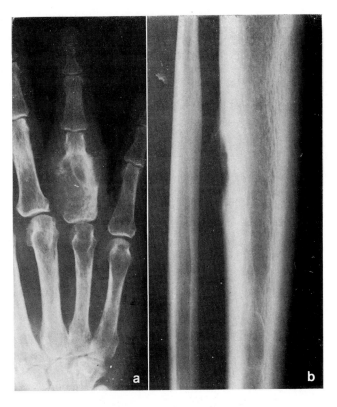

FIG. 560. - (a) Female aged 60 years. Metastases from carcinoma of the lung. (b) Male aged 38 years. Metastasis from carcinoma of the lung.

HEMATOCHEMICAL FINDINGS

Calcemia and calciuria are increased in multiple or extended

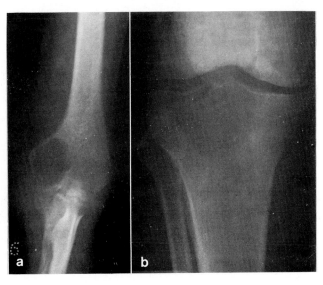

FIG. 561. - (a) Female aged 61 years. Metastasis of adenocarcinoma (origin not ascertained). (b) Male aged 50 years. Metastasis of adenocarcinoma (origin unknown).

and osteolytic M. The increase in calcemia may be enough to cause severe hypercalcemic syndrome and calcar impregnation of the kidneys, lungs and gastrointestinal mucosa. Hypercalcemia may be worsened by hormone therapy, particularly androgens in M. of breast cancer. Alkaline phosphatase increases in blastic M. (this increase may also be caused by cholostasis in case of M. in the liver). Acid phosphatase often increases in M. of prostatic carcinoma.

RADIOGRAPHIC FEATURES

Bone M. destroys the bone tissue provoking hypertransparency (**osteolytic** M.); otherwise it causes reactive hyperostosis with increase, which may even be eburneous, of skeletal radiopacity (**osteoblastic** M.) (Figs. 556-568). Lytic M. are due to cancer of kidney, lung, breast, thyroid, gastroenteric tract. Blastic M. par excellence are those of prostate carcinoma. Breast cancer, too, may cause osteosclerosis, which is often associated with osteolysis. Occasionally, M. of bronchial and enteric carcinoids, carcinomas of bladder, stomach, testicle, pancreas, lung, prove to be osteoblastic.

It must be recalled that a M. may extensively infiltrate the medullary spaces of the cancellous bone, without completely destroying the trabeculae (particularly if there is necrosis of the neoplastic tissue and of the bone). Thus, it may occur that a M. 2 or 3 cm in diameter is not at all visible on radiograms. The radiograms are negative even when, although causing complete osteolysis, the M. is too small (less than 0.5 cm in diameter if its site is in the vertebral bodies). This radiographic latency particularly concerns M. in cancellous bone, such as the vertebral bodies, where it is also due to the considerable thickness of the soft tissues, the meta-epiphyses of the long

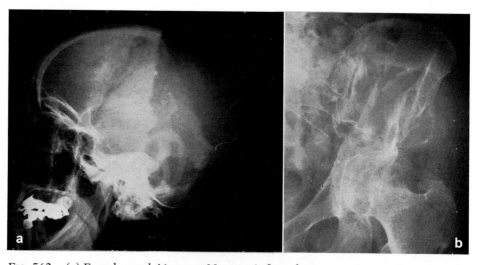

FIG. 562. - (a) Female aged 46 years. Metastasis from breast carcinoma destroying the posterior half of the cranium with no neurological symptoms. (b) Female aged 60 years. Metastasis of adenocarcinoma (origin not apparent).

bones, the pelvis, the scapula, the ribs. In prevalently cortical bones such as the cranium and in the diaphyseal compact bones, instead, even small osteolytic lacunae are visible on radiograms. Osteoblastic M. are manifested more clearly and thus earlier than osteolytic ones. In case of suspected or ascertained bone M., **total body bone scan** is of essential importance. This will not only reveal a lesion which is still not visible on radiograms but, in case of clinical and radiographically manifest metastasis, which is apparently unique, it may reveal any other metastatic localizations in the skeleton. Guided by clinical, radiographic and scintigraphic data, **CAT** and **MRI** are carried out. These will reveal the shape and the spatial relationships of the lesion better than radiograms, and furthermore, they may reveal the primary carcinoma (for example, renal or pulmonary).

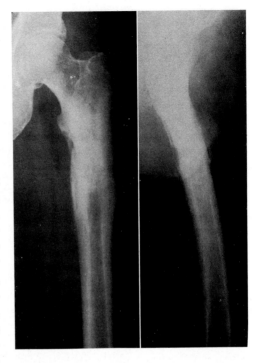

FIG. 563. - Male aged 70 years. Metastasis from adenocarcinoma (origin not apparent).

The lytic or blastic area may be single, or there may be numerous foci which are either separated or confluent. In any cases the boundaries tend to be faded. The cortex is generally infiltrated, eroded or cancelled. In exceptional blastic forms there is intense reactive periostosis, with images vaguely simulating an osteosarcoma. Vertebral lytic M. may appear late on radiograms and even on tomograms. More than central osteolysis, the first sign is constituted by an interruption or the cancelling of cortical borders of the vertebral body or of the pedicular «eye», or even by a pathologic collapse (Figs. 556, 573). In cases of fracture of the upper femoral end on M., the radiographic signs of M. may be hidden by the fracture. There are also normal fractures of the femoral neck which, due to the intense osteoporosis and external rotation of the diaphysis, may give the false impression of an osteolysis of the neck which does not exist. Some M., such as those of hypernephroma, may cause multiloculated or «bubbling» osteolyses, with thinning and ballooning of the cortex (Figs. 568a, 575). If **arteriography** is carried out M. of hypernephroma generally show a very rich blood supply (Fig. 565). In exceptional cases a lytic M. may have rather evident boundaries or it may be trabeculated, leaving the cortex intact, so that it mimics a benign tumor (Figs. 561a). In the diaphyses, rare M. which usually originate from lung cancer may be manifested by a small subperiosteal or intracortical osteolysis (Fig. 560b).

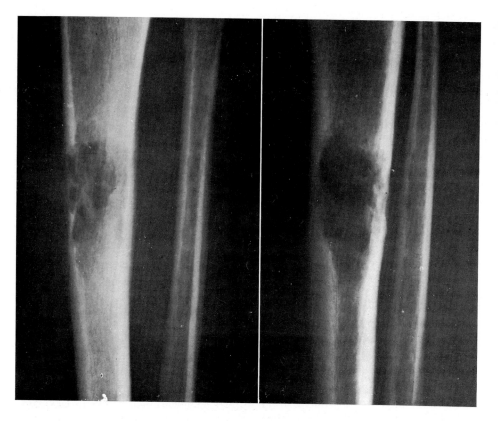

Fig. 564. - Male aged 53 years. Metastasis from adenocarcinoma (origin not apparent).

GROSS PATHOLOGIC FEATURES

The macroscopic picture obviously varies considerably. Consistency may be soft encephaloid, densely fibrous (scirrhus), or eburneous (intensely blastic forms). Color ranges from white to grayish, to hemorrhagic. M. due to hypernephroma are yellow, although such color is often hidden by the intense hyperemia and hemorrhagic changes; some cases of M. due to malignant melanoma are blackish or black (not necessarily all, not even within the same case). M. due to mucoid carcinomas may contain large cavities filled with mucoid fluid. At times the tissue is yellowish, deprived of blood, dry or diffluent, even frankly purulent, due to necrosis and to superimposed inflammation.

Even where it radiographically does not appear to be modified around the metastatic osteolysis, the bone may be friable and softened due to metastatic permeation and reactive inflammation. This explains the considerable frequency of pathologic fractures.

Even when there are extensive and/or multiple bone M., the primary carcinoma may remain very small, not apparent, and asymptomatic.

FIG. 565. - Male aged 59 years. (a) Metastasis from hypernephroma in the acromion. Intense angiographic injection. The metastasis had occurred in the form of swelling of the scapula which pulsated. Based on this clinical finding metastasis from hypernephroma was suggested, angiography of the renal arteries was obtained, thus revealing hypernephroma of the right kidney (b).

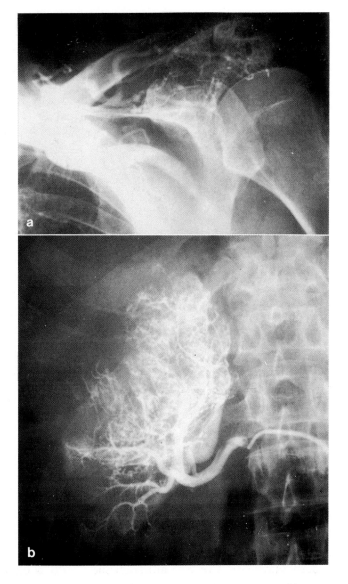

HISTOPATHOLOGIC FEATURES

Nearly always diagnosis is easy: to find neoplastic epithelial tissue inside the bone cannot but signify M. (Fig. 569). The metastatic tissue often repeats the cytology and the structure of the original carcinoma, but it may be anaplastic and/or modified by the reaction of the medullary and bone tissue. In rare cases (for example, of renal carcinoma) the cells are dispersed in the hyperplastic connective tissue and tend towards a spindle shape (Fig. 572c, d), so that the tumor may resemble poorly differentiated sarcoma. Similarly, rare cases of M. of small-cell carcinoma (lung, thyroid) may suggest Ewing's sarcoma or lymphoma (Fig. 571c, d). Very useful for a histological distinction between epitelial metatasis and sarcoma is trichromic staining for the connective tissue, argentic impregnation for the reticulum, and immunohistochemistry for the epithelial markers.

M. of hypernephroma generally maintains its typical organoid structure in cords and tubules, its cubico-cylindrical cells with «clear» cytoplasm, stuffed with lipoids and glycogen, with rounded and hyperchromic nuclei, its wide sinusoids among the tubules, its intense hyperemia and hemorrhagic effusions (Fig. 570a, b).

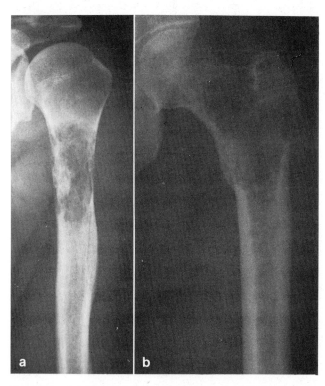

FIG. 566. - (a) Male aged 72 years. Metastasis from hypernephroma. (b) Female aged 49 years. Metastasis from breast carcinoma.

Not all clear-cell M. are due to hypernephroma. There are clear-cell carcinomas of the ovary and uterus.

Even M. of thyroid carcinoma often preserves a follicular structure and the ability to secrete colloid. These, too, are evidently differentiated and organoid, at times with little or minimum signs of cellular atypia (Fig. 570c, d).

M. of prostatic carcinoma (and at times mammary, pancreatic, etc.) are often characterized by epithelial cords and tubules scattered throughout an abundant reactive fibrous or bone tissue (scirrhus and osteoblastic forms, Figs. 571a, b; 572a). Even M. of prostate carcinoma may be well-differentiated enough to hypothesize the organ of origin. M. of pulmonary carcinoma may have a squamous epithelial aspect.

Generally, however, **the origin of M. cannot be determined by histological examination**.

Around the epithelial structures of M. there is a connective reaction and a leukocytary infiltration, which are usually greater than those observed in primary sarcomas.

PATHOGENESIS

M. of the skeleton oc-
cur by hematic route
(the presence of lym-
phatic vessels in the
bone is doubtless and
certainly rather scarce).

Although it is true
that most carcinomas
metastasize by lym-
phatic route, there are
some which do so by
hematic route, such as
those of the lung,
breast, kidney, prostate
and thyroid glands;
which are in fact those
most responsible for
bone M. As commonly
known, there are sub-
stantially three means
of metastasization by
hematic route. The first,
pulmonary, is that of
carcinomas of the lung
which, by means of the
pulmonary veins, the
left heart and the aorta
may be distributed to
any part of the body.
The second, **portal**, is
that of carcinomas of
the tributary organs of
the portal vein, which
metastasize in the liver.
The third, **caval**, is that
of carcinomas of the or-
gans and tissues tribu-
tary of the venae cavae
(including the liver)
which, via the right
heart and pulmonary
artery, metatasize in

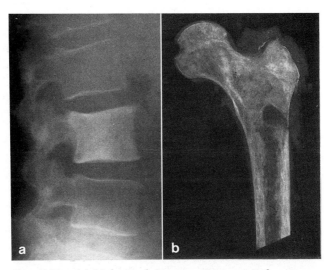

FIG. 567. - (a) Male aged 51 years. Metastasis from prostate carcinoma (ivory vertebra). (b) Female aged 61
years. Generalized and sclerosing bone metastases from
carcinoma of the pancreas. X-ray of anatomical specimen.

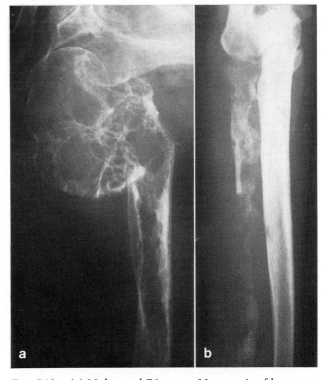

FIG. 568. - (a) Male aged 74 years. Metastasis of hypernephroma. (b) Male aged 58 years. Metastasis of adenocarcinoma (origin not apparent).

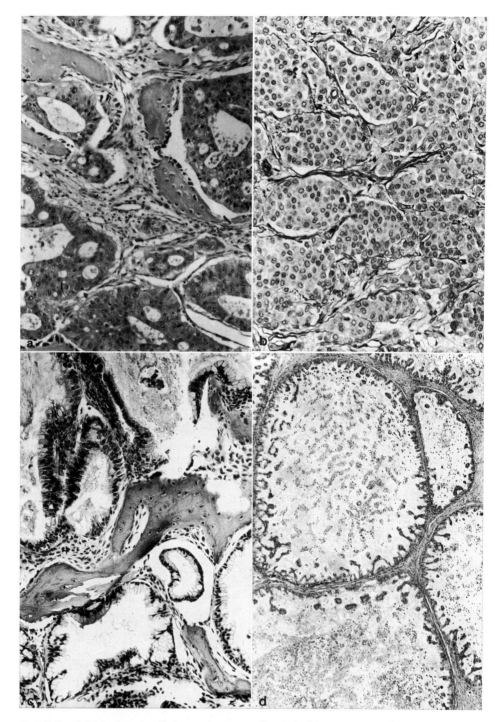

FIG. 569. - (a) Metastasis of adenocarcinoma (breast). (b) Metastasis of solid carcinoma (lung). (c) Metastasis of adenocarcinoma with mucin-secreting cells (of the biliary ducts). (d) Metastasis of mucin-secreting adenocarcinoma (origin not apparent) (*Hemat.-eos.*, 125, 200, 125, 50 x).

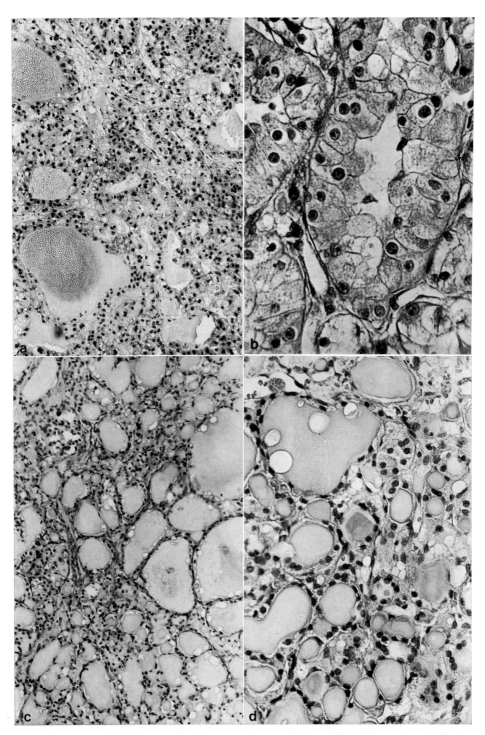

FIG. 570. - (a) and (b) Metastasis of hypernephroma. (c) and (d) Metastasis of follicular carcinoma of the thyroid in a female aged 23 years. (*Hemat.-eos.*, 125, 500, 125, 300 x).

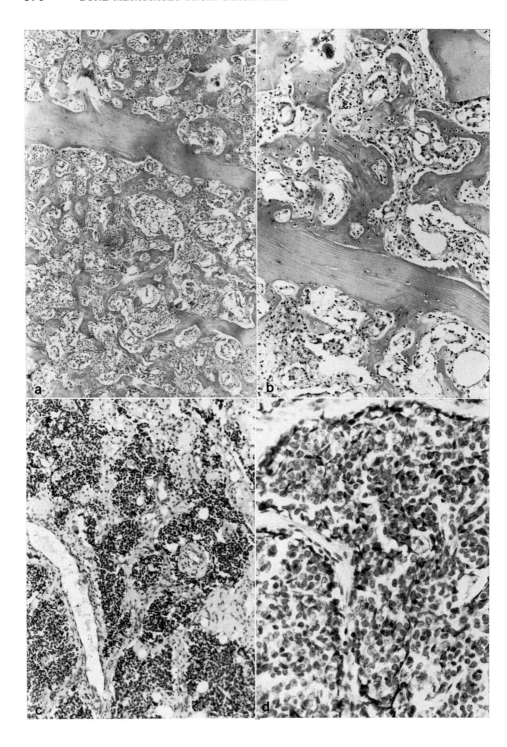

FIG. 571. - (a) and (b) Metastasis from carcinoma of the pancreas, osteoblastic: same case as in Fig. 567b. (c) and (d) Metastasis from medullary carcinoma of the thyroid in a male aged 22 years (*Hemat.-eos.*, 50, 125, 125 and 300 x).

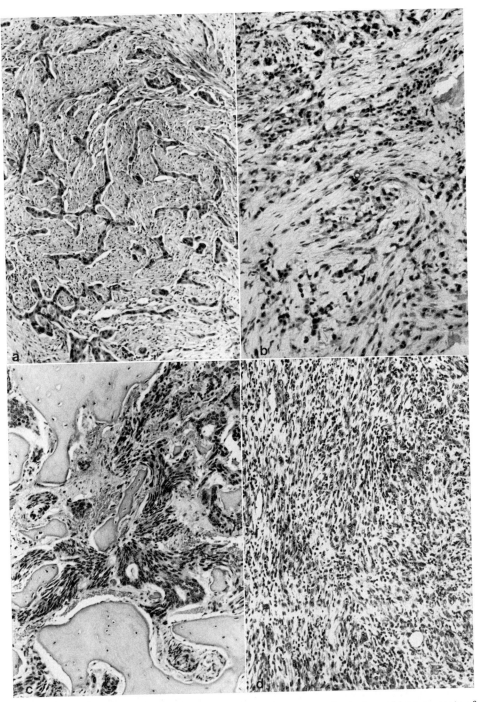

FIG. 572. - (a) Metastasis of adenocarcinoma with aspects of scirrhus. (b) Metastasis of carcinoma where the cells form rows and cords which could suggest hemangioendothelioma. (c) Metastasis of adenocarcinoma with spindling of the cell. (d) Metastasis of pulmonary carinoma where the cells are rather scattered and spindle-shaped enough to suggest a sarcoma (*Hemat.-eos.*, 125, 125, 125, 125 x).

the lungs. This scheme is, however, too simple, as shown by the fact that a carcinoma of a tributary organ of the portal vein or of the venae cavae frequently metastasizes in the bone and not in the liver or lungs. The hepatic filter may have «skipped» by means of the lymphatic vessels, the thoracic duct, and the upper vena cava. The «skip» of the pulmonry filter seems to be possible for small-cell carcinoma, but only rarely. Instead, there is a direct connection between the venous net (pertaining to the caval system) in the thoracic and abdominal wall, and the venous plexi of the vertebral column. This direct route is constituted by valveless anastomoses where, when abdominal and thoracic pressure increases, the flow is inverted, going from the thoracoabdominal walls towards the vertebral venous system, which, in turn, is connected to the veins of the cranium, the pelvis, the ribs, the proximal femur. This would explain M. of the skeleton of the trunk, in the absence of pulmonary M., due to carcinomas of the breast, prostate, kidney, thyroid, stomach, and the predilection of these M. for the skeleton of the trunk.

In addition to being invaded by hematic route, the bone may be more rarely invaded by adjacency: for example, from a carcinoma of the skin or of the mucosae covering the bone; or from carcinomatous M. in lymph nodes adjacent to the bone, such as the lumboaortic.

DIAGNOSIS

According to the relationships between symptoms due to bone M. and those due to primary carcinoma, there are three possibilities. 1) Bone M. occur unexpectedly, as the primary tumor is totally asymptomatic and not even suspected. This is a frequent occurrence, and the most common in orthopaedic practice. 2) The M. constitute the only current symptom, but the patient's history reveals previous diagnosis and treatment of the primary carcinoma. 3) The M. are manifested in association with an evident primary carcinoma and/or with its evident extraskeletal M.

Diagnosis may be a problem particularly in the first case. The possibility of bone M. must always be taken into consideration, when the patient is aged over 30 years, and moreso when he or she is of advanced age and the lesion is localized in the skeleton of the trunk, cranium or limb girdles, the radiographic aspect is lytic or blastic and aggressive.

The radiographic image of an osteolytic M. may not be distinguished from that of **osteolytic sarcomas** in the adult. Diagnosis of M. is more likely when the lesion is localized in the skeleton of the trunk, in the limb girdles, in the diaphyses. Multiple osteolytic M. may suggest **plasmacytoma**. In the vertebrae osteolytic M. rarely extends to the cancellous bone of the pedicle without modifying the cortex, unlike plasmacytoma. Moreover, isotope bone scan may be negative in plasmacytoma, hardly ever in M. Osteoblastic M. of the vertebral column (ivory vertebra) and of the pelvis (disseminated or diffused prostatic carcinoma) involve the radiographic differential problem of **Paget's disease**. A differential criteria is the fact that pagetic ivory vertebra

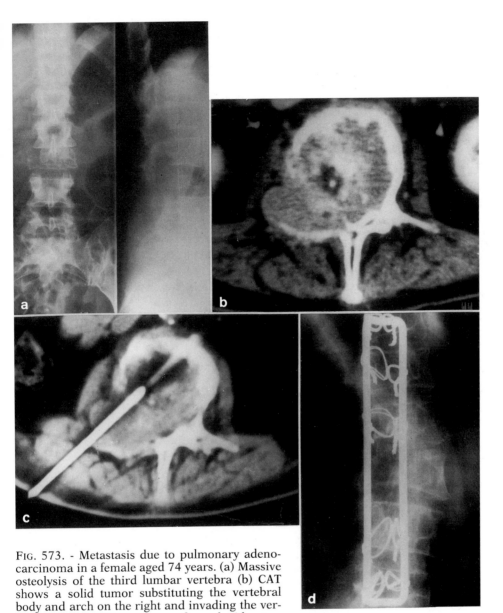

FIG. 573. - Metastasis due to pulmonary adeno-carcinoma in a female aged 74 years. (a) Massive osteolysis of the third lumbar vertebra (b) CAT shows a solid tumor substituting the vertebral body and arch on the right and invading the ver-tebral canal. (c) Biopsy was performed with a tro-car under CAT monitoring. (d) The patient was treated with decompressive laminec-tomy, stabilization with a Hartshill rectangle and radiation.

has more evident boundaries, at times revealing a hint of rough vertical trab-eculation and greater peripheral density (framelike vertebra) and, above all, it is increased in volume. Even in the pagetic pelvis the bone affected is often increased in volume, furthermore, the radiopacity and the borders of the bone have more evident boundaries and hardly ever is there not a hint of pagetic trabecular structure. In exceptional cases, osteoblastic M. in the long bones or in the clavicle may cause an exuberant periosteal reaction, enough to simulate an **osteosarcoma**. Finally, it must be recalled that even skeletal lesions due to **malignant lymphomas** and exceptionally to plasmacytoma may be partially blastic and sclerosing.

In conclusion, a radiographic diagnosis may be impossible and, when the existence of a primary carcinoma is not known, **biopsy must be performed without delay**. The insertion of a trocar or a simple surgical procedure allows for immediate and sound diagnosis where many complex instrumental and laboratory tests are often not conclusive, and time-consuming. More specific tests may be carried out after biopsy, guided by histological diagnosis.

The histological diagnosis of epithelial M. is nearly always easy. It is instead difficult to indicate the organ of origin. A certain or nearly certain indication is possible only in three conditions: **hypernephroma**, follicular carcinoma of the **thyroid**, and some adenocarcinomas of the **prostate**. In some other cases the organ of origin may be hypothesized: for example, small-cell (oat-cell) or squamous cell M. probably derive from a pulmonary carcinoma; mucus-secreting M. often derive from the gastroenteric tube.

It may in rare cases be difficult to recognize whether we are dealing with a M., or with a primary sarcoma (**angiosarcoma, lymphoma, malignant fibrous histiocytoma, fibrosarcoma**). In exceptional cases, epithelial M. may histologically simulate a **giant cell tumor** (see specific chapters).

«When the histology of a malignant tumor of the bone does not correspond to any of the known skeletal sarcomas in a satisfactory manner, always think of M.»: it is one of Lichtenstein's sayings which has been useful more than once (cf. histological finding).

Once the metastatic nature of the bone tumor has been diagnosed, its origin must be searched for. This search is always indicated, because of the prediction of prognosis, because of the therapeutic implications. Research will particularly focus on the lungs, breast, prostate, thyroid, kidneys and gastroenteric tube. Moreover, it must be recalled that the primary carcinoma may evade even the most complete and detailed study. It will end up being manifested later on, but exceptionally it may be and remain so small that not even autopsy will be able to determine it.

COURSE

Bone M. may occur even many years after ablation of the primary carcinoma (more than 10-15 years, for example, for carcinoma of the breast, for hypernephroma, for well-differentiated carcinoma of the thyroid, for malignant melanoma). Generally, the first M. is followed by other, skeletal and/or of the viscera, and death occurs within 1-2 years. In some cases, nonetheless (hypernephroma, well-differentiated follicular carcinoma of the thyroid, breast carcinoma responding to chemo-hormone therapy), the bone M. may remain solitary and/or relatively stationary even for several years.

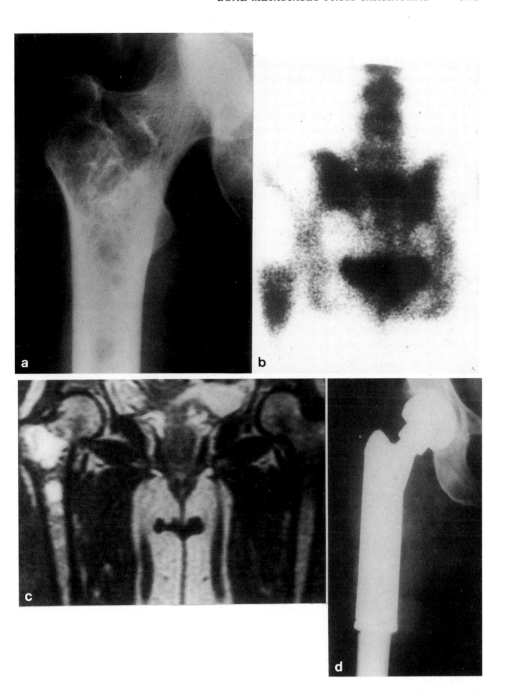

FIG. 574. - Metastasis due to adenocarcinoma in the breast in a female aged 52 years. Mastectomy 5 years earlier. (a) Painful osteolytic lesion occurring 1 year ago. (b) Bone scan shows the only localization in the proximal femur. (c) MRI shows extent of metastasis in the medullary canal. (d) Following needle biopsy, the patient was submitted to wide resection and cementless endoprosthesis. The patient had no signs of disease 16 months after surgery.

TREATMENT AND PROGNOSIS

Surgical treatment is nearly always palliative: nerve root decompression (with anthalgic purposes) and spinal cord decompression (in case of initial paraparesis) and surgical stabilization in vertebral M. (Fig. 573). Osteosynthesis with intramedullary nailing, screwed plates, acrylic cement, in M. of the long bones in order to prevent or treat fracture and allow for early function of the limb. At times resection, with or without endoprosthesis or arthroprosthesis (Figs. 574, 575). In case of hypernephroma and other very vascularized M., selective arterial embolization may be used, immediately prior to surgery in order to decreae hemorrhage, or as a palliative anthalgic treatment. Surgical treatment of the primary tumor is performed especially in those cases (renal, thyroid tumors) where the bone M. is solitary and a long survival rate may be hoped for.

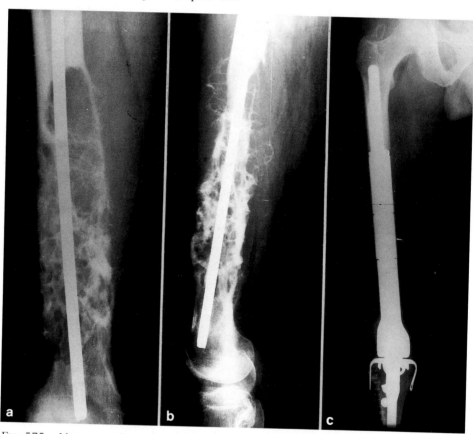

FIG. 575. - Metastasis due to hypernephroma in a male aged 70 years. Nephrectomy 16 years earlier. Metastasis, which had occured 5 years previously, apparently solitary, was treated with stabilization (inadequate) by intramedullary nailing and radiation (a, b). Observe the trabeculated and bubbly aspect of the osteolysis. (c) As pain, functional deficit and progression of osteolysis persisted, the patient was submitted to wide resection and cementless arthroprosthesis. Total remission of symptoms for one year. Then a new metastasis occurred in the periprosthetic soft tissues, which was treated by embolization.

Radiation treatment constitutes the weapon used most, particularly in the treatment of solitary or oligostotic M. of the skeleton of the trunk, in elderly patients. Its effectiveness is unpredictable, but often it is enough to reduce the neoplastic mass, to arrest or delay expansion, to diminish or abolish pain. It must be kept in mind that irradiation at strong doses may cause necrosis of the bone and make it more susceptible to fracture. Thus, even if radiographically the osteolytic area is not expanded, after radiation therapy the bone is probably more fragile than before.

An important place is that of **drugs**. Antiblastics, hormones (or surgery or irradiation of endocrine glands) in carcinomas of the breast and of the prostate, again hormones associated with antiblastics in hypernephroma. Strong doses of corticosteroids have also been used to reduce peritumoral reaction, pain, and to improve cenesthesia. I131 is used in thyroid carcinomas.

Finally, it is important to recall the **treatment of pain** with analgesics or narcotic, alcoholization or anesthetic blocks of the nerve paths and of the hypophysis, neurosurgery on the sensory pathways of the spinal cord.

Prognosis is constantly fatal. When bone M. occur, survival generally does not exceed 1-2 years. Survival is less if the bone M. are multiple. Nonetheless some exceptions do exist. For example, there are cases of hypernephroma where the bone M. is solitary ad may remain so for a long period of time. In cases such as these nephrectomy and extensive ablation of the M. may allow for prolonged survival. A considerable survival rate may be observed in M. of well-differentiated follicular carcinomas of the thyroid or of chemo-hormone responsive carcinomas of the breast.

Therapeutic planning of bone M. is absolutely interdisciplinary (oncologist, surgeon specialist of the organ of origin, orthopaedic surgeon, radiotherapist, etc.). It is important to evaluate the biological features of the neoplasm, the general state of the patient, the presumed survival rate, the risks of the various types of treatment, their succession in time. A correct balance should be found between a renouncing and an aggressive therapeutic attitude.

REFERENCES

1950 ABRAMS H. L., SPIRO R., GOLDESTEIN N.: Metastases in carcinoma. Analysis of 1000 autopsied cases. *Cancer*, **3**, 74-85.

1954 YOUNG J. M., FUNK J. F. Jr.: Incidence of tumor metastasis to the lumbar spine. A comparative study of roentgenographic changes and gross lesions. *Journal of Bone and Joint Surgery*, **35-A**, 55-64.

1960 SUM P. W., ROSWIT B., UNGER S. M.: Skeletal metastases from malignant testicular tumors. A report of 10 cases with osteolytic and osteoblastic changes. *American Journal of Roentgenology*, **83**, 704-708.

1960 TOOMEY F. B., FELSON B.: Osteoblastic bone metastasis in gastrointestinal and bronchial carcinoids. *American Journal of Roentgenology*, **83**, 709-715.

1966 MC CORMACK K. B.: Bone metastases from thyroid carcinoma. *Cancer*, **19**, 181-184.

1966 NORMAN A., LEVENTHAL E.: Skeletal metastases from latent primary carcinomas of gastrointestinal tract. *Journal of Medicine*, **66**, 2814-2817.

1967 BRIGGS R. C.: Detection of osseous metastases. Evaluation of bone scanning with strontium. *Cancer*, **20**, 392-395.

1967 MARCOVE R. C., YANG D. J.: Survival times after treatment of pathologic fractures. *Cancer*, **20**, 2154-2158.

1968 BARER M., PETERSON L. F. A., DAHLIN D. C., WINKELMANN R. K., STEWART J. R.: Mastocytosis with osseous lesions resembling metastatic malignant lesions in bone. *Journal of Bone and Joint Surgery*, **50-A**, 142-152.

1968 LEGIER J. F., TANBER L. N.: Solitary metastasis of occult prostatic carcinoma simulating osteogenic sarcoma. *Cancer*, **22**, 168-172.

1968 ROSAI J.: Carcinoma of pancreas simulating giant cell tumor of bone. Electron-microscopic evidence of its acinar cell origin. *Cancer*, **22**, 333-344.

1969 NORMAN A., ULIN R. A.: A comparative study of periosteal new-bone response in metastatic bone tumors (solitary) and primary bone sarcomas. *Radiology*, **92**, 705-708.

1969 SILVERBERG S. G., EVANS R. H., KOEHLER A. L.: Clinical and pathologic fractures of initial metastatic presentations of renal cell carcinoma. *Cancer*, **23**, 1126-1132.

1970 PARRISH F., MURRAY J. A.: Surgical treatment for secondary neoplastic fractures. A retrospective study of ninety-six patients. *Journal of Bone and Joint Surgery*, **52-A**, 665-686.

1971 BEALS R. K., LAWTON G. D., SNELL W. E.: Prophylactic internal fixation of the femur in metastatic breast cancer. *Cancer*, **28**, 1350-1354.

1971 GALASKO C. S. B.: Detection of skeletal metastases. *Journal of Bone and Joint Surgery*, **53-B**, 153-153.

1971 WHITE W. A., PATTERSON R. H. Jr., BERGLAND R. M.: Role of surgery in the treatment of spinal cord compression by metastatic neoplasm. *Cancer*, **27**, 558-561.

1972 MUGGIA F. M., HANSEN H. H.: Osteoblastic metastases in small-cell (oat-cell) carcinoma of the lung. *Cancer*, **30**, 801-805.'

1972 PEREX C. A., BRADFIELD J. S., MORGAN M. C.: Management et pathological fractures. *Cancer*, **29**, 684-693.

1972 TEMPLETON A. C., HUTT M. S. R., DODGE O. G.: Cryptogenic metastases in Uganda Africans. *Journal of Bone and Joint Surgery*, **54-B**, 122-124.

1973 DUPARC J., NORDIN J. Y., OLIVIER H.: Les fractures métastatiques du fémur. *Revue de Chirurgie Orthopedique*, **59**, 91-108.

1973 SCHURMAN D. J., AMSTUTZ H. C.: Treatment of neoplastic trochanteric fracture. Six cases treated with the Zickel nail. *Clinical Orthopaedics*, **97**, 108-113.

1973 SILVERBERG S. G., DE GIORGI L. S.: Osteoclastoma like giant-cell tumor of the thyroid. *Cancer*, **31**, 621-625.

1974 KATZNER M., PETIT R., SCHVINGT E.: Traitement chirurgical des métastases et des fractures métastatiques des os longs. A propos de 53 ostéosynthéses de confort. *Revue de Chirurgie Orthopedique*, **60**, 387-400.

1975 BLYTHE J. G., PTACEK J. J., BUCHSBAUM H. J., LATOURETTE H. B.: Bony Metastases from carcinoma of cervix. Occurrence, diagnosis, and treatment. *Cancer*, **36**, 475-484.

1976 DOUGLASS H. O. Jr., SHUKLA S. K., MINDELE E.: Treatment of pathological fractures of long bones excluding those due to breast cancer. *Journal of Bone and Joint Surgery*, **58-A**, 1055-1061.

1976 DUPARC J., DECOULX J.: *Le traitement des métastases osseuses*. Masson Ed., Paris.

1976 MEARY R., POSTEL M., TOMENO B., FOREST M., BROUT PH.: Fractures métestatiques du fémur. A propos de 100 cas. *Revue de Chirurgie Orthopedique*, **62**, 761-774.

1976 ZICKEL R. E., MOURADIAN W. H.: Intramedullary fixation of pathological fractures and lesions of the subtrochanteric region of the femur. *Journal of Bone and Joint Surgery*, **58-A**, 1061-1066.

1977 DURANDEAU A., GENESTE R.: Traitement chirurgical des fractures métastatiques et des métastases des os longs. A propos de 73 cas. *Revue de Chirurgie Orthopedique*, **63**, 501-517.

1977 OYASU R., BATTIFORA H. A., BUCKINGHAM W. B., HIDWEGI D.: Metaplastic squamous cell carcinoma of bronchus simulating giant cell tumor of bone. *Cancer*, **39**, 1119-1128.

1980   DEUTSCH A., RESNICK D.: Eccentric cortical metastases to the skeleton from bronchogenic carcinoma. *Radiology*, **137**, 49-52.

1982   SIMON M., KARLUK M.: Skeletal metastases of unknown origin. Diagnostic strategy for orthopaedic surgeons. *Clinical Orthopaedis*, **166**, 96-103.

1983   STOLL B.A., PARBHOO S.: *Bone metastasis: monitoring and treatment.* Raven Press, New York.

1986   GALASKO C.S.B.: *Skeletal metastases.* Butterworths, London.

1986   SIMON M., BARTUCCI E.: The search for the primary tumor in patients with skeletal metastases of unknown origin. *Cancer*, **58**, 1088-1095.

1987   LIBSON E., BLOOM R.A., HUSBAND J., STOCKER D.: Metastatic tumors of bones of the hand and foot. A comparative review and report of 43 additional cases. *Skeletal Radiology*, **16**, 387-392.

1987   NOTTEBAERT M., VON HOCHSTETTER A.R., EXNER G.U., SCHREIBER A.: Metastatic carcinoma of the spine. A study of 92 cases. *International Orthopaedics*, **11**, 345-248.

1988   GREENSPAN A., NORMAN A.: Osteolitic cortical destruction: an unusual pattern of skeletal metastases. *Skeletal Radiology*, **17**, 402-406.

1988   HARRINGTON K.D.: Anterior decompression and stabilization of the spine as a treatment for vertebral collapse and spinal cord compression for metastatic malignancy. *Clinical Orthopaedics*, **233**, 177-197.

1988   HARRINGTON K.D.: *Orthopaedic management of metastatic bone disease.* The C.V. Mosby Company, St. Louis.

1988   SIM F.H.: *Diagnosis and management of metastatic bone disease. A multidisciplinary approach.* Raven Press, New York.

1989   DUPARC J., HUTEN D., BENFRECH E.: Le traitement chirurgical des métastases du cotyle. *Revue de Chirurgie Orthopedique*, **75**, 1-10.

1989   HABERMAN E.T., LOPEZ R.A.: Metastatic disease of bone and treatment of pathological fractures. *Orthopaedic Clinics of North America*, **20**, 469-486.

1989   NOTTENBAERT M., EXNER G.U., VON HOCHSTETTER A.R., SCHREIBER A.: Metastatic bone disease from occult carcinoma: a profile. *International Orthopaedics*, **13**, 119-123.

1990   KATTAPURAM S.V., KHURANA J.S., SCOTT J.A., EL-KHOURY G.Y.: Negative scintigraphy with positive magnetic resonance imaging in bone metastases. *Skeletal Radiology*, **19**, 113-116.

1990   YAZAWA Y., FRASSICA F.J., CHAO E.Y.S., PRITCHARD D.J., SIM F.H., SHIVES T.C.: Metastatic bone disease. A study of the surgical treatment of 166 pathological humeral and femoral fractures. *Clinical Orthopaedics*, **251**, 213-219.

BONE METASTASES FROM NEUROBLASTOMA

Unique among non-epithelial tumors, N.B. (or sympathoblastoma) causes early and diffused skeletal metastases, which are of considerable clinical interest as they may occur prior to the clinical manifestation of the primary tumor or in any case dominate the clinical picture. N.B. is a malignant tumor which originates from the cells of the sympathetic nervous system. Thus, it generally develops in the retroperitoneal space, or in the posterior mediastinum, from the adrenal medulla, or from the sympathetic ganglia, but also from the sympathetic cells contained in the various tissues and organs.

N.B. is typical of **early childhood**, under 5 years of age, although it may be observed later and even during adult age. Bone metastases show predilection for the cranium, skeleton of the trunk, femur and humerus. Unlike osteolytic lesions in leukemia, these are rarely observed distal to the knee and elbow (Fig. 576).

The first **symptoms** may be caused by skeletal metastases. Often, they are

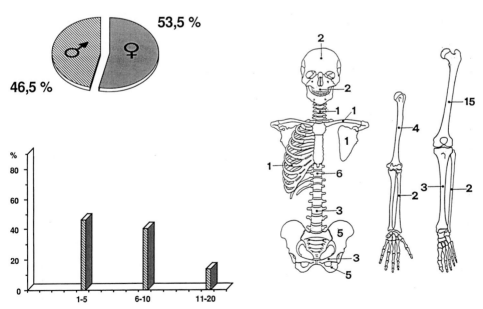

FIG. 576. - Sex, age and localization in 28 cases of bone metastases from neuroblastoma (56 localizations).

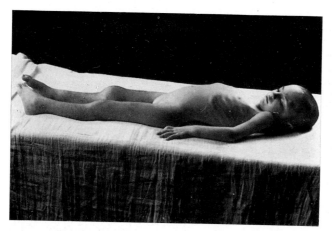

FIG. 577. - Female aged 5 years. Multiple metastases from neuroblastoma in the femurs, tibias, humerus and skull. Onset of symptoms 3 months previously. The patient died 5 months after this photograph was taken.

already multiple or diffused (at times, symmetrically), at diagnosis. In other cases the metastasis is initially solitary, particularly in a femur or a humerus. The most typical symptomatic association in advanced phases of the disease is constituted by soft swelling of the cranium, esophthalmus, enlargement of the preauricular and cervical lymph nodes, and those of other regions. The primary neoplastic mass may be symptomless for a long period of time. Metastases may occur in the liver, the kidney, and in the other organs, as well as in the skeleton and the lymph nodes. Often, there is fever and a worsening of the patients general state of health (Fig. 577).

The **radiographic aspect** of bone metastases is osteolytic and aggressive

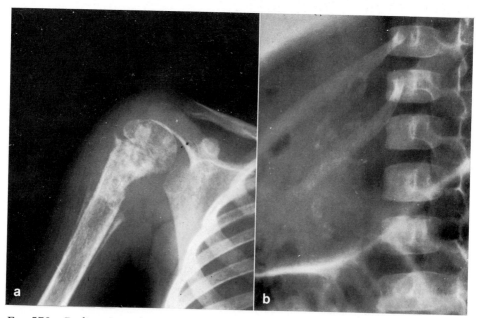

FIG. 578. - Radiograms of the same case as Fig. 577. (a) Metastasis in the proximal humerus. (b) Calcification in retroperitoneal primary tumor.

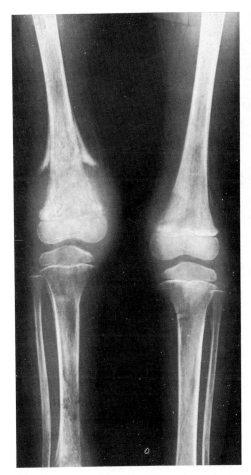

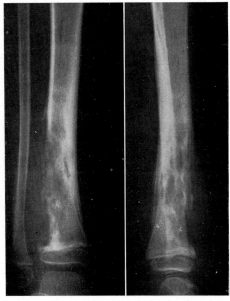

FIG. 580. - Female aged 3 years. Symptoms for the past 4 months. The radiographic aspect has suggested osteomyelitis. Shortly after this radiogram was obtained and biopsy was performed, other skeletal localizations occurred.

FIG. 579. - Metastases in the two femurs and in the tibias in the same case as that in Figs. 577, 578.

and it may resemble that of Ewing's sarcoma or even, more rarely, that of osteomyelitis or leukemia. When the neoplastic cells infiltrate the medullary spaces, the haversian canals, and the periosteum (as in Ewing's sarcoma) a faded moth-eaten aspect is observed, particularly of the metaphyseal cancellous bones, with porosity and small erosions of the cortical bone. In the diaphyses periosteal reaction is a frequent occurrence, which is in the form of laminae which may be superimposed on one another. This periostosis may be rather extended, even to the entire perimeter of an entire diaphysis. In diffused and polyostotic forms of the disease, faded osteoporosis of the metaphyses may be observed, similar to that of leukemia, but different in that it is mostly limited to the femurs and the humeri. In other cases there may be massive and expanded osteolysis, with cancelling of the cortices and periosteal reaction in the form of Codman's triangle (Figs. 578, 579). Faded osteolysis may also be observed in the cranium. Primary N.B. may appear on plain radiograms of the abdomen, as a suprarenal and retroperitoneal mass containing small faded areas of calcification (due to calcar precipitation in

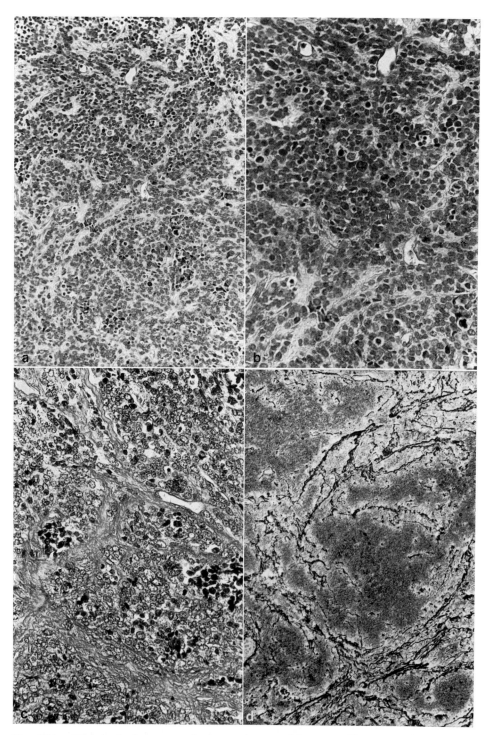

Fig. 581. - Histological aspects of metastatic neuroblastoma. The aspect is very similar to that of Ewing's sarcoma. Nonetheless, some large nuclei may be observed, as well as a certain amount of nuclear pleomorphism (*Hemat.-eos.* 200, 300 x; *Mallory* 300 x; *Argentic impregnation* 200 x).

the areas of necrosis, Fig. 578b). The abdominal or mediastinal mass is revealed by echography, angiography, CAT and MRI.

In order to diagnose N.B. it is important to show an increase in rinary **metabolites of catecholamine**.

Macroscopically, the tissue is encephaloid, at times hemorrhagic, at times liquescent and yellowish due to necrosis, possibly suggesting osteomyelitic pus.

Histologically, the aspect varies depending on the individual case and even within the same case, as the cells of the sympathoblastic line may show a different grade of differentiation from primary sympathoblast to gangliar cell. Nonetheless, in metastasizing N.B. more immature cellular aspects prevail or are exclusive. The tissue is densely cellular and the scarce fibro-vascular stroma delimits fields which are deprived of it (Fig. 581). The more immature cells are similar to lymphocytes, with scarce cytoplasm and a small round and dark nucleus. The less immature cells are somewhat larger, oval or piriform, with «flame-» or «tail-like» cytoplasmatic extensions, and their nuclei have a slightly vesicular aspect due to an evident nuclear membrane, distinct chromatin network, and evident nucleolus. Groups of cells at times appear to be surrounded and penetrated by bundles of parallel neurofibrillae, but the most typical aspect is constituted by rosettes. These are small round formations having nuclei at the periphery, and the center of which is formed by the intertwining of the cytoplasmatic fibrillary extensions. Often, these rather delicate fibrillae are damaged during fixation and resemble granular material, tenuously eosinophilic, or amorphous. The presence of the rosettes, however, is not constant. At times they are observed in the primary tumor and not in the metastasis; other times they are absent in both. The cytoplasms do not contain PAS positive granules of glycogen. Under electron microscopy intracytoplasmatic granules of neurosecretion (catecholamine) and neuritic processes are observed. In more immature forms, there is considerable cellular monomorphism. In less immature forms, instead, large cells are found alongside others which are lymphocyte-like. Mitotic figures are not frequently observed.

Histological differential **diagnosis** with Ewing's sarcoma is a classic and often difficult one to make. It is based on the rosettes, on the presence of bundles of neurofibrillae, on the presence of more differentiated sympathetic cells, on the absence of cellular glycogen, on electron microscopy, on age and clinical features, on the increase in urinary catecholamines (see diagnosis of Ewing's sarcoma).

The **prognosis** of N.B., even if metastasizing, is not invariably fatal. There are cases of long survival and perhaps healing obtained by radiation **therapy** and antiblastics. There are also undebatable cases of spontaneous regression: this nearly always occurs in patients aged under 6 months. Elements which seem to be associated with a less severe prognosis are: age under 2 years, scarce initial alteration of metabolism of catecholamines and rapid normalization with therapy, histological aspects of cellular differentiation.

REFERENCES

1968   REILLY D., NESBT M. E., KRIVIT W.: Cure of three patients who had skeletal metastases in disseminated neuroblastoma. *Pediatrics*, **41**, 47-51.

1970   GITLOW S. E., BERTANI L. M., RAUSEN A., GRIBETZ D., DZIEDZIC S. W.: Diagnosis of neuroblastoma by qualitative and quantitative determination of catecholamine metabolites in urine. *Cancer*, **25**, 1377-1383.

1971   EVANS A. E., D'ANGIO G. J., RANDOLPH J.: A proposed staging for children with neuroblastoma. *Cancer*, **27**, 374-378.

1972   MÄKINEN J.: Microscopic patterns as a guide to prognosis of neuroblastoma in childhood. *Cancer*, **29**, 1637-1646.

1973   GITLOW S. E., DZIEDZIC L. B., STRAUSS L., GREENWOOD S. M., DZIEDZIC S. W.: Biocemical and histologic determinants in the prognosis of neuroblastoma. *Cancer*, **32**, 898-905.

1973   LIEBNER E. J., ROSENTHAL I. M.: Serial catecholamines in the radiation management of children with neuroblastoma. *Cancer*, **32**, 623-633.

1975   KOOP C. E., SCHNAUFER L.: The management of abdominal neuroblastoma. *Cancer*, **35**, 905-909.

1976   EVANS A. E., ALBO V., D'ANGIO G. J., FINKLESTEIN J. Z., LEIKEN S., SANTULLI TH., WEINER J., HAMMOND G. D.: Cyclophosphamide treatment of patients with localized and regional neuroblastoma. A randomized study. *Cancer*, **38**, 655-660.

1976   EVANS A. E., ALBO V., D'ANGIO G. J., FINKLESTEIN J. Z., LEIKEN S., SANTULLI TH., WEINER J., HAMMOND G. D.: Factors influencing survival of children with nonmetastatic neuroblastoma. *Cancer*, **38**, 661-666.

1978   DOSIK G. M., RODRIGUEZ V., BENJAMIN R. S., BODEY G. P.: Neuroblastoma in the adult. Effective combination chemotherapy. *Cancer*, **41**, 56-63.

1978   ROMANSKY S. G., CROCKER D. W., SHAW K. N. F.: Ultrastructural studies on neuroblastoma. Evaluation of cytodifferentiation and correlation of morphology and biochemical and survival data. *Cancer*, **42**, 2392-2398.

1987   DAUBENTON J.D., FISHER R.M., KARABUS C.D., MANN M.D.: The relationship between prognosis and scintigraphic evidence of bone metastases in neuroblastoma. *Cancer*, **59**, 1586-1589.

1987   EVANS A.E., D'ANGIÒ G.J., PROPERT K., ANDERSON J., HANN H.L.: Prognostic factors in neuroblastoma. *Cancer*, **59**, 1853-1859.

1988   BROOK F.B., RAAFAT F., ELDEEB B.B., MANN J.R.: Histologic and immunohistochemical investigation of neuroblastomas and correlation with prognosis. *Human Pathology*, **19**, 879-888.

1988   OPPEDAL B.R., STORM-MATHISEN I., LIE S.O., BRANDTZAEG P.: Prognostic factors in neuroblastoma. Clinical, histopathological and immunohistochemical features and DNA ploidy in relation to prognosis. *Cancer*, **62**, 772-780.

1989   OPPEDAL B.R., STORM-MATHISEN I., KEMSHEAD J.T., BRANDTZAEG P.: Bone marrow examination in neuroblastoma patients. A morphologic, immunocytochemical and immunohistochemical study. *Human Pathology*, **20**, 800-805.

1990   HALL-CRAGGS M.A., SHAW D., PRITCHARD J., GORDON I.: Metastatic neuroblastoma: new abnormalities on bone scintigraphy may not indicate tumour recurrence. *Skeletal Radiology*, **19**, 33-36.

1990   TAYLOR S.R., LOCKER J.: A comparative analysis of DNA content and N-myc gene amplification in neuroblastoma. *Cancer*, **65**, 1360-1366.

PSEUDOTUMORS
OF BONE

BONE CYST
(Synonyms: simple, solitary, monocavitary, juvenile bone cyst)

DEFINITION

It is a cystic lesion characterized by serous contents, initiating from the metaphysis and developing during the growth age. Its nature is probably atrophic-degenerative and its etiopathogenesis unknown.

FREQUENCY

B.C. is a frequent occurrence, second only to histiocytic fibroma and exostosis.

SEX

Incidence is clearly greater in the male sex, at a ratio of more than 2:1 (Fig. 582).

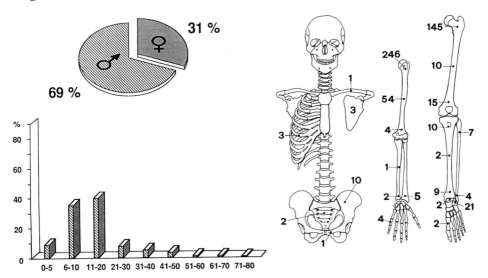

Fig. 582. - Sex, age and localization in 563 cases of bone cyst. In many typical localizations (proximal humerus and femur, calcaneus) diagnosis was only radiographic. In the other sites, diagnosis was surgical and histological.

AGE

It may be observed at any age (from a few months to 60 years of age). Nonetheless, when symptoms occur most patients are aged from 5 to 15 years. B.C. is rarely revealed — by radiographic examination carried out for other reasons or due to the presence of symptoms — prior to 5 and after 20 years of age (Fig. 582).

LOCALIZATION

Most cases of B.C. are localized in the proximal humerus or — less frequently — in the proximal femur. All of the other localizations are rare. Schematically, out of 100 cysts 55 are located in the proximal humerus, 25 in the proximal femur and 20 in other sites. Among the latter localization is as follows and in this order: the calcaneus, the other metaphyses of the long bones, the pelvis, the tubular bones of the hand and foot (Fig. 582).

In the long bones B.C. always initiates in the metaphysis, close to the growth cartilage of the epiphysis or of the apophysis (for example, the greater trochanter). With time it tends

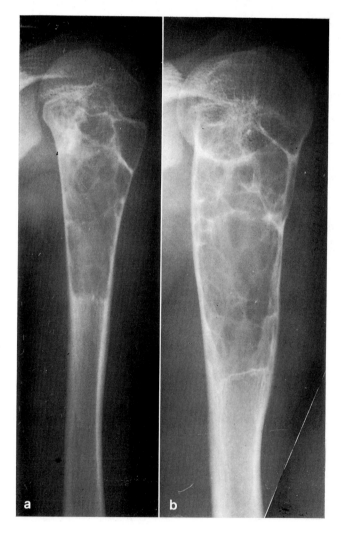

FIG. 583. - (a) Male aged 8 years. Four months earlier pathologic fracture had occurred. (b) The same case 5 years later. The cyst had been curetted and bone grafted and there had been recurrence.

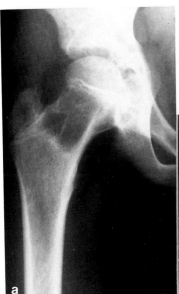

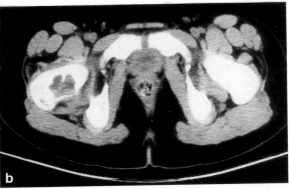

FIG. 584. - (a) and (b) Bone cyst in a girl aged 10 years.

to move farther away from the fertile cartilage and towards the diaphysis. B.C. which have migrated towards the center of the diaphyseal length are frequently observed in the humerus; in the femur, instead, B.C. rarely descends below the proximal diaphysis (Fig. 589). In the humerus, there is a relationship between age and the position of the B.C.: B.C. adjacent to the growth cartilage are more frequently seen during the first 5 years of age, while metadiaphyseal B.C. increase from 5 to 10 years of age, and those in the diaphysis from 10 to 15 years of age and during successive years. B.C. in the calcaneus is always localized in the anterior portion, where the trabecular system physiologically leaves a relatively empty space.

SYMPTOMS

B.C. is typically painless and thus symptomless until pathologic fracture occurs. This, in fact, occurs frequently (in approximately 80% of all diagnosed cases) due to the thinness of the cystic bony wall. Incomplete or complete fracture generally occurs after moderate trauma; in the humerus it may be the muscular effort of throwing a stone, in the femur simple weight-bearing.

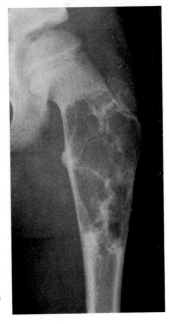

FIG. 585. - Male aged 7 years. Bone cyst, originating in the metaphysis of the greater trochanter.

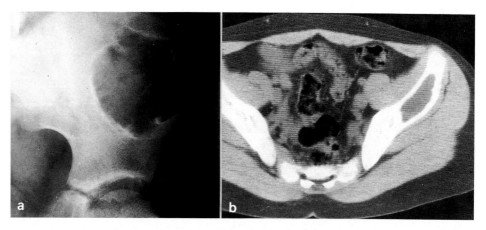

FIG. 586. - (a) and (b) Bone cyst in a boy aged 9 years. Diagnosis was ascertained histologically.

B.C. rarely causes a bone swelling (very expanded humeral cyst, cyst of the fibula, tibia, wrist, of a metacarpus or a metatarsus). At times, it remains symptomless until adult age or for an entire lifetime. B.C. of the calcaneus and of the iliac bone are usually discovered during adult age and/or by chance as they do not cause fracture. At times, there is shortening of the humerus or the femur, particularly in rather expanded B.C. and in cases previously operated (Fig. 591). The shortening may be unrelated to any previous surgery.

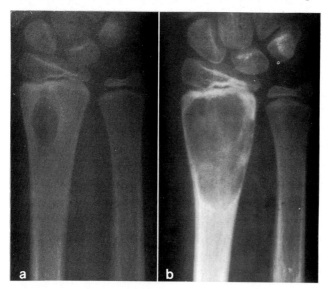

FIG. 587. - Female aged 8 years. (a) Initial bone cyst revealed by chance after trauma. (b) The same case 8 months later. Diagnosis was confirmed histologically.

RADIOGRAPHIC FEATURES

Only exceptionally is B.C. observed radiographically at the onset (Fig. 587), as it remains symptomless until it has so weakened the bone that fracture occurs. What we do know is the radiographic picture of expanded B.C. (Figs. 583, 584, 585, 586). It is a central osteolysis, which is intensely diaphanous, and which considerably attenuates and mildly expands the cortex for the entirety of its perimeter. Its limits are well-defined, but there is no or very thin osteosclerotic rim. Although the cortex is ten-uous, it is always continuous and there is no trace of periostal reaction unless fracture has occurred. The osteolytic cavity is generally traversed by «nerves» corresponding to thin parietal bone crests. Nonetheless, the cavity is not always unique. In some cases, as may be observed by injecting contrast medium in the cyst, the cavity is separated by fibrous or thin bony septa. In most cases which come to medical atten-tion, there is patholog-ic fracture with very little displacement, or incomplete fracture of the cystic wall. In ca-ses where there is frac-ture, a fragment of the thin bony wall may be observed to have «fal-len» inside the cavity (Fig. 599). B.C. only ex-ceptionally surpasses the growth cartilage and extends to the epi-physis; but this may occur during child-hood and with no pre-vious surgery (Fig. 590).

B.C. of the calca-neus rarely contains a radiopaque core simi-lar to that of necrotic bone sequester (Fig. 588b).

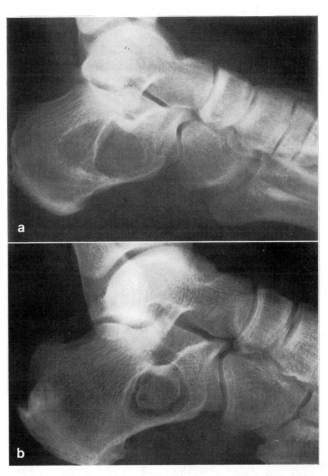

FIG. 588. - (a) Female aged 33 years. Chance radiographic finding, which remained unchanged for 6 years. (b) Fe-male aged 32 years. Asymptomatic lesion. Observe the island of radiopacity within the cystic area.

GROSS PATHOLOGIC FEATURES

The periosteum is always intact. It may be lacerated when there is a dis-placed pathologic fracture. After it has been incised and easily detached, the cortex appears slightly expanded and remarkably attenuated, and often blu-ish in color due to the serohematic content of the cyst. Often, the cortex is thin and as fragile as an eggshell or a sheet of paper; here and there there may be

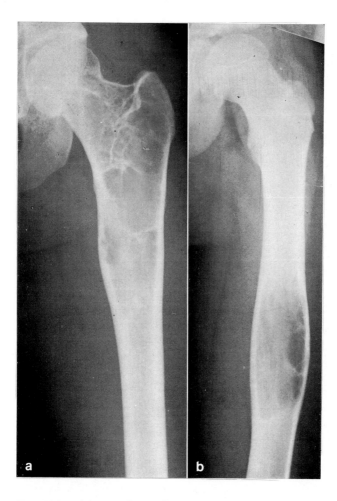

FIG. 589. - (a) Female aged 22 years. (b) Male aged 10 years. Diaphyseal migration of femoral cysts is a rare occurrence.

some small lacunae which allow the internal fluid to ooze.

At times, in cystic localizations which allow for surgery under hemostatic tourniquet, the bony wall of the B.C. may be observed to be poorly blood-supplied.

Within there is a single cavity, which may be septated, filled with fluid similar to serum (even chemically), if the B.C. is intact; serohematic or hematic fluid mixed with clots if there has been pathologic fracture.

The internal wall of the B.C. is matted everywhere (even towards the metaphyseal cancellous bone and the medullary canal of the diaphysis) by a thin, smooth connective membrane which is easily detached from the bone, soft and fragile, which may even form some septa. Usually, a rather expanded B.C. never gives more than two or three «curettesful» of this fibrous material. If pathologic fracture or surgery occurred much beforehand, the cavity tends to contain more abundant solid material, yellow-brown in color (due to the presence of lipoids and hemosiderin), which at times is gritty because it contains bony detritus and trabeculae. This material derives from the organization of the clots and from residues of previous bone grafts. Even in rare occasions of B.C. operated during adult age, the cavity may be found to be partially occupied by soft fibrous tissue, yellow-brown in color in some areas, subdividing it into multiple cavities with a fluid content.

HISTOPATHOLOGIC FEATURES

The membrane of the B.C. is made up of aspecific loose collagen the cells of which may assume a vaguely endotheliomorphous attitude at the surface (Fig. 592). In this connective tissue small hemorrhagic effusions and hemosiderin are observed, a few newly-formed bone trabeculae, few macrophages and multinucleate giant cells, scattered lymphomonocytary infiltrates. In short, this is the reactive and repair connective tissue that may be observed at the margins of skeletal lesions of varying nature.

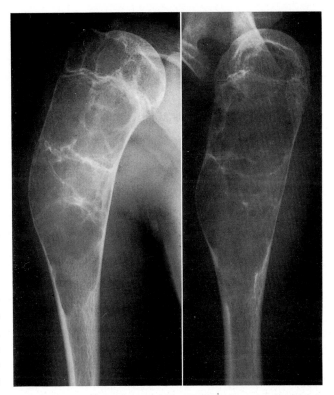

Fig. 590. - Female aged 13 years. The bone cyst, which was untreated, involved the epiphysis. This is an exceptional finding.

What is most typical — because it is observed in most cases and because it is nearly exclusive of B.C. — is the presence of globular to trabecular masses of a pseudofibrin material which does not contain cells and which is not bordered by osteoblasts. At times it calcifies, at times it gradually merges with osteoid trabeculae, at times osteoid-osteoblastic rims are deposited on its borders (Figs. 593, 594).

The bony wall of B.C. is constituted by newly-formed bone where, as it is expanded, the primary cortex no longer exists. It is a bone with rather wide haversian canals, generally not very vascularized (Fig. 592b).

In the site where the membrane of the B.C. is in contact with the metaphyseal cancellous bone, there is no reactive osteosclerosis. The metaphyseal trabecular fringe usually continues to grow even in contact with the B.C. In some cases, however, where the B.C. exerts considerable pressure on the cartilage, it may be disturbed in its normal growth.

In B.C. with an old pathologic fracture or in previously operated B.C., more abundant connective tissue occupies the cavity, with deposits of hemosiderin, bunches of cholesterin crystals, macrophages, and giant cells, bony detritus and rare newly-formed bone trabeculae (Fig. 595). In some aged forms in the adult, the tissue partially filling the cyst is similar to this, but more fibrous and mature.

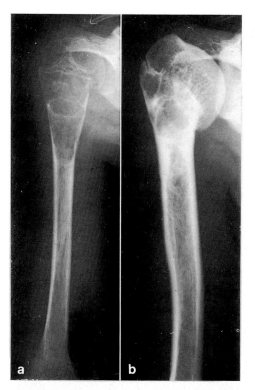

FIG. 591. - (a) Male aged 8 years. The patient was submitted to curettage and bone grafting. (b) After 7 years the cyst was repaired but there was early closing of the growth cartilage with marked shortening of the humerus.

◀

FIG. 592. - Histological aspects of the wall of the cyst (*Hemat.-eos.*, 50, 125 x).

▼

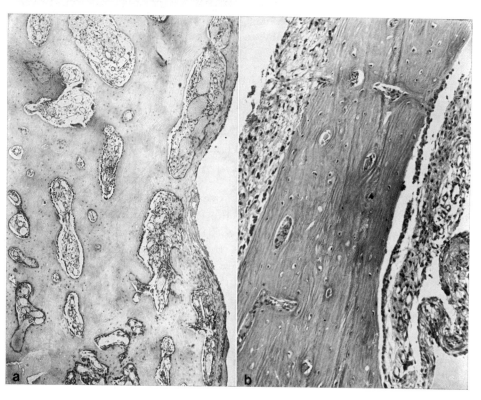

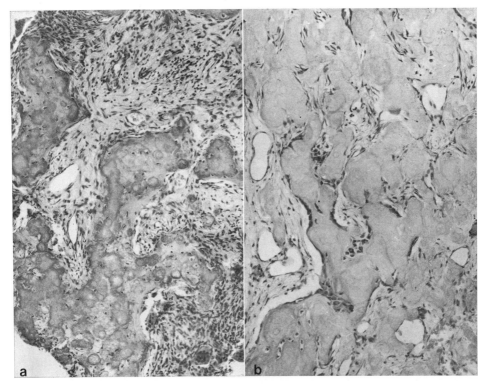

FIG. 593. - Histological aspects of the sui generis material produced by the bone cyst. Common opinion is that this is coagulated fibrin material (*Hemat.-eos.*, 125, 125 x).

PATHOGENESIS

The pathogenesis of B.C. remains a mystery. The probable cause should be searched for in an alteration in the circulatory regimen of the metaphysis during growth, which causes bone resorption and the accumulation of the serum fluid at the center of the metaphysis. No pathologic phenomenon of the bone is known, secondary to a definite cause, which may even slightly resemble B.C. Nor has a lesion similar to B.C. ever been reproduced experimentally. Probably, B.C. of the calcaneus, which are not adjacent to the growth cartilage of the greater tuberosity, have a different pathogenesis from that of metaphyseal B.C.

DIAGNOSIS

Diagnosis is generally easy, and it may even be based solely on clinical-radiographic data: age, localization in the proximal humerus (in the adult in the humeral diaphysis) or in the proximal femur, absence of symptoms until pathologic fracture, radiographic picture. Diagnosis is practically certain if serohematic fluid is extracted from the cavity with a needle, or if the typical

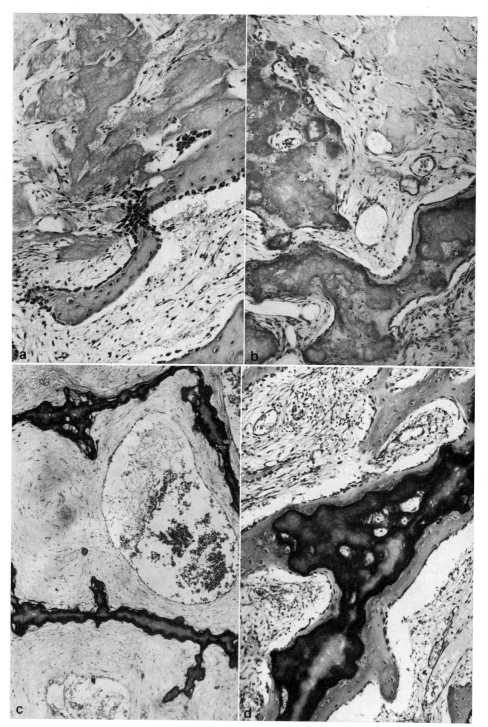

FIG. 594. - (a) and (b) Gradual passage of the fibrinoid material to newly-formed bone trabeculae. (c) Calcified fibrinoid material. (d) The same on which osteoid is laid (*Van Gieson*, 125 x, *Hemat.-eos.*, 125, 50, 125 x).

gross pathologic features are observed during surgery. A histological examination is a further confirmation. Another localization where B.C. is radiographically typical is in the calcaneus. In the other sites, rare ones, B.C. is not unequivocally suggested, and radiographic examination involves differential diagnosis with several other lesions. **Aneurysmal bone cyst**: it is eccentric and very expanding, often initiating subperiosteally; even when it is central, it may initiate far from the growth cartilage, unlike bone cyst. Nonetheless, rarely aneurysmal bone cyst may occupy the entire metaphysis and be totally identical to a B.C.; it more easily invades the epiphysis but this is also a possibility in B.C. There may still be doubts even after macroscopic and histological examinations have been carried out. In fact, there are

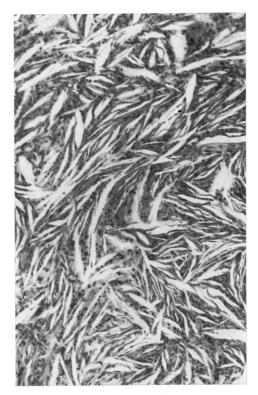

Fig. 595. - Bunches of cholesterin crystals in a fibrohistiocytary context (*Van Gieson* 125 x).

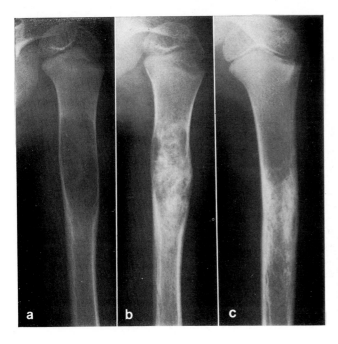

Fig. 596. - (a) Bone cyst in a child aged 6 years. Recurrence after curettage and bone grafting. (b) Six months after two cortisone infiltrations. (c) Healing after 2 years.

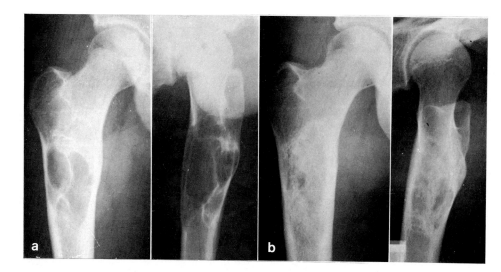

FIG. 597. - (a) Male aged 13 years. Bone cyst recurring after curettage bone grafting. The patient was treated with three injections of cortisone. (b) Result after 2 years.

fractured B.C. filled with blood clots which are partially organized, with numerous giant cells; and «mature» aneurysmal bone cysts containing only serous fluid and having scarce and thin fibro-hyalin walls (and septa), suggesting the membrane of B.C.

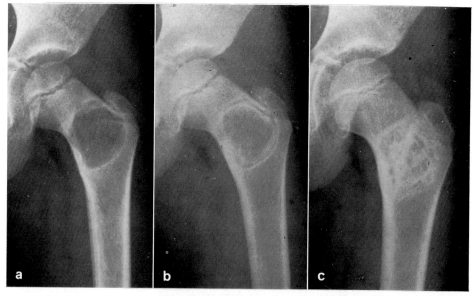

FIG. 598. - (a) Male aged 7 years. (b) Eight months later, after two injections of cortisone. (c) After 2 years. At 11 years of age there was nonetheless recurrence of the cyst.

In the adult, a circumscribed **fibrous dysplasia** may in all respects resemble ancient B.C. (see fibrous dysplasia).

ACTIVE AND INACTIVE CYSTS

Active cysts have the following features: age under 10-12 years; localization in contact with the fertile cartilage; radiographically, single cavity

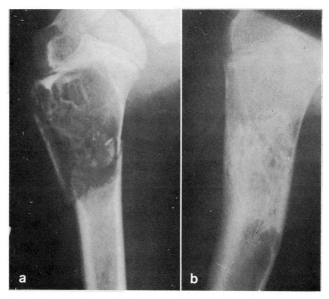

FIG. 599. - Male aged 11 years. (a) Untreated bone cyst. (b) Result 22 months after two injections of cortisone.

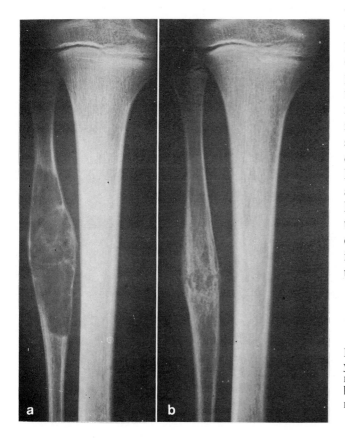

with very thin bony wall; high intracystic pressure (more than 30 cm of water) with a pulsating column; after injection of contrast medium in the cyst, rapid resorption of the same in the venous circulation. **Inactive cysts** have opposite features: age over 10-12 years; localization far from the fertile cartilage; radiographically the cavity appears to be multilocular with a thick

FIG. 600. - Male aged 10 years. (a) Bone cyst. Diagnosis was ascertained by biopsy. (b) Result 18 months after three injections of cortisone.

bony wall; intracystic pressure equal to venous pressure (6-10 cm of water) with a non-pulsating column; persistence of the contrast medium in the cyst for several seconds or minutes.

COURSE

B.C. probably initiates prior to 10-12 years of age, as a small metaphyseal area of central osteolysis. Then, it develops rather rapidly, as particularly revealed by the numerous observations of post-treatment recurrence, occupying all of the metaphysis within a few months-1 year.

As long as B.C. is active, with considerable accumulation of fluid, it compresses the metaphyseal growing trabeculae enough to resorb them as they form. Thus, the B.C. stays in contact with the fertile cartilage possibly altering it and causing shortening of the bone. When the activity of the B.C. decreases, the metaphyseal trabeculae are not completely resorbed and the B.C. moves farther away from the growth cartilage until it reaches (particularly in the humerus) the center of the diaphysis.

As previously observed, there is an evident relationship between age and the activity of the B.C., in the sense that, after 15 years, they are usually located far from the cartilage and more or less inactive. Even post-treatment recurrence never occurs after 15 years of age. **Thus, the activity of he B.C. is gradually exhausted as skeletal maturation occurs**.

Pathologic fracture in B.C. rapidly and constantly consolidates. The function of the periosteum is not impaired. Pathologic fracture has little influence on the development of the cyst. Only exceptionally does B.C. repair subsequent to a fracture treated nonsurgically.

TREATMENT AND PROGNOSIS

In the past B.C. was submitted to curettage and bone grafting. When this technique was used the incidence of recurrence was 20-30%. In order to have a higher probability of success, it would be necessary to remove more than half of the bony wall, considerably saucerizing the cavity, or even resecting the entire bone segment containing the cyst, preserving the periosteum alone.

This type of surgery has practically disappeared since the introduction (Scaglietti, 1973) of nonsurgical treatment with the infiltration of methyl-prednisolone acetate (Depomedrol).

Above all, the fact that B.C. does not require biopsy, that it does not cause any symptoms, and that it ends up healing spontaneously after puberty must not be overlooked. Thus, it is worth treating only those cases of B.C. which risk fracture during pre-puberal age. Those which do not run this risk because of localization (ilium, calcaneus), or because they are provided with a rather thick unloaded bony wall, or where it is presumed that the wall will spontaneously and soon become stronger because the cyst is inactive and age is close to or has surpassed the end of skeletal growth, do not require any type of treatment.

Treatment consists in penetrating the cavity wih two needles used for skeletal biopsy, extracting the fluid, using physiological solution to cleanse with pressure, finally removing one needle and with the other injecting a quantity of Depomedrol approximately equal to the fluid extracted. This treatment must be repeated every 2 months.

Generally, from 2 to 5 infiltrations are required. The first radiographic signs of repair are observed after approximately 6 months. They consist in a ground glass ossification of the cystic area, which gradually matures totally obliterate the cavity (Figs. 596, 597, 599, 600). At times some minor cavities remain (when the cyst was concamerated), or a radiolucent rim between the repair bone and the walls of the cyst (Fig. 598b). Recurrences of the cyst often originate from these residues. These recurrences, too, depending on expansion and age, may either be left untreated or further infiltrated.

Occasionally B.C. does not respond to local steroids. When this occurs, and particularly if the cyst appears to expand, a different diagnosis can be suspected and biopsy is indicated.

B.C. of calcaneus and those in adult age do not respond to local steroids. Treatment in such cases in usually unnecessary.

Generally, pathologic fracture does not change the indication. In conclusion, surgery is limited to exceptional cases of B.C. of the lower limb with displaced fracture, where reduction-osteosynthesis is indicated. Or, to rare cases with an anomalous site and radiographic progressiveness, where diagnosis is uncertain and biopsy is indicated.

In more than 90% of the cases B.C. is not a surgical disease. The action mechanism of cortisone is not known, but it has been shown that even simple repeated extractions of cystic fluid may have the same effect. In any case, even without treatment, B.C. ends up improving during adult age, with reinforcement of the bony wall which, providing mechanical strength, is equal to healing.

REFERENCES

1942 JAFFE H. L., LICHTENSTEIN L.: Solitary unicameral bone cyst. With emphasis on the roentgen picture, the pathologic appearance and the pathogenesis. *Archives of Surgery*, **44**, 1004-1025.

1948 JAMES A. G., COLEY B. L., HIGINBOTHAM N. L.: Solitary (unicameral) bone cyst. *Archives of Surgery*, **57**, 137-147.

1958 LODWICK G. S.: Juvenile unicameral bone cyst. A roentgen reappraisal. *American Journal of Roentgenology*, **80**, 495-504.

1959 FONTANILLAS J. L.: Necrosi avascolare asettica del calcagno. *Archivio di ortopedia*, **72**, 649-654.

1960 COHEN J.: Simple bone cysts. Study of cyst fluid in six cases with a theory of pathogenesis. *Journal of Bone and Joint Surgery*, **42-A**, 609-616.

1962 JOHNSON L., VETTER H., PUTSCHAR W. G.: Sarcomas arising in bone cysts. *Archives of Pathology*, **335**, 428-451.

1964 SADLER A. H., ROSENHAIN F.: Occurrence of two unicameral bone cysts in the same patient. *Journal of Bone and Joint Surgery*, **46-A**, 1557-1560.

1968 BRODER H. M.: Possible precursor of unicameral bone cysts. *Journal of Bone* and Joint Surgery, **50-A**, 503-507.

1969 FREIDMAN N. B., GOLDMAN R. L.: Cementoma of long bones. An extragnathic odontogenic tumor. *Clinical Orthopaedics*, **67**, 243-248.

1969 SPENCE K. F., SELL K. W., BROWN R. H.: Solitary bone cyst: Treatment with freezedried cancellous bone allograft. A study of one hundred seventyseven cases. *Journal of Bone and Joint Surgery*, **51-A**, 87-96.

1970 COHEN J.: Etiology of simple bone cist. *Journal of Bone and Joint Surgery*, **52-A**, 1493-1497.

1973 CAMPANACCI M., DE SESSA L., BELLANDO RANDONE P.: Cisti ossea. Revisione di 275 osservazioni. *Chirurgia degli Organi di Movimento*, **62**, 569-576.

1974 GRABIAS S., MANKIN H. J.: Chondrosarcoma arising in histologically proved unicameral bone cyst. *Journal of Bone and Joint Surgery*, **56-A**, 1501-1509.

1974 MOURGUES DE G., FISCHER L., CARRET J. P., MOYEN B.: Le kyste essentiel de l'os. A propos de huit observations revue après un long recul et d'une revue de 310 cas de la littérature. *Acta Orthopaedica Belgica*, **40**, 45-70.

1976 NELSON J. PH., FOSTER R. J.: Solitary bone cyst with epiphyseal involvement. A case report. *Clinical Orthopaedics*, **118**, 147-150.

1976 SPENCE K. F., BRIGHT R. W., FITZGERALD S. P., SELL K. W.: Solitary unicameral bone cyst: treatment with freeze-dried crushed cortical-bone allograft. *Journal of Bone and Joint Surgery*, **58-A**, 636-641.

1977 CAMPANACCI M., DE SESSA L., TRENTANI C.: Cura incruenta della cisti ossea con iniezioni locali di metilprednisolone acetato secondo Scaglietti. *Giornale Italiano di Ortopedia e Traumatologia*, **3**, 27-36.

1977 MCKAY D. W., NASON S. S.: Treatment of unicameral bone cysts by subtotal resection without grafts. *Journal of Bone and Joint Surgery*, **59-A**, 515-519.

1979 SANERKIN N. G.: Old fibrin coagula and their ossification in simple bone cysts. *Journal of Bone and Joint Surgery*, **61-B**, 194-199.

1979 SCAGLIETTI O., MARCHETTI P. G., BARTOLOZZI P.: The effects of methylprednisolone acetate in the treatment of bone cysts. Results of three years follow-up. *Journal of Bone and Joint Surgery*, **61-B**, 200-204.

1979 SCHNEPP J., MARCHETTI N., BARTAS J., BARTOLOZZI P., BEDOUELLE J., CARRÈ J. P., KOHLER R., NEZELOFF CH., SERINGE R.: Les kystes essentiels osseux (Table Ronde). *Revue de Chirurgie Ortopedique*, **65**, 3-10.

1980 WEISEL A., HECHT H.: Development of a unicameral bone cyst. Case report. *Journal of Bone and Joint Surgery*, **62-A**, 664-666.

1981 MCGLYNN F.J., MICKELSON M.R., EL-KHOURY G.: The fallen fragment sign in unicameral bone cyst. *Clinical Orthopaedics*, **156**, 157-159.

1982 CAPANNA R., DAL MONTE A., GITELIS S., CAMPANACCI M.: The natural history of unicameral bone cyst after steroid injection. *Clinical Orthopaedics*, **166**, 204-211.

1984 CAPANNA R., ALBISINNI N., CAROLI G.C., CAMPANACCI M.: Contrast examination as a prognostic factor in the treatment of solitary bone cyst by cortisone injection. *Skeletal Radiology*, **12**, 97-102.

1986 CAMPANACCI M., CAPANNA R., PICCI P.: Unicameral and aneurysmal bone cysts. *Clinical Orthopaedics*, **204**, 25-36.

1986 CAPANNA R., VAN HORN J., RUGGIERI P., BIAGINI R.: Epiphyseal involvement in unicameral bone cysts. *Skeletal Radiology*, **15**, 428-432.

1989 KAELIN A.J., MAC EWEN G.D.: Unicameral bone cysts. Natural history and the risk of fracture. *International Orthopaedics*, **13**, 275-282.

1989 MAKLEY J.T., JOYCE M.J.: Unicameral bone cyst (simple bone cyst). *Orthopaedic Clinics of North America*, **20**, 407-415.

1989 STRUHL S., EDELSON C., PRITZKER H., SEIMON L.P., DORFMAN H.D.: Solitary (unicameral) bone cyst. The fallen fragment sign revisited. *Skeletal Radiology*, **18**, 261-265.

1990 FARBER J.M., STANTON R.P.: Treatment options in unicameral bone cysts. *Orthopaedics*, **13**, 25-32.

ANEURYSMAL BONE CYST

DEFINITION

It is a pseudotumoral lesion of bone, which is expansive and hyperemic, frequently initiating from the surface of the bone. Its genesis is unknown and its nature is hyperplastic and hyperemic-hemorrhagic.

FREQUENCY

A.B.C. does not occur frequently. For example, it is twice less frequent than giant cell tumor.

SEX

There is predilection for the female sex (Fig. 601).

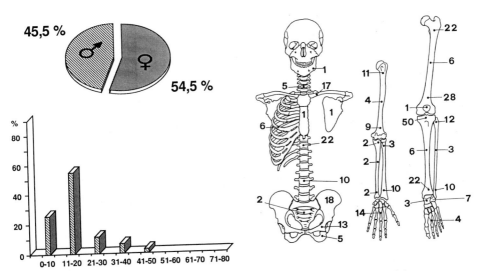

FIG. 601. - Sex, age and localization in 332 cases of aneurysmal bone cyst.

AGE

Although it may be observed at any age, it distinctly predominates from 10 to 20 years of age. Approximately 3/4 of all cases are observed under 20 years of age (in contrast with giant cell tumor which is rare before 20 years). It rarely occurs after 30 years of age, and it is exceptional after 50 years (Fig. 601).

LOCALIZATION

It has been observed in every site of the skeleton. Nonetheless, it shows evident predilection for the long bones and for the vertebral column. From 10 to 20% of cases are observed in the vertebrae and this constitutes an important peculiarity of the lesion (which is found among benign tumors of the skeleton only in osteoblastoma). The most common sites are, in this order: the long bones of the lower limb; the vertebral column; the long bones of the upper limb; the pelvis, clavicle (usually its medial end), tubular bones of the hand and foot, tarsus, cranio-facial bones (Fig. 601).

In the vertebral column it more often involves the posterior arch and the body together. As it expands, it may invade the nearby vertebrae. In the long bones it is preferably localized in the metaphysis or at one end of the diaphysis. Mid-diaphyseal localizations are not a frequent finding. It never originates in an epiphysis. It rarely surpasses the growth cartilage but, particularly during adult age, it may spread to the epiphysis. Wherever located, A.B.C. often seems to initiate at the surface of the bone and more precisely under the periosteum. From here it expands, bulging the periosteum and eroding the underlying cortical and cancellous bone.

SYMPTOMS

Pain and swelling are the main symptoms. Swelling, which may be more or less painful, is a frequent and important element in the clinical picture, due to the superficiality of the lesion, and its tendency to blow out. In approximately 1/3 of all cases the onset of symptoms is related to trauma; pathologic fracture, unlike what occurs in bone cyst, is rare. Not exceptionally (and this should not be surprising if we think of the hyperemic-hemorrhagic nature of the lesion) do symptoms occur or worsen during pregnancy.

In vertebral localizations of the disease there may be signs of myelo-radicular compression. At times, these signs are progressive, at other times they initiate suddenly when pathologic collapse of the vertebral body or rapid hemorrhagic expansion occur.

In expanded forms of the disease (particularly in the adult) and those extended as far as a joint surface, there may be limited range of movement and effusion of the joint.

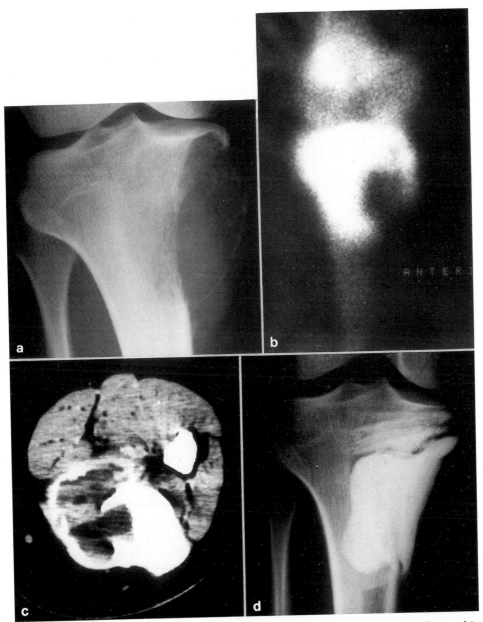

FIG. 602. - Aneurysmal bone cyst in a girl aged 17 years. (a) Typical radiographic aspect. (b) Bone scan shows a cold area at the center of the cyst. (c) CAT reveals expansion of the periosteum and the fluid content. (d) The patient was submitted to curettage, phenol, autogenous cortical grafting (from the tibial diaphysis) under the tibial plateau, and cement.

In rare cases, A.B.C. may become of monstruous size and give the clinical impression (and, as we shall see, radiographic, as well) of a malignant tumor.

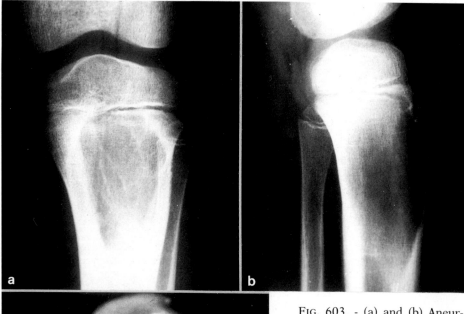

FIG. 603. - (a) and (b) Aneurysmal bone cyst in a boy aged 8 years. (c) CAT shows the typical horizontal level of the fluid content.

RADIOGRAPHIC FEATURES

If the radiographic progression of A.B.C. could be followed in its entire course, the radiographic diagnosis would often reveal rather typical elements enough to make it a sound diagnosis. On the contrary, the observation of the radiograms of an advanced and expanded A.B.C. may give the impression of a central tumor of the bone, even when the origin is subperiosteal; in other cases, a single radiogram may suggest the diagnosis of a malignant bone tumor.

Approximately half of all cases of A.B.C. radiographically show a subperiosteal origin (Fig. 604a); the others seem to initiate within the bone (Fig. 604b) although eccentrically, or they do not allow for recognition of ther origin as they are too expanded.

1) **Subperiosteal A.B.C.**

These are gener-ally localized in the dia-physis or the meta-diaphysis of a long bone (Figs. 602, 604a, 605, 609, 613b, 620, 623, 633). In the short and flat bones based on the radiographic picture it is generally difficult to establish whether the origin is central or subperio-steal. Nonetheless, there are cases in the vertebral column and

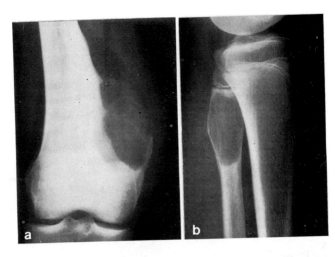

FIG. 604. - (a) Aneurysmal bone cysts. Female aged 16 years. (b) Female aged 13 years.

the pelvis where the lesion clearly appears to be oriented towards the skel-etal surface.

From the onset there is ballooning elevation of the periosteum, with un-derlying superficial erosion of the cortex (Fig. 605). At first the periosteal ele-vation may be invisible (unless ar-teriography, Figs. 606, 613b, or CAT or MRI are used) because there is not yet osteogenetic reaction; and, as erosion of the underlying cortex, which is also purely osteolytic, has rather fuzzy boundaries, a malig-nant neoplasm may be sugges-ted.

In a successive phase, the uplift-ed periosteum forms a thin and dis-

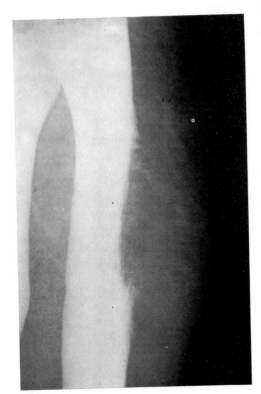

FIG. 605. - Aneurysmal bone cyst. Fe-male aged 26 years. For the past month swelling of the ulna, after trauma. The radiographic aspect, with faded osteol-ysis of the cortex, and having no demar-cation towards the soft tissues, had led to suspect a malignant tumor. The pa-tient is cured 17 years after extrape-riosteal and intralesional excision of the cyst.

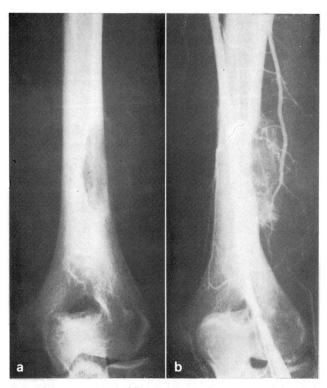

continuous «sheath» of tenuous radiopacity, at times with some slightly radiopaque and sparse streaks within the A.B.C. and perpendicular to the cortex. The osteolysis expands in the underlying cortex and cancellous bone, and often has faded boundaries, at times these boundaries are more evident due to the hyperostotic reaction to the advancing of the A.B.C. (Figs. 604a, 607, 609a, 620, 622).

As A.B.C. expands outwards and particularly inside the bone, and reaches a more advanced maturation stage, the periostotic shell becomes more evident and thicker, and it

FIG. 606. - Aneurysmal bone cyst. Male aged 44 years. (a) For the past 2 months swelling. (b) Arteriography more clearly reveals the periosteal swelling.

may give the false impression of being an expanded and thinned cortex. In this case, we have the radiographic impression of a central and expanding tumor of the bone, while in truth the A.B.C. originated under the periosteum and destroyed the cortex. In some more aggressive cases, instead, the reactive and repair osteogenesis remains rather scarce even when the A.B.C. is very expanded and advanced, enough to give the impression of a destructive and malignant tumor (Figs. 602, 614b, 625, 628, 630, 632, 633).

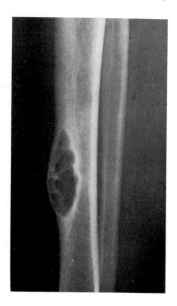

FIG. 607. - Aneurysmal bone cyst. Female aged 17 years. For the past 2 years swelling. In this case, the cyst activity was extinguished.

FIG. 608. - Aneurysmal bone cyst. Male aged 17 years. Pain and swelling for 6 weeks.

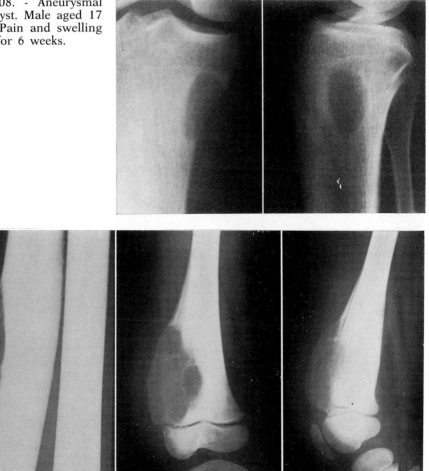

FIG. 609. - (a) Female aged 22 years. Diaphyseal aneurysmal bone cyst of the ulna 13 months after the onset of symptoms. (b) Female aged 4 years. Aneurysmal bone cyst of the distal metaphysis of the femur 1 month after the onset of symptoms.

2) Central A.B.C.

This is especially observed in the metaphyses. Even some A.B.C. of the short and flat bones have an apparently central origin.

A.B.C. initiates with a small spot of osteolysis, which is generally eccentric, in the metaphyseal cancellous bone. The osteolysis expands the perimeter of the bone attenuating the cortex. At times, the osteolysis tends to remain eccentric, at times, particularly in the thinner bones such as the fibula, radius, ulna, tubular bones of the hand and foot, it involves the entire cross-section of the bone (Figs. 603, 604b, 610, 612, 613a, 631a).

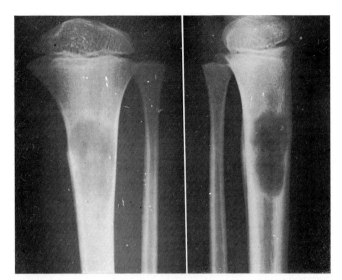

FIG. 610. - Boy aged 5 years. Aneurysmal bone cyst 2 months after the onset of symptoms. Typical radiographic aspect of the central variety.

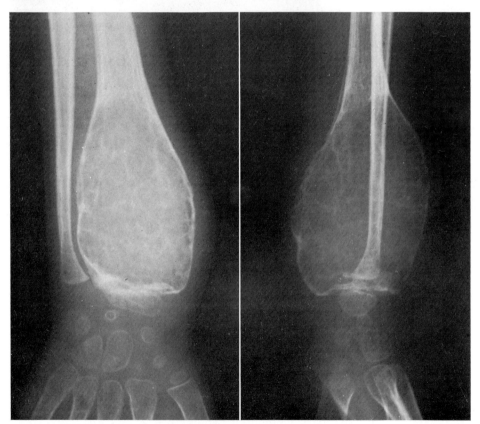

FIG. 611. - Aneurysmal bone cyst. Boy aged 6 years.

Generally, bone expansion is less in the metaphyseal areas, where the ligamentous and tendinous insertions substitute or reinforce the periosteum;

FIG. 612. - Aneurysmal bone cyst. Boy aged 11 years.

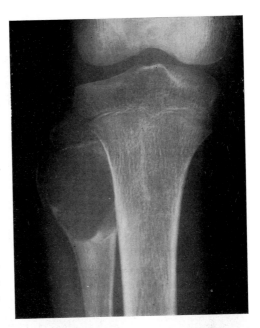

for the same reason, the expansion is scarce in the epiphyses, when these are invaded by the A.B.C. (Figs. 608, 613a).

In any case, due to the absence or the thinness of the periosteal bone layer, images of pseudosepimentation of the A.B.C. are rare and just hinted at (Figs. 602, 614a).

At times, particularly in subperiosteal lesions, the osteolysis is particularly expanded and «aggressive». The bone may be considerably invaded, one or both of the dia-

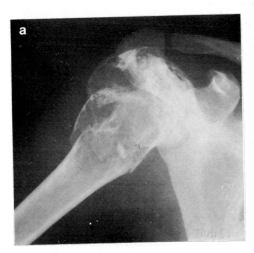

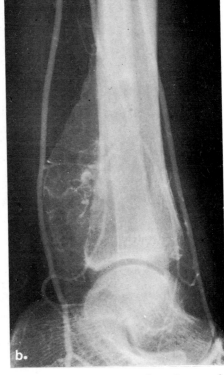

FIG. 613. - (a) Female aged 15 years. Aneurysmal bone cyst of the proximal humerus with pathologic fracture. The radiographic aspect and the localization could suggest bone cyst; nonetheless, the osteolysis invades the epiphysis, which is exceptional in bone cyst. (b) Male aged 15 years. Arteriography of subperiosteal aneurysmal bone cyst of the distal tibia 1 month after the onset of symptoms. Angiography designs the cyst, otherwise nearly invisible at this stage. Observe the absence of considerable afferent and efferent vascular branches.

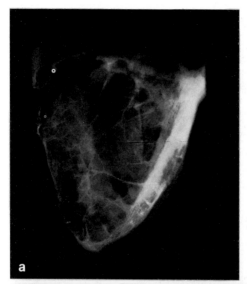

FIG. 614. - (a) Female aged 14 years. Aneurysmal bone cyst of the scapula. Anatomical specimen of resection of the scapular body. (b) Male aged 17 years. Aneurysmal bone cyst of the left pubis strongly swelling enough to move the bladder. The cyst was recent and yet did not reveal any ossification. Selective arteriography of the common iliac right and left. There was no increase in vascularity on the side where the cyst was located as compared to the contralateral one.

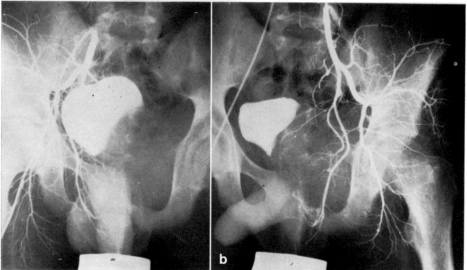

physeal cortices may appear to be cancelled. There is no radiopaque demarcation of A.B.C. (due to periosteal osteogenesis) and osteolysis is total, with faded boundaries, and no radiopacities within it (Figs. 614b, 625, 628, 532, 533).

In the vertebral column, the A.B.C. may expand the body and/or the posterior arch. There may be pathologic collapse of a vertebral body, at times with images of vertebra plana, and there may be subdislocation (Fig. 630). Particularly expanded forms may even extend to one or two adjacent vertebrae. The discs are left intact.

The radiographic picture is substantially modified when A.B.C., submit-

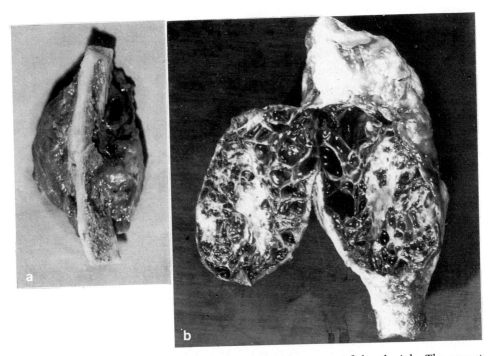

FIG. 615. - (a) Female aged 21 years. Aneurysmal bone cyst of the clavicle. The aspect is that of a soft sac containing blood which erodes the bone from the periosteal surface. (b) Male aged 16 years. Aneurysmal bone cyst of the proximal fibula. Typical aspect of the cut surface.

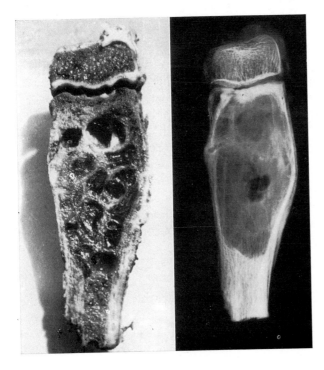

FIG. 616. - Female aged 13 years. Aneurysmal bone cyst of the proximal fibula. (Same case as in Fig. 604b).

ted to curettage or irradiation, infrequently even spontaneously, exhausts its progression and/or repairs. Then there is progressive ossification of the A.B.C. which takes on rather clear bony outlines and an internal radiopacity of structured or trabeculated bone which is more or less intense (Figs. 620-629).

With **angiography**, A.B.C. is injected rather intensely, and there is considerable persistance of the contrast medium. Rarely considerable afferent-efferent vessels are observed. There are neither direct or indirect signs of artero-venous shunt (Figs. 606, 613b, 614b, 623).

CAT may be used to more clearly reveal the expansion, relationships and contents of the A.B.C. The contents appear to be mostly liquid, at times there is a typical «level» image. Similar images are observed with MRI (Figs. 602, 603).

GROSS PATHOLOGIC FEATURES

If the clinical and radiographic pictures may suggest a malignant neoplasm, the intraoperative image of the lesion is much less worrisome and generally it clarifies diagnosis. Whether or not there is a bone layer around the A.B.C. there is a ballooning periosteum but one which is perfectly continuous. At times the wall of the A.B.C. is formed by periosteum alone, at times by a thin bone layer, which reveal by bluish color the hematic contents of the cyst. Often, in recent A.B.C., the cortex is absent in a central area which places the intraosseous part of the cyst in communication with the subperiosteal part.

Once the A.B.C. is opened there may be profuse bleeding, which is non-pulsating and relatively easy to control. Every time that a part of the tissue of the A.B.C. is removed, the hemorrhaging will start again. Thus, the curettage of a large A.B.C. and one located in areas where a tourniquet may not be used may result in a considerable loss of blood (large A.B.C. of the vertebral column, the pelvis, or the limb girdles). If the A.B.C. may instead be completely excised in an bloodless field, there will be very little bleeding when the tourniquet is removed. This observation agrees with arteriographic and anatomical ones, that is, that there are neither numerous nor large blood vessels penetrating the A.B.C. from the bone or from the outside of the bone. At times, instead, the A.B.C. contains serous liquid like that of bone cyst, even in large quantities and in tension. In cases such as these, the pathologic tissue of the cyst is represented by rather thin and fibrous walls and does not bleed much (less active A.B.C.).

On the cut surface, the structure is very typical (Figs. 615b, 616a). It is a sponge permeated with fluid blood and — in part — blood clots. The cavities are rather large and rounded as they are considerably distended by the blood. The septa dividing them are at times rather thick, reddish-gray, parenchymatous and soft; at other times they are thin, whitish and more fibrous. Some septa have a granulous consistency because they contain oste-

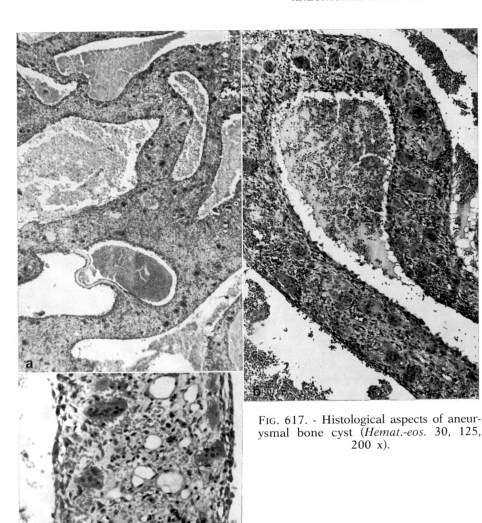

FIG. 617. - Histological aspects of aneurysmal bone cyst (*Hemat.-eos.* 30, 125, 200 x).

oid trabeculae. In quiescent and «mature» A.B.C. the cavities are larger and occupied by clots and serous fluid, and the tissue covering the walls and forming the septa is more fibrous and of a rusty color, not very bloody, and more or less ossified.

The boundaries of A.B.C. with the bone are always rather well-defined.

HISTOPATHOLOGIC FEATURES

Under low power the typical spongy structure is observed. If the A.B.C. is fixed without opening it (en bloc resections), the cavities appear to be roundish and completely filled and distended by blood and by serous fluid. When,

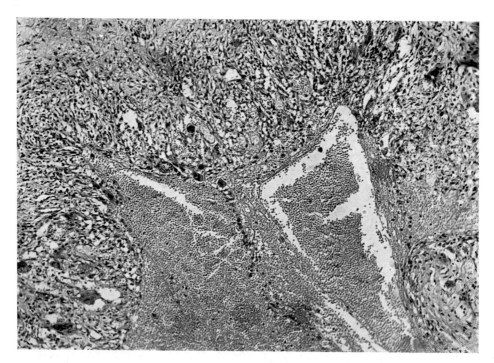

FIG. 618. - Finely spongy structure of the tissue of the aneurysmal bone cyst due to a great number of thin capillary vessels (*Hemat.-eos.* 125 x).

instead, the A.B.C. has been opened, the cavities collapse and appear as spaces and fissures with ondulated walls (Fig. 617). The cavities are of different size, from small to gigantic. In addition to blood, which is generally fluid, and serum, they may contain cellular and calcar debris. The cavities have neither vascular walls nor endothelial coating, rather they are «excavated» in the tissue of the A.B.C.

The actual tissue of the A.B.C., which forms the walls and septa of the hematic cavities, is a histio-fibroblastic tissue rich in thin blood capillaries and multinucleate giant cells. It also contains scattered red blood cells and some leukocytes (Figs. 617-619). Here and there it includes thin osteoid trabeculae. At times, this is a «dystrophic» osteoid, with a particular filamentous aspect, rarely there are fibrin-like globules like those of bone cyst. On the whole this tissue is clearly reactive and reparative and, as such, it tends to «mature» (Fig. 619d). In the septa and walls of the more ancient cysts, it may become dense fibro-collagen or fibro-hyalin, with few fibroblasts and mature fibrocytes. These are oriented at the surface of the cavities in an endotheliomorphous position, but there is no endothelial coating. The giant cells are rarefied. There is abundant hemosiderin.

Alongside and around this «specific» tissue of the A.B.C., within which the cavities are formed, there is aspecific repair tissue (Fig. 619c), made up of bland collagen tissue, with wide sinusoids (these are indeed blood vessels, but they are totally unrelated to the cavities of the cyst) and frequent newly-

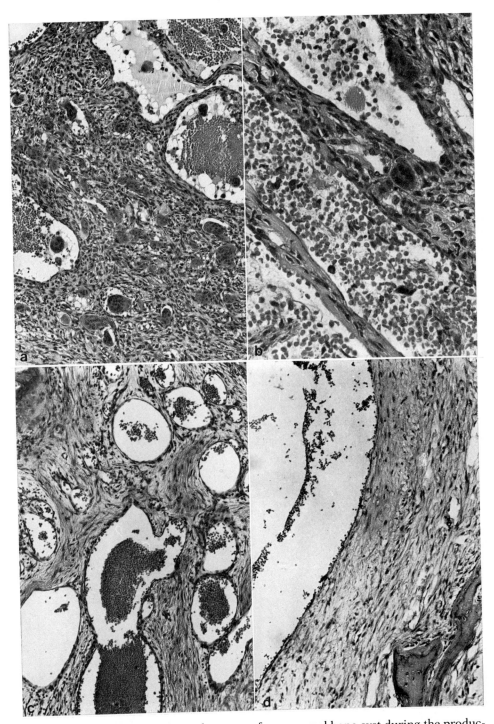

Fig. 619. - (a) and (b) Histological aspects of aneurysmal bone cyst during the productive stage. (c) «Aspecific» tissue of the cyst with ample sinusoids. In this tissue typical cavities of aneurysmal bone cyst are not formed. (d) Old or mature aneurysmal bone cyst (*Hemat.-eos.*, 125, 300, 125, 125 x).

formed osteoid trabeculae. This aspecific tissue is often infiltrated by inter-stitial hemorrhage in which the red blood cells are destroyed and the typical cavities of the A.B.C. are not formed (Campanacci and Zanoli, 1962).

HISTOGENESIS AND PATHOGENESIS

A.B.C. is not a neoplasm. Its histological features and course rather indi-cate a reactive and repair tissue consequent to a particular type of hemorrhage.

The primum movens of this hemorrhage remains obscure. Hematic cavi-tary images similar to those of A.B.C. may be observed in some areas of a giant cell tumor, of a brown tumor in hyperparathyroidism, of a fibrous dysplasia, of a chondroblastoma, of an osteoblastoma, of a hemangioendo-thelioma. This does not mean that A.B.C. constitutes the hemorrhagic trans-formation of some other pre-existing tumoral lesion, as previously affirmed. In our opinion, in genuine A.B.C. there should be no traces of any other le-sion; if this were so, it would not be an A.B.C., but rather another lesion with occasional cystic-hemorrhagic features. Furthermore, the anatomo-clinical features of A.B.C. are such that it is an entity in itself. All that which may be

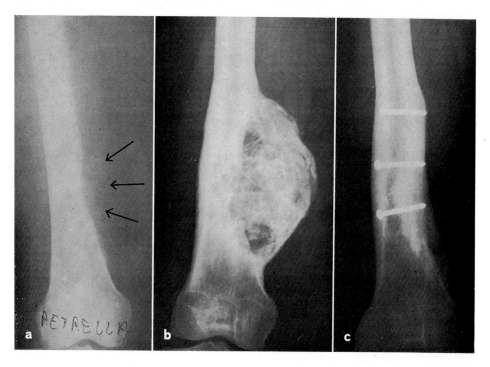

FIG. 620. - Female aged 49 years. (a) Aneurysmal bone cyst of the femoral diaphysis, subperiosteal, 4 months after the onset of symptoms. (b) One year after simple biopsy (example of nearly spontaneous maturation and repair). (c) Two years after tangen-tial resection and bone grafting.

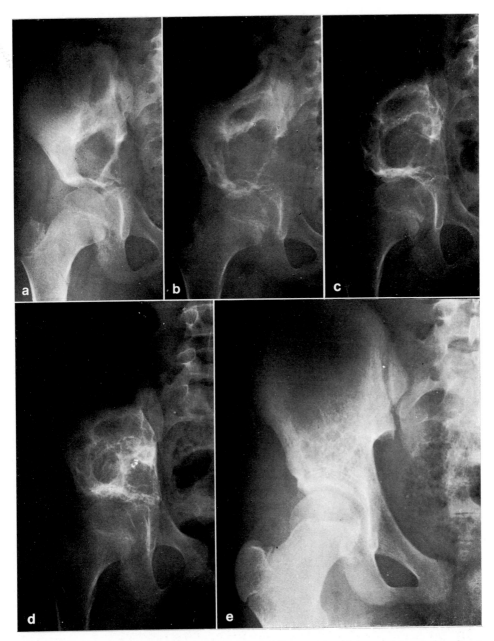

FIG. 621. - (a) Female aged 7 years. Aneurysmal bone cyst which was biopsied and not otherwise treated. (b) After 4 months expansion of the cyst. (c) After 3 more months a delimiting bony shell appeared, which was reinforced after 2 more months (d). (e) 5 years after biopsy, spontaneous healing of the cyst.

said based on the facts at hand is that A.B.C. probably begins due to some change in circulation and local hemorrhage. This produces a repair and

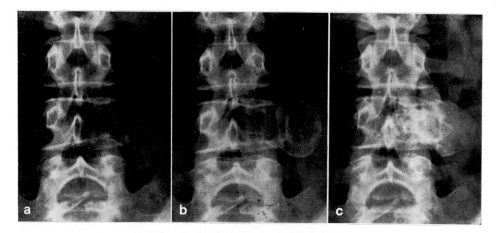

FIG. 622. - (a) Female aged 13 years with lumbar sciatic pain for the past 3 months. Aneurysmal bone cyst biopsied but not treated. (b) Initial ossification after 3 months. (c) Spontaneous healing of the cyst 1 and 1/2 years after biopsy.

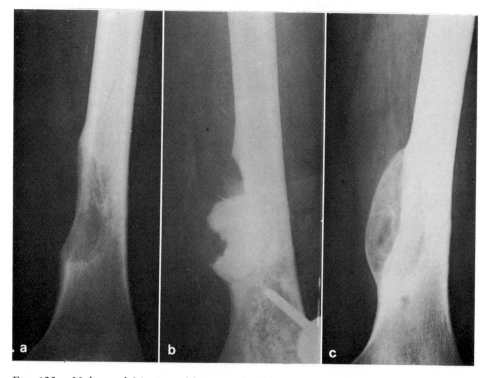

FIG. 623. - Male aged 34 years. (a) Aneurysmal bone cyst of the femoral diaphysis, of subperiosteal origin, 1 year after the onset of symptoms. (b) Transskeletal phlebography: observe intense and persistent accumulation of the contrast medium. (c) Five months after radiation therapy.

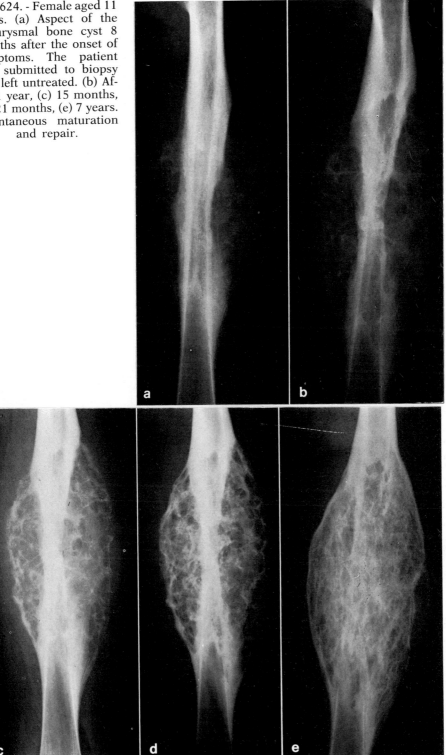

FIG. 624. - Female aged 11 years. (a) Aspect of the aneurysmal bone cyst 8 months after the onset of symptoms. The patient was submitted to biopsy and left untreated. (b) After 1 year, (c) 15 months, (d) 21 months, (e) 7 years. Spontaneous maturation and repair.

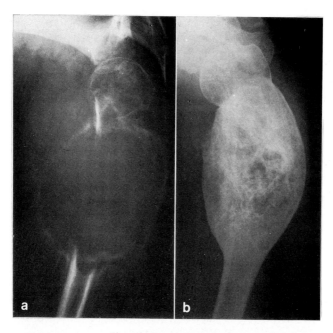

FIG. 625. - (a) Female aged 15 years. Pain for the past 6 months. Three months earlier pathologic fracture. Aneurysmal bone cyst biopsied and treated with radiation (4000 r). (b) Healing of the cyst after 2 years.

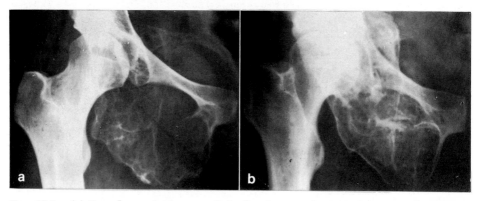

FIG. 626. - (a) Female aged 15 years. Pain for the past 2 years. Biopsy and radiation therapy (2000 r). (b) Healing of the aneurysmal bone cyst after 21 years.

osteolytic tissue, which in turn nourishes the hemorrhage. Thus, a vicious circle is produced, explaining the continuous and at times monstruous expansion of A.B.C. In some cases, instead, the phenomenon tends to slow down and become exhausted, and the A.B.C. «matures», stabilizes, and even spontaneously repairs. The facts which agree with this hypothesis are as follows. The cavities of the A.B.C. are not vessels. They do not communicate with either an arteriole or a venula, rarely with minute capillaries. The cavities originate as «small lakes» of red blood cells in the specific tissue of the A.B.C. and progressively dilate. It seems that the red blood cells ooze from the thin capillaries of the tissue itself, where perhaps there exists an open circulation

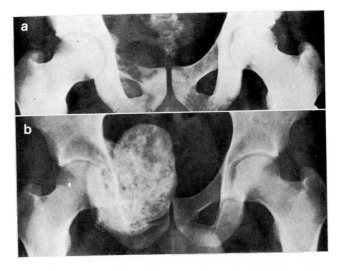

FIG. 627. - (a) Male aged 18 years. For the past month pain. Biopsy and radiation therapy (4000 r). Healing of the aneurysmal bone cyst after 7 years.

(Fig. 618). These facts may be demonstrated by means of the tridimensional reconstruction from seriated histological sections (Campanacci and Zanoli, 1962). Arteriography and surgical experience demonstrate that there are neither afferent nor efferent important vascular branches (Figs. 606, 613b, 614b, 623). The hemorrhage of A.B.C. is not pulsating and it may be dominated relatively well. Comparison with hyperparathyroidism brown tumor is particularly interesting; in this case, as well, it is a repair and reactive tissue which maintains itself and grows on its own, under the stimulus of continuous osteolysis and interstitial hemorrhage, in a vicious circle, as the hyperplasia of the tissue once again nourishes the osteolysis and the hemorrhage. Something similar probably happens here, as well. Except, unlike what occurs in brown tumor, we do not know either the initial cause or causes, and the hemorrhage plays a rather more preponderant part. As for the «maturation» of

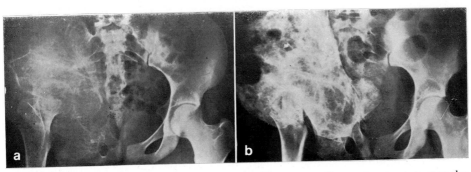

FIG. 628. - (a) Female aged 15 years. Aneurysmal bone cyst of monstruous extent to the entire right hemipelvis. The clinical and radiographic aspect had suggested a malignant tumor. Surgical curettage of the cyst was impossible due to profuse bleeding. Biopsy alone was performed. (b) Radiographic repair 4 years after radiation therapy (4000 r). Result is stable after 15 years.

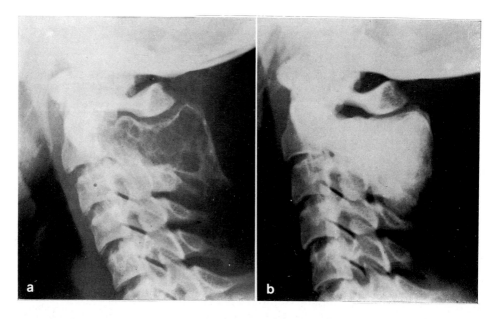

FIG. 629. - Female aged 15 years. (a) Aneurysmal bone cyst of the 2nd cervical vertebra 6 months after the onset of symptoms. (b) Five years after biopsy and radiation therapy (3000 r).

the A.B.C., old and stabilized forms of the disease may be observed, where the hematic cavities are reduced and the septa and walls are transformed into fibro-collagenous membranes, poor in cells. In time, the blood may coagulate and the A.B.C. gradually ossify, as occurs after embolization or radiation therapy (Figs. 620, 621).

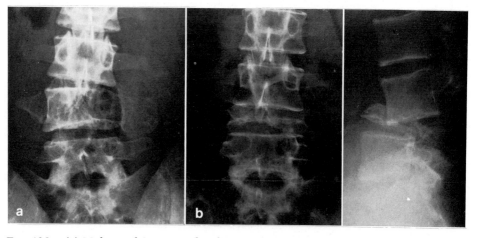

FIG. 630. - (a) Male aged 25 years, for the past 3 months bilateral lumbar crural pain. Biopsy and radiation therapy. (b) After 7 years there was complete flattening of the vertebra with dislocation. Thus, the patient was submitted to posterior fusion (Harrington) and anterior fusion. The tissue removed from the vertebra during these two operations showed no trace of the pre-existing aneurysmal bone cyst.

DIAGNOSIS

The radiographic image of osteolysis and subperiosteal ballooning is often sufficient for a founded diagnostic suspicion. In the vertebral site, the swelling is rather suggestive. At times, however, the osteolysis also involves a nearby vertebra and the expansion of the A.B.C. which is not delimited by an ossified layer may suggest a **cold abscess**. The vertebral localization may also suggest an **osteoblastoma**. Nonetheless, this is less swelling and it often contains a ground glass radiopacity. Let us recall that during surgery osteoblastoma may bleed as much as or even more than an A.B.C. In more central metaphyseal forms or those extended to the entire cross-

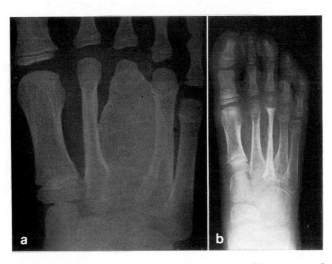

FIG. 631. - Boy aged 7 years. (a) Aneurysmal bone cyst of the 3rd metatarsal 3 months after the onset of symptoms. (b) A year and a half after marginal resection and allograft.

section of the bone, a **bone cyst** or a **chondromyxoid fibroma** may be suggested radiographically. With regard to bone cyst, site is also important: in fact, the bone cyst is rarely observed in sites other than the proximal humerus and the proximal femur. Furthermore, the bone cyst always begins at the center of the metaphysis and in contact with the fertile cartilage, has much less of a tendency to swell, a more defined cortical layer, is more septated, generally does not invade the epiphysis. Although chondromyxoid fibroma is eccentric in the metaphysis, it may cancel the cortex, but not blow out the periosteum; it often has polycyclical boundaries and bubbly sepimentation. **Giant cell tumor** may nearly be discarded when the osteolytic lesion is metaphyseal and the growth cartilage is still open. In the adult, instead, if the osteolysis extends as far as the epiphysis, radiographic differential diagnosis may be impossible. Finally, there are radiographically destructive forms of A.B.C., with a completely cancelled cortex and a «tumoral» mass totally deprived of radiopacity and boundaries. Here, the clinical and radiographical impression may decidedly be that of **malignant tumor**.

The macroscopic aspect of the tissue is generally enough to clarify the diagnosis with a good amount of approximation.

Histologically, there are considerable possibilities of error. First of all, the histological specimen must be large, because the diagnosis of A.B.C. requires

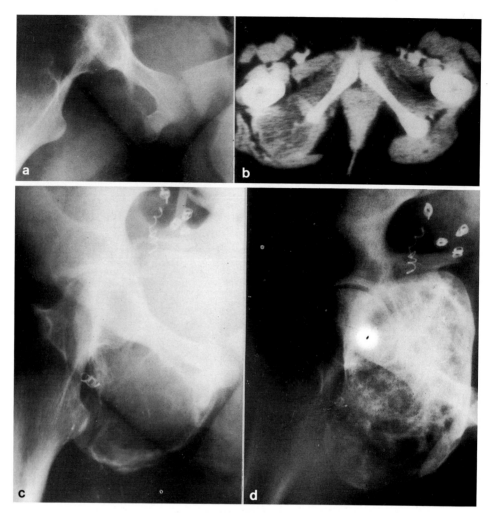

Fig. 632. - Aneurysmal bone cyst in a girl aged 15 years. Pain for the past 4 months after trauma with gradually increasing swelling and irradiated sciatic pain. Incisional biopsy (a, b). The patient was treated with three selective arterial embolizations. (c) Initial repair of cyst after 1 year. (d) Total ossification after 5 years. Total regression of symptoms.

an overall view. Furthermore, the cystic-hemorrhagic images which are similar or the same as that of A.B.C. may be observed in areas of a **giant cells tumor**, of **hyperparathyroidism brown tumor**, of a **fibrous dysplasia**, of a **chondroblastoma**, of an **osteoblastoma**, of a **hemangioendothelioma**. All of these possibilities may be ascertained by a thorough histological study and by an analysis of the clinical and radiographic data. Histological differential diagnosis with giant cell tumor may be particularly difficult. If this is vastly hemorrhagic and cavitated, the histological differences may be truly subtle and the clinical-radiographic picture will be of great help.

Finally, let us recall that some cases of **hemorrhagic osteosarcoma** may at times demonstrate a histological aspect which is similar to that of A.B.C. If the tissue septa of the hemorrhagic osteosarcoma are very thin, if we let ourselves be influenced by the presence of numerous reactive giant cells (not malignant), if nuclear atypiae of the few sarcomatous cells are not revealed, we may mistake hemorrhagic osteosarcoma for an A.B.C. Differential diagnosis may be particularly difficult in exceptional cases of low-grade malignancy hemorrhagic osteosarcoma.

This is why **when faced with a tissue which at first presents the typical structure of an A.B.C. we must routinely use high power to observe the stromal cells in order to exclude any malignant feature**.

A histological doubt may arise in rare cases of «mature» cysts where the tissue is very scarce and collagenized. At that point we might have a doubt between an ancient A.B.C. and a **bone cyst** with hemorrhage due to pathologic fracture. Favoring bone cyst are the site and radiographic aspect, the existence of pathologic fracture, the presence of typical globules of fibrin-like material.

COURSE

The course of the disease varies greatly. At times, the A.B.C. grows slowly; more often, growth is rather rapid and progressive, sometimes reaching enormous sizes (most cases at diagnosis complain of symptoms dating back less than 6 months). In some cases, even those left untreated, the growth of A.B.C. stops and initiates in a slow ossification of the cyst which, in 2-3 years, leads to stable healing. This «maturation» of the A.B.C. is induced by radiation therapy (Figs. 620-629) or by selective arterial embolization (Figs. 632, 633).

TREATMENT

The treatment of choice is extraperiosteal excision and complete curettage of the A.B.C., possibly associated with the use of local adjuvants (phenol, liquid nitrogen, cement) and bone grafting (Fig. 602). In some cases (fibula, ribs, metacarpals, metatarsals) segmental resection is preferable (Fig. 631). In order to reduce blood loss it is best to use a tourniquet or temporary closure of the main artery (for example, the common iliac for A.B.C. of the pelvis or of the proximal femur).

In sites such as the vertebral column, the pelvis, the proximal femur, selective arterial embolization is used successfully. This may be used immediately prior to surgery, in order to decrease surgical bleeding, and, particularly, as a treatment by itself. In fact, embolization, whether single or repeated, very often results in the healing of the A.B.C., without having to resort to surgery. Thus, this method is precious, particularly when surgery would be difficult and risky because of the site and/or the dimensions of the A.B.C. (Figs. 632, 633).

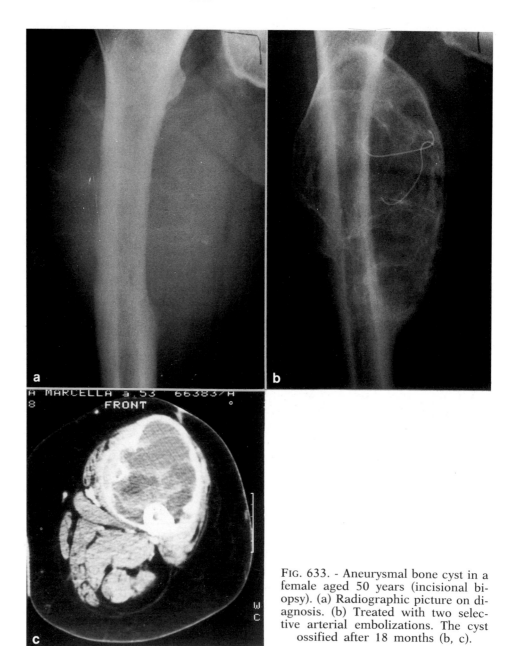

FIG. 633. - Aneurysmal bone cyst in a female aged 50 years (incisional biopsy). (a) Radiographic picture on diagnosis. (b) Treated with two selective arterial embolizations. The cyst ossified after 18 months (b, c).

Radiotherapy also obtains good results (Figs. 623, 625-629). The doses must be kept at a minimum of effectiveness (usually 3-5000 r) in order to decrease the risk of radiation-induced sarcoma. Radiation treatment matures and scars the tissue of the A.B.C., arrests its progression and induces extensive ossification. Nonetheless, radiation therapy must be limited to unoperable cases and where embolization has failed. This is because often A.B.C. is located close to fertile cartilage or sexual glands (lumbar column, pelvis), and because there is the risk of radiation-induced sarcoma.

In rare cases the expansion of the A.B.C. may be such as to advise resection of an important osteo-articular segment or, even more exceptionally, amputation.

PROGNOSIS

In the end A.B.C. nearly always heals, even if curettage was not complete, often associated with embolization, and exceptionally with no therapy. This is another element demonstrating that it is not a neoplasm. Nonetheless, recurrence is possible, after incomplete curettage (in 10-15% of all cases). Generally, radiation therapy is capable of «drying» the A.B.C. even if it is of enormous size. Neurological changes due to medullary compression regress with immediate surgical decompression.

REFERENCES

1957 LICHTENSTEIN L.: Aneurysmal bone cyst. Observations on fifty cases. *Journal of Bone and Joint Surgery*, **39-A**, 873-882.

1961 LINDBON A., SADERBERG G., SPJUT H. J., SUNNGVIST O.: Angiography of aneurysmal bone cyst. *Acta Radiologica*, **55**, 12-16.

1962 CAMPANACCI M., ZANOLI S.: Osservazioni morfologiche ed istomeccaniche sulla cisti aneurismatica dello scheletro. *Archivio di Anatomia e Istologia Patologica*, **36**, 251-273.

1967 ZUCCHI V., ALLEGRINI R.: Il reperto angiografico nella varietà eccentrica sotto-periostea della C.O.A. *Atti della Accademia Medica Lombarda*, **22**, 199-207.

1968 NOBLER M. P., HIGINBOTHAM N. L., PHILLIPS R. F.: The cure of aneurysmal bone cyst; irradiation superior to surgery in an analysis of 33 cases. *Radiology*, **90**, 1185-1192.

1968 TILLMAN B. P., DAHLIN D. C., LIPSCOMB P. R., STEWART J. R.: Aneurysmal bone cyst: an analysis of ninety-five cases. *Mayo Clinic Proceedings*, **43**, 473-495.

1971 CAMPANACCI M., CERVELLATI C.: Cisti aneurismatiche del bacino a sviluppo pseudosarcomatoso. *Chirurgia degli Organi di Movimento*, **60**, 105-112.

1976 CAMPANACCI M., CERVELLATI C., DONATI U., BERTONI F.: Cisti aneurismatica. Studio di 127 casi, 72 controllati a distanza. *Giornale Italiano di Ortopedia e Traumatologia*, **2**, 343-354.

1976 KOSKINEN E. V. S., VISURI T. I., HOLMSTRÖM T., ROUKKOLA M. A.: Aneurysmal bone cyst. Evaluation of resection and of curettage in 20 cases. *Clinical Orthopaedics*, **118**, 136-146.

1977 RUTTER D. J., VAN RIJSSEL TH. G., VAN DER VELDE E. A.: Aneurysmal bone cysts. A clinicopathological study of 105 cases. *Cancer*, **39**, 2231-2239.

INTRAOSSEOUS AND PERIOSTEAL MUCOUS CYST
(Synonyms: «ganglion» of the bone or periosteum, subchondral or juxta-articular bone cyst, synovial cyst of the bone)

DEFINITION

It is a M.C. which develops within the bone (in proximity of a joint) or under the periosteum (generally of the tibia). The anatomo-pathological nature of these cysts is the same as that of the more well-known and common M.C. of the soft tissues (joint capsules, tendinous sheaths, tendons, menisci).

GENERAL INFORMATION

This condition **does not occur rarely**. It is generally observed during adult **age** and there is predilection for the male **sex** (Fig. 634).

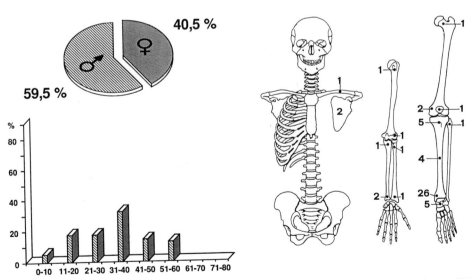

FIG. 634. - Sex, age and localization in 55 cases of mucous cyst of the skeleton (56 localizations).

FIG. 635. - Male aged 58 years. Mucous cyst of the internal malleolus. Symptoms date back 13 years with mild pain and swelling, aspirated several times. The patient was submitted to excision 5 years previously, and the cyst recurred.

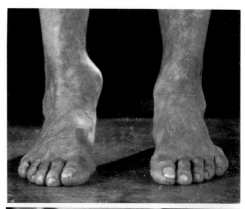

LOCALIZATION

Intraosseous M.C. occur much more frequently than periosteal ones. Intraosseous M.C. are observed with evident predilection for the **tibial malleolus** (fifty per cent of all cases); the remaining cases are distributed among the femoral or tibial condyles, the astragalus, rarer epiphyseal localizations (Fig. 634). In exceptional cases, M.C. is bilateral and symmetrical (Fig. 636). As may be observed, all intraosseous M.C. are located in proximity of a joint surface. Instead, subperiosteal M.C. are observed in the tibial diaphysis ([1]), in the tibial malleolus or in other epiphyses (in these last localizations the M.C. is part subperiosteal and part subligamentous).

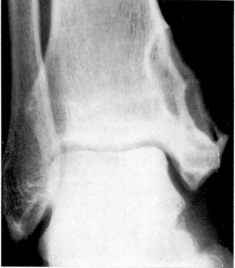

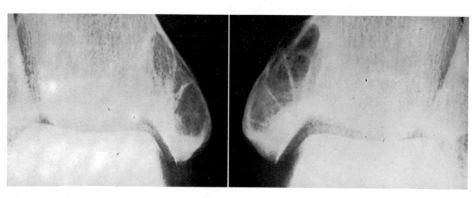

FIG. 636. - Male aged 48 years. Bilateral mucous cyst of the internal malleolus.

([1]) It is interesting to recall that the tibial lesions described by Ollier (1864) and by Poncet (1874) as «albuminous periostitis», characterized by the presence of a mucoid fluid under the periosteum, were probably M.C.

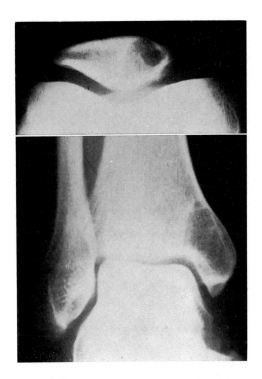

FIG. 637. - (a) Female aged 26 years. Mucous cyst of the patella. (b) Male aged 48 years. Mucous cyst of the internal malleolus.

SYMPTOMS

Symptoms for the most part consist in moderate pain. Swelling nearly exclusively occurs in periosteal M.C., as in intraosseous forms of the disease the cortex is rarely expanded (Fig. 635).

RADIOGRAPHIC FEATURES

In juxta-articular intraosseous M.C. there is an osteolytic cavity of moderate size (rarely more than 2 cm in diameter). The cavity is never at the center of the epiphysis, rather it is located close to a cortex which appears to be thinned. In most cases there is considerable thickness of bone between the cavity and the joint surface (Figs. 636-639). The cavity always has well-defined boundaries, marked by a radiopaque rim of reactive hyperostosis. Often it has a slightly polycyclical form and there is some cloistering due to osseous parietal crests. As previously stated, the cortex is generally thinned, at times slightly swollen, at times uplifted in the form of a subperiosteal «vesicle» having a very thin bony wall, which is radiographically hardly visible.

In periosteal forms (Fig. 641) the cortex may appear to be intact, so

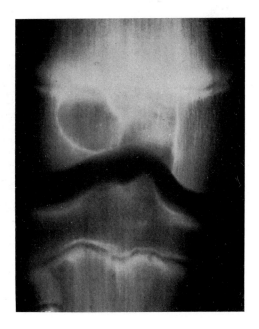

FIG. 638. - Boy aged 14 years. Mucous cyst of the posterior femoral condyle. This cyst protruded posteriorly in the intercondylar notch, covered by periosteum and synovial membrane.

FIG. 639. - Female aged 51 years. (a) Casual radiographic finding post-trauma. The lesion was completely asymptomatic. (b) Macroscopic aspect of the resected epiphysis.

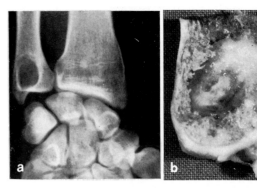

that the radiogram is totally negative. At other times, instead, it is excavated from the surface, with multiple «saucer-like» impressions, separated by crests and cloisters. The boundary of these excavations in metaepiphyseal localizations is marked by a rim of hyperostosis. The spindleshaped uplifting of the periosteum may be shown radiographically by a thin lamina of newly-

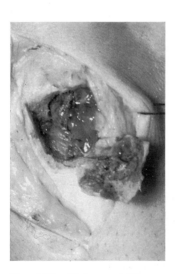

FIG. 640. - Male aged 48 years. Bilateral mucous cyst of the internal malleolus. Typical macroscopic aspect: the cyst has a thin fibrous membrane, which may be detached from the skeletal wall, and a mucoid content (same case as that in Fig. 636).

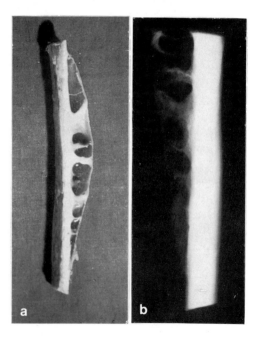

FIG. 641. - Female aged 40 years. For the past 2 years swelling of the tibial diaphysis. (a) Aspect of the resected diaphyseal cortex, with mucous cystic elevation of the periosteum. (b) X-ray of the segment.

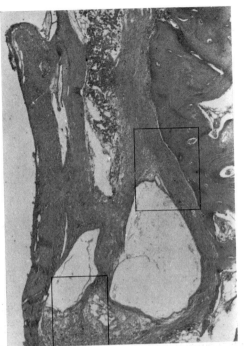

formed bone. Bone cloisters may originate from here, these too being of periosteal neoformation, perpendicular to the diaphyseal surface and separating multiple cystic cavities.

GROSS PATHOLOGIC FEATURES

The constant and pathognomic finding is the same as that of M.C. or «ganglia» of soft tissues. That is, these are globose, separate or confluent cystic cavities, containing transparent, colorless or yellowish, dense, viscid material, similar to mucus. The wall is formed by a yellowish-white connective membrane, which is more or less thick,

FIG. 642. - Wall of the mucous cyst under small enlargement (*Hemat.-eos.*, 30 x).

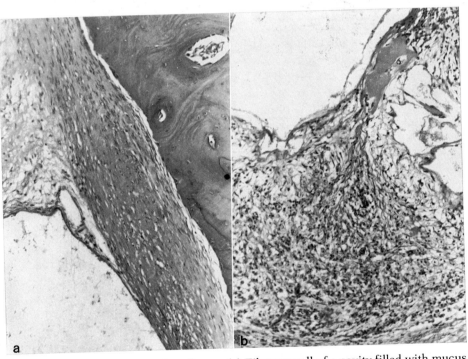

FIG. 643. - Details of the previous figure. (a) Fibrous wall of a cavity filled with mucus. (b) Myxoid cellular hyperplasia preceding the formation of the mucous cyst (*Hemat.-eos.*, 125, 125 x).

resistant and easily detached from the skeletal bed. The latter is smooth and compact (Figs. 640, 641).

In juxtacortical intraosseous forms of the disease, the M.C. is isolated from the periosteum by a thin layer of cortex. Generally, it is also isolated from the joint cavity, as may be shown intraoperatively by injecting me-thylene blue into the joint. In perio-steal forms, one has the clear impression that M.C. has developed within the periosteum.

HISTOPATHOLOGIC FEATURES

These features are the same as those for all M.C. of the connective tissue. The mucoid content is dissolved in the histological preparation, unless a few drops of acetic acid are added to the fixative liquid (so that the mucoid material hardens and is strongly reduced in volume, becoming macroscopically similar to the white part of a cooked egg). The mucoid material has the same chromatic reactions as mucin. The wall of larger and «mature» M.C. is formed by dense collagen in large parallel bundles (Figs. 642, 643a). Fibrocytes may on the surface be vaguely endotheliomorphous, but never enough to give the wall a simil-synovial aspect. The more external portion of the wall

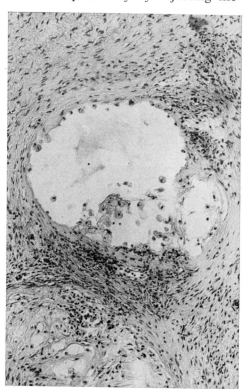

Fig. 644. - Formation of a small mucous cavity in which few cells with cytoplasm full of mucus float (*Hemat.-eos.*, 125 x).

often contains a few tufts of small newly-formed vessels, newly-formed bone trabeculae, at times small cartilaginous islands.

Small foci of hyperplasia and mucoid transformation of the connective tissue, representing new immature M.C., are often observed alongside the main mature M.C. (Figs. 643, 644). This mucoid transformation, the final result of which is that of M.C., may easily be reconstructed under microscopy. At first, a hyperplasia of fibroblasts is observed; they are numerous and swollen, and have abundant collagen. These cells secrete mucoid substance; the cytoplasms appear to be wide and well-stained, at times they are vesicular and foamy; the cells and the collagenous fibers are strewn about as the intercellular mucinous liquid increases; finally, the cells and fibers disappear, giving way to cystic cavities which are increasingly larger and more and more confluent. Foci of this type may open into a cavity which is already formed, and the cells, undergoing regression and necrosis, fluctuate scattered in the mucoid liquid. At the end, the wall of the M.C. is formed by fibrous and reactive bone tissue, which is compressed and mature.

HISTOGENESIS AND PATHOGENESIS

Thus, it may be concluded that intraosseous and periosteal M.C. are of the same nature and probably have the same pathogenesis as M.C. of other connective areas. Their nature is hyperplastic-regressive, and pathogenesis is the mucoid transformation of the connective tissue. The cause of this phenomenon remains obscure. The in situ transformation of the skeletal connective tissue or the periosteum also agrees with the possible recurrence after surgical removal. Recurrence is not caused by incomplete removal, but it may originate from the cystic transformation of the connective tissue surrounding the cysts.

The idea held by many that intraosseous M.C. is caused by microfractures of the joint cartilage and the penetration of synovial fluid or synovial tissue in the bone is totally unfounded. It neither explains periosteal M.C. nor juxta-cortical ones having no communication with the joint cavity, which are those most commonly observed. Furthermore, with regard to the rare intraosseous M.C. that would communicate with the joint cavity, it may be admitted that this communication is secondary to expansion of the M.C., rather than primary. On the other hand, even M.C. of the soft tissues do not generally communicate with the joint cavity and differ from synovial cysts. Finally, intraosseous M.C. are never observed in osteochondrosis dissecans, and rarely in arthrosis.

DIAGNOSIS

Site and radiographic features are often rather typical for a founded suspected diagnosis (particularly localizations in the tibial malleolus). The lesion cannot be confused with an **arthrosic geode**. First of all, in M.C. there is no radiographic sign of arthrosis. Age (often young) and localization, as well, are not those of arthrosis. Rather, the radiographic aspect may suggest **chronic infection**, either aspecific or specific; in some juvenile epiphyseal localizations **chondroblastoma** may be suggested, as compared to which M.C. has more evident boundaries and does not contain any calcification (Fig. 638).

The surgical and histological aspects are absolutely pathognomic and cannot be mistaken.

Intraosseous M.C. must also be distinguished from those M.C. (for example, of a meniscus) that dig into the bone (for example, on the border of the tibial plateau) due to external compression.

COURSE

The formation and growth of M.C. are rather slow. Often many years go by between the onset of the first symptoms and treatment. M.C. may remain asymptomatic for a long time. At times, it is revealed by a radiographic examination obtained for other reasons.

TREATMENT AND PROGNOSIS

Treatment of symptomatic cysts consists in surgical excision which is a rather simple procedure, due to the ease with which M.C. may be enucleated from the skeletal bed. In exceptional cases, there may be recurrence, even when excision was complete, due to mucoid transformation of the surrounding connective tissue.

REFERENCES

1961 WOODS C. G.: Subcondral bone cyst. *Journal of Bone and Joint Surgery*, **43-B**, 758-766.

1968 SALZER M., SALZER-KUNTSCHIK M.: Ganglien mit Knochenbeteilingung. *Archiv für Orthopädische und Unfallchirurgie*, **64**, 87-99.

1969 GOLDMAN R. L., FRIEDMAN N. B.: Ganglia (« synovial cysts ») arising in inusual locations. *Clinical Orthopaedics*, **63**, 184-189.

1970 BYERS P. D., WALDSWORTH TH. G.: Periosteal ganglion. *Journal of Bone and Joint Surgery*, **52-B**, 290-295.

1971 CAMPANACCI M., CERVELLATI C.: Cisti mucose periostee e intraossee. *Chirurgia degli Organi di Movimento*, **60**, 221-232.

1971 NIGRISOLI P., BELTRAMI P.: Sulle cisti ossee subcondrali. *Lo scalpello*, **1**, 65-75.

1971 SIM F. H., DAHLIN D. C.: Ganglion cysts of bone. *Mayo Clinic Proceedings*, **46**, 484-488.

1972 CAMPANACCI M., GULINO G.: Cisti mucosa intraossea bilaterale. *Chirurgia degli Organi di Movimento*, **61**, 367-370.

1979 SCHAJOWICZ F., CLAVEL SAINZ M., SLULLITEL J. A.: Juxta-articular bone cysts (intra-osseous ganglia). A clinicopathological study of eighty-eight cases. *Journal of Bone and Joint Surgery*, **61-B**, 107-116.

1981 ROSENTHAL D., SCHWARTZ A., SCHILLER A.: Case report 170: subperiosteal synovial cyst of knee. *Skeletal Radiology*, **7**, 142-145.

1987 YAGHAMAI I., FOSTER C.: Case report 404: intraosseous ganglion of the distal ulna with a pathologic result. *Skeletal Radiology*, **16**, 153-156.

1988 DALY P.J., SIM F.H., BEABOUT J.W., UNNI K.K.: Intraosseous ganglion cysts. *Orthopaedics*, **11**, 1715-1719.

1989 POPE T.L., FECHNER R.E., KEATS T.E.: Intra-osseous ganglion. Report of four cases and review of the literature. *Skeletal Radiology*, **18**, 185-187.

PROGRESSIVE TELANGIECTATIC OSTEOLYSIS
(Synonyms: massive idiopathic osteolysis, massive osteolysis due to hemangiomatosis, spontaneous acute resorption of bone, disappearing bone, phantom bone, Gorham's disease)

It is a regional lesion (skeleton and soft tissues) of unknown nature and origin, characterized by massive osteolysis and neoproduction of hematic and lymphatic capillaries. It is **very rare** (we have observed 8 cases); there is no predilection for **sex**, while it does show predilection for patients **aged** from 10 to 30 years (but it may be observed at any age).

LOCALIZATION

Distribution is generally not monostotic, but rather in several bones in an anatomical region (for example, the hip) or in adjacent anatomical regions (for example, the shoulder, vertebral column and chest). With the exception of the cranium, any bone may be affected. The highest incidence, in decreasing order, is observed in the shoulder, the hip, the long bones of the limbs, including the tubular bones of the hand and foot; it may also be observed in the vertebrae, ribs, carpus and tarsus, facial bones.

SYMPTOMS

Onset, which is often preceded by even slight trauma, may be acute, with pain, functional deficit, at times fever, at times pathologic fracture, chronic edema of the limb. At times soft swelling having indistinct boundaries of the subcutaneous and deeper soft tissues is associated; the latter may be covered with reddenned and telangiectatic skin.

Over months or years, the osteolysis expands, while pain and swelling decrease slowly. At the end, there is severe regional muscular atrophy, skeletal discontinuity, shortening and deformity, joint stiffness.

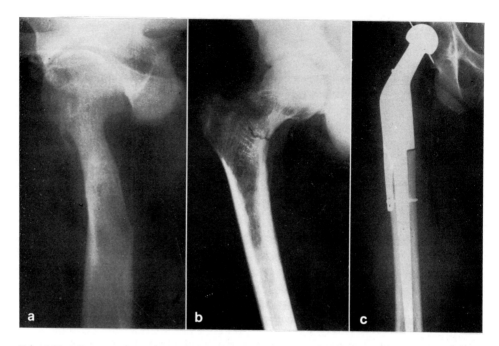

FIG. 645. - Progressive telangiectatic osteolysis of the proximal femur in a male aged 19 years. (a) Five months after repeated muscular tear and continuous pain, even during rest, the lateral view showed narrowing of the femoral neck. (b) One month later there was fracture due to movement in the bed, and progression of the faded osteolysis was observed. (c) The patient was submitted to resection and arthroprosthesis. A histological examination of the resected segment confirmed diagnosis (see Fig. 649) (Case of Prof. V. Zucchi).

RADIOGRAPHIC FEATURES

At first there is intense osteoporosis limited to a single bone; successively there is progressive osteolysis which, in the long bones, at the diaphyseal level, is manifested by concentric narrowing of the cortex, pathologic fracture and terminal formation of two skeletal segments «like the tip of a pencil» (Figs. 645, 647); in the metaepiphyseal site, instead, and in the flat and short bones, there is lacunar osteolysis with progressively confluent spots (Figs. 646, 648).

Arteriography and phlebography do not reveal any pathologic circulation (Fig. 646), or connections between the lesions and the surrounding vessels. If, instead, contrast medium is injected into the lesion, it stagnates for a long time. Occasionally lymphography has injected some of the swellings in the soft tissues.

Often, the disease extends to the adjacent bones without respecting the articular barrier. The final picture is that of complete skeletal resorption. Neither hyperostosis nor periostosis of a reactive nature have ever been observed. Any hint of spontaneous repair of the fractures by formation of bone

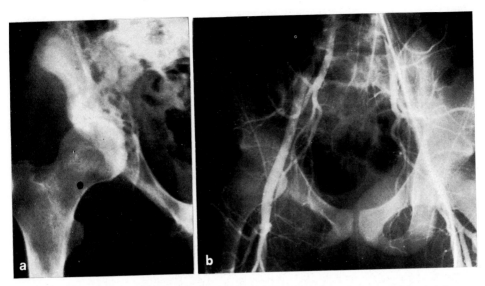

FIG. 646. - Progressive telangiectatic osteolysis of the pelvis in a male aged 17 years. For the past 1 and 1/2 years continuous pain and progressive severe functional deficit. There were two episodes of trauma in the patient's history: one contusive, initiating symptoms; a second episode, more intense, caused fracture of the ischium. For the past month soft swelling occurred in the homolateral inguinal region. The patient was treated for a long time for tubercular sacro-ileitis. (a) The radiogram shows the spotted osteolysis of the ilium and total osteolysis of the ischium. (b) Arteriography was negative. The intraoperative macroscopic picture and the histological picture clarified diagnosis.

callus is aborted by early callus resorption. The insertion of bone grafts during the active stage of the disease is also followed by their resorption.

Isotope scan is intensely hot in the active phase, tending to normalize when the disease becomes inactive.

LABORATORY FINDINGS

There are none in particular, except for a transitory increase in alkaline phosphatase during the acute phase.

GROSS PATHOLOGIC FEATURES

It is a disease of regional distribution; in fact, in addition to the bone, it involves the surrounding soft tissues (muscles, fasciae, subcutaneous tissue), which appear to be substituted and at times expanded by a soft, reddish or yellowish-red tissue, resembling a bunch of delicate lobules and grapes which, once opened, deflate, allowing sero-hematic fluid to flow out. At times, this fluid flows out in large quantites, revealing large empty cavities run through by a loose fibrous trabeculation resembling a «spider's web». Non-

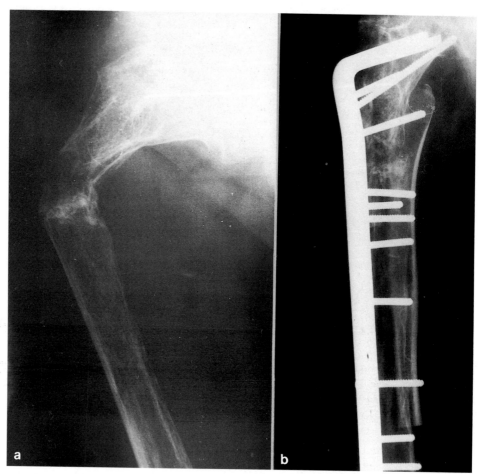

FIG. 647. - Progressive telangiectatic osteolysis in a male aged 21 years. Pain for the past 2 years. Nine months earlier pathologic fracture (a). (b) The patient was submitted to reduction and osteosynthesis with a hemicylindrical allograft.

tenacious adherences between the bone and the surrounding soft tissues, and between the different planes of the soft tissues may be observed. The muscular tissue surrounding the cavities filled with fluid may be degenerated and atrophic.

The bone, depending on the stage of the disease, may be severely porotic with intense bleeding, or vastly absent, substituted by wide smooth-walled cavities, filled with hematic or serous fluid, more often sero-hematic, delimited by a thin membrane, and run through by thin «spider-web» filaments of whitish collagen.

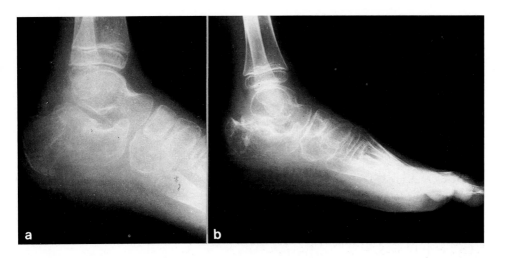

Fig. 648. - Progressive telangiectatic osteolysis in a boy aged 8 years (a) Initial radiographic picture: pain and swelling for the past 4 months; incisional biopsy. (b) Evolution after 6 months.

HISTOPATHOLOGIC FEATURES

It reveals the progressive disappearance of the skeletal structures, due to smooth resorption, substituted by rather loose collagen tissue, rich in hematic and sometimes lymphatic vascular spaces (dilated or cavernous capillaries), with an endothelium which may be hyperplastic (Fig. 649). At times, some lymphomonocytes and plasmacells are observed around the vessels. At the end, what remains is only a thin membrane of collagen tissue, with no endothelial coating, in the walling of the large cavities filled with sero-hematic fluid. Osteoblastic activity has never been observed; osteoclastic resorption is a rare finding. Frequently, in the adjacent soft tissues there is a mixture of lymphohematic capillary and cavernous spaces, vaguely reminiscent of the structure of some angiomas.

ETIOPATHOGENESIS

It is unknown; it has not been clarified whether P.T.O. may be likened to angiomatosis or rather to post-traumatic algo-dystrophy.

DIAGNOSIS

While diagnosis is easy in evident forms of the disease, it is less so during the early stages where, partially due to the rarity of the disease, **Sudeck's syndrome** or an **inflammatory or neoplastic process** are more easily suggested. In particular forms of the disease, differential diagnosis may involve **tu-

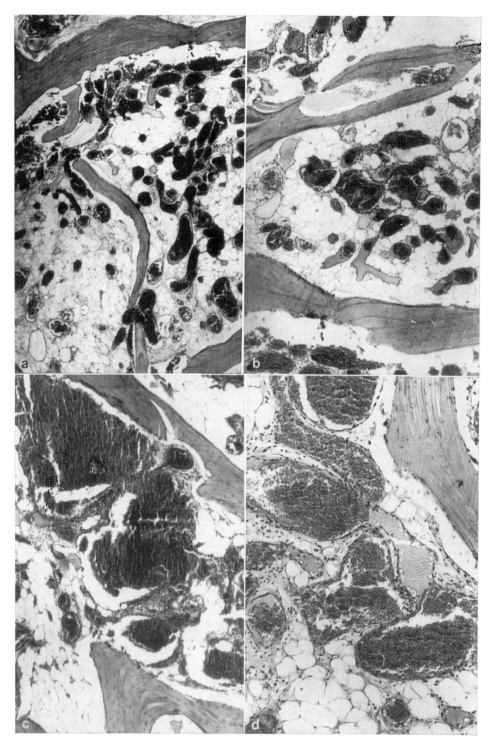

FIG. 649. - Histologic aspect of progressive telangiectatic osteolysis (*Hemat.-eos.*, 50, 50, 125, 125 x).

bercular osteoarthritis, **neurogenous osteo-arthropathy**, osteolytic forms of **rheumatoid arthritis**.

COURSE AND PROGNOSIS

Bone resorption progresses slowly over years, at the end, however, arresting spontaneously. Cases stabilized more than 10 years after clinical onset of the disease have been reported. There is no re-ossification of the osteolysis.

The most severe complications are of a neurologic nature, when the process is localized in the vertebrae (complications which are usually not fatal), or in the respiratory system, for vertebral and/or costal localizations; in cases such as these, due to possible chilo-, sero-, or hemothorax, which rapidly recurs even after thoracentesis, death may occur due to pulmonary atelectasia and/or pleuropulmonary infection.

TREATMENT

No treatment is capable of leading to healing or, at least, of arresting the progression of the pathologic process. It seems that radiation therapy may in some cases favor and/or accelerate arrest of the osteolysis. When the progressive stage of the osteolysis is extinguished, surgical reconstruction may be performed, if indicated (endoprosthesis, osteosynthesis with bone grafting) (Figs. 645, 647). If this type of surgery is performed during the progressive stage, it may fail, due to osteolysis at the interface with the prosthesis and due to resorption of the grafts.

REFERENCES

1955 GORHAM L. W., STOUT A. P.: Massive osteolysis (acute spontaneous absorption of bone, phantom bone, disappearing bone). Its relation to hemangiomatosis. *Journal of Bone and Joint Surgery*, **37-A**, 985-1004.

1958 HAMBACH R., PUJMAN J., MALY V.: Massive osteolysis due to hemangiomatosis. Report of a case of Gorham's disease with autopsy. *Radiology*, **71**, 43-47.

1958 JOHNSON P. M., MC CLURE J. G.: Observations on massive osteolysis. A review of the literature and report of a case. *Radiology*, **71**, 28-42.

1964 HALLIDAY D. R., DAHLIN D. C., PUGH D. G., YOUNG H. H.: Massive osteolysis and angiomatosis. *Radiology*, **82**, 637-644.

1965 TORG J. S., STEEL H. H.: Sequential roentgenographic changes occurring in massive osteolysis. *Journal of Bone and Joint Surgery*, **51-A**, 1649-1655.

1967 BACIN CL., TEMELIE AL., ROVENTRA N., FILIPESCO CH.: Ostéolyse essentielle massive du bassin. *Acta Orthopedica Belgica*, **33**, 788-796.

1967 STERN M. B., GOLDMAN R. L.: Disappearing bone disease. Report of a case and review of the literature. *Clinical Orthopedics*, **53**, 99-107.

1968 POIRIER H.: Massive osteolysis of the humerus treated by resection and prosthetic replacement. *Journal of Bone and Joint Surgery*, **50-B**, 158-160.

1968 TILLING G., SKOBOWYTSH B.: Disappearing bone disease, morbus Gorham. Report of a case. *Acta Orthopedica Scandinavica*, **39**, 398-406.

1970 FORNASIER V. L.: Haemangiomatosis with massive osteolysis. *Journal of Bone and Joint Surgery*, **52-B**, 444-451.

1970   KERY L., WOUTERS H. W.: Massive osteolysis. Report of two cases. *Journal of Bone and Joint Surgery*, **52-B**, 452-459.

1970   SCAPINELLI R., TURRA S.: L'osteolisi massiva segmentaria dello scheletro. *Clinica Ortopedica*, **22**, 230-244.

1974   IMBERT J. C., PICAULT C.: Ostéolyse massive idiopathique ou maladie de Jackson-Gorham. *Revue de Chirurgie Orthopedique*, **60**, 73-80.

1974   SAGE R. M., ALLEN P. W.: Massive osteolysis. Report of a case. *Journal of Bone and Joint Surgery*, **56-B**, 130-135.

1974   THOMPSON J. S., SCHURMAN D. J.: Massive osteolysis. Case report and review of the literature. *Clinical Orthopedics*, **103**, 206-212.

1975   CAMPBELL J., ALMOND H. G. A., JOHNSON R.: Massive osteolysis of the humerus, with spontaneous recovery. *Journal of Bone and Joint Surgery*, **57-B**, 238-240.

1976   PATRICK J. H.: Massive osteolysis complicated by chylothorax successfully treated by pleurodesis. *Journal of Bone and Joint Surgery*, **58-B**, 347-349.

1977   HEYDEN G., KINDBLOM L. G., MÖLLER NIELSEN J.: Disappearing bone disease. *Journal of Bone and Joint Surgery*, **59-A**, 57-61.

1977   SACRISTAN H. D., FERRANDEZ PORTAL L., CASTRESANA GOMEZ F., RODRIGUEZ P.: Massive osteolysis of the scapula and ribs. *Journal of Bone and Joint Surgery*, **59-A**, 405-406.

1983   GHERLINZONI F., ROCCO M.: Un caso di osteolisi progressiva teleangiectasica. *Giornale Italiano di Ortopedia e Traumatologia*, **9**, Suppl., 533-537.

1985   HARDEGGER F., SIMPSON L.A., SEGMUELLER G.: The syndrome of idiopathic osteolysis. Classification, review and case report. *Journal of Bone and Joint-Surgery*, **67-B**, 89-93.

1987   HEJGAARD N., ROSENKILDE P.O.: Massive Gorham osteolysis of the right hemipelvis complicated by chylothorax: report of a case in a 9-year-old boy successfully treated by pleurodesis. *Journal of Pediatric Orthopaedics*, **7**, 96-99.

1987   JOSEPH J., BARTAL E.: Disappearing bone disease: a case report and review of the literature. *Journal of Pediatric Orthopaedics*, **7**, 584-588.

1987   PASTAKIA B., HORVATH K., LACK E.E.: Seventeen-year-old follow-up and autopsy findings in case of massive osteolysis. *Skeletal Radiology*, **16**, 291-297.

1988   OSTERBERG P.H., WALLACE R.G.H., ADAMS G.A., CRONE R.S., DICKSON G.R., KANIS J.A., MOLLAN R.A.B., NEVIN N.C., SLOAN J., TONER P.G.: Familial expansile osteolysis. *Journal of Bone and Joint Surgery*, **70-B**, 255-260.

1989   MENDEZ A.A., KERET D., ROBERTSON W., MAC EWEN G.D.: Massive osteolysis of the femur (Gorham's disease): a case report and review of the literature. *Journal of Pediatric Orthopaedics*, **9**, 604-608.

HISTIOCYTOSIS X
(Synonyms: reticuloendotheliosis, histiocytary granuloma, eosinophilic granuloma of bone, Letterer-Siwe disease, Hand-Schuller-Christian disease)

DEFINITION

It is a reticuloendotheliosis of granuloma-like aspect and unknown etiology, which may involve the bone marrow, the internal organs, the skin and the mucosae. Depending on the age at which it initiates, on whether it is solitary, multicentric or generalized, on the tissues and organs involved, on whether progression is acute, subacute or chronic, H.X. causes different syndromes, with variations and intermediate forms. The most classic of these syndromes are eosinophilic granuloma of bone, Hand-Schuller-Christian disease and Letterer-Siwe disease [1].

CLASSIFICATION

Three main forms of the disease may be distinguished.
1. **H.X. localized in the skeleton**: solitary or multiple eosinophilic granuloma of bone.
2. **Chronic disseminated H.X.**: (including Hand-Schuller-Christian disease).
3. **Acute or subacute diffused H.X.** (including cases described as Letterer-K Siwe disease).

Schematically, it may be said that eosinophilic granuloma of bone occurs during late childhood and adolescence and heals completely. The chronic disseminated form (in the skeleton and outside the skeleton) initiates during early infancy and prognosis depends on the extent of the histiocytosis and on the involvement of vital organs such as the hypophysis and the lungs. The

---

[1] In 1953 Lichtenstein proposed temporarily defining this disease with the term histiocytosis X. By this, the author meant to indicate that it is a histiocytary proliferation, and to emphasize the need to search for the unknown (X) etiological agent.

acute form (prevalently extraskeletal) is observed before 3 years of age and nearly always has a severe prognosis. It must be recalled, however, that there is considerable variability from case to case, and that one form may even be transformed into the other.

Eponymic denominations should be abandoned. As there was no sound histological reference, cases of malignant lymphoma as well as leukemia have also been described under the name Letterer-Siwe disease. Hand-Schuller-Christian disease is based on the classic triad: multiple osteolysis («geography map cranium»), insipid diabetes and esophthalmus, which is rarely presented in cases of disseminated chronic H.X. Finally, it must be recalled that Hand-Schuller-Christian disease was at one time held to be lipoid thesaurismosis (cholesterin), similar to Gaucher and Niemann-Pick diseases [1].

FREQUENCY

H.X. is an infrequent occurrence but not a rare one. **Solitary eosinophilic granuloma** of bone represents the most common occurrence. Rarely, perhaps in 1 case out of 10, **multiple eosinophilic granuloma** of bone is observed.

Chronic disseminated H.X. is rare, and only exceptionally (in 1 case out of 10-20) is the symptomatic triad of Hand-Schuller-Christian observed therein.

Acute diffused H.X. is rare and observed only by pediatricians.

SEX

There is predilection for the male sex, at a ratio of approximately 2:1 (Fig. 650).

AGE

The acute diffused form is nearly always observed within the first 3 years of life. Eosinophilic granuloma of bone generally occurs before 20 years of age, with an evident peak in frequency between 5 and 10 years (Fig. 650). The chronic disseminated form is usually manifested early, between 3 and 5 years of age, rarely after 15.

---

[1] Genuine cholesterin lipoidosis is represented by multiple tuberous xanthoma of the soft tissues. On the contrary, the chronic disseminated form of H.X. has nothing in common with changes in the lipidic metabolism. The presence of intracellular lipoid, which had struck observers as the main feature, is instead a secondary finding, like fibrosis, and predominates in chronic forms of H.X. because it marks lesions which have aged (the only ones which at one time were histologically examined, on autopsy).

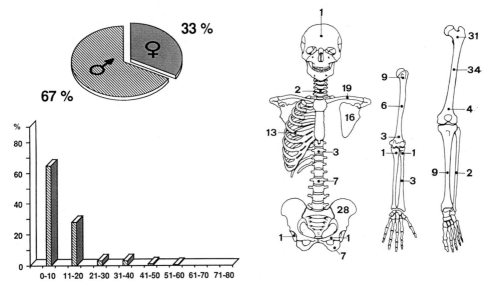

FIG. 650. - Sex, age and localization in 201 cases of solitary eosinophilic granuloma of bone (The series includes only lesions ascertained by biopsy, and thus vertebral localizations are not very represented).

LOCALIZATION

Eosinophilic granuloma of bone shows predilection for the flat and short bones of the trunk, in this order: cranium, ribs, pelvis, maxillary bones, vertebral column, clavicle, scapula. Furthermore, it may be observed in the long bones, among which the proximal half of the femur is preferred. This is followed by the humerus, the tibia, and then the other long bones. It hardly ever occurs in either the hand or the foot (Fig. 650).

In the cranium it is generally observed in the frontal or parietal bone; in the two maxillary bones it nearly always develops in the mandible; in the vertebrae it generally affects the body. In the long bones, diaphyseal localization is followed by the metadiaphyseal one. In exceptional cases, an epiphysis may be involved.

Eosinophilic granuloma occurring during adult age seems to clear-

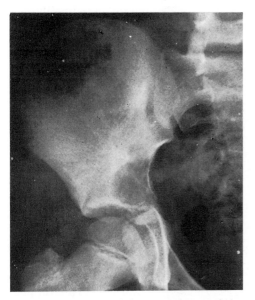

FIG. 651. - Eosinophilic granuloma of the ilium in a female aged 5 years.

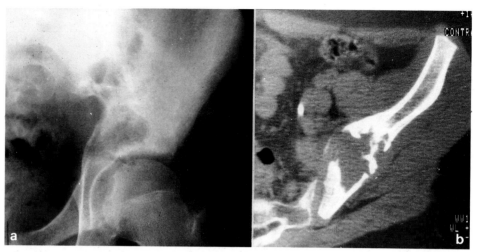

FIG. 652. - Eosinophilic granuloma in a boy aged 12 years. Observe osteolysis with irregular borders and destruction of the cortex in some areas.

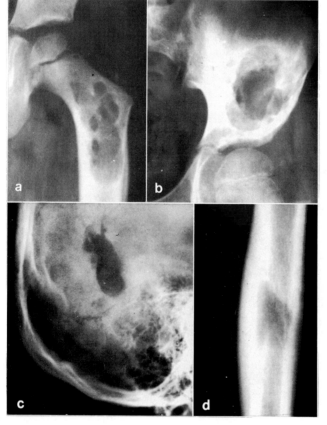

ly prevail in the cranium and in the skeleton of the trunk; it is rarely observed in the long bones.

Chronic disseminated H.X. nearly always involves the skeleton. Here, the most frequent localization is again the cranium, followed by the femur, pelvis, maxillary bones, vertebrae, ribs, tibia and humerus. In the cranium lesions extend to the vault and

FIG. 653. - Radiographic aspects of eosinophilic granuloma. (a) In a male aged 4 years. (b) In a female aged 7 years. (c) In a male aged 19 years (temporal bone). (d) In a female aged 17 years (humeral diaphysis).

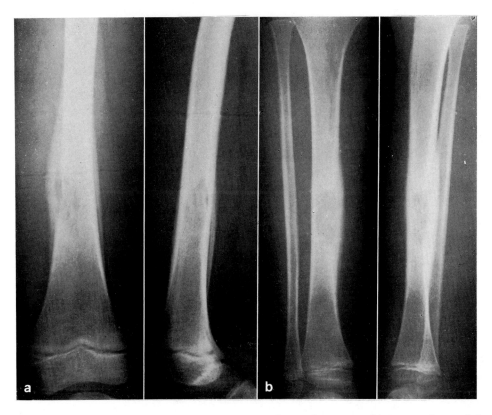

FIG. 654. - (a) Eosinophilic granuloma in a male aged 8 years. (b) In a male aged 3 years.

to the base. In addition to the skeleton, «target» tissues and organs include the skin, the oral and genital mucosae, the lungs, the lymph nodes, the liver, the spleen, the kidneys, the brain. Pulmonary localizations tend to be bilateral and diffused. The involved lymph nodes may be related to skin, mucosae, skeletal territories constituting the site of eosinophilic granuloma.

Acute and subacute H.X. is **diffused** or **generalized** to the reticuloendothelial system and thus to the lymph nodes, spleen, lungs, liver, thymus gland, skin and mucosae, bone marrow. Its localization in the skeleton is more easily documented by an anatomo-histological examination than a radiographic one, because the histiocytary proliferation is diffused and micronodular, and because the rapidly fatal course of the disease generally does not allow osteolysis to achieve the threshold of radiographic evidence.

SYMPTOMS

Eosinophilic granuloma of bone is manifested by pain and, in the superficial bones, by swelling which may be considerable. Pathologic fracture rare-

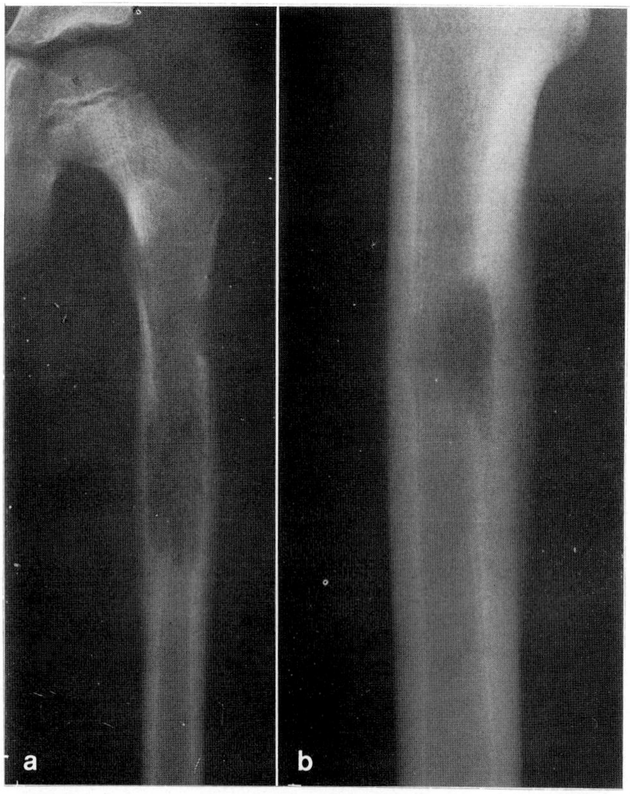

FIG. 655. - (a) Eosinophilic granuloma in a male aged 5 years. (b) In a male aged 20 years.

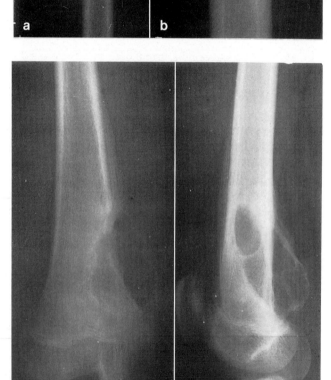

ly occurs. Vertebral eosinophilic granuloma may cause irradiated pain of the radicular type, more rarely, signs of medullary compression. Deformities of the column do not usually occur, as flattening of the vertebral body is uniform. At times, a mild increase in the sedimentation rate, in rare cases, mild eosinophilia, are observed.

In **chronic disseminated H.X.** the skeletal lesions cause the same symptoms as mentioned above, but often they are milder and occur later. In fact, skeletal changes, in addition to being disseminated, tend to be more slowly progressive. Nonetheless, in time they may become more extensive and expand-

FIG. 656. - Eosinophilic granuloma in a female aged 11 years; the radiographic aspect recalls that of aneurysmal bone cyst.

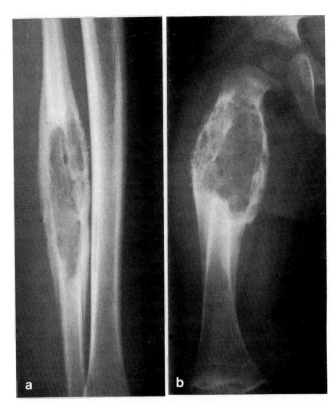

FIG. 657. - (a) Eosinophilic granuloma in a male aged 5 years. The radiographic aspect and clinical course, with some fever, had suggested Ewing's sarcoma. (b) Female aged 1 and 1/2 years. The patient was submitted to curettage. (c) Advanced repair after 2 years in the same case. (d) Twenty-two years after surgery.

ing, with extension of the newly-formed tissue even in the soft tissues. In some cases skeletal lesions occur late or not at all. Depending on the case, symptoms include some of the following. Frequent and early localizations in the maxillary bones and in the oral mucosa cause pain, swelling and ulcers of the gums, loosening of the teeth, purulent secretion and hemorrhage of the periodontal gums. Pulmonary localization is also frequent and early. At times, it is nearly asymptomatic and is discovered by chance during schermography or a radiographic examination of the skeleton. At times, symptoms (fever, asthenia, coughing) suggest a tubercular affection. In more severe and advanced stages of the disease, signs of emphysema, spontaneous pneumothorax may occur, as well as chronic heart and respiratory insufficiency. Cranioencephalic localizations may cause esophthalmus, polydipsia and pulyuria (insipid diabetes), somatic infantilism and genital hypoevolutism, mental retardation. Papulous skin eruptions and seborrhoic eczema, hepato-splenomegaly, enlargement of the lymph nodes may also be observed. Changes in the lymph nodes may occur in the lymphatic districts connected to skin, mucosae, skeletal areas involved. The famous Hand-Schuller-Christian triad (multiple osteolysis, particularly of the cranium, insipid diabetes and esophthalmus) may very rarely be observed.

Acute diffused H.X., nearly exclusively observed in the child aged under 3 years, is manifested by symptoms of a systemic reticulosis having a rapid and malignant course. Skeletal signs do not occur or decidedly take on secondary importance. There is fever, diffused painless enlargement of the lymph nodes, moderate or severe increase in the volume of the liver and of the spleen. Skin eruptions occur similar to those of seborrhoic eczema, there are ulcero-necrotic manifestations of the upper respiratory mucosae, otitis and recurring bacterial infections. Platelet-penic hemorrhagic diathesis is manifested, especially expressed by skin petechiae and progressive hypochromic anemia. There is an increase in sedimentation rate.

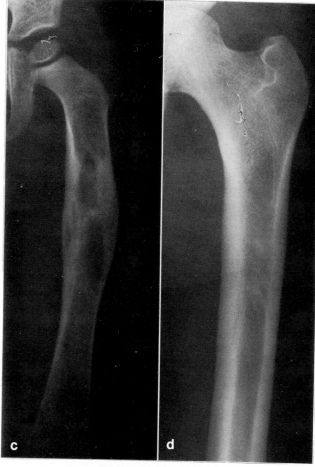

FIG. 657. (continued)

RADIOGRAPHIC FEATURES

Eosinophilic granuloma of bone (solitary or multicentric) is manifested by an area of osteolysis, which destroys the trabeculae and erodes the cortex

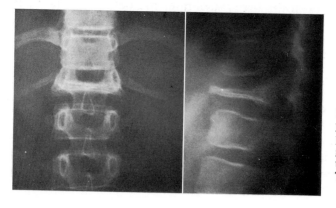

FIG. 658. - Female aged 7 years. Typical vertebral plana. The eosinophilic granuloma was ascertained histologically. There was a second skeletal localization.

from the inside (Figs. 651-659). In the diaphysis, the osteolysis may be central and involve the entire cortical shaft, or it may be eccentric, at the onset destroying only one side of the tubular compact bone. The osteolysis is homogeneous and complete, rounded in shape, often polycyclical. Its boundaries may be rather well-defined, they are rarely marked by a thin sclerotic rim (Fig. 653 a, b). This occurs in less active and less recent forms of the disease, where the process is less invasive and repair phenomena on the part of the surrounding bone are evident. On the contrary, in other cases, the osteolysis has indistinct boundaries (Figs. 651, 654), or small multiple and faded osteolyses are observed, located close together or confluent (Fig. 655a). These aspects denote an invasive process, that is, active and recent. It must be recalled that eosinophilic granuloma grows rapidly and has a fair

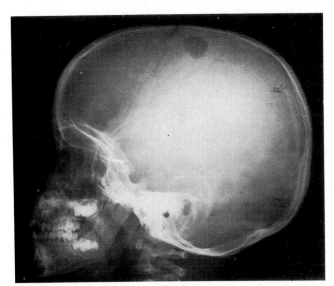

FIG. 659. - Male aged 2 years. Cranial lesion in a case of histiocytosis X disseminated in the skeleton.

capacity to infiltrate. Thus, it may erode and cancel an area of cortex, providing a **radiographic impression of malignancy** (Figs. 651, 654a, 657a). Particularly in diaphyseal localizations or in the clavicle, there is lively periosteal osteogenetic reaction (these are generally children or adolescents). This periostosis initially appears in thin, faded layers, at times superimposed «onion skin» like (Figs. 653d, 655b). In the vertebrae in the child and adolescent, uniform and rapid flattening of the vertebral body is typical (generally it has already occurred when the first radiograms are obtained). The vertebral body may be reduced to a lamina which is thinner than the discs (**vertebra plana**) (Fig. 658). The osteolysis may extend to the pedicle and to the vertebral arch. In the adult, instead, vertebral eosinophilic granuloma causes central and rounded osteolysis of the body, often without determining any collapse.

Total body isotope scan of the skeleton is indicated, in order to exclude multiple localizations. CAT and MRI show that the lesion is contained by the periosteum (Fig. 652) and, in the vertebral column, there is usually no expansion in the paravertebral soft tissues.

Chronic disseminated H.X. produces multiple osteolytic lesions of the type described now. Some of these lesions may be quite extensive. Due to the

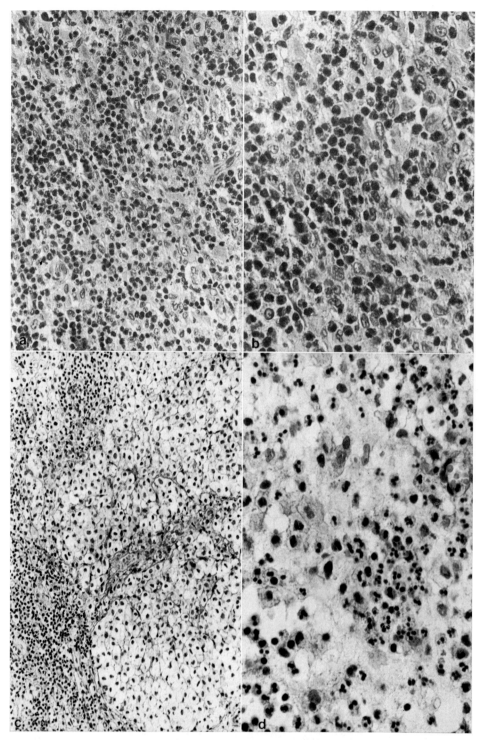

Fig. 660. - Histological aspects of eosinophilic granuloma. Foam cells are evident in (c) and (d) (*Hemat.-eos.*, 300, 500, 200, 500 x).

chronic progression of the lesions, well-defined boundaries due to considerable surrounding reactive hyperostosis may be observed (Figs. 661, 662a). In the cranium, larger and more confluent osteolyses have a polycyclical and uneven outline (like a «geography map»: Fig. 661a). In the cranial base, osteolysis of the sphenoid and walls of the orbit may be observed. There may be extensive destruction of the sella turcica. Osteolysis of the maxillary bones with erosion of the aveoli and the falling of teeth occur frequently. In the lungs there may be bilateral increase in finely reticulated opacity (Fig. 662b), at times dotted with small thickening nodules. This radiographic picture may be followed by that of marked interstitial fibrosis and of the polycystic lung. There is no enlargement of the hilar lymph nodes.

In acute diffused H.X. the radiographic picture of the skeleton is generally negative, as the diffused nature and the acute and rapidly fatal course of the disease does not allow for the skeletal lesions to become radiographically evident. Nonetheless, in some cases generalized and faded osteoporosis may be observed. In other cases, small disseminated osteolytic areas occur (particularly in the cranium, pelvis, and femurs). This last aspect is observed in subacute forms and in those exceptional cases characterized by long survival, and progression towards the disseminated chronic form.

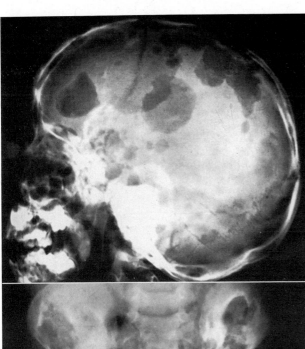
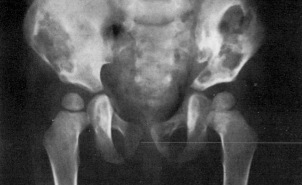

GROSS PATHOLOGIC FEATURES

As the tissue of **eosinophilic granuloma** is formed by histiocytes and leukocytes, it is rather soft, at times semi-liquid, and it is yellowish-gray or leathery-

FIG. 661. - Chronic disseminated histiocytosis X (Hand Schuller-Christian) in a male aged 5 years.

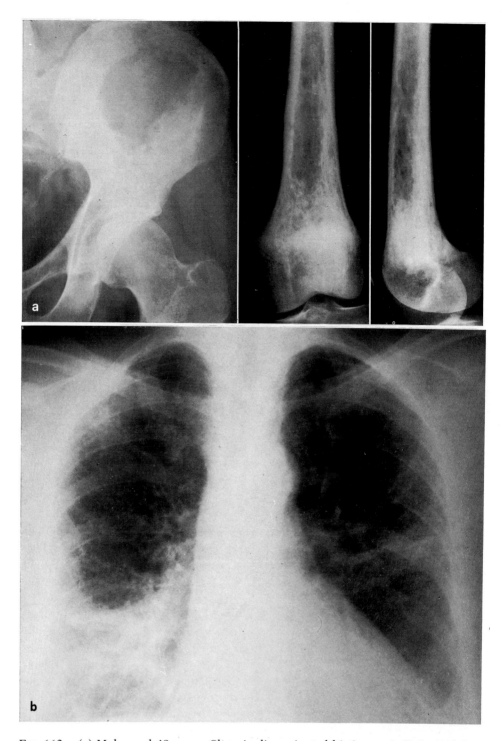

FIG. 662. - (a) Male aged 49 years. Chronic disseminated histiocytosis X. Insipid diabetes. (b) Female aged 60 years. Pulmonary changes in chronic disseminated histiocytosis X.

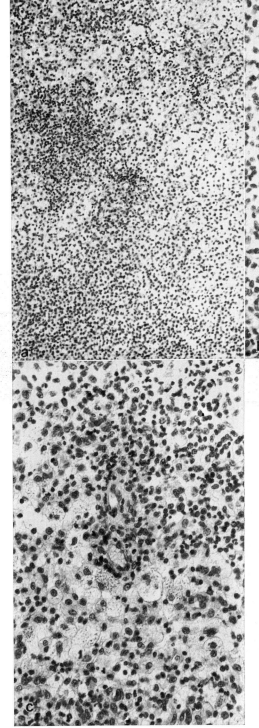

FIG. 663. - Histological aspects of chronic disseminated histiocytosis X. (a) and (b) Aspects the same as those of eosinophilic granuloma. (c) Abundant foam cells.

yellow in color. It often contains dull red areas of hemorrhage and other yellowish colliquative areas of necrosis.

Because of their abundant lipoid contents and greater amount of fibrosis, lesions in the **chronic disseminated form** are characterized by a more decidedly yellow or yellow-brown color and a firmer consistency. Nonetheless, these changes may also be observed in «aged» solitary eosinophilic granuloma; while more recent lesions in the disseminated chronic form ap-

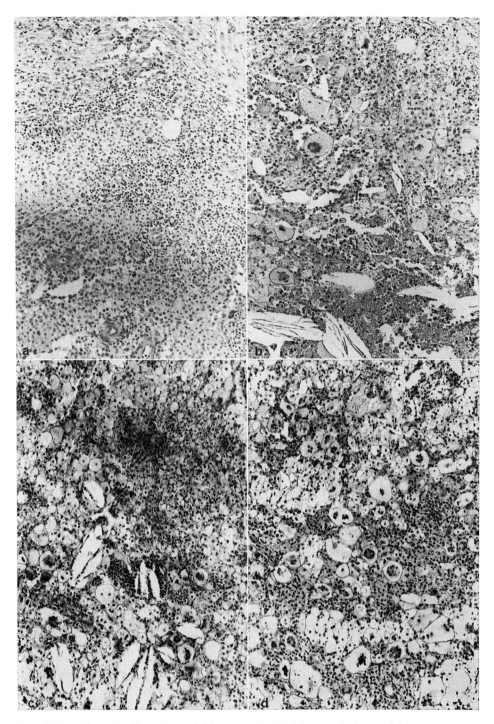

FIG. 664. - Chronic disseminated histiocytosis X. (a) Areas of initial fibrosis (upper part of photogram) surrounding granulomatous areas. (b) Foam cells at time gigantic and multinucleate, and bunches of cholesterin crystals. Similar aspects are observed in (c) and (d) (*Hemat.-eos.*, 125, 300, 300, 125, 125, 125, 125 x).

pear not unlike an eosinophilic granuloma. In the chronic form of the disease, the pulmonary lesions progress (as shown by autoptic findings) towards interstitial fibrosis and lead to emphysema, polycystic lung, chronic pulmonary heart. The use of pulmonary biopsy has shown that at an early stage these lesions are the same as eosinophilic granuloma.

HISTOPATHOLOGIC FEATURES

The histological feature common to H.X. is a hyperplastic production of histiocytes with infiltration of leukocytes among which eosinophilic ones dominate. Moreover, this infiltration is very variable: as we are dealing with a hyperplasia which tends to «mature», the histological features vary in time. Gradually, the eosinophiles decrease, the histiocytes are loaded with lipoids, fibrosis increases (Figs. 660, 664).

Eosinophilic granuloma of bone

A more or less loose net of large histiocytes is observed. The cytoplasms are wide, ramified, and have unclear boundaries; at times they are more intensely stained and have clear boundaries. The nuclei are globose, ovoid, indented or reniform, pale and having a small nucleolus. Mitotic figures may be observed. In some rare cases, these cells are rather numerous, constitute the pathologic tissue nearly by themselves, are collected in nests or nodules, and provide the impression of a neoplastic process. Generally, instead, they form a more rarefied pattern which acts as a background to the infiltration of eosinophilic granulocytes (Fig. 660a, b). These may be few and scattered, or very abundant, enough to constitute fields of thick and exclusive leukocytary composition. The eosinophiles cannot be mistaken, because of the small lobate and dark nucleus, and the cytoplasm stuffed with bright red granules [1]. Some eosinophiles have a globose and reniform nucleus (myelocytes). Neutrophiles and lymphocytes, although fewer in number, may be observed mixed in with the eosinophiles. This structure recalls that of an inflammatory granuloma. The stroma is made up of abundant reticulum surrounding small groups or single cells, or surrounding wider cellular areas having no intercellular reticulum. There are numerous newly-formed blood vessels having a thin wall. The histiocytes may fuse together and/or initiate intense macrophagic activity and lipoid accumulation. These aspects, in eosinophilic granuloma of recent formation, as in all recent lesions of H.X., are not con-

---

[1] Stained with eosin or floxin. It may be recalled that decalcification of the specimen may lead to loss of eosinophilia. Thus, it will be best to isolate the pathologic tissue from the bone when taking the specimen, so as to avoid decalcification. Acid and alcoholic fixatives act in the same manner as the decalcification. Thus, fixation in formalin is recommended.

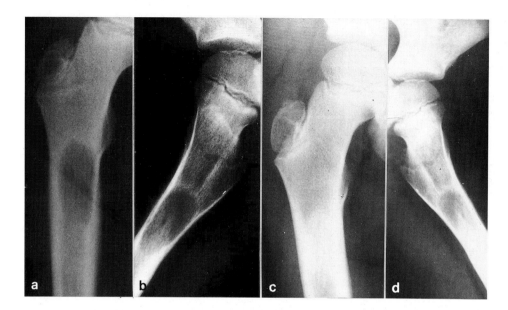

FIG. 665. - Eosinophilic granuloma in a boy aged 6 years. (a) and (b) Needle biopsy and two cortisone infiltrations. (c) and (d) Total repair after 18 months.

stant and sporadic. They consist in a few multinucleate giant cells with few nuclei, in cells with ample clear and foamy cytoplasm (stuffed with lipoid drops), or containing granules of hemosiderin. We rarely have the opportunity to observe an aged skeletal eosinophilic granuloma under microscopy (as the lesion tends to be rather destructive, enough to require earlier surgical treatment). When this occurs, the number of eosinophiles appears to have decreased, while foam and giant cells are more abundant (Fig. 660c, d). A gradually more extended and mature fibrosis also occurs, the expression of the development of scarring phenomena. These aspects are similar to those of the disseminated chronic form of the disease.

Chronic disseminated H.X.

As this is a lesion having a more torpid course than that of eosinophilic granuloma of bone, its histological aspect also differs, just as a productive tuberculosis differs from an exhudative one. But this difference is made even more apparent by related factors: due to the slow progression of the lesion, diagnosis is generally made late; furthermore, treatment is rarely surgical.

Thus, it is difficult to examine a recent lesion of disseminated chronic H.X. under microscopy. In rare cases in which this does occur (skeletal, pulmonary, skin, mucosa, lymph node, hepatic biopsy), the histological aspect is rather similar to that of eosinophilic granuloma (Fig. 663), even if often histiocytary production prevails over the quota of exhudative eosinophilia.

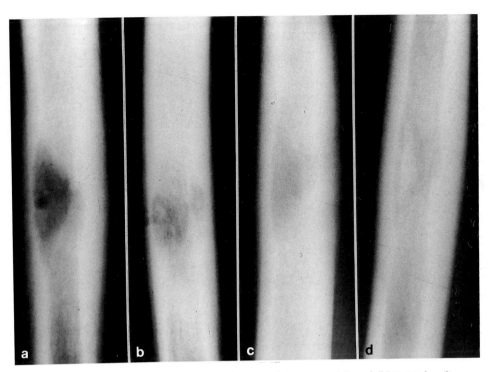

FIG. 666. - Eosinophilic granuloma in a boy aged 16 years. (a) and (b) Initial radiographic picture; observe the hole of the needle biopsy during which cortisone was introduced. Second infiltration after 1 month. (c) and (d) The lesion was repaired after 6 years.

The same identity is observed in those cases which initiate as solitary skeletal or pulmonary eosinophilic granuloma to then become the disseminated chronic form of the disease. But the tissue which is most commonly examined under microscopy, as a result of surgical or autoptic removal, is that of aged and extensive lesions. Large globose cells with ample foamy cytoplasm prevail, strongly stained with Sudan (Fig. 664b). Many cells are gigantic, with two or more nuclei, at times many nuclei arranged in a crown. The nuclei of the foam cells may be central or shifted towards the periphery, and appear to be smaller and darker than those of the proliferating histiocytes. Furthermore, there is considerable fibrosis, which is more or less mature, surrounding groups of cells and bunches of cholesterin crystals. Finally, the usual exhudative elements are observed, but this time at the background and not the foreground (eosinophiles, neutrophiles, lymphocytes). Areas of necrosis are also observed.

Acute and subacute diffused H.X.

The same finding may be observed in the lymph nodes, spleen, lungs, liver, thymus, bone marrow, skin and mucosae. It consists in a rich histiocytic

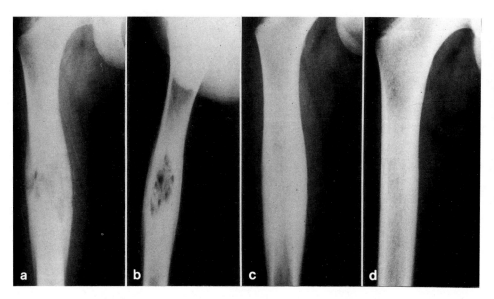

FIG. 667. - Eosinophilic granuloma in a boy aged 7 years (a, b). Pain for the past 2 months. Needle biopsy and two cortisone infiltrations. (c) Lesion repaired after 2 years. (d) Total bone remodelling after 2 more years.

production which diffusedly infiltrates the tissues and at times forms small nodules. The cells appear to be large, with mild pleomorphism and some mitotic figures. Numerous leukocytes are observed among which eosinophiles prevail. There may be some multinucleate giant cells and rare cells with foamy cytoplasm. Nonetheless, due to the speed of development, lipoid accumulation is very scarce or even absent.

In all forms of H.X., electron microscopy has revealed that in the histiocytary cells there are filaments and striated sticks having a swollen end in the shape of a vesicle (**Langerhans cells**).

ETIOLOGY AND PATHOGENESIS

Etiology is unknown, but a viral origin is supposed. The frequency of pulmonary localizations in chronic forms could indicate the principal entry of the virus in the respiratory path. Lesions of the lymph nodes, as well, which may be manifested as satellite lymphadenites, seem to confirm an infective nature of the disease. Nothing is known of its pathogenesis either. An allergic-hyperergic nature has been hypothesized. What is certain is that histiocytosis X is a pseudogranuloma hyperplastic process, not a neoplastic one. Arguments in favor of the gnosographic unit of the disease have already been discussed. As etiology is not known, these arguments are clinical and anatomo-pathological.

DIAGNOSIS

On a purely **radiographic** basis, because of its rapid osteolytic growth skeletal eosinophlic granuloma may simulate a **malignant tumor**: as we are generally dealing with children and localizations in the trunk or a diaphysis, the most probable impression is that of **Ewing's sarcoma** or (if there are multiple localizations) **metastatic neuroblastoma**. In some diaphyseal or clavicular localizations, with considerable periosteal reaction, the radiographic aspect may be the same as that of **osteomyelitis**. In some cases, particularly vertebral localizations and those in the long bones, the radiographic picture is typical enough to avoid biopsy. In the chronic disseminated form of the disease, the radiographic images of the lungs may suggest **Besnier-Boeck-Schaumann disease**, as compared to which there is no enlargement of the ilar lymph nodes.

The **macroscopic picture** of skeletal eosinophilic granuloma is rather suggestive, because of the soft yellowish-gray tissue. Nonetheless, it may be rather similar to the granulation tissue and pus of an **osteomyelitis**. Furthermore, yellowish areas of necrosis may also be observed in **Ewing's sarcoma** and in **lymphoma**.

The **histological** diagnosis of eosinophilic granuloma is generally easy, even if it requires good specimens (preferably not decalcified) and rather abundant samples, due to the frequent secondary modifications, such as hemorrhaging, necrosis, areas of fibrosis or lipidic storage. If the specimen has been decalcified or fixed in alcohol or in acid fixatives, the eosinophiles may not take up the eosin and may thus be difficult to distinguish from the neutrophiles. Thus, doubts may arise as to whether we are dealing with eosinophilic granuloma or osteomyelitis. In eosinophilic granuloma there is greater evidence of the histiocytary net, the eosinophiles have less «segmented» nuclei than those of the neutrophiles of a pyogenic process, and the plasmacells are absent. Histological differential diagnosis may also involve **Hodgkin's lymphoma**. This occurs in the case of a skeletal eosinophilic granuloma, and, even moreso, in lymph node localizations of chronic disseminated histiocytosis X at an early stage. Hodgkin's disease also has a granulomatoid structure, with reticular cells, lymphocytes, plasmacells, neutrophiles and, at times, a large number of eosinophiles. Nonetheless, the nuclei of the reticular cells, as compared to eosinophilic granuloma, are larger, pleomorphic, hyperchromic, with a large nucleolus, and more frequent mitotic figures. Sclerosis tends to be more intense and diffused. But, above all, there are the Sternberg cells. To this may be added that Hodgkin is usually observed in the adult, it is often associated with ondulating fever, enlargement of the lymph nodes, splenomegaly, relative neutrophilia. In the skeleton it tends to affect the vertebral column, pelvis and limb girdles. Radiographically, it causes images of osteolysis and often of osteosclerosis, characterized by very faded limits.

The histological diagnosis of chronic lesions of H.X. is generally unmistakeable. The aspect is very different from that of **Gaucher's disease**, where the foam cells are smaller, more uniform, mononucleate, and giant multinucleate cells, cholesterin crystals, fibrosis and the exhudative component are absent.

The histological aspect of the acute diffused form (and of some early lesions in eosinophilic granuloma of bone or in the chronic disseminated form) may present differential problems with respect to **lymphoma**, when histiocytic production with aspects of lively proliferation predominates, and eosinophiles are very scarce. The difference is based on the granulomatoid structure of the tissue (it is not a «matted» neoplastic proliferation), on the minor amount of pleomorphism, and on the absence of hyperchromia and atypia of the cells.

COURSE

Eosinophilic granuloma of bone has a relatively rapid course, causing rather ample osteolysis, enough to require treatment within a few months. Even if it is not treated, it tends towards spontaneous scarring maturation, with radiographic thickening of the surrounding bone and with those histological changes (lipoidosis, scarring sclerosis) previously recalled. At times the lesion repairs completely, with complete skeletal reconstruction. Spontaneous repair is well-known in cases of vertebra plana treated by immobilization in plaster, often healing with surprising reconstruction of the vertebral body.

Solitary eosinophilic granuloma of bone may be transformed into a multiple form, still localized in the skeleton. This is, however, a rare occurrence (perhaps in 1 case out of 10) and is always manifested within 1 year of the occurrence of the first lesion. Transformation into chronic disseminated H.X. is instead an exceptional occurrence.

Chronic disseminated H.X. may begin with a skeletal lesion, or a pulmonary one, or one of the oral mucosa. Thereafter, new localizations occur in different tissues and organs and the single lesions are extended, but considerably slowly, over the years. These lesions, too, as previously described, tend to mature with progressive lipoid accumulation and fibrosis.

Acute and subacute diffused H.X. has a rapid course and is generally fatal within a few months. In exceptional cases and under the action of therapy, it may transform into the chronic form of the disease.

TREATMENT

In **eosinophilic granuloma of bone**, the ideal treatment consists in injecting slowly absorbable cortisone in the lesion (Figs. 665, 666, 667). This is possible when the radiographic picture is diagnostic, or when diagnosis is already known (local recurrence, second localizations), and when the site favors injection. Usually from 1 to 3 injections are sufficient, and in 6-12 months there is first an arrest in development and then complete repair of the lesion.

When radiographic diagnosis is doubtful, surgery is performed with frozen section biopsy, curettage, local cortisone, possibly bone grafts. In vertebral localizations, if diagnosis is doubtful, needle-biopsy may be performed. Treatment may consist in simple immobilization with an external orthosis, or chemotherapy. Decompressive laminectomy is indicated in cases with extension of the lesion to the posterior arch and impingement on the nervous structures.

In some sites, such as the ribs or the fibular diaphysis, marginal resection may be used. In particular cases and during adult age, radiation therapy may also be used at minimum sufficient doses (2-3000 r). In multiple eosinophilic granulomas local or general cortisone treatment and antiblastic therapy may be used (see further on).

For **chronic disseminated H.X.** treatment is based on corticosteroids. Some skeletal lesions may be treated surgically (for example, femoral lesions compromising bone resistance) and/or with radiation therapy (cranial and vertebral lesions). Radiation is contraindicated on pulmonary fields as it favors fibrosis. In addition to corticosteroids, antiblastic products such as amethopterin (Methotrexate) and vinblastine (Velbe) have been used. Treatment also includes antibiotics (for ulcerated and infected lesions) and pitressin in order to control insipid diabetes.

For **acute diffused H.X.** treatment is based on corticosteroids and antiblastics, on antibiotics (because of a high susceptibility to bacterial infections), on hemostatics and transfusions.

PROGNOSIS

In **eosinophilic granuloma of bone** prognosis is always excellent. It is so also in the case of multiple lesions as long as there are no extraskeletal localizations. Rarely, when intralesional excision is made during the progressive phase of the disease, there may be local recurrence.

In **chronic disseminated H.X.** prognosis depends on the site and on the extent of the lesions. The worst outcomes are insipid diabetes and pulmonary fibrosis. These are irreversible changes and may lead to death. Skeletal lesions, even those which are rather extensive, may repair with radiation treatment.

The prognosis of **acute diffused H.X.** is usually fatal, within a few months to 1-2 years. The most unfavorable prognostic signs are: age under 3 years, splenomegaly, hemorrhagic diathesis, leukopenia, a high number of bones affected. If the patient survives more than 3 years after the onset of symptoms, prognosis becomes favorable.

REFERENCES

1953 LICHTENSTEIN L.: Histiocytosis X. Integration of eosinophilic granuloma of bone, « Letterer-Siwe disease » and « Schüller-Christian disease » as related manifestations of a single nosologic entity. *Archives of Pathology*, **56**, 84-102.

1960 Mc Gravan M. H., Spady H. A.: Eosinophilic granuloma of bone. A study of twenty-eight cases. *Journal of Bone and Joint Surgery*, **42**-A, 979-992.

1964 Lichtenstein L.: Histiocytosis X (Eosinophilic granuloma of bone, Letterer-Siwe disease and Schüller-Christian disease). Further observations of pathological and clinical importance. *Journal of Bone and Joint Surgery*, **46**-A, 76-90.

1966 Ochsner S. F.: Eosinophilic granuloma of bone. Experience with 20 cases. *American Journal of Roentgenology*, **97**, 719-726.

1967 Enriquez P., Dahlin D. C., Hayles A. B., Henderson E. D.: Histiocytosis X: a clinical study. *Mayo Clinic Proceedings*, **42**, 88-99.

1968 Manning C.: Eosinophilic granuloma. *Journal of Bone and Joint Surgery*, **50**-B, 232-232.

1969 Friedman B., Hanaoka H.: Langerhans cell granules in eosinophilic granuloma of bone. *Journal of Bone and Joint Surgery*, **51**-A, 367-374.

1969 Nesbit M. E., Kieffer S., D'Angio G. J.: Reconstitution of vertebral height in histiocytosis X: a long-term follow-up. *Journal of Bone and Joint Surgery*, **51**-A, 1360-1368.

1970 Bromberger N. A.: Eosinophilic granuloma in children. *Journal of Bone and Joint Surgery*, **52**-B, 802-802.

1970 Fevre M., Bertrand P.: Existence de granulomes éosinophiles épiphysaires. *Revue de Chirurgie Orthopedique*, **56**, 345-353.

1970 Fowles J. W., Bobechko W. P.: Solitary eosinophilic granuloma of bone. *Journal of Bone and Joint Surgery*, **52**-B, 238-243.

1970 Giunti G., Frizzera G., Giunti A., Bertoni F.: Sul granuloma eosinofilo dello scheletro. Dati clinico-anatomici e considerazioni istogenetiche su 41 casi. *Chirurgia degli Organi di Movimento*, **59**, 331-341.

1970 Shamoto M.: Langerhans cell granule in Letterer-Siwe disease. An electron microscopic study. *Cancer*, **26**, 1102-1108.

1971 Calandriello B.: Istiocitosi X dello scheletro. *Lo scalpello*, **1**, 9-25.

1971 Chacha P. B., Khong B. T.: Eosinophilic granuloma of bone. A diagnostic problem. *Clinical Orthopaedics*, **80**, 79-88.

1971 Cheyne C.: Histiocytosis X. *Journal of Bone and Joint Surgery*, **53**-B, 366-382.

1971 Imamura M., Muroya K.: Lymph node ultrastructure in Hand-Schüller-Christian disease. *Cancer*, **27**, 956-964.

1972 Basset F., Escaig J., Le Crom M.: A cytoplasmic membranous complex in histiocytosis X. *Cancer*, **29**, 1380-1385.

1972 Farine J., Onaknine G., Horoszowski H., Kosary I. Z., Katznelson A., Engel J., Rotem Y.: Granulomes éosinophiles vertébraux avec compression médullaire chez l'enfant. *Revue de Chirurgie Orthopedique*, **58**, 575-586.

1972 Kondi E. S., Deckers P. J., Gallitano L. A., Khung C. L.: Diffuse eosinophilic granuloma of bone. *Cancer*, **30**, 1169-1173.

1973 Schajowicz F., Slullitel J.: Eosinophilic granuloma of bone and its relationship to Hand-Schüller-Christian and Letterer-Siwe syndromes. *Journal of Bone and Joint Surgery*, **55**-B, 545-565.

1973 Smith D. G., Nesbit M. E., D'Angio G. J., Levitt S. H.: Histiocytosis X: role of radiation therapy in management with special reference to dose levels employed. *Radiology*, **106**, 419-422.

1973 West W. O.: Velban as treatment for diffuse eosinophilic granuloma of bone. Report of a case. *Journal of Bone and Joint Surgery*, **55**-A, 1775-1759.

1976 Stern M. B., Cassidy R., Mirra J.: Eosinophilic granuloma of the proximal tibial epiphysis. *Clinical Orthopaedics*, **118**, 153-156.

1977 Nezeloff C.: L'histiocytose X. *Revue de Chirurgie Orthopedique*, Suppl. II, **63**, 187-200.

1979 Bertoni F., Capanna R.: Granuloma eosinofilo atipico. Descrizione di 2 casi. *Giornale Italiano di Ortopedia e Traumatologia*, **5**, 367-378.

1979 Nezeloff C., Frileux-Herbert F., Cronier-Sachot J.: Disseminated histiocytosis X. Analysis of prognostic factors based on a retrospective study of 50 cases. *Cancer*, **44**, 1824-1838.

1980 Cohen H., Zornosa J., Cangir Ayten, Murray J.A., Wallace S.: Direct injection of methylprednisolone sodium succinate in the treatment of solitary eosinophilic granuloma of bone. *Radiology*, **136**, 289-293.

1980 KOTZ R.L., SILVA E.G., DE SANTOS L.A., LUKEMAN J.M.: Diagnosis of eosinophilic granuloma of bone by citology, histology and electron microscopy of
transcutaneous bone-aspiration biopsy. *Journal of Bone and Joint Surgery*,
62-A, 1284-1290.

1983 NAUERT C., ZORNOZA J., AYALA A., HARLE T.S.: Eosinophilic granuloma of bone:
diagnosis and management. *Skeletal Radiology*, **10**, 227-235.

1983 USUI M., MATSUNO T., KOBAYASHI M., YAGI T., SASAKI T., ISHII S.: Eosinophilic
granuloma of growing epiphysis. *Clinical Orthopaedics*, **176**, 201-205.

1984 ELEMA J.D., ATMOSOERODJO-BRIGGS A.: Langerhans cells and macrophages in
eosinophilic granuloma. An enzyme-histochemical, enzyme-cytochemical, and
ultrastructural study. *Cancer*, **54**, 2174-2181.

1984 IDE F., IWASE T., SAITO I., UMEMURA S., NAKAJIMA T.: Immunohistochemical
and ultrastructural analysis of the proliferating cells of histiocytosis X.
Cancer, **53**, 917-921.

1985 CAPANNA R., SPRINGFIELD D.S., RUGGIERI P., BIAGINI R., PICCI P., BACCI G.,
GIUNTI A., LORENZI E., CAMPANACCI M.: Direct cortisone injection in eosino-
philic granuloma of bone: a preliminary report on 11 patients. *Journal of
Pediatric Oncology*, **5**, 338-342.

1986 GOODMAN M.A.: Plasma cell tumors. *Clinical Orthopaedics*, **204**, 86-92.

1986 MAKLEY J.T., CARTER J.R.: Eosinophilic granuloma of bone. *Clinical Orthopaedics*, **204**, 37-44.

OSTEOSIS DUE TO PRIMARY HYPERPARATHYROIDISM

PHYSIOPATHOLOGY

The parathyroid hormone (PTH) controls the homeostasis of calcium. It raises calcemia and lowers phosphatemia (the product between ionized calcium and phosphate ions tends to remain constant). The increase in calcemia occurs because of the triple action of the PTH: mobilization of the phosphocalcic mineral from the bone with osteolysis, increase in the nephrotubular resorption of Ca, increase in the intestinal absorption of Ca (in the presence of vitamin D). The proportional decrease of phosphatemia (despite mobilization of the phosphates from the bone) occurs because the PTH inhibits resorption of the phosphates via the renal tubule.

The hyperincretion of PTH thus causes **hypercalcemia, hypophosphatemia, hyperphosphaturia**, and **hypercalciuria**. The latter depends on the fact that hypercalcemia produces a strong increase in $Ca++$ in the glomerular filtrate, which is not compensated by the increased calcic tubular resorption. In the skeleton, as an ineffective attempt to compensate for the intense osteolysis, diffused osteogenetic activity is revived, causing an increase in **serum alkaline phosphatase**.

In the long run, H.P.T. causes **hypercalcemic syndromes** including:

1) neuromuscular changes (let us recall the effect of $Ca++$ on neuromuscular excitability): psychological depression, drowsiness, irritability, apathy, at times actual psychosis; muscular hypotonia and asthenia, at times pseudomyopathic syndromes.

2) Digestive: anorexia, dyspepsia, stypsis; abdominal pains and vomiting; peptic ulcer; pancreatitis.

3) Cardiac: shortening of the Q-T interval in electrocardiogram.

4) Ocular: corneal calcification (band keratopathy).

5) Renal: polydypsia and polyuria (due to the increased urinary elimination of calcium and phosphates); renal calculosis of Ca phosphate and oxalate; interstitial nephrocalcinosis; hydronephrosis, pyelonephritis, and — at the end — chronic renal insufficiency.

6) Skeletal: osteoarticular pain and sometimes skeletal swellings, pathologic fracture, loosening of the teeth, osteolysis of the maxillae, «drumstick» fingers, deformity of the spine, of the pelvis and of the limbs. All of these symp-

toms depend on hyperparathyroid osteosis with diffused osteoporosis and «brown tumors».

7) Calcifications in the arteries, lungs, kidneys, pancreas, muscles and myocardium, in the articular and para-articular soft tissues.

These hypercalcemic syndromes vary greatly, depending on the association and intensity of symptoms, on the entity and duration of H.P.T., on the individual response, on the target organs which are more affected. As we are dealing with pseudotumoral lesions of the skeleton here, only **primary H.P.T.** will be discussed. **Secondary H.P.T.** (to hypocalcemia or hyperphosphatemia in osteomalacic syndromes, to vitamin D deficiency, to hyperazotemic chronic renal insufficiency, to congenital tubular nephropathies, to malabsorption syndromes) in fact cause skeletal changes which are weaker and more diffused, generally having no pseudotumoral aspects. In H.P.T. secondary to chronic renal insufficiency, which nowadays is more frequently observed as patients are kept alive by dialysis, pseudotumoral calcifications may be observed in the soft tissues (Fig. 673c).

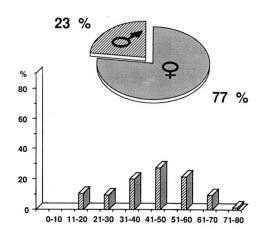

FIG. 668. - Sex, age in 65 cases of primary hyperparathyroidism with patent skeletal lesions.

DEFINITION

P.H.P.T. is a chronic disease due to hyperincretion of PTH due to: a) one or more parathyroid adenomas; b) primary and diffused hyperplasia of the parathyroid glands; c) secreting parathyroid carcinoma. In any case the result is chronic hypercalcemic syndrome, the clinical presentation of which varies. There are nearly exclusively renal forms, which are those occurring most frequently. There are renal and skeletal forms; prevalently skeletal foms; finally (more rarely) prevalently digestive or neuromuscular forms.

FREQUENCY

P.H.P.T. is erroneously considered to be rare. The fact is that many cases, characterized by weak symptoms but sometimes also having evident and even severe clinical pictures, go unrecognized, and are labelled renal calculosis, gastroduodenal affection, maxillary cyst or epulid, osteoporosis or osteo-malacia, fibrous dysplasia of bone, giant cell bone tumor, etc. Cases of P.H.P.T. characterized by prevalently extraskeletal clinical manifestations (particularly renal) occur more frequently. Those with evident and pseudotumoral lesions of bone are rarer (approximately 20% of the total number).

HEREDITY

This has been observed in some cases.

SEX

While when P.H.P.T. is considered overall it does not reveal significant predilection for sex, cases of the disease characterized by evident skeletal manifestations show clear predilection for the female sex, at a ratio of 3:1 (Fig. 668).

AGE

The disease is nearly always manifested after puberty, between 15 and 70 years of age (Fig. 668).

LOCALIZATION

Osteoporosis due to P.H.P.T. is diffused to the entire skeleton. Nonetheless, if in an advanced phase it tends to become evident throughout, at the onset it is particularly manifested in some areas, such as around the teeth, the hands, the cranium, the acromial ends of the clavicles, the pelvis, the metaepiphyses of the long bones. There is no constant rule: in one of our cases of P.H.P.T. going back 15 years and showing a very severe pseudo-osteomalacic picture of the skeleton of the trunk and of the long bones, with brown

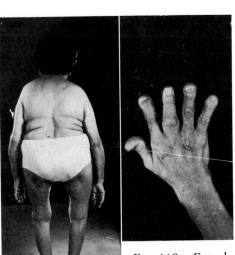

FIG. 669. - Female aged 56 years. Primary hyperparathyroidism with skeletal symptoms for the past 14 years. Observe deformity of the osteomalacic type in the skeleton and «drumstick» fingers.

tumors and pathologic fractures, the hands and cranium showed no evident lesions.

Brown tumors show predilection for the following and in this order: the metaepiphyses of the long bones, the pelvis, the diaphyses. They may be observed in the maxillary bones, the cranium, the ribs, the hand. They are hardly ever observed in the vertebral column.

SYMPTOMS

The patient affected with pseudotumoral skeletal lesions due to P.H.P.T. generally seeks orthopaedic advice for the following symptoms (in decreasing order of frequency). Chronic pain related to one or more brown tumors, which are usually para-articular, at times diaphyseal; sudden pain due to pathologic fracture of the wall of a brown tumor or in severe osteoporosis; diffused, chronic osteo-articular pain; slowly increasing swelling (when the brown tumor is characterized by a superficial site, such as the tibia, elbow, forearm, iliac crest, cranium, ribs). In exceptional cases there is tendinous avulsion (for example, of the patellar tendon) which may even be bilateral, or epiphysiolysis of the hip. At times the patient first turns to a stomatologist, for «cystic» lesion of a maxillary bone.

In these patients, **the clinical history** is very important, which nearly always reveals signs of considerable muscular and psychological asthenia, polydipsia and polyuria. Rather frequently there is nephrolithiasis or pyelonephritis, constipation, some digestive disorders or a peptic ulcer, weight loss (in more advanced stages). Pancreatic syndromes are rarely traced. Finally, cases (often hereditary) with pluriglandular adenomas are described, where the P.H.P.T. is associated with hyperthyroidism, acromegaly, Cushing's syndrome, Zollinger-Ellison syndrome.

An objective examination may reveal skeletal swellings, at times signs of fracture and, in the hands, «drumstick» fingers, with shortening of the last phalanx (Fig. 669b). In more severe and advanced cases there is anemia, weight loss, deformity of the chest, spine and pelvis as in severe osteomalacia (Fig. 669a), diffused skeletal pain, pathologic fractures. At times the patients may be unable to hold an erect position. Only rarely may the parathyroid adenoma be palpated.

RADIOGRAPHIC FEATURES

This may vary greatly, so much so that there hardly exist two similar cases. The radiographic picture is made up of two elements: lacunar osteoporosis and «brown tumor» images (Figs. 670-680).

Brown tumors appear to be rounded osteolytic areas, at times polycyclical (Figs. 670-674, 680, 687-690). The osteolysis may be central or eccentric and it may considerably attenuate or even partially cancel the cortex. It may tend to expand moderately (very large swelling is rare), but it never invades

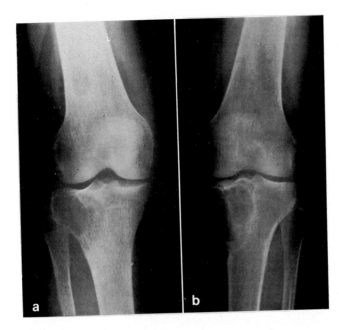

FIG. 670. - (a) Female aged 36 years. Brown tumors in the tibia and femur. Typical diffused lacunar osteoporosis. (b) Female aged 58 years. Brown tumor histologically exchanged for giant cell tumor and thus submitted to resection. Thereafter, parathyroid adenoma removed.

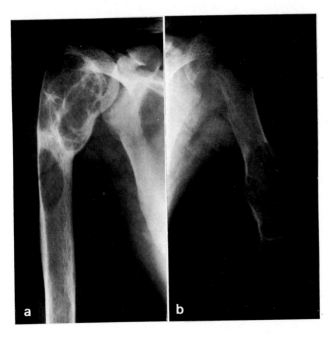

the soft tissues, nor does it cause periosteal reaction. Its boundaries may be relatively well-defined, or rather faded, but a delimiting rim of sclerosis is hardly ever observed. At times «brown tumor» osteolysis is veiled by a ground glass opacity due to neoproduction of osteoid tissue (Fig. 687a).

Osteoporosis is due to lively and diffused osteoclastic and periosteocytic osteolysis, both of the cancellous bone and of the compact bone (Figs. 675, 686). The consequence is progressive and consists in widening and confluence of the intraspongeose medullary spaces, uneven widening of the haversian canals, irregular endosteal (with widening of the medullary canal and narrowing of the

FIG. 671. - Male aged 22 years. (a) Brown tumors of the right humerus. (b) Left humerus in the same patient and at the same date, after immobilization in plaster. Observe the severe osteoporosis caused by immobilization.

diaphyseal compact bone) and subperiosteal resorption. Thus, at least at the beginning, we are dealing with actual «osteoporosis» due to widening of all of the «pores» of the bone. It may then turn into a rougher moth-eaten appearance, with all of the intermediate gradations between porosity and «brown tumor».

During the **initial stages** of the disease, in younger patients, when normal physical activity is still possible, alongside one or several «brown tumors» (the only cause of skeletal symptoms) there may only be moderate widening of the haversian canals and of the medullary spaces of the cancellous bone, the trabeculae of which preserve good thickness and normal radiopacity (Figs. 671a, 675, 689a, 690a).

Furthermore, there may be mild thinning of the diaphyseal compacts (particularly in the hands), mild «saucer-like» subperiosteal resorption in the intermediate phalanges, fine porosity of the cranium, moderate resorption of the hard lamina around the teeth.

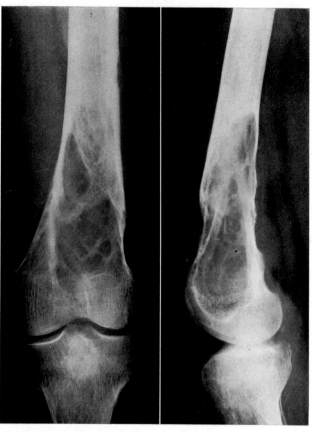

FIG. 672. - Female aged 38 years. Primary hyperparathyroidism. Observe the faded radiopacity of the lesion in the tibial epiphysis.

In **more advanced stages** of the disease, the general radiopacity of the skeleton decreases. Intense osteoporosis of a limb may occur after immobilization in plaster (Figs. 671b, 686b), while generalized osteoporosis is favored by immobilization in bed. Not only do the trabeculae of the cancellous bone become farther apart, but they also become thinner; the cortical bone becomes spongy and gradually loses its thickness (Figs. 671b, 673a, 676b). When skeletal resorption is slower, there is a rather regular and faded reduction in opacity; if, on the contrary, osteolysis is more intense and rapid, there is a diffused «moth-eaten» image, which is also extended to the diaphyses (Fig. 686b).

In the **cranium** there is fine or rough porosity. At times minute and regu-

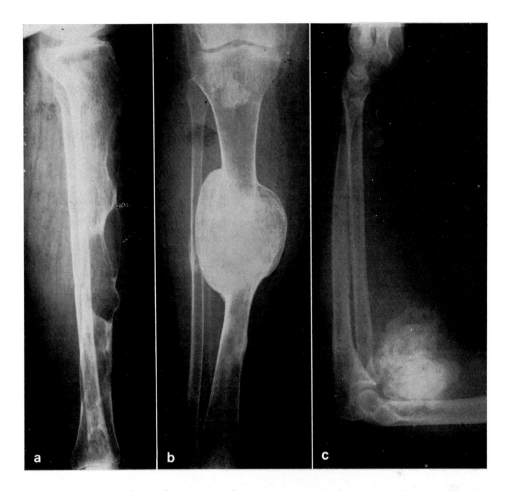

FIG. 673. - (a) Female aged 45 years. The patient wore a plaster cast. (b) Female aged 41 years. Two years earlier submitted to removal of the parathyroid adenoma. Large expanding brown tumor of the tibia ossified after parathyroidectomy. (c) Male aged 27 years. Secondary hyperparathyroidism in nephrodialysis. Pseudotumoral calcification in the soft tissues.

lar radiolucent and radiopaque spots coexist, suggesting a «thick snow-fall» (Fig. 679a). At times, there is thickening of the theca, with rough flakes of faded radiopacity (Fig. 679b). This aspect recalls Paget's disease. The image of puntiform («snow effect») or flaky opacity of the cranium is due to the intense osteogenesis which is associated with bone resorption.

Often, there is faded resorption of the **acromial end of the clavicle** (Fig. 678b). More rarely, due to subchondral resorption, there is faded widening of the sacroiliac joint space and of the pubic symphysis. Very typical is subperiosteal resorption of the tubular bones of the **hands**, particularly of the intermediate phalanges (Figs. 677, 691a). This resorption is more evident on the radial and palmar side of the phalanx, and it is in the form of a mild depression having a well-defined and regular surface (in less severe and less ad-

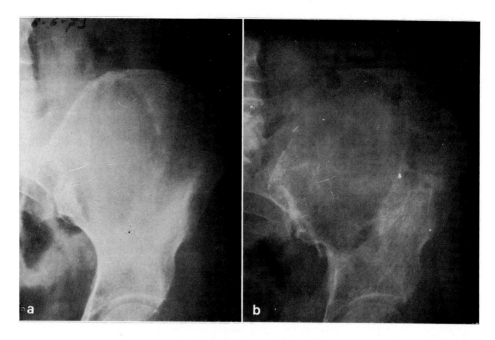

FIG. 674. - Female aged 62 years. (a) Iliac brown tumor. (b) The same after 4 months. The aspect and the rapid radiographic evolution could suggest a malignant tumor.

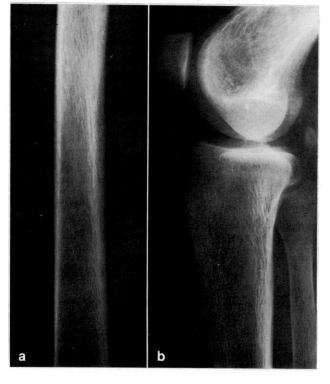

FIG. 675. - (a) Male aged 29 years. Typical microlacunar osteoporosis in the diaphysis of the femur. (b) Male aged 22 years. Diffused microlacunar osteoporosis.

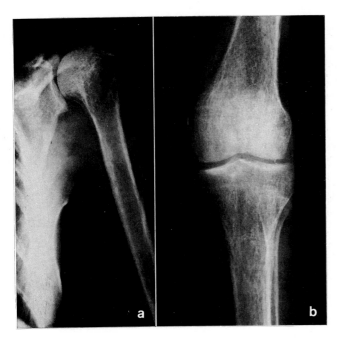

FIG. 676. - Female aged 30 years. (a) Observe subperiosteal resorption of the proximal metaphysis of the humerus, in its medial aspect. (b) Observe subperiosteal resorption in the metaphyses, particularly in the medial surfaces.

vanced cases), or faded or fringed. Similar resorption is observed on the tip of the last phalanx, where fibroblastic and osteoid hyperplasia associated with the osteolysis is the cause of «drumstick» finger deformity. Saucer-like, faded **subperiosteal osteolyses** are more rarely observed in the metaphyses of the long bones, too (Figs. 671b, 676). These subperiosteal resorptions have elective sites, such as the upper or lower surfaces of the femoral neck, the anterior aspect of the distal femur, the medial aspect of the proximal tibia, the medial aspect of the proximal humerus; they are exceptionally observed in the diaphyses.

The skeletal segment where radiographic changes are less evident is the **spine**. In more than half of all cases with evident osteopathy radiograms of the vertebral column are practically negative. Brown tumors are exceptionally observed in the vertebrae (Fig. 680b).

In **even more advanced forms** (when the P.H.P.T. goes back several years, when digestive and renal functions are modified, when the patient moves very little or may even be confined to bed, when we are dealing with females of post-climateric age) it is possible to observe radiographic pictures of extreme demineralization, similar to those of severe osteomalacia. These include intense and faded radiotransparence, considerable thinning of the cortices, «bell-like» deformity of the chest (with ribs which are thin, wavy, and fractured), «biconcave lens» or wedge-shaped vertebrae, distorted pelvis, multiple pathologic fractures.

The **presence and extent of «brown tumors»** are not at all related to the duration of the disease. There are juvenile cases where «brown tumors» are quite numerous and expanded, while osteoporosis is just hinted at. There are

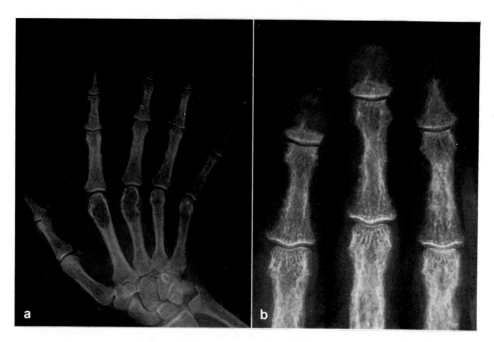

FIG. 677. - (a) Female aged 30 years (same case as in Fig. 676). (b) Female aged 56 years (same case as in Fig. 669).

cases which begin with a large «brown tumor» apparently solitary, associated with moderate osteoporosis and, within a few months or years, evolving with the occurrence of other «brown tumors» and progression of osteoporosis. Finally, there are others with severe diffused osteoporosis dating back several years and small and sporadic «brown tumors».

Osteoporosis takes on particular features in those rare cases which have just gone past **puberty**. There are bands of faded hypertransparence in all of the metaphyses and the skeletal areas adjacent to the nuclei of apophyseal ossification, like the plates delimiting the vertebral bodies, the iliac crest, the tuberosity of the ischium (Fig. 678)(¹).

While brown tumors vary considerably in terms of number and distribution (even if rarely they may appear to be nearly symmetrical in the metaepiphyses of the limbs), osteoporosis and subperiosteal resorption are nearly always diffused and symmetrical.

Rarely, radiograms reveal **calcification** in the form of thin lines in the joint cartilage, calcification of the menisci of the knee, of the intervertebral discs, of the ulno-carpic triangular fibrocartilage.

Infrequently, the **nephrocalcinosis** achieves the threshold of radiographic

---

(¹) Let us recall radiographic pictures of scurvy and renal scurvy, of which secondary H.P.T. is an important component.

evidence. Rarely, there are calcar renal calculi (Fig. 681). Even more rarely, there may be pancreatic calcification.

LABORATORY TESTS

Hypercalcemia

Calcemia (Ca ionized) is constantly increased. In many cases hypercalcemia (Ca total) is mild and discontinuous or totally absent, even in determina-

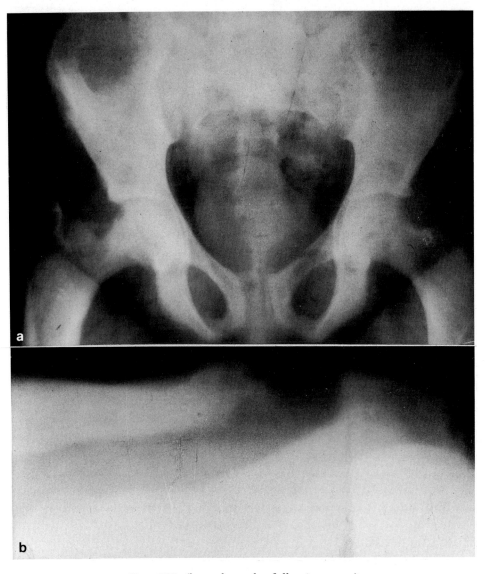

FIG. 678. (legend on the following page)

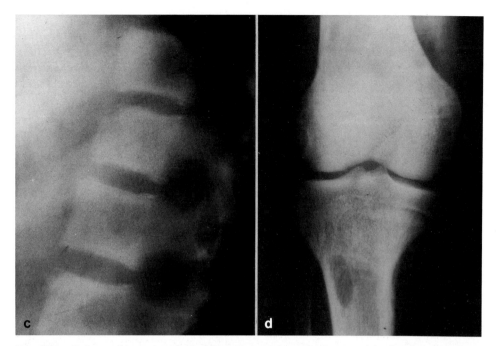

FIG. 678. - Primary hyperparathyroidism, in a girl aged 14 years. (a) Observe widening of the sacroiliac joint, the pubic symphysis and faded bone resorption under the secondary ossification centers of the iliac crest and of the ischiatic tuberosities, and of the upper border of the femoral necks. (b) Faded resorption of the acromial end of the clavicle. (c) Bone resorption under the apophyseal nuclei of the vertebral bodies. (d) Subperiosteal resorption of the medial aspect of the tibia and central metaphyseal area of osteolysis.

tions which are repeated several times and over time. Calcemia which is not very increased or normal may derive from phosphate retention (let us recall that the product $Ca++ \times HPO4--$ tends to remain constant, so that an increase in one of the two factors is associated with decrease of the other), due to insufficient glomerular filtration. It is particularly observed in long-lasting forms, when renal function is seriously compromised. But there are also cases characterized by nearly normal calcemia and preserved glomerular filtration. When this is the case, the test must be repeated and, above all, the ionized Ca must be dosed. However, the calcemia level probably depends on stages of differing parathyroid adenoma activity.

Hypophosphatemia

This finding, too, is not a constant one [1]. Phosphatemia may be normal or increased when glomerular filtration is reduced with phosphate retention.

---

[1] Phosphatemia is considerably influenced by diet.

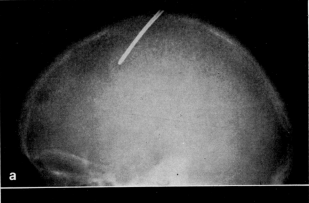

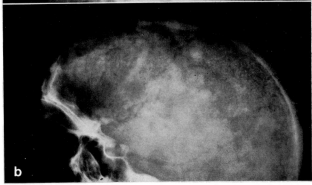

FIG. 679. - (a) Female aged 30 years. «Snow fall» image of cranium. (b) Aspect of cranium with osteolytic areas, other areas are cottony and sclerosed similar to those observed in Paget's disease; others still are «moth-eaten».

However, phosphatemia may also be decreased with normal calcemia and with a reduction in the glomerular filtrate.

Alkaline hyperphosphatasemia

It may be very evident and depend on the compensatory osteogenesis. Often there is a more moderate increase in the acid phosphatasemia, as well.

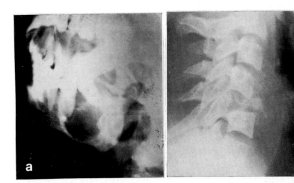

FIG. 680. - (a) Female aged 18 years. «Cyst» of the mandible. (b) Female aged 44 years. Large brown tumor in the 5th cervical vertebra (ascertained histologically). This H.P.T. was nonetheless secondary, in a patient in nephrodialysis.

Hypercalciuria

This is nearly constant.

Hyperphosphaturia

This is less marked and less constant than hypercalciuria.

Tests for renal function

These show the **reduced tubular resorption of the phosphates**. This finding is nearly always clearly positive, even when calcemia is normal. In more advanced forms complicated by nephrocalcinosis, interstitial nephrosclerosis, hydronephrosis, etc., there may be decrease in glomerular filtration.

Dosage of plasma PTH

This radioimmunological test is probatory when it reveals an evident increase in PTH.

GROSS PATHOLOGIC FEATURES

Parathyroid adenoma or adenomas occur more often in the lower glands and look like single, capsulated nodules from a chick pea to a walnut, of parenchymatous aspect. Adenoma is usually rounded or reniform, rather soft, yellow-brown in color; rarely, it is plurilobulated, harder and whitish (due to intense fibrosis). Sometimes adenomas occur in anomalous sites (intrathyroid, between the esophagus and the trachea, in the anterior or posterior mediastinum). In rare cases of primary parathyroid hyperplasia, all four of the glands appear to be fairly and not equally increased in volume. The

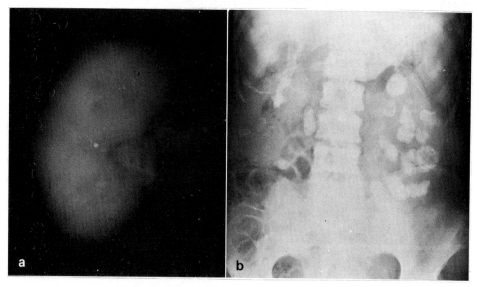

FIG. 681. - (a) Female aged 54 years. Kidney removed on autopsy. Nephrocalcinosis is observed. (b) Female aged 45 years. Both of the kidneys, which were very increased in volume, contain large calcar calculi.

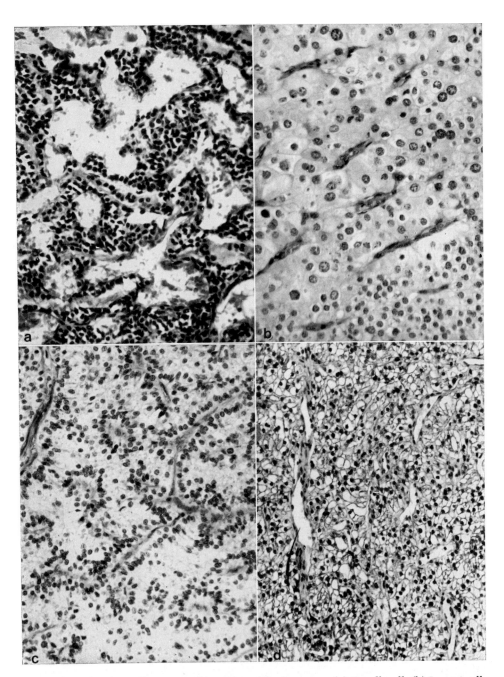

FIG. 682. - Histological aspects of parathyroid adenomas. (a) Small-cell. (b) Large-cell, with considerable nuclear pleomorphism. The large nuclei do not indicate malignancy, but only marked hyperfunction of the cell. (c) Cylindrical cells, with palisading of the nuclei. (d) Primary clear-cell hyperplasia. (*Hemat.-eos.*, 300, 300, 200, 200 x).

exceptional functioning carcinoma of a parathyroid looks like a hard, whitish, infiltrative mass, often with metastases in the lymph nodes of the neck.

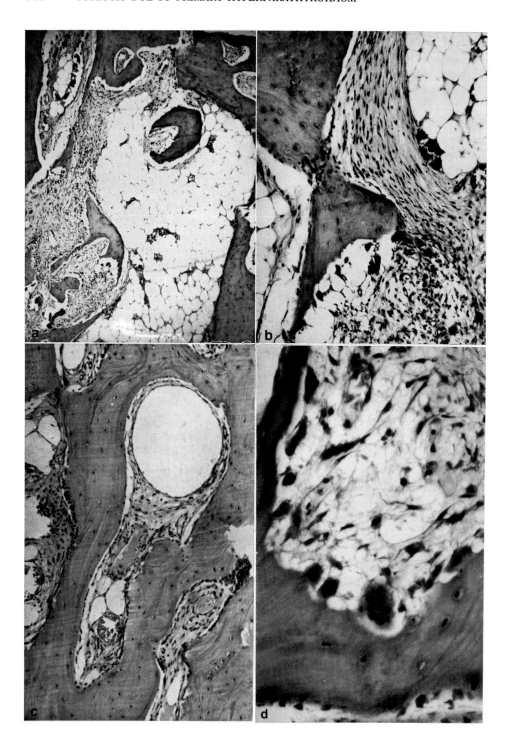

FIG. 683. - Hyperparathyroid osteosis. Intense osteoclastic resorption and typical medullary fibrosis (*Hemat.-eos.*, 50, 125, 125, 300 x).

«Brown tumors» of the skeleton are made up of a soft, reddish-brown tissue (hyperemic and often containing hemosiderin), with indistinct boundaries, always well-contained in the periosteum. In other areas of osteolysis the bone is substituted by a whitish fibrous tissue, which is gritty because of the osteoid content, similar to that of fibrous dysplasia. In both brown tumors and whitish fibrous tissue, cystic cavities are often included, which may even be multilocular, containing blood, coaguli, yellowish or yellow-brown serous fluid.

The kidneys may be characterized by calculi, hydronephrosis, parenchymal calcifications.

HISTOPATHOLOGIC FEATURES

Parathyroid adenoma maintains a certain organoid structure and is composed of principal cells which are much larger than normal ones, with a fair amount of pleomorphism of the nuclei (Fig. 682a, b). At times, clear cells are observed, so that it is difficult to distinguish adenoma from primary hyperplasia. The structure of the adenoma may be compact, tubulo-cordonal (Fig. 682c) or alveolar, at times with moderate colloid contents. There are also non-functioning adenomas made up of ossiphile cells. The boundaries of the adenoma are well-defined and circumscribed by a connective capsule. Alongside the adenomatous tissue generally there are residues of normal parathyroid tissue. The other parathyroids reveal hypotrophy from lack of function.

In primary hyperplasia the glands are made up of «water clear» cells which are rather large and regular, tending to form grapes, with nuclei oriented towards the base of the cell (Fig. 682d). More rarely, they are formed by principal cells and, in this case, the primary hyperplasia is histologically the same as the secondary hyperplasia (generally due to renal insufficiency).

The histopathologic picture of P.H.P.T. osteosis is dominated by four principal aspects.

1) Diffused bone resorption.

For the most part it is a lacunar resorption (osteoclastic), with niches of erosion, some osteoclasts on the bone surface, broken cement lines (Fig. 683). Nonetheless, there is also resorption caused by the osteocytes with widening of the bone lacunae. These aspects may be measured in bone biopsy («quantitative histology») and represent an important diagnostic parameter in non patent forms. In the cortex, resorption is often more intense under the periosteum. In the areas of diffused and moderate bone resorption aspects of osteogenesis are mild or absent: the osteoid is scarce or absent, the osteoblasts scattered and flattenend.

2) Fibrosis and medullary hyperemia.

Dilatation of the sinusoids, plasmostasis, neoproduction of capillary blood vessels associate the formation of a medullary fibrosis, which is at first loose and limited to the eroded bony surfaces, to then become more extensive, more consistent and richer in histio-fibroblasts with a plump nucleus (Fig. 683).

3) Fibro-cellular areas with osteogenesis.

In areas where the bone has been amply resorbed, there is tissue which is quite rich in fibroblasts with a swollen nucleus, associated with a dense collagen mesh. This tissue contains numerous small newly-formed osteoid trabeculae, bordered by osteoblasts which are fully active, and also by numerous osteoclasts. There is still evident hyperemia, with frequent small amounts of hemorrhaging and accumulation of hemosiderin (Fig. 684).

4) Pseudotumoral foci with giant cells.

These occur in the aforementioned fibro-osteoid tissue and are clearly visualized because of their darker stain due to a strong concentration of histio-

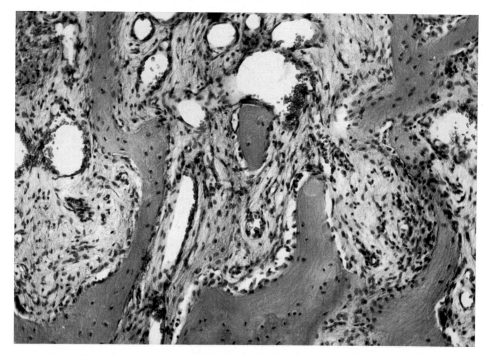

Fig. 684. - Fibrous and osteoid neoproduction in primary hyperparathyroidism (Hemat.-eos., 125 x).

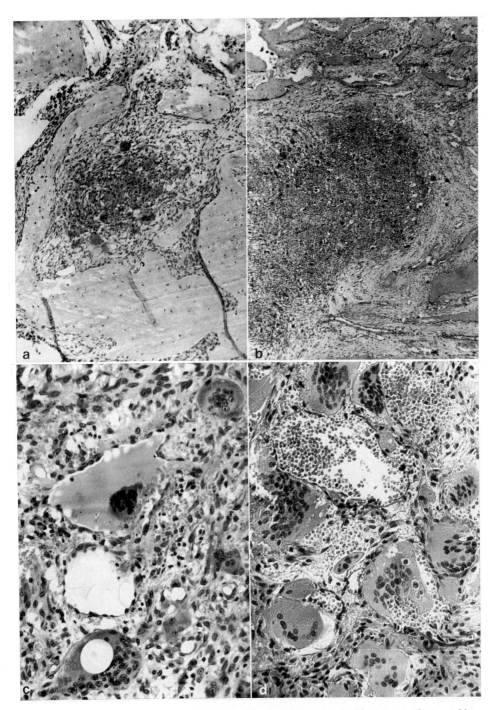

FIG. 685. - Brown tumor. (a) Development of a brown tumor as the accumulation of histiofibroblasts and giant cells at the center of an area of intense skeletal resorption.
(b) Brown tumor of larger size. (c) and (d) The histological details of a brown tumor
may appear to be very similar or identical to those of a giant cell tumor. (*Hemat.-eos.*,
125, 50, 300, 300 x).

FIG. 686. - (a) Male aged 32 years, with skeletal symptoms for the past 3 years. (b) The same humerus after 3 months of immobilization in plaster. (c) The same 1 and 1/2 year after excision of the parathyroid adenoma.

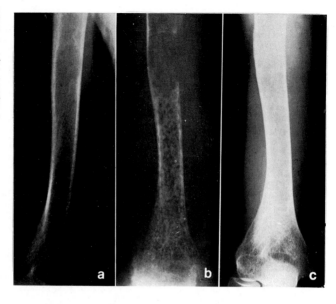

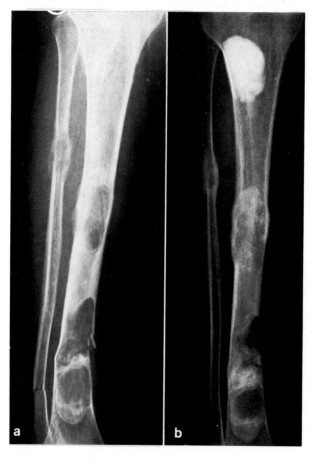

FIG. 687. - Female aged 51 years. (a) Two months after removal of a parathyroid adenoma. (b) Six months after removal.

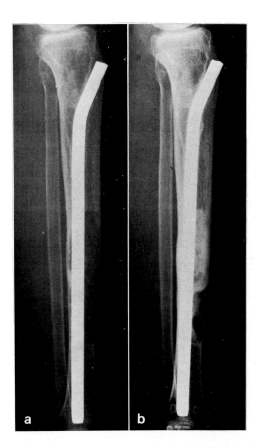

FIG. 688. - Female aged 28 years. (a) Before excision of the parathyroid adenoma. (b) Seven months after excision.

fibroblastic nuclei and a large number of multinucleate giant cells. At first, they are small multicentric nodes; they then expand and merge in large compact pseudotumoral masses (Fig. 685a, b). In this tissue («brown tumor») there is no trace of pre-existing bone and there is hardly any newly-formed osteoid. It is made up of histio-fibroblasts having a large oval or globose nucleus, not rarely in mitosis. The giant cells, which are usually numerous and diffused, are the same as the osteoclasts and as those of the giant cell tumor (Fig. 685c, d).

Histological aspects 1) and 2) correspond to the initial stages or

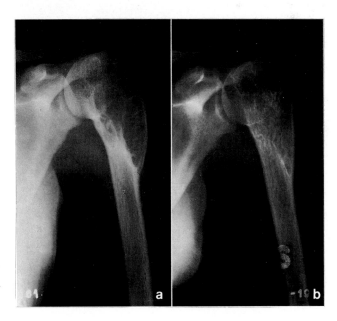

FIG. 689. - Female aged 18 years. (a) Before excision of the parathyroid adenoma. (b) Five years after excision.

to the slowly progressive forms, radiographically to microlacunar osteoporosis and to faded and diffused hypertransparence. Aspects 3) and 4) correspond instead to radiographic pictures of rough «moth-eaten» bone and of pseudotumoral or cystic osteolysis, to the more advanced stages of the disease and to the forms which are more rapidly progressive.

PATHOGENESIS AND HISTOGENESIS

P.H.P.T. is generally caused by adenoma of a single parathyroid, less often by two or more adenomas; at times by primary hyperplasia of the four glands; exceptionally by functioning carcinoma.

Skeletal changes are due to the direct action of the excess PTH, which causes intense osteoclastic and osteocytic osteolysis. The fibrous, fibro-osteoid and giant cell pseudotumoral tissue is hyperplastic, secondary to osteolysis, to attempts at osteogenetic repair, to microhemorrhaging. This hyperplasia is not «self-

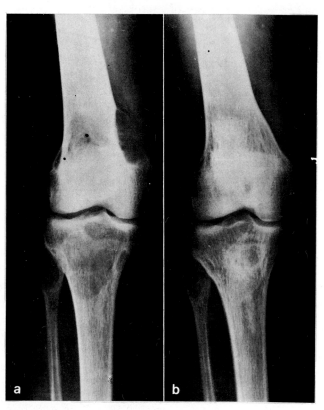

FIG. 690. - Female aged 24 years. (a) Before excision of the parathyroid adenoma. (b) Ten months after excision.

maintained», like that of aneurysmal bone cyst and pigmented villo-nodular synovitis, as removal of the adenoma is followed by repair of the skeletal lesions, which is generally rapid and complete.

DIAGNOSIS

Diagnosis is easy in patent skeletal forms. It may be difficult in initial forms.

Overall, diagnostic elements are the patient's history, as well as clinical, radiographic, histological, and laboratory data. **The patient's history** generally reveals polydipsia, polyuria, asthenia, nephrolithiasis, digestive disorders, tooth loss, maxillary cyst. A **clinical examination** may reveal «drum-stick» fingers, bone swellings, deformity of the spine, chest and pelvis. The **radiogram**, even if limited to the skeletal segment in which the first symptoms occur, usually suggests P.H.P.T., as it reveals an atypical pseudotumoral osteolysis (as compared to skeletal tumors) and/or multiple osteolyses and particularly associate with diffused and microlacunar osteoporosis of the adjacent bone. An x-ray of the chest, which is always obtained in cases of suspected tumor, often reveals fading of the lateral end of the clavicles. **Important diagnostic elements will be provided by radiograms of the entire skeleton.** Forms of pseudo-osteomalacic P.H.P.T. are radiographically distinguished from **osteoporosis** and **osteomalacia** due to the presence of brown tumors, subperiosteal erosions, changes in the hands and cranium. For information on radiographic differential diagnosis with **plasmacytoma**, see the specific chapter. **Skeletal biopsy** is more revealing in areas of osteoporosis than in brown tumors. In fact, fibroblastic areas with osteogenesis may resemble osteolytic **Paget's disease**; the tissue of brown tumors may be nearly identical to that of a **giant cell tumor**, rarely that of an **aneurysmal bone cyst**. Nonetheless, particularly when the specimen is extensive and includes in addition to the «tumor» bone tissue undergoing osteoclastic resorption, small

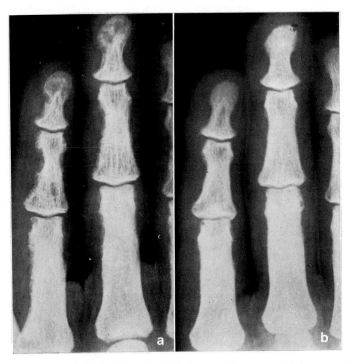

FIG. 691. - Male aged 42 years. (a) Typical radiographic image of parathyroid osteosis. (b) The same 1 year after excision of the adenoma. Complete *restitutio ad integrum*.

foci made up of giant cells, fibrocellular areas with osteogenesis, diagnosis may also be suggested **on a purely histological basis**. Among the laboratory elements, **the reduction of tubular resorption of phosphates and an increase in seric PTH are never absent. Normal calcemia does not exclude P.H.P.T.**. It may be observed, particularly in forms which date back several years, with severe osteomalacic syndrome and reduction in the glomerular filtrate. Ionized calcium is instead always increased in the blood.

There is no safe means to **reveal and localize parathyroid adenoma** prior to surgery. The radiographic visualization of the trachea and the esophagus, scan with marked seleno-methionine, selective arteriography have been used, but constant results have not been obtained. Today the most useful examinations are CAT and MRI of the thyroid region.

COURSE

P.H.P.T. has a discontinuous course, which is rather slow and progressive. Just like the clinical manifestations, the course may also be related to pathologic parathyroid incretion rate, age, sex, target organs, individual response to hormone action. Generally, osteopathy worsens over a few years time. At times progression is more rapid (favored by immobilization in plaster or in bed). At times, instead, the osteopathy remains nearly stationary for many years. The worsening of the skeletal lesions generally corresponds to a decay in the general conditions of the patient, and often considerable compromise of renal function.

TREATMENT

Treatment consists in excision of the adenoma or adenomas or (in the case of diffused hyperplasia) of three of the hyperplastic parathyroids. Because of the possibility of multiple adenomas, exploration must be bilateral. The topographic finding may be deceiving, as nodules which may even be separate from the thyroid are at times constituted by thyroid tissue, while some parathyroid adenomas are included in the capsule or even in the parenchyma of the thyroid. More valid is the macroscopic aspect of the nodule which, in the case of parathyroid adenoma, is perfectly and completely separate from the thyroid by a thin capsule, and is of a consistency (usually softer) and color (usually yellow-brown) which is different from that of the thyroid parenchyma. However, it is always best to carry out an intraoperative frozen section biopsy. When exploration of all of the posterior aspect of the thyroid is negative, the adenoma should be searched for in the sites of ectopia: intrathyroid, para- and retroesophagus, mediastinic.

Once the adenoma has been removed, pathologic fractures generally heal with non-surgical treatment. Only occasionally (diaphyseal fractures, fractures of the femoral neck) are osteosynthesis (Fig. 688) or endoprosthesis indicated.

In these patients there is often a certain amount of surgical risk, due to the instability of the renal, gastropancreatic, cardiocirculatory conditions, to the altered hydroelectrolytic balance, and to the decay of hematic crasis and general conditions. The hypercalcemia, which is aggravated by immobilization in bed or in plaster, may be the cause of severe intra- and postoperative complications: cardiac (arrest, changes in conduction), nervous (mental confusion, coma), renal (osmotic polyuria, dehydration, renal insufficiency), enteric (vomiting, diarrhea, dehydration).

For this reason, it is best to first perform excision of the adenoma. Surgery on the skeleton should be postponed to when the phosphocalcic metabolism has returned to normal values. In any case an accurate preoperative evaluation and careful postoperative monitoring are essential.

During the first weeks after parathyroidectomy, there is hypocalcemia, with possible tetanic and tachycardic crises. Thus, in these cases, intravenous calcium gluconate and vitamin D, at times PTH will be required.

PROGNOSIS

Prognosis depends on the earliness of diagnosis and of parathyroidectomy. In fact, skeletal lesions are amply reversible, even if severe and advanced (Figs. 673b, 686-691). Skeletal reconstruction begins after 4-6 months and occurs over 1-2 years, often in a complete manner. Immediately after parathyroidectomy laboratory tests show normal values and cenesthesia and general conditions rapidly improve. Instead, lesions of the kidneys are not reversible. When the disease goes unrecognized and is not treated in time, prognosis may become severe due to renal insufficiency. Another occurrence to be feared, although rare, is acute pancreatitis.

REFERENCES

1962 HELLSTRÖM J., IVEMARK B.: Primary hyperparathyroidism. Clinical and structural findings in 138 cases. *Acta Chirurgica Scandinavica*, **294**, 1-113.
1963 LIEVRE J. A., CHIGOT P. L., BLOCH M. H., CAMUS J. P., LIEVRE J. A.: L'hyperparathyroidisme primitif. Etude de 34 cas. *Presse Medicale*, **71**, 2233-2236.
1964 LICHTWITZ A., PARLIER R.: *Calcium et maladies metaboliques de l'os*. L'Expansion scientifique Francaise, Paris.
1966 LIEVRE J. A., KURC D:. Les manifestations articulaires de l'hyperparathyroidisme primitif. *Journal Belge de Rheumatologie et de Medecine Physique*, **21**, 351-360.
1968 DODDS W. J., STEINBACH H. L.: Primary hyperparathyroidism and articular cartilage calcification. *American Journal of Roentgenology*, **104**, 884-892.
1969 HOSHINO T., NOMURA T., SAKUMA T., MARIOKA S., KUDO K.: The osteocytic osteolysis in hyperparathyroidism. *Journal of the Japanese Orthopaedic Association*, **43**, 217-224.
1970 GUTTMANN G., STEIN I.: Fractured femur in a patient with parathyroid adenoma complicated by hypercalcemic crisis. *The Journal of Bone and Joint Surgery*, **52-A**, 1217-1221.
1970 LICHTENSTEIN L.: *Disease of Bone and Joints*. The C.V. Mosby Company, Saint Louis.

1970 RYCKEWAERT A.: *Physiopathologie des maladies des os et des articulations.* J. B. Bailliére & Fils, Paris.

1971 BLALOCK J. B.: The surgical treatment of hyperparathyroidism. *Surgery, Ginecology and Obstetrics,* **133**, 627-628.

1971 CZITOBER H., KEMINGER K., LECHNER G., POKIESER H., UMEK H., ZHUNBANER W.: Skeletveränderungen vor und nach Operation bei primären Hyperparathyroidismus. *Fortschritte auf dem Gebiete der Röntgenstrahlen und Nuklearmedizin,* **115**, 85-92.

1971 HAFF R. C., BALLINGER W. F.: Causes of recurrent hypercalcemia after parathyroidectomy for primary hyperparathyroidism. *Annals of Surgery,* **173**, 884-891.

1971 HATFIELD PH. M.: Palpable neck mass and multiple bone lesions. *Journal of the American Medical Association,* **215**, 1808-1809.

1971 LIEVRE J. A.: Étude sur 30 cas récents d'hyperparathyroidisme. *Revue du Rhumatisme,* **38**, 163-171.

1971 MARDSEN P., ANDERSON J., DOYLE D., MORRIS B. A., BURNS D. A.: Familial hyperparathyroidism. *British Medical Journal,* **3**, 87-90.

1972 JAFFE H. L.: *Metabolic, degenerative, and inflammatory diseases of bones and joints.* Urban and Schwarzenberg, München, Berlin, Wien.

1972 MEUNIER P., VIGNON G., BERNARD S., EDOUARD C., COURPRON P., PERTES: La lecture quantitative de la biopsie osseuse, moyen de diagnostic et d'étude de 106 hyperparathyroidies primitives, secondaires et paraneoplasiques. *Revue du Rhumatisme,* **39**, 635-644.

1972 RESTON E. T.: Avulsion of both quadriceps tendons in hyperparathyroidism. *Journal of the American Medical Association,* **221**, 406-407.

1973 CHIGOT P. L., FICAT C.: La main hyperparathyroidienne. Étude radiologique. *Revue de Chirurgie Orthopedique,* **59**, 309-319.

1973 GENANT H. K., HECK L., LAWRENCE H., ROSSMANN K., VANDER H., PALOYAN E.: Primary hyperparathyroidism. *Radiology,* **109**, 513-524.

1973 SCHANTZ A., CASTLEMAN B.: Parathyroid carcinoma. A study of 70 cases. *Cancer,* **31**, 600-605.

1973 STUBBS A. J., MYERS R. T.: Experience with hyperparathyroidism. *Surgery, Ginecology and Obstetrics,* **136**, 65-67.

1974 CHIROFF R. T., KENDRICK A. S., SLAUGHTER W. H.: Slipped capital femoral epiphyses and parathyroid adenoma. *Journal of Bone and Joint Surgery,* **56-A**, 1063-1067.

1974 HAFF R. C., ARMSTRONG R. G.: Trends in the current management of primary hyperparathyroidism. *Surgery,* **75**, 715-719.

1974 NGUYENK C., SENNOTT W. M., KNOX G. S.: Neonatal hyperparathyroidism. *Radiology,* **112**, 175-176.

1974 SAMAAN N. A., HICKEY R. C., STRATTON C. H., MEDELLIN H., GATES R. B.: Parathyroid tumors: preoperative localization and association with other tumors. *Cancer,* **33**, 933-939.

1974 WERNER S., HJERN B., SJÖBERG H. E.: Primary hyperparathyroidism. Analysis of findings in a series of 129 patients. *Acta Chirurgica Scandinavica,* **140**, 618-625.

1975 DEPLANTE J. P., DAUMONT A., BONVIER M., LEJEUNE E.: L'hyperparathyroidisme primitif. À propos de 50 cas personnels. *Revue du Rhumatisme,* **42**, 747-758.

1976 LATORZEFF S., DURROUX R., GAYRARD M., CARLES P., ARLET Ph., DEBROCK J.: Biopsie osseuse quantitative et hyperparathyroidie primitive. Interet pour le diagnostic. À propos de 45 cas. *Revue du Rhumatisme,* **43**, 497-502.

1980 CAMPANACCI M., GIUNTI A.: Osteosis in primary hyperparathyroidism. *Italian Journal of Orthopaedics and Traumatology,* **6**, Suppl., 100-113.

1982 CHARHON S.A., EDONARD C.H., ARLOT M.E., MEUNIER P.J.: Effects of parathyroid hormone on remodeling of iliac trabecular bone in patients with primary hyperparathyroidism. *Clinical Orthopaedics,* **162**, 255-263.

1985 LACHMANN M., KRICUN M., SCHWARTZ E.: Case report 310: primary hyperparathyroidism with patchy, diffuse sclerosis at multiple skeletal sites. *Skeletal Radiology,* **13**, 248-252.

1988 CHALMERS J., IRVINE G.B., Fractures of the femoral neck in elderly patients with hyperparathyroidism. *Clinical Orthopaedics,* **229**, 125-130.

PSEUDOTUMORAL PERIOSTEAL AND MUSCULAR OSSIFICATIONS
(Synonyms: localized or circumscribed myositis ossificans; hyperplastic bone callus: in periosteal forms)

This chapter includes different pathological conditions characterized by the neoformation of a hyperplastic bone tissue in muscular and/or periosteal sites. Hyperplastic ossification may be manifested as follows: 1) around a fracture or, more rarely, a dislocation; 2) after simple contusion or even when the patient's history does not record trauma. In the former case, we are dealing with hyperplastic fracture callus and hyperpastic para-articular ossification (in dislocations); in the second, with spontaneous or traumatic muscular and/or periosteal ossification (so-called circumscribed myositis and/or circumscribed periostitis ossificans.

In general, the degree of hyperplasia is inversely proportional to the age of the subject, so that **the most exuberant ossifications are observed in children and young adults**.

1) Hyperplastic bone callus or ossification of fracture or dislocation

This is nearly exclusively observed in **proximal segments of the limbs:** shoulder, humerus and elbow; hip, femur and knee. Hyperplasia of the fracture callus or hyperplastic periarticular ossification, at least in young patients, is a constant phenomenon when there is **severe cranial trauma** at the same time as fracture or dislocation (Fig. 692). It is less frequently observed in the paretic or paralytic limbs due to **cerebral lesion** (for example, vascular hemiplegia: Fig. 693) or **medullary lesion** (for example, traumatic or congenital: myelomeningocele: Fig. 694). It is rather common to observe hyperplasia of the fracture callus in spina bifida with myelomeningocele, as we are dealing with children or adolescents. Instead, it is never observed in poliomyelitic limbs, nor in cases of paralysis due to lesion of the peripheral nerves.

Finally, hyperplasia of the fracture callus may be manifested in cases of **osteogenesis imperfecta** (Fig. 695) and, although nowadays an exceptional occurrence, in those of **syphilis** (Fig. 696).

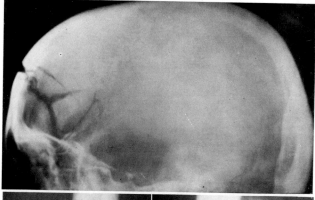

FIG. 692. - Hyperplastic fracture callus (femur) 15 days after trauma associated with cranial fracture in a man aged 25.

◀

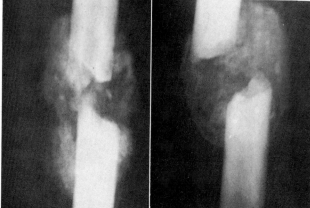

In all of these cases, the presence of fracture or traumatic dislocation excludes any problem of clinical and radiographic differential diagnosis with tumors. Nor is it probable that the histopathologist is involved, as generally biopsy is not performed. The histological aspect is the same as that of the forms that follow.

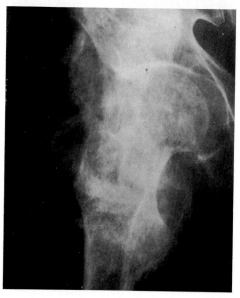

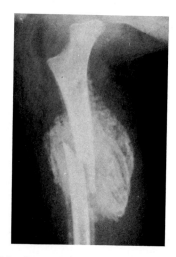

FIG. 693. - Male aged 59 years. Extensive periarticular muscular ossification in cerebral hemiplegia.

FIG. 694. - Boy aged 2 years. Paraplegia due to spina bifida. Hyperplasia of the bone callus after fracture of the femoral diaphysis. «Pennate» aspect of the myositis ossificans.

FIG. 695. - Female aged 11 years. Blue sclera. Previous multiple fractures, bilateral congenital dislocation of the radial heads, mild bowing of the femurs and tibias. Hyperplastic callus 2 months after fracture of the femur.

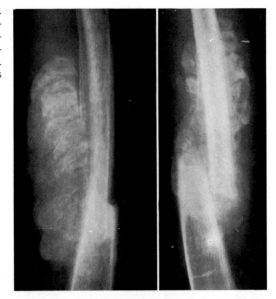

FIG. 696. - Female aged 8 years affected with congenital syphilis. Hyperplastic bone callus surrounding a fracture of the tibia which occurred with no apparent cause and without pain; often — as in this case — lesions of this type are multiple.

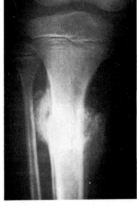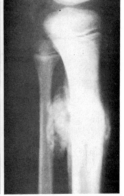

2) Pseudotumoral muscular and/or periosteal microtraumatic or spontaneous ossification

Traumatic muscular and/or periosteal ossification is an infrequent occurrence, but not a rare one. It is most often observed in the male **sex** and there is evident predilection for children, adolescents and **young** adults. The most common **localization** is the thigh (particular the quadriceps muscle), followed by the arm, shoulder, hip and knee (Fig. 697). It is rare in the muscles of the trunk, in the forearm and leg. The ossification may only be muscular, separated from the skeletal plane, but it often also involves the periosteum.

Symptoms generally initiate 2-4 weeks after trauma, which is generally contusive. At times there is repeated microtrauma[1], at times the patient does not recall any incidence of trauma. In the latter case the traumatic

---

[1] One of the first descriptions of pseudotumoral ossification in the delto-pectoral region (Hasse, 1832) referred to recruits of the Prussian infantry and was clearly related to prolonged use of a musket.

event was probably so mild that it went unobserved or was forgotten. The first clinical signs consist in deep, globose swelling of the soft tissue, having ill-defined limits, of firm consistency, and with slight pain (Fig. 699a). There may be an increase in local temperature and diffused edema of the surrounding soft tissues. The newly-formed mass grows during the first weeks, and it may become the size of a large orange. These clinical features easily led to suspicion of an inflammatory process or a sarcoma. Within 1-2 months the mass becomes of more definite boundaries and becomes of bony consistency. Edema and local warmth regress totally. At times it is mobile, at times fixed at the skeletal plane (when the periosteum is involved). In the meantime the mass has also become painless and, in the months thereafter, it tends to considerably decrease in volume (Fig. 10), at times almost totally regressing.

Radiographic examination at the onset (for 2-3 weeks after trauma) is completely negative. Then light and faded nubecolae of radiopacity in the soft tissues, and at times a thin lamina of osteogenetic elevation of the periosteum begin to appear. Within 1-2 months ossification is evident, then assuming its typical radiographic aspect. This consists in a globose mass, made up of a bundle of thin bony trabeculae (sometimes reproducing the direction of muscular bundles: feather-like or «pennate» feature — Figs. 694, 695), all contained within the muscle, or adhered to the periosteum which is uplifeted with regular and fusiform ossification. Radiopacity, which is at first tenuous and faded, gradually becomes denser and structured as the ossification matures (Figs. 10, 698-703). At this point the fact that the boundaries with the soft tissues are sharp and the radiopacity is more marked at the periphery than at the center is pathognomic (Fig. 701). This is the opposite of what occurs in osteogenic sarcomas. In successive months the mass is reduced (Fig. 10), gradually assuming the radiographic features of mature bone, and (when it adhered to the periosteum) it is completely fused with the implant cortex (Fig. 703). At times, in the area where the ossifying mass is adherent to the bone, excavation of the external aspect of the cortex is produced, which may accentuate the impression of a periosteal or parosteal tumor. Bone scan is clearly positive during the progressive stage, while it gradually becomes normal as ossification matures.

The **macroscopic aspect** also depends on the progressive stage. At the onset there is a hyperemic mass of edematous and fibrous aspect, at times containing traces of hematoma, characterized by unclear boundaries which fade into the edema and the degenerated muscular tissue. As it matures, the mass becomes more and more ossified, with boundaries which are more and more clear. At times there is an ossified «shell» and a softer center, at times containing blood.

The **histological findings** may be reconstructed in their development as follows (Figs. 11, 704-706). At first hematic effusion, edema and muscular degeneration, with richly proliferating repair connnective tissue which soon becomes osteogenetic. Fibroblasts, histiocytes, macrophages, some lymphocytes and plasmacells, newly-formed vessels begin to thicken between the degenerated and necrotic muscular cells (Fig. 704c). Attempts at muscular regeneration may give way to images which recall multinucleate giant cells.

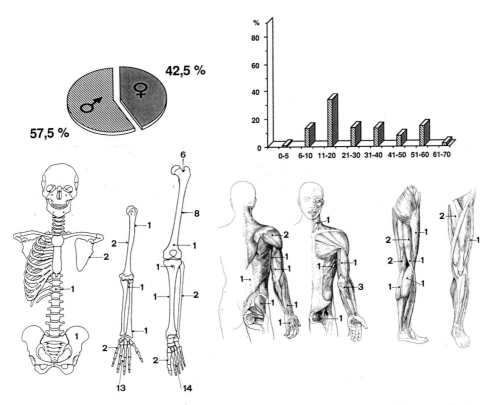

FIG. 697. - Sex, age and localization in 85 cases of myoperiostitis ossificans. Left the localizations involving the periosteum and adhered to the bone surface (59); right isolated localizations in the muscle (26).

Histio-fibroblastic proliferation is rather lively. The cells are large, with well-stained nuclei, of fairly variable shape and size, at times characterized by a large nucleolus, quite often in mitosis (Fig. 704d). Gradually, this tissue submerges the muscular cells, the fibroblasts may form wide streams with a vaguely fibrosarcomatoid aura, osteoblastic production begins. The first osteoid trabeculae are formed (Figs. 704a, 705a) which gradually widen and mature (Figs. 705b, 706). At the same time the intertrabecular connective tissue matures. Ossification may go through a cartilaginous stage, so that here and there the hyperplastic cartilage typical of repair callus is observed (Fig. 705c, d). In the mature stage, as well, residues of muscular cells trapped in the ossification are often observed.

If we examine a rather extensive specimen of a «ball-like» muscular ossification, we clearly see its structure in concentric or «zonal» layers (Ackerman, 1958) (Fig. 706). In fact, ossification and maturation begin and progress constantly from the «shell» inwards; so that from the center (soft, at times hematic, with immature connective cells) we go towards the periphery (evidently ossified and more mature) by intermediate gradations (cf. radiographic and macroscopic aspect).

The **pathogenesis** is generally related to trauma, even if often there is no

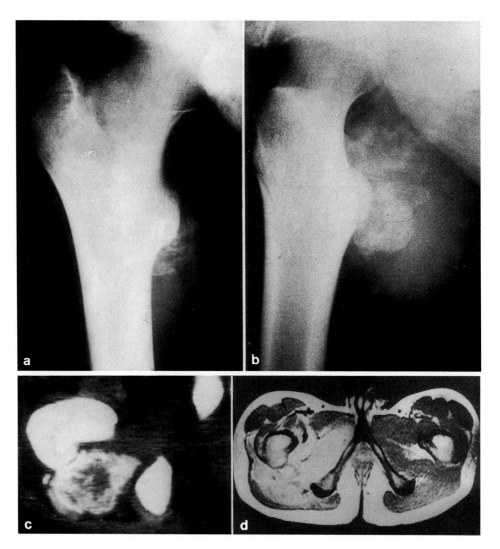

Fig. 698. - Myositis ossificans in a boy aged 19 years. (a) and (b) Radiographic picture. (c) CAT shows greater radiopacity of the peripheral zone and the sharp borders towards the soft tissues. (d) MRI reveals extensive alterations and faded limits of the gluteal and extrarotator muscles due to edema and diffused tissue reaction.

trace of this in the patient's history and even if the ossification occurs in a small number of muscular traumas. Age (childhood-youth), site (proximal segments of the limbs) and unknown individual factors are certainly of importance. Gnosographically, the circumscribed muscular ossification must be clearly distinguished from the **progressive fibrodysplasia ossificans** (generalized myositis ossificans, Munchmeyer disease), rare hereditary congenital dysplasia of the connective tissue, characterized by progressive and diffused ossification of the aponeuroses, tendons, ligaments and interstitial connective tissue of the muscles, associated with microdactylia.

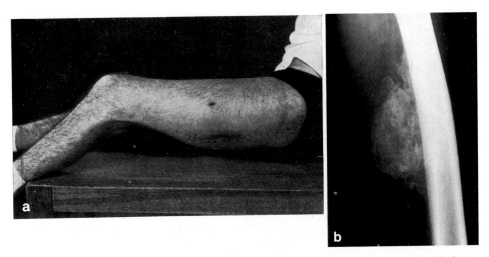

FIG. 699. - Myositis ossificans in a male aged 21 years. Incisional biopsy had led to a histological diagnosis of osteosarcoma and to the therapeutic proposal of hip disarticulation (a). (b) Radiographic picture is typical. Based on this and on a review of the slides, diagnosis was changed and the patient healed with no treatment.

Differential diagnosis should not present any problems. If muscular ossification is occasionally mistaken for osteosarcoma, this depends on the error of making a histological diagnosis without adequate clinical and radiographic data. In truth, the clinical and radiographic picture generally allows for diagnosis, without requiring biopsy. The histological error originates from

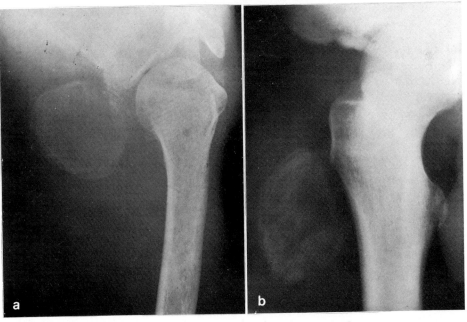

FIG. 700. - (a) «Ball-like» myositis ossificans in the posterior deltoid in a female aged 31 years. (b) Myositis ossificans in the vastus lateralis in a male aged 16 years.

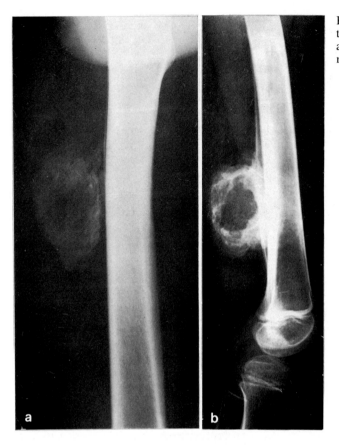

FIG. 701. - (a) Myoperiostitis ossificans in a male aged 20 years. (b) Myoperiostitis ossificans in a male aged 8 years.

the observation of a limited field of proliferating and osteogenetic tissue, where the cells are large, with well-stained nuclei, which are fairly pleomorphic and often in mitosis (Figs. 11, 704d). This error may easily be avoided, even on a purely histological basis, extending observation to include the histostructural features of the lesion: organoid structure and «zonal» architecture; bone trabeculae bordered by regular rows of osteoblasts (which does not occur in osteosarcoma); cartilage with very large cells, but with no nuclear atypia, closed within regular lacunae, with essentially well-formed ground substance. Clinical-radiographic elements are absolutely typical. Only during the first weeks can clinical and radiographic picture (negative, or with some initial radiopaque nubecolae) suggest sarcoma of the soft tissues. Let us recall that in **synovial sarcoma** (and other soft tissue tumors) calcification is more often granular, unstructured. Nonetheless, in exceptional cases synovial sarcoma may radiographically resemble the early phase of muscular ossification. **Osteosarcoma of the soft tissues** (very rare) may instead reveal nubecolae of faded radiopacity like very immature muscular ossification. In this case, differential diagnosis is clinical and histological. When ossification is more advanced (1-2 months after trauma) no mistake may be made. In particular, in myoperiosteal forms, the type of laminar periosteal reaction, the greater radiopacity of the «shell», clearly distinguish it from **parosteal osteosarcoma** (see relative chapter).

The complete **maturation** of the muscular ossification occurs within 6-12 months. This maturation, with reduction in the volume of the ossification, may be accelerated by **radiation therapy**, which may be used only in the adult in order to avoid injuring the growth cartilage. Complete maturation may also be judged by bone scan, as it corresponds to the exhaustion of increased

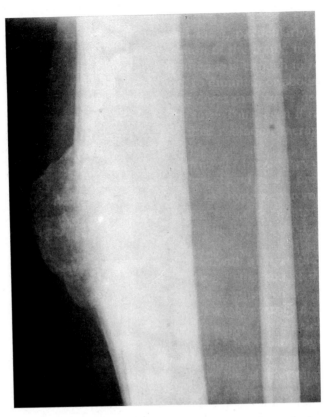

FIG. 702. - Myoperiostitis ossificans of the tibia in a female aged 9 years.

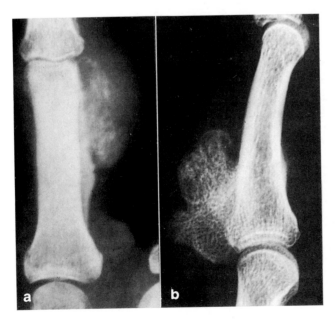

FIG. 703. - (a) Recent myoperiostitis ossificans, initiated over the past 3 months, after trauma, in a female aged 46 years. Excision was performed suspecting a neoplasm, there was no recurrence after 3 years. (b) Ancient (3 years earlier) and completely mature ossification in a female aged 36 years. Excision, with no recurrence after 2 years.

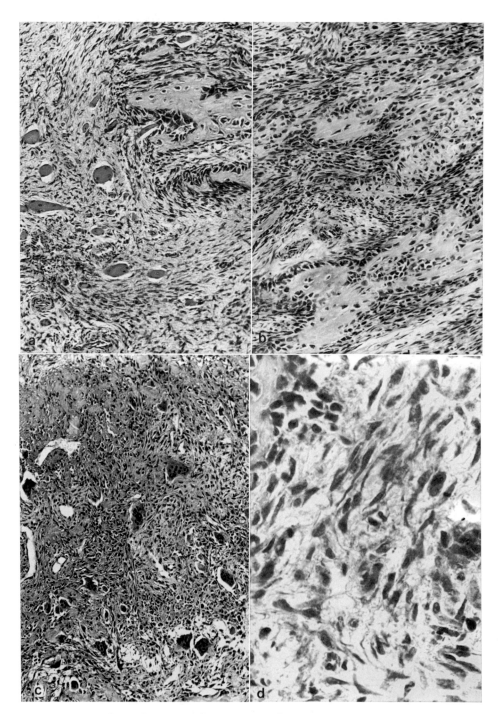

FIG. 704. - Histological aspects of myositis ossificans. In (a) and (b) there are newly-formed osteoid trabeculae, bordered by rows of osteoblasts. In (a) there are also muscular cells included. (c) There is histio-fibroblastic tissue with numerous giant cells. (d) Among the proliferating histio-fibroblastic cells there are two mitoses (*Hemat.-eos.*, 125, 125, 125, 500 x).

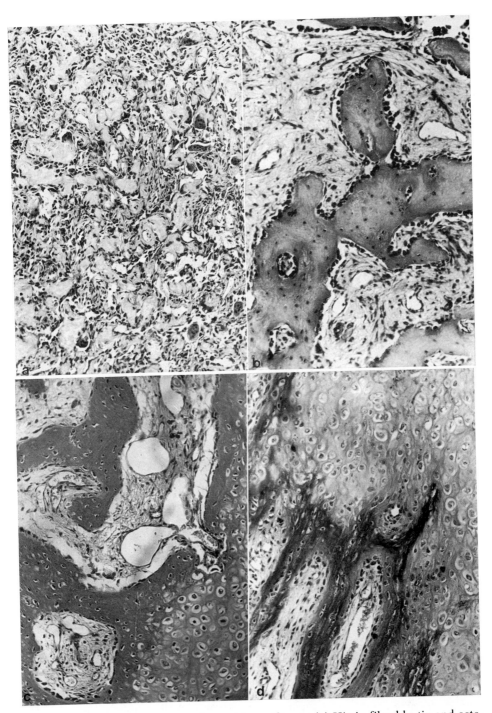

FIG. 705. - Histological aspects of myositis ossificans. (a) Histio-fibroblastic and osteoid proliferation which is rather immature (central part of the myositis). (b) Peripheral part of the same myositis. The cellular proliferation is very reduced and the fibrous and osseous tissue are more mature. (c) and (d) Cartilaginous production alongside that of osteoid tissue (*Hemat.-eos.*, 125, 125, 125, 125 x).

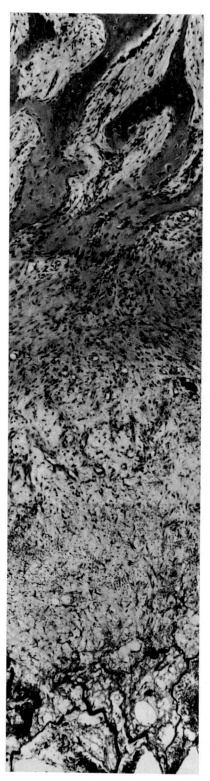

FIG. 706. - «Zonal» architecture of the myositis ossificans. From a central hematoma (below) we gradually move towards increasingly mature bone tissue at the periphery (above).

uptaking in the ossification. **Surgical excision** must not be performed prior to complete maturation, as otherwise ossification may easily recur. At times, within 1-2 years, the ossification is reduced so much in volume that surgery is no longer necessary (Fig. 10). If excision is performed when maturation has occurred, healing is complete and definitive.

3) Periosteal ossification of the small tubular bones of the hand and subungueal periosteal ossification (so-called subungueal osteoma or exostosis)

In the small bones of the hand, there may be periosteal and capsular ossification which evolves clinically and radiographically, like the periosteal ossification described in section 2). These are of traumatic or microtraumatic origin and are more often observed in the areas of capsular insertion at the phalanges or metacarpals (Figs. 707, 708).

Common to the hallux, more rarely to the other toes and fingers, is a reactive osteo-cartilaginous proliferation which protrudes under the nail and often raises from the ungueal fornix (Fig. 709). This is a small bony excrescence which is adhered to the surface of the ungueal phalanx. The nail is uplifted and shifted from the osseous nodule, which often raises at the surface. This lesion is secondary to mechanical or inflammatory stimuli («ingrown nail») and is prevalently observed in children and youths under 30 years of age. It is first associated with superficial inflammatory phenomena and pain, to then stabilize as a hard, dry and painless excrescence. **Radiographically**, it is constituted by a nodule of cancellous bone which is more or less mature, adhered to the cortex (no extroflexion of the latter, unlike true exostoses). **Histologically**, it has the structure of a fibro-osteo-cartilaginous callus, at times associating with inflammatory aspects. Although there may be a layer of chondroid tissue at the surface, its microscopic aspect is generally clearly distinguished from that of exostosis.

4) Pseudotumoral periosteal ossifications with a congenital base

In exceptional cases hyperplastic fracture callus (see Fig. 695) or pseudo-

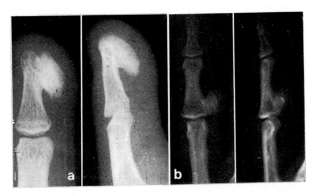

FIG. 707. - (a) Ossification occurred with no apparent cause at the apex of the index finger in a female aged 14 years, and recurrent after attempt at surgical removal. (b) Traumatic juxta-articular parosteal ossification in a female aged 30 years.

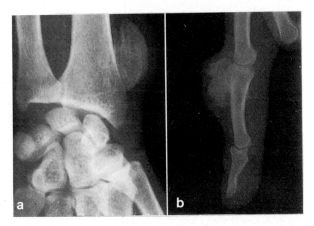

FIG. 708. - (a) Mature parosteal and juxta-articular ossification in a female aged 27 years. (b) Mature parosteal ossification in a female aged 30 year.

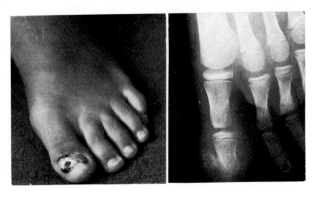

FIG. 709. - So-called subungueal exostosis of the hallux in a girl aged 9 years.

tumoral periosteal ossification may be observed after mild contusive trauma or when no trauma may be recorded, in relation with **osteogenesis imperfecta**. These ossifications are generally manifested during childhood, there is predilection for the male sex and they are prevalently localized in the femoral diaphysis (more rarely in another long bone). The familiarity of osteogenesis imperfecta has been observed. In rare cases, there may be «blue sclera», but often the patient's history reveals repeated fracture (moreover consolidated by non-hyperplastic callus); often, stature is smaller than normal, there may be thinning of the cortices, in some cases associated with bilateral congenital dislocation of the radial head (Fig. 710).

In half of all cases there are multiple and nearly symmetrical periosteal ossifications, particularly on the diaphyseal aspects facing the interosseous

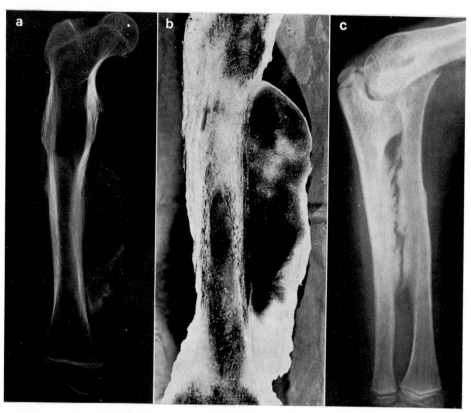

FIG. 710. - Pseudotumoral hyperplastic periosteal ossification in a male aged 13 years. Parosteal mass was present for the past 2 years. On biopsy it was interpreted as chondrosarcoma and hip disarticulation was performed. (a) Radiogram of the section of the anatomical specimen. In addition to the pseudotumoral mass of more recent formation there was rugose thickening of the proximal diaphysis indicating previous similar hyperplastic ossification which had already matured and decreased in volume. (b) Macroscopic aspect of the same specimen. (c) In the same case, congenital dislocation of the radial heads and typical ossification of the interosseous membranes. These cases generally present the stigmatae of osteogenesis imperfecta.

spaces of the forearm and leg, but also in the femur, pelvis, metacarpals and metatarsals. Some of these periostoses clearly originate from the maturation and reduction of a previous rather large pseudotumoral periosteal ossification.

Pseudotumoral **symptoms** are as follows. After trauma (which is usually mild, without fracture), but more often in an apparently spontaneous manner, deep swelling occurs, the site of election of which is the thigh. Swelling is often tender, at times characterized by fever, leukocytosis, increase in blood sedimentation rate and in serum alkaline phosphatase. At first the consistency of the newly-formed mass is firm with faded limits, but then it hardens and its limits become sharper, and it completely adheres to the bone. Its increase is rapid, at times achieving enormous size and becoming its largest in approximately 6 months. At this point the «tumor» begins to slowly decrease until, at times, it may totally regress within 1-2 years. At times the first pseudotumoral manifestation is followed by others, in different skeletal segments and having a similar development. Fever, increase in sedimentation rate and alkaline phosphatasemia regress when the mass stops growing, to then recur if other hyperplastic ossifications develop in other sites.

Radiographic picture: in the initial stage (1-2 months) a globose parosteal shadow may be observed, with the same density as the soft tissues. Diffused and faded radiopacity appears which gradually intensifies and acquires the features of mature bone. Here, too, as in muscular ossifications, maturation proceeds from the periphery to the center. The mass adheres with a large implant base to the cortex and seems to develop within the periosteum. When ossification is regressed, moderate periostotic knottiness and rugosity which are totally mature and confused with the cortex may be observed.

Anatomically we are dealing with an exuberant osteo-cartilaginous callus, characterized by organoid structure, considerable hyperemia, evident delimitation towards the soft tissues, complete fusion to the cortex, tendency to mature from the periphery to the center. At times, growth of the periosteal mass is such that it surrounds a large diaphyseal segment or even the entire diaphysis.

Histological **differential diagnosis**, the course, treatment and prognosis of the disease are the same as those described for muscular ossifications.

Hyperplastic myo-periosteal ossification is exceptionally observed in cases of **neurofibromatosis**, as well (see specific chapter).

In **melorheostosis** there may be ossifications in the soft tissues, particularly peri-articular, as well as hyperplastic periostoses which are bumpy and eburneous, which may radiographically suggest parosteal osteosarcoma.

REFERENCES

1958 ACKERMAN L. V.: Extra-osseous localized non-neoplastic bone and cartilage formation (so-called myositis ossificans). Clinical and pathological confusion with malignant neoplasms. *Journal of Bone and Joint Surgery*, **40-A**, 279-298.

1962 HUTTER R. V. P., FOOTE F. W., FRANCIS K. C., HIGINBOTHAM N. L.: Parosteal fasciitis. A self-limited benign process that simulates a malignant neoplasm. *American Journal of Surgery*, **104**, 800-807.

1967 LAURENT L., SALENIUS P.: Hyperplastic callus formation in osteogenesis imper-
      fecta. Report of a case simulating sarcoma. *Acta Orthopaedica Scandinavica*,
      38, 280-290.

1968 CAMPANACCI M., GIUNTI A.: Ossificazioni periostali a sviluppo pseudotumorale
      su base congenita. *Chirurgia degli Organi di Movimento*, **57**, 109-124.

1968 CAMPANACCI M., VELLANI G.: Iperplasia del callo osseo in fratture degli arti
      associate a gravi traumi cranici. *Chirurgia degli Organi di Movimento*, **57**,
      369-382.

1969 ANGERVALL L., STENER B., STENER I., AHREN C.: Pseudomalignant osseous tumor
      of soft tissue. *Journal of Bone and Joint Surgery*, **51-B**, 654-663.

1969 KAHN L. B., WOOD F. W., ACKERMAN L. V.: Fracture callus associated with
      benign and malignant bone lesions and mimicking osteosarcoma. *American
      Journal Clinical Pathology*, **52**, 14-24.

1969 SILVER J. R.: Heterotopic ossification. A clinical study of its possible relation-
      ship to trauma. *Paraplegia*, **7**, 220-230.

1970 NORMAN A., DORFMAN H. D.: Juxtacortical circumscribed myositis ossificans:
      evolution and radiographic features. *Radiology*, **96**, 301-306.

1971 BANTA J. V., SCHREIBER R. R., KULIK W. J.: Hyperplastic callus formation in
      osteogenesis imperfecta simulating osteosarcoma. *Journal of Bone and Joint
      Surgery*, **53-A**, 115-122.

1972 ROSEMEYER B.: Myositis ossificans traumatica im Bereich des Oberschenkels.
      Archiv für Orthopädische und Unfall-chirurgie, **73**, 136-148.

1975 CAMPANACCI M., GIUNTI A., LEONESSA C., PAGANI P. A., TRENTANI C.: Patholo-
      gical fractures in osteopathies and bony dysplasias. *Italian Journal of Ortho-
      paedic and Traumatology*, **1**, Suppl., 7-45.

1976 McCARTHY E. F., IRELAND D. C. R., SPRAGUE B. L., BONFIGLIO M.: Parosteal no-
      dular fasciitis of the hand. A case report. *Journal of Bone and Joint Surgery*,
      58-A, 714-716.

1976 ROBERTS J. B.: Bilateral hyperplastic callus formation in osteogenesis imper-
      fecta. A case report. *Journal of Bone and Joint Surgery*, **58-A**, 1164-1166.

1976 REDEGERDTS U., LENZE U., HERTEL E.: Zur Myositis ossificans localisata und
      ihrer operativen Therapie. *Archiv für Orthopädische und Unfall-Chirurgie*,
      84, 349-367.

1979 LONDON G. C., JOHNSON K. A., DAHLIN D. C.: Subungueal exostoses. *Journal of
      Bone and Joint Surgery*, **61-A**, 256-259.

1980 CAMPANACCI M., GARDINI G. F., GIUNTI A., DONATI U.: Ossificazioni muscolari
      e/o periostee pseudotumorali. (Studio di 57 casi). *Giornale Italiano di Orto-
      pedia e Traumatologia*, **6**, 379-386.

1980 OGILVIE-HARRIS D.J., HORES CH. B., FORNASIER V.L.: Pseudomalignant myositis
      ossificans: heterotopic new bone formation without history of trauma.
      Journal of Bone and Joint Surgery, **62-A**, 1274-1283.

1982 ZEANAH W.R., HUDSON T.M.: Myositis ossificans. Radiologic evaluation of
      two cases with diagnostic computed tomography. *Clinical Orthopaedics*, **168**,
      187-191.

1984 CAMPANACCI M., CAPANNA R.: Affezioni muscolari di natura metaplastica e
      circolatoria su base traumatica, in « *Trattato Italiano di Medicina Interna* ».
      Vol. XIII. USES, Firenze.

1987 SPENCER R.F.: The effect of head injury on fracture healing. *Journal of Bone
      and Joint Surgery*, **69-B**, 525-528.

1988 DULOYER PH., TOMENO B., FOREST H., BELLOIR C., WYBIER M.: La myosite ossi-
      fiante circonscrite non traumatique. A propos de 14 observations et revue
      générale. *Revue de Chirurgie Orthopedique*, **74**, 659-668.

1988 MILLER-BRESLOW A., DORFMAN H.D.: Dupuytren's (subungueal) exostosis.
      American Journal of Surgical Pathology, **12**, 368-378.

1989 SPENCER J. D., MISSEN G.A.K.: Pseudomalignant heterotopic ossification
      (« Myositis ossificans »). *Journal of Bone and Joint Surgery*, **71-B**, 317-319.

1990 SCHÜTTE H.E., VAN DER HEUL R.O.: Pseudomalignant, nonneoplastic osseous
      soft-tissue tumors of the hand and foot. *Radiology*, **176**, 149-153.

GIANT CELL REPARATIVE GRANULOMA
(Synonyms: giant cell reaction or lesion)

This pseudotumoral lesion is particularly observed in the maxillae, either under the gengival mucosa (epulid) with little or no penetration in the bone, or in the bone. A similar lesion is only rarely observed in other parts of the skeleton, and these particularly include the small tubular bones of the hand (Fig. 711).

Generally there is no indication of trauma in the patient's history, and symptoms are scarce.

Radiographically, there is an osteolytic lesion of small size, which is for the most part meta-epiphyseal (Figs. 712, 713). Osteolysis is eccentric at the onset, but thereafter it tends to involve the entire skeletal section, at times with thinning or even partial cancelling of the cortex, and characterized by boundaries which may be either faded or neater. At times it is constituted by a mass which is projected externally from the bone but which derives from the

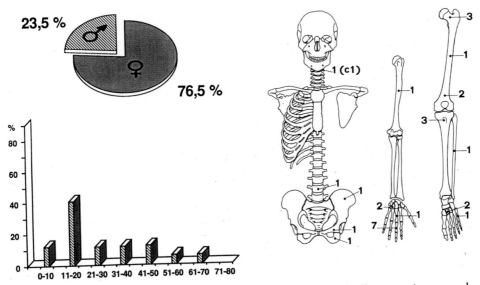

FIG. 711. - Sex, age and localization in 29 cases of giant cell reparative granuloma.

FIG. 712. - Giant cell reparative granuloma in a male aged 22 years, 3rd metarcarpal. The lesion was submitted to incomplete curettage and recurred after 1 year. The 3rd metacarpal was then resected and substituted with an autoplastic graft of the 4th metatarsal. Cured after 5 years.

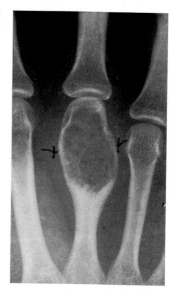

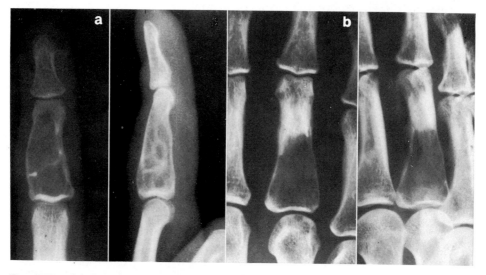

FIG. 713. - (a) Female aged 17 years. For the past 3 months pain and mild swelling. Cured 3 years after curettage and bone grafting. (b) Female aged 32 years. For 6 months pain and for 2 mild swelling. Cured 2 years after curettage and bone grafting.

bone. At times it contains a tenuous ground glass radiopacity.

Histologically it is a histio-fibroblastic tissue, whose structure may be similar to that of a histiocytic fibroma or of a fibrous dysplasia (Figs. 714, 715). The tissue contains numerous giant cells, but as compared to giant cell tumor it is more fibrous. At times there is focal calcification which recalls that of chondroblastoma, and osteoid production which, unlike that of fibrous

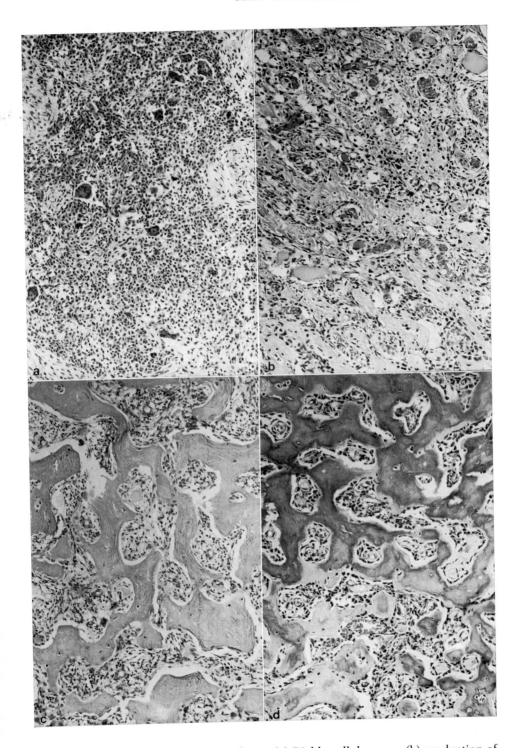

FIG. 714. - Giant cell reparative granuloma. (a) Richly cellular area; (b) production of scarce immature osteoid tissue; (c) and (d) newly-formed reticular bone (*Hemat.-eos.*, 125, 125, 125, 125 x).

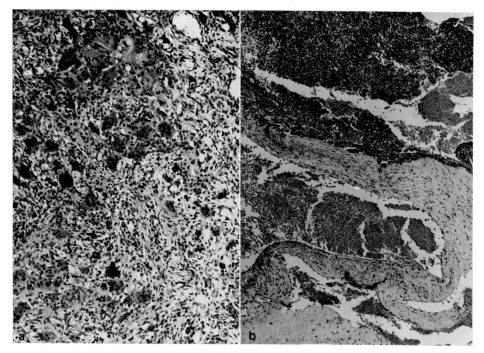

FIG. 715. - Giant cell reparative granuloma. (a) Area relatively rich in multinucleate giant cells; (b) cystic-hemorrhagic cavities recalling aneurysmal bone cyst (*Hemat.-eos.*, 125, 50 x).

dysplasia, is bordered by osteoblasts. Despite the fact that proliferation may appear to be lively, possibly with the presence of mitotic figures, the general aspect suggests a repair or hyperplastic process, more than a neoplastic one. It resembles a «solid» aneurysmal bone cyst, in which hematic cavities are absent (but not totally: Fig. 715b).

Differential diagnosis particularly involves giant cell tumor, histiocytic fibroma, fibrous dysplasia, chondroblastoma and osteoblastoma, pigmented nodular tenosynovitis.

The lesion is benign and usually heals with thorough curettage.

REFERENCES

1953 JAFFE P. L.: Giant cell reparative granuloma, traumatic bone cyst and fibrous (fibro-osseous) dysplasia of the jawbones. *Oral Surgery*, **6**, 159-175.

1972 D'ALONZO R., PITCOCK J. A., MILFORD L. W.: Giant-cell reaction of bone. Report of two cases. *Journal of Bone and Joint Surgery*, **54-A**, 1267-1271.

1972 SAPP J. P.: Ultrastructure and histogenesis of peripheral giant cell reparative granuloma of the jaws. *Cancer*, **30**, 1119-1129.

1980 CAMPANACCI M., LAUS M., BERTONI F.: Reazione a cellule giganti dell'osso. *Giornale Italiano di Ortopedia e Traumatologia*, **6**, 235-243.

TUMORS OF THE SOFT TISSUES

SUBDERMIC FIBROMATOSIS
(Synonym: fibrous hamartoma of infancy)

It is a hamartoma of mixed structure, fibro-myxo-adipose, which develops in the subcutaneous tissue.

It is a **rare** occurrence, observed in **young children**, under 3 years of age, at times at birth. There is evident predilection for the male **sex**. It nearly exclusively **occurs** in the regions of the shoulder, axilla, arm.

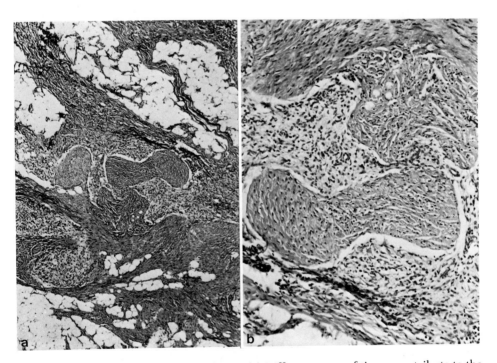

FIG. 716. - Fibrous hamartoma of infancy. (a) Different types of tissue contribute to the composite aspect of this lesion. Fibrous tissue, tissue constituted by immature round-oval cells immersed in mucoid substance, and mature adipose tissue. (b) Immature cells in loose aggregation are associated with fibrous tissue with spindle cells arranged in fascicles. (c) and (d) Organoid aspect of the lesion: alongside mature adipose tissue, fibrous tissue and islands of round-oval cells surrounded by mucoid ground substance (*Hemat.-eos.*, 60, 160, 250, 250 x).

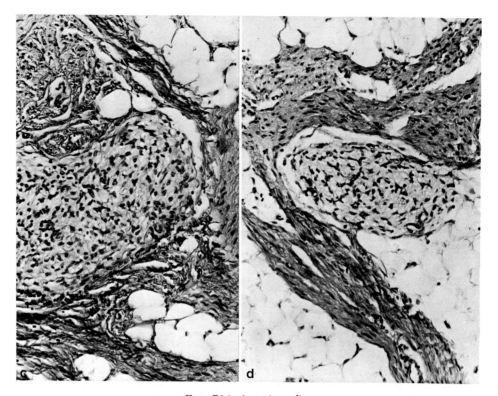

FIG. 716. (continued).

It is **manifested** as a single mass, at times growing with a certain vivacity and often achieving a size (greater than or equal to a walnut) which is considerable in relation to the size of the child. It is painless. Consistency varies from soft to firm, its limits are not very precise, the skin above it is unaltered, but generally adherent to the mass. The latter is instead mobile, but not in all cases, on the deep planes.

Macroscopically, the S.F. occupies the subcutaneous tissue and the deep layer of the derma. Its boundaries are not evident in relation to the surrounding fat, and it is characterized by a variegated aspect, which is partly fibrous or fibro-myxoid, and partly typically adipose. This adipose tissue (which, in larger tumors, exceeds in quantity the fat contained in the subcutaneous) is a component of tumoral growth.

Histologically there is an organoid structure, made up of three elements and which is very typical (Fig. 716). 1) There are long shoots of dense fibrocollagenous tissue, but which is relatively rich in cells, recalling the aspect of a fetal tendon. 2) There are immature and loose cellular areas, recalling the primitive mesenchyma, rich in capillaries. The cells are rounded-oval or stellate, often whorled or «ball-like» in orientation. The intercellular substance is mucoid, it takes up the mucin specific stains but not after hyaluronidase. 3) The third component is mature adipose tissue, in a variable quantity.

In time, growth of the tumor decreases and the tissue tends to mature (as do many hamartomas), with rarefaction of the cells and thickening of the collagenous bundles.

Complete **excision**, even marginal, is usually sufficient. The rare cases of local recurrence may be attributed to either incomplete excision or even to the ex novo origin of a hamartoma from surrounding and apparently normal subcutaneous tissue.

REFERENCES

1965 ENZINGER F.M.: Fibrous hamartoma of infancy. *Cancer*, **18**, 241.

1970 ROBBINS L.B., HOFFMAN S., KAHN S.: Fibrous hamartoma of infancy: Case report. *Plast. Reconstr. Surg.*, **46**, 197.

1974 IWASAKI H., ENJOJI M.: Fibrous hamartoma of infancy: Report of two cases. *Jpn. J. Cancer Clin.*, **20**, 216.

1979 KING D.F., BARR R.J., HIROSE F.M.: Fibrous hamartoma of infancy. *J. Dermat. Surg. Oncol.*, **5**, 482.

1982 MITCHELL M.L., DI SANT'AGNESE P.A., GERBER J.E.: Fibrous hamartoma of infancy. *Hum. Pathol.*, **13**, 586.

1984 GRECO A.M., SCHINELLA R.A., VULETIN J.C.: Fibrous hamartoma of infancy. An ultrastructural study. *Hum. Pathol.*, **15**, 717.

1988 FLETCHER C.D.M., POWELL G., VAN NOORDEN S., MCKEE P.H.: Fibrous hamartoma of infancy. A histochemical and immunohistochemical study. *Histopathology*, **12**, 65.

1989 PALLER A.S., GONZALES-CRUSSI F., SHERMAN J.O.: Fibrous hamartoma of infancy: eight additional cases and a review of the literature. *Archives of Dermatology*, **125**, 88.

DIGITAL FIBROMATOSIS
(Synonym: recurring digital fibrous tumor of infancy)

It is a **rare** lesion, occurring during the **first months of life**, or at birth, with no evident predilection for **sex**. It is **localized** in the second or third phalanx of a finger or toe, on the extensor or lateral aspect. At times more than one finger or toe is involved, or it may be bilateral, or it may involve both the hand and the foot.

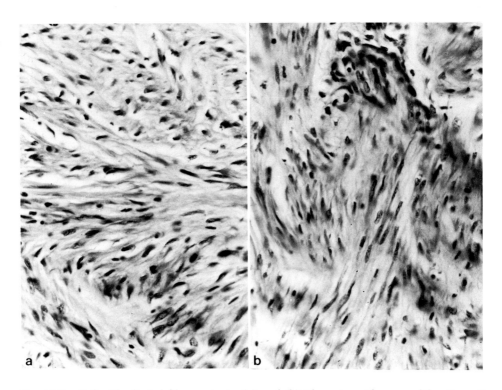

FIG. 717. - Infantile digital fibromatosis. (a) and (b) There is uniform proliferation of spindle cells, fibroblasts, and fibrocytes, immersed in collagen matrix. (c) and (d) Under higher enlargement in the paranuclear site of the cytoplasm there are rounded inclusions (*Hemat.-eos.*, 400, 400, 1000, 1000 x).

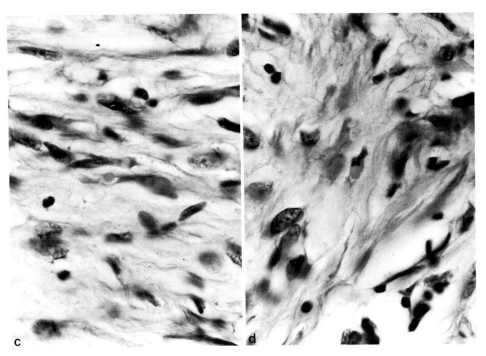

FIG. 717 (continued).

Macroscopically, it is a nodule (or nodules) the size of a pea or slightly larger, fibrous and compact, adherent to the skin and to the underlying fibrous and skeletal plane.

Histologically, it is made up of fibroblasts which are more or less swollen, and dense mesh of collagen (Fig. 717). The fibroblasts often present cytoplasmatic inclusions, near a nuclear pole, which are globose and eosinophilic, typical of this lesion. Histochemistry and electron microscopy have not as yet proven the meaning of these inclusions.

Incomplete and marginal **excision** is often followed by recurrence. Often, more than with actual recurrence, we are dealing with the occurrence of new nodules in adjacent tissue in the same finger or toe or in other fingers and toes. After a limited amount of growth, the nodules tend to arrest and at times they spontaneously regress. Thus, surgical treatment must be very conservative, and aimed more at preserving or restoring the axis and function of the digit than removing all of the pathologic tissue.

REFERENCES

1971 BATTIFORA H., HINES J.: Recurring digital fibromas of childhood. *Cancer*, **27**, 1530.
1972 ALLEN P.W.: Recurring digital fibrous tumours of childhood. *Pathology*, **4**, 215.

1974 BLOEM J.J., VUZEVSKI V.D., HUFFSTADT A.J.C.: Recurring digital fibroma of infancy. *J. Bone Joint Surg.*, **56/B**, 746.

1977 BECKETT J.H., JACOBS A.H.: Recurring digital fibrous tumors of childhood. A review. *Pediatrics*, **59**, 401.

1980 IWASAKI H., KIKUCHI M., MORI R. *et al.*: Infantile digital fibromatosis. Ultrastructural, histochemical and tissue culture observations. *Cancer*, **46**, 2238.

1981 FERRAGIANA T., CHURG J., STRAUSS L. *et al.*: Ultrastructural histochemistry of infantile digital fibromatosis. *Ultrastruct. Pathol.*, **2**, 241.

1982 MORTIMER G., GIBSON A.A.M.: Recurring digital fibroma. *J. Clin. Pathol.*, **35**, 849.

1984 PURDY I.J., COLBY T.V.: Infantile digital fibromatosis occurring outside the digit. *Am. J. Surg. Pathol.*, **8**, 787.

APONEUROTIC FIBROMATOSIS
(Synonyms: juvenile aponeurotic fibroma, calcifying aponeurotic fibroma)

It is a circumscribed and benign neoformation recalling histogenesis of the aponeurosis (from which it gets its name) and of the tendons and, like tendinous insertions at the bone, it has fibro-cartilaginous aspects. The presence of chondroid cells is associated with frequent focal calcification.

It is a **rare** occurrence, with predilection for the male **sex** and infant to juvenile **age**: most cases occur under 18 years of age. **Localization** is nearly exclusively in the hand and forearm, the foot and leg, with evident predilection for the palm of the hand (approximately half of all cases).

It is **manifested** by a deep mass, but it may also be subcutaneous, with unclear boundaries, of firm consistency. It is painless, characterized by slow growth, and it does not become of large size (it rarely surpasses the size of a walnut). In time it tends to become a nodule with more evident limits and of harder consistency.

Particularly during this late stage, **radiograms** may reveal a spray of tenuous calcar granules in the area of the neoformation.

Macroscopically compact, grayish-white tissue is observed, which infiltrates and surrounds the tendons, muscular fascicles, lobules of fat, vessels and nerves, and has no precise boundary (diffused fibromatosis). Generally at a later stage, there may be a more demarcated nodule, which is dense and fibrous and possibly speckled by calcar granules (calcifying fibroma). The neoformation may invade the subcutaneous tissue and adhere to the osteo-periosteal and capsular plane.

Histologically there is a *sui generis* proliferation of fibroblasts, which all seem to run in the same direction and surround muscular cells, adipose cells, tendons, vessels and nerves without invading or destroying them. The cells have large round-oval, well-stained nuclei, and rather swollen and vesicular cytoplasms. At times the cells are arranged in columns or palisades. There are foci of calcification and chondroid differentiation, the latter with ground substance rich in hyaluronidase-resistant mucopolysaccharides. Surrounding the calcified and necrotic chondroid areas the cells may be palisading, and scattered multinucleate giant cells may be observed. These areas may resemble a rheumatoid nodule. In more fibrous and «mature» forms the tissue may recall that of a palmar fibromatosis or a desmoid tumor. In the less

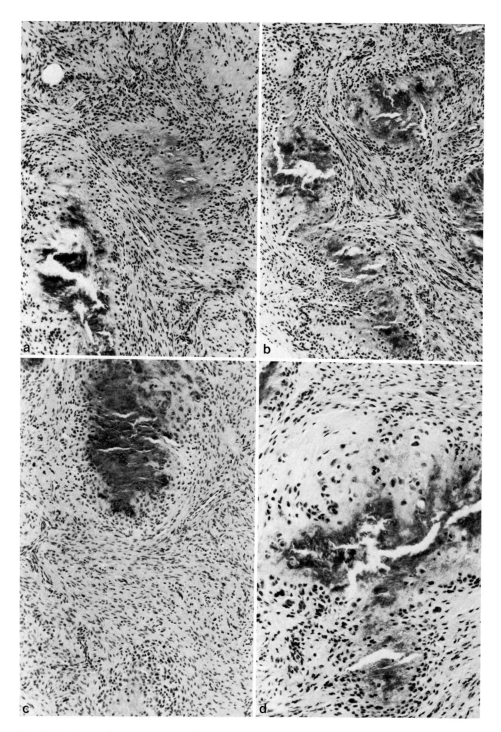

FIG. 718. - Juvenile aponeurotic fibromatosis. Lesion 1.5 x 1 x 0.6 cm in a male aged 8 years. Palm of the hand. The lesion recurred twice and a sarcoma was diagnosed. It was a spindle cell proliferation with areas of hyalinization and areas of calcified deposit surrounded by fibro-hyaline cartilage (Hemat.-eos., 160, 160, 400 x).

mature ones, it is rather cellular. However, mitotic figures are quite rare (Fig. 718).

It is important not to confuse this lesion **with a sarcoma or a desmoid tumor**. Despite its infiltrative attitude, A.F. is in fact characterized by limited growth, which seems to tend towards exhaustion with the end of body growth, and it has never caused important local disorders (such as joint limitation, vascular or nervous lesion).

Given the site and infiltrative features of the lesion, **surgical removal** is generally intralesional and incomplete. Recurrence is very frequent, particularly during childhood. Above 10-15 years of age, instead, the neoformation seems to slow down or arrest its growth, and recurrence after surgical excision becomes rare.

In conclusion, this lesion should be **operated on in a very conservative manner**, possibly when it has reached its mature, quiescent stage.

REFERENCES

1953 KEASBEY L.E.: Juvenile aponeurotic fibroma (calcifying fibroma). A distinctive tumor arising in the palms and soles of young children. *Cancer*, **6**, 338.

1961 KEASBEY L.E., FANSELAU H.A.: The aponeurotic fibroma. *Clin. Orthop.*, **19**, 115.

1964 LICHTENSTEIN L., GOLDMAN R.L.: The cartilage analogue of fibromatosis: A reinterpretation of the condition called «juvenile aponeurotic fibroma». *Cancer*, **17**, 810.

1970 ALLEN P.W., ENZINGER F.M.: Juvenile aponeurotic fibroma. *Cancer*, **26**, 857.

1970 GOLDMAN R.L.: The cartilage analogue of fibromatosis (aponeurotic fibroma). Further observations based on seven new cases. *Cancer*, **26**, 1325.

1972 DES MARCHAIS J., PAQUIN G., GUY R.: Fibromatose cartilagineuse calcifiante: Un cas de fibrome aponeurotique juvenile. *Union. Med. Can.*, **101**, 247.

1973 IWASAKI H., ENJOJI M.: Calcifying aponeurotic fibroma. *Fukuoka Aeta Med.*, **64**, 52.

1974 SUBBUSWAMY S., VYAS D., GADGIL R.: Cartilage analogue of fibromatosis. *Indian J. Cancer*, **11**, 476.

1975 SPECH E.E., KONKIN L.A.: Juvenile aponeurotic fibroma. The cartilage analogue of fibromatosis. *JAMA*, **234**, 626.

1975 ZAKI F.A., LIU S.K., KAY W.J.: Calcifying aponeurotic fibroma in a dog. *J. Am. Vet. Med. Assoc.*, **166**, 384.

1977 DUPRE A.: Keasbey's aponeurotic fibromatosis. *Ann. Dermatl. Venereol.*, **104**, 775.

1977 KARASICK D., O'HARA A.E.: Juvenile aponeurotic fibroma. A review and report of a case with osseous involvement. *Radiology*, **123**, 725.

1978 ZEIDE M.S.: Juvenile aponeurotic fibroma. Case report. *Plast. Reconstr. Surg.*, **61**, 922.

CONGENITAL FIBROMATOSIS:
SOLITARY, MULTIPLE, GENERALIZED
(Synonym: infantile myofibromatosis, solitary and multiple)

These tumors, which are probably hamartomas, are characterized as follows: 1) occurrence at birth or during the first months of life; 2) a peculiar histological aspect; 3) the localization. As for localization, there is a solitary form, a multiple one, and a generalized one. All are **very rare**.

The **solitary form** occupies the subcutaneous and the muscular planes, with a tumor which may be of considerable size, having poorly defined limits in relation to the surrounding tissues, which may contain satellite micro-

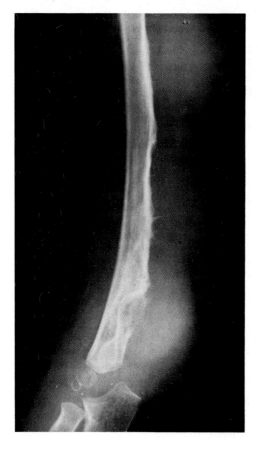

FIG. 719. - Boy aged 4 years. Congenital multicentric fibromatosis with repeated recurrence in the arm, and erosions of the adjacent skeleton. After several unsuccessful excisions and a final attempt at resection including the radial nerve, due to further recurrence which was threateningly close to the axilla, the patient was submitted to interscapulothoracic amputation. This treatment was excessive.

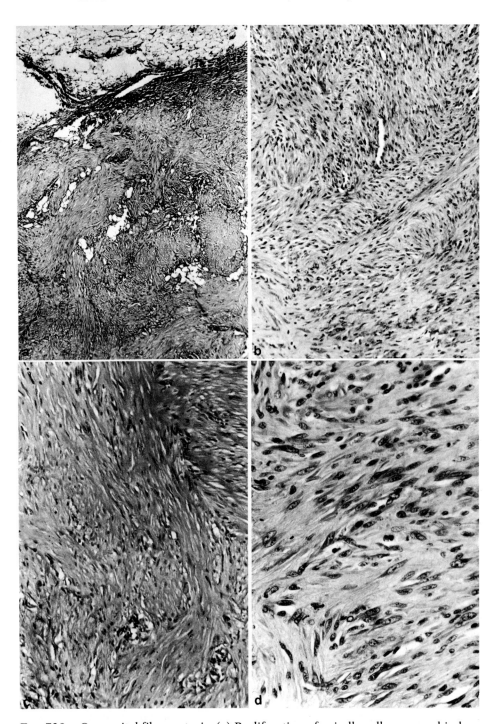

FIG. 720. - Congenital fibromatosis. (a) Proliferation of spindle cells arranged in bundles. Limits with the surrounding adipose tissue are not very neat. (b) and (c) Spindle cells of monomorphous aspect aggregated in bundles and separated by abundant quantity of collagen. (d) The cells have an ovoid nucleus, fine dispersed chromatin and a small nucleolus (*Hemat.-eos.*, 60, 160, 160, 400 x).

nodes around the principal mass. Nonetheless, a marginal excision is sufficient for healing, which may even occur spontaneously.

The **multiple form** involves the subcutaneous and the muscles with numerous nodes, but also the skeleton, where bubbly osteolytic areas occur (Fig. 719). This form often manifests spontaneous and complete regression of the nodules of the soft tissues and of the bones.

Finally, there is the **generalized form**, where the tumors involve not only the soft tissues and the skeleton, but the internal organs, as well. This form is fatal during the first days-months of life and in most cases.

Histologically, we are dealing with a proliferation which in some areas is richly cellular, made up of spindle cells with collagen fibers (Fig. 720). The histostructure at times recalls a leiomyoma, at times a neurofibroma, at times a hemangiopericytoma. There are areas with a chondroid aura, frequent areas of necrosis and minute calcar precipitations. In the more cellular fields plump nuclei and frequent mitotic figures may be observed.

In the multiple and generalized forms distribution of the lesions makes **diagnosis** easy. In the solitary form it is important to differentiate this congenital fibromatosis from fibrosarcoma, leiomyoma-leiomyosarcoma, neurofibroma and hemangiopericytoma.

REFERENCES

1958 SHNITKA R.K., ASP D.M., HORNER H.R.: Congenital generalized fibromatosis. *Cancer*, **11**, 627.

1961 BARTLETT R.C., OTIS R.D., LAAKSO A.O.: Multiple congenital neoplasms of soft tissues. Report of four cases in one family. *Cancer*, **14**, 913.

1973 BAER J.W., RADKOWSKI M.A.: Congenital multiple fibromatosis. Case report with review of the world literature. *Am. J. Roentgenol.*, **118**, 200.

1974 STOUT A.P.: Juvenile fibromatoses. *Cancer*, **7**, 953.

1977 KINDBLOM L.G., TERMEN G., SAVE-SODERBERGH J. *et al.*: Congenital solitary fibromatosis of soft tissues, a variant of congenital generalized fibromatosis. Two cases reports. *Acta Pathol. Microbiol. Scand.*, **85/A**, 640.

1981 CHUNG E.B., ENZINGER F.M.: Infantile myofibromatosis. A review of 59 cases with localized and generalized involvement. *Cancer*, **48**, 1807.

1981 LIEW S., HAYNES M.: Localized form of congenital generalized fibromatosis. A report of three cases with myofibroblasts. *Pathology*, **13**, 257.

1982 BRILL P.W., YANDOW D.R., LANGER L.O. *et al.*: Congenital generalized fibromatosis. Case report and literature review. *Pediatr. Radiol.*, **12**, 771.

1982 MODI N.: Congenital generalized fibromatosis. *Arch. Dis. Child.*, **57**, 881.

1982 WALTS A.E., ASCH M., RAJ C.: Solitary lesion of congenital fibromatosis. *Am. J. Surg. Pathol.*, **6**, 255.

1983 DIMMICK J.E., WOOD W.S.: Congenital multiple fibromatosis. *Am. J. Dermatopathol.*, **5**, 289.

1984 JENNINGS T., DURAY P.H., COLLINS F.S. *et al.*: Infantile myofibromatosis. Evidence for an autosomal-dominant disorder. *Am. J. Surg. Pathol.*, **8**, 529.

1984 SPRAKER M.K., STACK C., ESTERLY N.B.: Congenital generalized fibromatosis: a review of the literature and report of a case associated with porencephaly, hemiatrophy, and cutis mamorata telangiectatica congenita. *J. Am. Acad. Dermatol.*, **10**, 365.

1985 ALTEMAN A.M., AMSTALDEN E.I., FILHO J.M.: Congenital generalized fibromatosis causing spinal cord compression. *Hum. Pathol.*, **16**, 1063.

ABDOMINAL AND EXTRA-ABDOMINAL DESMOID TUMOR
(Synonyms: musculo-aponeurotic fibromatosis, aggressive fibromatosis)

DEFINITION

Desmoid tumor is an old term derived from the Greek «desmos» which means aponeurosis, tendon. By this term we mean an invasive, permeative and progressive tumor, uniformly composed of fibroblasts-fibrocytes and abundant collagen, frequently located on the deep soft tissues, and characterized by an age and localization differing from those previously listed (infantile fibromatoses) and from those of palmar and plantar fibromatosis (see pseudotumoral lesions). In other words, the histological aspect is not enough to characterize a D.T.: for example, the histological aspect of D.T. is the same as that of a Dupuytren's palmar fibromatosis.

Despite the fact the D.T. acts like a tumor having local malignancy, and thus similarly to a low-malignancy sarcoma, it is kept separate from fibrosarcoma for two reasons. First, because it does not manifest progression in malignancy; second, because it does not metastasize.

Nonetheless, the limit of separation in relation to grade 1 fibrosarcoma is sometimes faded and difficult to determine.

FREQUENCY, SEX, AGE

D.T. is not a rare occurrence. There is slight predilection for the male sex, except for its abdominal form which evidently shows predilection for females (after deliveries). It may be observed at any age, but it is more frequent in children and youths up to 40 years of age. In children it is rarely observed prior to 6 years of age (unlike congenital fibromatosis and those of early childhood).

LOCALIZATION

The most frequent localizations are in this order: the limbs, the trunk (those affecting the abdominal wall equal to less than 10% of the total), the head and neck. In the limbs it shows predilection for the proximal regions: particularly the shoulder and the buttock; these are followed by the posterior aspect of the thigh, the popliteal fossa and the sura, the arm and the forearm. It exceptionally occurs in the hand and foot. It may also be localized inside the pelvis, in the mesenteric and retroperitoneal site.

The tumor usually develops in the deep soft tissues; sometimes, however, it arises in the superficial fascia and from there it involves both the underlying muscle and the subcutaneous tissue (Fig. 723b). D.T. may be a part of Gardner syndrome, in association with polyposis of the large intestine and cranio-facial osteomas. There are rare cases of **multicentric D.T.**, in the same limb or in two limbs.

SYMPTOMS

These consist of a deep, painless mass, which may grow considerably in the course of several months, at times more slowly. It is not uncommon to see patients whose symptoms go back several years and who have already been operated on once or several times and present local recurrence. When the tumor achieves large size, there may be muscular retraction phenomena and limitations in joint function. If the tumor compresses a nerve trunk, irradiated pain and possibly paralysis occur.

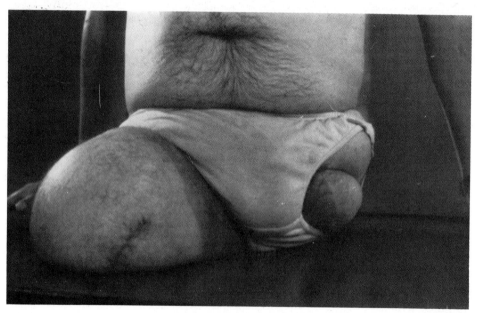

FIG. 721. - Male aged 20 years. Multicentric desmoid tumor, diffused and recurring in both of the lower limbs. The lesion began 8 years earlier in the right leg, and then extended proximally as far as the popliteal region. One year earlier, it occurred in the left leg, posterior aspect of the thigh and gluteal region. After numerous attempts at excision, followed by extensive local recurrences, the patient was amputated at the right thigh and hemipelvectomized on the left. This outcome was partially due to inadequate treatment at the onset and to overtreatment at the end: in any case it shows how extensive and aggressive the lesion can be. There were no signs of recurrence after 5 years.

The skin and subcutaneous are generally left intact; but they may be involved when the tumor develops or expands to the superficial fascia, or after repeated surgery followed by recurrence, or after radiation therapy.

The tumor is generally elongated in the direction of the muscles; rarely, it extends to include most of the length of the limb, with large masses disseminated along the muscles and joined together. Thus, it is not a «ball-like» tumor by concentric growth, rather it is a tumor which grows by infiltrative ramifications along the muscles, the aponeuroses and the tendons, and at times it is of multicentric origin (Fig. 721).

Its limits are typically not well-defined, consistency is typically firm to

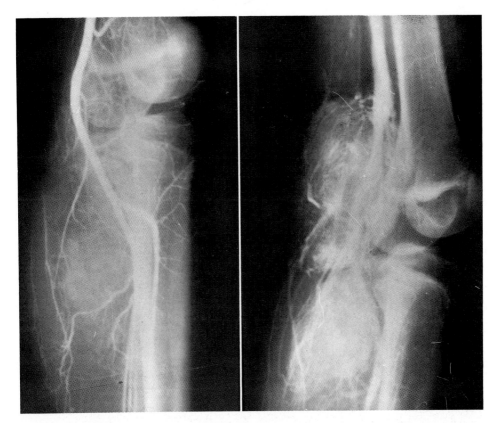

FIG. 722. - Female aged 13 years. Desmoid tumor observed 3 years earlier, operated on 1 year earlier by marginal excision, due to adherence to the popliteal vessels. Local recurrence after 10 months, arteriography. Observe the longitudinal extension in multiple nodes, the intense uptake of the contrast medium in the arterial phase and even more so in the venous one. This diffused uptake indicates a thick intratumoral capillary network, with scarce vessels of large caliber. At surgery for this recurrence, the tumor was found to englobe the popliteal vessels and the tibial nerve, and to adhere to the tibia and interosseous membrane. We then gave up the idea of excision, irradiating with 5000 rad. The mass remained unchanged after 4 years. Nonetheless, a new mass occurred more proximally, in the deep soft tissues of the posterior thigh. This mass was also excised marginally, and followed by radiation therapy at 5000 rad. The lesions stabilized after 8 more years, allowing for fair use of the limb.

FIG. 723. - (a) Female aged 43 years. Desmoid tumor of the gluteal region and upper/posterior thigh. The mass was observed for a few years, and was painful in a sitting position. CAT with intravenous contrast medium showed the neoformation, which intensely and diffusely took up the contrast medium and thus was easily distinguished from the surrounding muscles. The tumor was irregular in shape (not a single globose mass). Furthermore, it developed in the gluteus maximus muscle and outside it, in the aponeurosis, tendon and in the intermuscular spaces. Finally, it had faded boundaries and digitations. At surgery, it infiltrated the subcutaneous fat with nodules and digitations which it was necessary to excise widely. The surgical margins were questionably marginal in a couple of areas. Postoperative radiation was therefore given. No recurrence after 6 years. (b) Female aged 25 years. Desmoid tumor of the lumbar-gluteal region, recurring. CAT with and without contrast medium revealed the mass in two distinct and confluent nodes, mostly superficial in relation to the aponeurosis covering the lumbar muscles. Wide excision included, in addition to the subcutaneous tissue and the aponeurosis, a thick layer of the lumbar and glutei muscles, as well as a part of the spinous apophyses and of the posterior iliac crest. No further recurrence after 7 years.

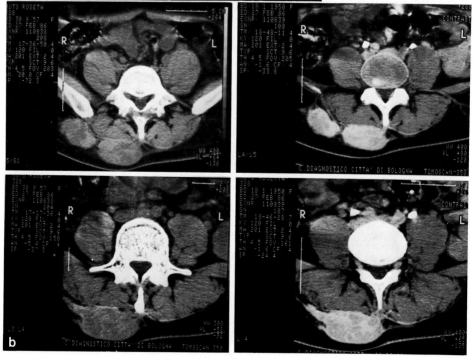

hard, and it does not change with muscular contraction. It is fixed to the musculo-aponeurotic plane. It may be free in relation to the skin plane and to the skeletal and capsular one, but at times it adheres to these planes, too.

RADIOGRAPHIC FEATURES

When arteriography is used the tumor may be injected very little or not at all; but in some cases (histologically rich in fibroblasts and not very collagenized) there is intense diffused uptake of the contrast medium (Fig. 722).

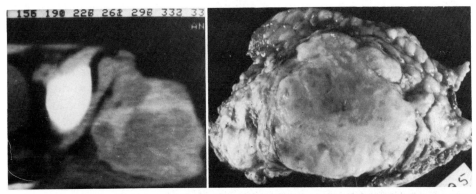

FIG. 724. - Boy aged 8 years. For the past year, a desmoid tumor in the gluteal region which was slightly painful was observed. CAT revealed the newly-formed mass in the gluteus maximus. The macroscopic picture of the specimen excised and transected showed compact, rosy tissue, vaguely fasciculated and fibrous, lobulated. The boundaries at times faded into the surrounding adipose and muscular tissue. Excision including most of the gluteus maximus was wide, there was no recurrence after 10 years.

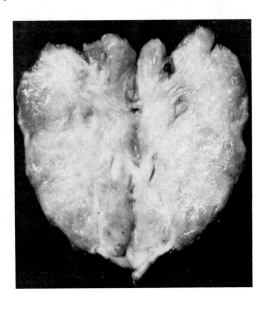

FIG. 725. - Male aged 32 years. Desmoid tumor of the thigh, submitted to wide excision. Macroscopic aspect. Observe the irregularly fasciculated, similtendinous aspect, and the limits which fade into the surrounding degenerated and compressed tissues. No recurrence after 6 years.

Even when CAT is used, D.T. is evident in the muscles due to an evidently higher and homogeneous density, after intravenous injection of contrast medium (Fig. 723). CAT and MRI are also diagnostic, when the tumor appears to be formed by multiple confluent masses, and shows digitations along the fascial and interstitial planes.

GROSS PATHOLOGIC FEATURES

D.T. may become of large or enormous size; it tends to infiltrate proximally and distally along the musculo-aponeurotic planes.

The features of the tumoral tissue, more clearly seen on its cut surface are those of a fibro-collagen tissue: this is less hard, paler pink in color, and juicy in less mature and more cellular forms (Fig. 724); harder, lucent-white, simil-tendinous, with rough shoots which are intertwined or convoluted, in more collagenized forms (Fig. 725). The tissue does not have well-defined limits; it infiltrates the muscles, where it fades into the degenerated and reactive muscular tissue. Satellite nodules may be scattered in proximity to the main tumoral mass. It firmly adheres to the aponeuroses, tendons, joint capsules, bone, subcutaneous or deep fat, vessels and nerves. These structures are compressed by the tumor, but rarely invaded. Rarely, the bone may be characterized by superficial excavations by effect of this compression *ab*

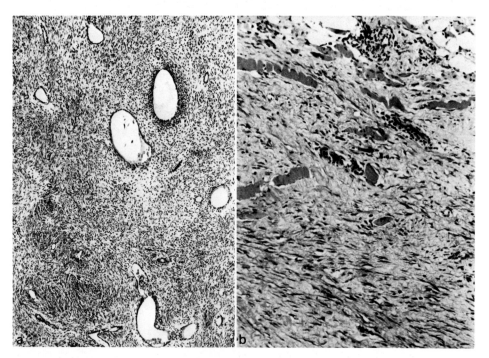

FIG. 726. - Desmoid tumor. (a) In the spindle cell proliferation ectatic vessels having a thin wall are visible. (b) Periphery of the lesion: spindle cell proliferation infiltrates the fibro-adipose and muscular tissue (*Hemat.-eos.*, 60, 160 x).

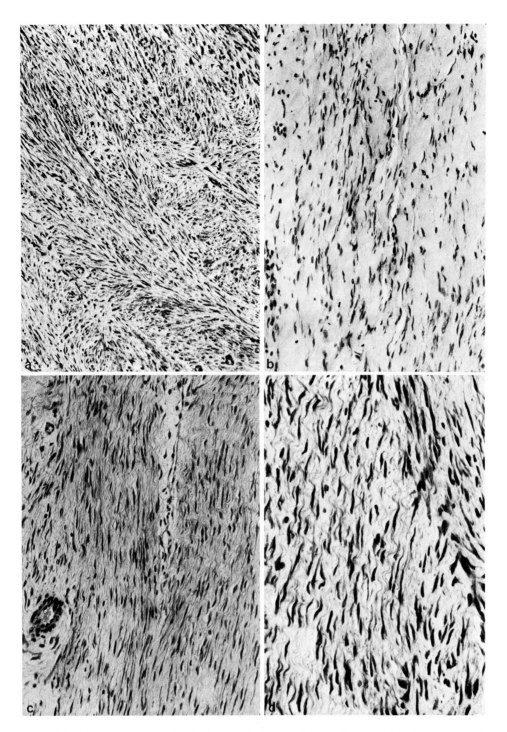

FIG. 727. - Desmoid tumor. (a) Spindle cells in parallel bundles. Fields with scarce collagen and considerable cellularity may be observed. (b) The lesion appears to be
richer in collagen and thus hypocellular. (c) and (d) There are elongated cells, with flattened dark nucleus, no mitotic figures (*Hemat.-eos.*, 160, 250, 250, 400 x).

estrinseco. In cases which were previously submitted to surgery, it is difficult or impossible to distinguish tumoral tissue from scar tissue.

HISTOPATHOLOGIC FEATURES

It is a compact tissue constituted by fibroblasts, fibrocytes and collagen fibers. These are arranged in intertwined bundles, which are wavy and have no particular order. The lesion is hardly ever very cellular. In some areas the fibroblasts are plumper and numerous, while in others they are quite scarce, mature and thin, with dark nuclei surrounded by thick fibro-hayline bundles. Even in the more cellular areas, the nuclei show finely dispersed chromatin, neither pleomorphism nor hyperchromia, minute or absent nucleoli, and rare mitotic figures. Vascularization is scarce, but despite this there are no areas of necrosis (Figs. 726, 727).

What is typical is the fact that this tumor infiltrates the muscle and the other surrounding tissues to a considerable extent. This infiltration is actually much more evident than what is observed in most sarcomas, and, in particular, in cases of fibrosarcoma.

HISTOGENESIS

In the history of D.T., it seems that trauma is of greater importance than it is in other tumors. In cases of D.T. of the abdominal wall trauma is constituted by delivery. Hormonal and genetic influences (such as in Gardner syndrome) have also been hypothesized.

DIAGNOSIS

Differential diagnosis with infantile fibromatosis, palmar and plantar fibromatosis, is based on age, localization, gross pathologic features and, for some types of fibromatosis, histological data. Differential diagnosis with **well-differentiated fibrosarcoma** (grade 1) may be difficult. Of the two forms, as previously stated, the limit of separation is not clear. In particular, D.T. occurring in early childhood resemble well-differentiated fibrosarcoma; however, this is characterized by «ball-like» and compressive growth, while D.T. diffusedly infiltrates the tissues.

COURSE

D.T. grows progressively and, if removed with marginal or even wide margins, it has a strong tendency to recur. Rapid growth and recurrence are variable and unpredictable (unrelated to the histological picture). Local recurrence is generally manifested after a few months and up to 3 years. Growth of the tumor is never very rapid: in some cases it may be rather lively, but in others it is nearly absent. There are exceptional cases in which the tumor remains unchanged or even regresses partially over several years.

Transformation in fibrosarcoma has never been observed. Even after many episodes of recurrence and many years, the histological aspect is always the same.

TREATMENT AND PROGNOSIS

Treatment is mainly surgical. Surgical removal must be decidedly wide. Every marginal or, worse yet, intralesional operation is usually followed by local recurrence. Given the anatomo-pathological features of the tumor, wide and conservative excision is often difficult or impossible. Surgery must be accurately planned with the help of CAT and MRI. Exclusively local malignancy leads us to be as conservative as possible.

In cases where wide excision is not possible, radiation therapy may be used which, particularly if carried out in addition to surgery, has obtained some favorable results. In other cases, where conservative and wide surgery is not possible, one may simply wait, as in some cases D.T. is arrested spontaneously or even partially regresses.

In exceptional cases, when the tumor compresses and surrounds main vessels and nerves of the limb, if it has recurred several times, if by pushing towards the limb girdle invasion of the pelvis or axilla is feared, wide amputation will be required (Fig. 721).

Metastases never occur, and thus prognosis *quoad vitam* is good. In rare cases of primary localization or secondary extension to the trunk, head and neck, nonetheless, the outcome was fatal as a result of local invasion of the vital organs.

REFERENCES

1954 STOUT A.P.: Fibrosarcoma, well-differentiated (aggressive fibromatosis). *Cancer*, **7**, 953.
1960 HUNT R.T.N., ACKERMAN L.V.: Principles in the management of extra-abdominal desmoids. *Cancer*, **13(4)**, 825.
1961 STOUT A.P.: The fibromatoses. *Clin. Orthop.*, **19**, 11.
1963 DAHN I., JONSSON N., LUNDH G.: Desmoid tumours. A series of 33 cases. *Acta Chir. Scand.*, **126**, 305.
1967 EZINGER F.M., SHIRAKI M.: Musculo-aponeurotic fibromatosis of the shoulder girdle (extra-abdominal desmoid), analysis of 30 cases followed up for 10 or more years. *Cancer*, **21**, 1131.
1969 DAS GUPTA T.K., BRASFIELD R.D., O'HARA J.: Extra-abdominal desmoids. A clinicopathological study. *Ann. Surg.*, **170**, 109.
1970 MÜLLER G., SCHWEIZER P., FLACH A.: Juvenile fibromatose. *Virchows Arch. (Pathol. Anat.)*, **349**, 138.
1973 BARBER H.M., GALASKO C.S.B., WOODS C.G.: Multicentric extra-abdominal desmoid tumours. Report of 2 cases. *J. Bone Joint Surg.*, **55B**, 858.
1975 BREWSTER R., IVINS J.: Extra-abdominal desmoid tumors. *J. Bone Joint Surg.*, **57A**, 1026.
1975 STILLER D., KATENKAMP D.: Cellular features in desmoid fibromatosis and well-differentiated fibrosarcomas. *Virchows Arch. (Pathol. Anat.)*, **369**, 155.

1976 DEHNER L.P., ASKIN F.B.: Tumors of fibrous tissue origin in childhood. A clinicopathologic study of cutaneous and soft tissue neoplasms in 66 children. *Cancer*, **38**, 888.

1977 ALLEN P.W.: The fibromatoses: A clinicopathologic classification based on 140 cases. *Am. J. Surg. Pathol.*, **1**, 305.

1979 MC DOUGALL A., MC GARRITY G.: Extra-abdominal desmoid tumors. *J. Bone Joint Surg.*, **61B**, 373.

1980 GOELLNER J.R., SOULE E.H.: Desmoid tumors. An ultrastructural study of eight cases. *Hum. Pathol.*, **11**, 43.

1981 ESCALONA-ZAPATA J.: Tumors of the soft tissue. Cytology and growth pattern of fibrosarcomas and related tumors. *Pathologica*, **73**, 119.

1984 DÖHLER J.R., HAMELMANN H., LASSON U.: Aggressive fibromatoses. *Chirurg.*, **55(3)**, 174-8.

1984 ROCK M.G., PRITCHARD D.J., REIMAN H.M., SOULE E.M., BREWSTER R.C.: Extra-abdominal desmoid tumors. *J. Bone Joint Surg.* **66A**, 1369

1985 GRIER H.E., PEREZ-ATAYDE A.R., WEINSTEIN H.J.: Chemotherapy for inoperable infantile fibrosarcoma. *Cancer*, **56**, 1507.

1985 HALL J., TSENG S.C.G., TIMPL R. *et al.*: Collagen types in fibrosarcoma. Absence of type III collagen in reticulum. *Hum. Pathol.*, **16**, 439.

1985 HUDSON T.M., BERTONI F., ENNEKING W.F.: Scintigraphy of aggressive fibromatosis. *Skeletal Radiol.*, **13(1)**, 26-32.

1986 NINANE J., GOSSEYE S., PANTEON E. *et al.*: Congenital fibrosarcoma. Preoperative chemotherapy and conservative surgery. *Cancer*, **58**, 1400.

1989 EASTER D.W., HALASZ N.A.: Recent trends in the management of desmoid tumors: summary of 19 cases and review of the literature. *Ann. Surg.*, **210**, 765.

FIBROSARCOMA

DEFINITION

The tumor is **exclusively** constituted by fibroblasts and collagen fibers; it is relatively monomorphous, with a «herring-bone» structure.

FREQUENCY, SEX, AGE

It occurs infrequently (approximately 10% of all sarcomas of the soft tissues). There is no clear predilection for sex, and it is observed at any age, with a higher incidence between 30 and 70 years of age. Average age is around 45 years. It is rare in children under 10 years of age and in some of these cases it is congenital.

LOCALIZATION

The most common localization is in the thigh; this is followed, approximately equally, by the trunk and the other segments of the limbs. The distal parts of the limbs, including the hand and foot, may be the site of F.S. in the child, but rarely in the adult.

SYMPTOMS

The tumor is nearly always deep, located under the superficial fascia (Fig. 728). It is a single, globose mass, at times lobate. It usually grows rapidly (but this is by no means the rule). At times the tumor doubles in just a few weeks. Some congenital forms of the tumor are of monstruous size at birth. Consistency is firm, limits rather well-defined. In advanced forms it may adhere to the skeleton and ulcerate the skin growing in a fungiform manner on the outside. It is nearly or totally painless, except when it compresses the nerve trunks.

RADIOGRAPHIC FEATURES

In exceptional cases it contains calcification. It may erode the adjacent

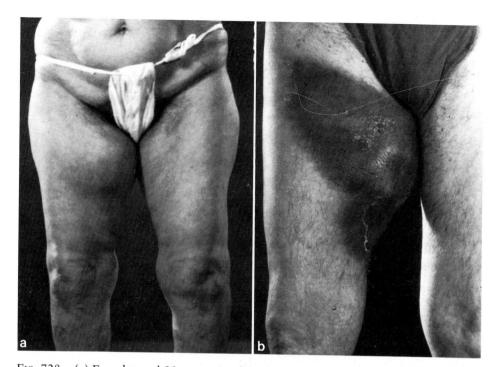

FIG. 728. - (a) Female aged 80 years. Grade 4 fibrosarcoma, swelling observed 3 years earlier. (b) Male aged 61 years. Grade 3 fibrosarcoma, swelling observed 4 months earlier. Red-brown discolored skin, adherent, warm. In both cases marginal excision was performed followed by radiation therapy at 4000 rad. In the first case there is no long-term follow-up (the patient died after 1 year of unrelated causes), in the second there was local recurrence after 4 months judged to be inoperable.

bone or bones. Angiography, CAT and MRI show the features common to most sarcomas (Figs. 729, 730).

GROSS PATHOLOGIC FEATURES

The tumor has a deep site. It is a globose mass with lobulated margins, at times (particularly in smaller tumors) having a pseudocapsule. On the cut surface, the aspect and consistency depend on the amount of collagen: it is soft encephaloid in more richly cellular forms (Figs. 729, 730, 731), firmer and more fibrous in collagenized ones (Fig. 732). However, it hardly achieves the similaponeurotic aspect of desmoid tumors. It may contain myxoid areas.

HISTOPATHOLOGIC FEATURES

The neoplasm is constituted throughout by spindle cells, having a nucleus with sharp ends and producing reticular and collagen fibers. Electron microscopy shows the intercytoplasmatic presence of collagen filaments. In less

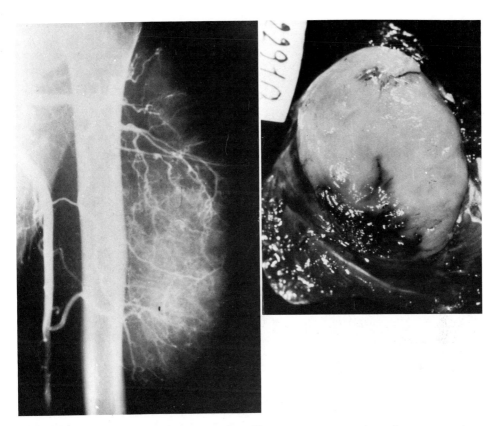

FIG. 729. - Female aged 44 years. Grade 3 fibrosarcoma, recurring after two previous excisions, over 1 year. Observe the angiographic aspects of malignancy: hypervascularity, ectatic, anomalous vessels, diffused uptake of the contrast medium. The patient was submitted to interscapulothoracic amputation and there were no signs of disease after 7 years. Macroscopically, on the cut surface, it is compact, homogeneous, whitish and juicy tissue, with a hemorrhagic area. The mass appeared to be pseudocapsulated. The boundaries are neater than those usually observed in desmoid tumor.

differentiated forms the collagen is limited to thin reticular fibers, which, moreover, surround each cell and are revealed by silver stain (Fig. 734d). In more differentiated forms, the collagen is more abundant, with rougher fibers which are stained blue by trichromic staining. Cells and fibers form bundles and currents, which may be parallel, and often intertwined and oriented like a «herring-bone».

There are different grades of malignancy in fibrosarcoma (from two to four according to the authors). Differentiation and histological malignancy are inversely proportional (Figs. 733, 734, 735, 736).

The histological elements useful in defining the grade of malignancy are: numerical density of the cells, cellular anaplasia, mitotic index, production of collagen. Thus, grade 1 is the most differentiated form, less cellular, with nuclei which are mildly enlarged and hyperchromic as compared to normal fibrocytes, scant mitosis, abundant collagen production. This form is that

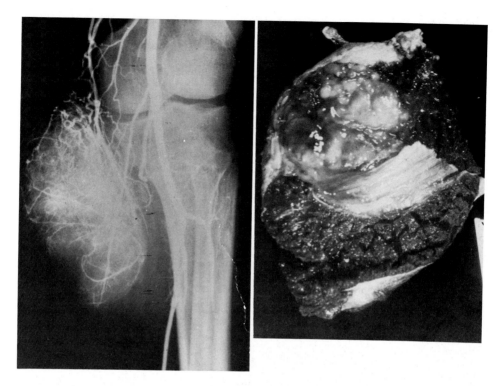

FIG. 730. - Male aged 55 years. Grade 3 fibrosarcoma, swelling for the past year. Angiographic aspect. The tumor is contained in the medial gastrocnemius and located far from the popliteal vessels. The patient was submitted to excision, and the transected specimen reveals the mass of soft tumor, having confluent nodes the color of light leather, with faded boundaries. The tumor was surrounded by healthy muscle or (above to the left) by an aponeurosis of compartmental delimitation. Thus, the surgical margin was wide. There were no signs of disease after 9 years.

which is closest to desmoid tumors. Grade 4 is the least differentiated form, the richest in cells, with highly anaplastic and at times monstruous elements, many mitoses, scant collagen production. It is the form which most resembles fibrous malignant histiocytoma. However, it must be recalled that intense pleomorphism, with giant or multinucleate sarcomatous cells, are rarely observed, even in the most undifferentiated F.S. Apart from these two extremes, which may be mistaken for desmoid tumors and pleomorphic sarcomas, respectively, the most frequent and typical aspect of F.S. (grades 2 and 3) is easily recognized by its monomorphous spindle cell composition and «herring-bone» structure.

Generally, the histological grade is the same throughout the entire tumor and does not change in local recurrences or metastases.

At times, the F.S. presents myxoid areas, with intercellular substance which takes on the colors of mucin but not after treatment with hyaluronidase. At the periphery of the tumor, in particular, inflammatory infiltration may be observed.

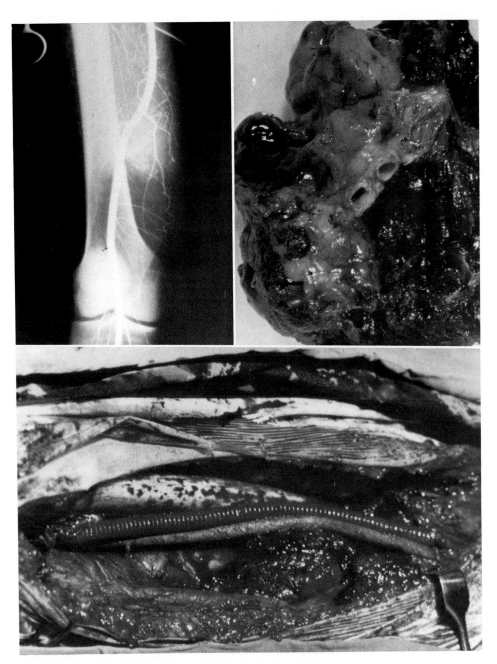

FIG. 731. - Male aged 43 years. Grade 3 fibrosarcoma, with swelling observed for the past 5 months. Angiography revealed the tumor (diffused uptake) adherent and shifting the superficial femoral artery. In order to obtain a wide surgical margin, the vastus medialis and the adductor muscles, the femoral vessels and the medial periosteum of the femur were resected en bloc with the tumor. The transected specimen shows the tumor (above to the left) which adheres to the vessels. The photo of the surgical field, after surgery has ended, shows the femur stripped of the periosteum, and vascular reconstruction obtained with a prosthesis in dacron for the artery and calf carotid for the vein. Circulation of the limb was good and there were no signs of disease after 5 years.

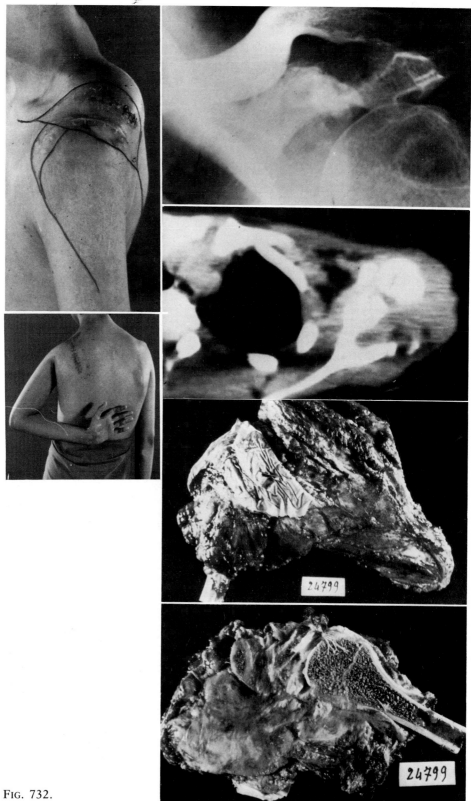

Fig. 732.

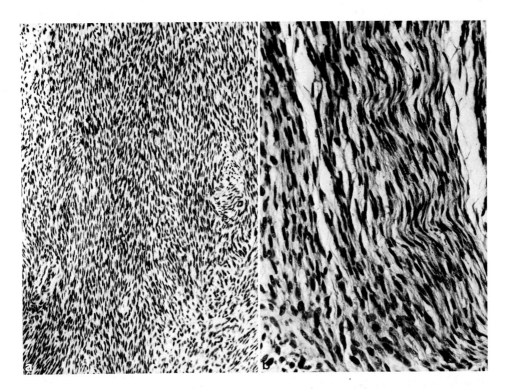

FIG. 733. - Grade 1 fibrosarcoma. (a) Proliferation of the spindle cells arranged in va-ryingly intersecting bundles. (b) Evident monomorphism. The cells are regularly ar-ranged in parallel bundles. The nuclei are spindling and chromatin is finely granular (*Hemat.-eos.*, 160, 400 x).

The attitude of F.S. as compared to the tissues is typically invasive and permeative (Fig. 736). The pseudocapsule, which may be apparent on macro-scopic examination, is always illusory.

◀

FIG. 732. - Male aged 13 years. Grade 3 fibrosarcoma. For the past 2 years pain and functional impairment of the shoulder. Because of an image of radiographic rarefac-tion of the humeral head, the patient was submitted to skeletal biopsy, with a nega-tive outcome. After 1 year, there was swelling in the region of the trapezius, submit-ted to a second biopsy with a correct diagnosis. Observe the two different bioptic scars which forced us to use an atypical incision for resection. X-ray shows erosion *ab estrinseco* of the acromion and the humeral head. CAT shows a mass in the supraspi-nous fossa, which adheres to the joint and to the head of the humerus. In order to ob-tain a radical surgical margin, the scapula, lateral half of the clavicle and proximal part of the humerus had to be resected en bloc with all of the scapular muscles (Ti-koff-Linberg operation). The humerus was substituted by an endoprosthesis and the cosmetic result was good 2 months after surgery. At resection there were pulmonary metastases so that the patient died after 2 and 1/2 years, with no signs of local recurrence.

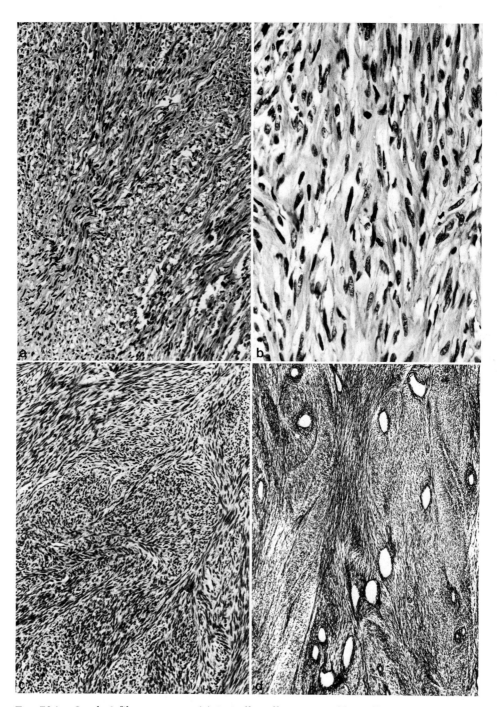

FIG. 734. - Grade 2 fibrosarcoma. (a) Spindle cells separated by collagen are arranged in intersecting bundles. (b) These are relatively monomorphous spindle cells; nuclei with narrowed ends and finely granular chromatin. (c) The neoplasm shows a fasciculated aspect which in several fields looks like a «herring-bone». (d) Among the cells there is collagen which is clearly revealed by silver impregnation (*Hemat.-eos.*, 160, 400, 60, x); *arg. impr.*, 60 x).

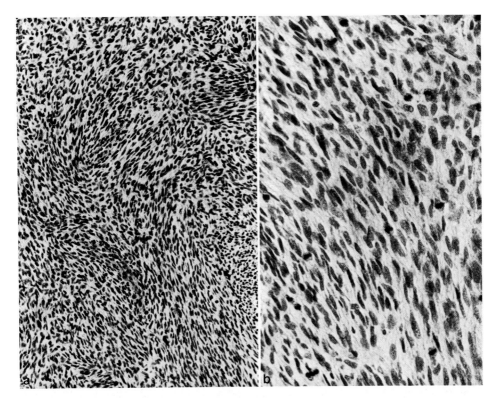

Fig. 735. - Grade 3 fibrosarcoma. (a) The spindle cells are arranged in bundles presenting varying orientation. (b) Under higher power more pleomorphism as compared to low grades of malignancy may be observed. The nucleo-cytoplasmatic relationship is shifted in favor of the nucleus, there are numerous mitotic figures and there is considerable nuclear hyperchromia. These are the cytological elements indicating the high grade of malignancy (*Hemat.-eos.*, 160, 400, x).

PATHOGENESIS

Cases of F.S. occurring on traumatic or burn scarring, osteomyelitic fistulae and, above all, after radiation treatment (at least 3 years after radiotherapy) have been described.

DIAGNOSIS

F.S. is characterized by a rather uniform histological picture. In order to exclude other tumors many extensive histological specimens are required.

Malignant fibrous histiocytoma involves a more advanced age, and it is histologically characterizd by a storiform structure, by the presence of giant and multinucleate tumoral cells with large intensely eosinophilic and at times foamy cytoplasms. Malignant fibrous histiocytoma may also have intensely collagenized areas, with a compact fibro-hyaline substance embedding

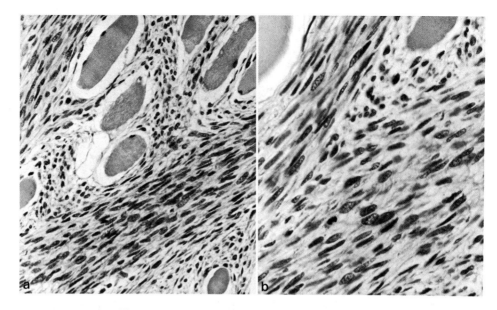

Fig. 736. - Grade 4 fibrosarcoma. (a) The spindle cell neoplasm, which is characterized by a relatively more pleomorphic aspect than that of grades 1, 2, 3 infiltrates the muscle. (b) Nuclear hyperchromia, relatively pleomorphic nuclei, many mitotic figures and coarse chromatin are indicative of a high grade of malignancy (*Hemat.-eos.*, 250, 400 x).

relatively scattered cells. Nonetheless, these areas demonstrate the storiform structure and are usually associated with areas richer in cells and having the aspects of cellular pleomorphism recalled above.

Differential diagnosis with **malignant neurinoma** may instead be more delicate (or impossible on a purely histological basis). Clinically malignant neurinoma is often painful and always originates from a nerve trunk or is associated with the stigmatae of neurofibromatosis. Histologically, the cells more rarely tend to form distinct bundles, arranged like a «herring-bone», rather they form whorls or palisades. Furthermore there may be aspects of transition from those of malignant neurinoma and benign neurofibroma.

Differential diagnosis involving **spindle cell monophasic synovial sarcoma** may also be difficult (see synovial sarcoma).

But these differential diagnoses, to which may be added that with **leiomyosarcoma** and practically all sarcomas having spindle cellular areas, are not of practical importance. Differential diagnosis with benign forms or those with local malignancy is instead essential. **Nodular fasciitis** is represented by a small nodule, it grows rapidly, it does not have a compact «herring-bone» structure, but rather it has a disorderly structure with a marked myxoid component and a certain amount of inflammation. The presence of mitotic figures does not influence diagnosis as mitotic figures are also frequent in nodular fasciitis, but the same may not be said for atypical mitoses.

Desmoid tumor has an aspect which is rather similar to that of a well-dif-erentiated grade 1 fibrosarcoma. In truth, it may be very difficult to decide between one and the other diagnosis. In favor of desmoid tumor are cellular-ity which is not thick, absence of hyperchromia of the nuclei, nearly total absence of mitotic figures, and abundant and dense collagen component. The distinction between desmoid tumor and grade 1 fibrosarcoma must include clinical data and course of the disease, and it must be based on numerous and extensive specimens, as histological aspects in favor of desmoid tumor or grade 1 fibrosarcoma may be associated within the same tumor.

PROGNOSIS AND TREATMENT

Prognosis depends on histological grade and age, as it is evidently better in children under 10 years of age. In the child local recurrence is nearly just as frequent as in the adult, but metastases are rarer, less than 10%.

In the adult local recurrence is common after marginal excision or ones which are not wide enough (most series report approximately 50% of local recurrence) and metastases occur in 60% of cases. After local recurrence, the incidence of metastases increases. Metastases are generally pulmonary, skel-etal, hepatic. Lymph node metastases are rare (less than 5% of cases). Ten-year survival rate is approximately 60% for grades 1 and 2, 30% for grades 3 and 4.

Treatment is prevalently surgical and must be aggressive in the adult, more conservative in the child. The surgical margin must always be wide. In the adult and in cases of grade 3 or 4 F.S. a radical surgical margin may be indicated (Figs. 730, 731, 732).

Radiotherapy and chemotherapy are of moderate or inconstant effective-ness, or as yet to be demonstrated. Thus, they are used as adjuvants, particu-larly in grade 3 and 4 forms.

REFERENCES

1950 IVINS J.C., DOCKERTY M.B., GHORMLEY R.K.: Fibrosarcoma of the soft tissues of the extremities. A review of 78 cases. *Surgery*, **28**, 495.

1962 STOUT A.P.: Fibrosarcoma in infants and children. *Cancer*, **15**, 1028.

1964 MAC KENZIE D.H.: Fibroma: A dangerous diagnosis. A review of 205 cases of fi-brosarcoma of soft tissues. *Br. J. Surg.*, **51**, 607.

1964 MORRIS J.M.: Fibrosarcoma within a sinus tract of chronic draining osteomye-litis. *J. Bone Joint Surg.*, **46**, 853.

1965 WERF-MESSING B. VAN DER, UNNIK J.A. VAN: Fibrosarcoma of the soft tissues. *Can-cer*, **18**, 1113.

1967 BALSAVER A.M., BUTLER J.J., MARTIN R.G.: Congenital fibrosarcoma. *Cancer*, **20**, 1607.

1968 SOULE E.H., MAHOUR G.H., MILLS S.D. *et al.*: Soft tissue sarcomas of infants and children. A clinicopathologic study of 135 cases. *Mayo Clin. Proc.*, **43**, 313.

1970 GANE N.F., LINDUP R.: Radiation-induced fibrosarcoma. *Br. J. Cancer*, **24**, 705.

1970 GONZALES-CRUSSI F.: Ultrastructure of congenital fibrosarcoma. *Cancer*, **26**, 1289.

1970 HAYS D.M., MIRABAL V.W., KARLAN M.S. *et al.*: Fibrosarcoma in infants and chil-dren. *J. Pediatr. Surg.*, **5**, 176.

1973 Castro E.B., Hajdu S.I., Fortner J.G.: Surgical therapy of fibrosarcoma of the extremities. *Arch. Surg.*, **107**, 284.

1973 Exelby P.R., Knapper W.H., Huvos A.G. *et al.*: Soft-tissue fibrosarcoma in children. *J. Pediatr. Surg.*, **8**, 415.

1974 Pritchard D.J., Soule E.H., Taylor W.F. *et al.*: Fibrosarcoma — a clinicopathologic and statistical study of 199 tumors of the soft tissues of the extremities and trunk. *Cancer*, **33**, 888.

1975 Pritchard D.J., Soule E.H.: Fibrosrcoma of the soft tissues of the extremities and limb girdles in children. *J. Bone Joint Surg.*, **57A**, 1026.

1976 Chung E.B., Enzinger F.M.: Infantile fibrosarcoma. *Cancer*, **38**, 729.

1977 Adam Y.G., Reif R.: Radiation-induced fibrosarcoma following treatment for breast cancer. *Surgery*, **81**, 421.

1977 Soule E.H., Pritchard D.J.: Fibrosarcoma in infants and children: A review of 110 cases. *Cancer*, **40**, 1711.

1978 Guber S., Rudolph R.: The myofibroblast. *Surg. Gynecol. Obstet.*, **146**, 641-649.

1978 Siegal A., Horowitz A.: Aggresive fibromatosis-infantile fibrosarcoma. Difficulty of diagnostic and prognostic evaluation. *Clin. Pediatr.*, **17**, 517.

1980 Gonzalez-Crussi F., Wiederhold M.D., Sotelo-Avila C.: Congenital fibrosarcoma. Presence of a histiocytic component. *Cancer*, **46**, 77-86.

1985 Hall J., Tseng S.C.G., Timpl R., Hendrix M.J.C., Stern R.: Collagen types in fibrosarcoma. Absence of type III colagen in reticulin. *Hum. Pathol.*, **16**, 439-446.

1986 Weiss S.W.: Proliferative fibroblastic lesions. From hyperplasia to neoplasia. *Am. J. Surg. Pathol.*, **10**, Suppl. 1, 14.

1989 Scott S.M., Reimah N.M., Pritchard D.J., Ilstrup D.M.: Soft tissue fibrosarcoma: a clinicopathologic study of 132 cases. *Cancer*, **64**, 295.

BENIGN FIBROUS HISTIOCYTOMA
(Synonyms: dermatofibroma, histiocytoma cutis, cutaneous fibrous histiocytoma, subepidermic nodular fibrosis, sclerosing angioma)

It is a benign tumor of the soft tissues which reveals moderate infiltrative capacity but limited growth potential.

A rather **frequent** occurrence, it is most often observed in the superficial skin planes, derma and subcutaneous tissue (Fig. 737), but it may be localized in the deep tissues.

There is predilection for adult **age**; it is frequently **localized** in the limbs. In a third of all cases cutaneous lesions are multiple. Size varies from a few millimeters to a few centimeters, and in general it does not exceed 3 cm. Deep forms of the disease may achieve larger size (5 cm).

Macroscopically a yellowish-white nodule is observed with rather defined limits, often containing hemorrhagic areas. In the skin the nodule is protrusive or pediculated and often, due to hemorrhage, it is of red-brown or dark color, which may suggest melanoma.

Histologically, in superficial and deep localizations, the limits of the tumor are not always well-defined even if there are no actual infiltrative aspects in relation to the surrounding tissues. There are spindle cells which varyingly intertwine in short fascicles, which often irradiate from

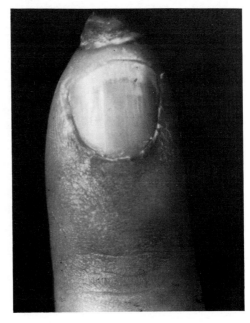

FIG. 737. - Benign fibrous histiocytoma. Male aged 33 years. The lesion was first noticed 2 1/2 years earlier. Skin nodule characterized by a reddish surface. Marginal excision and skin graft, cured after 6 years.

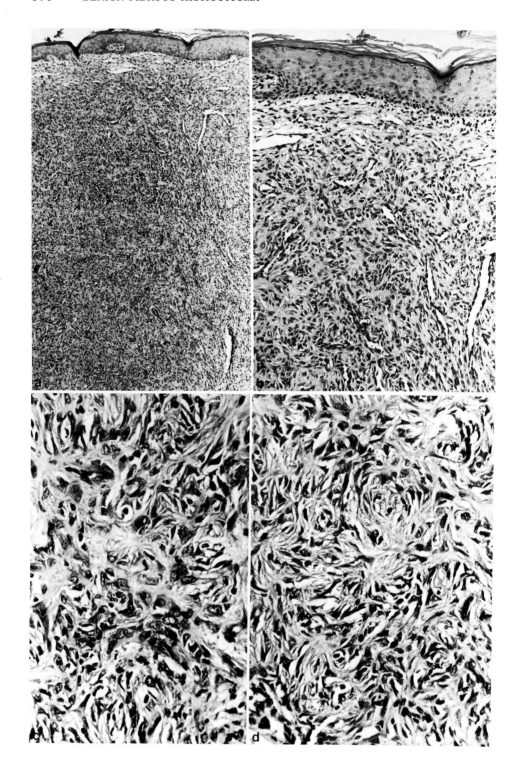

FIG. 738.

FIG. 738. - Benign fibrous histiocytoma. (a) The neoplasm extends on the surface until it comes up just below the epidermis. (b) Ovoid and spindle cells are arranged in short bundles. Observe the rich vascularization. (c) and (d) Central area of the neoplasm under high enlargement: observe globose cells and ovoid-spindle cells separated by collagen and irradiating in a storiform pattern from eosinophilic centers (storiform aspect). The cells present phagocytosis (*Hemat.-eos.*, 60, 160, 400, 400 x).

◀

central eosinophilic areas, producing the typical storiform or whorled aspect (Fig. 738). These elements are associated with cells of histiocytary features, with ample eosinophilic cytoplasm, nucleus which is often indented, macrophagic activity towards hemosiderin and lipids. Multinucleate giant cells, foam cells and lymphomonocytary and granulocytary phlogistic elements are often observed. In some areas the stroma appears to be more collagenized and rich in vessels (thus, the improper definition, sclerosing angioma). The stroma may assume a more abundant and hyaline aspect. In deeper localizations, this feature is associated with a more evident storiform aspect. Rarely groups of large histiocytes and giant cells are observed, which recall pigmented nodular synovitis.

Differential diagnosis, in superficial localizations, involves **dermatofibrosarcoma protuberans**: this has a more uniform cellular population, is constituted throughout by ovoid-spindle cells arranged in a storiform pattern, and its margins reveal a very evident infiltrative tendency.

In deep localizations B.F.H. must be differentiated from **malignant fibrous histiocytoma**, which reveals marked cellularity, evident pleomorphism and a high number of mitoses.

B.F.H. must also be distinguished from pseudosarcomatous lesions such as **nodular fascitis**, where very cellular areas are alternated with others of a myxoid aspect, with vessels having an «S» like pattern, and where cellularity and mitoses may be evident during the active stage.

B.F.H. is also differentiated from **leiomyoma** in which an evident fasciculated aspect prevails. The nuclei have rounded ends and there is longitudinal striation in the cytoplasm.

Treatment consists of marginal or wide surgical excision. It is a benign lesion, but recurrence is reported as occurring in 5% to 10% of all cases. The deeper forms are those which have a higher incidence of local recurrence.

REFERENCES

1970 NIEMI K.M.: The benign fibrohistiocytic tumours of the skin. *Acta Dermatoven.*, **50** (suppl. 63), 1.
1972 FLAM M., RYAN S.C., MAH-POY G.L. *et al.*: Multicentric reticulohistiocytosis: Report of a case with atypical features and electron microscopic study of skin lesions. *Am. J. Med.*, **52**, 841.
1973 HASHIMOTO K., PRITZKER M.S.: Electron microscopic study of reticulohistiocytoma. *Arch. Dermatol.*, **107**, 263.

1974 CARSTENS P.H.B., SCHRODT G.R.: Ultrastructure of sclerosing hemangioma. *Am. J. Pathol.*, **77**, 377.

1975 KATENKAMP D., STILLER D.: Cellular composition of the so-called dermatofibroma (histiocytoma cutis). *Virchows Arch. (Pathol. Anat.)*, **367**, 325.

1977 TAYLOR D.R.: Multicentric reticulohistiocytosis. *Arch. Dermatol.*, **133**, 330.

1978 MEISTER P., KONRAD E., KRAUSS F.: Fibrous histiocytoma: A histological and statistical analysis of 155 cases. *Pathol. Res. Pract.*, **162**, 361.

1982 DU BOULAY C.E.H.: Demonstration of alpha-l-antitrypsin and alpha-l-antichymotrypsin in fibrous histiocytomas using immunoperoxidase technique. *Am. J. Surg. Pathol.*, **6**, 559.

1982 GONZALES S., DUARTE I.: Benign fibrous histiocytoma of the skin: A morphologic study of 290 cases. *Path. Res. Pract.*, **174**, 379.

1982 KINDBLOM L.G., JACOBSEN G.K., JACOBSEN M.: Immunohistochemical investigation of tumours of supposed fibroblastic-histiocytic origin. *Hum. Pathol.*, **13**, 834.

1987 TAMADA S., ACKERMANN A.B.: Dermatofibroma with monster cells. *Am. J. Dermatopathol.*, **9**, 380.

DERMATOFIBROSARCOMA PROTUBERANS

It is composed of spindle cells in a storiform pattern. This monomorphous aspect is repeated in all parts of the neoplasm. Localization is generally cutaneous, its aspect is nodular.

It particularly involves the **age** group ranging from 30 to 50 years. There is predilection for the male **sex**. There is predilection for the following **localizations**: the trunk and the proximal parts of the limbs, but the tumor may occur everywhere.

The lesion is generally confined to the derma and subcutaneous tissue, it initiates as a lenticular growth of firm consistency, generally single and more rarely multiple. Growth is slow, but persistent; at times it is followed by more rapid growth. The lesion reveals protuberance, hence its name, only at an advanced stage. In this stage the **macroscopic aspect** is characterized by a large nodule, which is often single, or to which smaller nodules in the derma and subcutaneous may be associated (Fig. 740), with thinned, reddish overlying skin. Size is generally about 5 cm, but it may become of much larger volume. Growth generally occurs towards the surface, while lower down, and particularly beyond the fascia and in the muscles, it occurs rarely and only after repeated recurrences.

A **microscopic** examination reveals a neoplasm which at the periphery infiltrates the derma and the subcutaneous tissue (Fig. 739). The tumor is compact, thickly cellular and monomorphous. It is made up of spindle cells which may be plump or thin, arranged in a clearly storiform pattern throughout the neoplasm. Rarely, this aspect is not very evident, particularly if the stroma is substituted by a myxoid component. The cellular elements reveal moderate pleomorphism and mitotic activity is scarce. Overall, thus, evident monormorphism prevails, which at times is interrupted by rare xanthomatous cells, lymphocytary infiltrates and very scarce giant cells. In recurrences, in general, the morphological features of the initial lesion are repeated, but there may be **progression in malignancy**, with areas of a fibrosarcoma or malignant fibrous histiocytoma type (Fig. 740). In this case the lesion becomes more aggressive and it may metastasize. In initial lesions areas of necrosis are only rarely observed.

Differential diagnosis must first of all involve **malignant fibrous histiocytoma** which appears to be much more pleomorphic, with a more evident cytological malignancy, it reveals more evident mitotic activity and it presents areas of necrosis; furthermore, it is clinically characterized by more rapid growth and generally deeper localization.

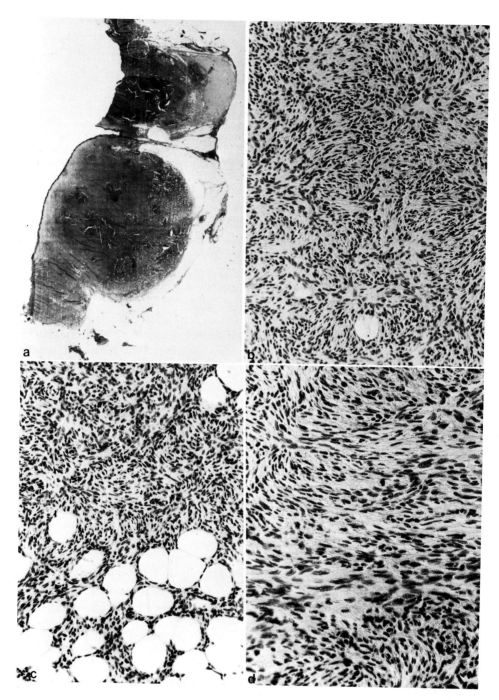

FIG. 739. - Dermatofibrosarcoma protuberans. (a) Overall view of the neoplasm involving the derma and subcutaneous. In its initial phase DFSP has a nodular aspect. (b) Spindle cells arranged in short bundles and characterized by a storiform pattern. (c) The lesion infiltrates the adipose tissue. (d) The cells are loosely arranged, there is no nuclear hyperchromia. It is a lesion with low-grade malignancy (*Hemat.-eos.*, 10, 250, 250, 400 x).

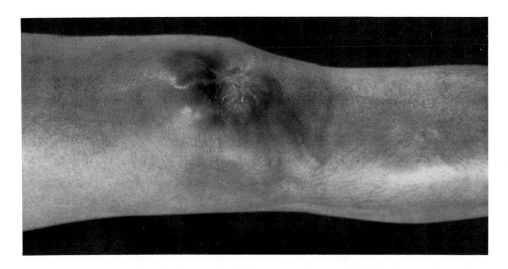

FIG. 740. - Dermatofibrosarcoma protuberans. Female aged 54 years. The lesion initiated 34 years earlier like a lentil. After that it was excised six times, irradiated twice. This was the seventh recurrence. It was widely excised with 2 cm of healthy skin surrounding it, the subcutaneous tissue, the fascia, part of the vastus medialis, the joint capsule, and grafted with a free skin flap. After 5 years, recurrence for the eighth time, with progression of malignancy to grade 4 malignant fibrous histiocytoma. Thigh amputation, no signs of disease after 2 years.

As compared to **benign fibrous histiocytoma**, differential diagnosis is based on the fact that this tumor does not infiltrate, has more numerous giant cells, foam cells and phlogistic cells, and does not reveal either hypercellularity or mitosis.

Forms of D.F.S.P. (particularly recurrences) with a rich myxoid component may suggest **myxoid liposarcoma**, as the storiform structure is hindered and the vascular component becomes more evident. Myxoid liposarcoma is localized in the deep structures, moreover, it presents lipoblasts.

D.F.S.P. is characterized by **local malignancy**, as revealed by local recurrence reported in 50% of all cases. This high tendency to recur is due to the infiltrative capacity of the lesion, which is often not recognized at surgery. When excision is wide recurrence is reported in a percentage of cases ranging from 20% to 30%. Local recurrence is manifested after 1-3 years, but at times even later. D.F.S.P. metastasizes in exceptional cases and only late, after repeated episodes of recurrence. There may be progression of malignancy in recurrence, which may prelude metastasis.

Treatment is surgical and consists of very wide excision, often completed by free or pediculated skin grafts. As there is a very low risk of metastasis, surgery is as conservative as possible. After repeated recurrence, however, and particularly if biopsy of the recurrence reveals progression in malignancy, more drastic types of surgery, or even amputation, are required.

REFERENCES

1961 Mc Gregor J.K.: Role of surgery in the management of dermatofibrosarcoma protuberans. *Ann. Surg.*, **154**, 255.

1962 Taylor H.B., Helwig E.B.: Dermatofibrosarcoma protuberans: A study of 115 cases. *Cancer*, **15**, 717.

1966 Burkhardt B.R., Soule E.H., Winkelmann R.K.: Dermatofibrosarcoma protuberans: Study of 56 cases. *Am. J. Surg.*, **111**, 638.

1967 Mc Peak C.J., Cruz T., Nicastri A.D.: Dermatofibrosarcoma protuberans: An analysis of 86 cases — five with metastasis. *Ann. Surg.*, **166** (suppl. 12), 803.

1968 Holm J.: Dermatofibrosarcoma protuberans: Report of a case with review of the literature. *Acta Chir. Scand.*, **134**, 303.

1972 Petkov I., Andreev V.C.: Dermatofibrosarcoma protuberans in seltener Lokalisation. *Hautarzt*, **23**, 508.

1974 Hagedorn M., Thomas C., von Kannen W.: Dermatofibrosarcoma protuberans mit Übergang in ein sogenanntes Fibrosarkom. *Dermatologica* , **149**, 84.

1974 Manalan S.S., Cohen I.K., Theogaraj S.D.: Dermatofibrosarcoma protuberans or keloid — a warning. *Plast. Reconst. Surg.*, **54**, 96.

1976 Ozzello L., Hamels J.: The histiocytic nature of dermatofibrosarcoma protuberans: Tissue culture and electron microscopic study. *Am. J. Clin. Pathol.*, **65**, 136.

1978 Alguacil-Garcia A., Unni K.K., Goellner J.R.: Histogenesis of dermatofibrosarcoma protuberans. An ultrastructural study. *Am. J. Clin. Pathol.*, **69**, 427.

1982 Kindblom L.G., Jacobsen G.K., Jacobsen M.: Immunohistochemical investigation of tumors of supposed fibroblastic-histiocytic origin. *Hum. Pathol.*, **13**, 834.

1982 Shelley W.B.: Malignant melanoma and dermatofibrosarcoma in a 60-year-old patient with lifelong acrodermatotitis enteropathica. *J. Am. Acad. Dermatol.*, **6**, 63.

1983 Frierson H.F., Cooper P.H.: Myxoid variant of dermatofibrosarcoma protuberans. *Am. J. Surg. Patholy.*, **7**, 445.

1984 Miyamoto Y., Morimatsu M., Nakashima T.: Pigmented storiform neurofibroma. *Acta Pathol. Jpn.*, **34**, 821.

1985 Robinson J.K.: Dermatofibrosarcoma protuberans resected by Mohs' surgery (chemosurgery): A 5-year prospective study. *J. Am. Acad. Dermat.*, **12**, 1093.

1986 Shneidman D., Belizaire R.: Arsenic exposure followed by the development of dermatofibrosarcoma protuberans. *Cancer*, **58**, 1585.

1989 Ding J., Hashimoto H., Enjoji M.: Dermatofibrosarcoma protuberans with fibrosarcomatous areas: clinicopathologic study of nine cases and comparison with allied tumors. *Cancer*, **64**, 721.

ATYPICAL FIBROXANTHOMA OF THE SKIN

It is a small nodular lesion of the derma, which is histologically nearly the same as a pleomorphic malignant fibrous histiocytoma. It is differentiated by its superficiality (it may just, but not extensively, extend into the subcutaneous tissue), by its absence of necrosis and, in particular, by its low aggressiveness.

It occurs in the regions of the body exposed to the sun in elderly subjects, more rarely in the skin of the trunk and of the proximal limbs in younger ones. It is a small nodule of derma, often ulcerated at the surface, but with no tendency to invade deeply.

Histologically, there are ovoid or spindle cells mixed with giant and foam cells arranged in a disorderly or moderately fasciculated pattern. Mitoses are not frequent and there is no necrosis. This lesion must be differentiated from **malignant fibrous histiocytoma**, which extends deeply, with marked pleomorphism, a high grade of malignancy and diffused necrosis. Furthermore, it must be differentiated histologically from **spindle-cell carcinoma** and from **malignant melanoma**.

A.F. must be treated conservatively. After wide removal recurrence is rare, metastases are nearly absent. Cases of progression in malignancy have been reported, with development of malignant fibrous histiocytoma.

REFERENCES

1964 KEMPSON R.L., MC GAVRAN M.H.: Atypical fibroxanthomas of the skin. *Cancer*, **17**, 1463.

1969 KROE D.J., PITCOCK J.A.: Atypical fibroxanthoma of the skin: Report of 10 cases. *Am. J. Clin. Pathol.*, **51**, 487.

1972 HUDSON A.W., WINKELMANN R.K.: Atypical fibroxanthoma of the skin: A reappraisal of 19 cases in which the original diagnosis was spindlecell squamous carcinoma. *Cancer*, **29**, 413.

1973 FRETZIN D.F., HELWIG E.B.: Atypical fibroxantoma of the skin. *Cancer*, **31**, 1541.

1973 VARGA-CORTES F., WINKELMANN R.K., SOULE E.H.: Atypical fibroxanthomas of the skin: Further observations with 19 additional cases. *Mayo Clin. Proc.*, **48**, 211.

1974 CAMMOUN M., TEMINE L., TABBANE F.: Fibroxanthomes atypique de la peau. *Ann. Anat. Pathol. (Paris)*, **19**, 327.

1975 JACOBS D.S., EDWARDS W.D., YE R.C.: Metastatic atypical fibroxanthoma of the skin. *Cancer*, **35**, 457.

1976 DAHL L.: Atypical fibroxanthoma of the skin. A clinicopathological study of 57 cases. *Acta Pathol. Microbiol. Scan.*, **84**, 183.

1977 ALGUACIL-GARCIA A., UNNI K.K., GOELLNER J.R. *et al.*: Atypical fibroxanthoma of the skin. *Cancer*, **40**, 1471.

1980 CHEN K.T.K.: Atypical fibroxanthoma of the skin with osteoid production. *Arch. Dermatol.*, **116**, 113.

1980 EVANS H.L., SMITH J.L.: Spindle cell squamous carcinoma and sarcoma-like tumors of the skin: A comparative study of 38 cases. *Cancer*, **45**, 2687.

1986 HELWING E.B.: MAY D.: Atypical fibroxanthoma of the skin with metastasis. *Cancer*, **57**, 368.

1989 WILSON P.R., STRUTTON G.M., STEWART M.R.: Atypical fibroxanthoma: two unusual variants. *J. Cutan. Pathol.*, **16**, 93.

MALIGNANT FIBROUS HISTIOCYTOMA

DEFINITION

M.F.H. is constituted by cells revealing histiocytary and fibroblastic differ-entiation. In recent years varieties of this tumor have been distinguished: pleomorphic storiform, myxoid, giant cell, inflammatory, angiomatoid. More than representing distinct anatomo-clinical entities having different prognoses and treatments, these variants must be considered to be part of the range in which M.F.H. may be manifested, and are particularly of diag-nostic value.

FREQUENCY

It is one of the most frequently-occurring malignant soft tissue tumors. Its number in recent times has increased as most of the lesions which were once classified as pleomorphic rhabdomyosarcoma, pleomorphic liposarcoma, and scarcely differentiated fibrosarcoma are now considered to belong to the M.F.H. group. In general, a re-examination of pleomorphic sarcomas with no specific aspects of cellular differentiation reveals the morphological features of M.F.H.

SEX

There is evident predilection for the male sex.

AGE

It affects advanced age, from 50 to 70 years, except for the angiomatoid form, which is observed before 20 years of age.

LOCALIZATION

There is preference for the limbs (particularly the lower limb, specifically the thigh) and the retroperitoneum. The inflammatory variety prevails in the retroperitoneum. In approximately 90% of all cases localization is deep, un-

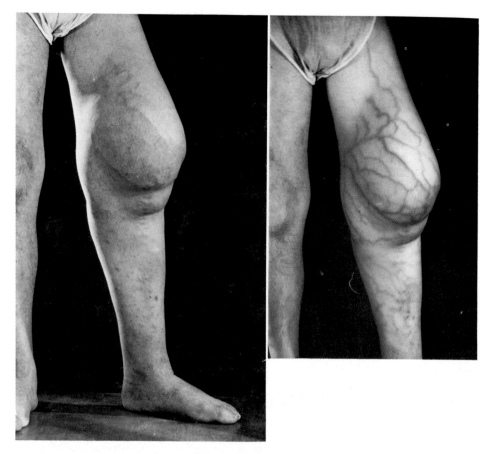

FIG. 741. - Grade 4 malignant fibrous histiocytoma. Male aged 49 years. Swelling occurring 19 years earlier and left untreated. Observe the subcutaneous venous reticulum in the infra-red photograph. Thigh amputation. The patient died 18 months later of pulmonary metastasis.

der the fascia, while in 10% it is suprafascial. This is not so in the angiomatoid variety, which shows predilection for the derma and subcutaneous tissue of the limbs.

SYMPTOMS

It is a deep, globose mass which grows gradually, at times slowly, at times more rapidly. Swelling is generally painless (Figs. 741, 742, 743). Usually the amount of time between the occurrence of swelling and diagnosis ranges from a few months to a few years. In retroperitoneal localizations diagnosis is made later and symptoms include anorexia, weight loss, symptoms of compression of the abdominal organs. In suprafascial localizations diagnosis is made earlier, when the tumor is still of moderate size.

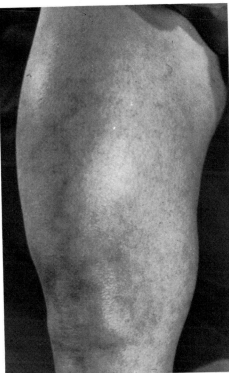

FIG. 742. - Grade 4 malignant fibrous histiocytoma. Female aged 51 years. Mass
present for an undetermined amount of
time, pain for the past month. The
swelling was globose and rather tense.
CAT showed liquid contents (the tumor
was in fact extensively hemorrhagic),
but a thick wall, with hyperdense nodules protruding inwards. Because of the
association of diffused pulmonary metastasis, surgical treatment was not
performed.

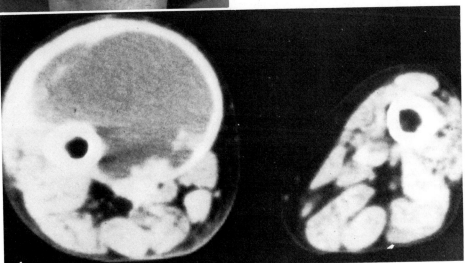

At times the tumor is extensively cystic and/or hemorrhagic, so that it
gives the false clinical and imaging impression of a hematoma (Fig. 742).

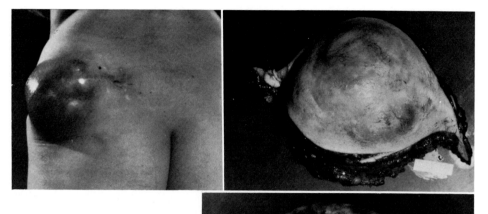

FIG. 743. - Grade 3 malignant fibrous histiocytoma. Female aged 36 years. The mass had occurred 7 years before. The tumor had been excised marginally and it recurred 4 times in 7 years. Wide excision was performed including the skin, subcutaneous tissue and gluteal muscles. On the cut surface, compact multilobular and encephaloid tissue, part of which whitish, part hemorrhagic or leather color, pseudocapsulated. No signs of disease after 2 years.

RADIOGRAPHIC FEATURES

Rarely, when the neoplasm is adjacent to the bone (Fig. 745), it may provoke images of superficial osteolysis or periosteal reaction. Bone scan is more sensitive in indicating skeletal reaction due to adjacency. Calcification and ossification are rarely observed, generally located peripherally, in the neoplastic mass. Angiography shows common changes occurring in malignant tumors, but even very large areas of the tumor may be avascular due to necrosis or hemorrhage. The major vessels may be displaced or compressed, but hardly ever infiltrated (Figs. 744, 745). CAT and MRI reveal a solid, non-homogeneous mass, at times ample cavities with fluid contents (Fig. 742).

GROSS PATHOLOGIC FEATURES

The mass is often plurilobated, grayish-white in color, at times yellowish or ocherous (lipids, hemosiderin) (Figs. 743, 745). There may be gelatinous areas, particularly in the myxoid variety. In angiomatoid forms a hemorrha-

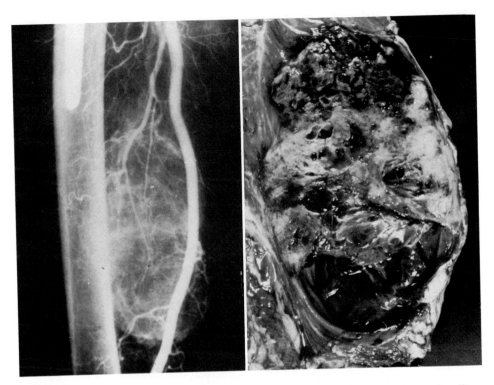

FIG. 744. - Grade 4 malignant fibrous histiocytoma. Female aged 77 years. Swelling observed 6 months previously. Angiographic aspect. Wide excision, the tumor was contained by the fascia of the vastus medialis and by the medial intermuscular septum, which divided it from the superficial femoral vessels. On the cut surface, the soft neoplastic tissue is modified by necrosis, hemorrhage, sero-hematic collections. No signs of disease after 2 years.

gic aspect prevails, with ample lacunae filled with blood. The yellowish color is particularly evident in the inflammatory variety. At times hemorrhage and necrosis (Fig. 744) are so extended that nearly the entire neoplastic mass is transformed into a sac with a liquid contents, similar to a cystic hematoma. Even when it seems to be circumscribed, the tumor infiltrates the surrounding tissues.

HISTOPATHOLOGIC FEATURES AND DIFFERENTIAL DIAGNOSIS

Pleomorphic storiform type

The histological picture is characterized by marked cellular pleomorphism (Fig. 746). In fact, spindle, ovoid and giant cells are observed. The latter may be benign or malignant. The pleomorphic aspect, the marked mitotic activity, the cellular atypia with hyperchromic nuclei, coarse chromatin and voluminous nucleoli are common in this lesion. At times, the giant cells and the mononucleate and spindle ones present an intensely eosinophilic cyto-

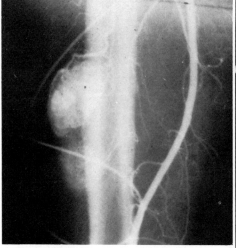

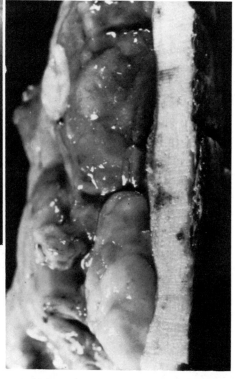

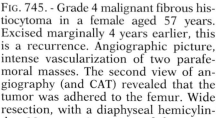

FIG. 745. - Grade 4 malignant fibrous histiocytoma in a female aged 57 years.
Excised marginally 4 years earlier, this
is a recurrence. Angiographic picture,
intense vascularization of two parafe-
moral masses. The second view of angiography (and CAT) revealed that the
tumor was adhered to the femur. Wide
resection, with a diaphyseal hemicylin-
der. Macroscopic picture of the transected specimen, with the multilobulated encephaloid tumor and the cortex of the femur, slightly excavated in its external surface.
New local recurrence after 1 year, hip disarticulation. No signs of disease after 2
years.

plasm, with a «myoid aura». But there is never transverse striation.

This pleomorphic component may form the predominant part of the lesion, but in truth it is always associated with the so-called storiform aspect
(Fig. 747). This consists in the fact that the spindle cells and collagen fibers
tend to be arranged in whorls or pinwheels, frequently irradiating from a
central eosinophilic area constituted by collagen or by a small vessel. Silver
stain reveals a particularly evident reticular pattern in the spindlecellular
areas, where it surrounds single cells, while in prevalently histiocytary areas
it surrounds small groups of cells. The argyrophilia appears to be particularly thick in the centers of storiform areas. Foam cells may be observed in
varying quantities as a result of their lipidic contents. At times acute and/or
chronic inflammatory infiltration appears.

PAS shows cytoplasmatic positiveness which is rather inconstant and
mostly diastase-resistant and hyaluronidase-sensitive (mucopolysaccharides, not glycogen). In the same tumor typical storiform and collagenized
aspects may be observed alongside others in which the pleomorphic aspect
dominates.

Differential diagnosis must include all of the neoplasms having marked

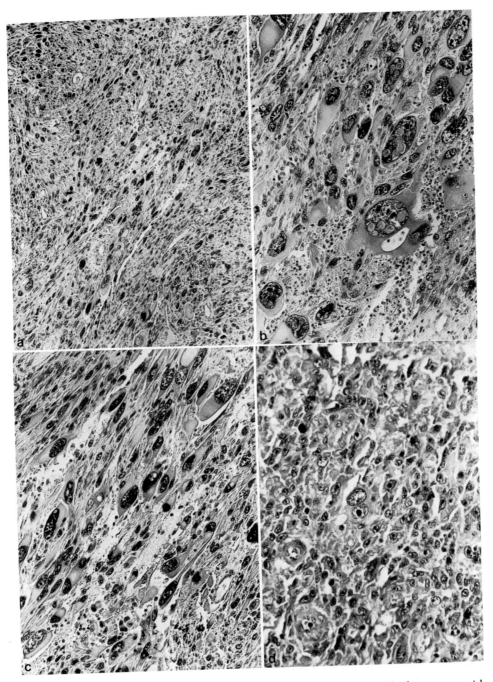

FIG. 746. - Pleomorphic storiform malignant fibrous histiocytoma. (a) There are ovoid, spindle and giant multinucleate cells arranged in bundles. (b) Under higher enlargement the cells reveal evident pleomorphism with atypical nucleo-cytoplasmatic features. (c) The nucleo-cytoplasmatic relationship is shifted in favor of the nucleus which presents evident hyperchromia, coarse chromatin. The cytoplasm is intensely eosinophilic (so-called «myoid aura»). (d) Areas with a prevalent round-ovoid cellular component (*Hemat.-eos.*, 250, 400, 400, 400 x).

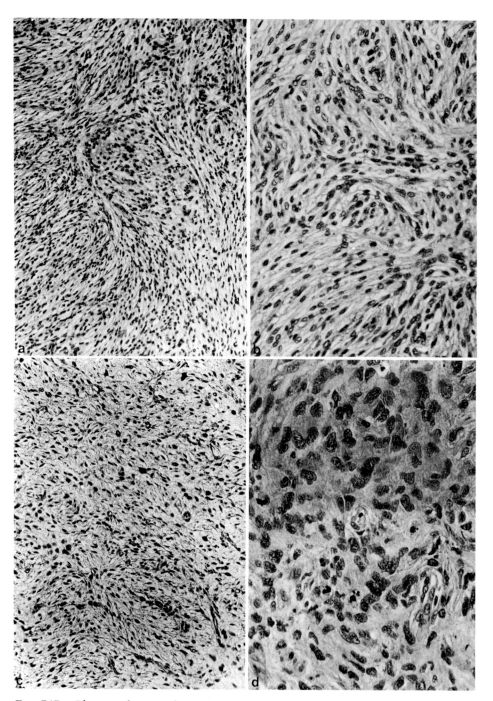

FIG. 747. - Pleomorphic storiform malignant fibrous histiocytoma. (a) Area in which the spindle cellular component predominates. The cells are aggregated in ondulated and intertwined bundles. (b) The spindle cells take on a storiform orientation. (c) At times a myxoid matrix is observed extensively separating the cells. There is evident pleomorphism. (d) The nucleo-cytoplasmatic features are atypical and the mitotic index is elevated (*Hemat.-eos.*, 160, 250, 160, 400 x).

pleomorphism, particularly **pleomorphic rhabdomyosarcoma**, which has become very rare. In the latter, transverse striation is hardly ever observed, and rhabdomyoblastic differentiation may be shown under electron microscopy; furthermore, the PAS positiveness sensitive to diastasis (glycogen) is constant and marked.

Differential diagnosis with **pleomorphic liposarcoma** is more difficult. In the latter there is no storiform aspect, while there is lipoblastic and lipocytic differentiation. Intracytoplasmatic vacuoles may be present in M.F.H., as well, but the vacuoles in the lipoblastic cell determine shifting of the nucleus to the periphery and flatten the nucleus. Furthermore, in vacuolated cells in M.F.H., there is mucopolysaccharide material. Staining for lipids does not discriminate, as it is positive in both neoplasms.

Aspects of M.F.H. may be present in undifferentiated and pleomorphic **carcinomas**. In these, special staining for glycogen and keratin, electron microscopy and a search for areas of epithelial differentiation orient diagnosis.

In **dermatofibrosarcoma protuberans** cutaneous localization and the clinical features, the diffused storiform aspect without pleomorphic cells, the low grade of histological malignancy, the absence of necrosis, all lead to diagnosis.

Atypical fibroxanthoma is histologically indistinguishable from M.F.H. from which it is differentiated by its exclusively cutaneous localization, small size and absence of necrosis.

Myxoid variant

According to Weiss and Enzinger (1977), one of the requirements of this variety is that the myxoid component constitutes more than half of the entire tumor (Fig. 748). Areas of myxoid aspect are arranged alongside areas with pleomorphic storiform features of M.F.H. At times, the two histological structures are clearly separated, while other times they are irregularly mixed together. The accumulation of intra- and extracellular mucopolysaccharides extensively modifies the aspect of the neoplasm. The fasciculated or storiform pattern decreases or totally disappears, the vessels become more visible, the cells contain vacuoles. In myxoid areas fasciculated storiform aspects cannot be recognized; the vessels may reveal plexiform aspects which make differential diagnosis with myxoid liposarcoma difficult; the vacuolated cells may recall lipoblasts, but they contain mucopolysaccharides.

Thus, differential diagnosis is made with **myxoid liposarcoma**, which is generally characterized by a lower grade of malignancy. In fact, the cellular pleomorphism is less marked and the plexiform vascularization more diffused and typical. In cases of myxoid liposarcoma with a higher grade of malignancy, or in those of pleomorphic liposarcoma, there are none of the storiform aspects typical of M.F.H.

Myxoid areas may be present in **fibrosarcoma** where however there is monormorphous proliferation of spindle cells arranged in a «herring-bone» pattern.

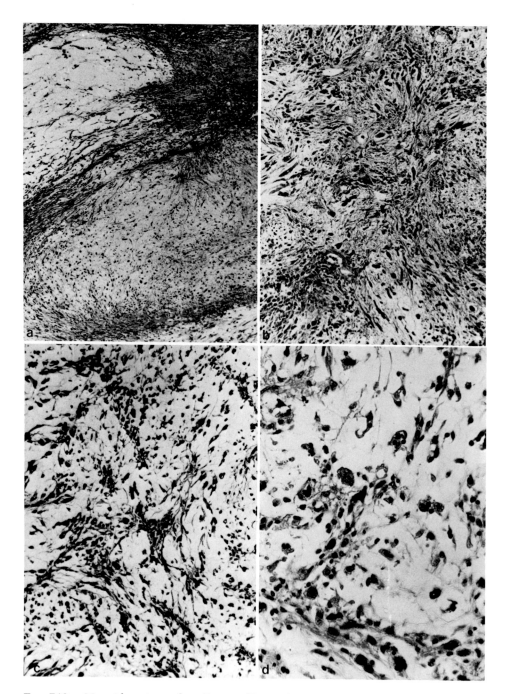

FIG. 748. - Myxoid variant of malignant fibrous histiocytoma. (a) The neoplasm presents markedly myxoid areas alongside more cellular areas. (b) In the more cellular areas the pleomorphic aspect dominates with arrangement of the cells in bundles and at times a storiform pattern. (c) and (d) There are cytological features proper to the pleomorphic malignant fibrous histiocytoma, but among the cells an abundant myxoid component may be observed. The nuclei are hyperchromic and have atypical features (*Hemat.-eos.*, 60, 160, 400, 400 x).

Among pseudosarcomatous lesions which may be characterized by myxoid aspects, **nodular fasciitis** must be recalled. In this case, the structure is similar to that of granulation tissue; the curvilinear aspect of the vessels (italic «S») and the absence of clearly atypical mitotic figures orient diagnosis.

Finally, **intramuscular myxoma** is distinguished from myxoid M.F.H. because it has no vascularization or cellular malignancy.

Giant cell variant

Described by Guccion and Enzinger in 1972, it is characterized by a marked giant cell component of the osteoclastic type (Fig. 749). The cellular proliferation is aggregated in multiple confluent nodules. The giant cells present both typical and atypical nuclear features. Marked inflammatory aspects dominate, which are more evident around the numerous areas of necrosis. At times, at the periphery of the neoplastic nodules there is osteochondroid metaplasia of the connective tissue.

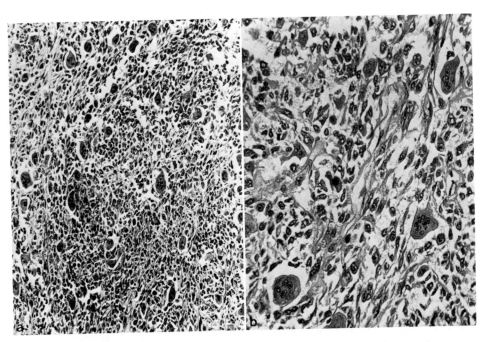

FIG. 749. - Malignant fibrous histiocytoma, giant cell variant. (a) The neoplasm presents marked pleomorphism: round, ovoid cells and numerous multinucleate giant cells. (b) Under higher power, the pleomorphic features may be observed. Some of the giant cells are reactive, not malignant (*Hemat.-eos.*, 160, 400 x).

Inflammatory variant

Described by Oberling in 1935 in the retroperitoneum under the name xanthogranuloma, it was defined by Kiriakos and Kempson (1972) as M.F.H.

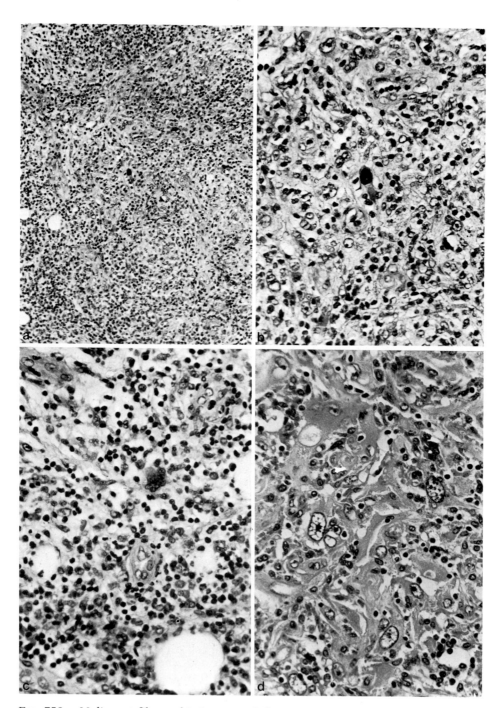

FIG. 750. - Malignant fibrous histiocyoma, inflammatory variant. (a) Rich inflammatory component made up of granulocytes and lymphocytes. The inflammatory infiltration is not related to areas of necrosis. (b), (c) and (d) Inflammatory cells appear to
be mixed with cells proper to malignant fibrous histiocytoma. Cells of varying shape
and size, with large eosinophilic cytoplasm and nucleus having a very evident nuclear membrane, often indented, with large nucleolus (*Hemat.-eos.*, 160, 400, 400,
400 x).

of the inflammatory type. The cellular elements are the same as those in the pleomorphic form, but in this case the xanthomatous and inflammatory components are preponderant (Fig. 750).

The histiocytary cells filled with lipids (xanthomatous cells) revealing various grades of pleomorphism and atypia, are varyingly mixed with inflammatory elements not associated with necrosis: these are prevalently lymphocytes, monocytes, and granulocytes. The vascular component is abundant, which may suggest granulation tissue. If the lesion is examined by means of numerous specimens, areas of pleomorphic storiform M.F.H. dictating diagnosis may be observed.

Differential diagnosis must include **storiform pleomorphic M.F.H.** and **fibrosarcomas** in which the inflammatory component is particularly evident. But in these two neoplasms the phlogistic component is in most instances associated with necrotic areas, and, above all, there is no extended xanthomatous component. Another differential diagnosis is made with **non-neoplastic inflammatory/granulomatous processes** and, thus, numerous specimens must be examined in order to determine the aspects of malignancy.

Angiomatoid variant

Of recent acquisition (Enzinger, 1979), it is encountered in children and young adults, and must be differentiated from malignant vascular lesions. Enzinger defines three typical aspects of this neoplasm: 1) solid areas of his-

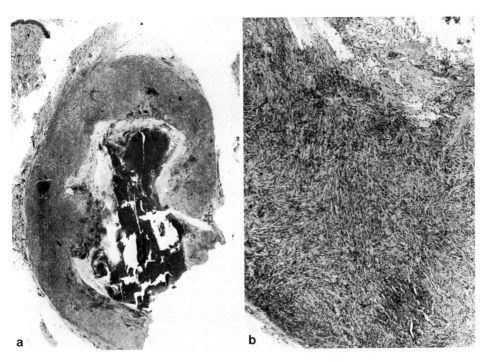

a   b

FIG. 751. (legend on the following page).

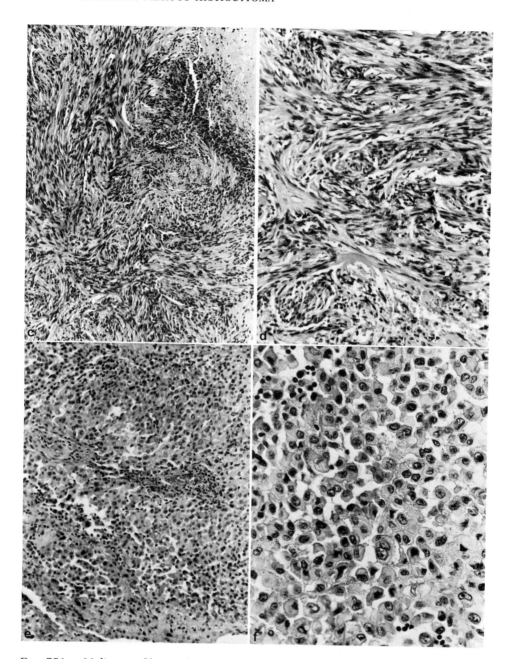

FIG. 751. - Malignant fibrous histiocytoma, angiomatoid variant. (a) and (b) It is a cystic mass with a diffusedly hemorrhagic central area. (c) and (d) The proliferation of spindle cells is arranged in small bundles with a storiform pattern. The cytological features do not show the usual pleomorphism of malignant fibrous histiocytoma, but the nuclear features are atypical (*Hemat.-eos.*, 10, 60, 160, 250 x). (e) and (f) Malignant fibrous histiocytoma, histiocytary variant. The proliferation has lost the pleomorphic features of the malignant fibrous histiocytoma. In fact, round-ovoid cells prevail with intensely eosinophilic, clearly marginated cytoplasm (f). The nucleus is large, hyperchromatic, central or eccentric, with an indented profile (*Hemat.-eos.*, 160, 400 x).

tiocytary cells in confluent fields, in cords or alveoli; 2) cystic-hemorrhagic areas recalling the structure of aneurysmal bone cyst; 3) diffused inflammatory infiltration (Fig. 751 a-d).

The inflammatory component generally constitutes a layer peripheral to the neoplasm. The vascular necrotic-hemorrhagic component makes up a large portion of the tumor and is often localized centrally. The vascular lacunae are not characterized by endothelial lining and the fundamental cells are the mononucleate and multinucleate histiocytes. Generally, there is a peripheral pseudocapsule.

Histiocytary variant

The neoplasm is mostly constituted by globose elements with a round nucleus having a well-designed membrane and sometimes indented. Generally, a voluminous nucleolus may be observed. The cytoplasm appears to be eosinophilic. The cells are characterized by phagic activity, and the storiform aspect appears rarely and sporadically. Mixed with these fundamental cells are giant, foam and spindle cells. There are numerous areas of necrosis associated with inflammatory lymphomonocytary infiltration (Fig. 751 e, f).

The histiocytary variant must be differentiated from **epithelioid sarcoma**, which in superficial localizations takes on the classic pseudo-granulomatous aspect centered by necrosis, while in deep localizations it presents cells in nodules and in strings. Furthermore, it must be differentiated from **metastasis due to undifferentiated carcinoma** and from large-cell **malignant lymphoma**.

HISTOGENESIS AND PATHOGENESIS

Although a controversial subject, it is believed that M.F.H. derives from undifferentiated mesenchymal cells which tend towards fibroblastic and histiocytary differentiation. M.F.H. of the soft tissues, like that in the skeleton, may be secondary to external radiations. In fact, it has been observed in areas irradiated for mammary carcinoma, malignant lymphoma, plasmacytoma and Hodgkin's disease.

COURSE AND PROGNOSIS

The different morphological aspects of the variants are particularly useful in diagnosis. In fact, there does not seem to be a clear relationship between variants and prognosis. The latter seems to be more correlated to clinical factors, such as site, size and localization of the tumor. For example, tumors localized in the subcutaneous tissue metastasize in 10% of cases, as compared to 40% of those of deeper localization. In the limbs, the distal localizations have a better prognosis than the proximal ones. The worst prognosis is that of retroperitoneal tumors.

TREATMENT

Surgery with wide or, better yet, radical margins is effective in locally controlling the neoplasm, but it is not capable of avoiding metastases. These occur early and are for the most part localized in the lungs (80%), lymph nodes (10%), liver and bone.

REFERENCES

1963 OZZELLO L., STOUT A.P., MURRAY M.R.: Cultural characteristics of malignant histiocytomas and fibrous xanthomas. *Cancer*, **16**, 331.

1972 GUCCION J.G., ENZINGER F.M.: Malignant giant cell tumor of soft parts. An analysis of 32 cases. *Cancer*, **29**, 1518.

1972 KEMPSON R.L., KYRIAKOS M.: Fibroxanthosarcoma of the soft tissue: A type of malignant fibrous histiocytoma. *Cancer*, **29**, 961.

1972 SOULE E.H., ENRIQUEZ P.: Atypical fibrous histiocytoma, malignant fibrous histiocytoma, malignant histiocytoma and epithelioid sarcoma. *Cancer*, **30**, 128.

1975 FU Y-S, GABBIANI G., KAYE G.I. *et al.*: Malignant soft tissue tumors of probable histiocytic origin (malignant fibrous histiocytoma) general considerations and electron microscopic and tissue culture studies. *Cancer*, **35**, 176.

1976 KYRIAKOS M., KEMPSON R.L.: Inflammatory fibrous histiocytoma: An aggressive and lethal lesion. *Cancer*, **37**, 1584.

1976 INADA O., YUMOTO T., FURUSE K. *et al.*: Ultrastructural features of malignant fibrous histiocytoma. *Acta Pathol. Jpn.*, **26**, 491.

1977 ALGUACIL-GARCIA A., UNNI K.K., GOELLNER J.R.: Malignant giant cell tumor of soft parts: Ultrastructural study of four cases. *Cancer*, **40**, 244.

1977 HUBBARD L.F., BURTON R.I.: Malignant fibrous histiocytoma of the forearm: Report of a case and review of the literature. *J. Hand Surg.*, **2**, 292.

1977 LEITE C., GOODWIN J.W., SINKOVICS J.C. *et al.*: Chemotherapy of malignant fibrous histiocytoma: A Southwest Oncology Group report. *Cancer*, **40**, 2010.

1977 TAXY J.B., BATTIFORA H.: Malignant fibrous histiocytoma: A clinico-pathologic and ultrastructural study. *Cancer*, **40**, 254.

1977 WEISS S.W., ENZINGER F.M.: Myxoid variant of malignant fibrous histiocytoma. *Cancer*, **39**, 1672.

1978 ALGUACIL-GARCIA A., UNNI K.K., GOELLNER J.R.: Malignant fibrous histiocytoma: An ultrastructural study of six cases. *Am. J. Clin. Pathol.*, **69**, 121.

1978 WEISS S.W., ENZINGER F.M.: Malignant fibrous histiocytoma: An analysis of 200 cases. *Cancer*, **41**, 2250.

1979 ENZINGER F.M.: Angiomatoid malignant fibrous histiocytoma: A distinct fibrohistiocytic tumor of children and young adults simulating a vascular neoplasm. *Cancer*, **44**, 2147.

1979 LAGACÉ R., DELAGE C., SEEMAYER T.A.: Myxoid variant of malignant fibrous histiocytoma: Ultrastructural observations. *Cancer*, **43**, 526.

1980 ENJOJI M., HASHIMOTO H., IWASAKI H.: Malignant fibrous histiocytoma: A clinicopathologic study of 130 cases. *Acta Pathol. Jpn.*, **30**, 727.

1980 KEARNEY M.M., SOULE E.H., IVINS J.C.: Malignant fibrous histiocytoma: A retrospective study of 167 cases. *Cancer*, **45**, 167.

1980 MEISTER P., NATHRATH W.: Immunohistochemical markers of histiocytic tumors. *Hum. Pathol.*, **11**, 300.

1982 DU BOULAY C.E.H.: Demonstration of alpha-1-antitrypson and alpha-1-antichymotrypsin in fibrous histiocytomas using immunoperoxidase technique. *Am. J. Surg. Pathol.*, **6**, 559.

1983 MAGNUSSON B., KINDBLOM L.G., ANGERVALL L.: Enzyme histochemistry of malignant fibroblastic histiocytic tumors. A light and electron microscopic analysis. *Appl. Pathol.*, **1(4)**, 223-40.

1984 FLETCHER C.D., MC KEE P.H.: Sarcomas: a clinicopathological guide with particular references to cutaneous manifestation. I. Dermatofibrosarcoma protuberans, malignant fibrous histiocytoma and the epithelioid sarcoma of Enzinger. *Clin. Exp. Dermatol.*, **9(5)**, 451.

1984 TRACY T. JR., NEIFELD J.P., DE MAY R.M., SALZBERG A.M.: Malignant fibrous histiocytomas in children. *J. Pediatr. Surg.*, **19(1)**, 81-3.

1984 WEISS L.M., WARHOL M.J.: Ultrastructural distinctions between adult pleomorphic rhabdomyosarcomas, pleomorphic liposarcomas, and pleomorphic malignant fibrous histiocytomas. *Hum. Pathol.*, **15(11)**, 1025-33.

1985 FISCHER H.J., LOIS J.F., GOMES A.S., MIRRA J.M., DEUTSCH L.S.: Radiology and pathology of malignant fibrous histiocytomas of the soft tissue: a report of ten cases. *Skeletal Radiol.*, **13(3)** 202-6.

1986 BRECHER M.E., FRANKLIN W.A.: Absence of mononuclear phagocyte antigens in malignant fibrous histiocytoma. *Am. J. Clin. Pathol.*, **86**, 344.

1987 LAWSON C.W., FISHER C., GATTER K.C.: An immunohistochemical study of differentiation in malignant fibrous histiocytoma. *Histopathology*, **11**, 375.

1989 EL-NAGGER A.K., RO J.Y., AYALA A.G.: Angiomatoid malignant fibrous histiocytoma: flow cytometric DNA analysis of six cases. *J. Surg. Oncol.*, **40**, 201.

1989 MIETTINEN M., SOINI Y.: Malignant fibrous histiocytoma: heterologous patterns of intermediate filament proteins by immunohistochemistry. *Arch. Pathol. Lab. Med.*, **113**, 1363.

LIPOMA

It is a benign tumor constituted by cells which are uniquely differentiated into lipocytes.

FREQUENCY

It is difficult to evaluate the incidence of this neoformation, which is often left unoperated and, when surgery is performed, may not be judged worthy of biopsy. However, it is a very common occurrence, and it is certainly the most frequent among the soft tissue tumors.

SEX

Superficial lipomas prevail in the female sex, deep and multiple ones in the male sex.

AGE

It hardly ever involves young age, it is more frequently observed between 40 and 60 years of age.

LOCALIZATION

L. are divided into **superficial and deep**. Superficial L. are contained in the subcutaneous tissue and show predilection for the dorsum, neck and proximal segment of the limbs (centripetal distribution). Deep L. (much less common) are observed within the muscles (intramuscular L.) or in the intermuscular space, or in the space between other structures (bones, tendons) or attached to a tendon, or adherent to the bone (so-called periosteal L.) or in proximity to the joints, or within a nervous trunk (intranervous L.).

Rarely (in 5% of cases) L. are multiple (Fig. 752). These are preferably localized in the dorsum and proximal segment of the upper limb: at times, distribution is symmetrical and the extensor aspect of the limbs is preferred.

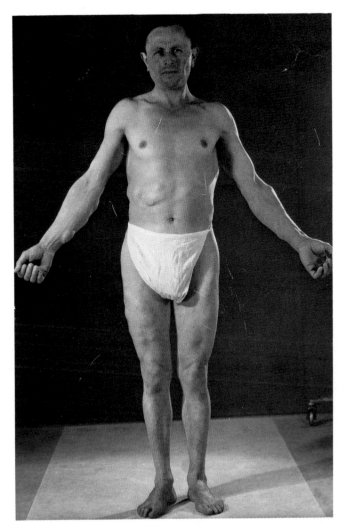

Fig. 752. - Multiple subcutaneous lipomas. Male aged 47 years.

SYMPTOMS

Growth is slow or very slow. L. seems to be more common in obese subjects and tends to increase during rapid increase in body weight, while it does not decrease during weight loss or even cachexia. This indicates that the fat in L. tends more to accumulate than to be mobilized and it is largely unused in the general metabolism.

Often, after a first growth phase, L. remains stationary. Often, the patient reports having observed the mass to remain unvaried for many years. Generally, it is painless (unless there is compression on nervous branches). Some deep L. may cause compression on a nerve (for example, the deep branch of the radial nerve in the forearm) and be manifested by progressive paralysis.

While superficial L. never grow large size (from 1 to 15 cm, average around 4 cm), deep L. tend to be of larger size (from 1 to 25 cm, average 8 cm).

Superficial L. is well-circumscribed and doughy, not painful, not adherent to the skin or the deep planes. Deep L. has the same features, but it is more difficult to palpate. Intramuscular L. is observed more easily with muscle contraction, which transforms it into a more spherical, fixed and firm mass.

Radiograms, CAT are typical in deep L., because they reveal a globose mass, having well defined and regular limits, with homogeneous density throughout, which is clearly hypertransparent in relation to the surrounding muscles (Fig. 753) and has the typical signal of fat in MRI. With angiography the mass is not injected.

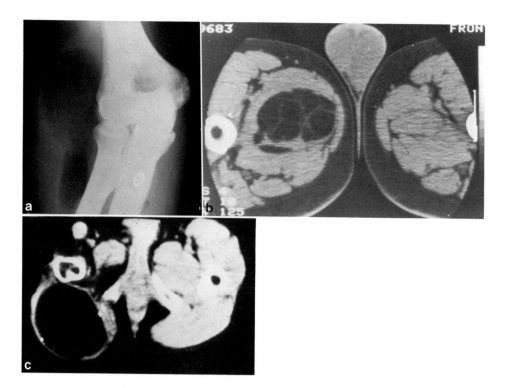

Fig. 753. - Intramuscular lipoma at the elbow. (a) Female aged 36 years. The tumor is lobulated, with a regular and clear perimeter, radiographic transparence typical of fat. The lipoma invades the supinator muscle causing compression of the deep branch of the radial nerve and resulting motorial palsy. (b) Male aged 38 years. Intramuscular lipoma of the long adductor muscle of the thigh. Observe on the CAT the cloistered aspect and the homogeneous hypertransparence. (c) Male aged 53 years. Lipoma observed 5 years earlier, intramuscular of the gluteus maximus (CAT).

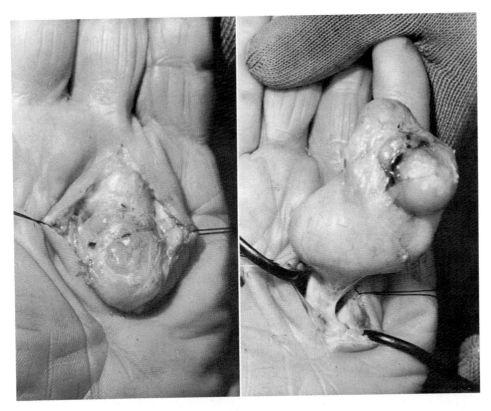

F<small>IG.</small> 754. - Female aged 71 years. Deep lipoma in the palm of the hand, excised 4 years earlier and recurring.

GROSS PATHOLOGIC FEATURES

Superficial L. is globose or lenticular. Deep L. assumes a shape which is conditioned by its growth within the surrounding structures; thus, it is often lobulated, or it has multiple masses united together by isthmi or pedicles (Fig. 754). Intramuscular L. is also globose and lobulated (Fig. 755), with the major axis parallel to the muscle, of which it may surpass the fascial boundary extending to several muscles and to the intermuscular spaces.

Each L. is often delimited by a very thin true capsule; this distinguishes L. from normal adipose tissue. External to the capsule, there may be a pseudocapsule, fibrous and thick and rather adherent to the surrounding tissues (as it is reactive to chronic compression and rubbing caused by L.). Consistency is soft on palpation. On the cut surface, it is pale yellow in color, with the typical aspect of well-differentiated fat (Fig. 755). In intramuscular L. there may be no capsule, the fat appearing to be interposed with the muscular fibers. Rarely in superficial forms, more often in deep ones, there are areas of hemorrhage or necrosis.

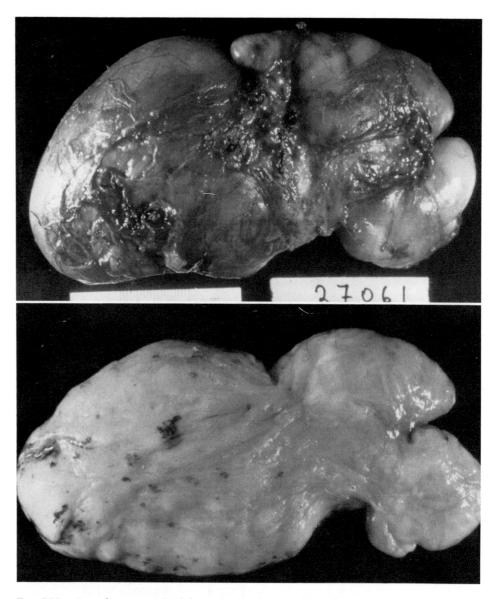

FIG. 755. - Deep lipoma excised from the thigh. Female aged 47 years. Observe the lobulated globose form, the thin capsule run through by a delicate vascular network. On the cut surface, the homogeneous aspect of mature fat, with some hemorrhagic spray.

HISTOPATHOLOGIC FEATURES

L. is constituted by mature adipose cells, lipocytes, of varying shape and size, at times greater than the normal lipocyte (up to 150 microns in diameter) (Fig. 756). In intramuscular L. the lipocytes diffusedly infiltrate the muscle («lipoma infiltrans»). The residual muscular cells are atrophized to then

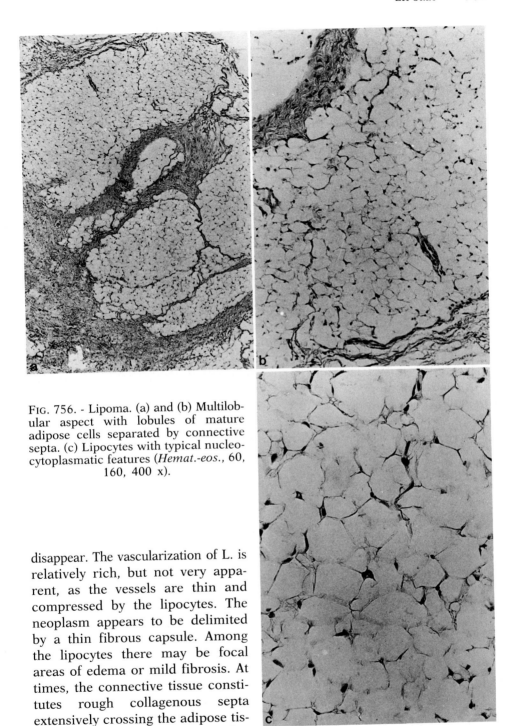

FIG. 756. - Lipoma. (a) and (b) Multilobular aspect with lobules of mature adipose cells separated by connective septa. (c) Lipocytes with typical nucleo-cytoplasmatic features (*Hemat.-eos.*, 60, 160, 400 x).

disappear. The vascularization of L. is relatively rich, but not very apparent, as the vessels are thin and compressed by the lipocytes. The neoplasm appears to be delimited by a thin fibrous capsule. Among the lipocytes there may be focal areas of edema or mild fibrosis. At times, the connective tissue constitutes rough collagenous septa extensively crossing the adipose tissue. Areas rich in mucopolysaccharides (myxoid) may be observed. These are intensely stained with halcian blue, a stain which is abolished after pre-treatment with hyaluronidase. Clusters of foam macrophages are frequently observed, the index of necrosis of the lipocytes, at times with multi-nucleate giant cells and sparse lymphocytes and plasmacells. Sometimes small bunches of embryonal or brown fat cells are seen.

PATHOGENESIS

Familiarity has been observed, particularly in multiple L.

L. are more frequent in obese subjects, in individuals aged over 45 years, in diabetics, in hypercholesterolemics.

DIAGNOSIS

Superficial L. is easily diagnosed by clinical examination, it does not cause any concern and it is generally left unoperated, unless it is large. Deep L., particularly if large and characterized by rapid growth, may cause one to suspect sarcoma. Even the slowness of its growth, the radiolucent homogeneous aspect, its delimitation by a thin capsule, the macroscopic adipose aspect, and the histological lipomatous picture of a limited specimen are not sufficient to exclude liposarcoma. In fact, there are liposarcomas which in some areas are well-differentiated and similar or identical to L. **In deep «lipomas» this requires an extensive anatomo-pathological study, with multiple specimens, in order to exclude malignancy**. Although reported, the cases of malignant transformation of L. most probably represent liposarcomas *ab initio*, unrecognized. The histological distinction between L. and well-differentiated liposarcoma is based on the absence in L. of lipoblasts and pleomorphic and hyperchromic nuclei. The histological distinction between L. with myxoid areas and myxoid liposarcoma is based on the absence in L. of rich plexiform vascularity and lipoblasts.

TREATMENT

Marginal excision is curative, recurrence is rare. The latter is more frequent in deep L. in which removal may have been incomplete.

SUBCUTANEOUS ANGIOLIPOMA

It is constituted by mature adipose tissue mixed with the proliferation of numerous vascular canals. Unlike lipoma, it occurs from 15 to 20 years of age, and is more frequent in males. The most frequent localization is the forearm, the trunk and arm are involved less frequently. S.A.L. is subcutaneous, small (it hardly ever exceeds 2 cm) and more often multiple than solitary. Unlike lipoma, it is painful, especially during the initial phases.

Macroscopically, a well-capsulated nodule is observed having a consistency which is more firm than that of lipoma and, on the cut surface, yellowish in color with reddish tones.

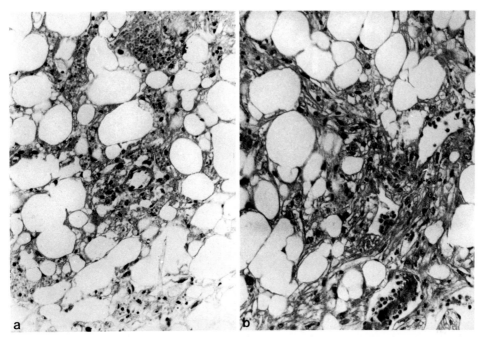

FIG. 757. - Angiolipoma. (a) and (b) The tumor consists in mature adipose cells and vessels of small caliber, around which there is proliferation of fibroblasts (*Hemat.-eos.*, 250, 250 x).

Histologically, it is constituted by mature lipocytes varyingly interspersed with a network of capillaries. This vascular network is more abundant in the subcapsular peripheral area where the mixture of mature lipocytes and narrow vascular channels is evident. In time, perivascular or diffused fibrosis may occur. The capillaries have empty and compressed lumi, or ones which are dilated and clogged by erythrocytes or fibrin. Microthrombi are frequently present. Lymphocytes, fibroblasts, mastocytes and undifferentiated mesenchymal cells are observed among the vessels (Fig. 757).

At times the vascular component overcomes the lipomatous one, enough to require differential diagnosis with spindle cell angiosarcoma and Kaposi's sarcoma.

Incidence of recurrence after marginal excision has not been reported.

SUBCUTANEOUS SPINDLE CELL LIPOMA

It is formed by mature adipose tissue mixed with fibroblasts. There is predilection for the male sex and advanced adult age, from 45 to 80 years. The sites of election are the dorsal region, the nucha and the shoulder. It remains circumscribed to the subcutaneous tissue, without surpassing the fascia. It is manifested as a painless, solitary mass of average size (1-13 cm, average 4 cm) which grows slowly.

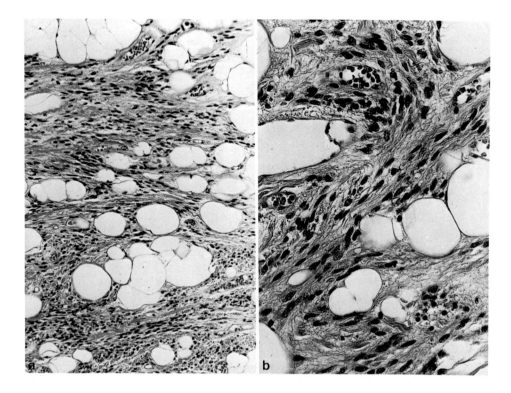

FIG. 758. - Spindle cell lipoma. (a) Spindle cells of uniform aspect and mature adipocytes are seen. Among the spindle cells there are collagen bundles. (b) Spindle cells of relatively monomorphous aspect with no atypical features are aggregated in bundles and closely adjacent to lipocytes (*Hemat.-eos.*, 160, 400 x).

Macroscopically, it is a nodule, of whitish-yellow color, well-capsulated, of firm or soft consistency, with a rich myxoid component. On the cut surface, a whitish color dominates (fibro-collagen component) with translucid aspects (myxoid component).

Histologically, there are various components: mature lipomatous tissue, spindle cells which may constitute a large part of the neoplasm, rough collagenous bands, myxoid alcian-positive matrix (positiveness which is abolished by pre-treatment with hyaluronidase), vessels with thick and hyalin wall. Mitotic figures are rare and there is no cellular pleomorphism (Fig. 758).

The lesion is benign and marginal excision is the treatment of choice.

SUBCUTANEOUS PLEOMORPHIC LIPOMA

It is a rare occurrence, with predilection for the male sex, the ages from 45 to 70 years, and the regions of the dorsum, shoulder, thigh and arm. Some

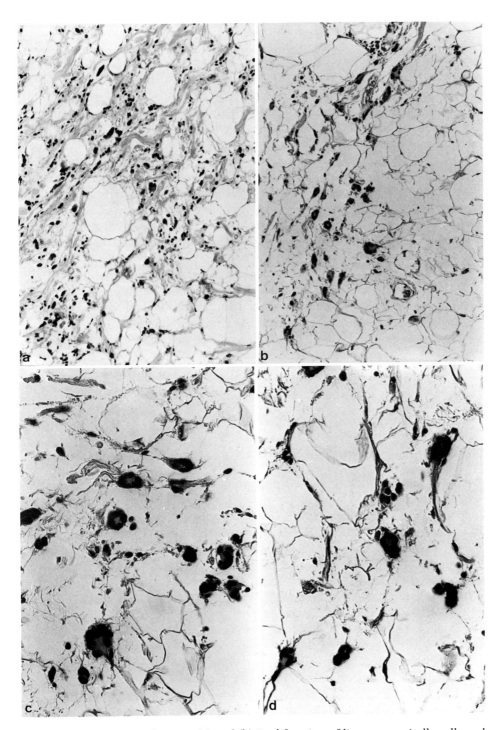

FIG. 759. - Pleomorphic lipoma. (a) and (b) Proliferation of lipocytes, spindle cells and giant cells with collagenous fibers. (c) and (d) Multinucleate giant cells, with «floret-like» aspect of the nuclei. These are hyperchromic and arranged crown-like around the eosinophilic cytoplasm (*Hemat.-eos.*, 160, 160, 400, 400 x).

authors consider P.L. to be a variation of spindle cell lipoma because the spindle cell aspect and the pleomorphic one may coexist.

Macroscopically it is a fibro-adipose mass, yellowish-white in color, well-circumscribed or capsulated. At times, on the cut surface, there is a myxoid aspect. Size varies from 1 to 15 cm.

Histologically, in addition to mature adipose tissue, spindle cells and collagen fibers, there are atypical pleomorphic and hyperchromic mononucleate cells (bizarre fibrocyte type) and bizarre multinucleate giant cells which may have nuclei arranged like the petals of a daisy (floret aspect) (Fig. 759). These are multiple hyperchromic nuclei which are concentrically arranged around an intensely eosinophilic cytoplasmatic area or one with small vacuoles. At times, lymphocytes and rare cells of brown fat are associated. Bizarre hyperchromic mononucleate cells, «floret-like» multinucleate giant cells and mature adipose tissue constitute constant morphological elements.

In some cases **differential diagnosis** with **well-differentiated liposarcoma** in its pseudo-lipomatous or sclerosing variants may be difficult. Useful elements in diagnosis are superficial localization, the circumscribed aspect of the lesion, the presence of «floret-cells» and spindle cells.

Rarely, there may be local recurrence, never metastases. When a doubt in diagnosis arises with regard to P.L. and well-differentiated liposarcoma, wide excision is recommended. In other cases, marginal excision is curative.

BENIGN LIPOBLASTOMA AND LIPOBLASTOMATOSIS

These are single or multiple lipomatous tumors typical of childhood. The first is capsulated and superficial, while the second is scarcely delimited and may extend to the deeper planes. These tumors are constituted by immature lipoblasts and in several sites closely resemble myxoid liposarcoma, thus, the adjective benign was added in order to emphasize the biological difference between the two lesions.

Benign lipoblastoma is very rare, observed at birth or during the first years of life (two-thirds of all cases occur under 2 years of age). There is predilection for the male sex. The preferred localizations are the limbs. Most of the lesions measure from 3 to 5 cm in diameter, even if in some rare cases a larger size may be achieved.

The circumscribed form (benign lipoblastoma) is a painless nodule localized in the subcutaneous tissue and which grows slowly. Lipoblastomatosis involves the subcutaneous tissue as well as the underlying muscle.

Macroscopically, the lesion is of lobulated aspect and on the cut surface it presents fields with a translucid aspect, whitish-yellow in color, solid or cystic.

Histologically, the aspect is the same in the two forms and appears to be unable to be distinguished from myxoid liposarcoma. Lobules of immature adipose tissue delimited by fibrous septa are observed, with ovoid, stellate or spindle cells, with single and multiple paranuclear vacuoles. Mature lipocytes are associated with these elements. Mitotic figures are not observed. A varying quantity of mucinous material which is stained by halcian blue is observed among the cells, but not after treatment with hyaluronidase. The proportion between immature lipoblasts, lipocytes and fibroblasts is the most variable, hence the differing aspect from field to field. Vascularization may be very evident, particularly in fields characterized by an immature cellular component. The vessels assume a plexiform aspect, a feature which contributes to making **differential diagnosis with myxoid liposarcoma** impossible on a solely histological basis, without knowing the age of the patient, which is the most important differential element.

The lesion is of benign nature. After marginal excision, localized forms rarely recur, more often diffused ones do, in which wide excision is thus indicated.

INTRANERVOUS AND PERINERVOUS FIBROLIPOMA (LIPOFIBROMATOUS HAMARTOMA OF THE NERVES)

This lesion is characterized by a mass of fibroadipose tissue which surrounds and infiltrates a major nerve and its branches.

It generally shows predilection for the male sex, it may be present at birth, its frequency is highest during childhood to young age (from birth to 30 years). Preferred sites are the volar region of the hand, the forearm and the wrist.

It is a slow-growing tumor, which causes pain and paresthesia. An increase in the volume of the neoplasm is generally associated with neuropathy due to compression.

Macroscopically, there is a whitish-yellow sausage-shaped mass which diffusedly infiltrates and substitutes a portion of a major nerve (the median nerve is preferred).

Histologically, it is a tissue which surrounds and infiltrates the nerve trunk, involving the epineurium and the perineurium.

This lesion must be differentiated from neurinomas and neurofibromas: in lipoma there is atrophy and compression of the nerve rather than proliferation of the nervous elements.

Because of the way in which the neoplasm grows and its localization is characterized by the destructive and infiltrative attitude toward the nerve, complete surgical excision may be contraindicated for the motor and sensory loss that it may cause. Sometimes partial excision or incision of the transverse carpal ligament and decompression of the median nerve are indicated. Microsurgical technique is advisable and nervous autografts may be used for reconstruction.

DIFFUSED LIPOMATOSIS

It is a scarcely circumscribed neoformation of mature adipose tissue which grows by infiltrating the superficial and deep soft tissues.

Early childhood is preferred. Extensive regions of the limbs and trunk are involved. The neoformation involves the subcutaneous tissue and the muscles. It is often associated with skeletal hypertrophy. Differential diagnosis must be made with intramuscular lipoma in cases where the lesion is limited to the muscular tissue or to intermuscular spaces, and with well-differentiated liposarcoma.

The lesion tends to recur and given the extreme extent that it may assume, although benign, it may require ablative surgery.

HYBERNOMA

It reproduces embryonal or brown fat, which is normally present in the adult in the interscapular areas, in the neck, the axilla, and in the retroperitoneum.

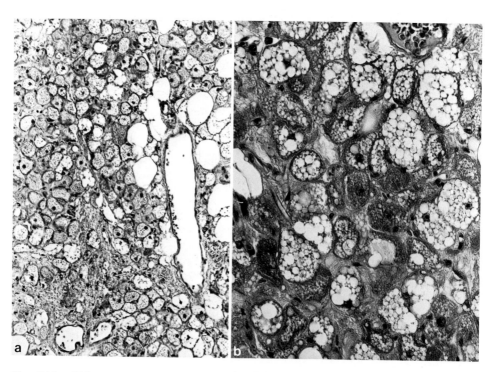

FIG. 760. - Hybernoma. (a) There are cells with a central nucleus and foam cytoplasm (similar to embryonal or brown fat) mixed with univacuolated cells (typical of the mature or white fat). (b) Finely vacuolated cells, at times with evident eosinophilia of the cytoplasm. The nucleus may be central or peripheral, but it is not flattened at the surface of the cell, like in mature lipocytes (*Hemat.-eos.*, 160, 400 x).

It occurs during adult age, but younger as compared to lipomas. It is an extremely rare occurrence. There is predilection for the interscapular area, the thigh, the thoracic wall, the axilla and the groin.

It is a slow-growing nodule, painless, which may grow to 5-15 cm in size. The duration of the patient's clinical history varies from a few weeks to several years. It involves the subcutaneous tissue but in some cases it penetrates the underlying planes.

Macroscopically, it is brownish-yellow in color and well-capsulated.

The histological aspect is dominated by a lobulated structure with round or oval cells, a central nucleus and intensely eosinophilic cytoplasm, which is uniformly granular, at times somewhat vacuolated, but without the vacuoles causing displacement and deformation of the nucleus (Fig. 760). Among these cells there are univacuolated or multivacuolated adipose elements. Based on the abundance of the latter, forms of transition with lipoma may be observed. Mitotic figures are practically absent, pleomorphism moderate, and vascularization is abundant.

Differential diagnosis is rather easy. It is differentiated from **rhabdomyoma** of the adult type, which reaches larger size, and the cells of which have cytoplasm with crystal-type inclusions, striations and are rich in glycogen. Another tumor which is included in differential diagnosis is **granular cell tumor**, where there is no cytoplasmatic lipidic vacuolization, and where structures suggesting a nervous origin are generally observed. **Sebaceous adenoma** may have features similar to those of H., but it is preferably localized in the derma. Finally, the granular cells of H. must not be mistaken for macrophages — foam-cells — in reactive lesions of the fat tissue.

H. is benign, but recurrence has been reported. Marginal surgery is curative.

REFERENCES

1956 SULLIVAN C.R., DAHLIN D.C., BRYAN R.S.: Lipoma of the tendon sheath. *J. Bone Joint Surg.*, **38A**, 1275.

1962 WHITE W.L., HANNA D.C.: Troublesome lipomata of the upper extremity. *J. Bone Joint Surg.*, **44A**, 1353.

1964 ANGERVALL L., NILSSON B.: Microangiographic and histologic studies in two cases of hibernoma. *Cancer*, **17**, 685.

1964 MORLEY G.H.: Intraneural lipoma of the median nerve in the carpal tunnel. Report of a case. *J. Bone Joint Surg.*, **46B**, 734.

1965 ANGERVALL L., BJÖRNTROP P., STENER B.: The lipid composition of hibernomas as compared with that of lipoma and mouse brown fat. *Cancer Res.*, **25**, 408.

1965 BOOHER R.: Lipoblastic tumors of the hands and feet; Review of the literature and report of 33 cases. *J. Bone Joint Surg.*, **47A**, 727.

1966 BARBER K.W. JR., BIANCO A.J. JR., SOULE E.H. *et al.*: Benign extraneural soft tissue tumors of the extremities causing compression of nerves. *J. Bone Joint Surg.*, **48B**, 781.

1969 BRASFIELD R.D., DAS GUPTA T.K.: Soft tissue tumors: Benign tumors of adipose tissue. *Cancer*, **19**, 3.

1969 JOHNSON R.J., BONFIGLIO M.: Lipofibromatous hamartoma of the median nerve. *J. Bone Joint Surg.*, **51A**, 984.

1970 BECKER J.A., WEISS R.M., SCHIFF M. *et al.*: Pelvic lipomatosis. A consideration in the diagnosis of intrapelvic neoplasms. *Arch. Surg.*, **100**, 94.

1971 NIXON H.H., SCOBIE W.G.: Congenital lipomatosis: A report of four cases. *J. Pediatr. Surg.*, **6**, 742.

1971 PHALEN G.S., KENDRIK J.I., RODRIGUEZ J.M.: Lipomas of the upper extremity, a series of 15 tumors in the hand and wrist and 6 tumors causing nerve compression. *Am. J. Surg.*, **121**, 298.

1972 LEVINE G.D.: Hibernoma. An electron microscopic study. *Human Pathol.*, **3**, 351.

1972 LEFFERT R.D.: Lipomas of the upper extremity. *J. Bone Joint Surg.*, **54/A**, 1262.

1972 PAARLBERG D., LINSCHEID R.L., SOULE E.H.: Lipomas of the hand. Including a case of lipoblastomatosis in a child. *Mayo Clin. Proc.*, **47**, 121.

1973 CHUNG E.B., ENZINGER F.M.: Benign lipoblastomatosis. An analysis of 35 cases. *Cancer*, **32**, 482.

1973 LOUIS D.S., DICK N.H.: Ossifying lipofibroma of the median nerve. *J. Bone Joint Surg.*, **55A**, 1082.

1974 DIONNE G.P., SEEMAYER T.A.: Infiltrating lipomas and angiolipomas revisited. *Cancer*, **33**, 732.

1974 KINDBLOM L.G., ANGERVALL L., STENER B. et al.. Intermuscular lipomas and intramuscular lipomas and hibernomas. A clinical, roentgenologic, histologic and prognostic study of 46 cases. *Cancer*, **33**, 754.

1974 LINN J.J., LIN F.: Two entities in angiolipoma. A study of 459 cases of lipoma with review of literature on infiltrating angiolipoma. *Cancer*, **34**, 720.

1974 RASANEN O, NOHTERI H., DAMMERT K.: Angiolipoma and Lipoma. *Acta Chir. Scand.*, **133**, 461.

1975 ENZINGER F.M., HARVEY D.J.: Spindle cell lipoma. *Cancer*, **36**, 1852.

1975 SEEMAYER T.A., KNAACK J., WANG N. et al.: On the ultrastructure of hibernoma. *Cancer*, **36**, 1785.

1976 ANGERVALL L., DAHL T., KINDBLOM L.G. et al.: Spindle cell lipoma. *Acta Pathol. Microbiol.*, **84**, 477.

1980 ALBA-GRECO R.L., VULETIN J.C.: Benign lipoblastomatosis. Ultrastructure and histogenesis. *Cancer*, **45**, 511.

1980 BOLEN J.W., THORNING D.: Benign lipoblastoma and myxoid liposarcoma. A comparative light and electron-microscopic study. *Am. J. Surg. Pathol.*, **4**, 163-174.

1980 GRECO M.A., GARCIA R.L., VULETIN J.C.: Benign lipoblastomatosis: ultrastructure and histogenesis. *Cancer*, **45**, 511.

1981 MYHRE-JENSEN O.: A consecutive 7-year series of 1331 benign soft tissue tumors. Clinicopathologic data. Comparison with sarcomas. *Acta Orthop. Scand.*, **52**, 287.

1981 SHMOOKLER B.M., ENZINGER F.M.: Pleomorphic lipoma: A clinico-pathologic analysis of 48 cases. *Cancer*, **47**, 126.

1982 WARKEL R.L.,REHME C., THOMPSON W.H.: Vascular spindle cell lipoma. *J. Cutan. Pathol.*, **9**, 113.

1982 PENOFF J.H.: Traumatic lipomas/pseudolipomas. *J. Trauma*, **22**, 63.

1983 RYDHOLM A., BERG N.O.: Size, site and clinical incidence of lipomas. Factors in differential diagnosis of lipoma and sarcoma. *Acta Orthop. Scand.*, **54**, 929.

1984 DEMOS D.C., BRUNO E., DOBOZI W.R.: Parosteal lipoma with enlarging osteochondroma. *A.J.R.*, **143**, 365.

1984 HOEHN J.G., FARBER H.F.: Massive lipoma of palm. *Ann. Plast. Surg.*, **11**, 431.

1984 MC DANIEL R.K., NEWLAND J.R., CHILES D.G.: Intraoral spindle cell lipoma: Case reported with correlated light and electron microscopy. *Oral Surg.*, **57**, 52.

1985 MUENCHOW T., SENITZ D., GOERTCHEN R.: Pleomorphic lipoma. *Zentralbl. All. Path.*, **130**, 13.

1986 JIMENEZ J.F.: Lipoblastoma in infancy and childhood. *J. Surg .Oncol.*, **32**, 238.

1989 BEHAM A., SCHMID C., HÖDL S., FLETCHER C.D.M.: Spindle-cell and pleomorphic lipoma: an immunohistochemical study and histogenic analysis. *J. Pathol.*, **158**, 219.

LIPOSARCOMA

DEFINITION

It is a malignant tumor of the soft tissues, the cells of which tend to differentiate in lipoblasts and lipocytes.

FREQUENCY

It is still considered to be the most frequent sarcoma of the soft tissues and of the adult, even if its incidence is reduced nowadays by the fact that many pleomorphic L.S. reported in older literature are classified as malignant fibrous histiocytomas.

SEX

There is mild predilection for the male sex in localizations in the limbs, not in retroperitoneal ones.

AGE

It is exceptional during infancy and very rare prior to 20 years of age. It is typical of adult and advanced age, with a maximum incidence between 50 and 60 years.

LOCALIZATION

There is predilection for the deep soft tissues, whether muscular or fibroadipose. L.S. originating from the subcutaneous tissue are very rare. The most frequent site is the thigh, particularly the quadriceps and the popliteal region. The second most frequent localization is the retroperitoneum. This is followed by the leg, shoulder, and arm. It is hardly every observed in the hand or foot.

SYMPTOMS

Symptoms consist in a mass which grows in a deep site and thus may be apparent only when it has become of considerable size. Retroperitoneal L.S. cause later symptoms and often are of very large or monstruous size. The duration of symptoms is difficult to evaluate because of the insidious growth of the lesion; doubtless there are cases where the newly-formed mass has been present for several years, with slow growth and with no significant disorders. The mass may be painful due to compression on the nerve trunks, or it may cause edema of the limb due to venous compression. Retroperitoneal L.S. may cause hydronephrosis, intestinal compression, inguinal hernia, edema of one or both of the lower limbs.

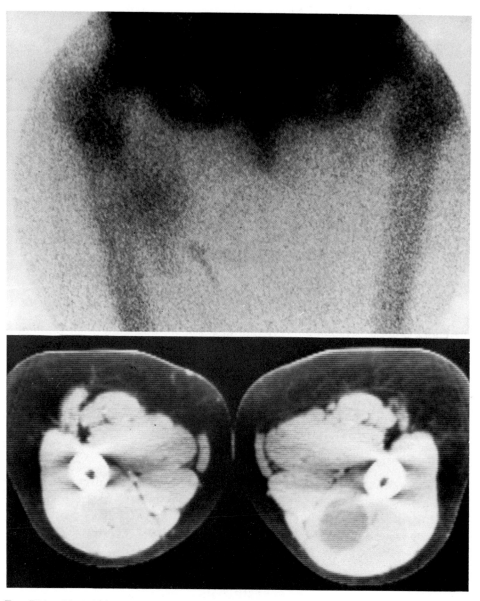

FIG. 761. - Myxoid liposarcoma (grade 2). Female aged 43 years. Bone scan with Tc99 reveals increased uptaking in the soft tissues during the vascular phase. CAT reveals a globose intramuscular mass, with a hypertransparence which is less intense and, furthermore, less homogeneous than that of lipomas.

RADIOGRAPHIC FEATURES

Generally, the radiopacity of the mass is similar to that of the muscle. The more the neoplasm is well-differentiated in mature adipose tissue, the more it becomes radiolucent. At times there are areas of radiopacity and radiolucency which are associated within the same tumor. Angiography (Fig. 763)

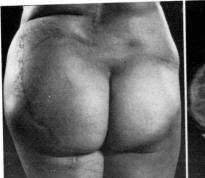
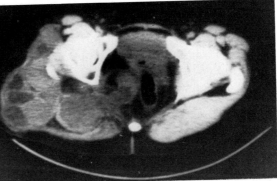

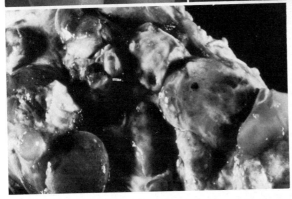

FIG. 762. - Myxoid L.S. (grade 2) of the gluteal region. Female aged 40 years. The symptoms began 6 years earlier with pain vaguely irradiated to the lower limb. Gluteal swelling was not observed at first, and the patient was submitted to explorative laparotomy, with a negative outcome. After a few months, as pain persisted, exploratory surgery was performed for disc herniation, with a negative outcome. After 4 years the gluteal swelling was finally observed, and submitted to marginal excision. The mass recurred after a few months, with progression of pain irradiated along the sciatic nerve. The patient was thus submitted to exploratory surgery with neurolysis of the sciatic nerve, but no attempt was made to resect the tumor. A photograph of the patient shows the vast gluteal swelling and the multiple scars from the last three operations. CAT shows the globose tumoral masses located under the atrophic gluteus maximus; some lobes are more translucent, and others more dense. The more lateral mass nearly reaches as far as the skin plane and surrounds the greater trochanter. The medial mass is expanded like an hour-glass outside and inside of the large ischiatic notch englobing the sciatic nerve and impressing the left wall of the rectum. Observe the mucoid aspect of the neoplastic nodes on the cut surface. The patient was submitted to atypical interilioabdominal disarticulation, removing the scars of previous surgery. After 4 years a local recurrence occurred located in front of the sacro-coccyx. This was widely excised resecting the caudal part of the sacro-coccyx below the third foramen. There were no signs of disease after 9 years.

particularly reveals with an intense uptake of the contrast medium the myxoid, pleomorphic and round-cell L.S., while the well-differentiated variant, so-called «lipoma-like», is scarcely injected. The extent and the relationships of the tumor are revealed by CAT (better still with intravenous contrast medium) and MRI (Figs. 761, 762).

GROSS PATHOLOGIC FEATURES

L.S. are usually large tumors, at times enormous (during advanced stages, in retroperitoneal localizations). Furthermore, they are multilobated tumors, which are usually delimited by a pseudocapsule (Figs. 762, 764, 765). This delimitation is an illusion, as the pseudocapsule is revealed by histological examination to be constituted by a layer of compressed, degenerated and reactive peritumoral tissue, and it is often penetrated by cells of the sarcoma, or nodules of these cells may be observed outside the pseudocapsule, in the tissues immediately surrounding the tumor (satellites). Furthermore, the pseudocapsule is thin and discontinuous.

L.S. are usually soft; consistency, color and aspect of the cut surface vary depending on the histological structure. The aspect is pale yellow and mucoid, translucid in the myxoid forms (Figs. 762, 764); it is yellowish or pale orange, soft, oily, friable, in the well-differentiated forms, or in any case rich in adipoblasts-adipocytes; whiter and firmer in forms having a larger spindle cell and collagen quota; softer, encephaloid, in scarcely differentiated forms (Fig. 765).

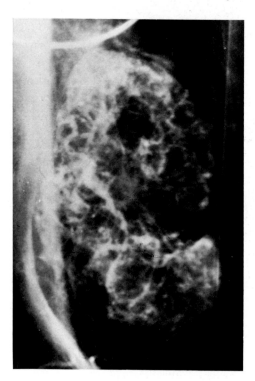

FIG. 763. - Myxoid liposarcoma (grade 3). Female aged 65 years. The tumoral mass was noticed in the posterior thigh 2 months earlier. Angiographic aspect: intense intra- and peritumoral neoangiogenesis. Marginal excision and radiation therapy. After 2 years, multiple pulmonary metastases.

HISTOPATHOLOGIC FEATURES

L.S. may be presented by different histologic subtypes repeating the different stage of evolution of the undifferentiated mesenchymal cell to the lipoblast and to the mature lipocyte. Thus, L.S. is classified as well-differentiated, myxoid round-cell and pleomorphic.

Well-differentiated liposarcoma

These represent approximately 30% of all cases of L.S. and are presented in two histological variants: lipoma-like L.S. and sclerosing L.S.

Lipoma-like L.S. is mostly constituted by mature lipocytes divided into fields of varying size by intervening collagen septa (Fig. 766). Somewhere there are atypical lipoblasts and lipocytes with hyperchromic and pleomorphic nuclei. Areas of well-differentiated L.S. may be identical to lipoma. Thus, it is important in deep lipomas to take numerous and extensive specimens for histology in order to exclude the presence of atypical cells. When, within the context of a lipoma-like L.S., an inflammatory component seems to be dominant, we are dealing with well-differentiated L.S. of the inflammatory variety. This picture may be confused with a phlogistic process of the fibroadipose tissue.

Sclerosing L.S. is less frequent in the soft tissues of the limbs than in the retroperitoneum and in the inguinal and scrotal regions. The lipoblastic and lipocytic components are associated with abundant collagen mesh which is intensely eosinophilic and which, at times, presents a myxoid aspect. Both the lipocytes and the fibroblasts may reveal hyperchromic nuclei and bizarre aspects (Fig. 767).

In well-differentiated L.S. the grade of malignancy is always low (grades 1-2 according to Broder) and mitotic figures are very scarce.

Nonetheless, there are rare cases in which, alongside the areas of well-differentiated L.S., in the

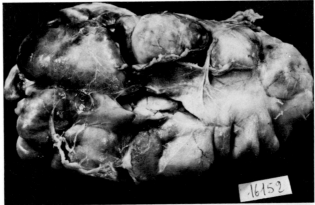
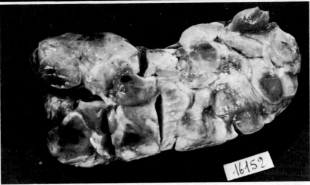

FIG. 764. - Myxoid L.S. (grade 3) of the thigh. Male aged 33 years. Marginal excision. Observe the lobulated aspect and the thin capsule, nearly identical to those of the lipomas. On the cut surface, the aspect is partially similar to fat, but more parenchymatous, and partially mucoid.

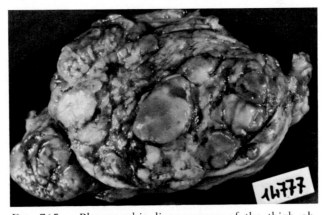

FIG. 765. - Pleomorphic liposarcoma of the thigh observed for the past year. Male aged 67 years. The patient was submitted to hip disarticulation. Observe the confluent multiple node aspect, with no capsule. On the cut surface, the tissue, although of yellow-orange color, is decidedly parenchymatous, encephaloid.

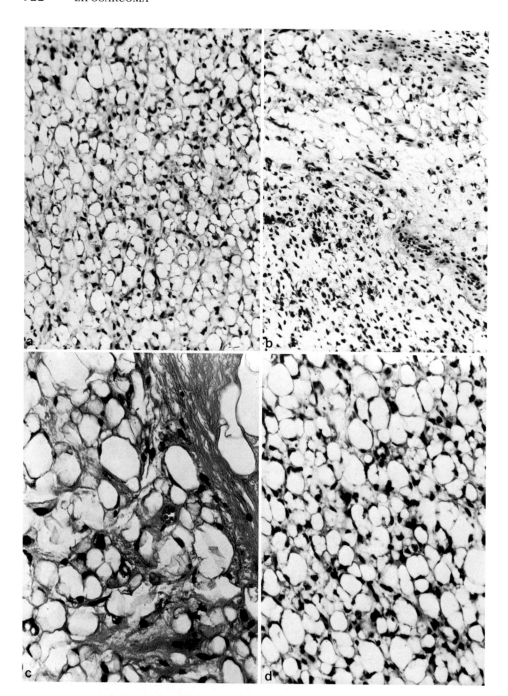

FIG. 766. - Well-differentiated lipoma-like L.S. (grade 1) . (a) and (b) Observe the lipoma-like differentiation, as lipocytes and lipoblasts constitute the entire lesion. (c)
and (d) Under higher power, there are well-differentiated lipocytes with extensive vacuoles dislocating the nucleus to the periphery. The cells generally reveal variations
in shape and size as compared to normal lipocytes. Isolated cells reveal hyperchromic
nuclei, which are often arranged close to collagen bundles (*Hemat.-eos.*, 250, 250, 400,
400 x).

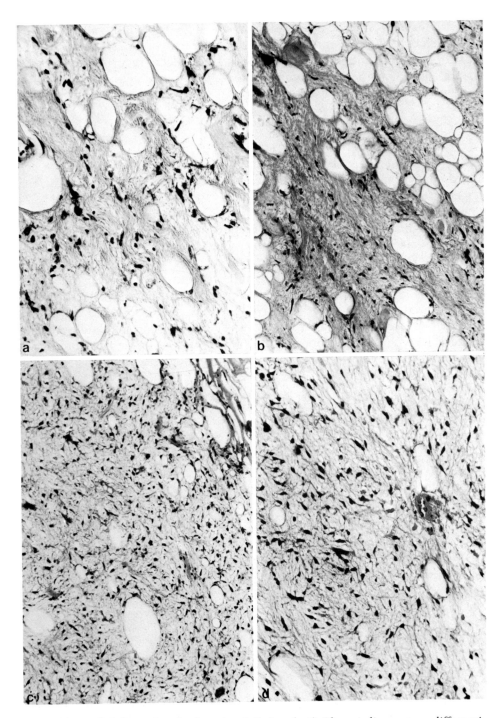

FIG. 767. - Well-differentiated sclerosing L.S. (grade 1). There is lipomatous differentiation of the cells which appear to be extensively vacuolized with a nucleus shifted to
the periphery. At times the nuclei are large and hyperchromic, with variations in
shape and size. The intercellular matrix may be constituted by loose or denser collagen (*Hemat.-eos.*, 250, 250, 250, 250 x).

same tumor areas may be observed, featuring high-grade L.S., or undifferentiated sarcoma, or malignant fibrous histiocytoma (grades 3-4). Such progression of malignancy may also be manifested in local recurrence or in metastases. By analogy with dedifferentiated chondrosarcoma, it has been defined **dedifferentiated liposarcoma**.

Myxoid liposarcoma

It is the most frequent L.S. in the soft tissues of the limbs (30-40%). Under microscopy it appears to be rather cellular, constituted by cells in various stages of lipoblastic differentiation, among which abundant myxoid substance is diffusedly present. Such myxoid substance is intensely stained by stains for mucopolysaccharides (not after treatment with hyaluronidase, which reveals that these are mucopolysaccharides rich in hyaluronic acid: Figs. 768, 769, 770).

Typical of this tumor is vascularization, constituted by a dense network of thin capillaries of uniform caliber (Figs. 768, 770). These capillaries are characterized by classic subdivision at an acute angle, so-called plexiform. The cells are regularly scattered in the myxoid substance. Spindle-stellate, round cells with one or more vacuoles arranged around the subcentral nucleus (lipoblasts), uni- or multivacuolated round cells having a nucleus

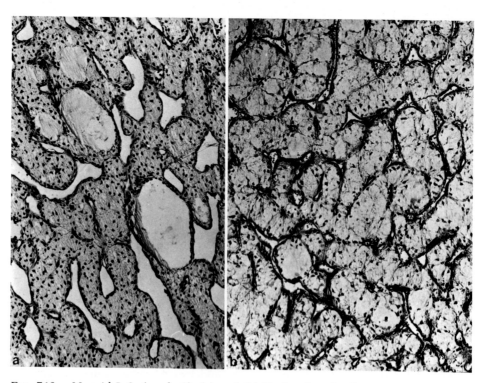

FIG. 768. - Myxoid L.S. (grade 2). (a) and (b) Notice the plexiform vascular pattern, amongst the diffusedly myxoid tissue (*Hemat.-eos.*, 160 x, *Mallory*, 160 x).

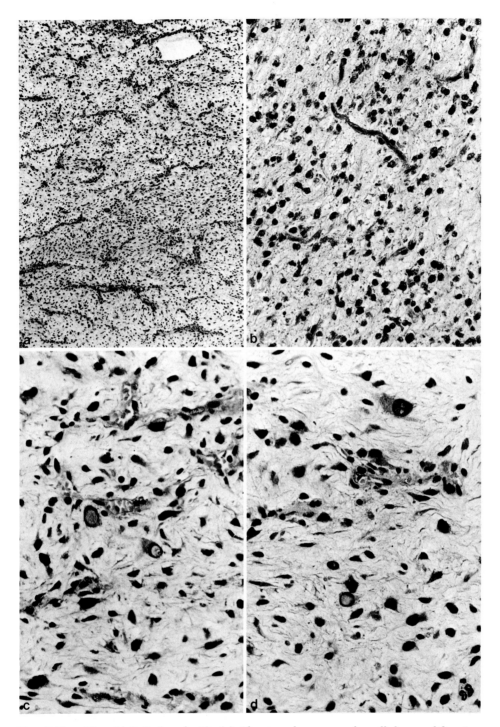

FIG. 769. - Myxoid L.S. (grade 3). (a) The neoplasm reveals cellular proliferation around a rich vascular network. (b) The cells appear to be located somewhat far apart due to interposition of myxoid substance. (c) and (d) At higher power atypical nucleocytoplasmatic aspects and nuclear hyperchromia may be observed (*Hemat.-eos.*, 60, 250, 400, 400 x).

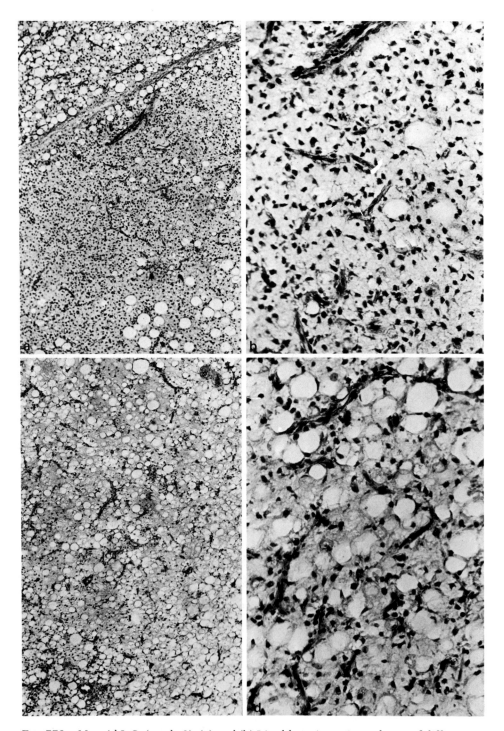

FIG. 770. - Myxoid L.S. (grade 2). (a) and (b) Lipoblasts in various phases of differentiation. (c) and (d) The plexiform aspect of the capillaries may be observed; there are numerous lipoblasts and lipocytes with the nucleus peripherally displaced and flattened. Among the cells there is abundant myxoid matrix (*Hemat.-eos.*, 60, 250, 60, 400 x).

which is pushed at the periphery and flattened (lipocytes) are observed (Fig. 770). Aspects of transition with well-differentiated L.S. (large mature lipocytes), with round-cell L.S. (globose cells similar to brown fat), with pleomorphic L.S. (giant and multinucleate lipoblasts, but usually few and sparse) may be observed.

Mitotic activity is generally scarce. The myxoid component may be abundant, enough to constitute actual lakes of mucoid substance (so-called pseudoglandular aspects), or rather scarce and dispersed among the cells; however, it is always well-represented.

Myxoid L.S. usually has a low grade of malignancy (1-2). Grade 3 myxoid L.S. are infrequently encountered; these are often transitional forms with the round-cell L.S.

Round-cell liposarcoma

It is an infrequent occurrence (approximately 10% of all liposarcomas). This variety, generally very cellular, is characterized by the proliferation of

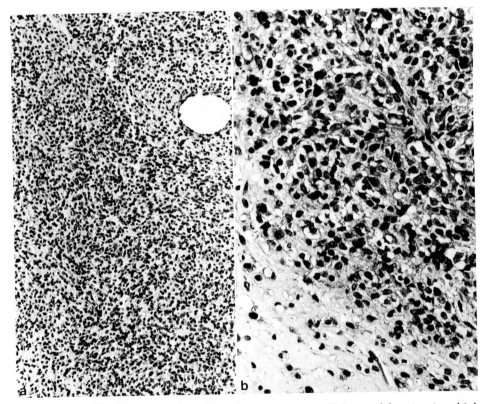

Fig. 771. - Round-cell L.S. (grade 3). (a) There is rich cellular proliferation in which there is no particular differentiation or preferential aggregation. (b) At higher power undifferentiated round-cells are mixed with others having vacuolized cytoplasm which may be referred to atypical lipoblasts. The nucleo-cytoplasmatic features and nuclear hyperchromia are indicative of a high grade of malignancy (*Hemat.-eos.*, 160, 400 x).

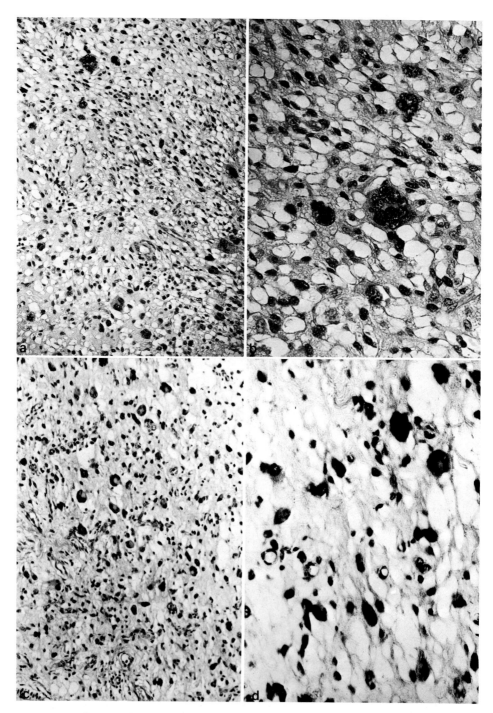

FIG. 772. - Pleomorphic L.S. (grade 2). (a) Marked pleomorphism of the cells is observed, and lipoblastic differentiation. (b) Cellular pleomorphism with nuclear hyperchromia and multinucleate giant cells are present in all areas of the neoplasm. (c) and (d) Vacuolized cells with an eccentric nucleus and giant cells with a hyperchromic nucleus (*Hemat.-eos.*, 160, 400, 250, 400 x).

ovoid-round cells, at times closely packed, at times separated by stroma which may be of myxoid aspect (Fig. 771). Here and there plexiform vascularization is observed. Among the undifferentiated cells, the lipoblasts and lipocytes, isolated or collected in small clusters are observed. There is neither evident nuclear pleomorphism, nor multinucleate giant cells, rather there is a somewhat undifferentiated aspect of the cells, with hyperchromic and atypical nuclei. In some cases large polyhedric, round cells prevail, with abundant eosinophilic cytoplasm, having well-defined limits and a large nucleus; other times the cells are nearly deprived of cytoplasm and have a pseudolymphocytary aspect. This is a high-grade (3-4) malignant tumor.

In some cases, the aspects of round cell L.S. are associated with those of pleomorphic L.S. There are numerous areas of necrosis and hemorrhage, at times it is possible to observe fields with a storiform or hemangiopericytomatous aspect. Thus, it is important to obtain numerous specimens from the entire tumor after surgical removal.

Pleomorphic liposarcoma

It represents about 20% of L.S.

It is characterized by pleomorphic cells among which lipoblasts with atypical and hyperchromic nuclei are recognized. The lesion is very cellular (Fig. 772). Alongside ovoid or round cells having a nucleus with a thick membrane, coarse chromatin and a very evident nucleolus, there are giant

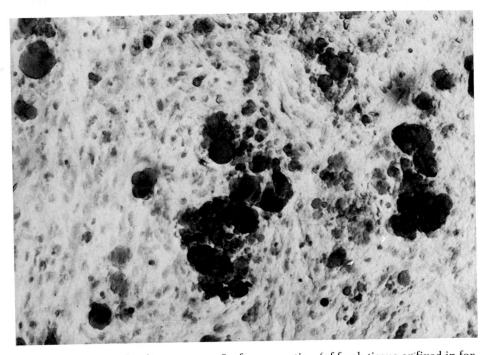

FIG. 773. - Pleomorphic liposarcoma. On frozen section (of fresh tissue or fixed in formalin) Sudan IV staining reveals abundant cytoplasmatic and extracytoplasmatic evidence of lipids (*Sudan*, IV, 250 x̄).

cells with intensely eosinophilic cytoplasm and a so-called «myxoid» aspect; these cells are not specific of pleomorphic L.S., as they may also be observed in pleomorphic rhabdomyosarcoma and in malignant fibrous histiocytoma. Lipoblasts with numerous vacuoles may be observed or, occasionally, mature lipocytes with large vacuole pushing the nucleus towards the periphery. Other times, instead of intensely eosinophilic cytoplasm, the giant cells reveal cytoplasm constituted by fine grape-like vacuoles, with monstruous, enormous, hyperchromic nuclei.

This is a neoplasm characterized by high-grade malignancy (3-4) with evident mitotic activity.

Mixed liposarcomas, dedifferentiated liposarcomas

As previously mentioned, there are L.S. in which alongside the well-differentiated or myxoid aspect, having a low histological grade, there are fields of higher malignancy; from this group, in 1979, Evans isolated dedifferentiated L.S., thus defined by analogy with dedifferentiated chondrosarcoma of bone. This is a neoplasm in which, alongside a low-grade L.S. (myxoid and/or lipoma-like) with a sharp «separation front», there is a high-grade malignant neoplasm. The latter may present the features of round-cell or pleomorphic L.S., or malignant fibrous histiocytoma. Rarely, L.S. presents **progression of malignancy** in local recurrence or in metastases.

These data emphasize just how **important it is to histologically examine deep lipomatous tumors using multiple and extensive samples.**

DIFFERENTIAL DIAGNOSIS

This must involve tumors or pseudotumors which present cells with cytoplasmatic vacuoles, an aspect which may be confused with lipoblasts. Staining for lipids (Fig. 773) is of relative importance, as cells which contain lipids are present not only in L.S., but also in many other sarcomas and in different carcinomas (kidney, liver, breast). On the contrary, in extremely undifferentiated L.S. the lipidic component may be very scarce and thus staining negative. Furthermore, lipoblasts and lipocytes must be distinguished from cells having vacuolated cytoplasm by contents in glycogen or in mucopolysaccharides.

Well-differentiated L.S. must be distinguished from inflammatory lesions (liponecrosis and reactions to silicone implants) and from varieties of lipoma, particularly from **pleomorphic lipoma**.

Myxoid L.S. has such abundant and typical vascularization that it may be easily distinguished from **intramuscular myxoma**. Confusion with **lipoblastoma** and lipoblastomatosis is avoided particularly by the age of the patient (childhood), as the histological aspect may be the same. In myxoid L.S., unlike what occurs in **myxoid chondrosarcoma** and **chordoma**, the mucoid substance does not stain for mucopolysaccharides after hyaluronidase pretreatment. Differential diagnosis with **malignant fibrous histiocytoma of the**

myxoid variant may be somewhat difficult. But in the latter, the cellular pleomorphism is generally more evident, mitotic figures are more frequent, giant cells are more numerous, and in non-myxoid areas the storiform aspect is observed, while cells rich in cytoplasmatic vacuoles contain mucinous rather than lipidic material.

Round-cell L.S. must be differentiated from vacuolized round-cell sarcomas, such as **embryonal rhabdomyosarcoma**, but in the latter recognition of the rhabdomyoblasts will orient diagnosis. **Malignant lymphoma** with vacuolated cells is distinguished from round-cell L.S. by the presence of indented nuclei. **Carcinoma with vacuolated cells** or generally undifferentiated carcinoma may be included in differential diagnosis with round-cell L.S., which may have pseudoepithelial aspects, but if specimens are extensive and multiple, the epithelial nature may be eliminated.

Pleomorphic L.S. must be differentiated from **malignant fibrous histiocytoma** (storiform aspect, absence of actual lipoblasts-lipocytes), and from **pleomorphic rhabdomyosarcoma** (cells containing abundant glycogen and positive for actin myoglobin).

COURSE

The subdivision of L.S. in well-differentiated, myxoid, pleomorphic and round-cell variants is important because of the different course. Well-differentiated and myxoid L.S. generally have a low grade of malignancy (1-2) while pleomorphic and round-cell L.S. are characterized by a high grade of malignancy (3-4).

Well-differentiated and myxoid L.S. recur locally even many years after excision. Metastases are exceptional in well-differentiated L.S., rare and late in myxoid L.S. Thus, multiple local recurrences may be observed over many years time, before metastases occur.

In round-cell and pleomorphic L.S., on the contrary, local recurrence tends to occur rapidly, within the first months or 1-2 years after excision, and metastases are frequent and relatively early. Metastases occur by hematogenous route, in the lungs, in the skeleton, and in other internal organs. Metastases in the regional lymph nodes are an exceptional occurrence. Metastases (or multicentric localizations?) in other areas of the soft tissues, such as in another limb or the retroperitoneum, are not exceptional.

TREATMENT

Even if this is so in only a small area of the surface of the tumor, marginal excision is followed by local recurrence in a high percentage of cases. It must thus be avoided as much as possible. The most suitable type of treatment, for myxoid and well-differentiated L.S., — nearly all stage I — is wide removal. For high-grade L.S. — stage II — radical removal may be preferred, as that which offers the highest guarantee. Radiotherapy is effective, particularly in myxoid L.S., and is thus widely used in association with surgery.

Pelvic and retroperitoneal L.S. are more difficult to treat and at times they cannot be excised with a wide surgical margin. When there are doubts as to whether surgery was marginal, even in a single site, it is best to associate postoperative radiotherapy. The usefulness of chemotherapy has not as yet been defined.

PROGNOSIS

It is very difficult to have reliable data as it would be necessary to be aware of the principal variables, which are the preoperative stage of the tumor, the surgical margins, the associated treatment. The largest case series report an overall ten-year survival rate in about 50% of cases, with a considerable difference between myxoid and well-differentiated forms (stage I) and pleomorphic and round-cell ones (stage II); and between retroperitoneal localizations (rarely wide excision) and localization in the limbs (removal which is more often wide or radical).

REFERENCES

1959 KAUFFMAN S.L., STOUT A.P.: Lipoblastic tumors of children. *Cancer*, **12**, 912.
1961 KIMBROUGH R.F., SOULE E.H.: Liposarcoma of the extremities. *Clin. Orthop.*, **19**, 40.
1962 ENZINGER F.M., WINSLOW D.J.: Liposarcoma: A study of 103 cases. *Virchows Arch. (Pathol. Anat.)*, **335**, 367.
1966 RESZEL P.A., SOULE E.H., COVENTRY M.B.: Liposarcoma of the extremities and limb girdles: A study of 222 cases. *J. Bone Joint Surg.*, **48A**, 229.
1968 EDLAND R.W.: Liposarcoma. A retrospective study of 15 cases, a review of the literature and a discussion of radiosensitivity. *Am. J. Roentgenol*, **103**, 778.
1969 GEORGIADES D.E., ALCALAIS D.B., KARABELA V.G.: Multicentric well-differentiated liposarcomas. A case report and a brief review of the literature. *Cancer*, **24**.
1970 SATO E.: Pathology of liposarcoma. Histological classification of 45 cases with emphasis on differential diagnosis. *Jpn. J. Cancer Clin.*, **16**, 690.
1971 SPITTLE M.F., NEWTON K.A., MAC KENZIE D.H.: Liposarcoma — a review of 60 cases. *Br. J. Cancer*, **24**, 696.
1972 QUINONEZ G.E.: Liposarcoma of the lower extremity. A review of 30 cases from the Ohio State University Hospital from 1955 to 1970. *Ohio State Med. J.*, **68**, 942.
1973 KINNE D.W., CHUE F.C.H., HUVOS A.G. *et al.*: Treatment of primary and recurrent retroperitoneal liposarcoma. Twenty-five year experience at Memorial Hospital. *Cancer*, **31**, 53.
1974 TANAKA M., HIZAWA K., TONEI M.: Liposarcoma — a clinicopathological study on 136 cases based on the histologic subtyping of WHO. *Gann.*, **20**, 1036.
1975 KINDBLOM L.G., ANGERVALL L., SVENDSEN P.: Liposarcoma. A clinicopathologic, radiographic and prognostic study. *Acta Pathol. Microbiol. Scand.*, **253**, 1.
1975 SAWHNEY K.K, MC DONALD M.J., JAFFE H.W.: Liposarcoma of the hand. *Am. Surg.*, **41**, 117.
1975 SHIU M.H., CHU F., CASTRO E.B. *et al.*: Results of surgical and radiation therapy in the treatment of liposarcoma arising in an extremity. *Am. J. Roentgenol.*, **123**, 577.
1978 DREYFUSS U., BEN-ARIEH J.Y., HIRSCHOWITZ B.: Liposarcoma — rare complication in neurofibromatosis. Case report. *Plast Reconstr. Surg.*, **61**, 287.
1978 KINDBLOM L.G., ANGERVALL L., JARLSTEDT J.: Liposarcoma of the neck. A clinicopathologic study of four cases. *Cancer*, **42**, 774.

1979 EVANS H.L., SOULE E.H., WINKELMAN R.K.: Atypical lipoma, atypical intramuscular lipoma, and well differentiated retroperitoneal liposarcoma. *Cancer*, **43**, 574.

1979 EVANS H.L.: Liposarcoma. A study of 55 cases with a reassessment of its classification. *Am. J. Surg. Pathol.*, **3**, 507.

1979 FELDMAN P.S.: A comparative study including ultrastructure of intramuscular myxoma and myxoid liposarcoma. *Cancer*, **43**, 512.

1979 KINDBLOM L., SÄVE-SÖDERBERGH J.: The ultrastructure of liposarcoma. A study of 10 cases. *Acta Pathol. Microbiol. Scand. (A)*, **87**, 109.

1979 SAUNDERS J.R., DARRELL A.J., CASTERLINE P.F. *et al.*: Liposarcomas of the head and neck. A review of the literature and addition of four cases. *Cancer*, **43**, 162.

1980 BATTIFORA H., NONEZ-ALONSO C.: Myxoid liposarcoma. Study of 10 cases. *Ultrastruct Pathol.*, **1**, 157.

1980 BOLEN J.W., THORNING D.: Benign lipoblastoma and myxoid liposarcoma. *Am. J. Surg. Pathol.*, **4**, 163.

1981 DE SANTOS L.A., GINALDI S., WALLACE S.: Computed tomography in liposarcoma. *Cancer*, **47**, 46.

1981 MACKENZIE D.H.: The myxoid tumors of soft somatic tissues. *Am. J. Surg. Pathol.*, **5**, 443.

1981 POPPER H., KNIPPING G.: A histochemical and biochemical study of a liposarcoma with several aspects on the development of fat synthesis. *Path. Res. Pract.*, **171**, 373.

1982 KINDBLOM L.G., ANGERVALL L., FASSINA A.S.: Atypical lipoma. *Acta Pathol. Microbiol. Scand.*, **90-A**, 27.

1982 SNOVER D.C., SUMMER H.W., DEHNER L.P.: Variability of histologic pattern in recurrent soft tissue sarcomas originally diagnosed as liposarcoma. *Cancer*, **49**, 1005.

1983 COCCHIA D., LAURIOLA L., STOLFI V.M. *et al.*: S-100 antigen labels neoplastic cells in liposarcoma and cartilaginous tumours. *Virchows Arch (Pathol. Anat.)*, **402**, 139.

1983 O'CONNOR M., SNOVERR D.C.: Liposarcoma. A review of factors influencing prognosis. *Am. Surg.*, **49**, 379.

1983 SHMOOKLER B.M., ENZINGER F.M.: Liposarcoma occurring in children. An analysis of 17 cases and review of the literature. *Cancer*, **52(3)**, 567-74.

1984 HASHIMOTO H., DAIMARU Y., ENJOJI M.: S-100 protein distribution in liposarcoma. An immunoperoxidase study with special reference to the distinction of liposarcoma from myxoid malignant fibrous histiocytoma. *Virchows Arch. (Pathol. Anat.)*, **405**, 1.

1984 VILMANT R., DAUPLAT J., FONCK Y.: Round cell liposarcoma. Histopathologic and ultrastructural study of a case developed within the framework of a lipomatosis. *Ann. Pathol.*, **4(5)**, 377-81.

1985 CHAUDHURI P.K., WALKER M.J., BEATTLE C.W., DAS GUPTA T.K.: The steroid hormone receptors in tumors of adipose tissue. *J. Surg. Oncol.*, **28(3)**, 87-9.

1985 DANIELL S.J.: Liposarcoma: a ten year experience. *Int. Orthop.*, **9(1)**, 55-8.

1985 LINDAHL S., MARKHEDE G. BERLIN O.: Computed tomography of lipomatous and myxoid tumors. *Acta Radiol.*, **26**, 709.

1985 ROSSOUW D.J., CINTI S., DICKERSIN G.R.: Liposarcoma. An ultrastructural study of 15 cases. *Am. J. Clin. Pathol.*, **85**, 649.

1986 CHAN J.K., LEE K.C., SAW D.: Extraskeletal chondroma with lipoblastlike cells. *Hum. Pathol.*, **17**, 1285.

1987 SANDBERG A.A., TURC-CAREL C.: The cytogenetics of solid tumors. Relation to diagnosis, classification and pathology. *Cancer*, **59**, 387.

1989 CHANG H.R., HAJDU S.I., COLLIN C., BRENNAN M.F.: The prognostic value of histologic subtypes in primary extremity liposarcoma. *Cancer*, **64**, 1514.

VASCULAR LEIOMYOMA
(Synonym: angiomyoma)

These are benign lesions which constitute most cases of superficial leio-myomas. There is predilection for the female sex, and age ranges from 30 to 60 years.

They are solitary lesions frequently located in the limbs, with preference for the leg. They are usually localized in the subcutaneous tissue, although the lesion may involve the derma. It is a globose mass which grows slowly, for years, characterized by pain in more than half of the cases.

Macroscopically, it is a well-circumscribed lesion, of firm consistency, and which on the cut surface reveals a grayish-white lucent aspect.

Histologically, there is a proliferation of smooth muscle cells around nu-

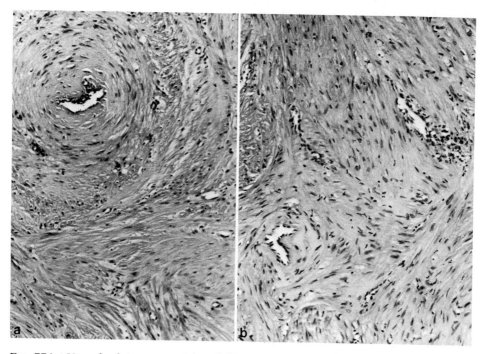

FIG. 774. - Vascular leiomyoma. (a) and (b) Proliferation of the spindle cells of smooth muscle aspect. These are arranged concentrically around the vessels (*Hemat.-eos.*, 160, 250 x).

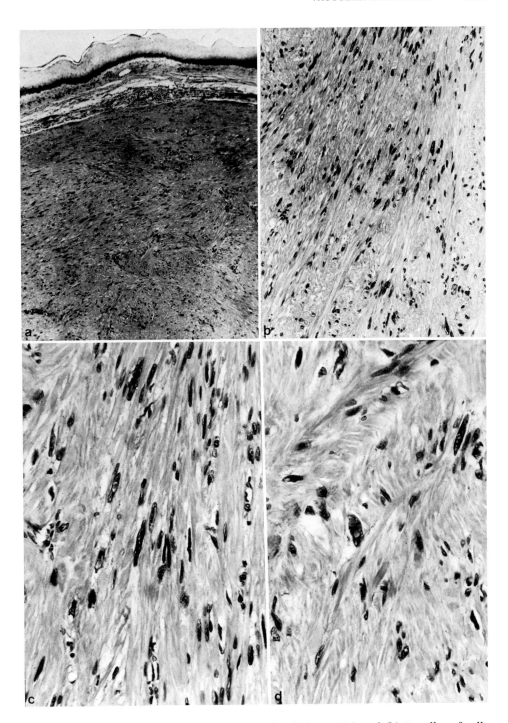

FIG. 775. - Leiomyoma localized in the superficial planes. (a) and (b) Bundles of cells arranged on an ordinate axis with intensely eosinophilic cytoplasm. The nuclei are elongated and have a rounded end. (c) and (d) Under higher power, the cells present an elongated nucleus whose ends are rounded and or indented by perinuclear cytoplasmatic vacuoles (Hemat.-eos., 60, 160, 400, 400 x).

merous vessels collected in nodules and/or diffused (Fig. 774). The vessels have thickened walls, recalling the structure of an arteriole, but there are no characteristic elastic components. The vessels are constituted by bundles of smooth muscle cells which are arranged circumferentially and which on the outside continue with the surrounding leiomyomatous tissue. Areas of fibrosis and myxoid areas are varyingly present. Around the vessels, spindle cells with a cylindrical nucleus having rounded ends (like a Havana cigar) are arranged in bundles forming wide and elegant waves (Fig. 775). The cytoplasm is eosinophilic with fucsinophile longitudinal striations, evident in trichromic stains and with PTAH. Van Gieson stain shows diffused yellowish tones revealing that these are muscle cells.

Treatment. It is a benign lesion in which marginal excision is curative; recurrence has not been reported.

DEEP LEIOMYOMA

It is a very rare occurrence and it is observed, with no preference for sex or age, in the muscular tissue of the limbs. It grows slowly, but it becomes larger in size than superficial forms of the disease, probably because it is treated later. Its radiographic feature may be calcification.

Histologically, it is constituted by intertwined bundles of smooth muscle cells. Cellularity may be considerable, but the cells are monomorphous. The cell bundles are intertwined and the nuclei may be palisading.

The cells are characterized by elongated cylindrical nuclei with a rounded end («Havana cigar»). In the cytoplasms fine longitudinal fibrillae are revealed (PTAH, Masson) as well as glycogen. Van Gieson stain reveals diffused yellowish staining. Some cytoplasms are vacuolated. Collagen is scarce but some areas may have considerable fibrosis. Furthermore, there may be myxoid areas with accumulation of mucopolysaccharides and dispersion of the cells. Regressive aspects are very frequent and diffused, where the calcium precipitates.

The cells have no pleomorphism, nor atypia, nor mitoses. Sporadic cells with a large and bizarre nucleus may be observed, which, as in neurinomas, are considered to be degenerative elements which do not indicate malignancy.

Differential **diagnosis** with **neurinoma** (palisading aspect) is also based on the features of the cells (glycogen, longitudinal fibrillae, fucsinophilia). The most important diagnosis involves the less rare **leiomyosarcoma** and it is above all based on the number of mitotic figures.

Deep L.M. is benign and **treatment** consists in marginal excision or, better yet, moderately wide excision.

REFERENCES

1959 DUHIG J.J., AYER J.P.: Vascular leiomyoma: A study of 61 cases. *Arch. Pathol.*, **68**, 424.

1965 GOODMAN A.H., BRIGGS R.C.: Deep leiomyoma of an extremity. *J. Bone Joint Surg.*, **47A**, 529.

1967 BULMER J.H.: Smooth muscle tumors of the limbs. *J. Bone Joint Surg.*, **49B**, 52.

1975 BARDACH H., EBNER H.: Das Angioleiomyoma der Haut. *Hautarzt*, **26**, 638.

1980 LEDESMA-MEDINA J., OH K.S., GIRDANY B.R.: Calcification in childhood leiomyoma. *Radiology*, **135**, 339.

1984 HACHISUGA T., HASHIMOTO H., ENJOJI M.: A clinicopathologic reappraisal of
562 cases. *Cancer*, **54**, 126.

1989 SMITH K., SKELTON H.G., BARRETT T.L., LUPTON G.P., GRAHAM J.H.: Cutaneous
myofibroma. *Mod. Pathol.*, **2**, 603.

LEIOMYOSARCOMA

This tumor constitutes approximately 7% of all sarcomas of the soft tissues. We will leave aside forms with retroperitoneal localization and discuss L.M.S. of subcutaneous and cutaneous localization, or those connected with large vessels of the limbs.

Cutaneous-subcutaneous L.M.S. constitute 2-3% of all superficial sarcomas. They are observed from 40 to 70 years of age. There is no specific predilection for sex.

Preferential localization is in the limbs, in relation to the piliferous areas. In general, these are solitary lesions, which in dermic forms never exceed 2 cm. Subcutaneous lesions may grow to larger size. A frequent symptom is pain. While when located in the derma the tumor has boundaries which are not very defined, in the subcutaneous tissue, growing and compressing the nearby fat, it gives origin to a pseudocapsule. On the cut surface a whitish-gray or pinkish color and fasciculated aspect may be observed. Rarely, there are necrotic and hemorrhagic areas.

L.M.S. originating from the vascular walls generally has a deep localization, involving the veins, exceptionally the arteries, in the lower limbs. The tumor may cause edema due to venous compression. At times it is difficult or impossible to ascertain the vascular origin of a L.M.S., if this is not clearly related to the wall of a large vessel. The macroscopic aspect may be polypoid or nodular, developed toward the inside or toward the outside of the vessel.

Histologically, independently of their localization, L.M.S. have a comparable aspect. It is a proliferation of spindle cells with an elongated nucleus having a rounded end and intensely eosinophilic cytoplasm (Fig. 776), positive for actin and myoglobin. Trichromic stain reveals longitudinal striations; there is cytoplasmatic PAS positiveness (glycogen) in the more differentiated forms.

Electron microscopy is diagnostic in well-differentiated forms (nuclei with deep indentations, myofilaments). At times in the cytoplasm, close to one end of the nucleus, there is a vacuole which produces a hollow in the nucleus itself, the convex extremity of which becomes concave. Multinucleate giant cells are rare. Generally, the cells have a spindle shape, they are arranged in bundles which form wide waves, at times they intersect with differing orientation. The orthogonal arrangement of the bundles is often observed, demonstrated by the fact that nuclei sectioned longitudinally are placed alongside nuclei sectioned transversally. These neoplasms do not produce

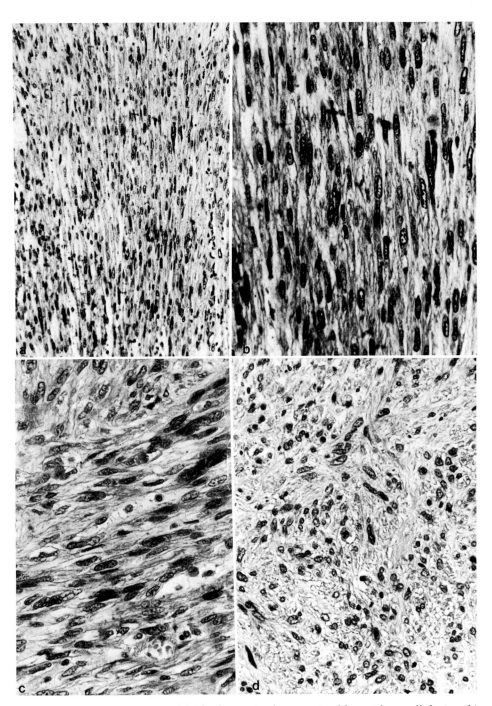

FIG. 776. - Leiomyosarcoma. (a) The lesion is characterized by evident cellularity. (b) and (c) The cells are arranged in parallel bundles and they are closely packed. The nucleus, when sectioned longitudinally, presents a «cigar-like» aspect, elongated with a rounded end. At times the chromatin is in fine granules, at times it is coarser. (d) The cells have perinuclear vacuoles and moderate pleomorphism (*Hemat.-eos.*, 160, 400, 400, 400 x).

collagen, but staining for the reticulum demonstrates a delicate argyrophilous mesh between the cells. At times the arrangement of the nuclei assumes a palisade-like aspect, similar to that which is observed in neurinoma. Areas of hyalinization may be present.

Rarely, in L.M.S. of the limbs, there are extremely pleomorphic aspects with giant cells having an intensely eosinophilic cytoplasm or highly anaplastic round cells, typical of localizations in the retroperitoneum. These so-called epithelioid aspects, in which the cells have a rounded shape with vacuolated cytoplasm (clear cells), are exceptional in L.M.S. of the limbs and, at most, they may occur in sporadic areas of the tumor.

In leiomyomas/leiomyosarcomas malignancy is indicated more by the mitotic index than the size of the tumor, the cellularity, the atypia, or necrosis. Five mitoses per 10 microscopic fields under high power are sufficient to consider the lesion malignant. From 1 to 4 mitoses indicate potential malignancy, particularly if extensive areas of necrosis and nuclear atypia are associated.

Superficial L.M.S., although followed by local recurrence in approximately 50% of cases, have a relatively good **prognosis**; the deep L.M.S. have a more severe prognosis, as the probability of metastasis increases. According to the evaluations of Fields and Helwig (1981), the neoplasms confined to the derma do not metastasize, while those which involve the subcutaneous tissue metastasize in a third of all cases.

Removal with a margin of healthy tissue (wide excision) is the **treatment** of choice. With local recurrence, the risk of metastasis increases, also because the superficial lesion tends to increase the volume and to involve the deeper structures.

REFERENCES

1962 PHELAN J.T., SHERER W., MESA P.: Malignant smooth muscle tumors (leiomyosarcomas) of soft tissue origin. *N. Engl. J. Med.*, **266**, 1027.

1963 DORFMAN H.D., FISHER E.R.: Leiomyosarcoma of the greater saphenous vein. *Am. J. Clin. Pathol.*, **39**, 73.

1964 STOUT A.P., HILL W.T.: Leiomyosarcoma of the superficial soft tissue. *Cancer*, **11**, 844.

1965 BOTTING A.J., SOULE E.H., BROWN A.L.: Smooth muscle tumors in children. *Cancer*, **12**, 711.

1970 JURAYJ M.N., MIDELL S., et. al.: Primary leiomyosarcoma of the inferior vena cava. Report of a case and review of the literature. *Cancer*, **26**, 1349.

1971 JOHANSEN J.K., NIELSEN R.: Leiomyosarcoma of the inferior vena cava: Report of a case. *Acta Chir. Scand.*, **137**, 181.

1973 KEVORKIAN J., CENTO J.P.: Leiomyosarcoma of large arteries and veins. *Surgery*, **73**, 39.

1974 DAHL I., ANGERVALL L.: Cutaneous and subcutaneous leiomyosarcoma — a clinicopathologic study of 47 patients. *Pathologia Europaea*, **9**, 307.

1975 PERTSCHUK L.P.: Immunofluorescence of soft tissue tumor with antismooth-muscle and antiskeletal-muscle antibodies. *Am. J. Clin. Pathol.*, **63**, 332.

1977 HEADINGTON J.T., BEALS T.F., NIEDERHUBER J.E.: Primary leiomyosarcoma of skin: A report and critical appraisal. *J. Cutan. Pathol*, **4**, 308.

1979 VARELA-DURAN J., OLIVA H. ROSAI J.: Vascular leiomyosarcoma: The malignant counterpart of vascular leiomyoma. *Cancer*, **44**, 1684.

1979 WOLFF M., SILVA F., KAYE G: Pulmonary metastases (with admixed epithelial elements) from smooth muscle neoplasms: Report of nine cases, including three males. *Am. J. Surg. Pathol.*, **3**, 325.

1981 FIELDS J.P., HELWIG E.B.: Leiomyosarcoma of the skin and subcutaneous tissue. *Cancer*, **47**, 156.

1981 MUKAI K., SCHOLLMEYER J.V., ROSAI J.: Immunohistochemical localization of actin. *Am. J. surg. Pathol.*, **5**, 91.

1981 WILE A.G., EVANS H.L., ROMSDAHL M.M.: Leiomyosarcoma of soft tissue: A clinicopathologic study. *Cancer*, **48**, 1022.

1983 ORELLANA-DIAZ O., HERNANDEZ-PEREZ E.: Leiomyoma cutis and leiomyosarcoma: a 10-year study and a short review. *J Dermatol. Surg. Oncol.*, **9**, 283.

1983 TAHERI S.A., CONNER G.W.: Leiomyosarcoma of iliac veins. *Surgery*, **94**, 516.

1986 HASHIMOTO H., DAIMARU Y., TSUNEYOSHI M., ENJOJI M.: Leiomyosarcoma of the external soft tissues. *Cancer*, **57**, 2077.

1986 LEU H.J., MAKEK M.: Intramural venous leiomyosarcomas. *Cancer*, **57**, 1395.

1989 NEUGUT A.I., SORDILLO P.P.: Leiomyosarcoma of the extremities (clinical discussion of 17 cases). *J. Surg. Oncol.*, **40**, 65.

RHABDOMYOMA

It is a very rare tumor, just 2% of all tumors having prevalent striated muscle differentiation. Furthermore, it hardly ever occurs in the soft tissues of the locomotor apparatus.

1) **Adult rhabdomyoma**. Occurring during adult-advanced age, it is localized in the oropharynx, the larynx, the muscles of the neck. It is constituted by large cells which resemble striated muscle cells which are completely differentiated: polygonal in transverse section, with vast intensely eosinophilic

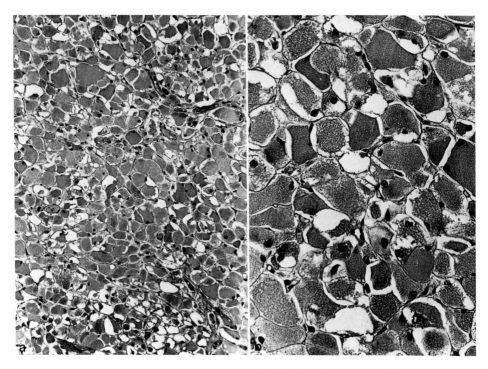

Fig. 777. - Adult rhabdomyoma. (a) Polygonal cells closely aggregated with ample intensely eosinophilic cytoplasm. The cytoplasms appear distinctly outlined. (b) and (c) At higher power the cytoplasm has a granulous and vacuolated aspect. The nuclei are small, vesicular, arranged eccentrically close to the cytoplasmatic membrane. (d) Transverse striation may be observed in the cytoplasm (*Hemat.-eos.*, 160, 400, 400 x; PTAH 400 x).

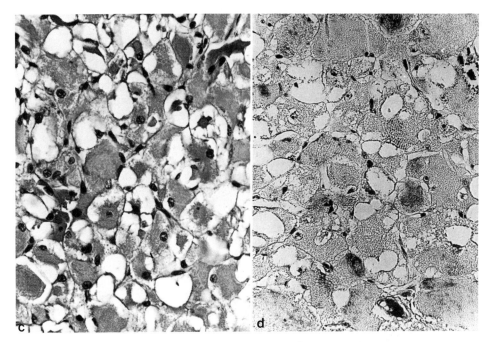

FIG. 777. (continued).

cytoplasm, longitudinal and transverse striations, small nuclei located at the periphery, abundant glycogen which at times dissolved in the course of histological preparation leaves multiple and large vacuoles (Fig. 777).

2) **Fetal rhabdomyoma**. It is observed in children under 4 years of age, in the subcutaneous tissue, in the head-neck, but rarely also in the limbs and in the trunk. It is constituted by rhabdomyoblasts at differing stages of differentiation, often more differentiated at the periphery than at the center of the tumor. The most interesting aspect of this rare tumor is constituted by the risk of mistaking it for an embryonal rhabdomyosarcoma. As compared to the latter, fetal rhabdomyoma is superficial, well-circumscribed, more differentiated at the periphery, with scarce cellular pleomorphism, rare mitotic figures, no necrosis.

3) **Genital rhabdomyoma**, which occurs in the vulvar or vaginal wall about the menopausal age.

4) **Cardiac rhabdomyoma**, occurring during childhood, is the only lesion for which a hamartomatous nature has been revealed.

REFERENCES

1963 GOLDMAN L.: Multicentric benign rhabdomyoma of skeletal muscle. *Cancer*, **16**, 1609.
1972 DEHNER L.P., ENZINGER F.M., FONT R.L.: Fetal rhabdomyoma. An analysis of nine cases. *Cancer*, **30**, 160.

1972 MIKULOWSKI P.: Extracardiac rhabdomyoma. *Acta Pathol. Microbiol. Scand.*, **80**, 222.
1976 DAHL I., ANGERVALL L., SÄVE-SÖDERBERGH J.: Foetal rhabdomyoma. *Acta Pathol. Microbiol. Scand.*, **84**, 107.
1980 DI SANT AGNESE P.A., KNOWLES D.M.: Extracardiac rhabdomyoma: A clinicopathologic study and review of the literature. *Cancer*, **46**, 780.
1980 SCRIVNER D., MEYER J.S.: Multifocal recurrent adult rhabdomyoma. *Cancer*, **46**, 790.
1982 KONRAD E.A., MEISTER P., HUEBNER G.: Extracardiac rhabdomyoma: report of different types with light microscopic and ultrastructural studies. *Cancer*, **49**, 898.
1982 LEHTONEN E., ASIKAINEN U., BADLEY R.A.: Rhabdomyoma: Ultrastructural features and distribution of desmin, muscle type, of intermediate filament protein. *Acta Pathol. Microbiol. Immunol. Scand.* (A) **90**, 125.
1983 GARDNER D.G., CORIO R.L.: Multifocal adult rhabdomyoma. *Oral Surg.*, **56**, 76.
1989 BLAAUWGEERS J.L.G., TROOST D., DINGEMANS K.P., TAAT C.W., VAN DEN TWEEL J.G.: Multifocal rhabdomyoma of neck, cases studied by FNA, light and electron microscopy, histochemistry and immunohistochemistry. *Am. J. Surg. Pathol.*, **13**, 791.

RHABDOMYOSARCOMA

DEFINITION

R.M.S. is a sarcoma with a tendency to differentiate towards the striated muscle cell. This tendency must be unique or prevalent: in fact, there are mesenchymal and epithelial malignant tumors (kidney, breast, lung, uterus, ovary) which present partial rhabdomyoblastic differentiation: just as rare cases of R.M.S. have foci of chondroid or osteoid differentiation.

R.M.S. is distinguished in **three varieties**: embryonal (of which the botryoid form is a sub-variety); alveolar; pleomorphic. This distinction is not always clear-cut and it is based on histological and (of the botryoid variety) macroscopic features.

R.M.S. is generally characterized by a rather variable histological picture, including a wide range which goes from the undifferentiated round cell to the rhabdomyoblast in its successive stages of differentiation.

FREQUENCY

R.M.S. is not rare, representing approximately 20% of all sarcomas of the soft tissues, and it is the most frequent sarcoma of the soft tissues in patients aged under 20 years. Embryonal R.M.S. is the most frequent type to occur, followed by the alveolar variety. Pleomorphic R.M.S. of advanced to adult age, a classic in the literature in the past, has today become a rarity, as its field is nearly totally impoverished by malignant fibrous histiocytoma.

SEX, AGE

There is predilection for the male sex and childhood-young age. The embryonal variety has the highest incidence from birth to 10-15 years of age, the alveolar variety from 10 to 25 years, and the pleomorphic variety during adult and advanced age.

LOCALIZATION

The most frequent sites are, in decreasing order, the head (orbit, mid-ear) and the neck, the uro-genital region (bladder, spermatic funiculus, prostate, vagina), the biliary ducts and the retroperitoneum, the soft tissues of the trunk and of the limbs. This last localization constitutes just 1/4-1/5 of the total number. The patient may thus be first observed by various specialists: pediatrician, pediatric surgeon, ear nose and throat specialist, oculist, urologist, general surgeon, orthopaedist.

Embryonal R.M.S. prevails in the head-neck, in the genito-rinary tract (botry-oid variety), in the retroperitoneum.

R.M.S. of the limbs are particularly of the alveolar type. The rare cases of pleo-morphic R.M.S. may also be observed in the large muscles of the limbs, particular-ly the thigh.

As for the localiza-tion of R.M.S. in the limbs, it affects the upper limb (particu-larly the forearm and hand) and the lower limb (particularly the foot) with more or less the same fre-quency.

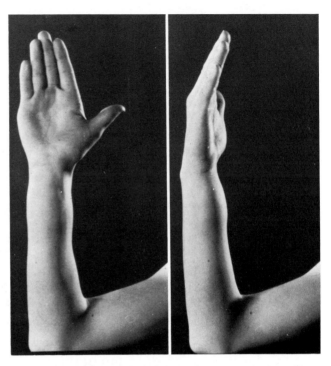

FIG. 778. - Embryonal rhabdomyosarcoma. Boy aged 15 years. Swelling observed 2 months earlier, growing ra-pidly, tense, painless. On diagnosis pulmonary metasta-ses were already present.

SYMPTOMS

It is a deep tumor and it is often located in relation to the muscles. Its growth is rapid, invasive and destructive. It easily grows out to the surface in the mucous cavities (botryoid aspect) and in the orbit. It usually does not grow to large size: because of the age group and site it affects, it is recognized and treated before this can happen. The mass is not painful, unless it compresses a nerve (Fig. 778).

RADIOGRAPHIC FEATURES

There is nothing typical about it; usually calcification is absent. The tumor may erode and cancel the adjacent bones, particularly in the cranium, forearm, hand and foot.

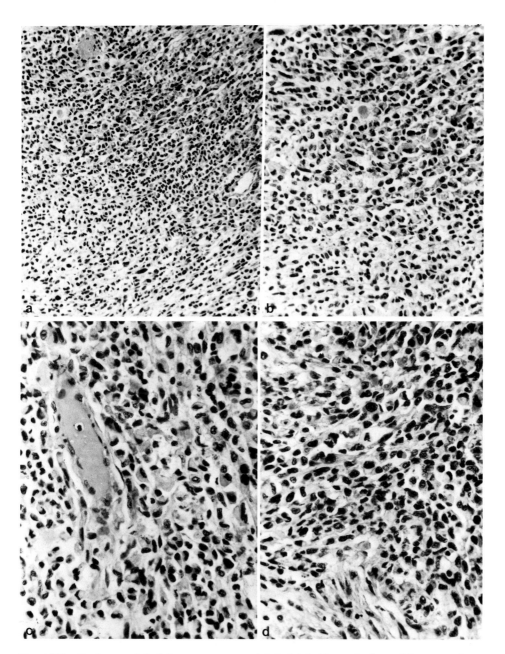

FIG. 779. - Embryonal rhabdomyosarcoma. (a) Solid field in which proliferation of undifferentiated round-oval cells is observed, which do not take on any particular
aspects or structural aggregation. (b) Undifferentiated round-oval cells with a hyperchromic nucleus and variable quantity of intensely eosinophilic cytoplasm. (c) and
(d) At higher power the various grades of rhabdomyoblastic differentiation are observed. The aspects vary from round-oval cells with hyperchromic nuclei and very
scarce cytoplasm, to cells in which the rhabdomyoblastic differentiation is recognizable. In the latter, a variable quantity of intensely eosinophilic cytoplasm is observed
which may have a ground glass aspect; round-oval cells are at times mixed with spindle cells (*Hemat.-eos.*, 160, 250, 400, 400 x).

Arteriography shows the aspects common to any well-vascularized malignant neoplasm.

CAT with contrast medium and MRI are the most important examinations as they reveal the situation, volume, boundaries and relationships of the tumor.

Other useful examinations may be bone scan of the skeleton (possible skeletal metastases) and lymphography (frequent lymphonodal metastases).

GROSS PATHOLOGIC FEATURES

The tumoral mass, whether single or plurilobulated, is generally soft due to its prevalently cellular composition, at times it contains myxoid or cystic areas. Color varies from gray-pink to light brown and there are frequent necrotic-hemorrhagic modifications. Its boundaries are not distinct, due to evident infiltration of the surrounding tissues.

When the tumor grows towards a mucous cavity (biliary tract, bladder, urethra, vagina, conjunctiva) it assumes a polypoid and myxoid aspect, which has been compared to a bunch of grapes and thus defined, from the Greek, «botryoid». The botryoid aspect is only a modulation of the embryonal variety, due to localization.

HISTOPATHOLOGIC FEATURES

Embryonal R.M.S.. It recalls the various stages of embryonal development of the striated muscle, with a considerable variability from case to case. In most cases undifferentiated cells prevail and only sporadic aspects of differentiation may be observed. In this case the tumor is characterized by **small round cells**. At other times, instead, it is more diffusedly and evidently differentiated, enough to recall the aspect of the fetal muscle (Fig. 779).

In all cases, densely cellular areas are alternated with others where the cells are more scattered and have a myxoid aura. Another constant feature is that the cells are distributed without order, and among them the reticular and collagen fibers are very scarce.

The undifferentiated cells are small, with a round-oval nucleus (rarely spindle), decidedly hyperchromic. The nuclear membrane is evident, the chromatin granules distinct; one or two nucleoli are clearly evident. As differentiation progresses, the volume of the cell increases. The nucleus becomes larger, tending towards being vesicular, with a large nucleolus. The cytoplasm is intensely eosinophilic, granular, there are filaments which may be wrapped around the nucleus; finally, transverse striations may be recognized. The less differentiated cells are globose with a thin perinuclear cytoplasmatic ring; as differentiation progresses cytoplasm is more ample, the shape is like a racket or a tad-pole and the nucleus is eccentric; finally, they take on a ribbon shape, at times long and angulated like broken straws of hay. In these last elongated cells with one or two nuclei, transverse striation may be observed.

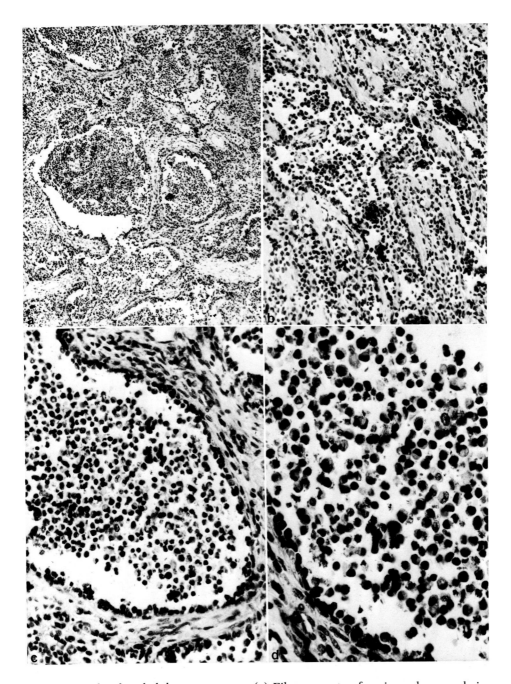

Fig. 780. - Alveolar rhabdomyosarcoma. (a) Fibrous septa of various shape and size circumscribe «alveolar» areas in which cells loosely arranged are observed. (b-c) The cells at the periphery of the alveolar spaces adhere to the fibrous septa. The cells at the center of the alveolar spaces are more scattered, with no intercellular matrix. (d) Round cells of varying size constitute the neoplasm. The nuclei are hyperchromic, the cytoplasm intensely eosinophilic may be extremely scarce or, if the cells are more differentiated, more abundant, granular, eosinophilic and it may push the nucleus towards the periphery (*Hemat.-eos.*, 60, 160, 250, 400 x).

Pleomorphism is considerable, or evident; mitotic figures are numerous.

At times the globose cells with ample cytoplasm appear to be vacuolated (due to dissolution of the glycogen during the histological preparation) and the cytoplasm may be reduced to filaments which from the nucleus irradiate to the periphery: «spider-web cells».

Alveolar R.M.S. It is made up of small round-oval cells (undifferentiated or scarcely differentiated) collected in solid islands or alveoli. The alveolar aspect is suggested by the fact that the cells of the peripheral border adhere to the wall, at times forming a row which recalls an epithelium, while the central ones are scattered and «fluctuate» in the lumen. Islands and alveoli are demarcated by rough bands of dense collagen, convoluted and ramified, containing dilated capillaries (Figs. 780, 781).

The aspects of differentiation (rhabdomyoblasts with ample eosinophilic, filamentous, and granulous cytoplasm) are much rarer as compared to embryonal R.M.S. Instead, multinucleate giant cells are present, with a pale central cytoplasm (never striated) and crown-like peripheral nuclei.

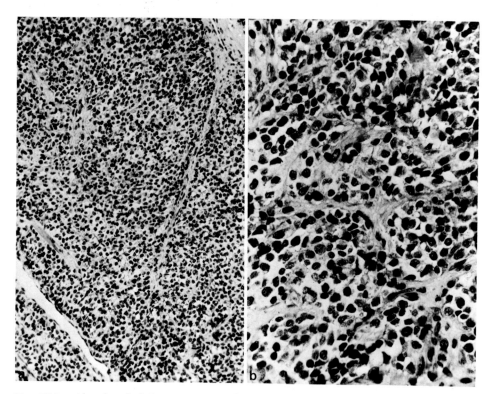

FIG. 781. - Alveolar rhabdomyosarcoma having solid areas. (a) Alongside areas of alveolar aspect, fields with a solid aspect are observed in which round cells of relatively monomorphous aspect appear to be closely aggregated. (b) Undifferentiated mesenchymal round cells are mixed with cells in which rhabdomyoblastic differentiation is recognizable: hyperchromic nucleus with scarce granular eosinophilic cytoplasm, at times abundant pale or vacuolized cytoplasm (*Hemat.-eos.*, 160, 400 x).

Pleomorphic R.M.S.. It is a very pleomorphic tumor, with globose and spindle cells, giant cells, racket and tad-pole cells. The cytoplasm is intensely eosinophilic, filamentous and granulous, but transverse striations are **rarely** observed (Fig. 782).

SPECIAL STAINING AND ELECTRON MICROSCOPY

PAS-diastasis. As differentiation increases, the cytoplasms become more and more PAS positive. As this positiveness is annulled by pre-treatment with diastasis, we are dealing with glycogen.

Ferric hematoxylin, phosphotungstic acid-hematoxylin (PTAH), Masson trichromic: these more effectively visualize the microfibrillae and the transverse striations (positive to these hematoxylins and to Masson fuchsin).

Silver stain for the reticulum. It shows the scarcity of reticular fibers and intercellular collagen.

Immunohistochemisty. The use of human antimyoglobin serums, both on fresh tissue examined under fluorescent light, and on tissue fixed in formalin with immunoperoxidase technique, reveals the rhabdomyoblastic nature of the more differentiated cells (Fig. 782d). These will also be positive for actin and myosin.

Electron microscopy. It reveals the filaments of myosin and actin and the transverse bands.

HISTOGENESIS

R.M.S. seems to originate from the undifferentiated mesenchymal cells or perhaps from areas of embryonal muscle tissue which remained excluded. This would explain the higher incidence during childhood and even the occurrence of the tumor in anatomical regions normally deprived of striated muscles.

DIAGNOSIS

It is above all based on the recognition of rhabdomyoblasts. For this, multiple and extensive samples, excellent specimens, supplementary staining, immunohistochemistry and electron microscopy are required and useful. The transverse striation must be searched for particularly in the more differentiated cells (ribbon-like). It is frequently observed in embryonal R.M.S., more rarely in alveolar R.M.S. (in this, however, diagnosis is favored by the alveolar structure and the characteristic giant cells); it is an exceptional occurrence in pleomorphic R.M.S.

Differential diagnosis, particularly in less differentiated R.M.S., may be difficult, and must be made with several small round cell or «blue cell» tumors: **Ewing's sarcoma, neuroblastoma, neuroepithelioma, malignant lymphoma, malignant melanoma**, and (in adult age) **small-cell carcinomas**. In some of these tumors glycogen is absent (neuroblastoma, lymphomas), in

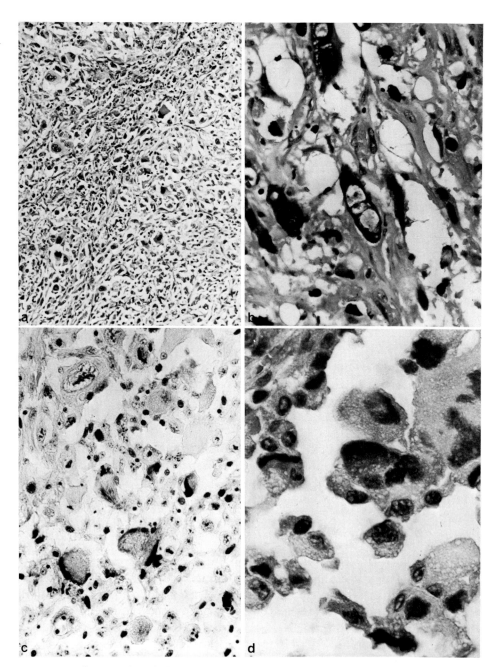

FIG. 782. - Pleomorphic rhabdomyosarcoma. (a) Evidently pleomorphic aspect of the cellular proliferation is observed: in fact, round-oval cells are mixed with giant, multinucleate cells and with spindle ones. In some cells intensely eosinophilic cytoplasm may be observed. (b) The cellular pleomorphism, hyperchromia and nuclear monstruosity are common cytological aspects in pleomorphic rhabdomyosarcoma. (c) Ample intensely eosinophilic cytoplasm with «crystalloid» structures and PAS positiveness are frequent. (d) The myoglobin which may be seen in the cytoplasm of a markedly pleomorphic neoplasm may be useful in identifying the rhabdomyoblastic differentiation (*Hemat.-eos.* 160, 400, 400 x; *PAP myoglobin*, 400 x).

others the reticulum abounds (lymphomas), in others specific markers may be detected.

Alveolar R.M.S. must not be confused with **alveolar sarcoma of the soft tissues**, which has a pseudo-endocrine structure and PAS positive, diastasis resistant crystals.

Pleomorphic R.M.S. is distinguished from **malignant fibrous histiocytoma** because in the latter the glycogen is variable and scarce and the collagen much more abundant.

COURSE

It is rather rapid and aggressive. There is a marked tendency towards local recurrence after inadequate surgical excision and without adjuvant therapy. Tendency to metastasize is very lively, in decreasing order in the lungs, lymph nodes, skeleton, internal organs, and brain. Lymph node metastases may occur early, and are more frequent in paratesticular R.M.S.

PROGNOSIS

As in Ewing's sarcoma, 30 years ago, with surgical and or radiation treatment alone, five-year survival rate was equal to approximately 10%. Nowadays, with combined surgery, radiation and chemotherapy, this percentage comes close to 80% for cases which at the onset of treatment do not have evidence of metastases. Alveolar R.M.S. has a worse prognosis than embryonal R.M.S. and thus localizations in the limbs — where the alveolar form predominates — tend to have a worse prognosis. Instead, the grade of histological differentiation and age are not of prognostic value.

STAGE CLASSIFICATION

The American Rhabdomyosarcoma Study Intergroup has proposed a 4-tage classification system: 1) localized tumor, surgically removed completely (wide excision), negative lymph nodes; 2) microscopic residues of tumor (marginal excision) and/or positive lymph nodes; 3) macroscopic residues of tumor (intralesional excision); 4) distant metastases. This classification system calls for CAT, skeletal bone scan, lymphography, systematic biopsy of the regional lymph nodes, macroscopic and histological study of the surgical margins.

TREATMENT

The treatment suggested is as follows: preoperative chemotherapy; surgical excision, possibly wide; better still with excision of the regional lymph nodes. When the excision is not wide, radiation therapy on the site of the primary tumor and on the lymph nodes (4000-6000 r). In all cases, cyclical polychemotherapy (vincristine, actinomycin-D, cyclophosphamide and adriamycin) for 2 years.

REFERENCES

1952 PACK G.T., EBERHART W.F.: Rhabdomyosarcoma of skeletal muscle. Report of 100 cases. *Surgery*, **32**, 1023.

1962 DITO W.R., BETSAKIG J.G.: Rhabdomyosarcoma of the head and neck: Appraisal of biologic behavior in 170 cases. *Arch. Surg.*, **84**, 582.

1965 JOHNSON W., JURAND J., HIRAMOTO R.: Immunohistologic studies of tumors containing myosin. *Am. J. Pathol.*, **47**, 1139.

1965 JONES I.S., REESE A.B., KROUT J.: Orbital rhabdomyosarcoma: An analysis of 62 cases. *Trans. Am. Ophthalmol. Soc.*, **63**, 223.

1965 LINSCHEID R.L., SOULE E.H., HENDERSON E.D.: Pleomorphic rhabdomyosarcomata of the extremities and limb girdles. A clinicopathological study. *J. Bone Joint Surg.*, **47A**, 715.

1965 MASSON J.K., SOULE E.H.: Embryonal rhabdomyosarcoma of the head and neck. Report of 88 cases. *Am. J. Surg.*, **110**, 585.

1967 MAHOUR G.H., SOULE E.H., MILLS S.D. *et al.*: Rhabdomyosarcoma in infants and children. A clinicopathological study of 75 cases. *J. Pediatr. Surg.*, **2**, 402.

1968 KEYHANI A., BOOHER R.J.: Pleomorphic rhabdomyosarcoma. *Cancer*, **22**, 956.

1968 McNEER G.P., CANTIN J., CHU F. *et al.*: Effectiveness of radiation therapy in the management of sarcoma of the soft somatic tussues. *Cancer*, **22**, 391.

1968 NELSON A.J.: Embryonal rhabdomyosarcoma. Report of 24 cases and study of the effectiveness of radiation therapy upon the primary tumor. *Cancer*, **22**, 64.

1969 ENZINGER F.M., SHIRAKI M.: Alveolar rhabdomyosarcoma. An analysis of 110 cases. *Cancer*, **24**, 18.

1969 SOULE E.H., GEITZ M., HENDERSON E.D.: Embryonal rhabdomyosarcoma of the limbs and limb-girdles. A clinicopathologic study of 61 cases. *Cancer*, **23**, 1336.

1970 HILGERS R.D., MALKASIAN G.D. JR., SOULE E.H.: Embryonal rhabdomyosarcoma (botryoid type) of the vagina: A clinicopathologic review. *Am. J. Obstet. Gynecol.*, **107**, 484.

1970 HORVAT B.L., CAINES M., FISHER E.R.: The ultrastructure of rhabdomyosarcoma. *Am. J. Clin. Pathol.*, **53**, 555.

1970 SUTOW W.W., SULLIVAN M.P., RIED H.L. *et al.*: Prognosis in childhood rhabdomyosarcoma. *Cancer*, **25**, 1384.

1971 EHRLICH F.E., HASS J.E., KIESEWETTER W.B.: Rhabdomyosarcoma in infants and children. Factors affecting long-term survival. *J. Pediatr. Surg.*, **6**, 571.

1972 BRADEL E.J., NEWTON W.A.: Electron microscopic analysis of rhabdomyosarcoma of children. *Am. J. Pathol.*, **66**, 25A.

1973 DONALDSON S.S., CASTRO J.R., WILBUR J.R. *et al.*: Rhabdomyosarcoma of the head and neck in children. Combination treatment by surgery, irradiation, and chemotherapy. *Cancer*, **31**, 26.

1973 GHAVIMI F., EXELBY P.R., D'ANGIO G.J. *et al.*: Combination therapy of urogenital embryonal rhabdomyosarcoma in children. *Cancer*, **32**, 1178.

1973 HOLTON C.P., CHAPMEN K.E., LACKEY R.W. *et al.*: Extended combination therapy of childhood rhabdomyosarcoma. *Cancer*, **32**, 1310.

1973 JAFFE N., FILLER R.M., FARBER S. *et al.*: Rhabdomyosarcoma in children. Improved outlook with a multidisciplinary approach. *Am. J. Surg.*, **125**, 482.

1973 KILMAN J.W., CLATWORTHY H.W., NEWTON W.A. *et al.*: Reasonable surgery for rhabdomyosarcoma. Study of 67 cases. *Ann. Surg.*, **178**, 346.

1974 EXELBY P.R.: Management of embryonal rhabdomyosarcoma in children. *Surg. Clin. North Am.*, **54**, 849.

1974 HEYN R.M., HOLLAND R., NEWTON W.A. *et al.*: The role of combined chemotherapy in the treatment of rhabdomyosarcoma in children. *Cancer*, **34**, 2128.

1975 ARIEL I., BRICENO M.: Rhabdomyosarcoma of the extremities and trunk. *J. Surg. Oncol.*, **7**, 269.

1975 BALE P.M., REYE R.D.: Rhabdomyosarcoma in childhood. *Pathology*, **7**, 101.

1975 FREEMAN J.E.: Changing concepts in the management of Wilms' tumor and rhabdomyosarcoma. *Proc. R. Soc. Med.*, **68**, 660.

1975 GHAVIMI F., EXELBY P.R., D'ANGIO G.J. *et al.*: Multidisciplinary treatment of embryonal rhabdomyosarcoma in children. *Cancer*, **35**, 677.

1975 HEYN R.M.: The role of chemotherapy in the management of soft tissue sarcomas. *Cancer*, **35**, 921.

1975 JOHNSON D.G.: Trends in surgery for childhood rhabdomyosarcoma. *Cancer*, **35**,
916.

1976 WEICHERT K.A., BOVE K.C., ARON B.S. *et al.*: Rhabdomyosarcoma in children. A
clinicopathologic study of 35 patients. *Am. J. Clin. Pathol.*, **66**, 692.

1977 LAWRENCE W. JR., HAYS D.M., MOON T.E.: Lymphatic metastasis with childhood
rhabdomyosarcoma. *Cancer*, **39**, 556.

1977 MAURER H.M., MOON T., DONALDSON M. *et al.*: The Intergroup Rhabdomyosarcoma Study: A preliminary report. *Cancer*, **40**, 2015.

1977 RANSOM J.L., PRATT C.B., SHANKS E.: Childhood rhabdomyosarcoma of the extremity. Results of combined modality therapy. *Cancer*, **40**, 2810.

1977 RAZEK A.A., PEREX C.A., LEE F.A. *et al.*: Combined treatment modalities of rhabdomyosarcoma in children. *Cancer*, **39**, 2415.

1977 TEFFT M., FERNANDEZ C.H., MOON T.E.: Rhabdomyosarcoma: Response with chemotherapy prior to radiation in patients with gross residual disease. *Cancer*,
39, 665.

1978 CHURG A., RINGUS J.: Ultrastructural observations on the histogenesis of alveolar rhabdomyosarcoma. *Cancer*, **41**, 1355.

1978 GREEN D.M., JAFFE N.: Progress and controversy in the treatment of childhood
rhabdomyosarcoma. *Cancer Treat. Rev.*, **5**, 7.

1979 DRITSCHILO A., WEICHSELBAUM R. CASSIDY J.R. *et al.*: The role of radiation therapy in treatment of soft tissue sarcomas of childhood. *Cancer*, **42**, 1192.

1979 MUKAI K., ROSAI J., HALLAWAY B.E.: Localization of myoglobin in normal and
neoplastic human skeletal muscle cells using an immunoperoxidase method.
Am. J. Surg. Pathol., **3**, 373.

1980 HAYS D.M.: Pelvic rhabdomyosarcomas in childhood. *Cancer*, **45**, 1810.

1980 MIERAU G.W., FAVARA B.E.: Rhabdomyosarcoma in children. Ultrastructural study of 31 cases. *Cancer*, **46**, 2035.

1981 CORSON J.M., PINKUS G.S.: Intracellular myoglobin — a specific marker for skeletal muscle differentiation in soft tissue sarcomas. An immunoperoxidase study. *Am. J. Pathol.*, **103**, 384.

1981 MUKAI K., SCHOLLMEYER J., ROSAI J.: Immunohistochemical localization of actin.
Applications in surgical pathology. *Am. J. Surg. Pathol.*, **5**, 91.

1984 FLAMANT F., HILL C.: The improvement in survival associated with combined
chemotherapy in childhood rhabdomyosarcoma. A historical comparison of
345 patients in the same center. *Cancer*, **53**, 2417.

1984 DONALDSON S.S., BELLI J.A.: A rational clinical staging system for childhood
rhabdomyosarcoma. *J. Clin. Oncol.*, **2**, 135.

1985 DONALDSON S.S.: The value of adjuvant chemotherapy in the management of
sarcoma in children. *Cancer*, **55**, 2184.

1985 SAKU T., TSUDA N., ANAMI M., OKABE H.: Smooth and skeletal muscle myosins
in spindle cell tumors of soft tissue. An immunohistochemical study. *Acta Pathol. Jpn.*, **35(1)**, 125-36.

1986 ALTMANNSBERGER M., DIRK T., OSBORN M., WEBER K.: Immunohistochemistry
of cytoskeletal filaments in the diagnosis of soft tissue tumors. *Semin.
Diagn. Pathol.*, **3**, 306.

1987 DE LONG A.S., VAN KESSEL-VAN VARK M., ALBUS-LUTTER C.E.: Pleomorphic rhabdomyosarcoma in adults: immunohistochemistry as a tool for diagnosis.
Hum. Pathol., **18**, 298.

1987 HAWKINS H.K., CAMACHO-VELASQUEZ J.V.: Rhabdomyosarcoma in children.
A correlation of form and prognosis in our institutions's experience. *Am. J.
Surg. Pathol.*, **11**, 531.

1989 DODD S., MALONE M., MC CULLOCH W.: Rhabdomyosarcoma in children: histological and immunohistochemical study of 59 cases. *J. Pathol.*, **158**, 13.

1989 GHAVIMI F., MANDELL R.L., HELLER G., HAJDU S.I., EXELBY P.: Prognosis in
childhood rhabdomyosarcoma of the extremity. *Cancer*, **64**, 2233.

1989 KODET R.: Rhabdomyosarcoma in childhood Immunohistological analysis
with Myoglobin, Desmin and Vimentin. *Pathol. Res. (Pract.)*, **185**, 207.

ANGIOMAS AND ANGIODYSPLASIAS

This chapter includes congenital modifications of the soft tissues of two types: 1) **vascular hamartomas** (angiomas), hematic or much more rarely lymphatic; 2) **congenital angiodysplasias**, particulaly venous anomalies and arteriovenous fistulae. The classification which we propose is as follows.

1) Isolated cutaneous and subcutaneous angiomas.
2) Single and localized deep angiomas.
3) Deep and extended angiomas.
4) Multiple angiomas (superficial and/or deep) in the same limb.
5) Angiomas (superficial and/or deep) diffused to one or more limbs.
6) Lymphangiomas.
7) Infantile angectatic osteohyperplastic syndromes.
8) Congenital arterovenous fistulae.

All of these pathological changes are not hereditary, they show predilection for the female sex, they initiate at birth or during childhood-young age.

Vascular angiomas or hamartomas are formed at the onset by capillary vessels (Fig. 787) which generally proliferate until body growth has ended. The capillary vessels tend to be transformed into caverns, pseudoveins and pseudoarterioles. Communication between the vessels of the hamartoma and the general circulation is scarce in single and localized angiomas, but it becomes more and more extensive the more extended, multiple and diffused the angiomas are.

ISOLATED CUTANEOUS AND SUBCUTANEOUS ANGIOMAS

We refer here to pseudotumoral angiomas, and not to simple discolorations of the skin. These angiomas are generally present at birth, or they may occur during childhood, and tend to grow slowly during the first years of life. They are reddish-wine in color if cutaneous, and hardly cause skin coloring if subcutaneous. They are not painful. Their histological structure may be capillary, cavernous, or pseudovenous.

SINGLE AND LOCALIZED DEEP ANGIOMAS

These constitute the most frequent benign tumor of the skeletal muscles.

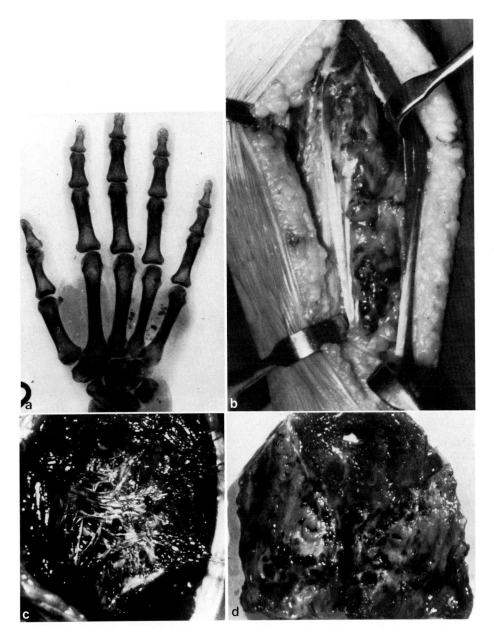

FIG. 783. - Cavernous angioma. (a) Female aged 20 years. Deep cavernous angiomas of the hand. Observe the radiographic image of the phlebolites, pathognomic for angioma. (b) Female aged 16 years. Muscular cavernous angioma extended to the deep flexor muscles of the forearm. Observe diffusion of the dark red spots and nodules, in the muscular bellies. (c) Male aged 15 years. Angioma circumscribed to the quadriceps, of the pseudovenous type. Observe the sponge of cavities characterized by a thick whitish fibrous wall, intercommunicating and empty of blood after aperture. (d) Female aged 18 years. Angioma circumscribed to the sublimis flexor muscle in the forearm, of the cavernous type. Observe multiple nodules dark red in color, scattered throughout the muscular tissue and surrounded by degenerated muscle and fibrous reactive tissue.

Nearly always the angioma is contained within the belly of a single muscle; it is only in the hand and foot that they extend between the aponeurosis, muscles, and tendons. There is evident predilection for the lower limb.

Rarely apparent at birth, angioma tends to manifest its first signs during childhood or adolescence, rarely between 20 and 30 years.

Symptoms consist of swelling, which often decreases when the limb is squeezed and increases with venous stasis, and particularly of pain, which may be sharp. As pain is accentuated by tension of the muscle containing the angioma, shortening of this same muscle often occurs, at first functional and then organic. Such shortening causes first limitation, then deformity of the joint (for example, limited flexion of the knee in angioma of the quadriceps, flexed knee in angioma of the flexor muscles, equinus foot in angioma of the sural triceps). In localizations in the hand and foot an increase in skin temperature and in the superficial venous reticulum, telangectasia, cyanosis and hyperhydrosis are observed.

Radiograms are often negative. At times there is mild localized periostotic reaction, or some phlebolite (small round grain of calcar opacity, having a smooth surface, at times characterized by aspects of concentric stratification, Fig. 783a), or faded calcification like «cigarette smoke». **Arteriography** is negative when it is a small or prevalently capillary angioma. Otherwise, it reveals thin arterial branches terminating in bunch-like faded opacities, which persist even after regression of the venous phase. Diagnostic typical images are produced by CAT (with contrast dye) and MRI (Fig. 784).

Macroscopically cavernous angioma, which is the most frequent to occur, resembles a bunch of scattered nodules, which may be very small or larger, dull red in color when the connective wall is thin, bluish when it is thicker, completely filled with blood, with internal cloistering which is not very visible (Fig. 783d). The areas of capillary angioma are more compact and pinkish. Pseudovenous angioma is like a sponge, with whitish fibrous cloisters and intercommunicating lacunae containing stagnant blood, thrombi and at times phlebolites (Fig. 783c). There is not much bleeding on surgical removal, as communication between the hamartoma and the circulation is scarce.

Histologically the most frequent finding is that of the caverns, bunches of extremely dilated dysplastic vessels having a very thin wall constituted by flattened endothelium and by a collagen membrane, filled with blood in tension (Fig. 788). There are also pseudoarterioles, convoluted and cylindrical vessels, with a thick pseudoarteriose wall which is deprived of internal elastic membrane. Furthermore, pseudoveins are observed: craggy ramified and labyrinthic cavities, with very irregular and poorly formed pseudovenous walls, containing very little blood, at times thrombi and phlebolites (Fig. 789). Finally, hamartomatous capillaries are observed, with all of the stages of transformation into caverns, pseudoveins and pseudoarterioles (Fig. 790).

Preoperative **diagnosis** is possible in most cases based on sharp pain localized in a restricted area, contraction-retraction of the muscle. When phlebolites are present in the x-ray, they are pathognomic. Arteriography, instead,

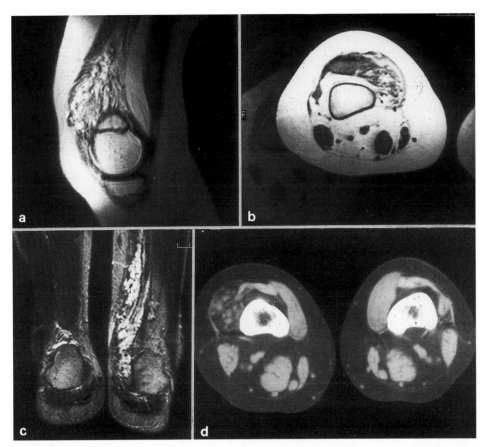

FIG. 784. - Cavernous angioma of the muscle. (a) and (b) Female aged 13 years. Cavernous angioma of the vastus medialis (MRI). (c) Female aged 26 years. Extended angioma which involves the muscles, subcutaneous tissue and surrounds the neurovascular bundle (MRI). (d) Female aged 27 years: contrast CAT shows typical spotted
aspect with dense spots separated by hypodense areas. The angioma is contained in the
vastus lateralis. (Publishing courtesy of Prof. J.M. Van Loon and Dr. J.R. Van Horn,
University Hospital, Nijmegen, Netherlands).

may be negative if the angioma is small and there is little communication
with the circulation. CAT (and MRI) is frequently diagnostic, showing multiple little dots taking the contrast dye and contained in an irregular area of
degenerated and fatty muscle.

The **course** of the disease is slow and variable. Worsening may be observed during puberty, pregnancy, or after a trauma.

Treatment is surgical. The angioma is nearly always made up of scattered
vascular bunches. Thus, if we wish to avoid recurrence, excision must be moderately wide. This is possible in angiomas contained within a muscle belly,
where a segment of the entire muscle may have to be removed. It is more difficult in angiomas localized in the hand and foot.

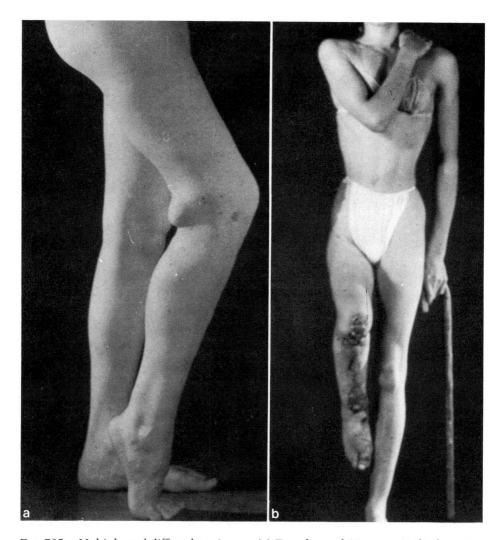

FIG. 785. - Multiple and diffused angiomas. (a) Female aged 16 years. Multiple angiomas of the posterior muscles of the thigh and leg. Observe the muscle swelling (painful) and muscular retraction causing flexed hip, flexed knee and equinus foot fixed deformities. Observe the small cutaneous angiomas in the knee, superficial venous dilatation in the foot and politeal region (large aneurysmal venous sac). There coexists elongation of the limb. (b) Female aged 16 years. Diffused angioma of the lower right limb. Observe the cutaneous angiomas, severe deformity (hip and knee flexed, equinus foot), irregular enlargement of the limb, trophic ulcers. The limb is shortened. In this case, the only type of treatment is amputation.

Prognosis depends on the age of the patient and on the site of the angioma. If the angioma was manifested during early childhood, it is more apt to grow, to recur after incomplete or even complete removal and to transform into an extended or multicentric form of the disease. Thus, during the first years of life, for the purposes of prognostic evaluation, it is important to exclude those initial and associated signs which indicate diagnosis of exten-

FIG. 786. - Diffused angioma. Male aged 23 years. Observe again the association of cutaneous angiomas and deformity in triple flexion of the limb. The patient was submitted to thigh amputation with surgical extension of the hip. The transection of the anatomical specimen reveals diffusion of the angiomas and of the venous varicosities to the superficial and deep tissues. Generally, the skeleton is not or very scarcely involved.

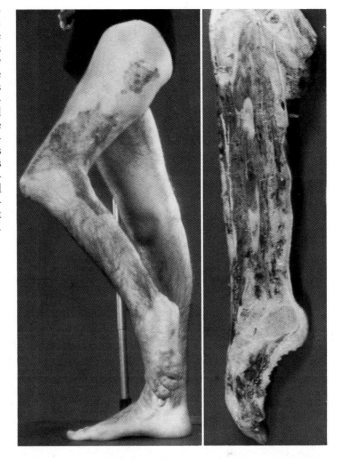

ded, multiple and diffused angioma (see further on). As for the site of the lesion, single and localized angiomas nearly always heal with excision, except for those in the hand and foot, which easily recur. Recurrence may be manifested even more than 5 years after excision.

SINGLE AND EXTENDED DEEP ANGIOMAS

These differ from the previous ones, as compared to which they occur more rarely, by size which is larger, and by extension to a muscular group or in any case to a vast area of tissue (Fig. 783b). Extended angiomas are generally manifested during early age and may nearly all be observed in the lower limb. The symptoms are those previously described, but more marked. There is always an increase in skin temperature; often there is accentuation of the superficial venous reticulum. At times there is mild elongation of the corresponding skeletal segment. Arteriography reveals evident injection of the angioma. Indirect signs (arteriographic, oxymetric) of arterovenous shunt are also frequently observed. Treatment must be planned based on arteriogra-

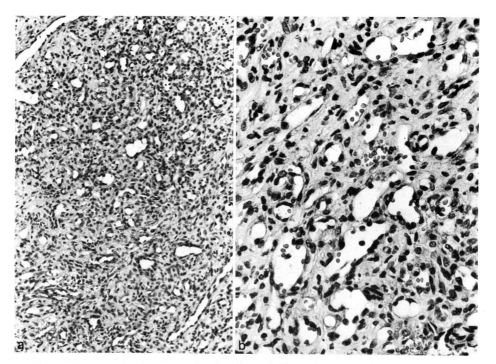

FIG. 787. - Capillary angioma. (a) The neoformation is constituted by numerous small vessels. (b) Capillary vessels are observed, regularly coated with flattened endothelium (*Hemat.-eos.*, 160, 400 x).

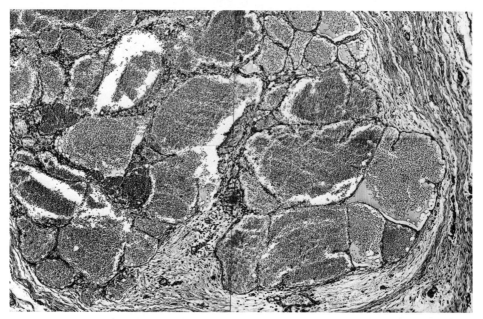

FIG. 788. - Cavernous angioma. This is an overall view of a well-capsulated lesion of lobulated aspect. Extensive lacunae filled with blood, and delimited by thin septa with mature endothelium are observed (*Hemat.-eos.*, 160 x).

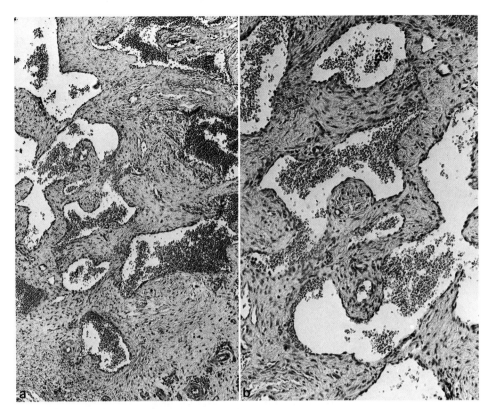

FIG. 789. - Pseudovenous angioma. (a) The neoformation presents wide irregular lacunae which are only partially filled with blood and delimited by thickened walls. (b) The thick walls have a pseudovenous fibromuscular structure (*Hemat.-eos.*, 40, 125 x).

phy. Complete excision of the angioma is hardly feasible without some functional loss.

MULTIPLE ANGIOMAS IN THE SAME LIMB

Whether localized or extended, they involve two or more different areas of the same limb and, in addition to the muscles, they often involve the subcutaneous tissue and the skin (Fig. 785a). The symptoms of deep angiomas are often associated with cutaneous angiomas in the same limb, elongation of the limb and, in particular, diffused venous dilation, at times large varices. An increase in skin temperature, pain, joint limitation and deformities are nearly always constant and progressive with age.

Angiography nearly always reveals multiple angiomas and furthermore it reveals indirect signs of arterovenous shunt and dysplastic venous dilatation (even aneurysmal).

Macroscopically, alongside multiple, localized or extended angiomas, there are often large venous, superficial or deep, tortuous and ectatic canals.

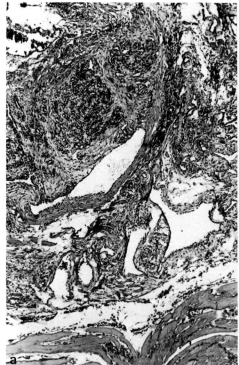
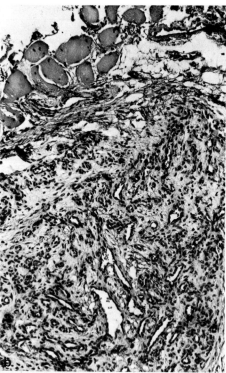
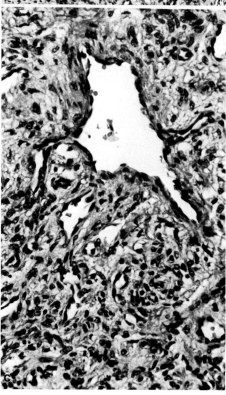

FIG. 790. - Intramuscular angioma. (a) In the muscles there is neoformation constituted by fibrous tissue containing vascular formations of various size. (b) and (c) Small vessels (pseudocapillary), and wider vessels are mixed together. A rather mature endothelium regularly coats the cavities (*Hemat.-eos.*, 60, 160, 400 x).

At times these have a fragile wall and, on surgery, they may cause problems involving difficult hemostasis. **Histologically** these dysplastic veins have an irregular and malformed wall, which may be surrounded by cavernous angiomatous bunches.

Treatment which is based on complete arteriographic and phlebographic examination may pose difficult problems. It consists of excision of the angiomas which is

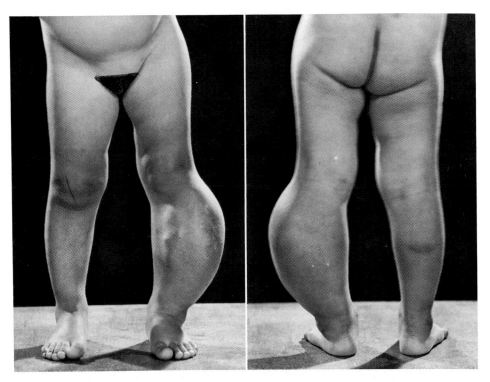

FIG. 791. - Congenital lymphangioma. Boy aged 2 years. Painless swelling, soft, having faded boundaries.

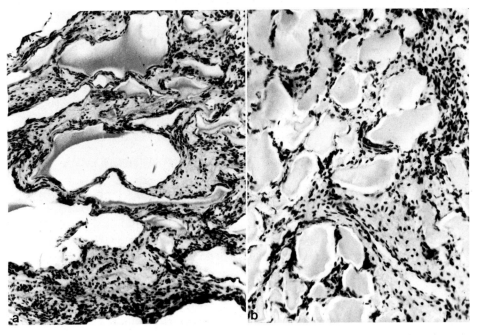

FIG. 792. - Cavernous lymphangioma. (a) and (b) Lymphatic spaces of cavernous aspect are immersed in collagen matrix characterized by rather cellular fields (*Hemat.-eos.*, 160, 250 x).

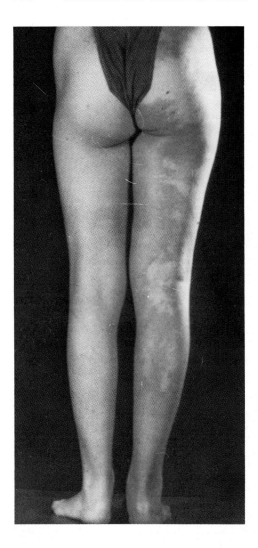

FIG. 793. - Female aged 12 years. In-fantile angiectatic osteohyperplastic syndrome. Observe the cutaneous angioma extended to the lower limb and to the right hemitrunk, elonga-tion and harmonic enlargement of the limb. During advanced age vari-ces are likely to occur. There are no deep swellings (angiomas), pain, muscle retraction and deformity. Arteriography is nearly normal, phlebography often reveals varicose dilatation of superficial and deep veins.

as complete as possible, and in ligature or excision of the vari-ces. This procedure may be diffi-cult or impossible when dealing with dysplastic vessels, which are very diffused at the surface and dilated deeper down, having fragile walls and being richly anastomized together. At times repeated surgical procedures are required. Complete healing is rarely obtained. Nonetheless, when the patient has completed growth, development of hamar-tomas seems to be arrested and the disease becomes chronic, with slow worsening of the vari-ces and of the circulatory, articu-lar and trophic symptoms.

ANGIOMAS DIFFUSED TO ONE OR MORE LIMBS

In this case angiomas are diffused at a maximum, to one or more limbs and to the soft tissues, both superficial and deep (Figs. 785b, 786). Further-more, the regional vascular alterations achieve their highest complexity as it is nearly impossible to determine the boundaries between the angiomas, the associated venous, arterovenous, and arterial dysplasias, and the vascular changes secondary to the altered hemodynamics of the region. Furthermore, there may coexist other dysplastic changes, as lymphangiomas, hyperplasia of the subcutaneous fat, enlargement of the nerve trunks. The site may be an entire lower limb, two limbs, or somatic territories which are even vaster.

The disease is nearly always evident at birth (particularly with cutaneous angiomas, enlargement, elongation of the limb, partial giantism). Pain, joint deformities, varices occur later. The greatest progression in the disease is often observed during puberty. In exceptional cases, in very diffused angiomas, **defects in coagulation** due to thrombocytopenia are associated (as if angiomas favored the destruction of the platelets stagnating in their cavernous spaces).

Differential diagnosis may involve some forms of elephantiasis and partial giantism in **neurofibromatosis**, but above all **infantile osteohyperplastic angiectatic syndromes**.

Effective surgical treatment is not possible. Deformities may be corrected by osteotomy or arthrodesis. At times amputation is required. Generally angiomas cease to grow after 20-25 years of age.

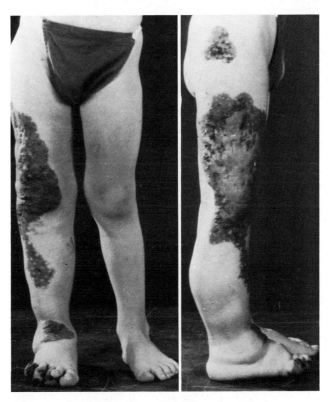

LYMPHANGIOMAS

They occur at birth and during the first years of life and there is no predilection for sex (Fig. 791).

The sites of election are the head-neck and axilla which represent those areas in which lymphatic vascularization is more diffused.

This lesion may be presented as a **cystic lymphangioma** in which few cystic lacunae are observed or as **cavernous lymphangioma** made up of

FIG. 794. - Male aged 12 years. Infantile angiectatic osteohyperplastic syndrome. The angiomas are superficial, there is neither pain nor joint deformity.

numerous confluent lacunae (Fig. 792).

Histologically, the lacunae are walled with round-ovoid cells arranged in a single endothelial layer. Collagen fibers or smooth muscle cells surround the lymphatic lacunae.

The lymphatic spaces are empty or full of serum with lymphocytes or rarely erythrocytes.

Treatment of choice is surgery. The size, localization in particular sites influence the type of surgery used.

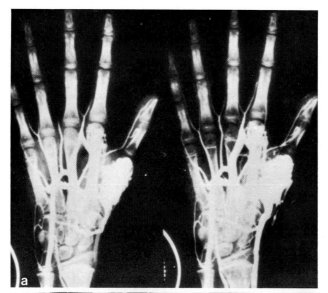

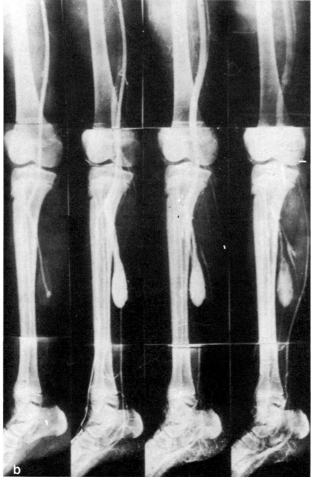

FIG. 795. - Congenital arterovenous fistulae. (a) Male aged 12 years. Congential arterovenous fistulae surrounding the first metacarpal. The first two metacarpals are elongated. Arteriography reveals a thick mesh of dilated vessels entangling the first metacarpal, dilatation of the arteries, immediate venous return, relative ischemia of the fingers. (b) Female aged 11 years. Single congenital arterovenous fistula of the tibialis posterior. Arteriography reveals the large fistula, the venous sac where the fistula enters, immediate venous return. The femoral artery and the femoral vein are dilated above the fistula. The arteries are instead filiform below.

INFANTILE ANGIECTATIC OSTEOHYPERPLASTIC SYNDROMES

These are dysplastic modifications diffused to a limb, characterized by flat cutaneous angiomas, skeletal elongation, and venous dilatation (Figs. 793, 794). There is still evident predilection for the female sex and the site nearly always corresponds to a lower limb. The syndrome is manifested at birth or during early childhood. The difference as compared with the previous forms is constituted by the **absence of deep angiomas**. Thus, there is no pain, no joint limitation, or deformities, no shortening of a limb. In addition to being elongated (up to 7-8 cm), the limb tends to increase in volume, due to harmonic hyperplasia of all of its tissues. Dilated or varicose veins are associated, at times clinical signs (even cardiocirculatory ones) of arterovenus fistulae. Apart from the eumorphic hyperplasia, radiographically the skeleton of the limb is normal. Angiography may reveal a nearly normal picture, or arteriose and/or venous anomalies, or better yet signs of diffused congenital arterovenous shunt.

Treatment consists in ligature and removal of the varices, at times made difficult by the thinness and the fragility of their walls; and in the ligature of the thin collateral arterial branches (never of the principal artery) afferent to the arterovenous fistulae. Skeletal elongation may be corrected with epiphysiodesis or with removal of a diaphyseal cylinder once growth has ended.

WIDE CONGENITAL ARTEROVENOUS FISTULAE

These include cases of simple arterovenous fistulae, of cirsoid aneurysm (in the hand and in the scalp) and of arterovenous angioma. They prevail in the upper limb, particularly the hand (Fig. 795). Symptoms generally begin during childhood or adolescence. They may, however, be manifested during adult age (compensated or latent arterovenous fistulae), mostly following trauma. Symptoms consist of pain (partially ischemic), pulsating swelling, increase in local warmth in the area of the fistulae and, on the contrary, cold skin, cyanosis and pallor distal to the fistulae, severe dilatation of the superficial veins, regional skeletal elongation (if the fistulae are active during fertile age), bruit on the fistulae. The heart is often enlarged and compression on the fistulae causes increase in systemic arterial pressure followed by a decrease in cardiac frequency. There are all of the angiographic and functional signs of a large arterovenous shunt. Treatment consists in ligature of the fistulae (rarely possible) or of the thin arterial branches afferent to it (not the principal artery, as this could worsen ischemia in the distal regions). At times, particularly in the fingers, amputation is required.

CAPSULO-SYNOVIAL ANGIOMA

There are two anatomo-clinical varieties: localized and extended. C.S.A. is a rare occurrence. There seems to be predilection for the female **sex**. **Age** ranges from birth to 20-30 years, but it is nearly always prepuberal, with a maximum frequency between 5 and 10 years.

Most cases of C.S.A. are observed in the **knee**; in exceptional cases localization may be in the elbow and ankle. It is exceptionally observed in the tendinous sheaths (particularly at the wrist or the ankle) or in a bursa mucosa.

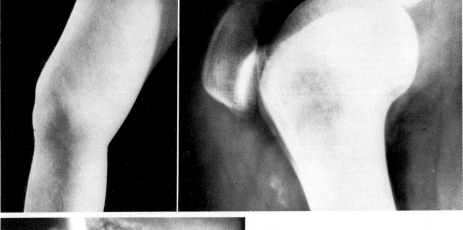

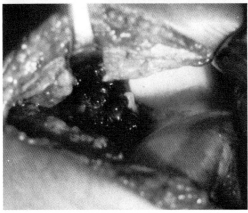

FIG. 796. - Angioma of the synovial membrane, circumscribed. Female aged 18 years. Observe medial parapatellar swelling, calcification in the suprapatellar pouch like «cigarette smoke», and the aspect in the arthrotomy like a bunch of purple grapes.

Symptoms include swelling, pain, hemarthrosis, functional limitation and deformity of the joint, increase in local skin temperature, cutaneous angiomas located close to the joint, dilatation of the regional superficial veins, muscular hypotrophy, alterations in the length of the limb (Figs. 796, 797).

Nonetheless, some of these symptoms are common to different joint lesions, others are only observed in extended joint angiomas.

Symptoms are characterized by a typical remittence or intermittence and may be practically reduced to nothing during the remission phase.

When joint effusion is present, it is nearly always hematic. Hemarthrosis is a rare occurrence in localized angiomas, very frequent in extended ones. These are generally recurring hemarthroses, the cause of diffused synovial hyperplasia.

Repeated episodes of joint blocking of the knee often occur (probably when the tumor remains pinched between the two joint surfaces in movement).

Generally, the **radiographic picture** is negative (apart from a possible diffused osteoporosis in cases with prolonged symptoms and repeated hemarthroses). Phlebolites or «cigarette smoke» calcification are rarely observed (Fig. 796).

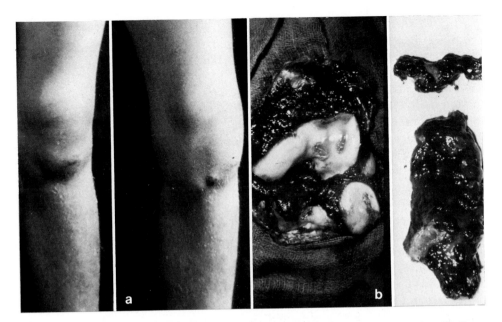

FIG. 797. - Extended synovial angioma. (a) Female aged 8 years. Observe the small cutaneous angiomas and the diffused swelling of the knee. The limb is elongated. (b) Arthrotomy shows thickness and red-brown color of the entire synovial membrane.

Arteriography is completely negative in the case of small localized angioma, or one with a prevalently capillary structure. It may instead reveal the angioma if this is wide and or extended, having a cavernous or pseudovenous structure. The contrast medium remains in the hamartomatous vessels for a long time. CAT and MRI may show the angioma in the capsule and synovial membrane.

Macroscopically, localized angiomas are the most frequent ones and look like one or more bluish-red nodules, at times contained within the thickness of the capsule, at other times slightly bulging on the synovial surface or protruding in the joint, sessile or pediculated (Fig. 796). On the cut surface, the angioma more often has a pseudovenous aspect than a cavernous one.

Extended angiomas are nodules with the same features as those mentioned above, but scattered throughout a wide region or nearly the entire synovial and capsular surface. Then, due to repeated hemarthroses, the synovial membrane tends to appear diffusedly thickened, red-brown or rusty in color (Fig. 797).

Removal of the extended angiomas by means of subtotal synovectomy tends to cause profuse bleeding, which however can always be kept under control.

Histologically, the capillary angiomas are very rare and probably observed only during early age, soon progressing towards the cavernous or pseudovenous forms. Cavernous angiomas are rare and are prevalently observed in the synovial membrane. Pseudovenous angiomas are more frequent and are particularly observed in the capsule.

In extended C.S.A. hyperplastic and diffused villous modifications of the synovial membrane are usually associated, secondary to repeated hemarthroses, with the accumulation of hemosiderin, hyperemia and small lymphocytary infiltrates.

Preoperative diagnosis is easy in extended angiomas, while it is difficult or impossible in localized ones (Table 7). Differential diagnosis of localized angiomas includes the **discoid meniscus** (childhood-young age, pain on the external joint space, signs of trigger phenomena), **mucous cysts of the meniscus** (swelling localized along the joint space of the knee, adult age), **traumatic lesion of the menisci** (young-adult age, evident relationship with distorsional trauma, sensation of an extraneous body and joint insufficiency, pain localized on the internal or external joint space, frequent joint blocking). Differential diagnosis of extended C.S.A. includes **hemophilic arthropathy** (male sex, heredity, signs of hemophilia, polyarticular hemarthroses, absence of every symptom of angioma except for hemarthrosis) and **pigmented villonodular synovitis** (adult or advanced age, progressive swelling, not frankly hematic effusion, anatomical aspects which are completely different).

Treatment consists of surgery and it must aim at complete removal of the angioma(s). This is easily obtained in localized angiomas. But in these lesions, as well, a wide synovial and capsular region must be explored, as angiomatous nodules are often multiple.

In extended angiomas complete removal is often difficult and we must limit our work to partial synovectomy, sometimes performing surgery with an anterior and posterior approach. Radiation therapy is not indicated.

The results of surgical treatment are rather satisfactory. Recurrence is infrequent, and it generally involves cases where excision was incomplete.

Table 7

	Localized synovial angioma	Extended synovial angioma
age at onset of symptoms	late childhood-adolescence	at birth or early childhood
swelling	localized or absent	diffused
hemarthrosis	rare	constant
increase in skin temperature	mild and localized	considerable and diffused to the joint
presence of cutaneous angiomas	—	frequent
superficial venous reticulum	—	constant
skeletal elongation	—	frequent
arteriography	more often negative	more often positive
increase in O_2 in the venous blood	at times slightly positive	often evidently positive

REFERENCES

ANGIOMAS AND ANGIODYSPLASIAS

1956 JOHNSON K.W., GHORMLEY R.K., DOCKERTY M.B.: Hemangiomas of the extremities. *Surg. Gynecol. Obstet.*, **102**, 531.

1956 MacCOLLUM D.W., MARTIN L.W.: Hemangioma in infancy and childhood. A report based on 6479 cases. *Surg. Clin. North. Am.*, **36**, 1647.

1961 BOOHER R.J.: Tumors arising from blood vessels in the hands and feet. *Clin. Orthop.*, **19**, 71.

1961 KASABACH H.H., MERRITT K.K.: Capillary hemangioma with extensive purpura: Report of a case. *Am. J. Dis. Child.*, **59**, 1063.

1962 GOIDANICH I.F., CAMPANACCI N.: Vascular hamartomata and infantile angioectatic osteohyperplasia of the extremities. *J. Bone Joint Surg.*, **44A**, 815.

1966 GONZALES-CRUSSI F., ENNEKING W.F., AREAN V.M.: Infiltrating angiolipoma. *J. Bone Joint Surg.*, **48A**, 1111.

1968 ANGERVALL L., NILSSON L., STENER B. *et al.*: Angiographic, microangiographic, and histologic study of vascular malformation in striated muscle. *Acta Radiol.*, **7**, 65.

1968 GOIDANICH I.F., CAMPANACCI M.: *Vascular hamartomas and angiodysplasias of the extremities.* Springfield, Ill., Charles Thomas Publisher.

1972 ALLEN P.W., ENZINGER F.M.: Hemangioma of skeletal muscle. An analysis of 89 cases. *Cancer*, **29**, 8.

1972 FERGUSSON I.L.: Hemangiomata of skeletal muscle. *Br. J. Surg.*, **59**, 634.

1972 TRIAS A., DILENGE D.: A new approach to the treatment of cavernous hemangioma of skeletal muscle. *J. Bone Joint Surg.*, **54B**, 770.

1974 GIRARD C., GRAHAM J.H., JOHNSON W.C.: Arteriovenous hemangioma (arteriovenous shunt). A clinicopathological and histochemical st dy. *J. Clin. Pathol.*, **1**, 73.

1975 SUTHERLAND A.D.: Equinus deformity due to hemangioma of calf muscle. *J. Bone Joint Surg.*, **57B**, 104.

1976 KOJIMA T., IDE Y., MARUMO E. *et al.*: Hemangioma of median nerve causing carpal tunnel syndrome. *Hand*, **8**, 62.

1978 EDGERTON M.T., HIEBERT J.M.: Vascular and lymphatic tumors in infancy, childhood and adulthood: Challenge of diagnosis and treatment. *Curr. Probl. Cancer*, **7**, 1.

1979 COOPER P.H., McALLISTER H.A., HELWIG E.B.: Intravenous pyogenic granuloma. A study of 18 cases. *Am. J. Surg. Pathol.*, **3**, 221.

1980 WOOD M.B.: Intraneural hemangioma: Report of a case. *Plast Reconstr. Surg.*, **65**, 74.

1981 BURGDORF W.C.H., MUKAI K., ROSAI J.: Immunohistochemical identification of Factor VIII — related antigen in endothelial cells of cutaneous lesions of alleged vascular nature. *Am. J. Clin. Pathol.*, **75**, 167.

1983 PASYK K.A., GRABB W.C., CHERRY G.W.: Ultrastructure of mast cells in growing and involuting stages of hemangiomas. *Hum. Pathol.*, **14**, 174.

1986 ALESSI E., BERTANI E., SALA F.: Acquired tufted angioma. *Am. J. Dermatopathol.*, **8**, 426.

LYMPHANGIOMA

1970 FISHER I., ORKIN M.: Acquited lymphangioma (lymphangiectasis). *Arch. Dermatol.*, **101**, 230.

1970 PEACHY R.O., LIMM C.C., WHIMSTER I.W.: Lymphangioma of skin: A review of 65 cases. *Br. J. Dermatol.*. **83**, 519.

1971 SINGH S., BABOO M.: Cystic lymphangioma in children: Report of 32 cases including lesions at rare sites. *Surgery*, **69**, 947.

1973 BARRANA K.G., FREEMAN N.V.: Massive infiltrating cystic hygroma of the neck in infancy. *Arch. Dis. Child*, **48**, 523.

1974 CHAIT D., YONGERS A.J., BEDDOE G.M. *et al*.: Management of cystic hygromas. *Surg. Gynecol. Obstet*, **139**, 55.

1974 FONKALSRUD E.W.: Surgical management of congenital malformation of the lymphatic system. *Am. J. Surg.*, **28**, 152.

1974 NGOC T., NINH T.X.: Cystic hygroma in children: A report of 126 cases. *J. Pediatr. Surg.*, **9**, 191.

1975 KUTARNA A.: Value of lymphangiography in the diagnosis and treatment of lymphangioma. *Neoplasma*, **22**, 81.

1975 SAIJO M., MUNRO I.R., MANCER K.: Lymphangioma: A long-term follow-up study. *Plast Reconstr. Surg.*, **56**, 642.

1977 FLANAGAN B.P., HELWIG E.B.: Cutaneous lymphangioma. *Arch. Dermatol.*, **113**, 24.

1978 CAUWELAERT V., GRUWEZ J.A.: Experience with lymphangioma. *Lymphology*, **11**, 43.

1983 TSYB A.F., MUKHAMEDZHANOV I.H.K., GUSEVA L.I.: Lymphangiomatosis of bone and soft tissue (results of lymphangiographic examinations). *Lymphology*, **16**, 181.

CAPSULO-SYNOVIAL ANGIOMA

1930 BURMAN M.S., MILGRAM J.E.: Hemangioma of tendon and tendon sheath. *Surg. Gynecol. Obstet*, **50**, 397.

1937 HARKINS H.N.: Hemangioma of a tendon sheath: Report of a case with a study of 24 cases from the literature. *Arch. Surg.*. **34**, 12.

1939 BENNETT G.W., COBEY M.C.: Hemangioma of joints. Report of five cases. *Arch. Surg.*, **38**, 487.

1943 COBEY M.C.: Hemangioma of joints. *Arch. Surg.*, **46**, 465.

1954 BATE T.H.: Hemangioma of the tendon sheath. *J. Bone Joint Surg.*, **36A**, 104.

1955 LICHTENSTEIN L.: Tumors of synovial joints, bursae, and tendon sheath. *Cancer*, **8**, 816.

1963 GOIDANICH I.F., CAMPANACCI M., BEDOGNI C.: Amartomi vascolari intrarticolari. Studio di 11 osservazioni. *Chir. Org. Mov.*, **52**, 351.

1978 MCINERNEY D., PARK W.M.: Thermographic assessment of synovial hemangioma. *Clin. Radiol.*, **29**, 469.

GLOMUS TUMOR

Generally, it is a small and capsulated organoid tumor, derived from arterovenous glomi and characterized by very sharp pain.

A rather rare occurrence, there is predilection for the female **sex** and during adult **age**. It is an exceptional occurrence during childhood. Its elective **localization** is the hand, particularly the ungueal bed (Fig. 798) and the subcutaneous tissue of the fingertips or the palm. Similar localizations in the foot and in the subcutaneous tissue of the limbs follow. Localizations in the deep soft tissues and multiple localizations are very rare.

Symptoms are characterized by pain, which is often burning and paroxystic. Pain is not continuous but reawakened or accentuated by pressure, at times by light brushing of the tumor; furthermore, by vasomotorial changes connected with changes in temperature, emotional state, menstruation. At times, pain is irradiated proximally or distally. The tumor may be so small that it cannot be identified with objective examination (Fig. 798). In one of our observations, with pain in the thumb irradiated to the upper limb, the patient had been operated on three times (exploration for suspected cervical disc herniation, syndesmotomy for suspected syndrome of the median nerve in the carpal tunnel, removal of a harmless lipomatous nodule in the arm) without obtaining any results. He was finally judged to be neurotic, until a very small bluish spot was observed in the nail of the thumb; the patient was then submitted to surgery which revealed a G.T. nested in the ungueal bed and as big as a peppercorn. In the subcutaneous sites, not to mention the deeper ones, the nodule may not be palpable. When it is very superficial and if it contains dilated vessels, it may lift up the skin and reveal its bluish color.

G.T. of the ungueal bed do not uplift the nail, rather they dig a niche in the nail bed and at times in the bone of the phalanx. In these cases, a **radiographic examination** may reveal a rounded osteolysis with well-defined boundaries, which is a saucer-like excavation in the dorsal aspect of the phalanx (Fig. 798). Radiographic differential diagnosis involves **dermoid cyst**.

Macroscopically it is a small nodule (Fig. 798), from the size of a peppercorn to a cherry, globose and not always capsulated. It is often compact, soft to firm in consistency and pinkish in color. If it contains dilated vessels, it may be reddish or bluish-red. At times it lifts up and attenuates the skin.

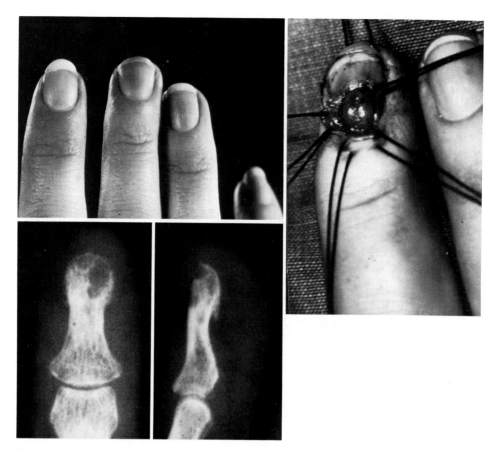

FIG. 798. - Glomus tumor. Female aged 33 years. For the past 20 years pain at the apex of the middle finger, occasionally acute, irradiated to the arm and shoulder. A bluish spot is hardly distinguished on the nail of the middle finger, sharply painful on pressure. After the nail was removed, the bluish-red neoformation was observed. The radiogram revealed saucer-like erosion of the phalanx.

Histologically it is made up of a thick mesh of thin vascular channels, with a normal endothelium. The wall of the vessels, outside the endothelium and the reticular basal membrane, is surrounded by a wide mantle of globose cells located close together, typically epithelioid. These have rather ample cytoplasm, which is light and finely granular, polyhedric in shape as a result of reciprocal contact, and their cytoplasmatic membranes resemble an elegant mosaic. The nuclei are round, well-stained, with an evident nuclear membrane which gives them a somewhat vesicular aspect. When the epithelioid cells are numerous, globose and located close together, the capillaries are collapsed and almost unable to be seen unless silver stain is used, the collagen stroma may be scarce and myxoid, so that there is nearly the impression of an epithelial tumor (Fig. 799). In other cases and in other areas the epithelioid cells take on a more spindle form, until they resemble smooth

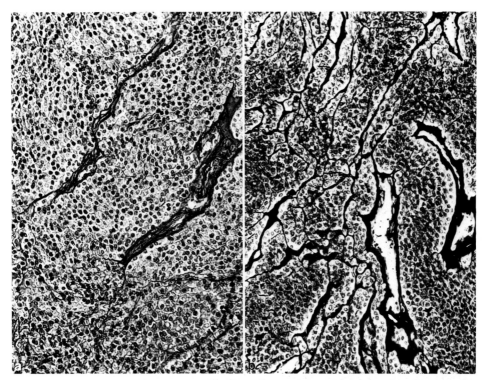

FIG. 799. - Glomus tumor. (a) The neoplasm is constituted by solid fields of «epithelio-morphous» cells aggregated in lobuli with interposition of vascular shoots. (b) Argentic impregnation shows the vasculo-connective pattern which «compartmentalizes» the lesion (*Hemat.-eos.*, 200 x; *argentic impregnation, 200 x*).

muscle cells (however they are deprived of myofibrillae and glycogen) and there is a greater collagen component. In these cases the myoepithelioid cells are dispersed and the aspect is more that of a vascular tumor. The vascular lumens may be collapsed or, on the contrary, dilated in a nearly cavernous shape. At times they have a thin endothelial wall and are filled with blood, at other times they have a thick collagen wall and an empty lumen. Elective staining always reveals a thick plexus of thin amyelinic nerve fibers irregularly running around the vessels and among the epithelioid cells. The nuclei are fairly monomorphous, the structure typically organoid, the boundaries of the tumor are usually evident.

G.T. derives from arterovenous glomi, arterovenous anastomoses having a highly differentiated structure. These glomi are present everywhere, but are particularly numerous in the ungueal bed, in the skin of the fingertips, of the palm of the hand, and of the sole of the foot. They are made up of an afferent arteriole, an efferent vein, and of a convoluted anastomotic vessel, where the endothelio-reticular wall is surrounded by a sheath of cells in several concentric layers known as myoepithelioid cells. These are pericytes or adventitial elements of considerable size, globose shape, abundant light cytoplasm, ovalar and vesicular nucleus. They do not contain myofibrillae, but they are provided with contractile activity.

G.T. heals with surgical excision which is easy, given its small size, the superficiality and the well-defined boundaries of the tumor. Recurrence is rarely observed.

REFERENCES

1924 MASSON P.: Le glomus neuromyoarteriel des regions tactiles et ses tumeurs. *Lyon Chir.*, **21**, 257.

1951 RIVEROS M., PACK G.T.: The glomus tumors — report of 20 cases. *Ann. Surg.*, **133**, 394.

1955 HORTON C., MAQUIRE C., NICHOLAS G. *et al.*: Glomus tumors: An analysis of 25 cases. *Arch. Surg.*, **71**, 712.

1961 KOHOUT E., STOUT A.P.: The glomus tumor in children. *Cancer*, **41**, 555.

1962 MacKENZIE D.H.: Intraosseous glomus tumors. *J. Bone Joint Surg.*, **44B**, 648.

1969 TOKER C.: Glomangioma: An ultrastructural study. *Cancer*, **23**, 487.

1971 SMYTH M.: Glomus cell tumors in the lower extremity: Report of two cases. *J. Bone Joint Surg.*, **53**, 157.

1972 CARROLL R.E., BERMAN A.T.: Glomus tumors of the hand: Review of the literature and report of 28 cases. *J. Bone Joint Surg.*, **54A**, 691.

1972 MULLIS W.F., ROSATO F.E., ROSATO E.F. *et al.*: The glomus tumor. *Surg. Gynecol. Obstet*, **135**, 705.

1980 HO K.L., PAK M.S.Y.: Glomus tumor of the coccygeal region. Case report. *J. Bone Joint Surg.*, **62-A**, 141.

1982 TSUNEYOSHI M., ENJOJI M.: Glomus tumor. A clinicopathologic and electron microscopic study. *Cancer*, **50**, 1601.

1983 MIETTININ M., LEHTO V.-P., VIRTANEN I.: Glomus tumor cells: Evaluation of smooth muscle and endothelial cell properties. *Virchow Arch. (Cell Pathol)*, **43**, 139.

1985 KISHIMOTO S., NAGATANI H., MIYASHITA A., KOBAYASHI K.: Immunohistochemical demostration of substance-P containing nerve fibers in glomus tumours. *Br. J. Dermatol.*, **113**, 213.

1989 DERVAN P.A., TOBBIA I.N., CASEY M., O'LOUGHLIN J., O'BRIEN M.: Glomus tumors: an immunohistochemical profile of 11 cases. *Histopathology*, **14**, 483.

EPITHELIOID HEMANGIOMA
(Synonyms: Kimura disease, histiocytoid hemangioma, angiolymphoid hyperplasia with eosinophilia)

It is a benign tumor characterized by angioblastic proliferation with an epithelioid aspect and associated with chronic inflammatory reaction where eosinophilic granulocytes prevail.

It is an infrequent occurrence, observed during **adult** age, and there is predilection for the female **sex**.

The lesion is generally **superficial** (derma and subcutaneous tissue), solitary or multiple in the same area, and it is particularly observed in the head and neck. It is rarely observed in the limbs and rarely in the deep soft tissues.

Clinically there are small bulging areas at the skin surface; these are reddish, itchy. These nodules may bleed and be confluent. In some cases there is enlargement of the regional lymph nodes and eosinophilia in the peripheral blood. In deep localizations, the proliferation may involve the wall of a vessel of average caliber.

Histologically there is a mixture of vascular channels, mostly capillary, matted by rather large endothelial cells, which at times protrude in the lumen «like gravestones», and at times tend to occlude it. These cells have the microscopic features of the angioblast and, although they are large, do not show signs of atypia. In addition to the capillaries, vessels of larger caliber may be observed, where the endothelial coating appears to be more mature. Surrounding the vessels is a rich phlogistic infiltration, where eosinophiles abound, but there are also lymphocytes, plasmacells, mastcells.

E.H. may recur after marginal excision, but it does not metastasize. It is fairly sensitive to radiation therapy.

REFERENCES

1948 KIMURA T., YOSHIMURA S.,ISHIKAWA E.: Unusual granulation combined with yperplastic change of lymphatic tissue. *Trans. Soc. Pathol. Jpn.*, **37**, 179.

1972 REED R.J., TERAZAKIS N.: Subcutaneous angioblastic lymphoid hyperplasia with eosinophilia (Kimura's disease). *Cancer*, **29**, 489.

1974 CASTRO C., WINKELMANN R.K.: Angiolymphoid hyperplasia with eosinophilia in the skin. *Cancer*, **34**, 1696.

1974 ROSAI J., AKERMAN L.R.: Intravenous atypical vascular proliferation: A cutaneous lesion simulating a malignant blood vessel tumor. *Arch. Dermatol.*, **109**, 714.

1979 ROSAI J., GOLD J., LANDY R.: The histiocytoid hemangiomas. A unifying concept embracing several previously described entities of skin, soft tissue, large vessels, bone and heart. *Hum. Pathol.*, **10**, 707-30.

1981 KONISHI N., TAMURA T., KAWAI C., SHIRAI T.: IgE associated nephropathy in a patient with subcutaneous eosinophilic lymphoid granuloma (Kimura's disease). *Virchows Arch.* [*A*], **392**, 127-34.

1983 HASHIMOTO H., DAIMARU Y., ENJOJI M.: Intravascular papillary endothelial hyperplasia. A clinicopathologic study of 91 cases. *Am. J. Dermatopathol.*, **5**(6), 539-46.

1984 KUNG I.T.M., GIBSON J.B., BANNATYNE P.M.: Kimura's disease: a clinicopathological study of 21 cases and its distinction from angiolymphoid hyperplasia with eosinophilia. *Pathology*, **16**, 39-44.

1984 ISHII Y., TAKAMI T., YUASA H., TAKEI T., KIKUCHI K.: Two distinct antigen systems in human B lymphocytes: identification of cell surface and intracellular antigens using monoclonal antibodies. *Clin. Exp. Immunol.*, **58**, 183-92.

1985 EISENBERG E., LOWLICHT R.: Angiolymphoid hyperplasia with eosinophils: a clinico-pathological conference. *J. Oral Pathol.*, **14**, 216-23.

1985 OLSEN T.G., HELWIG E.B.: Angiolymphoid hyperplasia with eosinophilia: a clinicopathologic study of 116 patients. *J. Am. Acad. Dermatol.*, **12**, 781-96.

1987 MORTON K., ROBERTSON A.J., HADDEN W.: Angiolymphoid hyperplasia with eosinophilia. Report of a case arising from the radial artery. *Histopathology*, **11**, 963.

1987 URABE A., TSUNEYOSHI M., ENJOJI M.: Epithelioid hemangioma versus Kimura's disease: a comparative clinicopathologic study. *Am. J. Surg. Pathol.*, **11**, 758-66.

HEMANGIOENDOTHELIOMA AND ANGIOSARCOMA

These are low-malignancy (H.E.) and high-malignancy (A.S.) tumors whose cells tend towards angioblastic differentiation.

The morphological features of these cells are ample well-stained PAS positive cytoplasm, the cytoplasmatic vacuoles which represent the primitive formation of the vascular lumen, the tendency to unite in syncytia. Electron microscopy reveals the basal lamina, the Weibel-Palade bodies, the pynocytotic vescicles. Immunohistochemistry with the peroxydase-antiperoxydase method reveals the antigene factor VIII.

These tumors rarely occur in the soft tissues.

EPITHELIOID HEMANGIOENDOTHELIOMA

It is a very rare tumor, observed during adult age and in the deep or superficial soft tissues, in relation to the wall of a large vein. It is a rather well-circumscribed and solid mass, pale, not hematic in color. Histologically, in fact, it is composed by solid cords, without any formation of vascular lumina, whose cells have endothelial features. These cords are surrounded by ground substance rich in mucopolysaccharides, which liken it to chondroid substance (Fig. 800 a-d).

The cells show nuclei which are not large, hardly pleomorphic, not hyperchromic, with dispersed and finely granular chromatin, and a small nucleolus or none at all. Mitotic figures are few (less than 1 x 10 fields under high power).

This tumor is considered to be characterized by low-grade malignancy, with scant potential for local recurrence and even less for metastasis.

Its acknowledgement is interesting from a conceptual point of view, but the distinction as compared to angiomas on one hand and to angiosarcoma on the other, and its biological behavior still need to be defined by a larger number of cases.

ANGIOSARCOMA

It is a very rare occurrence. It is more often observed in the skin-subcutaneous tissue than in the deep soft tissues.

A typical form occurs in the limbs affected by **chronic lymphedema** and

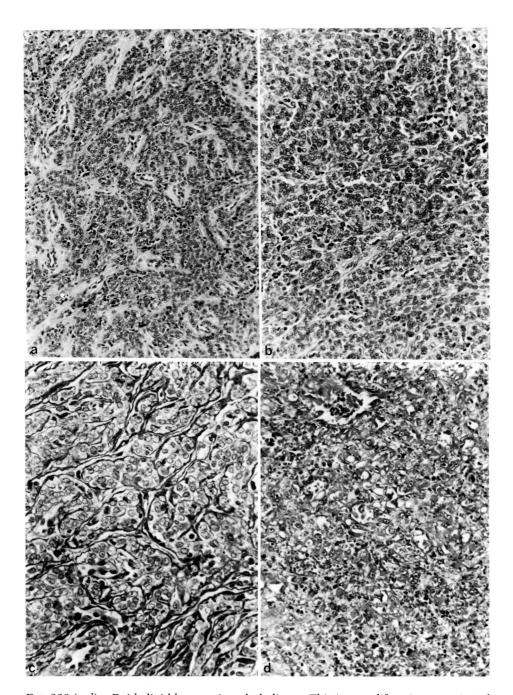

FIG. 800 (a-d). - Epithelioid hemangioendothelioma. This is a proliferation constituted by round-oval cells which aggregate in islands or short cords. (b) Sometimes the cellular proliferation seems to take on a solid aspect. The cells are round with eosinophilic cytoplasm and a round-oval monorphous nucleus. (c) A tenuous fibro-reticular pattern surrounds the single cells or groups of cells. (d) Cytoplasmatic vacuolization is observed, mimicking the formation of a vessel on the part of a single cell (a, b, d: *Hemat.-eos.*, 160, 250, 400 x; c: *Mallory-Vannucci*, 250 x).

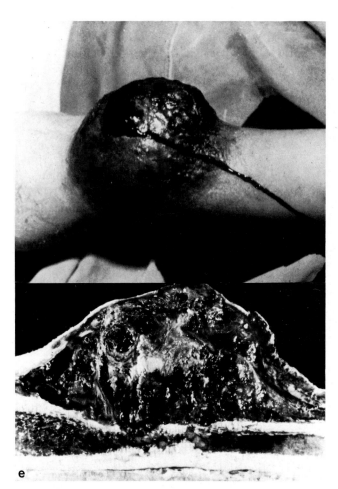

FIG. 800e. - Angiosarcoma in a male aged 68 years. The tumor occurred on an old necrotic calcific lesion of the soft tissues. At the age of 9 years the patient reported trauma which left a scar on the anterior aspect of the leg. Over the last year swelling occurred in the site of the old scar. Thigh amputation following frozen section biopsy. The tumor was ulcerated and bleeding; on the cut surface there was erosion of the underlying tibia.

after many years (mastectomized women, congenital and acquired lymphedemas). These A.S. (there is no proof that they originate from — or are differentiated in — lymphatic vessels rather than hematic ones) are cutaneous or subcutaneous, often in multiple nodes. As for pathogenesis, it has been hypothesized that the lymphedematous limb represents an area which has been subtracted from immunological surveillance monitoring cellular mutations, as would be indicated by the fact that skin grafts survive longer.

A.S. (apart from the post-mastectomy type) is more frequent in males and is observed at every age, but particularly during adult age.

Its **macroscopic** aspect is that of a globose mass which may be bumpy, at times characterized by a thin pseudocapsular delimitation. It is mostly a soft, encephaloid tissue, with vast areas which are very vascular or hemorrhagic (Fig. 800e). In forms of prevalently solid angioblastic proliferation the tissue may even appear to be compact and not particularly vascular.

Histologically A.S. is characterized by cells having large, intensely stained and slightly basophilic cytoplasm, often connected in syncytia, and vac-

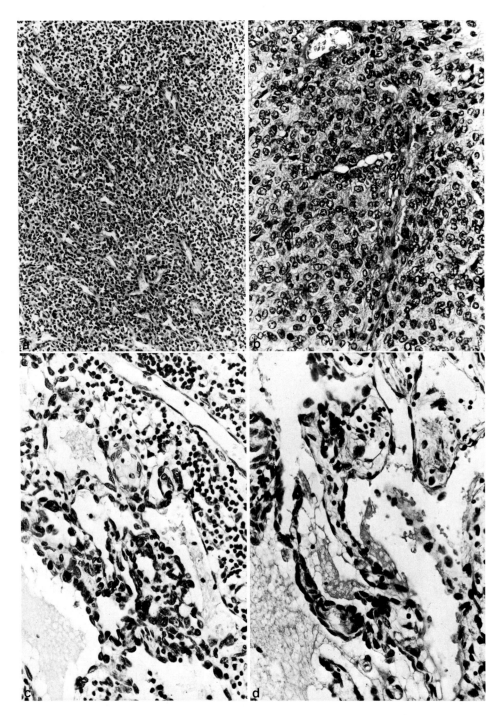

FIG. 801. - Angiosarcoma. (a) Prevalent solid aspect of the neoplasm. (b) Solid aspect with rich cellular proliferation having atypical features. (c) and (d) Other fields show vascular lacunae lined by swollen endothelial cells arranged in a single layer or in irregular groups with atypical nucleo-cytoplasmatic features (*Hemat.-eos.*, 160, 400, 400, 400 x).

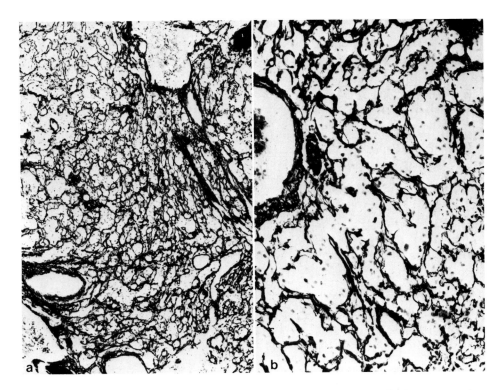

FIG. 802. - Angiosarcoma. (a) The argyrophilous reticulum surrounds the areas within which the cellular proliferation develops. (b) At higher power the neoplastic vascular lacunae are clearly delineated (*Silver stain*, 160, 400 x).

uolated; and large, globose, vesicular nuclei containing a large nucleolus (Fig. 801). These cells, which recall angioblasts, form solid fields and cords, or capillary tubules anastomized like a network, or mat the wall of craggy cavities. In those areas where they coat vascular spaces, they are arranged in one or more layers. At times they form cumuli or, surrounding a thin connective stem, typical small globose villosities protruding in the lumen. The larger cavities contain blood. In those areas where the structure is nearly entirely solid, the neoplastic cells may appear to be partly spindle and diagnostic suspicion originates particularly from the presence of dark cytoplasms and vesicular nuclei having a large nucleolus. In any case, diagnosis becomes more accurate with trichromic staining for the connective tissue and with argentic impregnation (Fig. 802). These clearly reveal the endothelial structure, with cells inside the delicate reticular membranes, delimiting the cords, tubules and vascular cavities.

A.S. is characterized by high malignancy and **treatment** must be early and radical. Metastases may occur by hematic route and not rarely by lymphatic route.

REFERENCES

1943 STOUT A.P.: Hemangioendothelioma: A tumor of blood vessels featuring vascular endothelial cells. *Ann. Surg.*, **118**, 445.
1948 STEWART F.W., TREVES N.: Lymphangiosarcoma in post-mastectomy lymphedema. *Cancer*, **1**, 64.
1953 TIBBS D.: Metastasizing hemangiomata: A case of malignant hemangioendothelioma. *Br. J. Surg.*, **40**, 465.
1961 KAUFFMAN S.L., STOUT A.P.: Malignant hemangioendothelioma in infants and children. *Cancer*, **14** 1186.
1962 TASWELL H.F., SOULE E.H., COVENTRY M.B.: Lymphangiosarcoma in chronic lymphedematous extremities. Report of 13 cases and review of the literature. *J. Bone Joint Surg.*, **44A**, 277.
1964 KHANNA S.K., MANCHANDA R.L., SEIGAL R.K. *et al.*: Hemangioendothelioma (angiosarcoma) of the breast. *Arch. Surg.*, **88**, 807.
1967 DANESE C.A., GRISHMAN E., OH C. *et al.*: Malignant vascular tumors of the lymphedematous extremity. *Ann. Surg.* **166**, 245.
1967 EBY C.S., BRENNAN M.J., FINE G.: Lymphangiosarcoma: A lethal complication of chronic lymphedema: Report of two cases and review of the literature. *Arch. Surg.*, **94**, 223.
1970 DI SIMONE R.N., EL-MAHDI A.M., HAZRA T. *et al.*: The response of Stewart-Treves syndrome to radiotherapy. *Radiology*, **97**, 121.
1971 SILVERBERG S.G., KAY S., KOSS L.G.: Post-mastectomy lymphangiosarcoma. Ultrastructural observation. *Cancer*, **27**, 100.
1972 WOODWARD A.D., IVINS J.C., SOULE E.H.: Lymphangiosarcoma arising in chronic lymphedematous extremities. *Cancer*, **30**, 562.
1976 PAIK H.H., KOMOROWSKI R.: Hemangiosarcoma of the abdominal wall following radiation therapy of endometrial carcinoma. *Am. J. Clin. Pathol.*, **66**, 810.
1976 ROSAI J., SUMNER H.W., KOSTIANOVSKI M. *et al.*: Angiosarcoma of the skin. A clinicopathologic and fine structural study. *Hum. Pathol.*, **7**, 83.
1979 CHEN K.T.K., HOFFMAN K.D., HENDRICKS E.J.: Angiosarcoma following therapeutic irradiation. *Cancer*, **44**, 2044.
1979 HODGKINSON D.J., SOULE E.H., WOODS J.E.: Cutaneous angiosarcoma of the head and neck. *Cancer*, **44**, 1106.
1979 SCHREIBER H., BARRY F.M., RUSSELL W.C. *et al.*: Stewart-Treves syndrome: A lethal complication of post-mastectomy lymphedema and regional immune deficiency. *Arch. Surg.*, **114**, 82.
1979 UNRUH H., ROBERTSON D.I., KARASEWICH E.: Postmastectomy angiosarcoma: Experience with three patients and electron microscopic observations in one. *Can. J. Surg.*, **22**, 556.
1980 NADIJ M., GONZALES M.S., CASTRO A. *et al.*: Factor VIII-related antigen: An endothelial cell marker. *Lab. Invest*, **42**, 139A.
1981 MADDOX J.C., EVANS H.L.: Angiosarcoma of skin and soft tissue: A study of 44 cases. *Cancer*, **48**, 1907.
1981 YAP B.S., YAP H.Y., MCBRIDE C.M. *et al.*: Chemotherapy for post-mastectomy lymphangiosarcoma. *Cancer*, **47**, 853.
1982 WEISS S.W., ENZINGER F.M.: Epithelioid hemangioendothelioma. A vascular tumor often mistaken for carcinoma. *Cancer*, **50**, 970.
1983 DAVIES J.D., REES G.J.G., MERA S.L.: Angiosarcoma in irradiated postmastectomy chest wall. *Histopathology*, **7**, 947.
1985 HUEY G.R., STEHAM F.B., ROTH L.M., EHRLICH C.E.: Lymphangiosarcoma of the edematous thigh after radiation therapy for carcinoma of the vulva. *Gynecol. Oncol.*, **20**, 394.
1989 MAC KAY B., ORDONEZ N.G., HUANG W.L.: Ultrastructural and immunocytochemical observations on angiosarcomas. *Ultrastru. Pathol.*, **13**, 97.
1989 MORGAN J., ROBINSON M.J., ROSEN L.B.: Malignant endovascular papillary angioendothelioma (Dabska tumor): case report and review of the literature. *Am. J. Dermatopathol.*, **11**, 64.

KAPOSI'S SARCOMA

It is a tumor characterized by endothelial, perithelial and fibroblastic differentiation. It is **very rare** in our regions, not so in central Africa where its clinical features and course are *sui generis*. It nearly exclusively occurs in the male **sex** and during adult-advanced **age**. It is prevalently **localized** in the

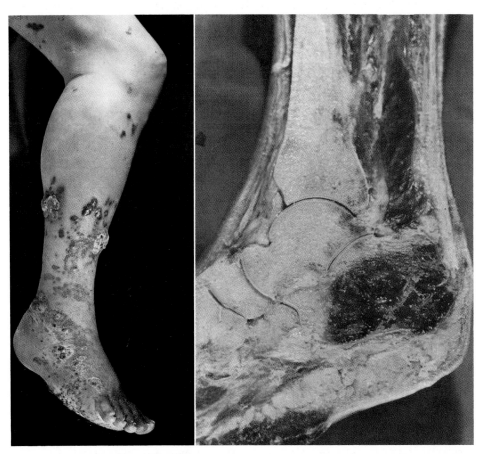

FIG. 803. - Kaposi's sarcoma. Male aged 77 years. The first skin dischromias occurred in both legs and in both hands-forearms 9 years earlier. For the last 7 months ulceration of the nodules in the right leg and foot, thigh amputation. Wine-red spots, flat or nodular, confluent, hyperkeratosic and ulcerated skin nodules, neoplastic invasion of the calcaneus were observed.

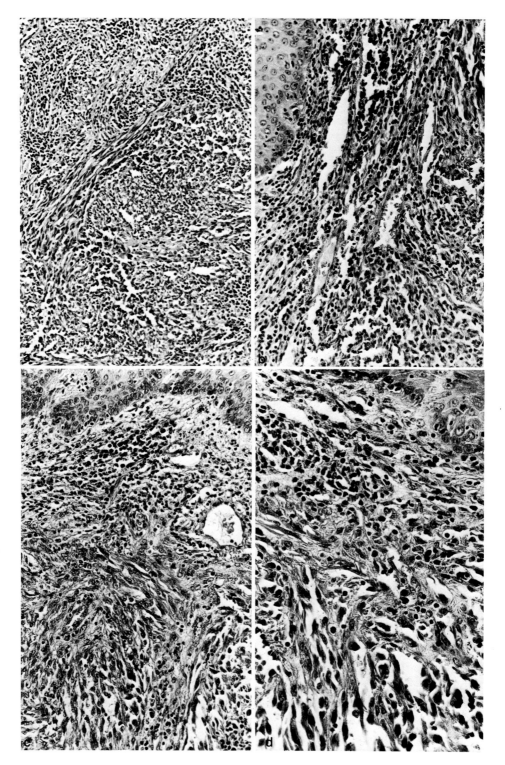

FIG. 804.

FIG. 804. - Kaposi's sarcoma. (a) Proliferation of spindle cells which are arranged in bundles around «vascular fissures» lined by endothelium. (b) The neoformation in volves the superficial layers of the derma, fissure-like vascular spaces and spindle cells may be observed, to which chronic lymphocytary phlogistic elements are associated. (c) In the derma spindle cells having a prevalently monomorphous aspect are observed, recalling fibrosarcoma, associated with vascular «fissures» and chronic lymphocytary phlogistic infiltrate. (d) The atypical nucleocytoplasmatic features of the spindle cells and the nuclear hyperchromia are observed (*Hemat.-eos.*, 160, 250, 250, 400 x).

◀

skin-subcutaneous tissue of the distal ends of the limbs, particularly the lower ones, in a multifocal and bilateral form.

Clinically it initiates with cutaneous nodules of a wine-red color which then becomes greenish, at times they ulcerate, tend to increase in volume and number, to merge together, to extend in a centripetal direction (Fig. 803). At times there is involvement of the regional lymph nodes, deep nodules (even in the skeleton), involvement of the internal organs.

Kaposi's sarcoma is often associated with another malignancy such as leukemia, lymphoma, plasmacytoma, and it seems to be related to **immunological alteration**.

Its **course** is very slow. Some lesions may regress spontaneously, while others progress.

The **histological picture** changes with the progressive stage of the single lesions (Fig. 804). At first tissue rich in neoformed vessels, histiofibroblasts and inflammatory infiltrates is observed, resembling granulation tissue. Nonetheless, the cells reveal features of proliferation which is so lively, if not actual atypia, that its neoplastic nature is indicated. In a more advanced phase, the inflammatory component decreases, the lesion becomes more nodular and more compact. It takes on the aspect of a well-differentiated fibrosarcoma, with scant pleomorphism and rare mitotic figures. This tissue contains vascular canals and fissures lined by swollen endothelium, which is also deprived of evident signs of atypia. In some cases, moreover, and in the long run, there is **progression in malignancy**, and when this is the case, histological aspects of a high-grade fibrosarcoma or angiosarcoma occur.

Given the multiplicity of the lesion, **treatment** prevalently involves radiation and chemotherapy. The prognosis depends on the stage of the disease and on its unpredictable evolution: it is good in forms which remain circumscribed, while it is less good in those which are locally aggressive with extent to ample skin regions and in depth, and poor in generalized forms with involvement of the lymph nodes, internal organs and metastases.

REFERENCES

1957   BLUEFARB S.M.: *Kaposi's Sarcoma*. Springfield, Ill., Charles Thomas Publisher.
1960   DUTZ W., STOUT A.P.: Kaposi's sarcoma in infants and children. *Cancer*, **13**, 684, 1960.
1963   LOTHE F.: Kaposi's sarcoma. *Acta Pathol. Microbiol. Scand.*, **161**, 1.

1964   DORFMAN R.F.: The ultrastructure of Kaposi's sarcoma. *Lab. Invest.*, **13**, 939A.

1969   SLAVIN G., CAMERON H.M., SINGH H.: Kaposi's sarcoma in mainland Tanzania: A report of 117 cases. *Br. J. Cancer*, **23**, 349.

1969   SIEGAL J.H., JANIS R., ALPER J.C., et al.: Disseminated visceral Kaposi's sarcoma. *JAMA*, **207**, 1493.

1971   TAYLOR J.F., TEMPLETON A.C., KYLAWAZI S., et al.: Kaposi's sarcoma in pregnancy: Two case reports. *Br. J. Surg.*, **58**, 577.

1972   D'OLIVERIA J.J., OLIVERIA T.F.: Kaposi's sarcoma in Bantu of Mozambique. *Cancer*, **30**, 533.

1972   TEMPLETON A.C.: Studies in Kaposi's sarcoma: Postmortem findings and disease patterns in women. *Cancer*, **30**, 854.

1975   STRACHLEY C.J., SANTOS J.I., DOWNEY D.M., et al.: Kaposi's sarcoma in a renal transplant recipient. *Arch. Pathol.*, **99**, 611.

1976   OLWENY C.L.M., MASABA J.P., SIKYEWUNDA W., et al.: Treatment of Kaposi's sarcoma with ICRD-159 (NSC-129943). *Cancer Treat. Rep.*, **60**, 111.

1978   HOLECEK M.J., HARWOOD A.R.: Radiotherapy of Kaposi's sarcoma. *Cancer*, **41**, 1733.

1978   KIEP O., DAHL O., STENWIG J.: Association of Kaposi's sarcoma and prior immunosuppressive therapy: 5 year material of Kaposi's sarcoma in Norway. *Cancer*, **42**, 2626.

1979   TANGE T.: Kaposi's sarcoma. Case report and review of Japanese cases. *Acta Path. Jap.*, **29**, 319.

1980   LO T.C.M., SALZMAN F.A., SMEDAL M.I., et al.: Radiotherapy for Kaposi's sarcoma. *Cancer*, **45**, 684.

1980   SAFAI B., MIKE V., GIRALDO G., et al.: Association of Kaposi's sarcoma with second primary malignancies: Possible etiopathogenic implications. *Cancer*, **45**, 1472.

1981   BOLDOGH I., BETH E., HUANG E.S. et al.: Kaposi's sarcoma. IV. Detection of CMV DNA, CMV RNA and CMNA in tumor biopsies. *Int. J. Cancer*, **28**, 469-74.

1982   JORGENSEN K.A., LAWESSON S.O.: Amyl nitrite and Kaposi's sarcoma in homosexual men. *N. Engl. J. Med.*, **307**, 893-4.

1984   BRODIE H., DREW W.I., MAAYAN S.: Prevalence of Kaposi's sarcoma in AIDS patients reflects differences in rates of cytomegalovirus infection in high risk groups. *AIDS Memorandum*, **1**, 12.

1985   BECKSTEAD J.H., WOOD G.S., FLETCHER V.: Evidence for the origin of Kaposi's sarcoma from lymphatic endothelium. *Am. J. Pathol.*, **119**, 294.

1988   CASTRO K.G., SELIK R.M., JAFFE H.W. et al.: Frequency of opportunistic diseases (OD) in AIDS patients, by race/ethnicity and HIV transmission categories — United States. Paper presented at the Twenty-eighth Interscience Conference on Antimicrobial Agents and Chemotherapy, Los Angeles, October 25.

1988   POLK B.F., MUÑOZ A., FOX R., et al.: Decline of Kaposi's sarcoma (KS) among participants in MACS. Paper presented at the Fourth International AIDS Conference, Stockholm, June 13.

HEMANGIOPERICYTOMA
(BENIGN AND MALIGNANT)

DEFINITION

It is made up of cells which are considered to be Zimmermann pericytes. The neoplastic pericytes accompany small blood vessels in which the endothelium is not neoplastic.

Even if electron microscopy has confirmed the pericytic nature of the tumor (particularly demonstrating the long cytoplasmatic processes), under the optic microscope the pericytes are not clearly distinguished from fibroblasts, endothelial cells, histiocytes. Thus, even in the forms of H.P. which are best differentiated, diagnosis is above all based on the histological structure of the lesion: a thick network of capillaries and sinusoids surrounded by the proliferation of neoplastic cells. Nonetheless, similar or identical structure may be observed in numerous other tumors, such as benign and malignant fibrous histiocytoma, dermatofibrosarcoma protuberans, synovial sarcoma, mesenchymal chondrosarcoma. What follows is that H.P. must be diagnosed when the typical histological structure is diffused to the entire tumor, when other tumors such as those listed above may be excluded by extensive and numerous sampling, and it should be confirmed by elective staining and electron microscopy.

Another difficult matter is the histological evaluation of the grade of malignancy of H.P. The well-differentiated and completely benign forms of the tumor are distinguished from clearly malignant ones, but there are intermediate forms, where it is very difficult to relate the histological grade and prognosis. For this reason, benign, malignant and intermediate forms are described in the same chapter.

GENERAL DATA

H.P. is an **infrequent** tumor. There is no predilection for **sex**, and it occurs nearly exclusively in the **adult**, uniformly distributed after 20 years of age. Its preferred **localization** is the lower limb (particularly the thigh), followed by the retroperitoneum and the pelvic region, and by the upper limb, trunk, head and neck. It is nearly always deeply located, within and between the muscles.

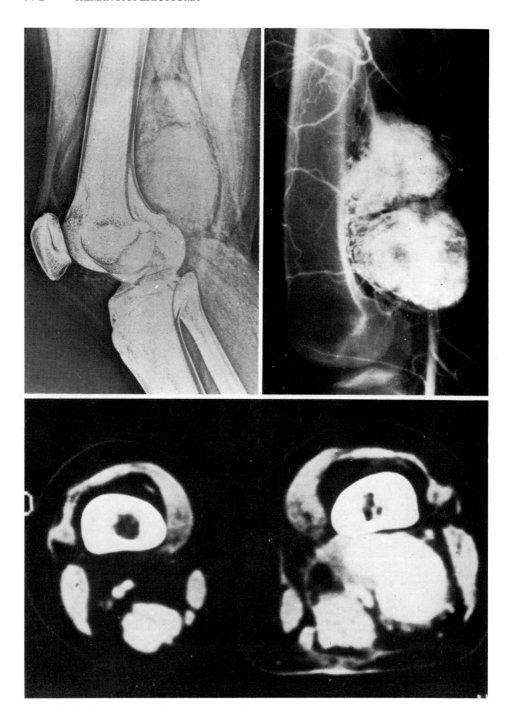

FIG. 805. - Hemangiopericytoma. Male aged 37 years. Arteriography and CAT with contrast medium reveal the intense and diffused vascularity of the tumor.

SYMPTOMS

The tumor, which is deep, grows slowly and does not usually cause any pain. The duration of symptoms prior to diagnosis may be months or years, even many years.

The rich vascularity of the tumor, which acts as an arterovenous shunt, may cause an increase in skin temperature and cutaneous telangiectasia *in loco*, dilatation of the regional veins. At times the tumor may be pulsating and a bruit may be perceived. In rare cases, hypoglycemia has been observed, or osteomalacia, the one and the other reversible after removal of the tumor.

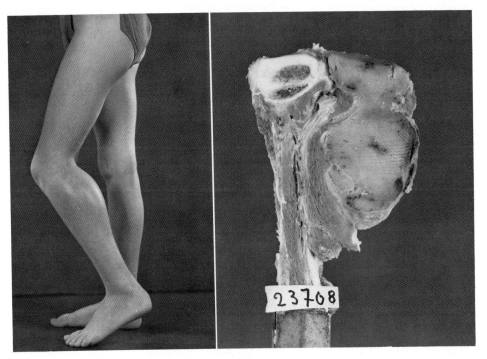

Fig. 806. - Hemangiopericytoma. Male aged 7 years. Swelling observed for 2 months. Thigh amputation. Observe the compact encephaloid tissue. No sign of disease after 7 years.

RADIOGRAPHIC FEATURES

The tumor does not contain calcar radiopacity (except in rare cases of many years duration) and thus the radiographic picture is not typical.

CAT with contrast medium and, above all, **arteriography** are instead indicative, revealing: rich vascularity of the tumor; at times one or more distinct vascular pedicles nourishing it; a rich network of peritumoral dilated and tortuous vessels; diffusion of the contrast medium in the tumor due to its rich capillary circulation; rapid arterovenous passage (Fig. 805).

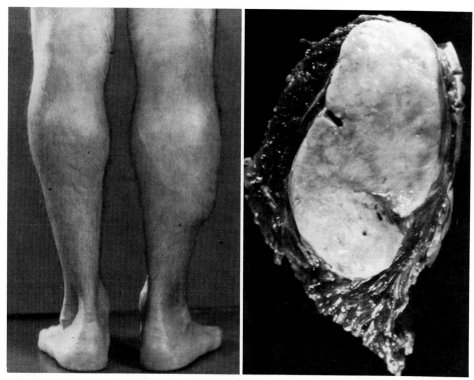

FIG. 807. - Hemangiopericytoma. Male aged 44 years. Swelling for the past 3 years. Preoperative radiotherapy at 4500 rad, then wide excision (necrosis of the neoplastic tissue exceeding 90%). No signs of disease after 9 years.

GROSS PATHOLOGIC FEATURES

It is a globose mass, single or multilobulated (in larger forms of the lesion). It may become of very large size in malignant forms (Figs. 806, 807).

Generally, it is surrounded by a thin pseudocapsule and run through by a network of dilated vessels. Surgical exposure of the tumor and its incision often cause heavy bleeding which may even be difficult to keep under control.

The tumor is soft or firm, at times cystic as a result of hemorrhagic or necrotic phenomena. Depending on the perviousness and dilatation of the capillaries, color ranges from pale to dull red or brownish red.

Larger size, softer consistency, more extensive areas of necrosis are observed in malignant forms of the tumor.

HISTOPATHOLOGIC FEATURES

Typical of H.P. is not the cytology, but the histological structure. A thick and diffused network of capillaries is observed, varying from those which are

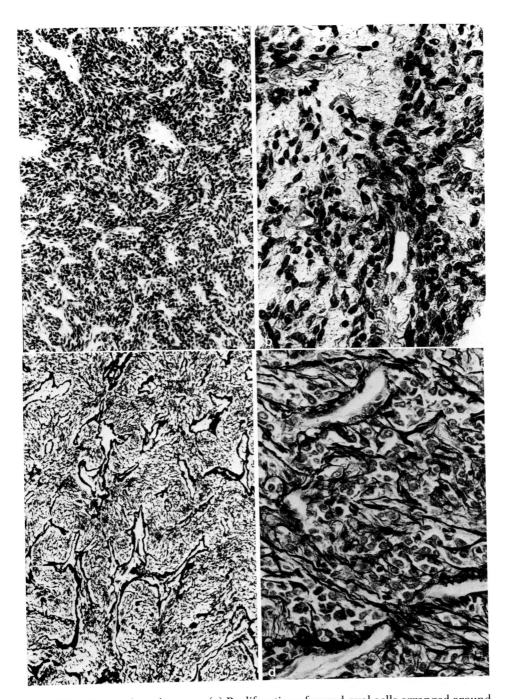

FIG. 808. - Hemangiopericytoma. (a) Proliferation of round-oval cells arranged around a thick vascular network. The vessels are wide, of varying caliber and anastomized together. (b) Among the vessels ovoid and spindle cells having indistinct cytoplasm are observed. The nuclei are hyperchromatic and have a relatively monomorphous aspect. (c) and (d) The neoplastic proliferation is constituted by cells which occupy an extravascular site. A fine reticular pattern which departs from the vessels surrounds the single cells (*Hemat.-eos.*, 60, 400 x; *argentic impregnation*, 250, 400 x).

totally collapsed to wide open sinusoids, surrounded by a usually compact cellular proliferation (Fig. 808). These cells, pericytes, have globose and oval nuclei, with a clearly distinct nuclear membrane, finely granular chromatin, a small nucleolus. The cytoplasm has no distinct limits and around the single cells there is a thick pattern of reticular and collagen fibers.

The endothelium lining the capillaries is monostratified and flattened, mature. Furthermore, the vessels branch out in typical fashion, with an «antler-like» shape. Rarely, in addition to the thin basal membrane, the vessels are surrounded by a thicker collagen layer. At times, due to accumulation of mucopolysaccharides, the myxoid aspect of areas of the tumor is observed.

Silver stain is important, because it reveals the capillary network even when the lumina are collapsed, the cellular proliferation around the vessels (not inside, as in angioendothelioma or angiosarcoma), and a thick and diffused reticulum surrounding the single pericytes (Fig. 808c, d).

In **benign** forms of the tumor, the nuclei are not too crowded, small, monomorphous, with pulverulent chromatin and without a nucleolus, with no mitotic figures.

In **malignant** forms of the tumor, in addition to the clinical and macroscopic features indicated above, there is hypercellularity, there are larger nuclei, which are more pleomorphic, hyperchromatic with coarse chromatin and at times evidence of a small nucleolus. But the most important element for an evaluation of the grade of malignancy seems to be the number of mitotic figures. H.P. is considered to be malignant if it contains more than 4 mitotic figures per 10 fields at high power.

There are, however, intermediate cases where an opinion on the grade of malignancy and thus prognosis is very difficult or even impossible.

DIAGNOSIS

As previously stated, the diagnosis of H.P. must be made with caution, based on extensive and numerous samples, where the typical structure is repeated throughout, the argyrophilous reticulum designs the vessels and surrounds the cells, and where aspects of other tumors may be excluded, particularly **benign and malignant fibrous histiocytoma, synovial sarcoma, mesenchymal chondrosarcoma.**

COURSE, PROGNOSIS AND TREATMENT

Benign forms seem to be more frequent than malignant ones. The latter are characterized by a considerable tendency to recur locally or to metastasize, particularly in the lungs and skeleton.

Treatment is surgical and consists in moderately wide removal for benign forms, wide for forms where malignancy is doubtful or intermediate, and very wide or radical for malignant forms. In order to prevent intraoperative hemorrhaging, it has been suggested that the principal vessels directed at the tumor be embolized or ligated, or that preoperative radiation therapy be used. It seems that H.P. responds to radiation to a fair extent.

REFERENCES

1942   STOUT A.P., MURRAY M.R.: Hemangiopericytoma. A vascular tumor featuring Zimmermann's pericytes. *Ann. Surg.*, **116**, 26.

1967   SUTTON D., PRATT A.E.: Angiography of hemangiopericytoma. *Clin. Radiol.*, **18**, 324.

1967   DE VILLIERS D.R., FARMAN J., CAMPBELL J.A.H.: Pelvic haemangiopericytoma: Preoperative arteriographic demonstration. *Clin. Radiol.*, **18**, 318.

1969   BREDT A.B., SERPICK A.A.: Metastatic hemangiopericytoma treated with vincristine and actinomycin D. *Cancer*, **24**, 266.

1970   BACKWINKEL K.D., DIDDAMS J.A.: Hemangiopericytoma. Report of a case and comprehensive review of the literature. *Cancer*, **25**, 896.

1971   KAUDE J., TYLEN U.: Angiographische symptomatic des Hamangiopericytoms. *Radiologie*, **11**, 345.

1973   BATTIFORA H.: Hemangiopericytoma. Ultrastructural study of five cases. *Cancer*, **31**, 1418.

1974   DUBE V.E., PAULSON J.F.: Metastatic hemangiopericytoma cured by radiotherapy. *J. Bone Joint Surg.*, **56/A**, 833.

1975   McMSTER M., SOULE E., IVINS J.: Hemangiopericytoma - a clinico-pathologic study and long-term follow-up of 60 patients. *Cancer*, **36**, 2232.

1975   WILBANKS G.D., SZYMANSKA Z., MILLER A.W.: Pelvic hemangiopericytoma. Report of four patients and review of the literature. *Am. J. Obstet. Gynecol.*, **123**, 555.

1976   ENZINGER F.M., SMITH B.H.: Hemangiopericytoma. An analysis of 106 cases. *Hum. Pathol.*, **7**, 61.

1977   MIRA J.G., CHU F.C.: The role of radiotherapy in the management of malignant hemangiopericytoma. Report of 11 new cases and review of the literature. *Cancer*, **39**, 1254.

1978   ANGERVALL L., KINDBLOM L.G., NIELSON J.M., et al.: Hemangiopericytoma, a clinicopathologic, angiographic and microangiographic study. *Cancer*, **42**, 2412.

1978   WONG P.P., YAGODA A.: Chemotherapy of malignant hemangiopericytoma. *Cancer*, **41**, 1256.

1978   YAGHMAI I.: Angiographic manifestations of soft-tissue and osseous hemangiperictyomas. *Radiology*, **126**, 653.

1979   PITLUK H.C., CONN J. JR.: Hemangiopericytoma. Literature review and clinical presentations. *Am. J. Surg.*, **137**, 413.

1981   NUNNERY E.W., KAHN L.B., REDDICK R.L., et al.: Hemangiopericytoma: A light microscopic and ultrastructural study. *Cancer*, **47**, 906.

1983   NEUMAN H. Morphologie und Klinik des Hemangioperizytoms. Eine Analyse von 84 Faellen mit einem eigenen Beitrag. *Pathologe*, **4**, 64.

1983   BEADLE G.F., HILLCOAT B.L.: Treatment of advanced malignant hemangiopericytoma with combination adriamycin and DTIC: A report of four cases. *J. Surg. Oncol.*, **22**, 167.

1984   TSUNEYOSHI M., DAIMARU Y., ENJOJI M.: Malignant hemangiopericytoma and other sarcomas with hemangiopericytoma-like pattern. *Pathol. Res. Pract.*, **178(5)**, 446-53.

1986   MITTAL K.R., GERALD W., TRUE L.D.: Hemangiopericytoma of the breast: Report of a case with ultrastructural and immunohistochemical staining. *Hum. Pathol.*, **17**, 1181.

1986   ROSAI J.: Vascular neoplasms. *Am. J. Surg. Pathol.*, **10**, 26.

1989   DARDICK I., HAMMAR S.P., SCHEITHAUER B.W.: Ultrastructural spectrum of hemangiopericytoma: a comparative study of fetal, adult and neoplastic pericytes. *Ultrastructu. Pathol.*, **13**, 111.

SYNOVIAL SARCOMA

DEFINITION

It is a sarcoma whose cells mimic the two types of cells (A and B) of the synovial membrane. As it is made up of two cellular types, it is called biphasic. When the biphasic aspect is totally absent, and the sarcoma is exclusively made up of fibroblastic cells (B), or epithelioid cells (A), diagnosis is difficult and doubtful (monophasic S.S.).

FREQUENCY

S.S. occurs relatively frequently, preceded only by malignant fibrous histiocytoma, liposarcoma, and rhabdomyosarcoma.

SEX, AGE

There is slight predilection for the male sex (1.2:1). It affects young-adult age, with a maximum peak between 15 and 35 years of age. It rarely occurs before 10 and after 60 years of age.

LOCALIZATION

Only less than 10% of all S.S. are observed within a joint cavity. Generally, the tumor, which is always deep and subfascial, is located close to a joint, but outside of this, adherent to the capsule, are the tendons, the fasciae, the synovial bursae. At times it is observed in areas far away from any normal synovial coating, such as the thigh and leg, the neck, the abdominal wall.

The most common localization is the region of the knee and distal of the thigh, followed by the foot and the ankle. These are followed, approximately equally, by the regions of the shoulder, arm and elbow, forearm and wrist, hip. It is rarer in the hand, trunk, head and neck.

Fig. 809. - Synovial sarcoma. Female aged 61 years. For the past 4 years pain and swelling. The patient was submitted to marginal excision, recurrence after 7 months. Below-knee amputation. The patient died after 9 years of pulmonary metastases.

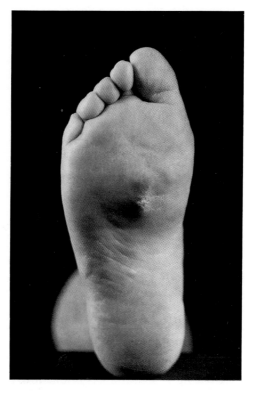

SYMPTOMS

In more than half of all cases of S.S. there is **pain**, occurring spontaneously and on palpation. In one of our cases the tumor was so small and pain so sharp that we suspected glomus tumor. At times symptoms initiate with pain although the newly-formed mass cannot as yet be palpated.

As observed, the mass is rather characteristically localized (Figs. 809, 810, 811, 814). When there is para-articular swelling in the knee, and particularly in the popliteal fossa, synovitis, bursitis, or synovial cyst are often suggested, neglecting the possibility of a S.S. Even the other para-articular or paratendinous forms may be clinically similar to a pigment-

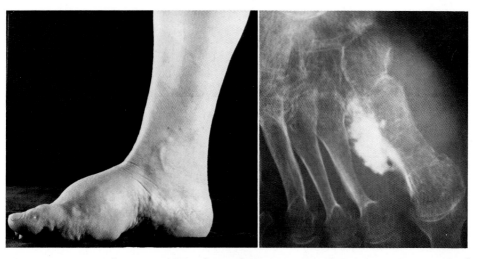

Fig. 810. - Synovial sarcoma. Female aged 65 years. For the past 3 years, pain and swelling. Observe the dense intratumoral calcification. Amputation and death after 3 years of pulmonary metastases.

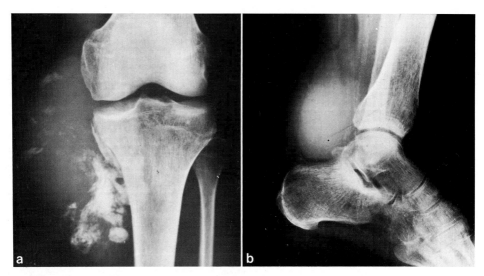

FIG. 811. - Synovial sarcoma. (a) Female aged 34 years. Painful mass which had oc-curred 3 years previously. Observe the intratumoral calcifications and ossifications. (b) Male aged 56 years. Synovial sarcoma. Painless swelling observed 6 months earlier.

ed nodular synovitis or a mucous cyst (ganglion). Rare intra-articular local-izations cause the symptoms of chronic synovitis.

Growth of the tumor is often slow or very slow. The time elapsed between the first symptoms and diagnosis generally ranges from 1 to 4 years, but there are cases in which it is much longer.

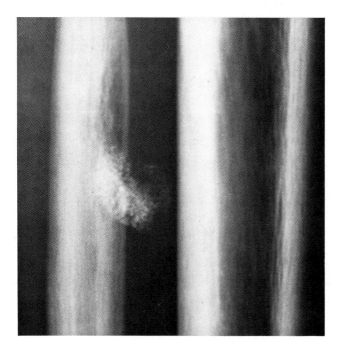

FIG. 812. - Synovial sar-coma. Female aged 10 years. For the past 3 months swelling and moderate pain. Observe the site, in the anterola-teral muscular compart-ment of the leg, located far from any joint, ten-dinous sheath, or bursa mucosa. Observe the in-tratumoral calcifica-tions in minute gran-ules. Marginal excision and postoperative radio-therapy at 4000 rad. The patient died after 3 and 1/2 years of pulmon-ary metastases.

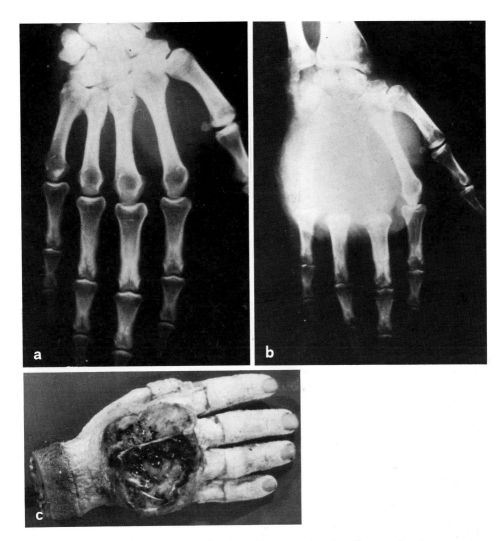

FIG. 813. - Synovial sarcoma. Male aged 31 years. (a) Swelling and pain occurring 2 months before. (b) After 11 months the tumor extensively destroyed the adjacent skeleton. (c) Forearm amputation. Section of the tumor, revealing encephaloid tissue which is extensively hemorrhagic and infiltrative.

RADIOGRAPHIC FEATURES

In approximately 40% of all cases S.S. contains **calcar radiopacities** (Figs. 810, 811, 812). At times it is a spray of very small amorphous specks, at other times a cloudy and faded shadow, others still a massive and dense radiopacity which is partially structured and thus osseous. As for the rest, apart from para-articular localization and frequent lobulated shape, radiographic and angiographic aspects do not differ from those of other richly vascular soft-tissue sarcomas (Fig. 815).

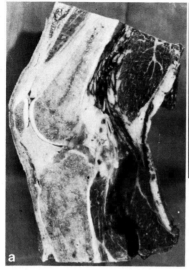
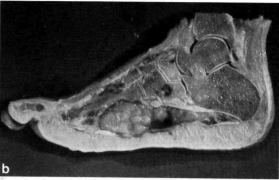

FIG. 814. - Synovial sarcoma. (a) Male aged 30 years. For the past 3 years a popliteal mass had been observed, for 1 year pain. Marginal excision was performed, with postoperative radiation therapy at 5000 rad, there was recurrence after a few months. Thigh amputation. Observe the deep popliteal site, adherent to the capsule but extra-articular, adherent to the vessels. No signs of disease after 6 years. (b) Female aged 63 years. Synovial sarcoma. For the past 8 years pain and then swelling. Below-knee amputation. No signs of disease after 12 years. In both cases wide excision would have been impossible.

In the knee, arthrography may exclude synovial cysts communicating with the joint, arteriography, CAT and MRI may exclude mucous cyst or bursitis, showing a solid tumoral mass.

GROSS PATHOLOGIC FEATURES

Size varies from very small (early surgery as a result of pain) to enormous. The mass is globose and often multilobulated. It may be apparently capsulated, but it is always a pseudocapsule.

S.S. is rarely characterized by a mass within a synovial membrane and rarely by a mass entirely contained within the muscle. It usually grows between and adheres to the tendons, joint capsules, bursae mucosae, fasciae, aponeuroses, skeleton, muscles, interosseous membranes. It models its shape and pushes its growth along these multiple planes. Here it infiltrates, creates intravascular plugs (even in the large vessels), erodes the skeleton (Figs. 813, 814).

These data explain how, except in specific cases and those observed during an early phase, wide conservative excision may be difficult or impossible.

On the cut surface, the tumor is soft (highly cellular forms which are not very differentiated) or firmer (more collagenized forms), pale or hemorrhagic, with areas of necrosis and cystic cavities.

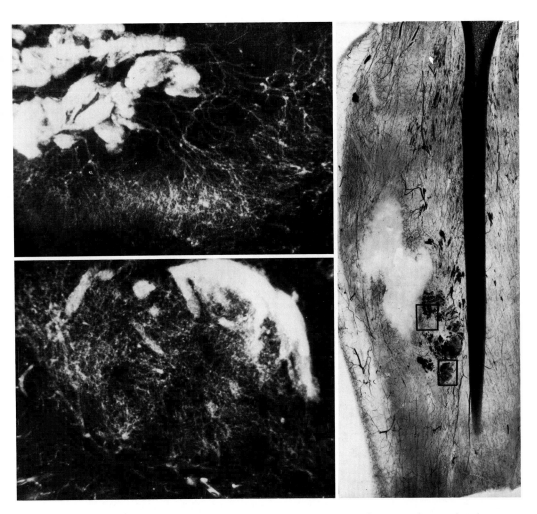

FIG. 815. - Synovial sarcoma. Male aged 20 years. Mass in the sura observed 4 years earlier, painless. Excised marginally, recurrence after 2 years. Thigh amputation. Injection of the amputated limb with intra-arterial micropaque. Observe the localization far from any synovial structure, and the vascularization of the tumor, which is partially formed by thin arborizations, partially by large cavernous lakes.

HISTOPATHOLOGIC FEATURES

They are characterized by a **biphasic structure**: pseudofibroblastic spindle cells, and pseudoepithelial cells (Figs. 816, 817, 818).

The epithelioid cells are globose, cubic or cylindrical, they have large vesicular nuclei and abundant pale cytoplasm characterized by rather well-defined limits. These cells form cords and laminae, nests and islands, tubules and alveoles, at times they cover villi and papillae. Their resemblance to the epithelial cells is such that at times cylindrical epithelial «glands» are observed, in exceptional cases even small keratin pearls, and under E.M. the cells

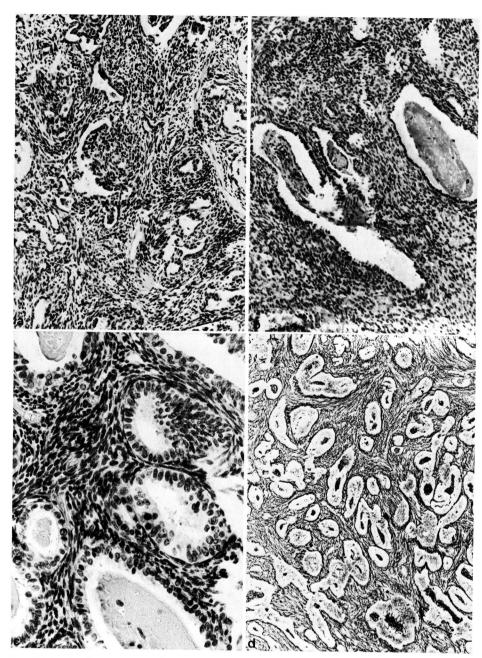

FIG. 816. - Biphasic synovial sarcoma. (a) The neoplasm appears to be constituted by pseudo-glandular and alveolo-cordonal structures (epitheliomorph component), surrounded by spindle cells arranged in bundles (pseudofibrosarcoma component). (b) The epitheliomorph component is represented by wide lacunae regularly coated with cubic cells. Spindle cells are observed among the «pseudo-glandular» structures. (c) Pseudoglandular tubes matted by cylindrical cells. (d) Argentic impegnation circumscribes the epitheliomorph formations. A fine argyrophilous net surrounds the single cells of the pseudofibrosarcomatous component (*Hemat.-eos.*, 60, 160, 400 x; *argentic impregnation*, 160 x).

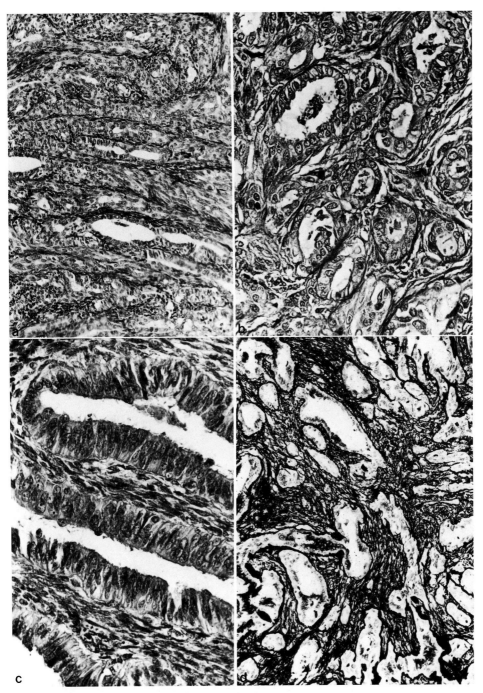

FIG. 817. - Biphasic synovial sarcoma. (a), (b) and (c) Two histostructural aspects are observed: glandular lumina and cords constituted by epitheliomorph cells; swollen spindle cells interposed between the «pseudoepithelial» structures. (d) Argentic impregnation reveals an argyrophilous reticulum surrounding each single cell in the pseudofibrosarcomatous area. The reticulum delimits «epitheliomorph» tubes (Hemat.-eos., 125, 250, 400 x; argentic impregnation, 125 x).

— unlike the A cells of the synovial membrane — have a basal lamina and intercellular junctions.

These epitheliomorphous structures are immersed in a very cellular tissue, which is nearly identical to a fibrosarcoma. It is made up of spindle cells with an oval nucleus which is rather plump and hyperchromatic. As compared to fibrosarcoma, the «herring-bone» pattern is less evident, while rounded «ball-like» whorls may be observed, and mitotic figures are scarcer.

In general, the fibroblastic phase appears to be more intensely stained than the epithelioid one, due to greater crowding of the nuclei and a greater concentration of their chromatin.

The spindle-cellular component is usually the predominant one. The epithelioid structures may be sporadic. At times the epithelioid phase is just hinted at, in the form of lighter cellular islands (more globose cells, more vesicular nuclei), in the pseudofibrosarcoma context. What is particularly helpful in these cases is argentic impregnation, which reveals a more abundant and diffused reticulum in the fibrosarcomatoid part, one which is scarcer or absent among the epithelioid cells (Figs. 816d, 817d).

At times, the S.S. is **scarcely differentiated**. Here, the cellularity is rather rich, with elements which are neither clearly fibroblastic nor epithelioid. Diagnosis in these areas is impossible; the aspect may recall that of Ewing's

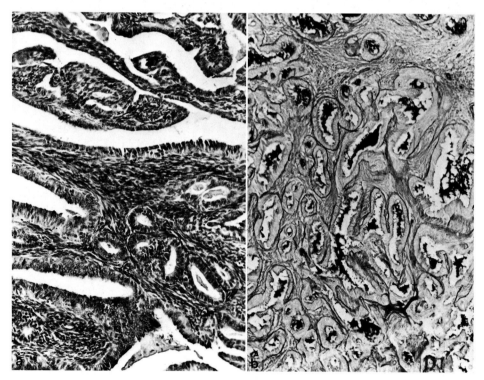

FIG. 818. - Biphasic synovial sarcoma. (a) Balanced distribution between the «biphasic» components. (b) The pseudoglandular tubules contain mucoid material which is intensely colored by PAS (*Hemat.-eos.*, 125x; *Halcian-Pas*, 125x).

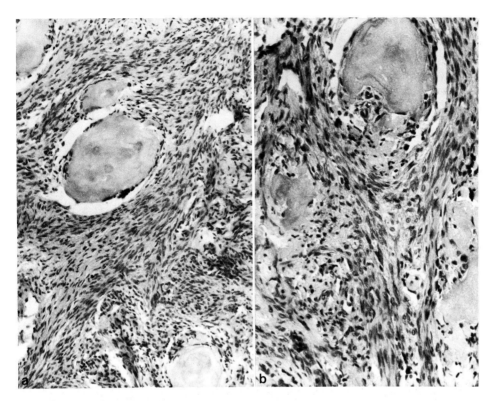

FIG. 819. - Biphasic synovial sarcoma with calcification. (a) and (b) In the epithelio-morph areas there are calcar precipitates. These may also be present in the spindle cell areas and originate from the hyalin stroma; rare epitheliomorph cells are present at the periphery of the calcific masses (*Hemat.-eos.*, 250, 400 x).

sarcoma, hemangiopericytoma, or poorly differentiated fibrosarcoma.

S.S. is always rather cellular, and the cells in both phases are relatively monomorphous. There are no giant or bizarre nuclei. Mitotic figures are not frequent.

The spindle-cellular areas may have myxoid modifications. Rather frequent is the formation of intertwined ribbons of dense and hyaline collagen, which divide and enclose the cells. The inflammatory component is rare or scarce, but sparse mastcells are often observed. Calcification is frequently associated with hyalinosis and necrosis, ossification is less frequent (this is a reactive bone, not a neoplastic one) (Fig. 819).

The epithelioid cells secrete a mucopolysaccharide material, PAS positive, resistent to diastasis and to hyaluronidase, not resistant to acid pH (Fig. 818b). This mucoid substance is present outside of the epithelioid cells and in the lumen of the tubules-alveoles, but it is scarce in the cytoplasm of the same cells. Intracellular glycogen is also scarce or absent.

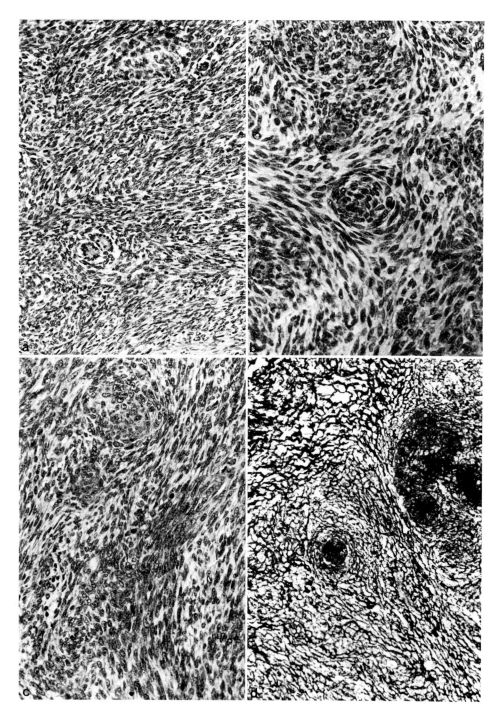

FIG. 820. - Monophasic spindle-cellular synovial sarcoma. (a) Proliferation of spindle cells in which rare «glandular» lumi are observed. (b) and (c) The neoplasm is totally constituted by spindle cells arranged in bundles. At times these cells are aggregated in a vaguely «ball-like» nodular pattern. (d) The argyrophilous reticulum is present between the single cells, even in the nodular areas (*Hemat.-eos.*, 100, 200, 200 x; *argentic impregnation*, 200 x).

HISTOGENESIS

Biphasic differentiation and mucin secretion from the epithelioid cells mimic the structure of synovial membrane.

DIAGNOSIS

The clinical diagnosis of the neoplasm is often delayed and sent off track by pain with no evident swelling, by para-articular localization of the swelling (which suggests synovial cyst, mucous cyst, pigmented nodular synovitis, or bursitis), by the slow or very slow growth of the mass.

Radiographic diagnosis, in case of intense calcification and ossification, may be oriented towards a myositis ossificans, or a cartilaginous tumor, or an osteosarcoma (which, however, is very rare in the soft tissues).

Histological diagnosis is easy in biphasic and well-differentiated forms, while it is difficult in those which are nearly totally monophasic and/or not very differentiated; it is impossible in those which are entirely monophasic.

Monophasic spindle-cellular forms. As compared to a fibrosarcoma, the herring-bone structure is less evident or even absent, while «ball-like» whorled structures are observed, the nuclei are more plump, mitotic figures less frequent (Fig. 820).

Monophasic epithelioid forms. These may be similar to annexial or metastatic carcinomas, malignant melanoma, malignant epithelioid neurinoma, epithelioid sarcoma (Fig. 821).

Poorly differentiated forms. The scarce and often rare epithelioid differentiation must be searched for, particularly with the help of silver stain and mucopolysaccharide staining. Otherwise, the histological picture may be difficult to distinguish from that of a scarcely differentiated fibrosarcoma or a hemangiopericytoma. Sometimes the tumor is composed of small cells and it may considerably resemble a Ewing's sarcoma or a neuroblastoma.

Supporting diagnostic elements are age, localization, pain, calcifications, mast cells, fibro-hyaline bands.

It remains, however, that **without a demonstration of the biphasic structure, the diagnosis of S.S. is not certain but rather presumed. This limit is generally of little practical importance, as prognosis and treatment do not change depending on whether S.S. or poorly differentiated sarcoma is diagnosed.**

COURSE

S.S. has a high tendency to recur locally after conservative treatment. Recurrence is mostly manifested within the first 2 years, but there are cases of recurrence 10 years and more after excision.

The tendency to metastasize is also high, and even metastases may be early or late. The sites preferred are, in this order, the lungs, lymph nodes, skel-

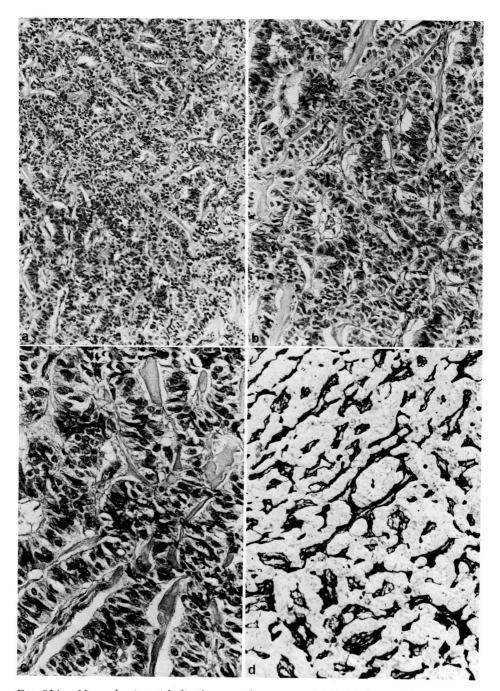

FIG. 821. - Monophasic epithelioid synovial sarcoma. (a) Epitheliomorph aspect: the cells are aggregated in cords and tubes which are closely packed, with the interposition of vascular stroma. (b) Cells with an epithelial aspect and a relatively monomorphous nucleus are aggregated in cords. (c) Under higher power the structural and cytological epitheliomorph aspect may be observed. (d) Argentic impregnation delineates spaces having no reticulum occupied by cells which constitute solid cords and islands (*Hemat.-eos.*, 160, 250, 400 x; *argentic impregnation*, 160 x).

eton. Metastases are often histologically less differentiated than the primary tumor.

PROGNOSIS

Due to the frequently slow growth of the tumor and to the possibly late recurrence and metastases, prognosis must be evaluated at least 10 years after treatment. Prognosis is rather severe, with ten-year survival rate equal to 15-30%. Unfavorable prognostic factors are: 1) size of the tumor (>5 cm); 2) a poorly differentiated histological aspect; 3) the number of mitotic figures; 4) the presence of intravascular plugs. A favorable prognostic sign would instead be an extended and intense calcification-ossification of the tumor.

TREATMENT

Surgical removal must aim at obtaining very wide margins. If this means sacrificing functionally important structures, or even amputation, one should not hesitate to do so, considering the severe prognosis of S.S. In the regions preferred by S.S. (knee, foot/ankle, elbow/wrist) an adequate wide en bloc excision can often be made and repaired by a vascularized muscle and/or skin flap. It may be useful to associate pre- or postoperative radiotherapy and chemotherapy (adriamycin), as long as one or the other does not constitute an excuse for inadequate surgery.

Excision of the regional lymph nodes, particularly when they are enlarged, is appropriate given the fair tendency of the tumor to metastasize by lymphatic route.

REFERENCES

1950 PACK G.T, ARIEL I.M.: Synovial sarcoma (malignant synovioma): A report of 60 cases. *Surgery*, **28**, 1047.

1955 CRAIG R.M., PUCH D.G., SOULE E.H.: The roentgenologic manifestations of synovial sarcoma. *Radiology*, **65**, 837.

1955 LICHTENSTEIN L.: Tumors of synovial joints, bursae and tendon sheaths. *Cancer*, **8**, 816.

1959 CROCKER D.W., STOUT A.P.: Synovial sarcoma in children. *Cancer*,**12**, 1123.

1960 GREISSINGER H.: The clinical aspects and therapy of synovialoma. *Brun. Beitr. Klin. Chir.*, **200**, 326.

1961 ANDERSON K.J., WILDERMUTH O.: Synovial sarcoma. *Clin. Orthop.*, **19**, 55.

1963 ARIEL I.M., PACK G.T.: Synovial sarcoma. *N. Engl. J. Med.*, **268**, 1272.

1965 CADMAN N.L., SOULE E.H. KELLY P.J.: Synovial sarcoma: An analysis of 134 tumors. *Cancer*, **18**, 613.

1966 MACKENZIE D.H.: Synovial sarcoma. A review of 58 cases. *Cancer*, **169**.

1968 HAMPOLE M.K., JACKSON B.A.: Analysis of 25 cases of malignant synovioma. *Can. Med. Assoc. J.*, **99**, 1025.

1968 MOBERGER G., NILSONNE U., FRIBERG S.: Synovial sarcoma. *Acta Orghop. Scand. (Suppl.)*, **111**, 3.

1971 GABBIANI G., KAYE G.I., LATTES R., *et al.*: Synovial sarcoma. Electronmicroscopic study of a typical case. *Cancer*, **28**, 1031.

1973   Horowitz A.L., Resnick D., Watson R.C.: The roentgen features of synovial sarcomas. *Clin. Radiol.*, **24**, 481.

1974   Bahners W., Burkhardt K.: Klinisches Bild, Verlauf und Prognose maligner Synovialome. *Chirurg.*, **45**, 507.

1974   Cameron H.U., Kostuik J.P.: A long-term follow-up of synovial sarcoma. *J. Bone Joint Surg.*, **56B**, 613.

1974   Lee S.M., Hajdu S.I., Exelby P.R.: Synovial sarcomas in children. *Surg. Gynecol. Obstet.*, **138**, 701.

1975   Roth J.A., Enzinger F.M., Tannenbaum M.: Synovial sarcoma of the neck. A followup study of 24 cases. *Cancer*, **35**, 1243.

1976   Fernandes B.B., Hernandes F.J.: Poorly differentiated synovial sarcoma. A light and electron microscopic study. *Arch. Pathol.*, **100**, 221.

1977   Hajdu S.I., Shiu M.H., Fortner J.G.: Tendosynovial sarcoma. A clinicopathological study of 136 cases. *Cancer*, **39**, 1201.

1977   Mackenzie D.H.: Monophasic synovial sarcoma - a histological entity? *Histopathology*, **1**, 151.

1977   Murray J.A.: Synovial sarcoma. *Orthop. Clin. North. Am.*, **8**, 963.

1978   Dische F.E., Darby A.J., Howard E.R.: Malignant synovioma: Electron microscopical findings in three patients and review of the literature. *J. Pathol.*, **124**, 149.

1979   Kuhl J., Kuhner U., Wunsch P.H.: Synovialsarkom im Kindesalter: Probleme der Therapie un prognostische Faktoren. *Z. Kinderchirug*, **27**, 9.

1979   Shiu M.H., McCormack P., Hajdu S.I., *et al*.: Surgical treatment of tendosynovial sarcomas. *Cancer*, **43**, 889.

1980   Evans H.L: Synovial sarcoma: A study of 23 biphasic and 17 probable monophasic examples. *Pathol. Annu.*, **15**, 309.

1980   Mickelson M.R., Brown G.A., Maynard J.A., *et al*.: Synovial sarcoma. An electron microscopic study of monophasic and biphasic forms. *Cancer*, **45**, 2109.

1981   Krall R.A., Kostianovsky M., Patchefsky A.S.: Synovial sarcoma. A clinical, pathological, and ultrastructural study of 26 cases supporting the recognition of a monophasic variant. *Am. J. Surg. Pathol.*, **5**, 137.

1982   Shmookler B.M., Enzinger F.M., Brannon R.B.: Orofacial synovial sarcoma. A clinicopathologic study of 11 new cases and review of the literature. *Cancer*, **50**, 269.

1984   Zito R.A.: Synovial sarcoma: an Australian series of 48 cases. *Pathology*, **16(1)**, 45-52.

1985   Salisbury J.R., Isaacson P.G.: Synovial sarcoma: An immunohistochemical study. *J. Pathol.*, **147**, 49-57.

1986   Bolen J.W., Hammar S.P., McNutt M.A.: Reactive and neoplastic serosal tissue. A light microscopic, ultrastructural, and immunocytochemical study. *Am. J. Surg. Pathol.*, **10**, 34-47.

1987   Cagle L.A., Mirra J.M., Storm F.K., Roe D.J., Eilber F.R.: Histologic features relating to prognosis in synovial sarcoma. *Cancer*, **59**, 1810

1987   Ghadially F.N.: Is synovial sarcoma a carcinosarcoma of connective tissue? *Ultrastructu. Pathol.*, **11**, 147.

1989   Rooser B., Willen H., Hugoson A., Rydholm A.: Prognostic factors in synovial sarcoma (24 cases, clinical review). *Cancer*, **63**, 2182.

1989   Sumitomo M., Hirose I., Rudo E., Sano T., Shinomija S., Hizawa I.: Epithelial differentiation in synovial sarcoma. Correlation with histology and immunophenotypic expression. *Acta Pathol. Jpn.*, **39**, 381.

1989   Wrba F., Fertl H., Amann G., Tell E., Krepler R.: Epithelial markers in synovial sarcoma. An immunohistochemical study on paraffin embedded tissues. *Virch. Arch. A.*, **415**, 253.

1990   Ordoñez S.M., Mahfouz S.M., Mc Kay B.: Synovial sarcoma: an immuno-histochemical and ultrastructural study. *Hum. Pathol.*, **21**, 733.

BENIGN TUMORS OF THE PERIPHERAL NERVES

This chapter includes neurinoma and neurofibroma. Although many authors tend to consider the two lesions as part of the same pathologic process, clinical and histological differences lead us to describe them separately. Neurofibroma involves a younger age group and patients affected with von Recklinghausen's disease. Neurinoma rarely involves the deep nerves and the internal organs more frequently involved in von Recklinghausen's disease, and hardly ever undergoes malignant transformation. Malignant evolution is a rare occurrence in solitary neurofibroma, but it is a more frequent one in cases associated with von Recklinghausen's disease. From a histological point of view, neurinoma is generally well-capsulated, with clearly recognizable organized structures (Antoni's types A and B), while neurofibroma is never capsulated and it may be localized, diffused or plexiform.

NEURINOMA
(neurilemmoma or schwannoma)

Made up of cells having schwannic differentiation, it occurs on a nerve, is well-capsulated and present typical histology. All **ages** may be involved, but it prevails during adult age (between 20 and 50 years). There is no specific predilection for **sex**. It is particularly **localized** in the spinal roots (Fig. 822), in the nerves of the mediastinum and of the retroperitoneum. It is nearly always a single nodule; multiple nodules or association with von Recklinghausen's disease are rarely observed.

N. of the spinal roots is generally contained in the dural sac, it originates from a root, and it causes liquoral block, compression of the other roots of the cauda equina, or of the spinal cord in the more cranial sites. Symptoms are of long duration as a result of the slow or very slow growth of the tumor. Rachialgia, positive liquoral signs, nocturnal increase in pain, stiffness and spinal contractures, signs of nerve root or medullary irritation or compression (often pluriradicular and bilateral) prevail.

Clinical differential diagnosis in relation to lumbar and lumbosacral disc herniation is based on the more subtle and progressive onset of symptoms, on the nerve root symptoms which are not limited to a single root (usually L5 or S1). Diagnosis is supported by myelography and CAT-myelography, and especially by MRI.

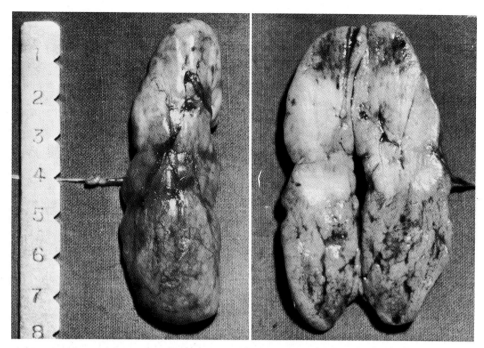

FIG. 822. - Male aged 37 years. Neurinoma of the 4th lumbar nerve root.

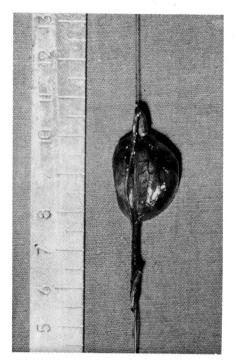

FIG. 823. - Female aged 29 years. Neurinoma of the 5th lumbar nerve root, partially cystic.

When it is localized in a peripheral nerve, N. may be sharply painful, particularly with pressure, and at times cause algodystrophic syndromes of the limb. It may be palpated and its palpation may cause sharp, irradiated pain with paresthesiae.

In the intradural site, N. **macroscopically** appears to be a globose «sausage-like» nodule elongated in the direction of the length of the sac. The nodule is on both sides connected to a nerve root (Fig. 822). At times the other roots, the arachnoid and the dura, or the cord may adhere slightly to the surface of the nodule, but this is always well-delimited by a thin capsule and enucleable. Coloring is grayish, often bluish-red; consistency is soft, at times partially or to a great extentcystic, as a result of the ser-

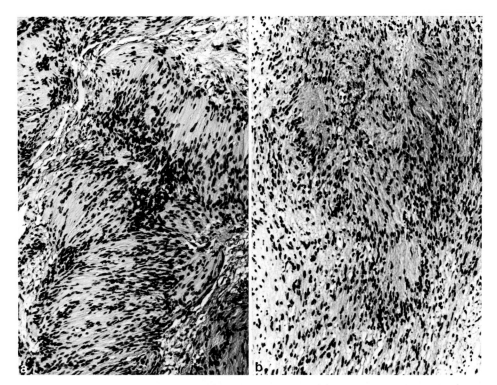

FIG. 824. - Neurinoma. (a) and (b) There is palisading of the nuclei with formation of the Verocay's bodies (*Hemat.-eos.*, 125, 160 x).

ous or sero-hematic fluid contents. Rarely intradural N. are multiple, like rosary beads along the roots. In rare cases N. is extradural, and it expands like an hour-glass inside and out of the intervertebral root foramen. N. of the peripheral nerves may be totally contained in the nerve, which may appear to be enlarged «like an onion bulb» (Fig. 823); or protrude externally attached to a nerve like a piece of fruit to its stem (in the smaller nerves). In both cases, the N. is well-capsulated. Unlike intradural N., those of the peripheral nerves are more solid, whitish in color.

The size of N. rarely surpasses that of a walnut. Occasionally, however, N. reaches large or very large size, particularly in the sacrum, where it may cause vast osteolyses and bulge inside the pelvis (see N. of bone).

Histologically an overall examination reveals a periphery delimited by a fibrous capsule. N. is characterized by a particular cellular arrangement: Antoni areas A and B. Antoni's area A is characterized by the proliferation of spindle cells with indistinct cytoplasm which are arranged in intersecting bundles. Often, the nuclei tend to be arranged in palisades around eosinophilic areas towards which the cytoplasmatic processes are oriented (Verocay's bodies) (Fig. 824). At times the cells tend to be arranged in whorls, surrounding hyaline centers. The cells are positive for protein S 100.

Some tumors are exclusively constituted by Antoni's A areas. In others, instead, the A areas associate with B areas. Antoni's B areas are characterized by less cellularity, with an «edematous» aspect, cells loosely distributed, widely apart from each other.

The vessels are open, at times thrombized, they have a thickened wall, fibrohyalin.

Some N. present unusual and alarming cytological aspects characterized by cells with rather voluminous, bizarre and hyperchromatic nuclei. These cells are more often associated with degenerative phenomena (cysts, necrosis, hemorrhage, calcification, hyalinization), there are no mitotic figures, and these are considered to be «degenerative aspects».

N. is a benign lesion the simple excision of which is curative. At times surgery must be repeated because incomplete excision or the presence of a second nodule which was not excised result in recurrence of the symptoms. Malignant transformation is very rare.

SOLITARY NEUROFIBROMA AND NEUROFIBROMA ASSOCIATED WITH VON RECKLINGHAUSEN'S DISEASE

It is the same lesion which may be presented as a single localization or within von Recklinghausen's disease. When it is associated with the latter N.F. may take on the various morphological aspects which are typical of von Recklinghausen's disease. The latter is classified as a neurocutaneous or facomatose syndrome and is a dominant autosomic disease with a high grade of penetration. It occurs more frequently in the male sex and clinically there is a peripheral form and a central one. The disease is associated with café au lait skin spots, due to increased melanic pigmentation in the basal layer of the epidermis (Figs. 825, 826).

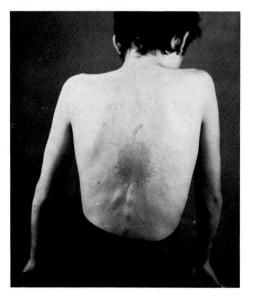

Solitary N.F. generally involves patients aged from 20 to 40 years, while that associated with von Recklinghausen's disease involves a younger age group. As for site, solitary N.F. is nearly limited to subcutaneous tissue and to the

FIG. 825. - Neurofibromatosis. Female aged 14 years, with painful subcutaneous swellings in the forearm, dorsum and thigh. Café au lait skin spots with uneven margins.

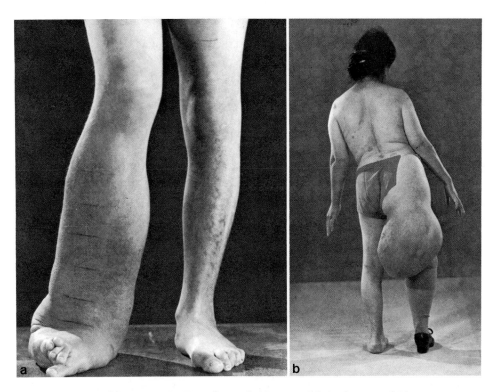

FIG. 826. - Neurofibromatosis. Female aged 44 years. (a) At the age of 13 years, aspect of the right leg and foot, the swelling of which initiated at 5 years of age. Because of the lesion the patient was amputated below the knee. (b) At the age of 44 years, swelling of the thigh on the same side (prosthetized) which progressively increased over recent years. The histological aspect is that of a neurofibroma with areas of evident cellularity, but no signs of malignancy. Swelling was excised; no signs of local recurrence after 3 years.

derma, while that in Recklinghausen's disease may occur in all sites and in all of the organs.

Macroscopically solitary N.F. is a spindle mass within the context of the nerve, of moderately firm consistency, on the cut surface it is grayish in color with pink areas. **Histologically** its structure varies depending on the quantity of cells, collagen and myxoid component (Fig. 827). Intersecting bundles are observed, constituted by spindle cells and having an ondulated pattern. These cells are associated with collagen fibers and varying quantities of mucine. There may be scattered xanthomatous cells and/or lymphocytes. The differing quantity of mucine conditions the differing aspect of N.F.: when mucoid substance is scarce, the lesion is very cellular and, at times, areas with nuclear hyperchromia may lead to suspicion of sarcomatous evolution, which may be excluded by the rarity of mitotic figures and the absence of necrosis. In general, there is no fibrous capsule and there are no Antoni's A and B areas, so that differential diagnosis with neurinoma is easy.

The typical histological picture of localized N.F. is the same as that of N.F. associated with von Recklinghausen's disease. Here, N.F. may become

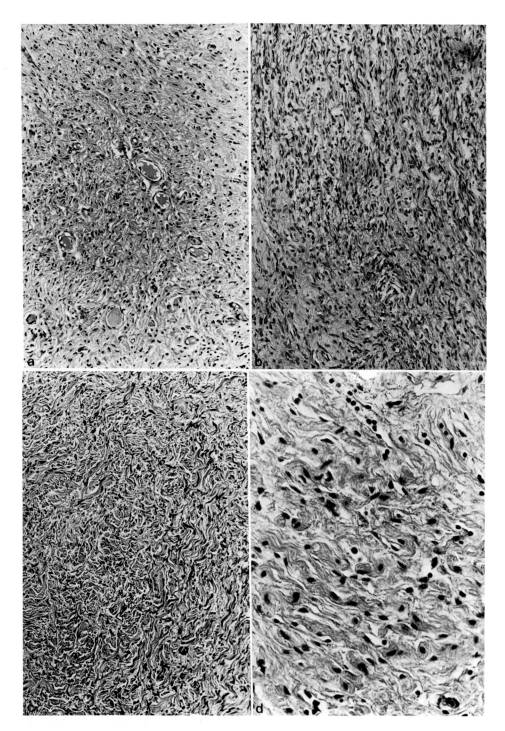

FIG. 827. - Solitary neurofibroma. (a), (b) and (c) There are bundles of intersecting cells. The cells are spindle, have a wavy profile, hyperchomic nuclei and they are mixed with collagen fibers. (d) Spindle Schwann cells associated with collagen fibers (*Hemat.-eos.*, 125, 125, 125, 400 x).

FIG. 828. - Female aged 61 years. Plexiform neurofibroma of the median nerve at the wrist.

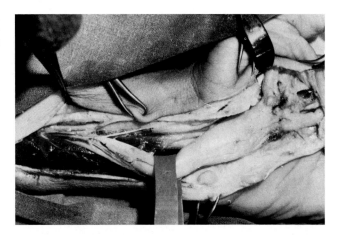

of larger size, and more frequently undergo malignant evolution, particularly of the deeply localized N.F.

During the course of von Recklinghausen's disease, the N.F. assumes other typical aspects which are absent in the solitary form. These are represented by plexiform N.F. and diffused N.F.

Plexiform neurofibroma. It occurs in nerves of larger caliber which it transforms into cordonal masses of convoluted aspect (Fig. 828). At times,

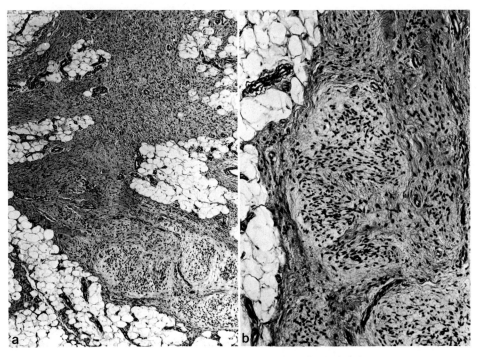

FIG. 829. - Diffused neurofibroma. (a), and (b) The ramified proliferation is diffused in the fibro-adipose tissue. There is a uniform fibrillary matrix with Schwann cells arranged in small groups (*Hemat.-eos.*, 50, 125 x).

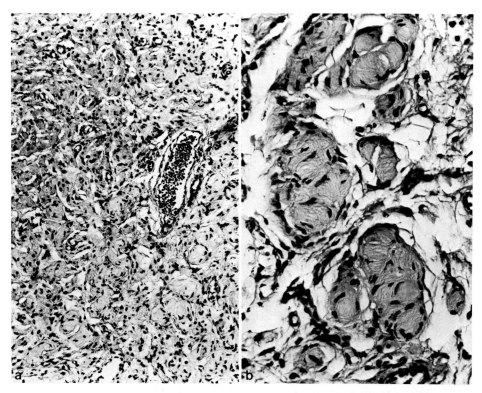

FIG. 830. - Diffused neurofibroma in von Recklinghausen's disease. (a) There are Schwann cells with organoid organization immersed in fibrillary stroma. (b) Under higher power there is a tendency towards organoid organization of the cells which look like Wagner Meissner's bodies (*Hemat.-eos.*, 160, 400 x).

the neoformation may be widely extended and involve an entire limb (neurofibromatous elephantiasis). Histologically there is a mixture of nerve trunks of differing shape and size crossing each other along various planes of orientation. In some cases, the individuality of the nerve fibers is respected, while in others there is a proliferation of Schwann cells and of fibroblasts producing collagen.

Diffused neurofibroma. In general it is localized in the area of the head and neck in the subcutaneous tissue, and it resembles a plaque-like thickening of the skin. Macroscopically the subcutaneous tissue and the derma appear to be thickened and transformed into a whitish tissue. The term diffused refers to the way in which the lesion grows, as it is diffused along the connective septa and among the cells of the adipose tissue. The subcutaneous structures are surrounded by the neoplasm which in its growth does not lead to their destruction. Histologically, diffused N.F. differs from circumscribed N.F. by a less evident fibrillary collagen matrix. The Schwann cells are immersed in a finely fibrillary homogeneous matrix, they appear to be more ovoid or round, with a monomorphous aspect (Fig. 829). At times the cells tend to aggregate in structures recalling Meissner's bodies (Fig. 830). The sarcomatous evolution of diffused N.F. rarely occurs, the extension of which sometimes makes effective surgical treatment impossible.

·Sarcomatous evolution of neurofibroma

While neurinoma exceptionally evolves into sarcoma, this evolution is observed in neurofibroma and, particularly, in neurofibroma in von Recklinghausen's disease. The incidence of the malignant evolution is difficult to determine and the literature reports that it varies from 2 to 30%. High-risk patients are those in whom the disease has been present for a longer time and is localized in a deep site.

REFERENCES

NEURINOMA

1967 WHITE N.B.: Neurilemomas of the extremity. *J. Bone Joint Surg.*, **49/A**, 1605.
1969 CARSTENS H., SCHRODT G.: Malignant transformation of a benign encapsulated neurilemoma. *Am. J. Clin. Pathol.*, **51**, 144.
1969 DAS GUPTA T.K., BRASFIELD R.D., STRONG E.W., et al.: Benign solitary schwannomas (neurilemomas). *Cancer*, **24**, 355.
1969 STENER B., ANGERVALL L., NILSSON L., et al.: Angiographic and histological studies of the vascularization of peripheral nerve tumors. *Clin. Orthop.*, **66**,113.
1971 DINAKDAR I., RAO S.B.: Neurilemomas of peripheral nerves. *Int. Surg.*, **55**, 15.
1973 HYBBINETTE C.H.: Solitary benign nerve sheath tumors around the knee joint: Report of four cases. *Acta Orthop. Scand.*, **44**, 296.
1975 CHANDRA S., JERVA M.J., CLEMICS J.D.: Ultrastructural characteristics of human neurilemoma cell nuclei. *Cancer Res.*, **35**, 2000.
1976 WHITAKER W.G., DROULIAS C.: Bening encapsulated neurilemoma: A report of 76 cases. *Am. Surg.*, **42**, 675.
1981 SIAN C.S., RYAN S.F.: The ultrastructure of neurilemoma with emphasis on Antoni B tissue. *Hum. Pathol.*, **12**, 145.
1984 DAHL I., HAGMAR B., IDVALL I.: Benign solitary neurilemoma (Schwannoma). A correlative cytological and histological study of 28 cases. *Acta Pathol. Microbiol. Immunol. Scand.*, **92**, 91.
1986 WEIDENHEIM K.M., CAMPBELL W.G.: Perineurial cell tumor. Immunocytochemical and ultrastructural characterization. Relationship to other peripheral nerve tumors with a review of the literature. *Virchows Arch. Pathol. Anat.*, **408**, 375.
1987 FLETCHER C.D.M., DAVIES S.E., MC KEE P.H.: Cellular schwannoma. A distinct pseudosarcomatous entity. *Histopathology*, **11**, 21.
1988 KAWAHARA E., ODA Y., ODI A., KATSUDA S., NAKANISHI I., UMEDA S.: Expression of glial fibrillary acidic protein (GFAP) in peripheral nerve sheath tumors. A comparative study of immunoreactivity of GFAP, vimentin, S-100 protein, and neurofilaments in 38 schwannomas and 18 neurofibromas. *Am. J. Surg. Pathol.*, **12**, 115.
1989 KAO G.F., LASKIN W.B., OLSEN T.G.: Solitary cutaneous plexiform neurilemmoma (schwannoma): clinicopathologic, immunohistochemical and ultrastructural study of 11 cases. *Mod. Pathol.*, **2**, 20.

NEUROFIBROMA

1956 CROWE F.W., SCHULL W.J., NEEL J.V.: *A Clinical, pathological, and genetic study of multiple neurofibromatosis.* Springfield, Ill., Charles C. Thomas Publisher.

1956   McCarroll H.R.: Soft tissue neoplasms associated with congenital neurofibromatosis. *J Bone Joint Surg.,* **38,** 717.

1966   Rodriquez H.A., Berthrong M.: Multiple primary intracranial tumors in von Recklinghausen's neurofibromatosis. *Arch. Neurol.* **14,** 467.

1971   Sane S., Yunis E.: Subperiosteal or cortical cyst and intramedullary neurofibromatosis: Uncommon manifestations of neurofibromatosis. *J. Bone Joint Surg.* **53,** 1194.

1972   Brasfield R.D., Das Gupta T.K.: Von Recklinghausen's disease: A clinicopathological study. *Ann. Surg.* **175,** 86.

1974   Greene J., Fitzwater J., Burgess J.: Arterial lesions associated with neurofibromatosis. *Am J. Clin. Pathol.* **62,** 481.

1975   Weiser G.: An electron microscope study of «Pacinian neurofibroma». *Virchows Arch (Pathol Anat)* **366,** 331.

1977   Adkins J.C., Ravitch M.M.: The operative management of von Recklinghausen's neurofibromatosis in children, with special reference to lesions of the head and neck. *Surgery* **82,** 342.

1977   Lassmann H., Jurecka W. Lassmann V., *et al.:* Different types of benign nerve sheath tumors: Light microscopy, electron microscopy, and autoradiography. *Virchows Arch. (Pathol Anat)* **375,** 197.

1978   Akwari O.E., Payne W.S., Onofrio B.M., *et al.:* Dumbbell neurogenic tumors of the mediastinum. *Mayo Clin. Proc.* **53,** 353.

1979   Guccion J.G., Enziger F.M.: Malignant schwannoma associated with von Recklinghausen's neurofibromatosis. *Virchows Arch. (Pathol. Anat)* **383,** 43.

1981   Riccardi V.M.: Von Recklinghausen neurofibromatosis. *N. Engl. J. Med.,* **305,** 1617.

1982   Friedman J.M., Fialkow P.J., Greene C.L., Weinberg W.N.: Probable clonal origin of neurofibrosarcoma in a patient with hereditary neurofibromatosis. *J. Natl. Cancer Inst.,* **69,** 1289.

1986   Sorensen S.A., Mulvihill J.J., Nielsen A.: Long-term follow-up of von Recklinghausen neurofibromatosis: Survival and malignant neoplasms. *N. Engl. J. Med.,* **314,** 1010.

1987   Barker D., Wright E., Nguyen L.: Gene for von Recklinghausen neurofibromatosis is in the pericentromeric region of chromosome 17. *Science,* **236,** 1100.

MALIGNANT TUMORS OF THE PERIPHERAL NERVES

MALIGNANT NEURINOMA
(malignant neurilemmoma, malignant schwannoma)

What we mean by malignant neurinoma is a sarcoma which originates from a peripheral nerve or occurs within neurofibromatosis. These clinical and anatomo-surgical criteria are essential, as there are no constant and undebatable histological elements which distinguish this sarcoma from a fibrosarcoma.

Solitary M.N. occurs during advanced adult **age** (40 years and up) while that associated with von Recklinghausen's disease (Fig. 831) occurs on the average at an earlier age (30 years). There is no predilection for **sex**. Important clinical signs are the occurrence of pain and a progressive increase in

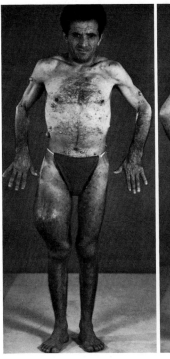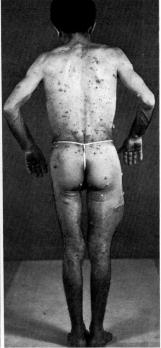

FIG. 831. - Malignant neurinoma in von Recklinghausen's disease. Male aged 44 years, affected with neurofibromatosis. Observe the typical café au lait spots and the cutaneous and subcutaneous nodules, particularly diffused in the trunk. For the past 4 months there was a rapidly increasing mass in the right thigh. Biopsy revealed spindle cell sarcoma characterized by a high grade of malignancy. The patient was submitted to interileo-abdominal amputation, and died after 3 years of metastases.

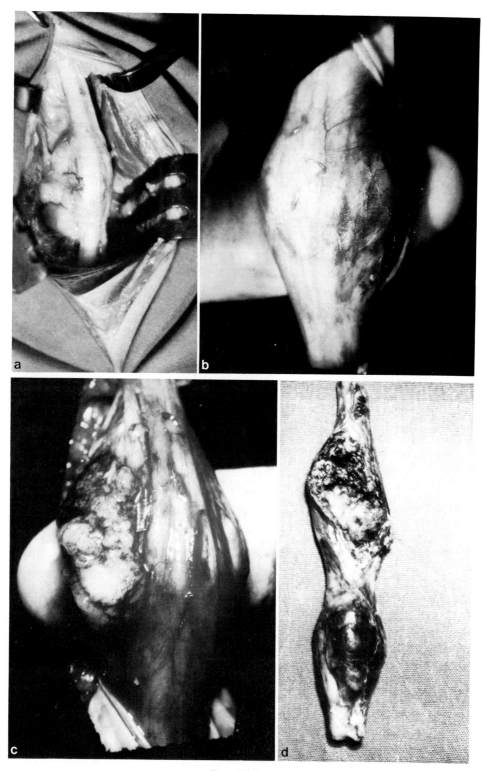

FIG. 832.

the volume of the neoplasm. These two elements are sufficient to raise suspicion as to a malignant transformation, and to perform biopsy. The sites most frequently involved are the major nerve trunks such as the sciatic nerve, the brachial plexus, and the sacral plexus.

Macroscopically M.N. is a mass connected with a nerve and which is often eccentric in relation to it (Fig. 832). As previously stated, anatomical dissection is essential to diagnosis, as connection between the tumor and the nerve (or the association with von Recklinghausen's disease) is an essential diagnostic element. Areas resembling rosary beads in the nerve in the proximal or distal site in relation to the principal tumoral mass indicate diffusion of the neoplasm along the epineurium or the perineurium. Localization is generally deep although there may be rare superficial sites. The lesion often has a diameter exceeding 5 cm. On the cut surface it is of whitish aspect, like fishmeat or encephaloid, with diffused necrotic-hemorrhagic areas.

The **histological aspect** is partially comparable to that of fibrosarcoma (Figs. 833-836). The cells may be distinguished by the fibroblast as the nuclei have a wavy, «curly» profile. In transverse section they appear to be oval. The cytoplasm has indistinct margins. An overall view reveals areas with thicker cellularity interspersed with others in which the cellularity is poorer. This aspect of variation in the cellular distribution is a rather distinct feature as compared to what is observed in fibrosarcoma. At times myxoid areas modify the fasciculated and parallel assemblage of the cells. The ovoid or spindle cells may take on a nodular or pin-wheel aspect suggesting a rudimentary tactoid differentiation of the Meissner or Pacini body type. Palisading of the nuclei may be seen, but not constanly. At times, fibrohyaline bands bordered by ovoid cells are observed. Cellular proliferation around the vessels uplifts the parietal constituents so that the neoplastic cells seem to make a hernia inside the lumen.

Cartilaginous and osseous metaplasia, or differentiation in rhabdomyoblasts and in pseudoglands which secrete mucin may be observed in these tumors. When rhabdomyoblasts are observed we speak of malignant «**triton tumor**». When glandular elements secreting mucin are present, the tumor is defined **malignant glandular neurinoma**. The tumoral cells may also assume epitheliomorphous aspects. When the entire tumor is constituted by epithe-

◄

FIG. 832. - Malignant neurinoma of the sciatic nerve. (a) Male aged 40 years. Surgical finding. Observe the lobulated mass of compact, whitish, encephaloid tissue originating from the nerve. The patient was submitted to hip disarticulation and died after 2 months of metastases. (b) Male aged 26 years. Malignant neurinoma of the sciatic nerve. At surgery, fusiform enlargement of the nerve was seen. (c) The nervous sheath was incised, to reveal protrusion of the soft tumoral tissue, which was friable and encephaloid. (d) The nerve presented a second similar and more proximal neoplastic node. Surgery consisted of a marginal resection of the nerve. The tumor recurred after 1 year, and it was treated by atypical thigh amputation removing the posterior compartment of the thigh (skin, muscles and sciatic nerve) as far as the ischiatic tuberosity. Chemotherapy. Died after 3 years of pulmonary metastases.

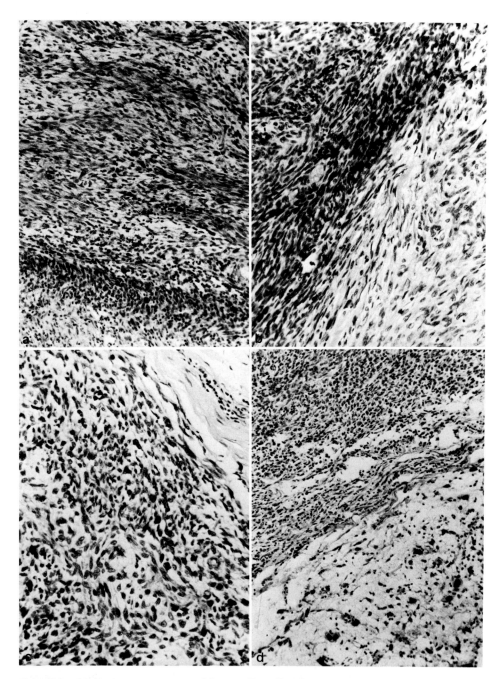

FIG. 833. - Malignant neurinoma. (a) Spindle cells of monomorphous aspect arranged
in closely aggregated bundles. (b) Hypercellular tumoral areas side by side with
hypocellular ones. (c) Areas in which the spindle cells reveal arrangement in wavy
bundles. The nuclei present moderate pleomorphism with a curved profile. (d) Areas
with spindle cells arranged in bundles and with a monormophous aspect are alternated with areas in which there is myxoid aspect and evident pleomorphism (*Hemat.-
eos.*, 160, 250, 250, 160 x).

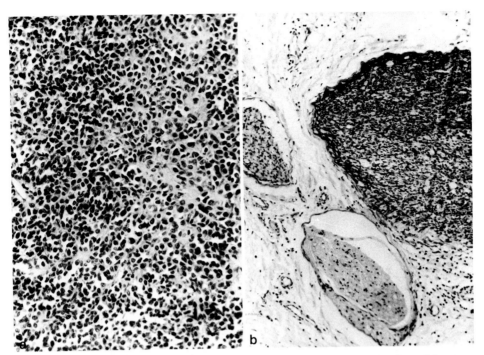

FIG. 834. - (a) Malignant neurinoma with prevalent round and oval cell proliferation. (b) Nerve trunk invaded by a proliferation of oval and spindle cells having a high grade of malignancy (*Hemat.-eos.*, 250, 160 x).

liomorphous cellular elements it is defined **malignant epithelioid neurinoma**.

Overall, M.N. manifests a wide range of grades of malignancy and differentiation, from highly undifferentiated and malignant forms where it is difficult to recognize the nervous differentiation unless electron microscopy is used or the protein S 100 is identified, to more differentiated and less malignant forms, where the aspect is similar to that of neurofibroma, but with evident mitotic activity, cellular pleomorphism and greater cellularity.

Differential diagnosis involves spindle-cell sarcomas, such as monophasic synovial sarcoma, fibrosarcoma and leiomyosarcoma. **Fibrosarcoma** and **spindle-cell monophasic synovial sarcoma** present a monomorphous cytology with uniformly distributed nuclei; while in M.N. the quantitative distribution of the nuclei varies and the aspect is generally more pleomorphic. The presence of protein S 100 is supportive for diagnosis. **Leiomyosarcoma** presents cells with clearly defined eosinophilic cytoplasm, cytoplasmatic vacuoles, nuclei with rounded ends. Special staining methods may reveal the longitudinal striations and contents in glycogen.

It is sometimes a problem for the histologist to decide whether during the course of von Recklinghausen's disease a specific lesion is an innocent neurofibroma, or whether it is a neurofibroma with areas in sarcomatous evolu-

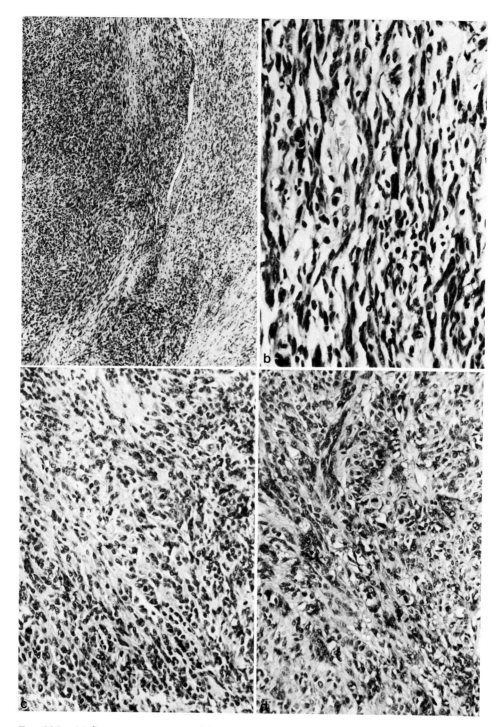

FIG. 835. - Malignant neurinoma. (a) In some areas spindle cells are closely packed, in others loosely arranged. (b), (c) and (d) The neoplasm is characterized by a high grade of malignancy and a specific differentiation cannot be distinguished (*Hemat.-eos.*, 60, 400, 400, 400 x).

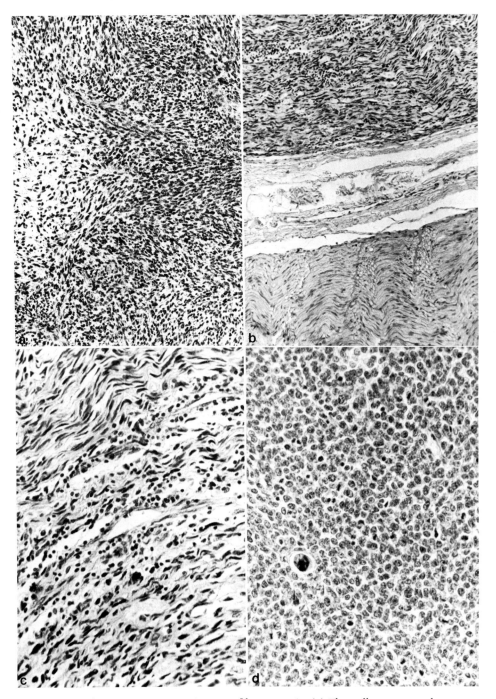

FIG. 836. - Malignant neurinoma in neurofibromatosis. (a) The cells appear to be organized in bundles with densely cellular areas recalling the aspect of fibrosarcoma, associated with other hypocellular areas. (b) and (c) Adjacent to the nerve trunk there are cells of malignant neurinoma with a wavy pattern and hyperchromatic nuclei. (d) Malignant neurinoma with vast areas constituted by round-oval cells having atypical nucleocytoplasmatic features (*Hemat.-eos.*, 125, 125, 250, 250 x).

tion. Important criteria are the presence of mitotic activity, cellular pleomorphism and areas of necrosis.

The **prognosis** of M.N. associated with von Recklinghausen's disease (30% five-year survival rate) is worse than that of solitary M.N. (75% five-year survival rate). Similarly, in sarcomas associated with von Recklinghausen's disease the percentage of local recurrence and metastases is higher. It seems that the worse prognosis in sarcomas in von Recklinghausen's disease is also related to their deep localization.

The **treatment** of M.N. is mainly surgical and, as we are generally dealing with a high grade and extracompartmental tumor (stage IIB), it requires very wide or radical margins. Its often multicentric origin and the diffusion of the tumor along the nerves at times make even radical surgery uneffective. There is little information with regard to chemotherapy.

PERIPHERAL NEUROEPITHELIOMA
(peripheral neuroblastoma)

It is a primitive neuroectodermic tumor which originates in the peripheral nerves. In 1918 Stout first described this unusual entity, demonstrating that cultivated in vitro the tumor cells developed features suggesting their neu-

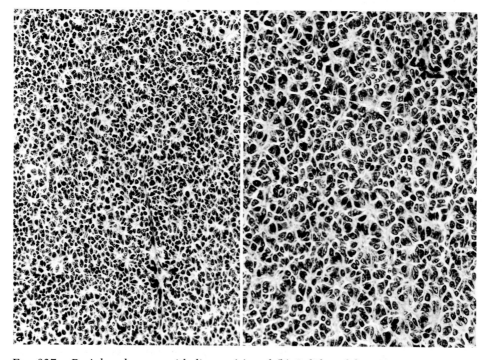

FIG. 837. - Peripheral neuroepithelioma. (a) and (b) Solid proliferation constituted by undifferentiated round cells. The nuclei are hyperchromatic, ovoid or round. The cells are arranged «rosette-like» with extensions of cytoplasms converging at the center. This finding is similar to that of neuroblastoma (*Hemat.-eos.*, 160, 400 x).

roblastic nature. The tumor originates from the large nerves and histologically it resembles neuroblastoma. In fact, solid fields or lobules constituted by small round cells having an intensely hyperchromatic round-oval nucleus may be observed (Fig. 837). Cytoplasm is scarce, with indistinct margins. At times rosette formations are observed, in the central part of which the filiform cytoplasmatic extensions converge. These rosettes repeat the features of the neuroblastoma.

While differential diagnosis in the child must include **metastasis due to neuroblastoma**, in the adult it involves **small-cell carcinoma**, both primary and metastatic. In these cases electron microscopy is useful as it reveals the cytoplasmatic processes of the neuroepithelial cells.

The peripheral neuroepithelioma is highly malignant, with an elevated propensity to metastasize and to diffuse locally.

REFERENCES

MALIGNANT NEURINOMA

1963 D'AGOSTINO A.N., SOULE E.H., MILLER R.H.: Primary malignant neoplasm of nerves (malignant neurilemomas) in patients without manifestations of multiple neurofibromatosis (von Recklinghausen's disease). *Cancer,* **16**, 1003.

1971 WHITE H.R.: Survival in malignant schwannoma: An 18-year study. *Cancer* **27**, 720.

1973 GHOSH B.C., GHOSH L., HUVOS A.G., *et. al.:* Malignant schwannoma: A clinico-pathologic study. *Cancer* **31**, 184.

1973 WOODRUFF J.M., CHERNIK N.L., SMITH M.C., *et. al:* Peripheral nerve tumors with rhabdomyosarcomatous differentiation (malignant «Triton» tumors). *Cancer* **32**, 426.

1975 GIANNESTRAS N.J., BRONSON J.L.: Malignant schwannoma of the medial plantar branch of the posterior tibial nerve (unassociated with von Recklinghausen's disease). *J. Bone Joint Surg.* **57/A**, 701.

1976 WOODRUFF J.M.: Peripheral nerve tumors showing glandular differentiation (glandular schwannoma). *Cancer* **37**, 2399.

1978 KRUMERMAN M.S., STINGLE W.: Synchronous malignant glandular schwannomas in congenital neurofibromatosis. *Cancer* **41**, 2444.

1978 McKEEN E.A., BODURTHA J., MEADOWS A.T., *et. al.:* Rhabdomyosarcoma complicating multiple neurofibromatosis. *J. Pediatr.* **93**, 992.

1979 GUCCION J.G., ENZINGER F.M.: Malignant schwannoma associated with von Recklinghausen's neurofibromatosis. *Virchows Arch. (Pathol. Anat.)* **383**, 43.

1979 MENNEMEYER R.P., *et al.*: Melanotic schwannoma, clinical and ultrastructural studies of three cases with evidence of intracellular melanin synthesis. *Am. J. Surg. Pathol.,* **3**, 3.

1979 TSUNEYOSHI M., ENJOJI M.: Primary malignant peripheral nerve tumors (malignant schwannomas): A clinicopathologic and electron microscopic study. *Acta Pathol. Jpn.* **29**, 363.

1980 STORM F.K., EILBER F.R., MIRRA J., *et al.:* Neurofibrosarcoma. *Cancer* **45**, 126.

1981 TAXY J.B., BATTIFORA H.B.: Epithelioid schwannoma: Diagnosis by electron microscopy. *Ultrastruc Pathol.* **2**, 19.

1984 BOJSEN MOLLER M.; MYHRE-JENSEN O.: A consecutive series of 30 malignant schwannomas. Survival in relation to clinico-pathological parameters and treatment. *Acta Pathol. Microbiol. Immunol. Scand.,* **92**, 147.

1984 NAMBISAN R.N.; RAO U.; MOORE R.: KARAKOUSIS C.P.: Malignant soft tissue tumors of nerve sheath origin. *J. Surg. Oncol.,* **25**, , 268.

1985   BROOKS J.S., FREEMAN M., ENTERLINE H.T.: Malignant "Triton" tumors. Natural history and immunohistochemistry of nine cases with literature review. *Cancer*, **55**, 2543.

1986   DUCATMAN B.S., SCHEITHAUER B.W., PIEPGRAS D.G.: Malignant peripheral nerve sheath tumors: A clinicopathologic study of 120 cases. *Cancer*, **57**, 2006.

1987   WICK M.R., SWANSON P.E., SCHEITHAUER B.W., MANIVEL J.C.: Malignant peripheral nerve sheath tumor. An immunohistochemical study of 62 cases. *Am. J. Clin. Pathol.*, **87**, 425.

1989   HIROSE T., SUMITOMO M., RUDO E., HASEGAWA T.: Malignant peripheral nerve sheath tumor (MPNST) showing perineurial cell differentiation (case). *Am. J. Surg. Pathol.*, **13**, 613.

PERIPHERAL NEUROEPITHELIOMA

1973   NINFO V., ZILIOTTO G.R.: Il neuroepitelioma maligno dei nervi periferici (cosiddetto medulloblastoma dei nervi periferici). *Pathologica* **65**, 393.

1975   SEEMAYER T.A., THELMO W.L., BOLAND R., *et al.:* Peripheral neuroectodermal tumors. *Perspect. Pediatr. Pathol.* **2**, 151.

1980   BOLEN J.W., THORNING D.: Peripheral neuroepithelioma: A light and electron microscopic study. *Cancer* **46**, 2456.

1981   HARPER P.G., PRINGLE J., SOUHAMI R.L.: Neuroepithelioma — A rare malignant peripheral nerve tumor of primitive origin: Report of two new cases. *Cancer*, **48**, 2282.

1983   HASHIMOTO H., ENJOJI M., NAKAJIMA T., *et al.:* Malignant neuroepithelioma (peripheral neuroblastoma): A clinicopathologic study of 15 cases. *Am. J. Surg. Pathol.*, **7**, 309.

1984   VOSS B.L., PYSHER T.J., HUMPHREY G.B.: Peripheral neuroepithelioma in childhood. *Cancer*, **54**, 3059.

1989   LLOMBART-BOSCH A., TERRIER-LACOMBE M.J., PEYDRO-OLAYA A., CONTESSO G.: Peripheral neuroectodermal sarcoma of soft tissue (peripheral neuroepithelioma): a pathologic study of ten cases with differential diagnosis regarding other small, round-cell sarcomas. *Hum. Pathol.*, **20**, 273.

CHONDROSARCOMA

Chondrosarcoma of the soft tissues is a rare occurrence. Unlike chondrosarcoma of the skeleton, the tumors constituted by well-differentiated cartilage are limited to exceptional cases of synovial chondrosarcoma. The near totality of chondrosarcomas of the soft tissues is instead constituted by myxoid forms and by mesenchymal chondrosarcomas.

MYXOID CHONDROSARCOMA
(extraskeletal myxoid chondrosarcoma, chordoid sarcoma)

It is a rare tumor, which shows predilection for the male **sex** and is nearly exclusively observed during adult and advanced **age**. Its **localization** is deep (even if exceptional cases localized superficially have been described). It is especially observed in the limbs and particularly in the lower limb.

Symptoms are not typical and they are generally of long duration due to the slow growth of the tumor. Despite its cartilaginous nature, the **radiographic picture** is completely aspecific, lacking images of calcification or ossification.

Macroscopically it is a mass which is usually provided with a thin pseudocapsular delimitation. Its consistency is tense and on the cut surface there is a tissue of mucoid aspect, partly translucid, altered by frequent areas of hemorrhage. At times, the accumulation of liquid mucoid material and/or hemorrhages may be the cause of extensive cystic transformation of the tumor. The tumor may become of average to large size.

Histologically M.C. has a lobular structure. The blood vessels are exclusively observed in the cloisters alternating with the lobules. The tumor is more or less cellular, more or less differentiated in a chondroblastic sense. Nonetheless, this differentiation hardly ever achieves the stage of well-differentiated hyaline cartilage. Cells are arranged mostly in intertwined strings and cords, among which there is abundant mucoid substance (Fig. 838). The cells have rounded or oval nuclei and little intensely eosinophilic cytoplasm (with PAS its glycogen content is revealed). The nuclei are intensely stained, with moderate pleomorphism and few mitotic figures. In the less differentiated areas the cells do not produce mucoid material, they are larger, and they have paler nuclei and a higher number of mitotic figures. Rarely, some areas of

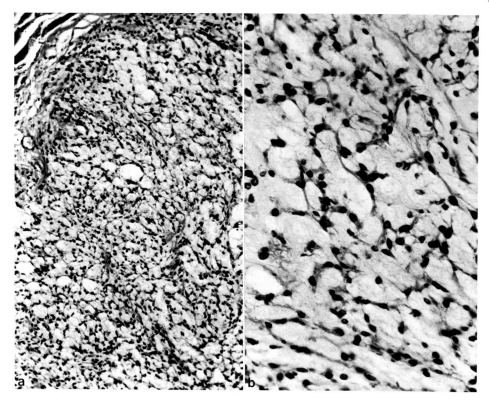

FIG. 838. - Myxoid chondrosarcoma. (a) The cells are dispersed in a myxoid matrix. (b) The spindle or stellate cells are regularly assembled in cords or strings separated by abundant material of myxoid aspect (*Hemat.-eos.*, 160, 400 x).

greater differentiation are observed with cells closed in lacunae and surrounded by a more homogeneous and compact ground substance.

As in other tumors which produce mucoid substance, the intercellular substance of C.M. takes the halcian blue and the colloidal iron and is stained metachromatically with toluidine blue. However, unlike other myxoid tumors, staining occurs at a lower pH and, in particular, it is not annulled by pre-treatment with hyaluronidase.

Myxoid liposarcoma is distinguished by its plexiform vascular pattern, by the presence of lipoblasts, and because the mucoid substance is not colored after treatment with hyaluronidase. **Myxoma** is distinguished because the cells are dispersed, they do not have the aspect of chondroblasts (plump nuclei and intensely eosinophilic cytoplasm), and they are not arranged in cords. Furthermore, in myxoma as well the mucin loses its tingibility after treatment with hyaluronidase. **Chordoma** is that tumor which most resembles M.C. and its mucoid substance has the same tintorial characteristics as those of M.C. The distinction is based on the presence, in the chordoma, of physaliphore cells and on the anatomo-clinical situation (origin in the sacrococcyx, in the vertebrae or in the cranial base).

Prognosis of M.C. of the soft tissues is like to that of most skeletal chondrosarcomas. The tumor usually grows slowly, but it has a considerable tendency to recur locally and it is capable of metastasizing. Given the rareness of this tumor it is not clear whether a grade of histological malignancy correlated with prognosis may be established as it is in the skeletal chondrosarcomas. In the same manner, nearly nothing is known as to the sensitivity of this tumor to radiation and chemotherapy. The most suitable type of **treatment** appears to be wide surgical excision.

MESENCHYMAL CHONDROSARCOMA

It is rare in the soft tissues, even more rare than in the skeleton. There is no predilection for **sex** and, unlike myxoid chondrosarcoma, it is observed during young-adult **age**, from 15 to 40 years. It prefers the following **localizations**: the neck and lower limb, with a deep site.

Clinically, again unlike myxoid chondrosarcoma, Mes. C. has rather rapid growth and, if left untreated it easily becomes of very large size. **Radiogra-**

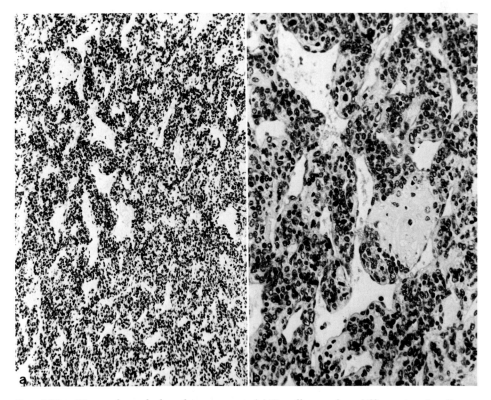

FIG. 839. - Mesenchymal chondrosarcoma. (a) Small round undifferentiated cells are aggregated around wide vascular lacunae conferring a pseudo-hemangiopericytoma aspect on the lesion. (b) The biphasic aspect of the lesion may be observed: areas of low-grade malignancy cartilaginous differentiation are immersed in fields of undifferentiated highly malignant cells (*Hemat.-eos.*, 160, 400 x).

phically it is often sprayed by calcifications having faded boundaries or by ossifications. With angiography the tumor is injected intensely in virtue of its rather rich and dilated capillary circulation.

Macroscopically it is a hardly circumscribed tumor, of parenchymatous and compact aspect. There are no mucoid or cystic aspects. On the cut surface, instead, hyperemic-hemorrhagic areas and areas of calcification and ossification may be seen.

The **histological aspect** is characterized by a rather richly cellular tissue made up of undifferentiated cells and frequently having intense vascularization constituted by fissures and dilated sinusoids which confer onto the tissue a typical pseudohemangiopericytoma pattern. The cells are globose-oval and they rarely have a spindle form; they contain scarce intracytoplasmatic glycogen. The feature which allows for diagnosis is represented by the presence of foci of cartilaginous differentiation (Fig. 839). This cartilage is usually well-differentiated, with cells which are not very anaplastic and often having calcification, at times ossification. In conclusion, the histological aspect is the same as that described for Mes. C. of the skeleton.

Differential diagnosis above all involves **hemangiopericytoma**: this has a greater quantity of intercellular reticulum and, in particular, it does not present areas of cartilaginous differentiation.

Mes. C. is a tumor characterized by high malignancy. Its growth is rapid, tendency to metastasize is also high; **prognosis** is very severe. Metastases occur particularly in the lungs. Surgical **treatment** must be immediate and aggressive, preferably involving radical or compartmental removal. The tumor seems to respond rather well to radiation therapy, thus, radiation and chemotherapy may be associated with surgical treatment.

SYNOVIAL CHONDROSARCOMA

There are exceptional cases where a synovial chondromatosis gives birth to a chondrosarcoma, or where a chondrosarcoma originates in the joint. In this last case it may be difficult to establish whether the tumor originated from the epiphyseal bone or from the capsulo-synovial structures. The clinical, radiological and macroscopic features are similar to those which we will describe for aggressive and tumor-like synovial chondromatosis. It is a soft and compact cartilaginous tissue filling the joint cavity, eroding the capsule, invading the soft tissues, digging into and infiltrating the joint bones, and continuously expanding.

Histologically the features which distinguish chondrosarcoma from synovial chondromatosis are that there is no cluster-like arrangement: the cells are scattered without any particular order among the ground substance. The chondrosarcoma may be well-differentiated, or myxoid. Furthermore, the features of giantism, pleomorphism and nuclear hyperchromia are more accentuated than those which may be observed in synovial chondromatosis.

In some of the few cases reported in the literature it is difficult to establish whether it was truly a chondrosarcoma or an aggressive and tumor-like synovial chondromatosis. In fact, the patient was treated by amputation and there were no metastases. In only very few cases the diagnosis of chondrosarcoma was proven by the occurrence of pulmonary metastases. In conclusion, synovial chondrosarcoma must be considered to be possible but absolutely exceptional. In most cases we are dealing with aggressive and tumor-like synovial chondromatosis. Before accepting the diagnosis of synovial chondrosarcoma and undertaking aggressive and demolitive surgery, the features of the course of the disease, the clinico-radiographic picture, and the histological picture will have to be carefully evaluated, keeping in mind that aggressive synovial chondromatosis occurs more frequently than synovial chondrosarcoma and that in most cases surgical treatment must thus be conservative.

REFERENCES

1953 STOUT A.P., Verner E.W.: Chondrosarcoma of the extraskeletal soft tissues. *Cancer*, **6**, 581.

1960 UEHARA H., BECKER F.P.: Extraskeletal cartilaginous tumors: Report of two cases with review of the literature. *AMA Arch. Surg.* **80**, 319.

1963 KAUFMANN S.L., STOUT A.P.: Extraskeletal osteogenic sarcomas and chondrosarcomas in children. *Cancer*, **16**, 432.

1964 GOLDMAN R.L., LICHTENSTEIN L.: Synovial chondrosarcoma. *Cancer*, **17**, 1233.

1965 MULLINS F., BERARD C., EISENBERG S.H.: Chondrosarcoma following synovial chondromatosis. A case study. *Cancer*, **18**, 1180.

1966 CHAVES E.: Mesenchymal chondrosarcoma. *Arch. Ital. Pat. Clin. Tumori*, **9**, 97.

1967 BRANDENBURG J.H., HARRIS D.D., BENNET M.: Chondrosarcoma of the larynx. *Laryngoscope*, **77**, 752.

1967 GOLDENBERG R., COHEN P., STEINLAUF P.: Chondrosarcoma of the extraskeletal soft tissues: A report of seven cases and review of the literature. *J. Bone Joint Surg.* **49/A**, 1487.

1967 GOLDMAN R.L.: «Mesenchymal» chondrosarcoma, a rare malignant chondroid tumor usually primary in bone: Report of a case arising in extraskeletal soft tissue. *Cancer*, **20**, 1494.

1967 KING J.W., SPJUT H.J., FECHNER R.E., et al.: Synovial chondrosarcoma of the knee joint. *J. Bone Joint Surg.*, **49/A (7)**, 1389.

1967 KORNSORNS M.E.: Primary chondrosarcoma of extraskeletal soft tissue. *Arch. Pathol.* **83**, 13.

1969 GUCCION J.G., FONT R.L., ENZINGER F.M., et al.: Extraskeletal mesenchymal chondrosarcoma. *Arch. Pathol.*, **95**, 336.

1969 THOMPSON J., ENTIN S.D.: Primary extraskeletal chondrosarcoma. *Cancer*, **23**, 936.

1972 ENZINGER F.M., SHIRAKI M.: Extraskeletal myxoid chondrosarcoma: An analysis of 34 cases. *Hum. Pathol.* **3**, 421.

1973 ANGERVALL L., ENERBACK L., KNUTSON H.: Chondrosarcoma of soft tissue origin. *Cancer*, **32**, 507.

1973 MARTIN R.F., MELNICK P.J., WARNER N.E., et al.: Chordoid sarcoma. *Am. J. Clin. Pathol.* **59**, 623.

1973 STEINER G.C., MIRRA J.M., BULLOUGH P.G.: Mesenchymal chondrosarcoma. A study of the ultrastructure. *Cancer*, **32**, 926.

1974 MOORE J.P., SHANNON E.: Extraskeletal chondrosarcoma. *Tex. Med.* **70**, 65.

1974 DAHLIN D.C., SALVADOR A.H., Cartilaginous tumors of the soft tissues of the hands and feet. *Mayo Clin. Proc.* **49**, 721.

1976   KLEIN H., SPINELLI M.: Mesenchymales Chondrosarkom (Bericht ueber 2 extra-ossäre Fälle). *Zentralbl. Allg. Pathol.*, **120 (1)**, 51.

1976   SMITH T., FARINACI J., CARPENTER A., *et al.:* Extraskeletal myxoid chondrosar-coma - a clinicopathologic study. *Cancer*, **37**, 821.

1980   WU K.K., COLLON D.J., GUISE E.R.: Extraosseous chondrosarcoma. Report of five cases and review of the literature. *J. Bone Joint Surg.* **62/A**, 189.

1981   HARWOOD A.R., KRAJBICH J.I., FORNASIER V.L.: Mesenchymal chondrosarcoma: A report of 17 cases. *Clin. Orthop.*, **158**, 144.

1981   PARDO-MINDAN G., GUILLES F.J., VILLAS C.: A comparative ultrastructural study of chondrosarcoma, chordoid sarcoma, and chordoma. *Cancer*, **47**, 2611.

1982   JESSURUN J., ROJAS M.E., ALBORES-SAAVEDRA J.: Congenital extraskeletal em-bryonal chondrosarcoma. Case report. *J. Bone Joint Surg.*, **64-A**, 293.

1982   SILBERT J.E.: Structure and metabolism of proteoglycans and glycosamino-glycans. *J. Invest. Dermatol.*, **79**, 31s.

1983   BERTONI F., PICCI P., BACCHINI P., CAPANNA R., INNAO V., BACCI G., CAMPANACCI M.: Mesenchymal chondrosarcoma of bone and soft tissues. *Cancer*, **52**, 533.

1983   KINDBLOM L.G., ANGERVALL L.: Myxoid chondrosarcoma of the synovial tissue. A clinicopathologic, histochemical, and ultrastructural analysis. *Cancer*, **52**, 1886.

1983   NAKAMURA Y., BECKER L.E., MARKS A.: S-100 protein in tumors of cartilage and bone. *Cancer*, **52**, 1820.

1985   HINRICHS S.H., JARAMILLO M.A., GUMERLOCK P.H.: Myxoid chondrosarcoma with a translocation involving chromosomes 9 and 22. *Cancer Genet. Cyto-genet*, **14**, 219.

1985   LOUVET C., DE GRAMONT A., KRULIK M., *et al.*: Extraskeletal mesenchymal chondrosarcoma: case report and review of the literature. *J. Clin. Oncol.*, **3**, 858.

1985   POVYSIL C., MATEJOVSKY Z.: A comparative ultrastructural study of chondro-sarcoma, chordoid sarcoma and chordoma periphericum. *Pathol. Res. Pract.*, **179**, 546.

1986   FLETCHER C.D.M., POWELL G., MC KEE P.H.: Extraskeletal myxoid chondrosar-coma. A histochemical and immunohistochemical study. *Histopathology*, **10**, 489.

1986   NAKASHIMA Y., UNNI K.K., SHIVES T.C., SWEE R.G., DAHLIN D.C.: Mesenchymal chondrosarcoma of bone and soft tissue. A review of 111 cases. *Cancer*, **57**, 2444.

1986   REIMAN H.M., DAHLIN D.C.: Cartilage and bone forming tumors of the soft tissues. *Sem. Diagn. Pathol.*, **3**, 288.

OSTEOSARCOMA

It is a malignant mesenchymal tumor whose cells produce osteoid substance. It is very **rare** and may be primary, or it may occur in an irradiated area. Unlike skeletal osteosarcoma it is observed during adult and advanced **age** and seems to prefer the female **sex**. The **sites** most involved are the thigh, the muscles of the pelvic girdle, and the shoulder.

Radiographically there may be areas or nodules of faded radiopacity, due to tumoral osteogenesis (Fig. 840). Bone scan reveals uptaking in the lesion.

Macroscopically there is a mass in the soft tissues which may have a pseu-

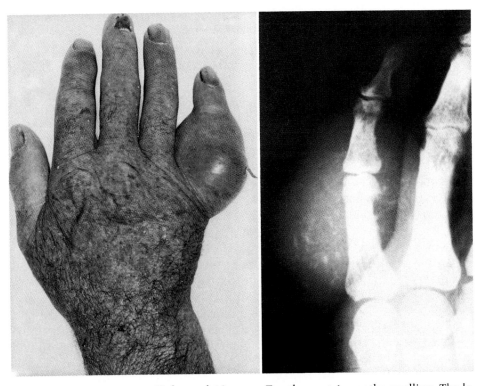

FIG. 840. - Osteosarcoma. Male aged 68 years. For the past 6 months swelling. The lesion, which contains small faded areas of radiopacity, surrounded the phalanx, but originated in the soft tissues.

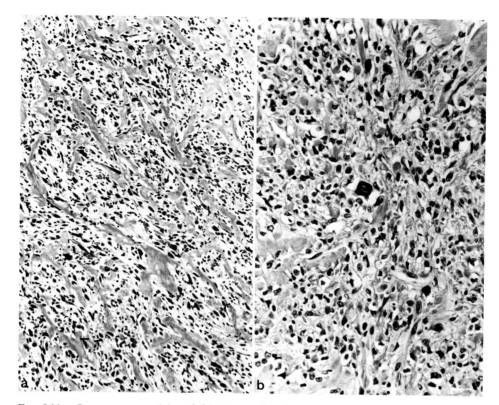

FIG. 841. - Osteosarcoma. (a) and (b) Among the pleomorphic cells with hyperchromatic nuclei, there are shoots of osteoid.

docapsulated aspect or an infiltrative growth. On the cut surface it is granular whitish and gritty with foci of necrosis and hemorrhage.

Microscopically extraskeletal O.S. is prevalently osteoblastic, but chondroblastic and/or fibroblastic areas may be present. Cytology may be so pleomorphic that it recalls malignant fibrous histiocytoma, or it may be relatively monomorphous, thus recalling fibrosarcoma. The cell's osteoid production orients diagnosis (Fig. 841). The osteoid tissue may appear lace-like almost surrounding the single cells, or rather form larger islands or trabeculae. Mitotic figures are numerous, and signs of cytological malignancy are
evident. In general, these are high-grade malignant neoplasms.

Differential diagnosis must include osteoproductive lesions, benign or
malignant. Among benign lesions the distinction must be made with **myositis ossificans**, in which a zonal aspect may be observed (immature areas in
the center of the lesion and more mature areas, with ossification, at the periphery). Differential diagnosis is less easy if biopsy is performed at the initial
stage of the myositis ossificans, in which proliferating and immature cells
prevail. It must be noted that the clinical and imaging features of myositis
ossificans are usually so typical that any histological confusion with O.S.
should be impossible, and indeed biopsy itself may be avoided.

Osteogenesis of a metaplastic nature may be present in **carcinomas or sarcomas**. In these cases differential diagnosis is based on the recognition of the reactive nature of the osteogenesis and of the basic pathological picture.

The **prognosis** of extraskeletal O.S. is severe, as pulmonary metastases frequently occur. **Treatment** is the same as that of skeletal O.S.: preoperative chemotherapy, wide or radical surgery, and maintenance chemotherapy.

REFERENCES

1956 FINE G., STOUT A.P.: Osteogenic sarcoma of the extraskeletal soft tissues. *Cancer*, **9**, 1027.

1963 KAUFMAN S.L., STOUT A.P.: Extraskeletal osteogenic sarcomas and chondrosarcomas in children. *Cancer*, **16**, 432.

1968 DAS GUPTA T.K., HAJDU SI, FOOTE F.W. Jr.: Extraosseous osteogenic sarcoma. *Ann. Surg.*, **168**, 1011.

1971 ALLAN C.J., SOULE E.H.: Osteogenic sarcoma of the somatic soft tissues. Clinicopathologic study of 26 cases and review of the literature. *Cancer*, **27**, 1121.

1972 NISHIMURA H., ISHIKAWA T., ISHIKI T.: Extraskeletal osteogenic sarcoma. A light microscopic and ultrastructural study of a case. *Acta Pathol. Jpn*, **22**, 195.

1972 WURLITZER F., AYALA A., ROMSDAHL M.: Extraosseous osteogenic sarcoma. *Arch. Surg.* **105**, 691.

1973 ALPERT L.I., ABACI IF., WERTHAMER S.: Radiation-induced extraskeletal osteosarcoma. *Cancer*, **31**, 1359.

1973 PATIL S.D., TALIS V.H., SULTANA Z., *et al.*: Extraosseous osteogenic sarcoma. Report of two cases. *Indian J. Cancer*, **10**, 479.

1974 MILLER W.B. Jr., WIRMAN J.A., McKINNEY P.: Extraosseous osteogenic sarcoma of forearm. *Arch. Pathol.*, **97**, 246.

1974 SHAHIN W., CHAIMOFF C., DINTSMAN M.: Extraosseous osteogenic sarcoma. *Clin. Orthop. Rel. Res.*, **101**, 151.

1975 HASSON J., HARTMAN K.S., MILIKOW E., *et. al.*: Thorotrast-induced extraskeletal osteosarcoma of the cervical region. Report of a case. *Cancer*, **36**, 1827.

1975 LEE W., LAURIE J., TOWNSEND A.: Fine structure of a radiation-induced osteogenic sarcoma. *Cancer*, **36**, 1414.

1978 RAO U., CHENG A., DIDOLKAR M.S.: Extraosseous osteogenic sarcoma. *Cancer*, **41**, 1488.

1979 LORENTZON R., LARSSON S.E., BOQUIST L.: Extra-osseous osteosarcoma. A clinical and histopathological study of four cases. *J. Bone Joint Surg.*, **61/B**, 205.

1981 MEISTER P., KONRAD E.A., STOTZ S.: Extraskeletal osteosarcoma. Case report and differential diagnosis. *Arch. Orthop. Traumat. Surg.*, **98**, 311.

1981 WAXMAN M., YULETIN J.C., SAXE B.I., *et al.*: Extraskeletal osteosarcoma: Light and electron microscopic study. *Mt. Sinai J. Med.*, **48**, 322.

1982 BHAGAVAN B.S., DORFMAN H.D.: The significance of bone and cartilage formation in malignant fibrous histiocytoma of soft tissue. *Cancer*, **49**, 480.

1983 SORDILLO P.P., HAJDU S.I., MAGILL G.B., GOLBEY R.B.: Extraosseous osteogenic sarcoma. A review of 48 patients. *Cancer*, **51**, 727.

1986 HUVOS A.G.: Osteogenic sarcoma of bones and soft tissues in older persons. A clinicopathologic analysis of 117 patients older than 60 years. *Cancer*, **57**, 1442.

1986 REIMAN H.M., DAHLIN D.C.: Cartilage and bone forming tumors of the soft tissues. *Sem. Diagn. Pathol.*, **3**, 288.

1987 CHUNG E.B., ENZINGER F.M.: Extraskeletal osteosarcoma. *Cancer*, **60**, 1132.

INTRAMUSCULAR MYXOMA

It is a uniformly myxoid tumor, an absolutely benign one, which must be distinguished from mucous cyst or «ganglia» as well as from myxoid sarcomas of the soft tissues.

It is a **rare** occurrence, showing no evident **sex** predilection, and it is particularly observed in patients **aged** over 40 years. As for **site**, it is generally observed in the large muscles of the limbs, in decreasing order: in the thigh, shoulder, gluteal region and arm.

M. occurs as an oblong intramuscular mass, having very well-defined boundaries and tense, hard consistency; it is mobile and painless. Its growth is very slow, but it may grow to very large size, up to 15 cm or more. CAT and NMR reveal a hypodense image as compared to the muscle, of regularly globose shape, having very evident boundaries, and homogeneous content. Arteriography shows the absence of intra- and peritumoral vascularity.

Macroscopically it may be totally surrounded by muscle or it may adhere to the deep aspect of the muscular fascia. It is a single, globose-oval mass, which is often delimited by a thin pseudocapsule which is however confused with a small layer of surrounding degenerated muscle. The surface is smooth, consistency tense, it has a whitish, pearly, translucid aspect. On the cut surface the typical mucoid aspect is observed, resembling a jelly-fish, nearly bloodless (Fig. 842).

Histologically it is a uniform, myxoid tissue, which is scarcely cellular. The cells are widely sparse, spindle-stellate, with thin nuclei, dense chromatin, nearly pyknotic. They are immersed in abundant semi-fluid mucoid substance, which takes the color of mucin (halcian blue, PAS, and colloidal iron), but not after treatment with hyaluronidase. In the mucoid substance there is a sparse and thin argentophilous reticulum, there are few collagen fibers, rare and thin blood vessels. Cystic spaces may be present but they never constitute a predominant finding, which differentiates M. from mucous cysts. The boundaries of the tumor are not always evident, rather they often fade into the edematous and degenerated muscle (Fig. 843).

Histogenesis is uncertain. At times intramuscular M. which may even be multiple are associated with **fibrous dysplasia of the skeleton**.

The most important differential diagnosis includes **myxoid sarcomas**, such as **myxoid liposarcoma, myxoid malignant fibrous histiocytoma, myxoid chondrosarcoma, botryoid rhabdomyosarcoma**. In addition to their differing

FIG. 842. - Myxoma in a female aged 69 years. Mass in the posterior aspect of the thigh, observed for the past month, painless. The mass, of globose shape and very regular surface, of firm-elastic consistency, was contained in the belly of the biceps. Marginal excision and typical aspect of the tumor, capsulated and mucoid.

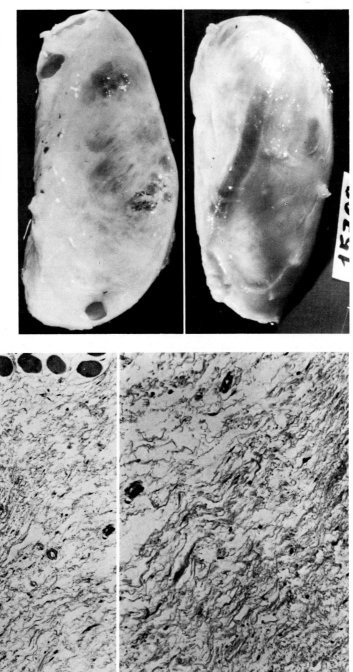

FIG. 843. - Myxoma. (a) Spindle or stellate cells are dispersed in an abundant myxoid substance. Vascularization cannot be seen. Proliferation tends to infiltrate the skeletal muscle. (b) Spindle cells with small hyperchromic nuclei are immersed in a rich myxoid component. Thin ondulating collagenous fibers are observed. Vascularization is at a minimum (*Hemat.-eos.*, 160, 250 x).

clinical features, these sarcoma reveal a) hypercellularity, cellular pleomorphism, b) greater vascularity, c) specific cellular elements (lipoblasts, histioblasts, chondroblasts, rhabdomyoblasts); d) myxoid chondrosarcoma is differentiated histochemically, as well, as the mucoid material is hyaluronidase-resistant.

Prognosis of M. is excellent: local recurrence is very rare, even after marginal or sometimes intralesional excision.

REFERENCES

1965 ENZINGER F.M.: Intramuscular myxoma. *Am. J. Clin. Pathol.*, **43**, 104.
1967 MAZABRAUD A., SEMAT P., ROZE R.: A propos de l'association de fibromyxomes des tissues mous a la dysplasie fibreuse des os. *Presse Med.*, **75**, 2223.
1971 WIRTH W.A., LEAVITT D., ENZINGER F.M.: Multiple intramuscular myxomas. Another extraskeletal manifestation of fibrous dysplasia. *Cancer*, **27**, 1167.
1973 IRELAND D.C., SOULE E.H., IVINS J.C.: Myxoma of somatic soft tissues. A report of 58 patients, 3 with multiple tumors and fibrous dysplasia of bone. *Mayo Clin. Proc.*, **48**, 401.
1974 KINDBLOM L., STENER B., ANGERVALL L.: Intramuscular myxoma. *Cancer*, **34**, 1737.
1976 LOGEL R.J.: Recurrent intramuscular myxoma associated with Albright's syndrome. Case report and review of the literature. *J. Bone Joint Surg.*, **58/A**, 565.
1979 FELDMAN P.: A comparative study including ultrastructure of intramuscular myxoma and myxoid liposarcoma. *Cancer*, **43**, 512.
1981 EKELUND L., HERRLIN K., RYDHOLM A.: Computed tomography of intramuscular myxoma. *Skeletal Radiol.*, **7**, 15.
1981 MacKENZIE D.H.: The myxoid tumors of somatic soft tissues. *Am J. Surg. Pathol.*, **5**, 443.
1984 FELDMAN R.H.; LEWIS M.M.; ROBBINS H.: KLEIN M.: Intramuscular myxoma. Case report and review of the literature. *Bull. Hosp. Jt. Dis.*, **44**, 76.
1985 MIETTINEN M.; HÖCKERSTEDT K.; REITAMO J.: TÖTTERMAN S.: Intramuscular myxoma - a clinicopathological study of twenty-three cases. *Am. J. Clin. Pathol.*, **84 (3)**, 265-72.
1986 BLASIER R.D., RYAN J.R., SCHALDENBRAND M.E.: Multiple myxomata of soft tissue associated with polyostoic fibrous dysplasia. A case report. *Clin. Orthop.*, **206**, 211.
1986 HASHIMOTO H., TSUNEYOSHI M., DAIMARU Y., ENJOJI M., SHINOHARA N.: Intramuscular myxoma. A clinicopathologic, immunohistochemical and electron microscopic study. *Cancer*, **58**, 740.

GRANULAR CELL TUMOR

It is made up of typical cells characterized by ample granular cytoplasm; histogenesis is uncertain. It is nearly always small and benign.

G.C.T. is a **rare** occurrence, there is predilection for the black **race**, the female **sex** and **age** from 30 to 60 years. It is generally observed in the derma/mucous chorion, in the subcutaneous/submucous tissue, but at times in the striated or smooth muscles. It is most frequently observed in the following **sites**: the tongue, thoracic wall and upper limb; these are followed by the lower limb, the respiratory tree, the digestive system, the ano-genital region.

At times the lesion is **multicentric**, with nodules which vary in number, and which may occur synchronously or successively.

Macroscopically it is a nodule (or several nodules) which is generally superficial, characterized by slow growth and of small size. Diameter generally does not exceed 3 cm, the nodule has unclear boundaries with the surrounding tissues, it is of firm or hard consistency (in sclerosing forms), and on the cut surface it is typically pale yellow-brown in color.

Histologically the lesion is made up of globose or polyhedric cells, with ample roughly granular cytoplasm and a small central nucleus, which tends to be vesicular, and having a minute nucleolus (Fig. 844). Cytoplasms and nuclei are uniform. The cytoplasmatic granules are eosinophilic and reveal a weak diastasis-independent PAS positiveness, thus they do not contain glycogen.

These cells are arranged in nests or cords, separated by reticular and collagen shoots. At times the collagen is thickened in large bands and fields, which embed small nests of granular cells. At times the granular cells surround a small nerve, or they form cylindrical cords surrounded by concentric spindle cells thus recalling an amputation neuroma. These aspects suggest a nervous histogenesis. When the G.C.T. is superficial, the epithelium located above may reveal aspects of hyperplasia which could lead to suspicion of a squamous carcinoma. Instead, these are aspects of reaction to the G.C.T.

Under electron microscopy the cytoplasmatic granules appear to be vacuoles, probably autophagic ones, containing cellular debris. These aspects are typical and have been interpreted as an index of nervous **histogenesis**. This is the most accredited, so much so that the term granular cell schwannoma (neurinoma, neurofibroma) has been used. Some, however, believe a

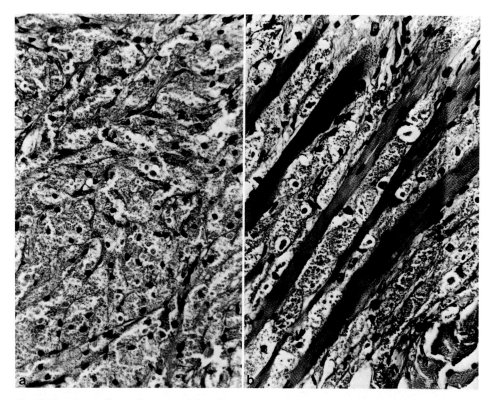

FIG. 844. - Granular cell tumor. (a) Cells having a round polygonal aspect with eosino-philic granular cytoplasm. The nucleus is round and of uniform shape and size. (b) Islands and cords of granular cells appear to be separated by striated muscle fibers. This «pseudo-infiltrative» aspect must not suggest a malignant nature of the tumor (*Hemat.-eos.*, 250, 400 x).

histiocytic nature of the lesion to be more probable, while the hypothesis of a muscular histogenesis (from which the old term granular cell myoblastoma, or Abrikossoff tumor) has been abandoned.

Diagnosis in relation to benign tumors is simple. As compared to **rhabdo-myoma** there are no striations or glycogen; as compared to **hybernoma** there are no lipidic drops.

Differential diagnosis between benign G.C.T. and very rare forms of **malignant G.C.T.** is instead very difficult or even impossible. The latter has never been observed in children, reaches larger size at times characterized by rapid growth. In any other feature, it is nearly indistinguishable from the benign form. As compared to the benign form, however, histology may reveal a certain amount of hypercellularity, mild nuclear pleomorphism, some mitotic figures. Mitotic figures are scarce, so much so that two or more in 10 high power fields are considered to be an index of malignancy.

Benign G.C.T. heals easily with wide excision. The malignant variety, instead, often metasta sizes, even much later, despite aggressive surgical and radiation treatment.

REFERENCES

1962 FISHER E.R., WECHSLER H.: Granular cell myoblastoma - a misnomer. Em and histochemical evidence concerning its Schwann cell derivation and nature (granular cell schwannoma). *Cancer*, **15**, 936.

1970 STRONG E.W., McDIVITT R.W., BRASFIELD R.D.: Granular cell myoblastoma. *Cancer*, **25**, 415.

1971 AL SARRAF M. LOUD A., VAITKEVICIUS V.: Malignant granular cell tumor. *Arch. Pathol.*, **91**, 550.

1971 KÜCHEMANN K.: Malignes granulaeres Neurom (Granularzellmyoblastom). Fallbericht und Literaturuebersicht. *Zentralbl Allg. Pathol.*, **114**, 426.

1972 HARRER W.V., PATCHEFSKY A.S.: Malignant granular cell myoblastoma of the posterior mediastinum. *Chest*, **61**, 95.

1972 PASKIN D.L., HULL J.D.: Granular cell myoblastoma. A comprehensive review of 15 years' experience. *Ann. Surg.*, **175**, 501.

1973 SOBEL H.J., SCHWARZ R., MARQUET E.: Light and electron microscopic study of the origin of granular cell myoblastoma. *J. Pathol.*, **109**, 101.

1974 CADOTTE M.: Malignant granular cell myoblastoma. *Cancer*, **33**, 1417.

1975 COMPAGNO J., HYAMS V.J., STE-MARIE P.: Benign granular cell tumors of the larynx: A review of 36 cases with clinicopathologic data. *Ann. Otol. Rhinol. Laryngol.*, **84**, 308.

1978 TYAGI S.P., KHAN M.H., TYAGI N.: Malignant granular cell tumor. *Indian J. Cancer*, **15**, 77.

1979 DONHUIJSEN K., SAMTLEBEN V., LEDER L.D., *et al.:* Malignant granular cell tumor. *J. Cancer Res. Clin. Oncol.*, **95**, 93.

1980 LACK E.E., WORSHAM G.F., CALLIHAN M.D., *et al.:* Granular cell tumor. A clinicopathologic study of 110 patients. *J. Surg. Oncol.*, **13**, 301.

1981 ROBERTSON A.J., McINTOSH W., LAMONT P., GUTHRIE W.: Malignant granular cell tumor (myoblastoma) of the vulva. Report of a case and review of the literature. *Histopathology*, **5**, 69.

1982 STEFANSSON K., WOLLMANN R.L.: S-100 protein in granular cell tumors (granular cell myoblastoma). *Cancer*, **49**, 1834.

1982 STEFFELAAR J.W., NAP M., VAN HAELST U.J.G.M.: Malignant granular cell tumor. Report of a case with special reference to carcinoembryonic antigen. *Am. J. Surg. Pathol.*, **6**, 665.

1983 BEDETTI C.D., MARTINEZ A.J., BECKFORD N.S. *et al.:* Granular cell tumors arising in myelinated peripheral nerves. Light and electron microscopy and immunoperoxidase study. *Virchows Arch. (Pathol. Anat.)*, **402**, 175.

1983 DHILLON A.P., RODE J.: Immunohistochemical studies of S 100 protein and other neural characteristics expressed by granular cell tumour. *Diagn. Histopathol.*, **6**, 23.

1984 MIETTINEN M., LEHTONEN E., LEHTOLA H., EKBLOM P., LEHTO V., VIRTANEN I.: Histogenesis of granular cell tumor. An immunohistochemical and ultrastructural study. *J. Pathol.*, **162**, 221.

1985 KHANSUR T., BALDUCCI L., TAVASSOLI M.: Identification of desmosomes in the granular cell tumor. Implications in histologic diagnosis and histogenesis. *Am. J. Surg. Pathol.*, **9**, 898.

1985 SMOLLE J., KONRAD K., KERL H.: Granular cell tumors contain myelin-associated glycoprotein. An immunohistochemical study using Leu 7 monoclonal antibody. *Virchows Arch.*, **406**, 1.

1986 NATHRATH W.B.J., REMBERGER K.: Immunohistochemical study of granular cell tumours. Demonstration of neuron specific enolase, S-100 protein, laminin and alpha-1-antichymotrypsin. *Virchows Arch.*, **408**, 421.

1989 THUNOLD S., VON EYBEN F.E., MAEHLE B.: Malignant granular cell tumour on the neck: immunohistochemical and ultrastructural studies of a case. *Histopathology*, **14**, 655.

EWING'S SARCOMA

Ewing's sarcoma, characterized by clinical and morphological features very similar to those of Ewing's sarcoma of bone, may be observed in the soft tissues.

It is a **rare** occurrence, there is predilection for the male **sex**, and for those **aged** between 10 and 30 years. As for **site**, there is predilection for the paravertebral and thoracic soft tissues and the lower limb (Fig. 845).

The tumor has a deep site and develops rapidly. More often it is painless and the duration of symptoms is generally less than 1 year.

Macroscopically the tumor is often multilobulated and soft. On the cut surface, the typical encephaloid aspect is observed. Areas of colliquative necrosis and hemorrhage are frequently observed.

Histologically the aspect is the same as that of Ewing's sarcoma of the bone: uniform fields of small round cells (Fig. 846). Cytoplasms are scarce, pale, at times vacuolated and containing glycogen. The nuclei are round, small, and have a well-defined membrane and a finely granular chromatin, as well as minute nucleoli. Pleomorphism and mitotic figures are scarce, even if there are forms with more ample and irregular nuclei and numerous mitotic figures. Argentic impregnation reveals the absence or scarcity of reticular fi-

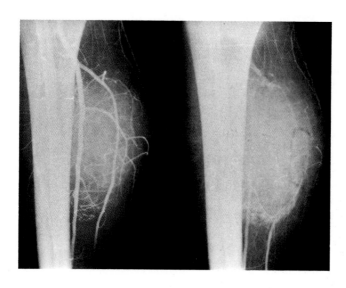

FIG. 845. - Ewing's sarcoma. Male aged 22 years. Swelling for 2 months. Marginal excision, recurrence after 3 months. The patient was submitted to wide excision of the recurrence, followed by radiation therapy at 4000 rad. and adjuvant chemotherapy with the same protocol as that used for skeletal Ewing's sarcoma. There were no signs of disease after 8 years.

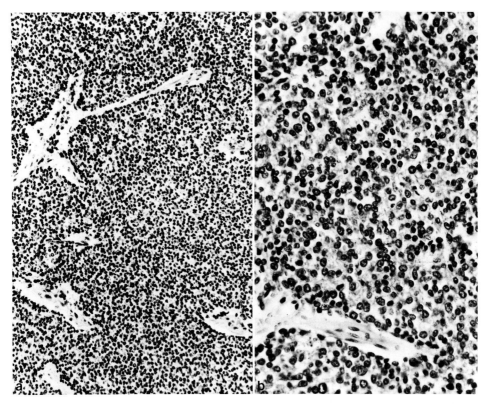

FIG. 846. - Ewing's sarcoma. (a) There is monomorphous proliferation of round cells in extended solid fields interrupted by sparse vessels or collagenous septa. (b) The cells have evident monomorphism. Cytoplasm is scarce, the nucleus is round, and the chromatin is finely granular. Among the cells there is no evident stroma (*Hemat.-eos.*, 160, 400 x).

bers between the cells. PAS stain and electron microscopy reveal cytoplasmatic glycogen. There are frequent areas of necrosis, with the persistence of haloes of vital cells surrounding the numerous vessels.

Differential diagnosis must include **neuroblastoma** (in paravertebral or retroperitoneal localizations: younger age, rosette images, absence of glycogen, presence of neurosecretory granules in electron microscopy, presence of metabolites of the catecholamines in the urine). But above all, differential diagnosis must include **embryonal or alveolar rhabdomyosarcoma**, the clinical features of which are similar or identical to those of Ewing's sarcoma of the soft tissues. In rhabdomyosarcoma the nuclei are more hyperchromatic and pleomorphic, there may be an alveolar structure, multinucleate giant cells are seen, and eosinophilic cytoplasms typical of the rhabdomyoblast are revealed. Finally, as for Ewing's sarcoma of the bone, and particularly in patients aged over 30/40 years, differential diagnosis includes **malignant lymphoma** (which in exceptional cases involves the soft tissues without involving the lymph nodes) and **metastasis of small-cell carcinoma** (particularly pulmonary).

Prognosis and **treatment** seem to be very similar to what is indicated for Ewing's sarcoma of the skeleton. Unlike the latter, there are not enough cases submitted to homogeneous protocols of treatment and having an adequate long-term follow-up.

REFERENCES

1969   TEFFT M., VAUTER G.F., MITUS A.: Paravertebral «round cell» tumors in children. *Radiology,* **92**, 1501.

1974   SZAKACS J.E., CARTA M., SZAKACS M.R.: Ewing's sarcoma, extraskeletal and of bone. *Ann. Clin. Lab. Sci.,* **4**, 306.

1975   ANGERVALL L., ENZINGER F.M.: Extraskeletal neoplasm resembling Ewing's sarcoma. *Cancer,* **36**, 240.

1977   WIGGER H.J., SALAZAR G.H., BLANC W.A.: Extraskeletal Ewing's sarcoma. An ultrastructural study. *Arch. Pathol.,* **101**, 446.

1978   MAHONEY J.P., BALLINGER W.E. Jr., ALEXANDER R.W.: So-called extraskeletal Ewing's sarcoma. Report of a case with ultrastructural analysis. *Am. J. Clin. Pathol.,* **70**, 926.

1978   MEISTER P., GOKEL J.M.: Extraskeletal Ewing's sarcoma. *Virchows Arch. (Pathol. Anat.),* **378**, 173.

1978   SOULE E.H., NEWTON W. Jr, MOON T.E., *et al.:* Extraskeletal Ewing's sarcoma. A preliminary review of 26 cases encountered in the Intergroup Rhabdomyosarcoma Study. *Cancer,* **42**, 259.

1979   GILLESPIE J.J., ROTH L.M., WILLS E.R., *et al.:* Extraskeletal Ewing's sarcoma. Histologic and ultrastructural observations in three cases. *Am. J. Surg. Pathol.,* **3**, 99.

1983   CHEN K.T.; PADMANABHAN A.: Extraskeletal Ewings sarcoma. *J. Surg. Oncol.,* **23**, 70.

1984   TSOKOS M., LINNOILA R.I., CHANDRA R.S., *et al.:* Neuron-specific enolase in the diagnosis of neuroblastoma and other small, round-cell tumors in children. *Hum. Pathol.,* **15**, 575.

1985   DONNER L., TRICHE T.J., ISRAEL M.A., *et al.:* A panel of monoclonal antibodies which discriminate neuroblastoma from Ewing's sarcoma, rhabdomyosarcoma, neuroepithelioma, and hemopoietic malignancies. *In*: EVANS A.E., D'ANGIÒ G.J., SEEGER R.C. (eds): Advances in Neuroblastoma Research. New York, Liss p. 347.

1985   SHIMADA H., AOYAMA C., CHIBA T. *et al.:* Prognostic subtypes for undifferentiated neuroblastoma; immunohistochemical study with anti-S-100 protein antibody. *Hum. Pathol.,* **16**, 471.

1986   DEHNER I.P.: Peripheral and central primitive neuroectodermal tumors: a nosologic concept seeking a consensus. *Arch. Pathol. Lab. Med.,* **110**, 997.

1986   DICKMAN P.S., TRICHE T.J.: Extraosseous Ewing's sarcoma versus primitive rhabdomyosarcoma. Diagnostic criteria and clinical correlation. *Hum. Path.,* **17**, 881.

1986   KAWAGUCHI K., KOIDE M.: Neuron-specific enolase and Leu-7 immunoreactive small round-cell neoplasm: the relationship to Ewing's sarcoma in bone and soft tissue. *Am. J. Clin. Pathol.,* **86**, 79.

1988   SHIMADA H., NEWTON W.A., SOULE E.H., *et al.:* Pathologic features of extraosseous Ewing's sarcoma: a report from the intergroup rhabdomyosarcoma study. *Hum. Pathol.,* **19**, 442.

ALVEOLAR SARCOMA

It is a malignant tumor of the soft tissues of unknown histogenesis and with a histological structure *sui generis*, which is alveolar, pseudo-endocrine, organoid.

A.S. is a **rare** occurrence, there is predilection for the female **sex** and young-adult **age** between 15 and 35 years. It may also be observed in children. As for **site** there is predilection for the deep soft tissues, particularly of the lower limb and thigh.

It is **presented** as a deep, globose mass, at times a multinodular one, which generally increases slowly and is painless. At diagnosis, thus, it may have reached a large size and have been present for several years. Because of its rich vascularization, there may be pulsation or bruit on the mass. In some cases, metastases (pulmonary, cerebral or skeletal) may constitute the first symptom of the tumor which is still unrecognized in its primary site. With CAT and angiography, there is intense uptake of the contrast medium. Furthermore, with angiography there is intense intra- and peritumoral neoangiogenesis and indirect signs of artero-venous shunt.

Macroscopically the tumor is often surrounded by numerous and ectatic vessels, which may cause heavy intraoperative bleeding. It is a globose mass, at times plurinodular, poorly delimited by a thin pseudocapsule. Its color is yellowish-white or gray-red-purple, with areas of necrosis and hemorrhage. Its consistency is soft, encephaloid.

Histologically what becomes immediately apparent under lower power is the typical pseudoendocrine alveolar structure (Fig. 847). Round-polyhedric islands of tumoral cells are separated by blood sinusoids whose wall is constituted by mature endothelium and by a thin reticular lamina. The alveoli tend to be smaller and more solid at the periphery of the tumor and in children. In areas where they are larger, the cells lose their cohesion, they disperse and degenerate at the center of the alveolus, which appears to be partially empty. The cells making up the alveoli are epitheliomorphous as there is no trace of reticular or collagen fibers between them. They are large cells, globose-polyhedric, with ample eosinophilic granular cytoplasm, which may be vacuolated. The nucleus (possibly two or more nuclei) is vesicular, the nucleolus is very evident, there is fair or considerable pleomorphism and hyperchromia, mitotic figures are rare. Sporadic gigantic elements having monstruous nuclei may be observed.

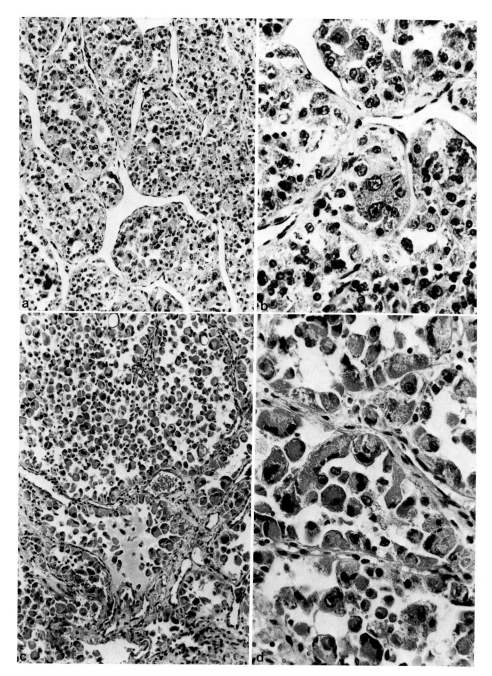

FIG. 847. - Alveolar sarcoma. (a) The neoplasm presents pseudoendocrine organoid pattern with cellular islands separated by dilated sinusoids. (b) The latter have a thin wall and a flattened endothelium. (c) The cells are large, they have intensely stained cytoplasm. In the islands the cells may be closely aggregated together, at other times they lose cohesion, they even appear to be dispersed, producing a «pseudo-alveolar» aspect. (d) Among the «alveoli», endocrine type circulation may always be observed. The cells have hyperchromatic nuclei with a prominent nucleolus (*Hemat.-eos.*, 160, 400, 160, 400 x).

The cytoplasms contain varying quantities of glycogen and, moreover, intensely PAS positive diastasis-resistant crystals. These crystals, which have a typical aspect under electron microscopy, are typical of A.S.

A last important histological aspect is represented by the intense neoangiogenesis and peritumoral vascular dilatation, and by the frequent vascular invasion on the part of neoplastic cells. This last aspect could be related to possible early metastasis of A.S.

Diagnosis is generally easy. On a histological level, A.S. may be mistaken for a **metastatic renal carcinoma** (alveoli of clear cells surrounded by sinusoids). It is differentiated by cytoplasms of differing aspect, the presence of crystals, age under 30-40 years. **Paraganglioma** has a pseudoendocrine structure like A.S., but it is never observed in the limbs, rarely before 40 years of age; the cells contain neither glycogen nor crystals. **Granular cell tumor** does not have a pseudoendocrine structure, the cells do not contain glycogen or crystals, it is generally observed after 40 years of age, its site is more superficial than deep.

The **histogenesis** of A.S. is unknown. The strongest hypothesis is that it derives from chemoreceptorial specific nerve endings.

Prognosis is that of a high-grade malignancy sarcoma. Metastases occur frequently and, as previously stated, they may occur before diagnosis of the primary tumor has been made. At times, instead, they occur very late, even tens of years after diagnosis. Metastases are generally pulmonary, skeletal and (another peculiarity of this tumor) cerebral.

Surgical **treatment** must be wide or radical and associate adjuvants (radiation and chemotherapy) as for other sarcomas of the soft tissues characterized by a high grade of malignancy.

REFERENCES

1952 CHRISTOPHERSON W.M., FOOTE F.W. Jr., STEWART F.W.: Alveolar softpart sarcoma. Structurally characteristic tumors of uncertain histogenesis. *Cancer*, **5**, 100.

1959 MARTIN F., PLAUCHU M., CABANE F.: Une tumeur en quete d'une appellation d'origine: le sarcoma alveolaire de parties molles. *Ann. Anat. Pathol. (Paris)*, **4**, 390.

1964 SHIPKEY F.H., LIEBERMAN P.H., FOOTE F.W., *et al.*: Ultrastructure of alveolar soft part sarcoma. *Cancer*, **17**, 821.

1966 LIEBERMAN P.H., FOOTE F.W., STEWART F.W., *et al.*: Alveolar soft part sarcoma. *JAMA*, **198**, 1047.

1971 ROSENBAUM A.E., GABRIELSEN T.O.: Cerebral manifestations of alveolar soft part sarcoma. *Radiology*, **99**, 109.

1971 RUBENFELD S.: Radiation therapy in alveolar soft part sarcoma. *Cancer*, **28**, 577.

1972 WELSH R.A., BRAY D.M. III, SHIPKEY F.H., *et al.*: Histogenesis of alveolar soft part sarcoma. *Cancer*, **29**, 191.

1975 UNNI K., SOULE E.: Alveolar soft part sarcoma. *Mayo Clin. Proc.*, **50**, 591.

1977 BERENZWEIG M.S., MUGGIA F.M., KAPLAN B.H.: Chemotherapy of alveolar soft part sarcoma. A case report. *Cancer Treat. Rep.*, **61**, 77.

1978 WEBBES T.J.: Alveolar soft part sarcoma. *J. Surg. Oncol.*, **10**, 201.

1979 EKFORS T.O., KALIMO H., RANTAKOKKO V., *et al.*: Alveolar soft part sarcoma. A report of two cases with some histochemical and ultrastructural observations. *Cancer*, **43**, 1672.

1981 BAUM E.S., FICKENSCHER L., NACHMAN J.B., *et al.:* Pulmonary resection and che-
      motherapy for metastatic alveolar soft part sarcoma. *Cancer,* **47,** 1946.
1982 De SCHRYVER-KECSKEMETI K., KRAUS, F.T., ENGLEMAN B.A.: Alveolar soft-part sar-
      coma - a malignant angioreninoma. Histochemical, immunocytochemical, and
      electron-microscopic study of four cases. *Am. J. Surg. Pathol.,* **6,** 5.
1983 MUKAI M., IRI H., NAKAJIMA T., HIROSE S., TORIKATA C., KAGEYAMA K. UENO N., MU-
      RAKAMI K.: Alveolar soft-part sarcoma. A review on its histogenesis and fur-
      ther studies based on electron microscopy, immunohistochemistry, and bio-
      chemistry. *Am. J. Surg. Pathol.,* **7 (7),** 679-89.
1984 MUKAI M., TORIKATA C., SHIMODA T., IRI H.: Alveolar soft part sarcoma. Assess-
      ment of immunohistochemical demonstration of desmin using paraffin sec-
      tions and frozen sections. *Virch. Arch. A. Pathol. Anat.,* **414,** 503.
1985 EVANS H.L.: Alveolar soft-part sarcoma. A study of 13 typical examples and
      one with a histologically atypical component. *Cancer,* **55,** 912.
1986 MUKAI M., TORIKATA C., IRI H. *et al.:* Histogenesis of alveolar soft part sar-
      coma. An immunohistochemical and biochemical study. *Am. J. Surg. Pathol.,*
      10, 212.
1987 AUERBACH H.E., BROOKS J.J.: Alveolar soft part sarcoma. A clinicopathologic
      and immunohistochemical study. *Cancer,* **60,** 66.
1989 LIEBERMAN P.H., BRENNAN M.F., KIMMEL M., ERLANDSON R.A., GARIN-CHESA P.,
      FLEHINGER B.Y.: Alveolar soft-part sarcoma: a clinico-pathologic study of
      half century. *Cancer,* **63,** 1.

EPITHELIOID SARCOMA

It is a **rare** occurrence, but it is among the most frequent sarcomas occurring in the hand and forearm.

There is evident predilection for the male **sex** and **age** from 20 to 30 years (with extremes at 5 and 60 years of age).

Its initial **localization** is typical: the hand (particularly in its palmar aspect) and the forearm (particularly in its dorsal aspect). It is observed less

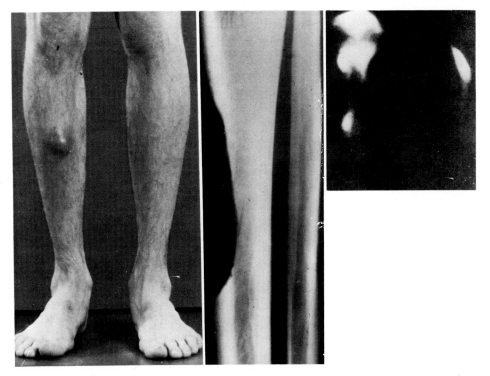

Fig. 848. - Epithelioid sarcoma. Male aged 21 years. Nodule occurring 8 years earlier, painless, with slow growth. One year earlier marginal excision, this is a local recurrence. Bone scan reveals intense uptaking in the adjacent tibia. The patient was submitted to excision including the skin and the anterior cortex of the tibia. After 2 years, further recurrence, and further excision. No signs of disease after 2 more years.

frequently in the foot (plantar aspect), the leg (anterior aspect), and in the more proximal segments of the limbs.

Clinically it begins with one or more small, hard, superficial nodules, adherent to the derma, slightly elevated on the skin (Fig. 848). The nodules grow slowly and often ulcerate the skin surface (Fig. 849). At other times one or more of the nodes are deep, and they become of larger size (like an egg or larger). The nodes are nearly painless, unless they compress or surround a nerve trunk. Their consistency is always hard, nearly woody, and the tumor tends considerably to adhere and become fixed at the surrounding planes. Regional lymph node metastases are frequent.

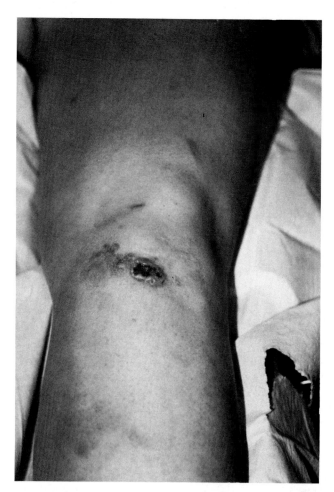

FIG. 849. - Epithelioid sarcoma. Female aged 38 years. Observe the superficial and ulcerated lesion of the knee. (Case kindly provided by Dr. J. Makley, Cleveland).

The **radiograph** is generally negative: intratumoral calcification is hardly ever observed, erosion of the adjacent bone rarely.

Macroscopically the tumor is usually multinodular, whitish, hard, and it tends to be disseminated, to tenaciously adhere to the skin, subcutaneous tissue and fascia, tendinous sheaths and tendons, aponeuroses and muscles, vessels and nerves, periosteum.

Histologically it is a proliferation of large cells of polygonal shape, having ample eosinophilic cytoplasm, a large vesicular nucleus, a clearly evident nucleolus (Fig. 850). These cells form nodules which, particularly in superficial localizations, contain a central area of necrosis, which may lead to confusion with rheumatoid granuloma and necrotizing granuloma. At the periphery or more rarely inside the nodules there is a transition between epithe-

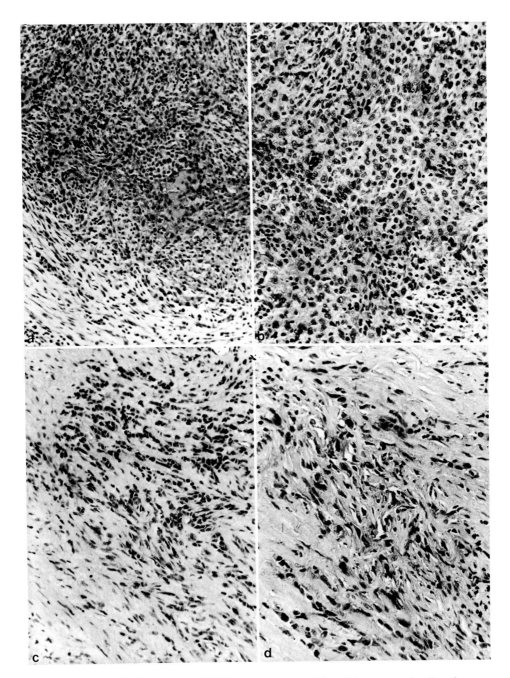

Fig. 850. - Epithelioid sarcoma. (a) Nodular aggregation of the tumoral cells. The central area of the nodule contains necrotic tissue. (b) The cells are ovoid or polygonal in shape. They present intensely eosinophilic cytoplasm and evident boundaries. There is minimal pleomorphism. (c) In the deeply located tumors the cells become prevalently spindle. Frequently they are arranged in strings separated by abundant collagen stroma. (d) The nuclei are hyperchromatic and the nucleo-cytoplasmatic features are atypical (*Hemat.-eos.*, 160, 250, 160, 250 x).

lioid cells and spindle cells. The latter maintain the same nucleo-cytoplasmatic features of the epithelioid cells and tend to be arranged in bundles. An argyrophilous reticulum may be observed between the single cells in the «granulomatous» nodule and it continues among the spindle cells.

In the deep localizations of the tumor the infiltrative aspect prevails: strings and thin cords of epithelioid cells permeate the collagen and muscular tissues. The cells have more marked pleomorphism as compared to superficial localizations and at times they aggregate in a pseudoglandular or pseudovascular form. Rarely, in deep localizations there is the nodular aspect. At times, in both superficial and deep localizations, there are multinucleate giant cells.

Histogenesis is uncertain; a resemblance with synovial sarcoma and malignant fibrous histiocytoma has been suggested.

Differential diagnosis includes **necrotizing granuloma** in general, and **rheumatoid nodule** in particular. E.S. shares topography and a painless onset with the latter, but in the rheumatoid nodule the central necrotic area is constituted by fibrinoid necrosis, well-documented by blue staining with phosphotungstic acid hematoxylin. Amongst tumors, E.S. must be distinguished from **malignant fibrous histiocytoma**, when the proliferation of pseudoepithelial cells is abundant and associated with a moderate necrotic component. In the cases of E.S. with prominent permeation of the adipose, collagenous and muscular tissues, differential diagnosis must include infiltration due to **squamous carcinoma**. Furthermore, common to both neoplasias is ulceration, but the age of the patient (squamous carcinoma rarely involves patients of young age) and the fields of squamous differentiation, with the possible presence of intercellular bridges, orient diagnosis. Sometimes the pseudoglandular arrangement of the epithelioid cells of E.S. may simulate a **synovial sarcoma**. But the absence of a definite biphasic aspect and the presence of an argyrophilous pattern among the cells of E.S. help to exclude synovial sarcoma, in which the argyrophilous pattern is absent among the epitheliomorphous cells. Masson-Fontana staining, which demonstrates the absence of melanin, will be sufficient to exclude **melanoma**. Finally, the cellular aspect of E.S. (ample eosinophilic cytoplasm and large nucleolus) and the presence of artefacts may suggest a diagnosis of **angiosarcoma**. But the reticulum, present between the single cells in E.S. and surrounding the vascular cavities or cords in angiosarcoma, and the presence of factor VIII in the cytoplasm of the cells of the angiosarcoma will differentiate the two lesions.

The **course** is slow or very slow. At times years go by between the onset of the first symptoms and diagnosis; and there are cases which were literally operated tens of times over 15 to 20 years. The tumor tends to diffuse in the limb in a proximal direction along the tendinous sheaths and the tendons, aponeuroses and muscles, neurovascular bundles. Its tendency to diffuse through the lymphatic network of the derma, as it creates multiple superficial ulcerated nodules, is a peculiar one. Regional lymph node metastases occur frequently. Distant metastases are above all pulmonary.

Treatment is surgical and must be very aggressive from the start, with very wide or radical margins and with dissection of the regional lymph nodes. With less aggressive surgery, local recurrence is the rule.

Prognosis in the cases reported up to now has been severe, but the treatment, too, of these cases has generally been inadequate and late.

REFERENCES

1968   BLISS B.O., REED R.J.: Large cell sarcomas of tendon sheath. *Am. J. Clin. Pathol.*, **49**, 776.

1970   ENZINGER F.M.: Epithelioid sarcoma: A sarcoma simulating a granuloma or a carcinoma. *Cancer*, **26**, 1029.

1972   FISHER E.R., HORVAT B.: The fibrocytic derivation of the so-called epithelioid sarcoma. *Cancer*, **30**, 1074.

1972   GABBIANI G., FU, Y.S., KAYE G.I., et al.: Epithelioid sarcoma. A light and electron microscopic study suggesting a synovial origin. *Cancer*, **30**, 486.

1972   HEPPENSTALL R.B., YVARS M.F., CHUNG S.M.K.: Epithelioid sarcoma. Two case reports. *J. Bone Joint Surg.*, **54/A**, 802.

1972   SANTIAGO H., FEINERMAN L.K., LATTES R.: Epithelioid sarcoma. A clinical and pathological study of nine cases. *Hum. Pathol.*, **3**, 133.

1972   SOULE E.H., ENRIQUEZ P.: Atypical fibrous histiocytoma, malignant histiocytoma, and epithelioid sarcoma. A comparative study of 65 tumors. *Cancer*, **30**, 128.

1973   FRABLE W.J., KAY S., LAWRENCE W., et al.: Epithelioid sarcoma. An electron microscopic study. *Arch. Pathol.*, **95**, 8.

1973   LINELL F., MYHRE-JENSEN O., OSTBERG G., et al.: Epithelioid sarcoma. Report and review of two cases. *Acta Pathol. Microbiol. Scand.*, **236**, 21.

1974   AHMED M.N., FELDMAN M., SEEMAYER T.A.: Cytology of epithelioid sarcoma. *Acta Cytol.*, **18**, 459.

1974   BRYAN R.S., SOULE E.H., DOBYNS J.H., et al.: Primary epithelioid sarcoma of the hand and forearm. *J. Bone Joint Surg.* **56/A**, 458.

1976   ROITZSCH E., IRMSCHER J.: Das epithelioide Sarkom. Bericht ueber 3 Faelle mit Literatuerebersicht. *Zentralbl. Allg. Pathol.*, **120**, 417.

1977   LO H.H., KALISHER L., FAIX J.D.: Epithelioid sarcoma: Radiologic and pathologic manifestations. *Am. J. Roentgenol.*, **128**, 1017.

1977   PATCHEFSKY A.S., SORIANO R., KOSTIANOVSKY M.: Epithelioid sarcoma. Ultrastructural similarity to nodular synovitis. *Cancer*, **39**, 143.

1977   SAXE N., BOTHA J.B.C.: Epithelioid sarcoma. A distinctive clinical presentation. *Arch. Dermatol.*, **113**, 1106.

1978   BOYES J.G.: Epithelioid sarcoma of hand and forearm. *Hand*, **10**, 302.

1978   PRAT J., WOODRUFF J.M., MARCOVE R.C.: Epithelioid sarcoma: An analysis of 22 cases indicating the prognostic significance of vascular invasion and regional lymph node metastasis. *Cancer*, **41**, 1472.

1980   TSUNEYOSHI M., ENJOJI M., SHINOHARA N.: Epithelioid sarcoma: A clinicopathologic and electron microscopic study. *Acta Pathol. Jpn.*, **30**, 411.

1982   MACHINAMI R., KIKUCHI F., MATSUSHITA H., Epithelioid sarcoma: Enzyme histochemical and ultrastructural study. *Virchows Arch. (Pathol. Anat.)*, **397**, 109.

1984   CHASE D.R.; ENZINGER F.M.; WEISS S.W.; LANGLOSS J.M.: Keratin in epithelioid sarcoma. An immunohistochemical study. *Am. J. Surg. Pathol.*, **8**, 435.

1985   CHASE D.R.; ENZINGER F.M.: Epithelioid sarcoma. Diagnosis, prognostic indicators, and treatment. *Am. J. Surg. Pathol.*, **9 (4)**, 241-63.

1985   MUSCIANESE V., SIMONI R., CAVALIERI R., MUSCARDIN L.M.: Epithelioid sarcoma. *Dermatologica*, **170**, 43.

1987   DAIMARU Y., HASHIMOTO H., TSUNEYOSHI M., ENJOJI M.: Epithelial profile of epithelioid sarcoma. An immunohistochemical analysis of eight cases. *Cancer*, **59**, 134.

1987   MANIVEL J.C., WICK M.R., DEHNER L.P., SIBLEY R.K.: Epithelioid sarcoma. An immunohistochemical study. *Am. J. Clinic. Pathol.*, **87**, 319.

CLEAR-CELL SARCOMA
OF THE TENDONS AND APONEUROSES
(Synonym: malignant melanoma of the soft tissues)

It is a **very rare** tumor. There seems to be predilection for the female **sex**. **Age** ranges from 10 to 60 years, and the average age is about 25 years. The most frequent **site** is the foot and ankle, followed by the knee and the upper limb. It is hardly ever observed at the limb girdles or in the trunk.

Clinically it is a mass of generally moderate size, painless, single and globose, which grows slowly. In most cases many years go by between the first occurrence of the tumor and surgery.

Macroscopically the tumor is considerably adherent to a tendon or to an aponeurosis, but not to the subcutaneous tissue or to the skin. Its consistency is rather firm, it is globose or slighly lobulated in shape and it has well-defined boundaries, with a capsulated appearance. On the cut surface, it is whitish in color, at times varied by reddish or blackish areas; its consistency is solid, rather firm, it rarely contains mucoid areas.

Microscopic aspect. It is constituted by round, ovoid, spindle cells, generally having clear cytoplasm, at times mildly or intensely eosinophilic (Fig. 851). The nuclei may be round, ovoid or elongated, with fine chromatin and — a salient feature — a very large nucleolus. Mitotic activity is scarce. These cells, which are fairly monomorphous, are aggregated in nodules or bundles, which are clearly designed by a fine reticular stroma (argentic impregnation). At times there are rough collagen bands from which the delicate argyrophilous fibers depart.

The cytoplasms reveal a variable grade of PAS positiveness which is annulled by diastasis (glycogen). Among the cells halcian-blue stain reveals the presence of hyaluronidase-sensitive mucopolysaccharides, diffused or collected in lacunae. At times Masson-Fontana staining reveals scarce small granules of melaninic pigment — an aspect which is confirmed under electron microscopy with the evidence of melanosomes. Sometimes, however, cells containing iron pigment (Prussian blue) or iron and melaninic pigment together may be seen.

The fact that melanosomes and melanin have been observed in a good number of C.C.S. has led to consider this tumor to be a particular type of melanoma, or more generally a tumor derived from cells of the neurocrest.

Diagnosis. Because of its fasciculated aspect with fissures or lacunae filled with mucopolysaccharides, C.C.S. must be differentiated from **synovial**

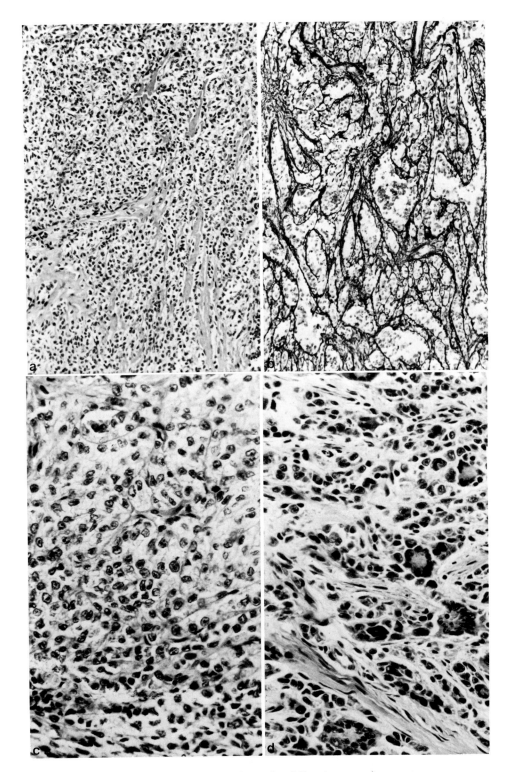

FIG. 851. (legend on the following page).

FIG. 851. - Clear-cell sarcoma. (a) Observe the compact islands of relatively monomor-phous cells. (b) Argentic impregnation reveals a stroma pattern surrounding cellular cords and islands. (c) The cells present a regular aspect. The nuclei are round-oval with a vesicular aspect, with a large nucleolus. The cytoplasm is generally pale or te-nuously eosinophilic. (d) In some fields the mononucleate cells are associated with multinucleate giant cells having nuclei arranged in a crown at the periphery of the cell (*Hemat.-eos.*, 160 x; *argentic impregnation* 160 x; *Hemat.-eos.*, 400, 400 x).

◀

sarcoma. There is no biphasic aspect in C.C.S.: the cells bordering on the mu-cous lacunae have the same features as the surrounding cells. The fascicula-ted structure may suggest a **fibrosarcoma** but there is no «herring-bone» aspect and the monomorphism of fibrosarcoma is absent. As compared to **epithelioid sarcoma**, in C.C.S. there is no nodulo-granulomatous aggregation centered by areas of necrosis and there is no perinodular fibrosis. The nodu-lar aggregation and the prevalent clear-cell component of C.C.S. must be dif-ferentiated from other tumors having a nodular structure and having cyto-plasm of varying tingibility, such as **paraganglioma** and **alveolar sarcoma**. Paraganglioma is easily differentiated by the classic «Zellballen» aggrega-tion and by the presence of Grimelius-positive granules. The alveolar sar-coma has features which are similar to C.C.S. with eosinophilic cells, but it is differentiated by its pseudo-endocrine structure. Furthermore, in alveolar sarcoma the cytoplasms contain PAS positive diastasis-resistant crystals. Fi-nally, when the cells of C.C.S. contain melaninic pigment, **melanoma** may be suspected. It is differentiated because it has a relationship with the epider-mis and because there is hyperplasia of the melanocytes in the areas superfi-cial to the neoplasm.

Treatment and prognosis. C.C.S. nearly always recurs after marginal excision, usually within 1 year. At times recurrence involves multiple nodes, along tendons and aponeuroses. Metastases particularly occur in the regio-nal lymph nodes and the lungs; they are often late (even after 30 years, with an average of 6 years) but they are very frequent. Moreover, this frequency is due to the fact that most cases are treated inadequately, due to the apparent-ly not very aggressive clinical presentation. Thus, indicated treatment is very wide surgical ablation, possibly with excision of the regional lymph nodes.

REFERENCES

1965   ENZINGER F.M.: Clear cell sarcoma of tendons and aponeuroses. An analysis of 21 cases. *Cancer*, **18**, 1163-1174.
1968   ENZINGER F.M.: Clear cell sarcoma of tendons and aponeuroses. An analysis of 21 cases. *Cancer*, **18**, 1163.
1969   ANGERVALL L., STENER B.: Clear-cell sarcoma of tendons. A study of four cases. *Acta Pathol. Microbiol. Scand.*, **77**, 589.
1969   KUBO T.: Clear celll sarcoma of patellar tendon studied by electron microsco-py. *Cancer*, **24**, 948.

1970   DUTRA F.R.: Clear cell sarcoma of tendons and aponeuroses. Three additional cases. *Cancer*, **25**, 942.

1973   HOFFMAN G.J., CARTER D.: Clear cell sarcoma of tendons and aponeuroses with melanin. *Arch. Pathol.*, **95**, 22.

1974   MACKENZIE D.H.: Clear cell sarcoma of tendon and aponeuroses with melanin production. *J. Pathol.*, **114**, 231.

1975   BEARMAN R.M., NOE J., KEMPSON R.: Clear cell sarcoma with melanin pigment. *Cancer*, **36**, 977.

1977   ALITALO K., PAAVOLAINEN P., FRANSSILA K., *et al.*: Clear cell sarcoma of tendons and aponeuroses. Report of two cases. *Acta Orthop. Scand.*, **48**, 241.

1977   HAYDU S.I., SHIU M.H., FORTNER J.G.: Tendosynovial sarcoma. A clinicopathologic study of 136 cases. *Cancer*, **39**, 1201.

1978   BOUDREAUX D., WAISMAN J.: Clear cell sarcoma with melanogenesis. *Cancer*, **41**, 1387.

1978   CHUNG E.B., ENZINGER F.M.: Clear cell sarcoma of tendons and aponeuroses. Further observations, abstracted. *Lab. Invest*, **38**, 338.

1978   GUPTA S.C., MEHROTRA T.N., GUPTA R.C., *et al.*: Clear cell sarcoma from tendinous part of quadriceps muscle. *Clin. Oncol.*, **4**, 369.

1978   TOE T.K., SAW D.: Clear cell sarcoma with melanin. Report of two cases. *Cancer*, **41**, 235.

1978   TSUNEYOSHI M., ENJOJI M., KUBO T.: Clear cell sarcoma of tendons and aponeuroses. A comparative study of 13 cases with provisional subgrouping into the melanotic and synovial types. *Cancer*, **42**, 243.

1979   EKFORS T.O., RANTAKOKKO V.: Clear cell sarcoma of tendons and aponeuroses: malignant melanoma of soft tissue. Report of four cases. *Pathol. Res. Pract.*, **165**, 422.

1979   RADSTONE D.J., REVELL P.A., MANTELL B.S.: Clear cell sarcoma of tendons and aponeuroses treated with bleomycin and vincristine. *Br. J. Radiol.*, **52**, 238.

1979   RAYNOR A.C., VARGAS-CROTES F., ALEXANDER R.W., *et al.*: Clear-cell sarcoma with melanin pigment: a possible soft-tissue variant of malignant melanoma. Case report. *J. Bone Joint. Surg.*, **61/A**, 276.

1980   PARKER J.B., MARCUS P.B., MARTIN J.H.: Spinal melanotic clear-cell sarcoma: A light and electron microscopic study. *Cancer*, **46**, 718.

1983   ECKHARDT J.J., PRITCHARD D.L., SOULE E.H.: Clear cell sarcoma. A clinicopathologic study of 27 cases. *Cancer*, **52**, 1482.

1983   KINDBLOM L.G., LODDING P., ANGERVALL L.: Clear-cell sarcoma of tendons and aponeuroses. An immunohistochemical and electron microscopic analysis indicating neural crest origin. *Virchows Arch.*, **401**, 109.

1984   KATENKAMP D., PEREVOSHCHIKOV A.G., RAIKHLIN N.T.: Soft tissue clear cell sarcoma. Morphology, differential diagnosis and tumor classification. *Zentralbl. Allg. Pathol.*, **129**, 521.

1984   RAMDHANE B.K., LACOMBE M.J., SEVIN D., *et al.*: Les sarcomes a cellules claires des tissus mous. Reévaluation des sarcomes a cellules claires des tendons et de gaines. A propos de 14 cas. *Ann. Pathol.*, **4**, 349.

1985   BENSON J.D., KRAEMER B.B., MacKAY B.: Malignant melanoma of soft parts. An ultrastructural study of four cases. *Ultrastruct. Pathol.*, **8**, 57.

1989   HASEGAWA T., HIROSE T., RUDO E., HIZAWA R.: Clear-cell sarcoma. An immunohistochemical and ultrastructural study. *Acta Pathol. Jpn.*, **39**, 321.

1989   SWANSON P.E., WICK M.R.: Clear-cell sarcoma: immunohistochemical analysis of six cases. Comparison with other epithelioid neoplasms of soft tissue. *Acta Pathol. Lab. Med.*, **113**, 55.

PSEUDOTUMORS OF
THE SOFT TISSUES

PALMAR (Dupuytren's disease)
AND PLANTAR (Ledderhose's disease)
FIBROMATOSIS

Dupuytren's disease occurs too frequently and is too well-known for us to have to recall its features here (Fig. 852). Suffice it to emphasize that the nodules which enlarge the palmar aponeurosis initially have a histological structure which is nearly the same as that of a desmoid tumor or even a well-differentiated fibrosarcoma (grade 1), with numerous plump fibroblasts, and some mitotic figures (Fig. 853). Thereafter, the nodules «mature» in a dense, pseudotendinous, collagenous tissue, retracting and adhering to the derma.

Plantar fibromatosis occurs more **rarely** and may be associated with Dupuytren's disease and to dorsal digital nodules at the metacarpo-phalangeal and interphalangeal level. Like Dupuytren's disease, plantar fibromatosis shows predilection for the male **sex**, it may be hereditary and more frequent

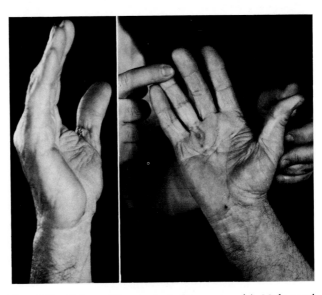

FIG. 852. - Palmar fibromatosis (Dupuytren's). Male aged 66 years. Initial retraction of the palmar aponeurosis along the fourth ray.

in epileptics and diabetics. Unlike Dupuytren's disease, it may also be observed in childhood-young **age**.

It is manifested as a globose mass, which at times is bumpy, located in the plantar aponeurosis. It may become of considerable size (5 or 6 cm in diameter). It may be painful and it generally does not cause flexor retraction of the toes.

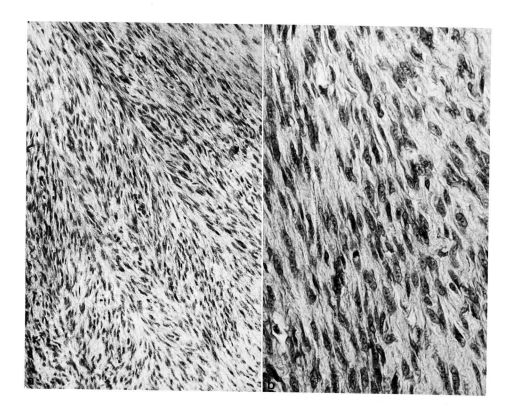

FIG. 853. - Cellular (early) phase of Dupuytren's disease. (a) Spindle cells in fasciculated pattern which at times mimick fibrosarcoma. (b) At higher power, ovoid-spindle cells with a plump nucleus, and a small nucleolus. The features are those of the «myofibroblast». A mitotic figure may be seen (*Hemat.-eos.*, 120, 250 x).

Macroscopically it is a fibrous tissue, pinker and fleshier as compared to the normal aponeurosis (white and lucent). It is similar to Dupuytren's nodules in their early stage. Plantar fibromatosis infiltrates the aponeurosis and may adhere to the skin. It tends to mature in dense collagen form. Its histological aspect is the same as that of Dupuytren's disease.

In conclusion, plantar fibromatosis has a more pseudotumoral aspect than Dupuytren's disease and it may be painful. Both probably mean hyperplastic proliferation due to unknown causes. Both easily recur if excision is not complete and does not include the entire aponeurosis. Recurrence probably does not only depend on residues of fibromatous tissue left *in situ*, but also on the possibility that other parts of the normal aponeurosis develop the same proliferative alteration. In the sole of the foot excision of the entire aponeurosis is hardly ever performed. For this reason, as well, recurrence is more frequent than in Dupuytren's disease.

Histologically, if we examine a fibromatous nodule during an early stage, a distinction in relation to desmoid tumor is impossible. Differential diagnosis is based on clinical data and on extensive histological sampling. The latter demonstrates a gradual transition from the nodules to a dense pseudotendinous connective tissue and the normal aponeurosis.

REFERENCES

1955 ALLEN R.A., WOOLNER L.B., Ghormley R.K.: Soft tissue tumors of the sole. With special reference to plantar fibromatosis. *J. Bone Joint Surg.*, **37/A**.

1956 LAGIER R., RUTISHAUSER E.: Anatomie pathologique et pathogenie de la maladie de Dupuytren. *Presse Med.*, **64**, 1212.

1958 LARSEN D., POSCHE L.: Dupuytren's contracture: with special reference to pathology. *J. Bone Joint Surg.*, **40/A (4)**, 773.

1959 LUCK J.V.: Dupuytren's contracture. A new concept of pathogenesis correlated with surgical management. *J. Bone Joint. Surg.*, **41/A**, 635.

1960 LARSEN R.D., TAKAGISHI N., POSCH J.L.: The pathogenesis of Dupuytren's contracture: experimental and further clinical observations. *J. Bone Joint Surg.*, **42/A**, 993.

1962 EARLY P.E.: Population studies in Dupuytren's contracture. *J. Bone Joint Surgery.*, **44/B**, 602.

1963 LING R.S.M.: The genetic factor of Dupuytren's disease. *J. Bone Joint Surg.*, **45/B**, 708.

1965 CURTIN J.W.: Fibromatosis of the plantar fascia: Surgical technique and design of skin incision. *J. Bone Joint. Sug.*, **47/A**, 1605.

1970 MILLESI H.: Die Stellung der Dupuytrenschen Kontraktur in der Pathologie. *Handchirurgie*, **1**, 15.

1973 WARTHAN T.L., RUDOLPH R.I., GROSS P.R.: Isolated plantar fibromatosis. *Arch. Dermatol.*, **108**, 823.

1975 KREBS H.: Erfahrungen bei 350 operativ behandelten Dupuytrenschen Kontracturen. *Arch. Chir.*, **338**, 67.

1976 NEMETSCHEK T., MEINEL A., NEMETSCHEK-GANSLER H., *et al.:* Zur Aetiologie der Kontraktur beim Morbus Dupuytren. *Virchows Arch. (Pathol. Anat.)*, **372**, 57.

1980 JAMES W.D., ODOM R.B.: The role of the myofibroblast in Dupuytren's contracture. *Arch. Dermatol.*, **116**, 807.

1982 VANDE BERG J.S., RUDOPH R., GELBERMAN R., *et al.*: Ultrastructural relationship of skin to nodule and cord in Dupuytren's contracture. *Plast. Reconstr. Surg.*, **69**, 835.

1984 IWASAKI H., MULLER H., STUTTE H.J., BRENNSCHEIDT U.: Palmar fibromatosis (Dupuytren's contracture) ultrastructural and enzyme histochemical studies of 43 cases. *Virchows Arch (Pathol. Anat.)*, **405**, 41.

1984 KISCHER C.W., SPEER D.P.: Microvascular changes in Dupuytren's contracture. *J. Hand Surg.*, **9-A**, 58.

NODULAR FASCIITIS
(Synonyms: proliferative fasciitis, infiltrative fasciitis, pseudosarcomatous fasciitis, pseudosarcomatous fibromatosis)

DEFINITION

It is a nodular neoformation of a probably hyperplastic nature, which because of its rapid growth, cellularity and presence of mitotic figures, may be mistaken for a malignant neoplasm.

FREQUENCY

It is a rather frequent lesion, the most frequent among tumors and pseudotumors of a fibroblastic nature in the soft tissues.

SEX

There is no difference with regard to sex.

AGE

There is predilection for young adult age, between 20 and 40 years. It infrequently occurs in children and it is rare in the elderly.

LOCALIZATION

N.F. shows evident predilection for the upper limb, particularly the volar aspect of the forearm. This is followed by the thoracic wall and the dorsum. Localizations in the head and neck are more common during childhood. It is a rare occurrence in the lower limb and decidedly rare in the hand and foot.

SYMPTOMS

It is a nodule, which is always or nearly always solitary, usually superficial (in the subcutaneous tissue, in the superficial fascia); at times it is deeper

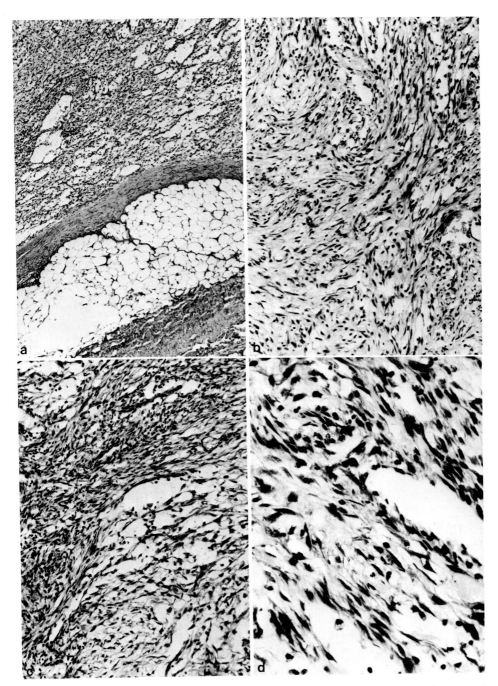

FIG. 854. - Nodular fasciitis. (a) Undefined boundaries characterize the proliferation of nodular aspect. (b) Vaguely fasciculated proliferation of the spindle cells, with rich vascularization. (c) Areas in which the cells appear to be closely packed alternate with others in which the cells are loosely arranged. Observe the vessels having thin walls, lymphocytary infiltration and foamy histiocytary cells. (d) The cytological features may appear to be rather alarming as alongside a moderate pleomorphism there is hyperchromia of the nuclei (*Hemat.-eos.*, 60, 160, 160, 400 x).

(in the muscle). The nodule is **formed rapidly** and in less than 1 month it achieves maximum size which generally does not exceed 3-4 cm in diameter. Often, the nodule is moderately painful, particularly on pressure.

GROSS PATHOLOGIC FEATURES

The nodule may be localized within the subcutaneous tissue, starting from the superficial fascia or, more rarely, it may be contained within a muscle. In all cases it is round or oval, at times moderately lobulated, usually well-circumscribed. At times it tends to expand along the fascia and from here along the septa between the lobules of fat in the subcutaneous tissue or between the bundles of muscular fibers, with a slightly stellate form. On the cut surface, the tissue is rather soft, whitish-gray, often having a myxoid aura. In veterate forms (where the tissue, following its hyperplastic nature, tends to mature in a collagenous tissue) the nodule becomes more whitish, hard and fibrous and it may contain cystic cavities filled with mucus.

HISTOPATHOLOGIC FEATURES

N.F. is made up of bundles of fibroblasts which are rather numerous and which resemble those of a granulation tissue or of an in vitro culture (Fig. 854). The fibroblasts have rather plump nuclei, with dispersed chromatin and an evident nucleolus. Mitotic figures are rather frequent, but atypical mitoses are never observed. The fibroblasts are arranged in intertwining bundles with no particular order and among these there is abundant mesh of reticular fibers, while mature collagen fibers are scarce. In advanced or veterate stages of the lesion, the quantity of collagen fibers increases, which become rougher and collected in hyalin bands, while fibroblasts rarefy and mature. The ground substance rich in hyaluronic acid (PAS and halcian-positive annulled by pre-treatment with hyaluronidase) is also abundant. The abundance of this ground substance may confer a myxoid aura on the tissue, with dissociation of the fibroblasts and fibers and at times the formation of small lakes full of mucoid substance. Among the fibroblasts it is possible to observe sparse erythrocytes, lymphocytes, some macrophages, some multinucleate giant cells.

HISTOGENESIS AND PATHOGENESIS

Pathogenesis is unknown. As for the histogenesis, it seems to be a proliferation of fibroblastic origin and of hyperplastic nature. This is shown by its rapid growth, tendency to mature, the fact that the nodule hardly ever becomes of considerable size, the benign behaviour of the lesion even without adequate surgical treatment.

DIAGNOSIS

As is the case for so-called myositis ossificans, N.F. too draws a good part of its interest, for the clinician and the pathologist, from the fact that it may be erroneously diagnosed sarcoma.

Malignant fibrous histiocytoma, whether in its usual variety or in its myxoid one, is differentiated by its storiform structure, by the greater nuclear pleomorphism and hyperchromia, by the presence of multinucleate giant and sarcomatous cells, by the presence of atypical mitoses. On a clinical level, moreover, malignant fibrous histiocytoma is often observed in adults and elderly patients, it does not grow as rapidly as N.F. and it frequently becomes of a size which is greater than that of N.F. Certainly, differential diagnosis is more difficult with regard to rare cases of low-grade malignant fibrous histiocytoma.

Desmoid tumor or aggressive fibromatosis is distinguished by its slow growth and rather large size, by its infiltrative attitude in relation to the surrounding tissues, by its compact and densely fibrous structure.

Fibrosarcoma is distinguished by its cellularity, by its typical herringbone structure, by the greater amount of hyperchromia and pleomorphism in the nuclei, by the presence of mitoses which may even be atypical, and again by its clinical features (deep site, long duration, progressive growth, large size).

Finally, **intramuscular myxoma** is distinguished by its completely myxoid structure with rather scarce cells scattered in an abundant mucoid substance.

COURSE

As previously mentioned, N.F. forms and grows rapidly, whereupon it stops growing and tends to mature spontaneously with hardening and fibrosis of the nodule. These features indicate the hyperplastic nature of the lesion, similar to a nodule of granulation tissue.

TREATMENT AND PROGNOSIS

N.F. is a benign lesion. It usually heals after even marginal or intralesional excision. In some cases spontaneous regression of the nodule has been observed. Recurrence after surgical excision is rare and evidently corresponds to cases excised incompletely while the lesion was still developing. Treatment of choice is thus marginal excision.

REFERENCES

1961   Stout A.P.: Pseudosarcomatous fasciitis in children. *Cancer,* **14**, 1216.

1962   Hutter R.V., Stewart F.W., Foote F.W. Jr.: Fasciitis.: a report of 70 cases with follow up proving the benignity of the lesion. *Cancer,* **15**, 992.

1962   Soule E.H.: Proliferative (nodular) fasciitis. *Arch. Pathol.,* **73**, 437.

1966   Mehregan A.H.: Nodular fasciitis. *Arch. Dermatol.,* **93**, 204.

1968   Kleinstiver B.J., Rodriguez H.A.: Nodular fasciitis - a study of 45 cases and review of the literature. *J. Bone Joint Surg.,* **50/A**, 1204.

1976   Wirman J.A.: Nodular fasciitis, a lesion of myofibroblasts. An ultrastructural study. *Cancer,* **38**, 2378.

1977   Dahl I., Angervall L.: Pseudosarcomatous proliferative lesions of soft tissue with or without bone formation. *Acta Pathol. Microbiol. Scand.,* **85**, 577.

1978   Meister P., Bückmann F.W., Konrad E.: Nodular fasciitis (analysis of 100 cases and review of the literature). *Pathol. Res. Pract.* **162**, 133.

1980   Lauer D., Enzinger F.M.: Cranial fasciitis. *Cancer,* **45**, 401.

1981   Dahl I., Ackerman M.: Nodular fasciitis. A correlative cytologic and histologic study. *Acta Cytol.,* **25**, 215.

1981   Patchefsky A., Enzinger F.M.: Intravascular fasciitis. *Am. J. Surg. Pathol.,* **5**, 29.

1982   Bernstein K.E., Lattes R.: Nodular (pseudosarcomatous) fasciitis, a nonrecurrent lesion. *Cancer,* **49**, 1668.

1984   Pasquier B., Keddari E., Pasquier D., et al.: Fasciite crânienne de l'enfant. A propos d'un cas à révélation neonatale avec extension dure-mèrienne. *Ann. Pathol.,* **4**, 371.

1984   Shimizu S., Hashimoto H., Enjoji M.: Nodular fasciitis. An analysis of 250 patients. *Pathology,* **16**, 161.

1986   Weiss S.W.: Proliferative fibroblastic lesions. From hyperplasia to neoplasia. *Am. J. Surg. Pathol.,* **10** (suppl.), 14.

PROLIFERATIVE FASCIITIS AND
PROLIFERATIVE MYOSITIS

These terms indicate nodular lesions whose anatomo-clinical presentation and nature are similar to that of nodular fasciitis (Fig. 855).

The main difference consists in the histological picture where, alongside a fibroblastic proliferation with some myxoid aspect which is totally analogous to that of a nodular fasciitis, there are large cells of pseudogangliar or

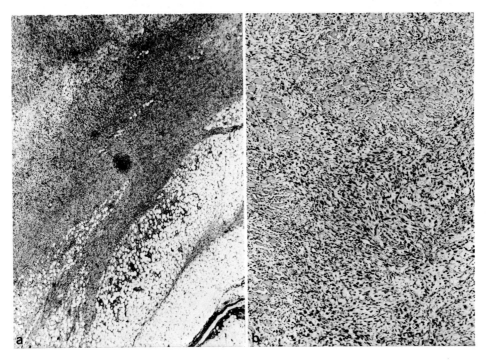

FIG. 855. - Proliferative myositis. (a) The margins of the lesion seem to be indistinct and at times infiltrative. (b) Rather pleomorphic cellular proliferation infiltrates the muscle tissue. (c) Disorderly proliferation of the spindle cells immersed in myxoid matrix. The nuclei are large with an evident nucleolus. The cytoplasm is eosinophilic without evident boundaries. (d) Infiltrative aspect in the muscle: the proliferating cells are associated with lymphocytes and rich vascularization (Hemat.-eos., 25, 60, 400, 250 x).

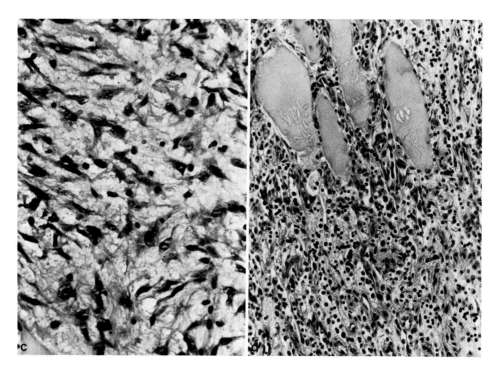

FIG. 855. (continued).

pseudomyoblastic aspect; these cells have a rather large and intensely basophilic cytoplasm, in which there may be inclusions with the tintorial affin-
ities of collagen. Moreover, these cells have very large nuclei with a vesicular
aura, an evident nuclear membrane and a large or gigantic nucleolus. These
cells probably represent modified fibroblasts.

In proliferative myositis, moreover, the fibroblastic proliferation including these peculiar cells tends to infiltrate among the muscular cells, as if the
proliferation derived from the sheets of the muscular cells and muscular
bundles.

The presence of such giant cells results in differential diagnosis with **gan-
glioneuroblastoma** and **pleomorphic rhabdomyosarcoma**.

REFERENCES

1967   ENZINGER F.M.: Proliferative myositis. Report of 33 cases. *Cancer*, **20**, 2213.
1974   ROSE A.G.: An electron microscopic study of the giant cells in proliferative
        myositis. *Cancer*, **33**, 1543.
1975   CHUNG E.B., ENZINGER F.M.: Proliferative fasciitis. *Cancer*, **36**, 1450.
1980   HEFFNER R.R. JR., BARRON S.A.: Denervating changes in focal myositis, a be-
        nign inflammatory pseudotumor. *Arch. Pathol. Lab. Med.*, **104**, 261.
1983   ORLOWSKI W., FREEDMAN P.D., LUMERMAN H.: Proliferative myositis of the
        masseter muscle. A case report and a review of the literature. *Cancer*, **52**,
        904.
1983   PAGES A., DOSSA J., PAGES M.: La myosite proliferante, un pseudosarcome
        musculaire. A propos d'un cas avec examen ultrastructural. *Ann. Pathol.*,
        3, 161.

ELASTOFIBROMA
(Synonym: elastofibroma dorsi)

It is a **rare** pseudotumoral lesion which is observed nearly exclusively during advanced age (over 55 years) and in the tissues between the lower angle of the scapula and the thoracic wall. There is predilection for the female **sex** and for individuals who do heavy manual labor.

It is presented as a globose mass, which grows slowly or very slowly, and which is nearly painless. As previously stated, it is localized nearly always

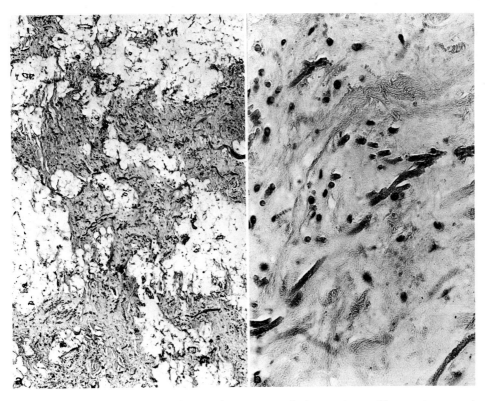

FIG. 856. - Elastofibroma. (a) Observe the mixture of adipose tissue, fibrous shoots and refracting material which may be related to elastic fibers. (b) Fragments of highly re-fracting elastic fibers are immersed in collagen mesh (*Hemat.-eos.*, 60, 400 x).

between the muscles of the scapulothoracic region and generally adheres to the costal wall. The mass may become of considerable size (up to 10 cm in diameter), it has poorly defined limits and it is of firm consistency. On the cut surface it has a fibrous aspect, at times variegated by lobules of fat or some more hyperemic areas.

Histologically it is a scarcely cellular tissue, with scattered fibrocytes of mature aspect, alternating with a dense mat of collagen fibers and rough elastic fibers. The latter are swollen and segmentated, and they take the elective colors for elastin (not after treatment with elastasis and pepsin: Fig. 856).

E. is a hyperplastic and self-limiting growth, as indicated by incidence during advanced age, in individuals who have carried out heavy manual labor for many years, in an area where there is continuous confrication between the scapula and the thoracic wall. This pathogenesis is also suggested by the rare bilateral incidence of the lesion.

Thus, it is an absolutely non-aggressive lesion, which may not require any treatment in less expanded forms, or which may be treated successfully by marginal excision and, it seems, even radiation treatment.

REFERENCES

1965 DELVAUX T.C., LESTER J.P.: Elastofibroma dorsi. *Am. J. Clin. Pathol.*, **43**, 72.

1966 BARR J.R.: Elastofibroma. *Am. J. Clin. Pathol.*, **45**, 679.

1966 BROWN R.K., CLEARKIN K.P., NAKACHI K., *et al.*: Elastofibroma dorsi. *N. Engl. J. Med.*, **275**, 154.

1971 COSTANZI G., EUSEBI V.: Elastofibroma dorsi. *Tumori*, **57**, 349.

1973 RENSHAW T.S., SIMON M.A.: Elastofibroma. *J. Bone Joint. Surg.*, **55/A**, 409.

1977 AKHTAR M., MILLER R.M.: Ultrastructure of elastofibroma. *Cancer*, **40**, 728.

1980 DIXON A.Y., LEE S.H.: An ultrastructural study of elastofibromas. *Hum Pathol.*, **11**, 257.

1981 MADRI J.A., DISE C.A., LIVOLSI V.A., *et. al.*: Elastofibroma: An immunohistochemical study of collagen content. *Hum. Pathol.*, **12**, 186.

1982 KINDBLOM L.G., SPICER S.S.: Elastofibroma. A correlated light and electron microscopic study. *Virchows Arch. (Pathol. Anat.)*, **396**, 127.

1982 NAGAMINE N., NOHARA Y., ITO E.: Elastofibroma in Okinawa. A clinicopathologic study of 170 cases. *Cancer*, **50**, 1794.

1983 BENISCH B., PEISON B., MARQUET E., *et al.*: Pre-elastofibroma and elastofibroma (The continuum of elastic-producing fibrous tumors). A light and ultrastructural study. *Am. J. Clin. Pathol.*, **80**, 88.

1986 NAKAMURA Y., OKAMOTO K., TANIMURA A., KATO M., NORIMATSU M.: Elastase digestion and biochemical analysis of the elastin from an elastofibroma. *Cancer*, **58**, 1070.

1987 FUKUDA Y., MIYAKE H., MASUDA Y., *et al.*: Histogenesis of unique elastinophilic fibers of elastofibroma. Ultrastructural and immuno-histo-chemical studies. *Hum. Pathol.*, **18**, 424.

XANTHOMA

It is a histiocytary production with the accumulation of lipids, particularly cholesterids, in the cytoplasm (foam cells) and outside (cholesterid crystals) (Fig. 857). It is associated with hyperlipidemia (which may be hereditary) and it is secondary to it. X. are generally multiple. The most typical forms are xanthelasma (in the palpebral subcutaneous tissue), tuberous X. (in the subcutaneous tissue of the elbows, buttocks, knees, fingers) and X. of the tendons, particularly the Achilles tendon.

In tendinous localizations there are bumpy masses which protrude from the surface of the tendon. On the cut surface, they have a typical canary-yellow color and infiltrate the tendinous tissue.

Treatment must tend to correct the dyslipidemia and, if surgical, it must be as conservative as possible.

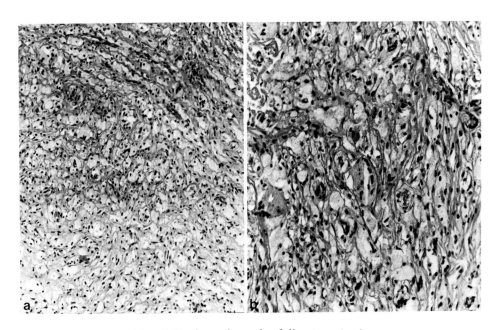

FIG. 857. (legend on the following page).

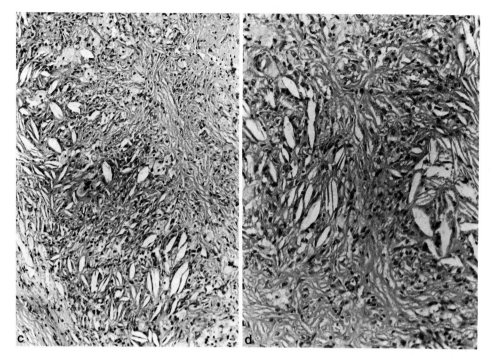

FIG. 857. - Xanthoma. (a) and (b) Solid fields constituted by histiocytes having a small, pyknotic, subcentral or peripheral nucleus in finely foamy cytoplasm. Among the cells there is a delicate fibrous pattern. (c) and (d) Alongside cells with foamy cytoplasm there are negative images of cholesterol crystals, surrounded by multinucleate giant cells (*Hemat.-eos.*, 160, 250, 160, 250 x).

REFERENCES

1971 GATTEREAU A., DAVIGNON J., LEVESQUE H.P.: Roentgenological evaluation of Achilles-tendon xanthomatosis. *Lancet*, **2**, 705.

1972 PALMER A.J., BLACKET R.: Regression of xanthomata of the eyelids with modified fat diet. *Lancet*, **1**, 67.

1972 SIEGELMANN S.S., SCHLOSSBERG I., BECKER N.H., *et al.*: Hyperlipoproteinemia with skeletal lesions. *Clin. Orthop.*, **87**, 228.

1973 FAHEY J.J., STARK H.H., DONOVAN W.F., *et al.*: Xanthoma of the Achilles tendon: Seven cases with familial hyperbetalipoprotemia. *J. Bone Joint. Surg.*, **55/A**, 1197.

1973 WALTON K.W., THOMAS C., DUNKERLEY D.J.: The pathogenesis of xanthomata. *J. Pathol.*, **109**, 271.

1975 HAMILTON W.C., RAMSEY P.L., HANSON S.M., *et al.*: Osseous xanthoma and multiple hand tumors as a complication of hyperlipidemia. *J. Bone Joint Surg.*, **57/A**, 551.

1977 WILKES L.L.: Tendon xanthoma in type IV hyperlipoproteinemia. *South. Med. J.*, **70**, 254.

1984 BERGINER V.M., SALEN G., SHEFER S.: Long-term treatment of cerebrotendinous xanthomatosis with chenodeoxycholic acid. *N. Engl. J. Med.*, **311**, 1649.

INFANTILE XANTHOGRANULOMA

It is a cutaneous lesion, which is presented after birth and up to 3 years of age, with small nodules, and spontaneously regresses within a few years. Rarely the nodules also occur in the deep soft tissue, in the eye, in the internal organs.

Histologically, it is formed by histiocytes, foam cells, giant cells (Touton), and inflammatory cells including eosinophilic granulocytes.

It is probably a hyperplastic production of unknown etiology. It is different from histiocytosis X and it is not associated with seric lipid modifications.

REFERENCES

1966 WEBSTER S.B., REISTER H.C., HARMAN L.E.: Juvenile xanthogranuloma with extra-cutaneous lesions: a case report and review of the literature. *Arch. Dermatol.*, **93**, 71.

1970 GONZALEZ-CRUSSI F., CAMPBELL R.J.: Juvenile xanthogranuloma. Ultrastructural study. *Arch. Pathol.*, **89**, 65.

1972 ESTERLY N.B., SAHIHI T., MEDENICA M.: Juvenile xanthogranuloma: an atypical case with a study of ultrastructure. *Arch. Dermatol.*, **105**, 99.

1973 NEWELL G.B., STONE O.J., MULINS J.F.: Juvenile xanthogranuloma and neurofibromatosis. *Arch. Dermatol.*, **107**, 262.

1985 SONODA T., HASHIMOTO H., ENJOJI M.: Juvenile xanthogranuloma: Clinicopathologic analysis and immunohistochemical study of 57 patients. *Cancer*, **56**, 2280.

MUCOUS CYST
(Synonym: ganglion)

These are very frequent lesions and they rarely involve problems in differential diagnosis with tumors. We discuss them here for the sake of completeness and in order to compare them to intraosseous and periosteal M.C. M.C. of the soft tissues are particularly observed adherent to the tendinous sheaths and in the peritendinous and fascial tissues, in the wrist, hand, foot and ankle. But at times they develop inside a tendon (Fig. 858), within a joint capsule or at the periphery of the menisci of the knee (Fig. 859). In exceptional cases a M.C. develops in the sheath (epineurium) of a peripheral nerve, in areas submitted to mechanical stress, such as the popliteal nerve near the neck of the fibula.

M.C. originate from a mucoid transformation *in situ* of the connective tissue. If we histologically examine numerous cysts it is possible to reconstruct

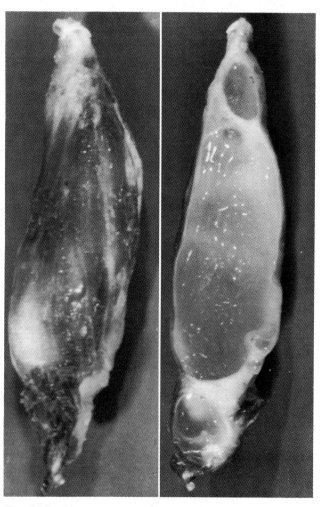

FIG. 858. - Mucous cyst at the musculotendinous junction of the long peroneal muscle.

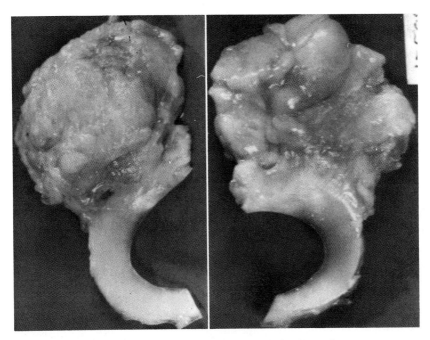

FIG. 859. - Parameniscal mucous cyst of the lateral meniscus.

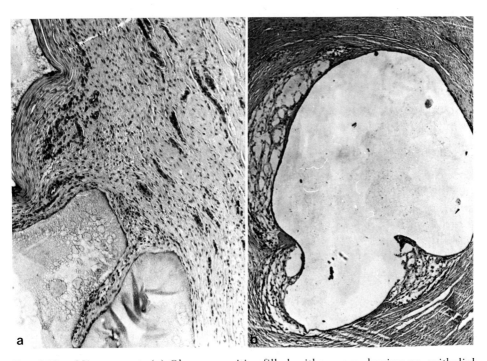

FIG. 860. - Mucous cyst. (a) Observe cavities filled with mucus, having no epithelial coating. (b) In the wall, among the fibrous cells of the stroma, observe deposit of mucous material which at first tends to separate the cells to then flow into more ample lacunae until the cystic space is formed (*Hemat.-eos.*, 50, 150 x).

their histogenesis. At first the connective cells are rarefied because a semili-quid mucoid substance forms between them and the collagen fibers surround-ing them (Fig. 860). This mucoid transformation, which probably represents a localized regressive process, associates with moderate cellular hyperplasia, expressed by the fact that the cells are initially numerous and plump.

This hyperplasia is particularly evident in the tendons, where the cells are normally rather scarce. Gradually the mucoid substance increases and the cells disappear. Thus, single or multiple cysts are formed, which tend to become larger and to flow together.

When the cyst is formed, it has a fibrous wall and viscous content, which is transparent and colorless. The wall is formed by parallel collagenous bun dles, poor in cells. At times there are residues of myxoid tissue which dis-solves towards the lumen of the cyst.

The mucoid liquid is mostly dissolved during histological preparation, unless acetic acid is added to the fixative solution. In this case, the mucoid becomes similar to the white of a hardboiled egg. Histologically, it is mildly foamy and basophile. Outside of the cystic wall there is a fair amount of vas-cular hyperplasia, with a crown of small newly-formed vessels.

M.C. usually do not communicate with the joint or tenovaginal synovial cavities and do not derive from hernias of the synovial membrane. True synovial cysts, which are particularly observed in the popliteal region, are a different lesion.

REFERENCES

1943   GHORMLEY R.K., DOCKERTY M.B.: Cystic myxomatous tumors about the knee: Their relation to cysts of the menisci. *J. Bone Joint Surg.* **25**, 306.

1961   McEVEDY V.: Simple ganglia. *Br. J. Surg.*, **49**, 585.

1963   BARRETT R., CRAMER F.: Tumors of the peripheral nerves and so-called ganglia of the peroneal nerve. *Clin. Orthop.*, **27**, 135.

1964   BARNES W.E., LARSEN R.D., POSCH J.L.: Review of the ganglia of the hand or wrist with analysis of surgical treatment. *Plast. Reconstr. Surg.*, **34**, 570.

1965   BECTON J.L., YOUNG H.H.: Cysts of semilunar cartilage of the knee. *Arch. Surg.*, **90**, 708.

1965   GURDJIAN E.S., LARSEN R.D., LINDNER D.W.: Intraneural cyst of the peroneal and ulnar nerves: Report of two cases. *J. Neurosurg.*, **23**, 76.

1974   COBB C.A. III., MOIEL R.N.: Ganglion of the peroneal nerve. Report of two cases. *J. Neurosurg.*, **41**, 255.

1986   OERTEL Y.C., BECKNER M.E., ENGLER W.F.: Cytologic diagnosis and ultra-structure of fine-needle aspirates of ganglion cysts. *Arch. Pathol. Lab. Med.*, **110**, 938.

AMPUTATION NEUROMA

This is a hyperplastic lesion characterized by the proliferation of all of the elements constituting the nerve. After amputation or resection of the nerve trunk, when proximal nervous regeneration cannot be channeled in the distal nerve segment, it constitutes «hanks» of cells and fibers. It is the disorderly proliferation of nerve fibers, with their myelinic coating, Schwann cells and fibroblasts, deriving from the proximal segment of the nerve, and which is exhausted within a few months. The lesion is painful.

Macroscopically the amputation neuroma is a nodule of firm consistency, and it occurs in the area corresponding to a traumatized or transected nerve.

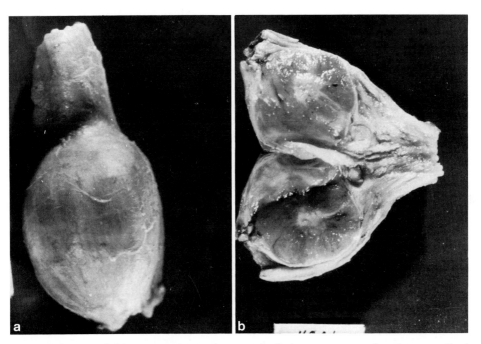

FIG. 861. - (a) and (b) Amputation neuroma: the lesion appears to be circumscribed, nodular, in continuity with the nerve trunk. (c) and (d) There are richly proliferative nervous fascicles cloistered by collagenous septa. Proliferation of the nerve fibers, Schwann cells and fibrocytes is observed (*Hemat.-eos.*, 160, 250 x).

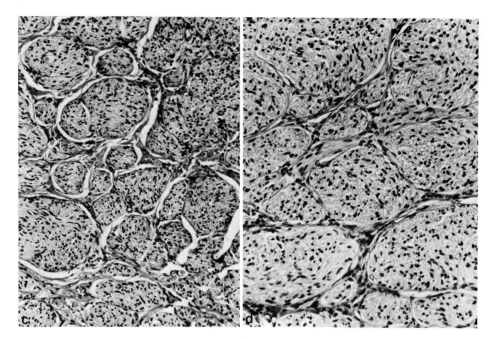

FIG. 861. (continued).

Histologically there are convoluted and intertwined bundles of nerve fibers and Schwann cells, which are more or less mature depending on the amount of time which has passed since nervous dissection (Fig. 861).

MORTON NEUROMA

It originates from the digital plantar nerve in the area corresponding to the head of the third and fourth metatarsal and is caused by microtrauma on the nerve, compressed between the heads of the metatarsals.

Macroscopically the nerve appears to be increased in volume, particularly in the area corresponding to its bifurcation.

Microscopically it dominates fibrosis and edema of the nerve trunk. The fibrosis surpasses the epineurium and perineurium and spreads to the surrounding tissues.

REFERENCES

1946 CIESLAK A.K., SOUT A.P.: Traumatic and amputation neuromas. *Arch. Surg.*, **53**, 646.

1965 SNYDER C.C., KNOWLES R.P.: Traumatic neuromas. *J. Bone Joint. Surg.*, **47/A**, 641.

1973 REED R.J., BLISS B.O.: Morton neuroma. Regressive and productive intermetatarsal elastofibrositis. *Arch. Pathol.*, **95**, 123.

1976 LASSMANN G., LASSMANN H., STOCKINGER L.: Morton's metatarsalgia: Light and electron microscopic observations and their relations to entrapment neuropathies. *Virchows Arch. (Pathol. Anat.)*, **370**, 307.

1984 GREENFIELD J., REA J. Jr., ILFELD F.W.: Morton's interdigital neuroma. Indications for treatment by local injections versus surgery. *Clin. Orthop.*, **185**, 142-4.

SYNOVIAL CHONDROMATOSIS
(Synonyms: synovial osteochondromatosis; extraskeletal chondroma; chondroma of the soft tissues)

DEFINITION

It is a neoformation of well-differentiated hyaline cartilage, occurring within the joint synovial membrane or, outside of the joints, within the tendinous sheath or the bursae mucosae.

GENERAL INFORMATION

S.C. is a relatively rare occurrence. There is predilection for the male **sex** and for adult-advanced **age**. It is hardly ever observed prior to puberty and it is frequently observed between 30 and 50 years of age. In more than half of all cases it is **localized** in the knee, and this is followed by the elbow and the other large joints (shoulder, wrist, hip, ankle) and, more rarely, by small joints such as the metacarpo-phalangeal. The extra-articular form of S.C. is observed in most cases in the fingers, and more rarely in the hand, the wrist, the foot and the ankle; this form is nearly always related to a tendon and thus it presumably originates from the synovial membrane of the tendinous sheaths. In exceptional cases, S.C. has been observed in two symmetrical joints or in two paratendinous extra-articular localizations.

SYMPTOMS

In joint S.C. symptoms are moderate, recurring and very slowly progressing. Generally, the amount of time between the first symptoms and treat- is a few years. Symptoms include pain, limited joint motion, a sensation of joint crackling. Blocking and synovial effusion are rarely observed. At times the loose endoarticular bodies may be palpated.

In aggressive, pseudotumoral forms of the lesion, a plurilobulated mass may develop, which expands in the peri-articular tissues and which has the hard-elastic consistency of cartilage.

Even the nodules of the fingers and toes grow slowly, are nearly painless, and hardly ever become of large size (Fig. 867).

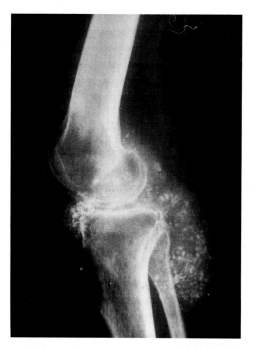

FIG. 862. - Synovial chondromatosis in a 60-year-old man. Discontinuous pain in the last 5 years worsened in the last year. Prevalently popliteal swelling and marked functional impairment. An arthrodesis was performed with no attempt at excising the posterior chondromatous mass. The latter was practically unchanged at 4-year-follow-up.

RADIOGRAPHIC FEATURES

The radiographic picture is completely negative if the cartilaginous nodules are not calcified or ossified. In this case diagnosis of articular S.C. may be suspected with CAT an MRI and confirmed by arthroscopy or arthrotomy. When calcification begins, minute faded radiopaque granules are observed in the capsulo-synovial soft tissues (Figs. 863, 864, 865). In paratendinous S.C. of the hand and foot, as well, calcification-ossification is a frequent finding (Fig. 868). When the calcification-ossification of the intrasynovial nod-

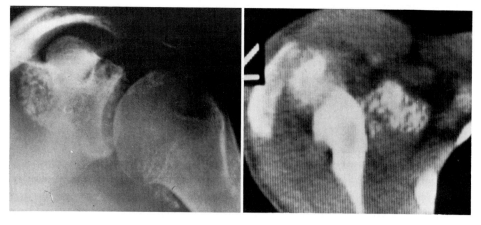

FIG. 863. - Male aged 40 years. Synovial chondromatosis of the shoulder.

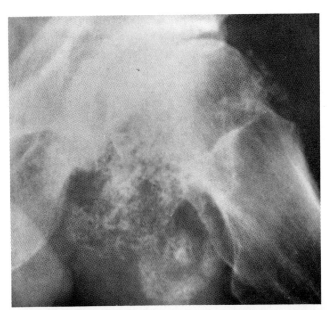

Fig. 864. - Male aged 76 years. Synovial chondromatosis of the hip, which initiated 25 years earlier.

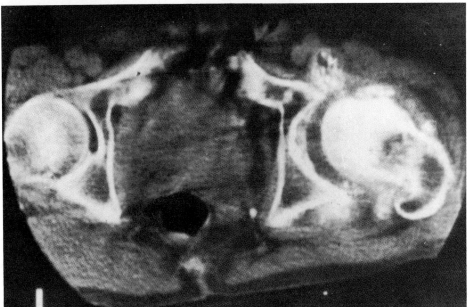

ules and of the loose bodies is more intense and mature, numerous round and intensely radiopaque bodies are seen (at times the radiopacity is more intense at their periphery) which occupy and at times distend all of the synovial recesses. The joint skeleton is generally not altered. In some inveterate forms there may be some signs of arthrosis.

In aggressive pseudotumoral forms of S.C., there are para-articular tumoral masses with the same radiopacity as the soft tissues, but which are often sprayed by minute tenuous and faded calcifications (Fig. 862). In these cases, furthermore, it is possible to observe even severe erosion of the joint bone ends. This erosion may reach as far as the metaphysis and the diaphyseal end, as the pseudotumoral masses, by climbing along the capsular insertions and invading the pericapsular soft tissues, surround and dig from the outside the metadiaphysis.

GROSS PATHOLOGIC FEATURES

In typical cases, once the joint has been opened, there are a large number of loose bodies, up to many tens of them, of size varying from that of a peppercorn to a cherry (Fig. 866). They are white, smooth, lucent, with the aspect of mature hyaline cartilage, the smaller ones globose in shape, the larger ones bumpy, deriving from the fusion of many nodules together.

In more recent forms and having no calcification-ossification of the nodules, the loose bodies are smaller, of translucid cartilaginous aspect, and relatively soft.

The synovial membrane is thickened and seeded with cartilaginous nodules which are located close together or confluent, other contained within the membrane, other arising at the surface, other pediculated and ready to fall in the joint. Even these smaller nodules have the aspect of immature, grayish, translucid and relatively soft cartilage; the larger ones are white, lucent and harder. The synovial membrane may appear to be thickened, velvety and hyperemic.

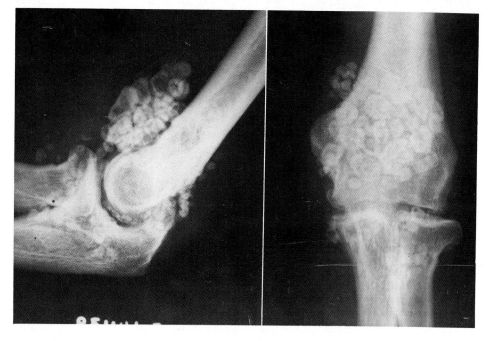

FIG. 865. - Male aged 42 years. Synovial chondromatosis of the elbow.

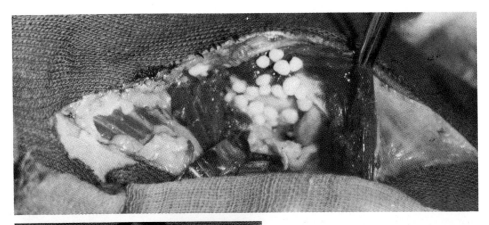

FIG. 866. - Female aged 35 years. Synovial chondromatosis of the elbow.

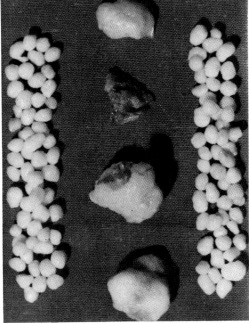

On the cut surface, calcified loose bodies and intrasynovial nodules contain hard, granular, yellowish-white and opaque areas; the ossified ones include areas of bony aspect and consistency. The articular surfaces are normal; only in inveterate forms of the lesion can they present degenerative changes of the arthrosic type.

In paratendinous extra-articular forms, the cartilaginous nodule is single, lobulated, it generally does not exceed 3 cm in diameter. It is a nodule of cartilaginous aspect which often contains calcifications and/or ossifications, at times mucoid areas.

In aggressive pseudotumoral articular forms, the joint capsule may be thinned or lacking in places. Inside and around the joint there are solid masses, which are usually multiple and which may become of considerable size (5-10 in diameter). These masses are globose, with a lobulated surface and limited by a rather thin pseudocapsule. They may surround the joint and push towards the metaphysis and the diaphysis of the articular bones, surrounding them and digging the bone from the outside. Despite the fact that they invade the peri-articular soft tissues and the skeleton, these cartilaginous masses generally have rather well-defined boundaries. They have the appearance of well-differentiated cartilaginous tissue, rather soft and friabile, with some areas which are more transparent and grayish. The joint is completely filled with this tissue which has the gross aspect of well-differentiated chondrosarcoma. In these cases there are no loose bodies.

HISTOPATHOLOGIC FEATURES

There are two pathognomic findings: 1) the presence of cartilaginous nodules within the synovial membrane; 2) the typical aspect of cartilaginous tissue (Fig. 869).

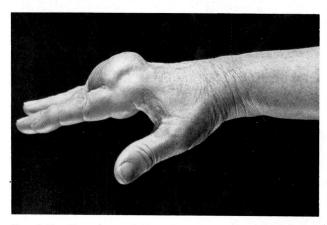

FIG. 867. - Female aged 51 years. Paratendinous synovial chondromatosis of the hand.

The synovial membrane — and at times the capsule, too — contains isolated or confluent nodules of actively proliferating hyaline cartilage. At the onset, the cartilaginous nodules are formed by direct metaplasia of the synovial connective tissue.

The typical histological aspect of S.C. is that of a well-differentiated rather cellular hyaline cartilage. The cells are typically collected in small bunches, divided by bands and areas of ground substance. In addition to being numerous, the cells are often large, with a plump nucleus, considerable nuclear pleomorphism, with frequent cells having a double nucleus.

These cytological aspects are often the same as those observed in a grade 1 chondrosarcoma. At times the number, size, pleomorphism of the nuclei are such as to correspond to that which in another anatomo-clinical situation we will define grade 2 chondrosarcoma. The difference in relation to chondrosarcomas is based on clinical and imaging data, on the histological structure with cells in bunches, on the well-defined boundaries of the cartilaginous lobuli at their periphery, on the intrasynovial localizations of the lobuli.

The calcification of this cartilage is a frequent occurrence with necrosis of the cells and ossification of the cartilage itself. When the loose bodies are ossified, this ossification evidently occurred prior to their being detached from the synovial membrane, when penetration of the blood vessels within the cartilage was possible. In the loose bodies, the proliferative aspects of the cartilage are attenuated or absent, and the bony areas often appear to be necrotic.

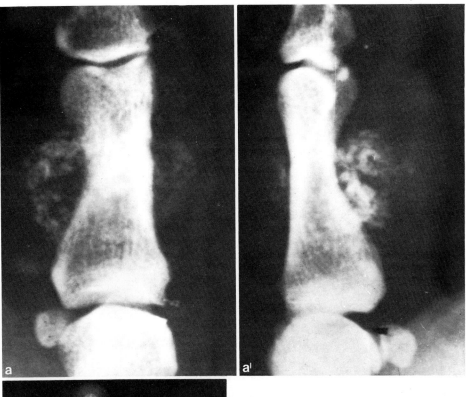

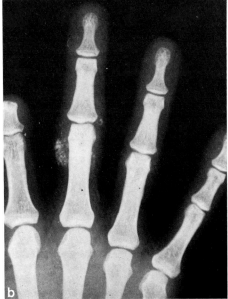

FIG. 868. - Two cases of tendinous synovial chondromatosis. In (a) there is erosion from the outside of the phalanx of the thumb and the lesion recurred twice after intralesional excision, so that thumb disarticulation was performed.

HISTOGENESIS AND PATHOGENESIS

The cartilage seems to form by metaplasia of the synovial connective tissue. This metaplasia is not surprising if we consider that in the embryo the

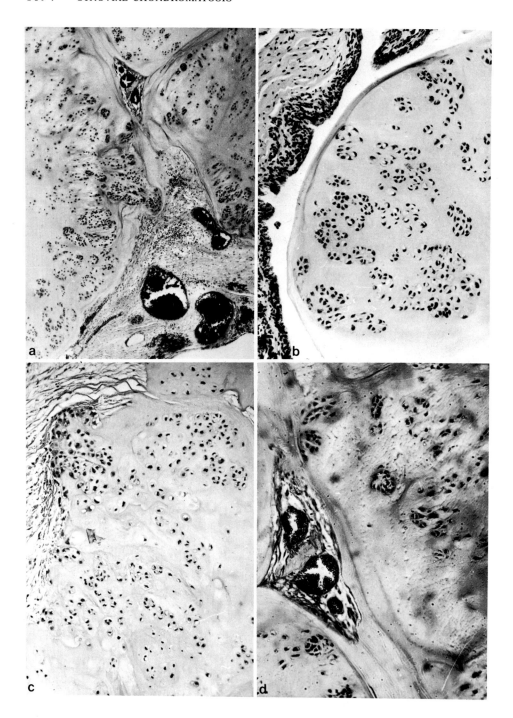

Fig. 869. - Synovial chondromatosis. (a) and (b) Within the synovial membrane there is cartilaginous metaplasia. (c) and (d) The cartilage reveals evident proliferative activity, with large pleomorphic nuclei, which tend to be arranged in small bunches (*Hemat.-eos.*, 60, 160, 160, 250 x).

cartilage and the synovial membrane originate from the same skeletogenous mesenchyma. In our opinion, this is not a neoplasm. What contrasts with the neoplastic nature is the multicentric origin with disseminated nodules, the possible insurgence of the lesion in two joints, the spontaneous maturation and exhaustion of the cartilaginous proliferation in many cases with ossified loose bodies. Also in agreement with the metaplastic-hyperplastic nature is the fact that limited foci of synovial chondroid metaplasia are observed in different chronic synovial alterations such as arthrosis, Charcot joints, rheumatoid arthritis. Certainly, in the rare aggressive pseudotumoral forms of S.C. it is difficult to avoid the impression of a tumor, even a malignant one. Nonetheless, this behavior is rather similar to that which is observed in pigmented villonodular synovitis. Also of interest is the analogy between S.C. and pigmented villonodular synovitis with regard to involvement of the joints and of the tendinous sheaths of the hand and foot.

DIAGNOSIS

Preoperative diagnosis is difficult when the radiogram is completely negative. In these cases, as indicated, diagnosis may be above all arthroscopic or obtained at arthrotomy. Diagnosis is certain when the radiogram and/or arthrotomy reveal intra-articular loose bodies and when cartilage nodules are also observed within the synovial membrane.

When the loose bodies are single or few and there are no intrasynovial nodules, we are generally dealing with an **osteochondrosis dissecans**, an **arthrosis** or a **neurogenous arthropathy**. In these situations the radiographic and anatomical lesions common to arthrosis are observed. Histologically, the synovial membrane presents hyperemia, chronic edema, inclusions of necrotic osteo-cartilaginous debris, activated macrophages, lymphocytes, and plasma cells. These degenerative synoviopathies may present microscopic foci of cartilaginous metaplasia, but with an aspect which differs from that of chondromatosis: these are minute and sporadic areas where few cells are surrounded by homogenous and scarcely basophile ground substance.

The most important differential diagnosis is that with **chondrosarcomas**, in the more aggressive and pseudotumoral forms of S.C. Radiographically, the presence of large masses in the para-articular soft tissues, containing some tenuous and faded sprays of calcification, and the excavation of the adjacent epiphyses and at times of the metadiaphyses may lead to diagnosis of chondrosarcoma. S.C. is indicated by the absence of signs of a pre-existing exostosis, the aspect of skeletal excavation suggesting that this occurred due to compression from the outside, the well-defined limits of these skeletal excavations, the fact that the cartilaginous growth fills the joint cavity and expands starting from the joint. The slowness of its course, which is prolonged over years, is not a fundamental element because it may also be quite slow in chondrosarcomas. Macroscopically, S.C. will have to be suspected when cartilaginous tissue is found to fill the joint cavity and the synovial recesses, from these surrounding and compressing the adjacent bone. Histologically, the fundamental feature is the bunch-like pattern of the cartilaginous cells and the always well-differentiated aspect of the cartilage, despite the possible evident grade of nuclear pleomorphism.

Paratendinous localizations must be distinguished from **juvenile aponeurotic fibroma** (younger age, localization in the hand and forearm rather than in the fingers, fibromatous tissue with small foci of chondroid differentiation and calcification).

COURSE, TREATMENT AND PROGNOSIS

The course of the lesion is very slow. The cartilaginous nodules tend to mature, calcify and ossify, the proliferative potential tends to be exhausted. In some cases the smaller intrasynovial cartilaginous nodules may spontaneously regress. In rare aggressive pseudotumoral forms, instead, the mass of cartilaginous tissue, as indicated in the previous description, reveals more aggressive pseudotumoral growth, but this too is very slow and probably not indefinite.

The paratendinous nodules of the fingers have a more limited growth as they hardly ever exceed 3 cm in diameter. In this respect, as well, S.C. singularly resembles pigmented nodular synovitis.

Treatment of the articular forms of the lesion consists in removal of the loose bodies and synovectomy which is as complete as possible. Nonetheless, it seems that even when synovectomy is only partial, recurrence is infrequent and not very important. For this reason it is probably not worth being too aggressive in dealing with the lesion, for example performing synovectomy with two incisions, anterior and posterior to the knee, or constantly dislocating the proximal femoral epiphysis at the hip. In aggressive pseudotumoral forms of the lesion, treatment must be as conservative as possible. It must aim at excision of the cartilaginous masses with intralesional surgery which is as complete as possible. When the skeletal surfaces appear to be completely worn or excavated, particularly at the hip joint, arthroprosthesis is indicated.

In exceptional cases, such as in the hip when the pelvic aspect of the joint is considerably excavated as well, extra-articular resection of the proximal femur and acetabulum may be indicated. In rare particularly aggressive forms of the lesion, amputation was performed, probably dictated by the impression that we were dealing with a chondrosarcoma. In truth, amputation is hardly ever necessary.

In paratendinous forms of the lesion, the treatment of choice is simple marginal excision of the nodule.

S.C. is a benign lesion which rarely recurs even after marginal, intralesional or even incomplete excision, and which grows very slowly.

Exceptional cases have been described in which there was transformation from S.C. to chondrosarcoma. Nonetheless, most of the aggressive tumor-like forms of S.C. respond well to conservative treatment and do not metastasize.

Radiation therapy is not indicated, as it has little effect on cartilaginous proliferation.

REFERENCES

1958 MURPHY A.F., WILSON J.N.: Tenosynovial osteochondroma in the hand. *J. Bone Joint Surg.*, **40/A**, 1236.

1962 MURPHY F.P., DAHLIN D.C., SULLIVAN C.R.: Articular synovial chondromatosis. *J. Bone Joint. Surg.*, **44/A**, 77.

1964 LICHTENSTEIN L., GOLDMAN R.L.: Cartilage tumors in soft tissue, particularly in the hand and foot. *Cancer, 17*, 1203.

1973 DUNN A.W., WHISTLER J.H.: Synovial chondromatosis of the knee with associated extracapsular chondroma. *J. Bone Joint. Surg.*, **55/A**, 1747.

1974 DAHLIN C., SALVADOR H.: Cartilaginous tumors of the soft tissues of the hands and feet. *Mayo Clin. Proc.*, **49**, 721.

1974 DUNN E.J., McGAVRAN M., NELSON P., *et al.*: Synovial chondrosarcoma: Report of a case. *J. Bone Joint. Surg.*, **56/A**, 811.

1977 SIM F.H., DAHLIN D.C., IVINS J.C.: Extraarticular synovial chondromatosis. *J. Bone Joint Surg.*, **59-A**, 492.

1978 DELLON A., WEISS S.W., MITCH W.E.: Bilateral extraosseous chondromas of the hand in a patient with chronic renal failure. *Am. Soc. Surg. Hand.*, **3**, 139.

1978 SOMEREN A., MERRITT W.H.: Tenosynovial chondroma of the hand: A case report with a brief review of the literature. *Hum. Pathol.*, **9**, 476.

1979 DE BENEDETTI M.J., SCHWINN C.P.: Tenosynovial chondromatosis in the hand. *J. Bone Joint. Surg.*, **61/A**, 898.

1985 MINSINGER W.E.: BALOGH K.: MILLENDER L.H.: Tenosynovial osteochondroma of the hand. A case report and brief review. *Clin. Orthop.*, **196**, 248-52.

1988 MAURICE H., CRONE M., WATT I.: Synovial chondromatosis. *J. Bone Joint Surg.*, **70-B**, 807.

1988 PATTEE G.A., SYNDER S.J.: Synovial chondromatosis of the acromioclavicular joint: a case report. *Clin. Orthop.*, **233**, 205-207.

1988 PERRY B.E., McQUEEN D.A., LIN J.: Synovial chondromatosis with malignant degeneration to chondrosarcoma. *J. Bone Joint Surg. (Am)*, **70**, 1259-1261.

1988 VON ARX D.P., SIMPSON M.T., BATMAN P.: Synovial chondromatosis of the temporomandibular joint. *Br. J. Oral Maxillofac. Surg.*, **26**, 297-305.

1988 WILSON W.J., PARR T.J.: Synovial chondromatosis. *Orthopedics*, **11**, 1179-1183.

PSEUDOTUMORAL CALCINOSIS

It is a fibrohistiocytary proliferation which surrounds masses of calcium. Because of its tendency to grow it resembles a tumor. There are no changes in the metabolism of calcium.

It is rare and prefers the male **sex**. There is predilection for **ages** from 10 to 30 years. The **sites** most involved are the joint and/or peri-articular tissues of the hip, shoulder, elbow. At times the lesion appears to be multiple, bilateral and symmetrical.

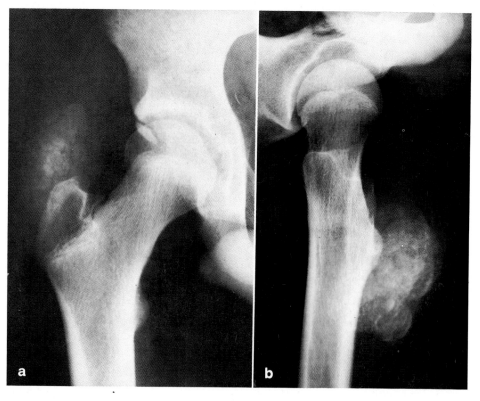

FIG. 870. - Pseudotumoral calcinosis. Male aged 14 years. For the past year paratrochanteric swelling, mildly painful (a). The patient was submitted to excision, after 6 months there was more distal and posterior swelling, in the same thigh (b).

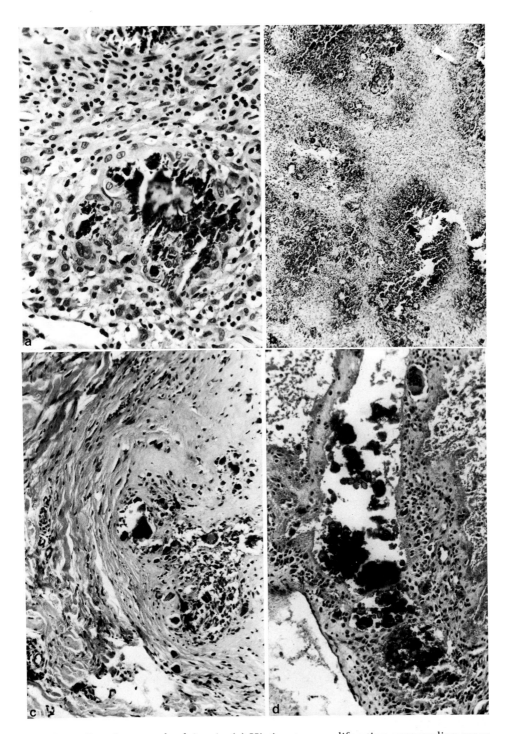

FIG. 871. - Pseudotumoral calcinosis. (a) Histiocytary proliferation surrounding areas of calcific deposit. (b) Multifocal aspect with central area constituted by calcific material. (c) and (d) At the margins of the calcific deposits, histiocytes, macrophages, giant cells and fibrosis are observed (*Hemat.-eos.*, 400, 60, 400, 400 x).

Radiographically there are numerous ovoid opaque areas, constituted by calcium deposits, located far apart or tending to mass together (Fig. 870). The skeleton is not characterized by changes in the mineral component.

Macroscopically in the peri-articular tissues there are whitish nodules of paste-like consistency, of varying size from a few cm to 20 cm. On the cut surface, the nodules, which are of granular chalky white aspect, at times cystic, are surrounded by tissue of fibrous aspect.

Histologically there is amorphous, granular, calcific, intensely basophilic material, which is arranged in small masses or in vast fields. Surrounding these there is a regular layer of macrophagic histiocytes, multinucleate giant cells, and chronic inflammatory elements. In other fields, surrounding the calcific material, fibroblastic proliferation and the production of collagen bundles prevails (Fig. 871).

P.T.C. must be differentiated from other lesions with calcium salt precipitations in the tissues: **hyperparathyroidism**, particularly secondary, chronic renal insufficiency, hypervitaminosis D and hypercalcemic conditions secondary to skeletal metastases or paraneoplastic syndromes. In these cases, the age of the patient is more advanced than it is in P.T.C., often there are intra-parenchymal calcifications, and calcium and phosphorus ions are often altered in the blood and urine.

Intratissutal calcific deposits associated with normal hematic levels of calcium and phosphorus are observed in calcar tendinitis in which calcification is of small size and localized at the superficial planes, and in **universal calcinosis**. The latter occurs more frequently during childhood and is often associated with diseases of the collagen. The calcifications are deposited extensively and, when they involve the joints, they cause stiffness and ankylosis.

Treatment of choice is surgery. This obtains good results when the lesion may be completely removed, during initial stages of the disease. When the calcific masses become of considerable size, the possibility of complete removal may be compromised and in this case recurrence is more frequent.

REFERENCES

1961   BARTON D.L., REEVES R.J.: Tumoral calcinosis. Report of three cases and review of the literature. *Am. J. Roentgenol*, **86**, 351.
1967   HARKESS J.W., PETERS H.J.: Tumoral calcinosis. *J. Bone Joint. Surg.*, **49/A**, 721.
1967   SMIT G.G., SCHMAMAN A.: Tumoral calcinosis. *J. Bone Joint. Surg.*, **49/B**, 698.
1969   BALDURSSON H., EVANS E.B., DODGE W.F., *et al.*: Tumoral calcinosis with hyperphosphatemia. A report of a family with incidence in four siblings. *J. Bone Joint. Surg.*, **51/A**, 913.
1971   WAGHMAI I., MIRBOD P.: Tumoral calcinosis. *Am J. Roentgenol*, **111**, 573.
1972   BERG D.: Tumoral calcinosis. *Br. J. Surg.*, **59**, 570.
1973   VASUDEV K.S., TAPP L., HARRIS M., *et al.*: Tumoural calcinosis in Britain. *Br. Med. J.*, **1**, 676.
1976   VERESS B., MALIK O.A., EL HASSAN A.M.: Tumoural lipocalcinosis: a clinicopathological study of 20 cases. *J. Pathol.*, **119**, 113.

1977   Brown M.L., Thrall J.H., Cooper R.A., *et al.:* Radiography and scintigraphy in tumoral calcinosis. *Radiology,* **124**, 757.

1978   Hacihanefioglu U.: Tumoral calcinosis. A clinical and pathological study of 11 unreported cases in Turkey. *J. Bone Joint. Surg.* **60/A**, 1131.

1980   Balachandran S., Abbud Y., Prince M.J., *et al.:* Tumoral calcinosis: Scintigraphic studies of an affected family. *Br. J. Radiol.,* **53**, 960.

1980   Lufkin E.G., Wilson D.M., Smith L.H., *et al.:* Phosphorus excretion in tumoral calcinosis: response to parathyroid hormone and acetazolamide. *J. Clin. Endocronol. Metab.,* **50**, 648.

1980   Mitnick P.D., Goldfarb S., Slatopolsky E., *et al.:* Calcium and phosphate metabolism in tumoral calcinosis. *Ann. Int. Med.,* **92**, 482.

1983   Knowles S.A.S., Declerck G., Anthony P.P.: Tumoral calcinosis. *Br. J. Surg.,* **70**, 105.

1986   Di Giovanna J.J., Helfgott R.K., Gerber L.H., *et al.:* Extraspinal tendon and ligament calcification associated with long-term therapy with etretinate. *N. Engl. J. Med.,* **315**, 1177.

PIGMENTED VILLONODULAR SYNOVITIS, TENOSYNOVITIS, BURSITIS
(Synonyms: xanthoma, xanthogranuloma, benign synvialoma, giant cell tumor of the tendinous sheaths, fibrous histiocytoma of synovium)

DEFINITION

Pigmented villonodular synovitis (tenosynovitis, bursitis)[1] is a hyperplastic production of synovial tissue of the joints, the tendinous sheaths, the mucous bursae, or the fibrous tissue adjacent to the tendons.

P.V.N.S. may present: 1) in a diffused villous or villonodular form, 2) in a localized nodular form. In the tendinous sheaths and peritendinous tissue the localized nodular form is almost exclusively observed. In the joints, instead, the diffused villous or villonodular form and the localized nodular form are observed approximately with equal frequency.

FREQUENCY

Paratendinous nodular synovitis (particularly of the hand) is frequent. Joint localizations, on the contrary, are relatively rare. Those in the bursae are an exceptional occurrence[2].

---

[1] The term P.V.N.S. was coined by Jaffe, Lichtenstein and Sutro in 1941, in order to express the «inflammatory» or at least non-neoplastic nature, the villous and and nodular structure, the hemosiderin pigmentation of the lesion. This term was widely accepted as the most suitable to define an affection the etiopathogenesis of which is not known. Nonetheless, there are still other names given to the lesion, among which xanthoma, xanthogranuloma, giant cell tumor, and synvialoma. The term xanthoma is derived from the presence of macrophages loaded with cholesterids, but it is definitely inappropriate as the foam cells do not at all represent the main feature of the lesion, nor are they a constant finding; it is also inappropriate because it causes confusion with multiple tuberous xanthoma, a lesion of another nature. The term giant cell tumor is just as inappropriate, as the giant cells, like the foam cells, are a secondary and inconstant component of the lesion; it is also inappropriate because it causes confusion with true giant cell tumor of the skeleton. The term synvialoma would be appropriate only if we were dealing with a synovial neoplasm, which, in our opinion, is improbable. In any case, the adjective «benign» would have to be added in order to avoid confusion with actual and more well-known synovial neoplasm, that is, synovial sarcoma.

[2] At least the diffused villonodular bursitis which manifests clinically, as the localized nodular form of a bursa generally remains asymptomatic.

SEX

There is no predilection for sex.

AGE

P.V.N.S. is typical of adult age. Despite the fact that age may range from 10 to 75 years, most patients are aged over 20, with the highest incidence of the disease occurring between 20 and 40 years of age.

LOCALIZATION

Pigmented tenosynovitis (nearly always nodular and localized) is prevalently observed in the fingers and above all in the sheath of a flexor tendon. Less frequently it occurs in the palm of the hand (close to a metacarpo-phalangeal joint), or in the wrist, or on the dorsum of a finger, in relation to an extensor tendon. It is not very common in the foot, in relation to the flexor or extensor tendons. Pigmented synovitis of the joints (diffused or localized nodular) is observed, in more than 75% of all cases, in the knee. The following sites follow at a considerable distance: the hip, wrist, ankle, shoulder. Even more rare is localization in other joints. Localization in the bursae is very rare.

Multiple localizations of P.N.V.S. are exceptional. In some advanced and extensive villonodular forms of the lesion, for example of the wrist or of the ankle, the lesion invades both the tendinous sheaths and the joint spaces of one or more joints. Nonetheless, very expanded and tumor-like forms of the lesion are usually of articular origin.

SYMPTOMS

a) Extra-articular nodular P.S.

The patient complains of a nodule which has formed and grown, over a few years, in the hand (more rarely in the foot, wrist or ankle), in relation to a tendinous sheath or peritendinous fibrous tissue. The nodule rarely grows rapidly due to microtraumatic and hemorrhagic phenomena, but it never exceeds 4 cm in diameter. It is generally painless. Only when it achieves its greatest size, compressing the surrounding structures and exposed to microtrauma, does it cause some pain. Tendinous and joint function is hardly or not at all impaired, or dysfunction may be moderate and late. The nodule is usually softer and more mobile in its initial stages of growth. Thereafter, due to the fibrous scarring evolution, it becomes harder, adherent to the tendon and possibly to the bone.

b) Extra-articular P.V.N.S.

In these very rare cases, symptoms may be those of a hyperplastic and

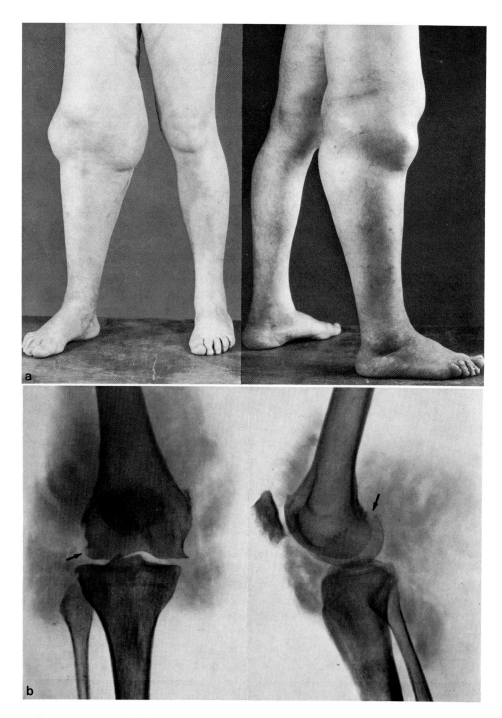

FIG. 872. - Pigmented villonodular synovitis. Female aged 53 years. (a) Swelling of the knee which initiated 17 years earlier, mobility fairly preserved, pain scarce. The patient was submitted to synovectomy, the tissue mass removed weighed 1800 kg. (b) Observe little erosions on the skeletal borders of insertion of the synovial membrane.

moderately exhudative tenovaginitis, possibly associated with the presence of nodules. Or they may include tumor-like swelling, which may even be extensive and expanded. Villous or villonodular tenosynovitis, in fact, is usually extended to the palm of the hand and to the wrist, to the foot and ankle, surrounding various tendons. At times it progresses via the interosseous spaces, and it may involve the palm and the dorsum of the hand.

c) Intra-articular nodular P.S.

In this case, as well, symptoms may last years; or (it nearly always involves the knee) clinical onset may be acute, with pain, blocking and effusion. Symptoms include intermittent pain, at times in the meniscal site, at times related to trauma; episodes of mild, serous (rarely sero-hematic) joint effusion; lack of extension, or joint blocking; subjective or objective sensation of loose intra-articular body. Localized nodular synovitis may remain asymptomatic and represent a chance arthroscopic/surgical finding.

d) Intra-articular P.V.N.S.

Symptoms are initially mild, of long duration. Often diagnosis is made a few years after the onset of symptoms. The main symptom is joint swelling, with diffused synovial thickening and — particularly in the knee — repeated episodes of effusion (Fig. 872). The liquid which is extracted is typically sero-hematic, reddish or brown and contains cholesterids. Pain varies in intensity and may be discontinuous. It increases during effusion and may be associated with joint blocking phenomena (in the knee) due to the entrapment of synovial villi or nodules between the joint surfaces. As a rule, the joint is slightly warm, it is stable and **it moves widely**. There is little or no muscular hypotrophy, as there is no considerable compromise in joint function. After many years the joint swelling may become of large or enormous size and it may expand to the para-articular tissues (Figs. 872, 873, 876c). Even in this case, however, joint mobility remains relatively preserved.

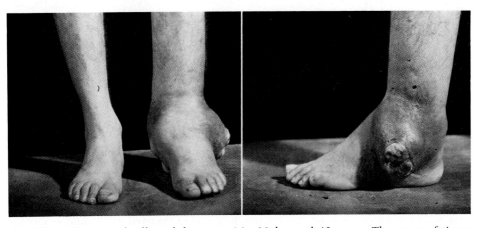

FIG. 873. - Pigmented villonodular synovitis. Male aged 43 years. The mass of tissue (soft and yellow-brown) surrounds the ankle and ulcerates the skin. Amputation was performed.

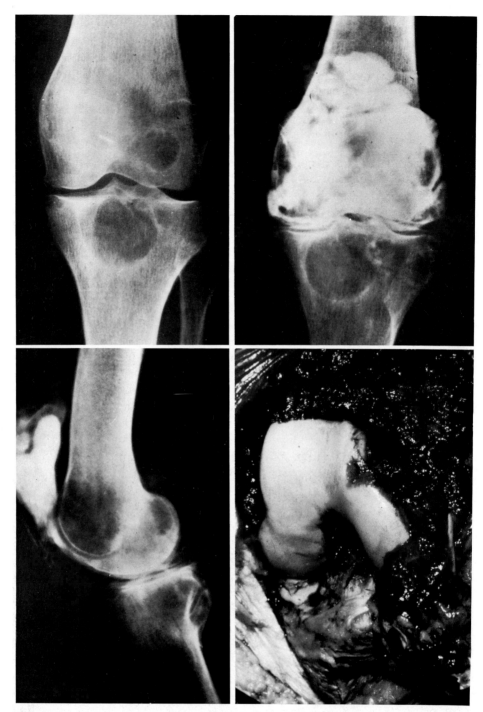

FIG. 874. - Pigmented villonodular synovitis. Female aged 40 years. Swellling for the past 6 years. Observe roundish skeletal excavations in the tibia and femur, where the contrast medium does not penetrate because they are filled with synovitic tissue. Arthrography shows nodules of the thickened synovial membrane. On arthrotomy, typical hyperplastic aspect and brown color of the synovial membrane.

e) In exceptional cases of **villonodular or localized nodular bursitis**, symptoms include pain, swelling, effusion. At times nodular bursitis is asymptomatic and constitutes a chance surgical finding (in two of our observations we discovered a nodule in the subscapular bursa, during surgery for recurring dislocation of the shoulder).

RADIOGRAPHIC FEATURES

Often radiograms are negative, or they reveal some thickening of the synovial membrane, diffused or nodular. This amount of thickening has the same density as the soft tissues and does not contain calcifications. In particularly expanded forms, the mass of «soft» tissue may be in multiple nodes or lobes. These are revealed by arthrography, but particularly by CAT and MRI, which often provides pathognomic findings in joint P.V.N.S. (Figs. 874, 875, 876c).

Sometimes, skeletal erosions due to compression are observed. In **localized nodular tenosynovitis**, this phenomenon occurs in 10-20% of all cases. It is manifested by «saucer-like» erosion of the phalanx, usually on the palmar or plantar aspect (Fig. 877). The cortex is cancelled and osteolysis may have polycyclical boundaries. In anteroposterior projection the osteolysis may well appear to be central and cloistered, and thus it gives the false impression of a lesion which has developed within the bone. The boundaries of the osteolysis are rather well-defined. In joint **diffused villonodular synovitis** skeletal erosion occurs only in particularly advanced and neoplastiform forms (Figs.

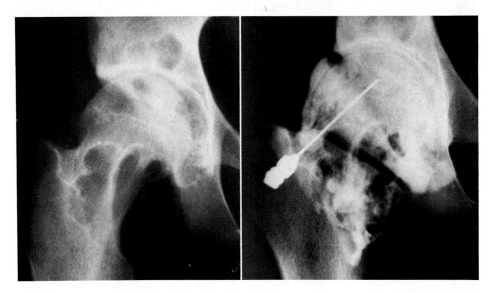

FIG. 875. - Pigmented villonodular synovitis. Female aged 21 years. Coxalgia for the past 5 years, mobility of the hip fairly preserved. Observe multiple bubbly excavations in the femur and acetabulum, where the contrast medium does not penetrate as they are filled with synovitic tissue. Arthrography shows synovial nodules.

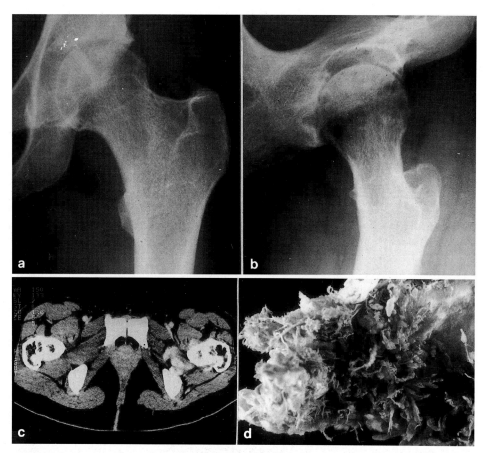

FIG. 876. - Pigmented villonodular synovitis in a woman aged 33, who for one year has had pain in the left hip with only a slight decrease in range of motion of the joint. (a) and (b) The x-rays show narrowing of the articular space and several subchondral «cysts» with well-defined limits, both in the femur and the acetabulum. (c) The CAT shows lobulated newly formed tissue in the joint area with considerable uptake of the contrast dye. (d) Gross aspect of the removed synovial tissue, showing the typical villous rusty-coloured features.

872, 874), or more precociously in those joints where synovial proliferation has little space to expand (Figs. 875, 876a-c). Thus, it is more easily observed in the hip or ankle than in the knee. Radiographic images consist in rounded osteolyses, at times polycyclical, with relatively neat boundaries, usually initiating in the areas of insertion of the synovial membrane to the bone, that is, on the perimeter of the articular cartilage. In a more advanced phase, the newly-formed masses of the synovitis dig ample cavities in the epiphyis, creating osteolyses of not very intense radiolucency (the cavities are rather superficial), bubbly, and polycyclical. Even when there are wide bony erosions, the joint space may maintain normal width for a long period of time. Eventually, and particularly in the hip joint, it progressively reduces.

GROSS PATHOLOGIC FEATURES

a) Extra-articular nodular P.S.

As previously stated, the nodule is single and of moderate size: it never exceeds 4 cm in diameter.

In «younger» stages of the lesion it is a roughly lobulated nodule, having a

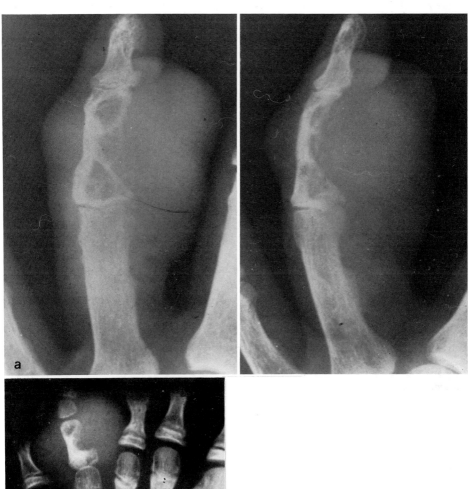

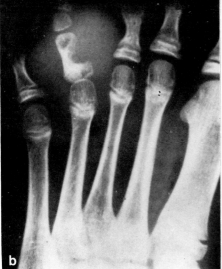

FIG. 877. - Extra-articular nodular tenosynovitis. (a) Lesion of unusually large size, which erodes the phalanges from the outside. (b) Large lesion in the toe of a boy aged 10 years, with erosion of the phalanx from the outside.

smooth surface, of relatively soft to elastic consistency. The cut surface is compact and variegated, because of the closely-packed and confluent lobules and the color which goes from yellow to white to pale brown. The nodule is part of the tendinous sheath, but it does not adhere much to the surrounding adipose tissue, to the tendon or to the bone.

In more «veterate» stages of the disease, the nodule tends to **mature in a fibrous scarring form**. Thus, it becomes harder, until it takes on a fibro-cartilaginous consistency. It always appears to be made up of a group of closely-packed lobules, but it is more compact, and the dominant color is white, with some yellowish or brown bands. It adheres to the surrounding tissues, to the tendon and to the bone. Nonetheless, even when it digs a niche in the bone, it may easily be enucleated.

b) Extra-articular P.V.N.S.

Within the tendinous sheaths there is a diffused villous synovial hyperplasia, which is rather soft, poultice-like, greasy and of a typical rusty color. Furthermore, there are usually multiple nodules of differing size.

c) Intra-articular nodular P.S.

The nodule is generally single, not of large size, sessile or pediculated. In its usual site, the knee, it often originates from the synovial membrane in proximity of a meniscus, or it protrudes in the intercondylar notch; but it may be observed in any part of the joint cavity. It is globose and it may be

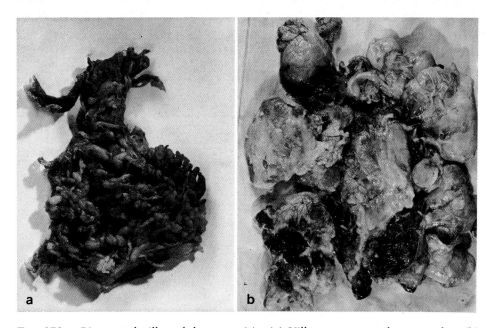

FIG. 878. - Pigmented villonodular synovitis. (a) Villous aspect and rusty color. (b) Compact and nodular masses of soft, greasy tissue, brown, ochre, light yellow in color.

vaguely lobulated. Its aspect is similar to that of paratendinous nodules, and, like these, it tends towards fibrous maturation. At times, a pediculated nodule, due to traumatic and vascular phenomena caused by joint movement, may present hemorrhagic and/or necrotic changes.

d) Intra-articular P.V.N.S.

Its aspect varies depending on the nodular quota and the phase of development. That which always dominates the picture and characterizes it in relation to all inflammatory, reactive and neoplastic lesions of the synovial membrane, is the intense hyperplasia and the rusty and yellowish color.

The joint cavity often contains sero-hematic liquid of red-brown or brown color. The synovial membrane appears throughout to be very thickened, leathery-yellow in color, often matted by long large villi (Figs. 874, 876d, 878). At times, the villi are so developed that the surface resembles a «ruffled beard». Often the villi are associated with numerous nodules, of varying size, single or lobulated, contained within the synovial membrane. The nodules are soft, elastic, yellowish and yellow-brown in color. The villi, which grow in the limited joint space, tend to fuse into compact masses. On the cut surface, these often reveal a spongy structure, due to the coalescence of the villi. The surface of the villi and of the nodules may be covered here and there by fibrin membranes.

In more advanced and neoplastiform lesions, all of the joint space is filled with a soft, pasty, friabile and yellow-brown tissue. This tissue may dig rounded niches in the bone, particularly at the periphery of the joint surfaces. Nonetheless it may easily be enucleated from these niches, which have a smooth bony wall. The tissue, moreover, may invade the joint capsule and expand outside of it, in the muscles, between the tendons, as far as the subcutaneous tissue. The pseudotumoral mass, which is generally lobulated, may adhere to the surrounding tissues, but it never infiltrates them. The cut surface of the tissue, due to its lipid contents, is often greasy.

The joint cartilage may be degenerated (sometimes of brown-greenish color), undermined and eroded in the more expanded forms and those of longer duration.

Thus, the diffused villonodular form, as compared to the localized nodular one, has little or no tendency towards fibrous scarring «maturation». Thus, hyperplasia continues indefinitely, even for tens of years, and it may, although very slowly, become of neoplastiform aggressive proportions.

HISTOPATHOLOGIC FEATURES

The histological aspect of P.V.N.S. is composite, but in its entirety very typical. The basic elements are as follows:

   1) histio-fibroblastic and capillary hyperplasia;

   2) formation of villi and/or cavities having a synovial cell coating;

   3) intense macrophagic activity of the cells, which particularly englobe the hemosiderin pigment;

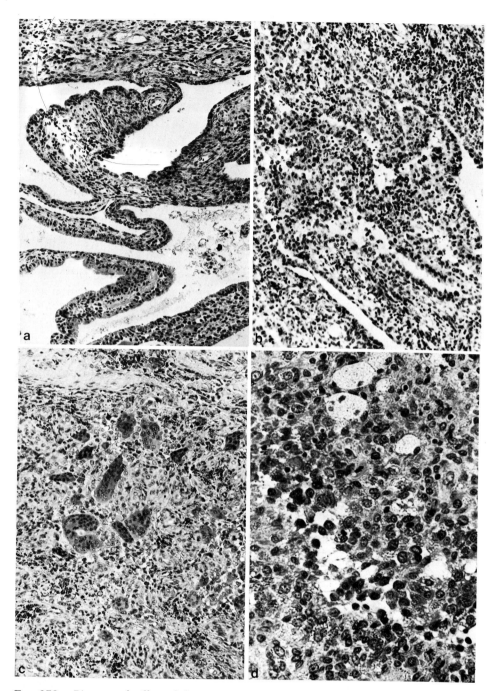

FIG. 879. - Pigmented villonodular synovitis. (a) Alongside areas of solid aspect there are areas with villous digitations which tend to flow together. (b) In the solid areas and in the villous ones the cellular constituent is the same: histiocytary cells, multicleate giant cells, macrophages, lymphocytes and fibroblasts. (c) Histiocytes and giant cells in nodular pattern. (d) Foam cells surrounded by cells with intensely eosinophilic cytoplasm, oval nucleus, clear, with a small nucleolus. Amongst these histiocytary cells there may be mitotic figures (*Hemat.-eos.*, 60, 160, 250, 400 x).

4) presence — inconstant — of foam cells with lipoid content;

5) presence — incostant — of multinucleate giant cells;

6) tendency — particularly in localized nodular forms — towards collagen sclerosis (fibro-hyalin).

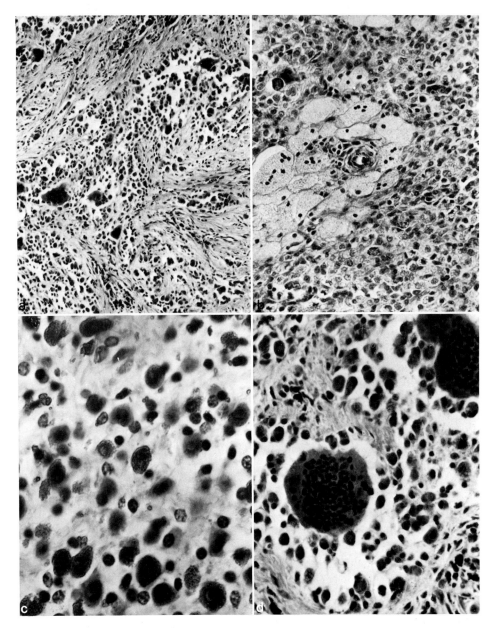

FIG. 880. - Pigmented villonodular synovitis. (a) Overall view: formation of cavities having simil-synovial coating, with numerous giant cells. (b) Xanthomatous modifications, with foam cells having lipoid contents. (c) Detail of cells with macrophagic activity that englobe hemosiderin pigment. (d) Detail of multinucleate giant cells (*Hemat.-eos.*, 160, 250, 400, 400 x).

The histological aspect varies considerably, due to the association and prevalence of the aforementioned elements, depending on whether we are dealing with the diffused villous and villonodular form, or the localized nodular form, and on the evolution stage of the lesion.

a) Diffused villous and villonodular form.

The histological aspect is the same in the joints and in the tendinous sheaths and bursae (Figs. 879, 880).

During the initial stages, there is villous hyperplasia of the synovial membrane with epithelioid coating in several layers and histio-fibroblastic hyperplasia of the chorion, which is so intense as to form thick and compact cellular fields. There is also intense capillary hyperplasia, the cause of hyperemia and continuous interstitial and articular micro-hemorrhaging. There is abundant hemosiderin pigment among the cells and particularly in the swollen cytoplasm of the histiocytes. Here and there, there are multinucleate giant cells with central or peripheral nuclei, identical to foreign body cells and to osteoclasts. Infiltration of lymphomonocytes and plasmacells may appear, mild and sporadic. The very initial histological aspects may present similarities with those of simple synovial hyperplasias reactive to joint degenerative processes, trauma, inflammation.

In a more advanced stage, the hyperplasia of the villi increases, the villi tend to coalesce, until they fuse into spongeose and compact tissue areas. At times the macrophages, loaded with hemosiderin, form a thick mat, spotted with some multinucleate giant cells. At times there are cavities with cells oriented towards the wall. These cavities may result from the partial fusion of the villi, but they may also be newly-formed embryos of synovial cavities. At times, there are nests or vast fields of large foam cells. At times the collagen stroma becomes more consistent and thickened in fibro-hyaline form, separating and embedding groups of cells. This fibrous maturation, moreover, is not very intense in diffused villonodular forms. The nodules which alternate with the villi are none other than globose and lobular masses of histiocytary and fibroblastic hyperplastic tissue, as previously described. There may be rare mitotic figures.

b) Localized nodular form.

If we compare a specimen of initial villous form with one of localized nodular form at an advanced stage of sclerosis, one has the impression of a great difference. But if we recall the development cycle of villonodular synovitis, which we have tried to summarized above, we may see how the nodule has the same structure as the villous form with a more evident prevalence of fibrous scarring maturation phenomena. The nodule generally maintains a lobulated compact structure. The histio-fibroblastic hyperplasia is the same as that previously described. There is no trace of villi, but generally there are small areas of disgregation, with an empty space at the center, epithelioid and multinucleate giant cells surrounding it, probably constituting embryos of synovial spaces (Fig. 881).

Generally, there are large shoots and compact areas of fibro-hyaline colla-

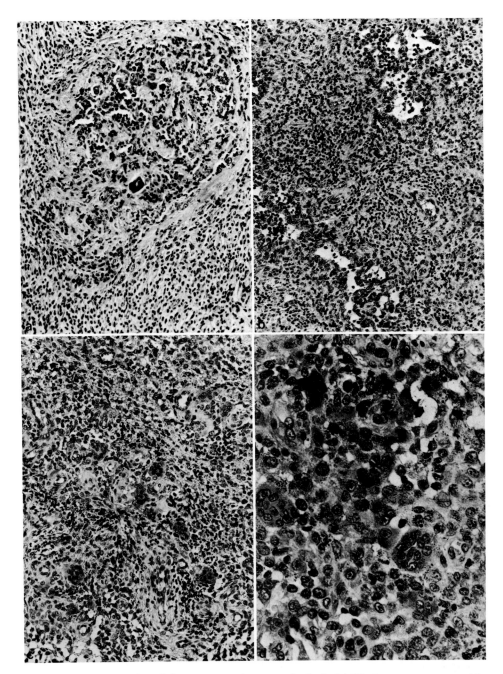

FIG. 881. - Pigmented nodular synovitis (extra-articular). (a) Histiocytes aggregated in cords and nests associated with giant cells are arranged in nodules surrounded by sclerohyaline stroma. (b) Histiocytary and inflammatory cells. The former circumscribe irregular lacunae recalling embryos of synovial spaces. (c) Multinucleate giant cells, histiocytes, and lymphocytes with collagen stroma. (d) Under higher power cytological features of the mononucleate cells may be seen with ample eosinophilic cytoplasm, nucleus having fine chromatin with a very evident nucleolus. Multinucleate giant cells are associated (*Hemat.-eos.*, 160, 250, 250, 400 x).

gen tissue, within which single cells or groups or cells are embedded. At first sight, this connective tissue may even give the impression of osteoid substance and the cells may resemble osteoblasts. But experience makes the picture unmistakable. The hemosiderin pigment is not so abundant as in the villous form; at times it is rather scarce. The foam cells are observed in some cases.

HISTOGENESIS AND PATHOGENESIS

It remains a controversial subject. Some facts related to diffused villonodular synovitis have suggested a neoplastic genesis. The mass may become of such enormous size, and recurrence after incomplete excision may occur. These phenomena are not exclusive of the neoplasms, for example they are the same as those observed in aneurysmal bone cyst. On the contrary, there are all of the elements to hold that P.V.N.S. constitutes a hyperplastic process. Such is diffusion (in villous forms) to the entire synovial membrane; the type of proliferation including different cellular stems in which macrophages prevail; the organoid structure with the formation of synovial villi; the histological aspects of transition between common hyperplastic synovites and initial pigmented villonodular synovitis; the tissue's tendency towards fibrous maturation; the fact that P.V.N.S. never transforms into sarcoma.

To continue with the example of aneurysmal bone cyst, even in P.V.N.S., as in A.B.C., it is possible to reconstruct the histogenesis of the hyperplastic lesion, but not to guess the primary cause. In our opinion, the most probable histogenesis is the following one. The hyperplasia, which begins from synovial chorion, when it is nodular and localized, grows slowly and moderately and tends to mature in a fibro-hyaline form. It acts similar to the polyp of a mucosa. In diffused villous forms, on the contrary, the rich capillary hyperplasia is important. This could provoke repeated micro-hemorrhage, with the effect of maintaining and increasing the hyperplasia of the macrophages which are loaded with hemosiderin. Thus, a vicious circle would be established, with the hyperplasia which increases the vascular and hemorrhagic quota, and the hemorrhage which maintains and increases the hyperplasia. This could explain the constant and at times enormous growth of some diffused villonodular synovites. Intra-articular hemorrage alone is not, however, capable of causing P.V.N.S. In fact, this is never observed in the joints of hemophiliacs nor in synovial angiomas (with repeated hemarthrosis).

DIAGNOSIS

Clinically speaking, it is easy to be oriented towards **extra-articular nodular P.S.** when it is localized in the hand. But, if the tendinous nodules are multiple (hands, feet, elbows, Achilles tendons) we are generally dealing with **multiple tuberous xanthoma** which is mostly presented in association with skin xanthelasms and hypercholesterolemia. The surgical finding of extra-articular nodular P.S. is nearly pathognomic and the histological finding is ab-

solutely unmistakable. We will only mention the fact that the compact fibro-hyaline areas may recall osteoid substance, so that a superficial examination of the specimen and not having any knowledge of the clinico-radiographic data could suggest osteogenetic production.

In articular **nodular forms** diagnosis can only be arthroscopic, or intra-
and postoperative. The macro- and microscopic aspects are typical.

In **diffused villous and villonodular synovites** clinical diagnosis may be
suspected based on the patient's history (symptoms going back years, repeated effusions), on the type of effusion (sero-hematic or red-brown with the
presence of cholesterids), considerable synovial hyperplasia with preserved
joint motion and little pain, at times the radiographic, arthrographic and
particularly CAT and MRI pictures (saucer-like skeletal erosion of the two
joint ends, with joint space relatively preserved, sometimes lobulated soft
tissue masses filling the joint space and projecting from the joint into the
surrounding anatomical compartments) (Fig. 876c).

Once the joint has been opened, faced with a diffused synovial hyperplasia rusty in color, where there are no large villi or nodules (initial forms)
doubts may arise with regard to **extended synovial angioma** or with a synovial hyperplasia in **repeated hemarthrosis (traumatic and hemophilic)**.
Extended synovial angioma begins during childhood, the joint is more painful and warmer, with severe muscular hypotrophy, there is often an increase
in the superficial venous reticulum, at times skin angiomas and lengthening
of the limb are observed. Macroscopically, the angioma presents, besides diffused pigmented synovial hyperplasia produced by repeated blood effusions,
the typical angiomatose nodules. The histological examination will dispel
any doubt, as the picture of synovial angioma and that of P.V.N.S. are completely different.

The more advanced forms of P.V.N.S. are easily diagnosed in the macroscopic picture, which is unmistakable.

From a histological point of view, P.V.N.S. cannot be mistaken for any
other lesion. Nonetheless, there are cases where **malignant tumor** has been
suspected, due to the neoplastiform and enormous development of the lesion,
its expansion outside of the joint or (exceptional forms originating from a
synovial bursa) far from any joint, because of the very cellular and actively
proliferative histological aspect.

COURSE

As previously observed, the growth of P.V.N.S. is very slow and gradual.

Localized nodular forms (thus nearly all paratendinous forms) never become of large size and always tend towards fibrous maturation.

Diffused villonodular forms (nearly always articular), on the contrary,
may become of enormous size. In one of our observations, in the knee, the tissue removed weighed 1.8 kg (Fig. 872). In another, in the ankle, the «tumor»

was so expanded that it had ulcerated the skin and required amputation (Fig. 873).

These monstruous and neoplastiform expansions occur slowly, over 10-20 years.

TREATMENT AND PROGNOSIS

Treatment is not a problem in localized nodular forms, whether paratendinous or articular: marginal excision is easy, and, if complete, there is no recurrence.

In diffused villonodular forms of the joint, on the contrary, complete surgical excision may be difficult or impossible. In the knee synovectomy with a double incision, anterior and posterior, is often indicated. In the hip, total synovectomy requires a wide approach and dislocation of the epiphysis. Thus, these cases risk recurrence. Radiation therapy may be indicated as a complement to surgical excision, but we do not know whether it is capable of decreasing the incidence of recurrence. In forms where there is a greater amount of osteocartilaginous joint modification, an arthroprosthesis or arthrodesis may be required (particularly in the hip).

REFERENCES

1941   JAFFE H.L., LICHTENSTEIN L., SUTRO C.J.: Pigmented villonodular synovitis, bursitis, and tenosynovitis: A discussion of the synovial and bursal equivalents of the tenosynovial lesion commonly denoted as xanthoma, xanthogranuloma, giant cell tumor or myeloplaxoma of the tendon sheath, with some consideration of the tendon sheath lesion itself. *Arch. Pathol.*, **31**, 731.

1951   WRIGHT C.J.E.: Benign giant cell synovioma. An investigation of 85 cases. *Br. J. Surg.*, **38**, 257-271.

1956   ATMORE W.G., DAHLIN D.C., GHORMLEY R.K.: Pigmented villonodular synovitis: a clinical and pathologic study. *Minn. Med.*, **39**, 196.

1958   BREINER C.W., FREIBERGER R.H.: Bone lesions associated with villonodular synovitis. *Am. J. Roentgenol.*, **79**, 618-629.

1959   PHALEN G.S., McCORMACK L.J., GAZALE W.J.: Giant cell tumor of tendon sheath (benign synovioma) in the hand: evaluation of 56 cases. *Clin. Orthop.*, **15**, 140.

1960   Mc MASTER P.E.: Pigmented villonodular synovitis with invasion of bone. *J. Bone Joint Surg.*, **42/A**, 1170-1183.

1962   SMITH J.H., PUGH D.G.: Roentgenographic aspects of articular pigmented villonodular synovitis. *Am. J. Roentgenol.*, **87**, 1146-1156.

1965   CHUNG S.M.K., JANES J.M.: Diffuse pigmented villonodular synovitis of the hip joint: review of the literature and report of four cases. *J. Bone Joint Surg.*, **47/A**, 293.

1968   BYERS P.D., COTTON R.E., DEACON O.W., *et al.*: The diagnosis and treatment of pigmented villonodular synovitis. *J. Bone Joint Surg.*, **50/B**, 290.

1968   SCHAJOWICZ F., BLUMENEELD I.: Pigmented villonodular synovitis of the wrist with penetration into bone. *J. Bone Joint Surg.*, **50/B**, 312-317.

1968   SCOTT P.M.: Bone lesions in pigmented villonodular synovitis. *J. Bone Joint Surg.*, **50/B**, 306-311.

1969   GEWHEILER J.A., WILSON V.W.: Diffuse biarticular pigmented villonodular synovitis. *Radiology*, **93**, 845-851.

1969   JONES F.E., SOULE E.H., COVENTRY M.B.: Fibrous histiocytoma of synovium (giant cell tumor of tendon sheath, pigmented nodular synovitis). *J. Bone Joint Surg.*, **51/A**, 76.

1972   ARTHAUD J.B.: Pigmented nodular synovitis: report of 11 lesions in nonarticular locations. *Am. J. Clin. Pathol.,* **58**, 511.

1972   GAMBERT J.: Villonodular synovitis of the knee in children. *Ann. Chir.,* **26**, 1011.

1972   SALM R., SISSONS H.A.: Giant cell tumors of soft tissues. *J. Pathol.,* **107**, 27.

1976   GRANOWITZ S.P., D'ANTONIO J., MANKIN H.J.: The pathogenesis and longterm end results of pigmented villonodular synovitis. *Clin. Orthop.,* **114**, 335.

1977   BROWN-CROSBY E., INGLIS A., BULLOUGH P.G.: Multiple joint involvement with pigmented villonodular synovits. *Radiology,* **122**, 671.

1978   ALGUACIL-GARCIA A., UNNI K.K., GOELLNER J.R.: Giant cell tumor of tendon sheath and pigmented villonodular synovitis: An ultrastructural study. *Am. J. Clin. Pathol.,* **69**, 6.

1978   KINDBLOM L.G., GUNTERBERG B.: Pigmented villonodular synovitis involving bone. *J. Bone Joint Surg.,* **60/A**, 830.

1978   JERGESEN H.E., MANKIN H.J., SCHILLER A.L.: Diffuse pigmented villonodular synovitis of the knee mimicking primary bone neoplasm. *J. Bone Joint. Surg.,* **60/A**, 825.

1980   MYERS B.W., MASI A.T., FEIGENBAUM S.L.: Pigmented villonodular synovitis and tenosynovitis: A clinical epidemiologic study of 166 cases and literature review. *Medicine,* **59**, 223.

1982   DANZIG L.A., GERSHUNI D., RESNICK D.: Diagnosis and treatment of diffuse pigmented villonodular synovitis of the hip. *Clin. Orthop.,* **16**, 42-47.

1988   ANDERSEN J.A., LADEFOGED C.: A case of aggressive pigmented villonodular synovitis. *Acta. Orthop. Scand.,* **59**, 464-470.

1988   GOLDMANN A.B., DI CARLO E.F.: Pigmented villonodular synovitis: diagnosis and differential diagnosis. *Radiol. Clin. North Am.,* **26**, 1327.

1988   WEISZ G.M., GAL A., KITCHENER P.N.: Magnetic resonance imaging in the diagnosis of aggressive villonodular synovitis. *Clin. Orthop.,* **236**, 303-306.

1989   GITELIS S., HELIGMAN D., MORTON T.: The treatment of pigmented villonodular synovitis of the hip: a case report and literature review. *Clin. Orthop.,* **239**, 154-160.

INDEX

---

* s.t. = soft tissues